Food and Nutrients in Disease Management

Food and Nutrients in Disease Management

Edited by
Ingrid Kohlstadt

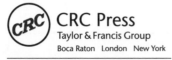

CRC Press
Taylor & Francis Group
Boca Raton London New York

CRC Press is an imprint of the
Taylor & Francis Group, an **informa** business

CRC Press
Taylor & Francis Group
6000 Broken Sound Parkway NW, Suite 300
Boca Raton, FL 33487-2742

© 2009 by Taylor & Francis Group, LLC
CRC Press is an imprint of Taylor & Francis Group, an Informa business

No claim to original U.S. Government works
Printed in the United States of America on acid-free paper
10 9 8 7 6 5 4 3 2 1

International Standard Book Number-13: 978-1-4200-6762-0 (Hardcover)

Library of Congress Cataloging-in-Publication Data

Food and nutrients in disease management / editor, Ingrid Kohlstadt.
    p. ; cm.
  "A CRC title."
  Includes bibliographical references and index.
  ISBN 978-1-4200-6762-0 (hardcover : alk. paper)
  1. Diet therapy. I. Kohlstadt, Ingrid.
  [DNLM: 1. Nutrition Therapy. WB 400 F686 2009]

RM216.F677 2009
615.8'54--dc22

2008035787

Visit the Taylor & Francis Web site at
http://www.taylorandfrancis.com

and the CRC Press Web site at
http://www.crcpress.com

To medical students and physicians,
who desire to make a difference
in the lives of their patients
and the practice of medicine

Contents

SECTION I Disorders of the Ears, Eyes, Nose, and Throat

SECTION II Cardiovascular and Pulmonary Diseases

SECTION III   Gastrointestinal Diseases

SECTION IV   Endocrine and Dermatologic Disorders

SECTION V   Renal Diseases

SECTION VI   Neurologic and Psychiatric Disorders

SECTION VII   Musculoskeletal and Soft Tissue Disorders

SECTION VIII   Neoplasms

SECTION IX   Reproductive Health

Preface

Throughout time, food has been used in healing. In recent decades food and medicine have taken divergent paths. Food has become bereft of nutrients, and modern medicine has sought to heal with technical advances that initially seem dazzlingly more powerful than food. Consequently, the healing potential of food is underutilized in modern medicine.

After decades of journeying on different paths, food and medicine are now located far from each other in the health care system. The current gap between food and medicine is illustrated in our terminology, which considers food and nutrients to be alternative and complementary to modern medicine. Not only do such terms contradict the obvious—we must eat to live—they imply the opposite of what has taken place. Food and nutrients are the original medicine. They are the molecules of biochemistry, physiology, and immunology, and the shoulders on which modern medicine stands.

This textbook was developed to help physicians reunite food and medicine in clinical practice. With food deviating from what the human body was designed to eat, with the population's health challenged, and with emerging technologies creating new clinical tools, this is a time like no other to restore food and nutrients to their vital clinical roles.

FOR MEDICAL DOCTORS

Apple-a-day prevention is supposed to keep the doctor away! So why is this book on nutrition written for doctors? Food and nutrients not only keep people healthy, they are clinical tools powerful enough to make sick people well.

Optimal nutrition as understood by recent advances in molecular science has the potential to unfetter patients bound by chronic disease. Once disease is present, dietary counseling may be insufficient. Treatment may require diagnosing associated medical conditions, screening genetic factors, minimizing nutrient-drug interactions, ordering blood tests, referring patients to appropriate specialists, and modifying prescriptions. In other words, this book is not intended to add another responsibility to ever-shrinking office visits. It is about the practice of medicine. Each chapter was written by medical doctors for medical doctors.

ABOUT HELPING TODAY'S PATIENTS

This book is written by physicians on the front lines of disease management. It is written for doctors who want the latest treatment approaches that benefit today's patients.

This book does not represent guidelines, recommendations, or the current standard of medical care as defined by medical law. Neither does it contain patient-sensitive information.

PERTAINING TO BOTH FOOD AND NUTRIENTS

One who considers individual nutrients and biochemistry, but not food, is likely to miss the big picture. It matters how food tastes, how much time it takes to prepare, and how enjoyable it is to eat. Food is more than the sum of its nutrients. When it is eaten, with what other foods it is eaten, how it is prepared, and who is eating it all matter.

On the other hand, if you consider only food, you are forfeiting important knowledge such as how nutrient needs vary with disease and how the nutrient content of food varies greatly in modern agriculture. Nutrients can overcome toxicant exposure, compensate for disease, overcome predisposing genetics and epigenetics, and repair medication-induced nutrient deficiencies. In addition, this book reviews the medical literature on effectiveness of supplemental nutrients in treating disease. The quality of supplemental nutrients varies greatly and is also discussed.

BY A TEAM OF EXPERTS

People want to do what it takes to get better. However, information on nutrition tends to be incomplete, confusing, and often dangerously not applicable to the patient using it. As a result, food and nutrients are seldom used to their full healing potential.

Food and Nutrients in Disease Management gives complete, clear, and patient-specific answers. Its 64 author experts come from extremely diverse backgrounds such as food anthropology, industry, clinical practice in medical subspecialties, international health, academic medicine, and biochemical research. While awaiting the first chapter manuscripts, I nervously wondered what I would do if one chapter concluded "black" and the other said "white." That never happened! Instead this large, diverse, and highly regarded team has spoken with remarkable convergence. Each chapter supports the others with varying shades of pearl, dove, and silver.

WITH MUCH EVIDENCE

Medical doctors have a professional duty to carefully consider the appropriateness of a therapy for their patients. To closely examine potential treatments for diseases of muscle, fat, and bone metabolism, I developed *Scientific Evidence for Musculoskeletal, Bariatric, and Sports Nutrition* (Kohlstadt, I., editor, CRC Press, Boca Raton, FL, 2006). The evidence for food and nutrients in disease treatment was compelling and complex.

Food can be used for healing, but food is not medicine in the same way a drug is medicine. Foods that heal have gotten acquainted with human genes for millennia. They have evolved together. Eating food is not elective. It is not a matter of food or no food, the way a physician must decide whether or not to prescribe a drug. Food anthropology is compelling information. When food contents, agriculture, processing, and preparation change, health conditions change with them.

Interpreting nutritional studies poses an often overlooked challenge. Unlike medications that are foreign to the body, everyone has preexisting levels of nutrients. Generally it is only people with suboptimal levels who benefit from supplemental dosing. Yet many nutrients cannot be measured in a laboratory. Dietary assessment is often inadequate to determine preexisting levels of nutrients since medications, diseases, modern food practices, and environmental toxins place additional burdens on the body's nutrient levels. Even if a dietary assessment indicates that a person eats sufficient nutrients, their nutrient levels may still be inadequate. In this book clinical experts share their insights on interpreting clinical studies.

AND EXPERIENCE

The authors present solutions. They share the clinical approaches they have developed as experts in the field. Yes, nutritional medicine needs better diagnostics, a detailed understanding of food reactivities and obesity, and uniformly high-quality supplemental nutrients. However, your patient is in your office today!

Thank you for caring for your patients. May the knowledge in this book extend your healing reach.

Acknowledgments

Thanks to the team! This book is a gift from its 64 authors, who have given the project long hours after clinical practice and other professional duties. They have freely shared their clinical *pears*, fruits from years of patient care and research. Their work enables physicians everywhere to maximize the healing potential of food and nutrients.

Writing is a discovery process, which is a gentle way of saying it invariably takes longer than expected. I thank the families of the authors, including my own dear Ellis and Raeha, for giving time and support to this project. As the book's editor I am deeply appreciative.

About the Editor

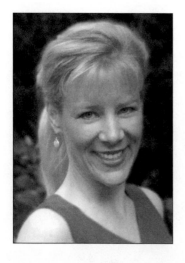

Ingrid Kohlstadt, MD, MPH, FACN, is an FDA Commissioner's Fellow at the U.S. Food and Drug Administration, Office of Scientific and Medical Programs. There she works toward improving communication on food and drug interactions. She has been elected a Fellow of the American College of Nutrition and is an associate at the Johns Hopkins School of Public Health. She is the founder and chief medical officer of *INGRID*ients™, Inc., which provides medical nutrition information to colleagues, clients, and consumers.

Dr. Kohlstadt is a graduate of Johns Hopkins School of Medicine, Class of 1993. She earned her bachelor's degree in biochemistry at the University of Maryland and as a Rotary Club scholar at Universität Tübingen, Germany, in 1989.

Board-certified in General Preventive Medicine and with a graduate degree in epidemiology, Dr. Kohlstadt became convinced that nutrition is powerful and underutilized in preventing disease. She therefore focused her career on nutrition through fellowships at Johns Hopkins and the Centers for Disease Control and Prevention. She worked as a bariatric physician at the Johns Hopkins Weight Management Center and the Florida Orthopaedic Institute.

As a congressional intern and later with the FDA, USDA, local health departments, USAID, and United States Antarctic Program, Dr. Kohlstadt studied the rugged terrain of health policy, specifically how food and nutrients can be incorporated into primary care medicine. Prior to developing *Food and Nutrients in Disease Management,* she edited *Scientific Evidence for Musculoskeletal, Bariatric, and Sports Nutrition* (CRC Press, Boca Raton, FL, 2006).

Dr. Kohlstadt resides with her husband, Ellis Richman, and their daughter Raeha in historic Annapolis, Maryland.

Contributors

Shoma Berkemeyer, Ph.D.
Ruhr-Universität Bochum
Klinik für Altersmedizin und Fruehrehabilitation
Marienhospital Herne
Herne, Germany

Roger Billica, M.D., F.A.A.F.P.
Tri-Life Health, PC
Center for Integrative Medicine
Fort Collins, Colorado

Keith I. Block, M.D.
Medical and Scientific Director,
Block Center for Integrative Cancer Treatment
Institute for Cancer Research and Education
Evanston, Illinois

**Kenneth Bock, M.D., F.A.A.F.P.,
F.A.C.N., C.N.S.**
Rhinebeck Health Center
Rhinebeck, New York

Annette L. Cartaxo, M.D.
Newton Memorial Hospital/
Hackensack University Medical Center
Kinnelon, New Jersey

Gary Chan, M.D.
Department of Pediatrics
University of Utah
Salt Lake City, Utah

Michael Compain, M.D.
Rhinebeck Health Center
Rhinebeck, New York

Richard C. Deth, Ph.D.
Northeastern University
Boston, Massachusetts

**Geovanni Espinosa, N.D., M.S.,
L.Ac., R.H. (A.H.G.)**
Department of Urology
Columbia University Medical Center
New York, New York

Laura Flagg, C.N.P.
Veterans Affairs Medical Center
Cincinnati, Ohio

Majid Fotuhi, M.D., Ph.D.
Assistant Professor of Neurology,
Johns Hopkins University School of Medicine
Director, Center for Memory and Brain
Health, Sinai Hospital of Baltimore
Baltimore, Maryland

Lynda Frassetto, M.D.
Associate Professor of Medicine
Medical Director,
UCSF CTSI Clinical Research Center
University of California San Francisco
San Francisco, California

Sheila George, M.D.
Center for Metabolic Wellness
New York, New York

**Leah Gramlich, M.D.,
F.R.C.P. (Canada)**
Royal Alexandra Hospital
University of Alberta
Edmonton, Alberta, Canada

Erminia M. Guarneri, M.D., F.A.C.C.
Director,
Scripps Center for Integrative Medicine
La Jolla, California

Charlotte Gyllenhaal, Ph.D.
Block Center for Integrative Cancer Treatment
Evanston, Illinois

Georges M. Halpern, M.D., Ph.D.
Distinguished Professor of Pharmaceutical
Sciences,
Hong Kong Polytechnic University
Portola Valley, California

Mary L. Hardy, M.D.
Medical Director, Simms/Mann–UCLA
Center for Integrative Oncology
David Geffen School of Medicine at UCLA
Los Angeles, California

Geoffrey R. Harris, M.D.
Private Practice
Ventura County, California

Marty Hinz, M.D.
Neuroresearch Clinics, Inc.
Duluth, Minnesota

Alan R. Hirsch, M.D., F.A.C.P.
Smell & Taste Treatment and
Research Foundation, Ltd.
Chicago, Illinois

Michael F. Holick, M.D., Ph.D.
Boston University
School of Medicine
Boston, Massachusetts

**Mark C. Houston, M.D., M.S.,
F.A.C.P., F.A.H.A.**
Associate Clinical Professor of
Medicine, Vanderbilt University
School of Medicine
Director, Hypertension Institute
Nashville, Tennessee

Mark Hyman, M.D.
Institute of Functional Medicine
Lenox, Massachusetts

Russell Jaffe, M.D., Ph.D.
PERQUE, LLC
ELISA/ACT Biotechnologies, LLC
Health Studies Collegium Foundation
Sterling, Virginia

Patricia C. Kane, Ph.D.
NeuroLipid Research Foundation
1st Health Centers
Millville, New Jersey

Aaron E. Katz, M.D.
Department of Urology
Columbia University Medical Center
New York, New York

Ingrid Kohlstadt, M.D., M.P.H., F.A.C.N.
Associate, Johns Hopkins University
Baltimore, Maryland
Founder and Chief Medical Officer,
INGRIDients, Inc.
Annapolis, Maryland
FDA Commissioner's Fellow
(October 2008–October 2010)
Office of Scientific and Medical Programs
Rockville, Maryland

Cindy A. Krueger, M.P.H.
Preservion, Inc.
Tampa, Florida

Joseph J. Lamb, M.D.
Director of Intramural Clinical Research,
Functional Medicine Research Center
MetaProteomics, LLC
Metagenics, Inc.
Gig Harbor, Washington

Linda A. Lee, M.D.
Director, Johns Hopkins Integrative
Medicine and Digestive Center
Johns Hopkins University School of Medicine
Baltimore, Maryland

Jayashree Mani, M.S., C.C.N.
PERQUE, LLC
Sterling, Virginia

Alexander Mauskop, M.D.
New York Headache Center
New York, New York

Dennis Meiss, Ph.D.
President/CEO,
ProThera, Inc.
Reno, Nevada

Payam Mohassel, M.D.
Johns Hopkins School of Medicine
Baltimore, Maryland

Joseph A. Molnar, M.D., Ph.D., F.A.C.S.
Department of Plastics and
Reconstructive Surgery
Wake Forest University, Baptist Medical Center
Winston-Salem, North Carolina

Gerard E. Mullin, M.D., M.H.S., C.N.S., C.N.S.P., F.A.C.N., F.A.C.P., A.G.A.F., A.B.H.M.
Director,
Division of Gastroenterology and Hepatology
Johns Hopkins University School of Medicine
Baltimore, Maryland

Melissa A. Munsell, M.D.
Division of Gastroenterology and Hepatology
Johns Hopkins University School of Medicine
Baltimore, Maryland

David Musnick, M.D.
Private Practice
Bellevue, Washington
Faculty, Institute for Functional Medicine
Gig Harbor, Washington
Clinical Instructor
Department of Orthopaedics and Sports
Medicine
University of Washington Medical School
Bellevue, Washington

Chailyn Nelson, R.D.
Utah State University
Logan, Utah

**Trent William Nichols, Jr., M.D.
F.A.C.N., C.N.S., Diplomate A.B.I.M.,
Gastroenterology**
Kaiser Permanente—Mid-Atlantic
Hanover, Pennsylvania

Stephen Olmstead, M.D.
Chief Science Officer,
ProThera, Inc.
Reno, Nevada

**David Perlmutter, M.D., F.A.C.N.,
A.B.H.M.**
Medical Director,
Perlmutter Health Center
Naples, Florida

Octavia Pickett-Blakely, M.D.
Johns Hopkins School of Medicine
Baltimore, Maryland

Valencia Booth Porter, M.D., M.P.H.
Chopra Center for Wellbeing
Carlsbad, California

**Steven G. Pratt, M.D., F.A.C.S.,
A.B.H.M.**
Scripps Memorial Hospital
La Jolla, California

Stuart Richer, O.D., Ph.D., F.A.A.O.
Chief, Optometry Section,
Department of Veterans Affairs
Medical Center
North Chicago, Illinois

Rebecca Roedersheimer, M.D.
Division of Urology
University of Cincinnati College of Medicine
Cincinnati, Ohio

Jyotsna Sahni, M.D.
Canyon Ranch Health Resort
Tucson, Arizona

**Ron N. Shemesh, M.D., F.A.C.O.G.,
A.B.H.M.**
Mindbodyspirit Care, Inc.
Tampa, Florida

Stephen T. Sinatra, M.D., F.A.C.C., C.N.S.
University of Connecticut
School of Medicine
Farmington, Connecticut

Isaac Soo, M.D.
Internal Medicine Resident,
Department of Medicine
University of Alberta
Edmonton, Alberta, Canada

Allan E. Sosin, M.D.
Medical Director,
Institute for Progressive Medicine
Irvine, California

Paula Stuart, M.M.S., P.A.-C., R.D., L.D.N.
Wake Forest University,
Baptist Medical Center
Winston-Salem, North Carolina

Christina Sun-Edelstein, M.D.
New York Headache Center
New York, New York

Frederick T. Sutter, M.D., M.B.A.,
F.A.A.P.M.R.
Center for Wellness Medicine
Annapolis, Maryland

Jacob Teitelbaum, M.D.
Medical Director,
Fibromyalgia and Fatigue Centers
Kailua-Kona, Hawaii

Sherri J. Tenpenny, D.O., A.O.B.N.M.M.
Executive Director,
Sanoviv Medical Institute
Rosarito, Mexico

David R. Thomas, M.D., F.A.C.P.,
A.G.S.F., G.S.A.F.
Professor of Medicine,
Saint Louis University Health Sciences Center
Saint Louis, Missouri

Valori Treloar, M.D., C.N.S.
Integrative Dermatology
Newton, Massachusetts

Douglas W. Triffon, M.D., F.A.C.C.
Scripps Center for Integrative Medicine
La Jolla, California

Elizabeth R. Volkmann, M.D.
Department of Rheumatology
David Geffen School of Medicine
University of California
Los Angeles, California

Heidi Wengreen, R.D., Ph.D.
Assistant Professor,
Department of Nutrition and Food Sciences
Utah State University
Logan, Utah

Susan E. Williams, M.D., M.S., R.D.,
C.N.S.P., C.C.D., F.A.C.P., F.A.C.N.
Director, Center for Nutrition and
Metabolic Medicine
Assistant Professor of Clinical Medicine,
Wright State University,
Boonshoft School of Medicine
Dayton, Ohio

Section I

*Disorders of the Ears, Eyes,
Nose, and Throat*

1 Age-Related Macular Degeneration

Geoffrey R. Harris, M.D., Steven G. Pratt, M.D., and Stuart Richer, O.D., Ph.D.

I. INTRODUCTION

Age-related macular degeneration is an eye disease characterized by a gradual loss of central vision in people over the age of 55. While medical treatments for macular degeneration have demonstrated limited success, nutritional interventions can make a marked difference in the prevention of disease progression. Understanding these nutritional and lifestyle measures that have shown benefit against this disabling disease is important for managing an expanding older population that is at risk for developing age-related macular degeneration.

II. BACKGROUND

Age-related macular degeneration (AMD) is the leading cause of blindness in the United States in people over the age of 55 [1]. In 1992, the Beaver Dam Eye Study, a large, longitudinal study of over 5000 individuals in Wisconsin, found that the prevalence of AMD increases with age from 14.4% in patients 55 to 64 years old, to 19.4% in patients 65 to 74 years old, and to 36.8% in patients over 75 years of age [2]. With the population of individuals over the age of 55 reaching more than 66 million in the United States in 2006, the estimated number of cases of AMD has grown to over 1.6 million [3, 4]. As the number of people over the age of 55 continues to grow, the number of cases of AMD will also continue to rise. It is estimated that there will be almost 3 million cases of AMD by 2020 [5].

AMD primarily affects the foveal area of the retina, which is used for sharp, central vision. There are two forms of AMD: atrophic (dry) and exudative (wet). Atrophic AMD is the more common and milder form, accounting for 85% to 90% of cases. It develops gradually over time and typically causes only mild vision loss. The exudative form is less common but more threatening to vision and is considered an advanced form of AMD. Wet AMD accounts for only 10% to 15% of AMD cases, but causes 90% of the severe vision loss associated with AMD [4].

To understand the pathophysiology of AMD, it is helpful to first review the pertinent anatomy. The macula is a small part of the retina, approximately 5 mm in diameter, which contains the fovea at its center. The center of the fovea is the thinnest part on the retina and is typically free of any blood vessels or capillaries. The macula, particularly the fovea, is responsible for detailed central vision and has a preponderance of cone-type photoreceptive cells. There are two functional layers to the macula: the photosensitive layer of rods and cones that gather light and convert it to nerve impulses, and the underlying retinal pigment epithelium with its basal lamina (Bruch's membrane) that maintains the division between the retina and the choroidal vasculature [6].

Although the exact etiology of AMD is unknown, understanding the pathophysiology helps to explain the current medical and nutritional therapies for AMD. Clinically, the symptoms of early AMD are subtle, with the patient complaining of blurring and distortion of the central vision. Blurring can progress to central scotoma and severe loss of vision. Examination of the eye in early atrophic AMD reveals the accumulation of cellular debris between the retinal pigment epithelium and the basement membrane in the form of pale spots called drusen. Atrophic AMD causes atrophy of photoreceptors and changes to the retinal pigment epithelium, Bruch's membrane, and choroidal blood flow with calcification of the choriocapillaris. Over time, these changes worsen and can damage the macula and fovea through retinal pigment epithelium detachment, which destroys the overlying photoreceptors. The more severe exudative (wet) AMD is characterized by neovascularization of the fovea, which leads to capillary leakage and exudative damage to the macula. It is hypothesized that neovascularization occurs after the integrity of Bruch's membrane is compromised [6–10]. It is not uncommon for a patient to have both atrophic and exudative changes in a single retina. Clinically, patients with atrophic AMD can develop exudative AMD at a later time, although this progression is not well understood. The onset and progression of AMD do not seem to follow a pattern and further research is needed [10].

The symptoms of early AMD are subtle, with the patient complaining of disturbances in glare-readaptation (photo-stress recovery), a drop in contrast sensitivity (i.e., decreased vision of medium and large objects), and the requirement of more light when reading. Regrettably, most eye doctors do not evaluate these early changes. Central visual acuity changes occur later in the disease process compared to the early stealth-like changes that affect cultural vision such as driving and reading ability. Eventually, when central foveal acuity is affected, severe loss of Snellen vision occurs in a gradual or abrupt manner.

As AMD progresses, patients indicate worsening vision ability and reduced quality of life. Central vision is critical for reading, performing basic manual tasks, driving, and even walking in an unfamiliar environment. Indeed, AMD is associated with an increased risk for hip fracture [11]. Individuals with AMD and visual impairment rate themselves lower on quality-of-life surveys and questionnaires that assess activities of daily living when compared to matched, unaffected controls [12].

AMD is also a risk factor for poorer survival and cardiovascular morbidity. Data from the Copenhagen City Eye Study identified an increased risk (RR = 1.59 with 95% CI of 1.23–2.07) for all-cause mortality in women with early and late-stage macular degeneration [13]. In this study, men did not have a significantly increased risk, but the Age-Related Eye Disease Study (AREDS) research group found an increased risk for mortality in their group of men and women with advanced AMD with a relative risk of 1.44 with a 95% confidence interval of 1.08 to 1.86 [14]. AMD is also associated with a higher risk for developing a myocardial infarction, even when controlling for other factors like smoking and age [15]. Furthermore, the 2006 Atherosclerosis Risk in Communities Study found that middle-aged individuals with AMD have an increased risk for stroke, independent of other stroke risk factors [16]. While AMD may not be the direct cause of mortality or cardiovascular disease, it is a marker for other processes and diseases that affect mortality.

III.   DIAGNOSIS OF MACULAR DEGENERATION

Signs of early AMD run the gamut from difficulty reading small type without bright lighting, color vision disturbances, and glare readaptation delays to severe central scotomas and actual loss of visual acuity on a Snellen eye chart. Early screening for AMD can be performed using an Amsler grid, which looks like graph paper made from dark lines on a white background. Patients focus their vision on a small central spot about 14 inches from their face. If any of the straight lines appear wavy, broken, or distorted, a patient should be referred for a timely dilated retinal examination [17]. An eye professional will perform an assessment of visual acuity and a full retinal examination. Examination of the fundus will identify any atrophy or neovascularization. Exudative AMD is typically examined with retinal and choroidal angiography using fluorescein dyes, optical coherence tomography, or indocyanine dyes that show the architecture of the retinal vascular tree and identify any leakage. Serial funduscopic imaging with a camera can help identify changes and at-risk areas of the macula [6].

IV. MEDICAL TREATMENTS FOR MACULAR DEGENERATION

Currently, there are no medical treatments for atrophic AMD; the only successful management of atrophic AMD is nutritionally related and will be discussed below. The existing current medical treatments for AMD address only exudative AMD and focus on inhibiting the neovascularization that leads to capillary leakage of blood and fluid in the macula. Managing neovascular AMD is a difficult, long-term process that aims to slow vision loss by preventing vessel formation. Treatments must be instituted early to prevent exudative damage and extensive neovascularization [18].

Thermal photocoagulation with a laser was the first effective therapy to show promise in neovascular AMD [6, 9]. Unfortunately, thermal laser was only found to be helpful when used on vessels outside of the foveal avascular zone so as to prevent any collateral damage to the crucial foveal photoreceptive cells by the laser [19]. Newer techniques have focused on foveal neovascularization using a nonthermal laser and a photosensitizing drug (verteporfin) that is more selective to blood vessels and causes less collateral photoreceptor damage [6]. Radiotherapy using fractionated radiation has also been shown to provide benefit in preserving near vision and contrast sensitivity [20]. Other treatments being tested involve anti-angiogenic compounds (anecortave acetate and triamcinolone acetonide) injected intravitreally or administered periocularly. Recent research has focused on slowing vision loss by neutralizing epithelial growth factor using a monoclonal antibody (ranibizumab) or modified oligonucleotide (pegaptanib sodium) injected directly into the vitreous [9, 21]. Another promising molecule is pigment-epithelium-derived growth factor, which prevents angiogenesis and may improve the health of the retinal pigment epithelium and restore the blood-retinal barrier [18, 22, 23]. Currently, no treatments are available for advanced AMD or the associated severe central vision loss.

V. RISK FACTORS FOR AMD

MEDICAL RISK FACTORS FOR AMD

To effectively manage and prevent both the development and progression of AMD in patients, a physician must have an understanding of the associated risk factors for AMD (Table 1.1). The unmodifiable risk factors for AMD include age, gender, race, eye color, previous AMD in one eye, and genetic predisposition or family history. As previously discussed, the risk for developing AMD increases with age, and individuals over 75 years of age have the highest risk [2]. Females are also at a higher risk for developing AMD, though many authors suggest that this may be because women have a longer life expectancy and survive to develop AMD [24, 25]. Blue or green iris color and Caucasian race are also risk factors for developing AMD. Caucasians are at a much higher risk of losing vision to AMD than African Americans. This risk may be related to a decrease in melanin pigments or other protective mechanisms in the iris and retina that prevent high-energy light from damaging the macula [26]. Another unmodifiable risk factor for developing AMD in an eye is having AMD in the other eye, indicating that the disease is not a random occurrence, but may be related to an individual's genetic and environmental predispositions [27, 28].

Genetic studies have shown that there is a hereditary susceptibility to developing AMD [10, 29, 30]. Monozygotic twin studies have identified an increased risk for developing AMD in individuals whose identical twins have AMD, even when environmental factors are not shared [31]. Other studies support this shared genetic predisposition for AMD among siblings and twins [32, 33]. While the development of AMD is likely multifactorial, there is particular interest in the ABCR gene, associated with autosomal recessive Stargardt macular dystrophy. It is hypothesized that heterozygotes for ABCR mutations are at a higher risk for developing AMD [34]. Other genes, including the complement factor H (CFH) gene are being studied as potential predisposing factors for AMD [35–38].

Modifiable risk factors for AMD are more clinically relevant because they can be altered through medical intervention. The most well-established modifiable risk factors for the development of AMD are smoking and obesity. Smoking may be the most well-established modifiable risk factor for developing AMD, with many studies reporting a two- to three-fold higher risk for current smokers compared with nonsmokers [24, 39–41]. Past smoking is also a risk, one which drops each

TABLE 1.1
Risk Factors for AMD

Unmodifiable Risk Factors
Advancing age
Female gender
Caucasian race
Blue or light-colored iris
AMD in one eye
Family history of AMD
Previous cataract surgery [217, 218]
Modifiable and Cardiovascular Risk Factors
Smoking
Obesity
High blood pressure
Elevated serum cholesterol
Physical inactivity
Coronary artery disease
Atherosclerosis
Diabetes
History of stroke
Elevated hsCRP
High serum homocysteine
Increased serum levels of IL-6
Ocular Risk Factors
Excessive sunlight and blue light exposure
Low macular pigment optical density (MPOD)
Nutritional Risk Factors
Low dietary intake of lutein and zeaxanthin
Eating <2 servings of fish on a weekly basis
Low long-chain omega-3 PUFA intake
High dietary omega-6 to omega-3 PUFA ratio
High fat diet
Low serum vitamin D

year after quitting, although it never returns to that of age-matched individuals who never smoked [41]. Obesity has emerged as the second main modifiable risk factor behind smoking. Obesity, BMI greater than 30, higher waist circumference, and elevated waist-to-hip ratio have all been associated with a greater than two-fold risk for the development and progression of AMD [42–44].

Another main set of medical risk factors associated with AMD are cardiovascular-related risks. Physical inactivity is one cardiovascular risk that is also a risk for AMD. Physically active individuals have a lower risk for developing exudative AMD (OR = 0.3, CI = 0.1 − 0.7) [45]. In addition, hypertension, elevated total cholesterol, coronary artery disease, atherosclerosis, diabetes, history of stroke, elevated C-reactive protein (specifically high-sensitivity C-reactive protein, hsCRP), high serum homocysteine, and increased levels of the systemic inflammatory marker, IL-6, are each risk factors for the development of AMD [46–53]. The association of AMD with elevated serum homocysteine, hsCRP, and IL-6 suggests that AMD is both an inflammatory and oxidative process [54–56].

OCULAR RISK FACTORS FOR AMD

Light exposure has a significant effect on ocular tissue. The sun creates full-spectrum light, from ultraviolet through the visual spectrum to the infrared wavelengths. The higher energy light in the ultraviolet and blue spectrum can injure eye tissue through oxidative damage from the generation of free radicals.

Ultraviolet light is absorbed by the human lens, so the only high-energy light that reaches the retina and macula is blue light [57–59]. There are many studies showing that exposure to blue light is toxic to retinal cells and retinal pigment epithelial cells in cell culture [60], rats [61, 62], and monkeys [63, 64].

Epidemiological studies of light exposure and AMD in human populations have produced conflicting results. The Pathologies Oculaires Liees à l'Age (POLA) study from France found no relationship between self-reported history of light exposure and the development of AMD [65]. However, in the Beaver Dam Eye Study, older participants who indicated that they had been exposed to the sun for more than 5 hours a day during their teenage years and young adulthood had a higher risk of developing AMD (RR = 2.20, CI = 1.02 – 4.73). In this study, participants who indicated that they had the same, high level of summer sun exposure but used hats and sunglasses at least half the time during their teenage and young adult years had a decreased risk of developing the early signs of AMD [66]. Similarly, in the Chesapeake Bay Waterman Study, men exposed to increased levels of blue light were more likely to develop advanced AMD [67]. Overall, it does seem that there is an association between sunlight and blue light exposure and AMD.

Research has revealed that the retinal pigments that absorb high-energy blue light also have a protective effect and reduce the risk of developing AMD [68]. The macula, or macula lutea (lutea means yellow in Latin), has a yellow coloration that is attributable to the macular pigments, which consist of the carotenoid xanthophyll isomers: lutein and zeaxanthin [69, 70]. Xanthophylls are a type of carotenoid. There are over 600 known carotenoids, and between 40 and 50 carotenoids are available in a typical Western diet [71], although only 14 of these carotenoids have been detected in human blood [72–74]. The two large groups of carotenoids are xanthophylls, which contain oxygen molecules in their molecular structure, and carotenes, which typically consist of only carbon and hydrogen. The most common xanthophylls in foods are lutein and zeaxanthin, while the most common carotenes are alpha-carotene, beta-carotene, and lycopene [75].

Lutein and zeaxanthin are yellow pigments that reach their greatest concentration in the fovea (the center of the macula) with zeaxanthin being the predominant carotenoid [76–78]. There is controversy regarding the specific role of these pigments in the retina, but it is generally accepted that they protect the delicate macular photoreceptors and improve vision. The suggested functions of these pigments include reduction of light scatter and color abnormalities [79, 80], direct absorption of high-energy blue light that can damage the macula [81], and protection against free radicals created from photochemical reactions in the photoreceptor cells through lutein's and zeaxanthin's antioxidant abilities [82–85]. It is likely that these carotenoids perform each of these functions to protect the retina and preserve central vision [85, 86].

The risk for developing AMD is related to the carotenoid levels in the macular pigment. A 2008 Japanese study identified that macular carotenoid levels decrease with age in both normal subjects and individuals with AMD. They also found that macular pigment carotenoid levels are significantly lower in patients with early AMD when compared with individuals without signs of AMD [87]. This study confirms previous work that found macular pigment optical density (MPOD) is inversely related to the risk of developing AMD [88–90].

Nutritional Risk Factors for AMD

Intrinsic production of carotenoids does not occur in mammals, and thus macular pigment must be traced to dietary intake. Studies have shown that high dietary intake of lutein and zeaxanthin and of fruits and vegetables high in the xanthophyll carotenoids is associated with a lower risk for developing AMD [91–95]. Numerous studies have also shown that dietary intake of lutein and zeaxanthin has a direct association with serum levels of lutein and zeaxanthin [96–101]. Furthermore, MPOD is directly related to dietary intake of the xanthophyll carotenoids and serum levels of lutein and zeaxanthin [96, 97, 102, 103].

Other dietary and nutritional risk factors for the development of AMD include low fish consumption, high-fat diet, and low vitamin D levels. Increased intake of fish, at least two or more servings per week, reduces the risk for developing AMD [39, 104]. Furthermore, dietary omega-3 fatty acids, which are found in high levels in fish, are also associated with a lower risk for developing AMD [39, 104, 105]. This reduced risk seems to be related to increased dietary intake of omega-3 polyunsaturated fatty acids (PUFAs) [106].

Docosahexaenoic acid (DHA) is the predominant PUFA in brain and retinal tissue, and retinal concentrations of DHA are dependent on dietary concentrations [107]. Animal studies have shown that dietary deprivation of DHA leads to lower retinal DHA levels, abnormal electroretinograms, and visual impairment [108, 109]. Higher fish intake is associated with a lower risk for developing AMD in part because of the high concentrations of preformed DHA in fish [104]. In order to achieve optimal retinal levels of DHA, the following dietary considerations are proposed:

1. A diet high in omega-6 PUFAs can inhibit omega-3 usage [110]. Due to the pervasive use of vegetable oils that are high in omega-6 PUFAs like corn and soybean oil, the relative ratio of omega-6 to omega-3 in a typical Western diet has risen to approximately 10 to 1 [111–113]. In non-Westernized diets and historic diets, the ratios have been estimated to be 2 to 1 and 1 to 1, respectively [114]. A 2003 study confirms that high dietary intake of omega-6 PUFAs in the form of vegetable fat increases the risk of developing AMD [43]. Vu et al. reported that individuals who ate more than 7.17 mg a day of the essential omega-6 fat linoleic acid (LA) had an increased risk of developing AMD [106]. The study found that lutein and zeaxanthin were protective for the development of AMD when LA levels were low. However, with high intake of LA, higher lutein and zeaxanthin levels increased AMD risk, suggesting that a poorly understood inflammatory response may be present as is the case with beta-carotene in smokers.

2. Omega-6 fats from vegetable oils often undergo partial hydrogenation, which produces *trans* fats. *Trans* fats interfere with synthesis of DHA in several ways. One mechanism that has been well studied is the ability of *trans* fats to inhibit the rate-limiting enzyme delta-6-dehydrogenase. Zinc deficiency also inhibits this enzyme, presenting another mechanism by which zinc may prevent AMD.

3. Fats and oils that are processed through hydrogenation, partial hydrogenation, and several other methods lose a substantial amount of fat-soluble vitamins such as vitamin D, vitamin E, beta-carotene, lutein, and zeaxanthin. Enriched fats are those that have had the many different tocopherols and tocotrienols removed and replaced with alpha-tocopherol. Beta-oxidation within the body is an oxidative process that requires diverse antioxidants to protect sensitive tissues like the retina. Separating fats from their antioxidant companions impairs the body's ability to safely achieve optimal DHA for retinal health. How fats are processed can explain why a diet high in fat increases AMD. Consuming nuts, an unprocessed high-fat food, lowers risk for developing AMD [43].

The combination of high omega-6 content in the Western diet, introduction of *trans* fats, and processing fats to remove the natural antioxidants appears to have created a shortage of DHA usable for the retina, which can be mitigated with supplemental DHA.

Finally, vitamin D deficiency is related to the development of AMD. Serum levels of vitamin D have been shown to be inversely associated with early AMD. Furthermore, in a group of people who did not consume milk, which is fortified with vitamin D, patients who consistently took a vitamin D supplement were at lower risk (OR = 0.67, 95% CI = 0.5–0.9) of developing early AMD than individuals who did not take a vitamin D supplement [115].

VI. TESTING FOR AMD IN HIGH-RISK PATIENTS

Screening for AMD is important after the age of 55. Patients can use an Amsler grid on a weekly basis to self-test for any central vision changes. An Amsler grid can easily be printed from the Internet and demonstrated in the office in only a few minutes. Unfortunately, the Amsler grid has a sensitivity of less than 50% and can miss a number of patients with AMD [116]. Sensitivity of the Amsler grid is even lower for detecting patients with early AMD [117]. Additionally, many patients with early AMD have 20/20 vision by Snellen eye chart. The best way to diagnose early AMD is through a thorough dilated retinal exam by an eye professional.

After the age of 55, patients should have a dilated eye examination by an eye professional at least every 3 years and Snellen visual acuity (eye chart) testing on at least a yearly basis. The American Academy of Ophthalmology recommends that patients have a dilated eye examination every 1 to 2 years starting at the age of 65 [118]. Ideally, individuals over 55 years old should have a dilated eye examination every year by an eye professional, and this should be strongly recommended for at-risk patients.

Yearly routine physical examinations of patients over 55 years of age should include questions about visual changes, problems with adapting after bright light exposure, difficulty reading, perception issues while driving, or vision loss. In addition to a thorough family history that includes eye diseases, the history should also include a social history that addresses sun exposure, utilization of sunglasses and hats, supplement usage, and dietary habits with an emphasis on fruit, vegetable, and fish consumption. Further testing should be recommended for high-risk patients. In addition to routine screening for cardiovascular disease with lipid panels, hsCRP levels, homocysteine levels, and renal and liver function panels, patients with multiple risk factors for AMD may benefit from serum carotenoid levels and ocular testing for MPOD.

Serum quantification of carotenoids is available for clinical usage [119–121]. LabCorp offers a beta-carotene level that only identifies beta-carotene [122], while Quest Diagnostics offers a frac-tionated carotene test that measures serum levels of alpha-carotene, beta-carotene, lutein, and zeax-anthin [123]. The Quest Diagnostics test is performed by the Associated Regional and University Pathologists, Inc. (ARUP) and requires an overnight fast (12 hours) and abstinence from alcohol for at least 24 hours prior to the test. The charge for the test is around $150, with the price varying based on the local laboratory [124]. Check with your laboratory about the availability of carotenoid testing before ordering the test to ensure the proper evaluation is performed.

MPOD testing is becoming a more widely available tool for evaluating AMD risk [96, 125–127]. Typically performed by an eye professional, MPOD testing is accomplished by a machine that measures lutein and zeaxanthin levels in the macula. Check with your local eye professionals as to whether they are performing MPOD determinations prior to referring a patient at high risk for developing AMD. MPOD testing and serum carotenoid levels can help guide a therapeutic plan for lowering risks and preventing AMD. Counseling and education about dietary habits, nutrient supplementation, and high-energy light avoidance and protection are part of preventing and slowing the progression of AMD.

VII. DIETARY AND NUTRITIONAL MANAGEMENT OF AMD

Nutritional management and prevention of AMD can be divided into two approaches: first, increas-ing dietary antioxidants; and second, augmenting the macular pigment by increasing the intake of xanthophyll carotenoids. Research has shown that the prevalence of AMD is higher in individuals with low antioxidant intake and low lutein intake [128]. Clearly, there is overlap between antioxidant and xanthophyll carotenoid intake because carotenoids are able to act as antioxidants, and antioxi-dants can increase intestinal absorption of lutein and zeaxanthin by protecting these pigmentary carotenoids [129]. However, this division is helpful when considering the scientific literature and counseling patients to make dietary changes.

ANTIOXIDANT INTAKE

Oxidative stress has been linked to AMD, and the earliest nutritional studies of AMD focused on the effects of antioxidant intake. The most commonly recognized antioxidants include vitamin C, vitamin E, and beta-carotene. Vitamin C, l-ascorbic acid, is a water-soluble, essential nutrient that can scavenge free radicals and be regenerated (reduced) by glutathione. Vitamin E, which usually appears in supplements as alpha-tocopherol, is only one molecule in the tocopherol antioxidant family. In fact, the tocopherols, and the closely related tocotrienols, all have vitamin E activity. Tocopherols and tocotrienols are fat-soluble nutrients. The main compounds with vitamin E activity are alpha-, beta-, gamma-, and delta-tocopherol, and alpha-, beta-, gamma-, and delta-tocotrienols. Nuts, seeds, olive oil, whole grains, and green leafy vegetables are all excellent sources of tocopherols and tocotrienols. Oxidized vitamin E, which is formed after vitamin E absorbs a free radical, is reduced back to its active form by vitamin C [130, 131].

Beta-carotene is the most extensively studied of the carotenoids and serves as an example of both the benefit and potential risk of antioxidants. Early nutritional research found a positive correlation between consumption of foods high in beta-carotene and a lower cancer risk. This correlation led to many studies using beta-carotene supplementation as a potential means for preventing cancer. However, results of beta-carotene supplementation have been mixed, and in two large studies, beta-carotene supplementation was actually shown to increase lung cancer risk and increase mortality in smokers [132, 133].

While most of the early studies of beta-carotene supplementation looked for a single nutritional compound for effective cancer prevention, subsequent research has identified that the antioxidant benefit of beta-carotene involves a complicated relationship between vitamin C, vitamin E, glutathione, and other antioxidants [134]. Beta-carotene requires other antioxidants to regenerate itself and prevent the development of its pro-oxidant form. To clarify this process, free radicals that are generated by oxidative stress can be absorbed by antioxidants to prevent these reactive free radicals from damaging DNA or cellular proteins and enzymes. When antioxidants absorb a free radical, they become oxidized (a pro-oxidative state) and must be reduced (regenerated). It is hypothesized that exclusive beta-carotene supplementation in individuals with low intake of other antioxidants actually causes a pro-oxidative state with oxidized beta-carotene causing further cellular damage [135].

Since antioxidants work in concert, the first antioxidant studies in AMD used a mix of compounds. One of the most publicized research studies of antioxidant supplementation in AMD is from the AREDS (Age-Related Eye Disease Study) group, which is sponsored by the National Eye Institute. In their study, 11 retinal centers enrolled individuals from 55 to 80 years of age and divided them into four groups based on their degree of AMD. Category 1 had no AMD, and categories 2 through 4 had increasing degrees of AMD. Using a randomized, double-blinded, placebo-controlled design, participants in each category of AMD were assigned to one of four study groups: antioxidants, 80 mg of zinc (with copper to prevent anemia), antioxidants plus zinc (and copper), or placebo. In this study, the antioxidant mix included 500 mg of vitamin C, 400 IU of vitamin E, and 15 mg of beta-carotene. Average follow-up for the study was 6.3 years, with only 2.4% lost to follow-up. The outcomes that the study measured were AMD progression and change in visual acuity.

AREDS found no benefit of supplementation in patients with no AMD (category 1), but it did identify benefits to categories 2, 3, and 4. When categories 2, 3, and 4 were combined for analysis, there was a statistically significant decrease in risk of progression to advanced AMD for the zinc groups (when adjusted for age, sex, race, AMD category, and baseline smoking status) with an OR of 0.71 (CI = 0.51 − 0.98) and the antioxidant plus zinc groups with an OR of 0.72 (CI = 0.52 − 0.98). The risk of progression to advanced AMD was even lower when just the moderate and severe AMD groups (subjects in category 3 and 4) were analyzed. When the study looked at visual acuity loss in category 3 and 4 subjects, the only statistically significant risk decrease was achieved by subjects in the groups who took antioxidants plus zinc (OR = 0.73, CI = 0.54 − 0.99). It is important to note that trends toward lower risk for progression to advanced AMD and loss of visual acuity were found in categories 2, 3, and 4, for antioxidants, zinc, and antioxidants plus zinc, though these did not reach statistical significance. Unfortunately, the study may not have been adequately powered to identify a benefit in the group with no AMD (category 1) [136]. Alternatively, the lack of benefit in category

1 patients may be because participants without AMD were zinc and antioxidant replete prior to supplement use.

Since recent research has identified the added benefit of the pigmentary carotenoids and the advantage of diets with high intake of antioxidant-rich foods, studies using isolated antioxidants have been replaced by those evaluating more comprehensive supplements and dietary approaches [137]. The AREDS has started the AREDS II trials that will evaluate the effects of supplemental lutein and zeaxanthin and/or omega-3 long-chain PUFAs, in combination with the original antioxidant formulation, on the development of AMD.

BETA-CAROTENE

As mentioned above, beta-carotene supplementation has been associated with an increased risk for developing lung cancer in smokers [138]. Smokers, individuals with a history of smoking, and people with a higher risk for developing lung cancer, should not take beta-carotene supplements or multivitamins that contain beta-carotene. Furthermore, asbestos workers as well as individuals who abuse alcohol should avoid beta-carotene supplements. The AREDS II trial will also evaluate the effect of removing beta-carotene from the antioxidant formulation.

ZINC

Zinc is an antioxidant that has shown benefit in preventing the progression of AMD and has been included in antioxidant supplements for AMD. Zinc has antioxidant properties that protect proteins and tissues against free radical damage [139]. However, taking too much daily zinc can be a problem. High zinc intake can suppress copper absorption and lead to copper deficiency with subsequent immunosuppression and anemia [140, 141]. The National Academy of Sciences–National Research Council's (NAS–NRC) Recommended Dietary Allowance (RDA) for zinc is 8 mg/day of elemental zinc for women and 11 mg/day for men. The NAS–NRC has indicated that zinc supplementation should be limited to 40 mg/day and that zinc supplements should include copper to prevent copper deficiency [142].

Zinc is found in the protein component of plant and animal matter and is found in a variety of foods. The food sources of zinc include shellfish (especially oysters), red meat, poultry, fortified cereals, whole grains, legumes, greens, and nuts. Oysters have the highest amount of zinc per serving, but in a typical American diet most of the zinc comes from red meat and poultry. Zinc absorption is higher from animal protein than plant protein, because plants contain organic acids like phytic acid and oxalic acid that bind elements like zinc and calcium and prevent their absorption; this differential absorption is more pronounced in individuals with high dietary fiber intake. Consequently, vegetarians have a higher risk for zinc deficiency than omnivores [143–145]. Alcohol also decreases the absorption of zinc and increases urinary zinc excretion, and zinc deficiency is common in alcoholics [146]. Diarrhea also results in loss of zinc and zinc deficiency. Chronic diarrhea and malabsorption from celiac sprue, Crohn's disease, short bowel syndrome, and bariatric surgery are risk factors for zinc deficiency [147]. Furthermore, one of the physiologic responses to emotional and physical stress is higher urinary excretion of zinc, which results in increased need of this trace mineral.

Zinc is available as a supplement, and daily multivitamins typically contain 15 mg of elemental zinc. Nutritional supplement shakes such as Ensure and Boost also contain zinc. When counseling patients about zinc intake and supplementation, it is important to understand the symptoms of zinc toxicity [148]. High doses of zinc are associated with stomach upset, vomiting, headaches, diarrhea, fatigue, exhaustion, and a metallic taste [149], while copper deficiency typically presents with anemia symptoms [150]. Studies have also identified that supplementation with high levels of zinc can cause prostate enlargement [151] and increase the risk for developing Alzheimer's [152]. Continued high-dose therapy with zinc may also accelerate the development of atherosclerosis and heart disease by increasing total cholesterol and LDL, elevating serum triglycerides, and lowering HDL [153, 154]. Zinc may also interfere with angiotensin-converting enzyme inhibitors, antibiotics, hormone replacement therapy, and nonsteroidal anti-inflammatories [149]. Zinc status can be difficult to assess in patients, and physicians must rely on a thorough dietary history and questions about supplementation to ensure patients are getting an adequate amount of zinc and avoiding excessive zinc consumption. Depleted zinc may also be suspected with certain rashes, frequent colds or viral infections, and lack of ability to taste zinc. If zinc cough drops or zinc challenge liquid tastes neutral or even tastes good, it is an indication that zinc stores are low. As zinc becomes replete the same cough drops and liquid taste bitter.

While zinc is a beneficial antioxidant and an important element in the diet, long-term high-dose zinc therapy may not be necessary to manage AMD. Patients should be encouraged to take a daily supplement with antioxidants including zinc and copper, but dosages above 40 mg a day are unnecessary and potentially harmful due to the side effects and lipid effects mentioned above. The AREDS II trial will also test a lower level of zinc supplementation (25 mg) against the original high-dose zinc (80 mg) that was used in the original AREDS trial.

Alpha-Lipoic Acid

Alpha-lipoic acid is a thiol antioxidant with an active cyclic disulfide bond that has been shown to be beneficial to retinal tissue by preventing oxidative stress and regenerating other antioxidants like glutathione, vitamin C, and vitamin E [155–157]. Alpha-lipoic acid is soluble in water and lipids due to its small size and chemical structure. In cell culture, retinal pigment epithelial cells are protected from oxidative damage by alpha-lipoic acid and its ability to scavenge reactive molecules [158]. Good sources of alpha-lipoic acid include broccoli and spinach. Both broccoli and spinach are also high in other antioxidants that work synergistically with alpha-lipoic acid. For example, sulforaphane, an isothiocyanate found in cruciferous vegetables like broccoli, has been shown to defend retinal tissue by working with other antioxidants to protect the macular cells from light-induced damage [159]. Furthermore, flavonoids, like luteolin, which is found in leafy vegetables like spinach, have been shown to protect retinal pigment epithelial cells from oxidative damage and decrease corneal neovascularization [160, 161].

Alpha-lipoic acid is available as a supplement; however, recommended dosages have not been clearly established. As a nutritional supplement, the typical dosage of alpha-lipoic acid is 100–200 mg/day, although higher doses have been shown to be effective in treating liver disease and diabetic neuropathy. The No Observable Adverse Effect Level (NOAEL) for alpha-lipoic acid is considered to be 60 mg per kg of body weight per day [162, 163].

Lutein and Zeaxanthin Intake

Early studies revealed that increasing the dietary intake of lutein and zeaxanthin augmented the MPOD in study participants [164, 165]. Furthermore, lutein supplementation of only 10 mg/day was shown to increase MPOD in individuals by 4% to 5% during a 4-week study published in 2000 [166]. Since these studies were published, the interest in the effect of lutein and zeaxanthin on AMD has generated a large amount of exciting research.

In 2004, the LAST (Lutein Antioxidant Supplementation Trial) study published results showing improvement in visual function and MPOD in veterans with AMD taking either 10 mg of lutein alone or in combination with an antioxidant supplement [167]. In 2007, the LAST II showed that individuals with the lowest MPOD were the most likely to benefit from supplementation with lutein alone or lutein plus antioxidants [168]. The LAST II study results suggest that individuals with low MPOD can benefit from supplementation and actually improve their MPOD. Furthermore, the LUXEA (Lutein Xanthophyll Eye Accumulation) study published in 2007 found that supplementation with lutein (10 mg) causes pigment accumulation in the fovea, and zeaxanthin supplementation (10 mg) causes pigment accumulation over a wider area of the retina. Both xanthophyll carotenoids improved

MPOD, but a mixture of lutein and zeaxanthin (10 mg/10 mg) resulted in the greatest statistically significant increase in MPOD [169]. The TOZAL (Taurine, Omega-3 Fatty Acids, Zinc, Antioxidant, Lutein) study tested a multivitamin supplement that included vitamin C, vitamin E, lutein (8 mg), zeaxanthin (400 μg), beta-carotene, zinc (70 mg), copper, and long-chain omega-3 PUFAs (120 mg DHA and 180 mg eicosapentaenoic acid [EPA]) in patients with atrophic AMD. It found stabilization and improvement in visual acuity in 76.7% of the subjects who took the supplement over a 6-month period [170].

One potentially contradictory study published in 2007 found that 6 mg of lutein supplementation in a group of 15 patients did not significantly improve contrast sensitivity in a group of AMD patients during a 9-month trial [171]. However, the small size of the study and low relative dose of lutein create more questions about the necessary study size, lutein dosage, and time to show benefit in supplement trials and AMD. The AREDS II trial will help clarify the appropriate supplement therapy because it is a very large, long-term (6 year) study.

For now, it is reasonable to recommend an antioxidant supplement. Since many people at risk for AMD take multivitamins, the antioxidant supplement could be a multivitamin that contains lutein, zeaxanthin, alpha-lipoic acid, zinc with copper, and a full spectrum of vitamin E. This supplement should be combined with a fish oil supplement or other source of preformed DHA and EPA. We recommend patients take a total of 1 to 2 g of a fish oil supplement daily.

THE SYNERGY OF WHOLE FOODS

To appropriately achieve a healthy dietary mix of antioxidants, carotenoids, and omega-3 PUFAs, AMD patients should receive nutritional counseling about incorporating beneficial foods and limiting harmful foods in their diet.

Whole foods are very important to the management and prevention of AMD. As scientific research expands the number of crucial nutrients that are included in the latest antioxidant AMD supplements, whole foods seem increasingly significant. Whole foods contain a mix of vitamins, minerals, and phytonutrients that act as antioxidants and anti-inflammatories. Phytonutrients are plant nutrients that work with the traditionally recognized vitamins and minerals and have therapeutic benefit. The common families of phytonutrients include carotenoids such as lutein, zeaxanthin, lycopene, beta-carotene, and alpha-carotene; and polyphenols, which include the isoflavones, flavonoids, and tannins. The flavonoid group includes anthocyanins and catechins. Whole fruits and vegetables contain an extensive mix of these phytonutrients [75].

Early studies that established the benefit of antioxidants and carotenoids on AMD examined food questionnaires in epidemiological studies. The focus on individual nutrients was borne out of these studies when researchers tried to identify single vitamins, minerals, or phytonutrients from the whole foods that might be providing the benefit for AMD. Trying to discover one beneficial compound in the complicated mix of nutrients in whole foods may not be reasonable. Identifying the fruits and vegetables that prevent and slow the progression of AMD is the important issue, not the possible individual nutrients.

Intake of foods high in lutein and zeaxanthin is important to preventing AMD and slowing its progression. Studies have revealed an inverse relationship between both the volume and the frequency of carotenoid-rich food consumption and risk of developing macular pigment abnormalities [172]. A partial list of foods that are high in lutein and zeaxanthin can be found in Table 1.2. Spinach is an excellent food for AMD because it is high in lutein and zeaxanthin, contains a mix of tocopherols, and has alpha-lipoic acid and other carotenoids and phytonutrients. Broccoli contains the xanthophyll carotenoids, alpha-lipoic acid, and sulforaphane, a phytonutrient that protects retinal cells from high-energy light-induced free radicals [159]. Egg yolks are another good source of lutein, with a higher bioavailability than lutein supplements, lutein ester supplements, or spinach [173].

Furthermore, many flavonoids found in whole foods have shown benefit in protecting retinal pigment epithelial cells from oxidative stress. Fisetin found in strawberries, luteolin in oranges and spinach, quercetin from apples and red onions, and epigallocatechin gallate (EGCG) from green tea

TABLE 1.2
Lutein and Zeaxanthin Content in Select Foods

Fruit, Vegetable, or Food Source	Lutein and Zeaxanthin Amount (micrograms/100 grams edible portion)
Kale, raw	39,550
Kale, boiled and drained	15,798
Spinach, raw	11,938
Spinach, boiled and drained	7,043
Lettuce, romaine, raw	2,635
Broccoli, boiled and drained	2,226
Corn, sweet, yellow, boiled and drained	1,800
Peas, green, canned	1,350
Carrots, baby, raw	358
Oranges, raw	187
Egg, raw	55

Source: Adapted from USDA-NCC Carotenoid Database for U.S. Foods [219].

all have a protective effect against free radicals in retinal cells [160]. By including the whole food source for these phytonutrients in a typical diet, a patient will increase dietary levels of many other vitamins and minerals that may help prevent AMD, including vitamin C, tocopherols, carotenoids, and zinc. Whole fruits and vegetables offer a nutrient synergy due to their complex mix of many vitamins, minerals, and phytonutrients, which is difficult to recreate.

By increasing fruit and vegetable intake, and limiting high-fat, high-calorie, and low-nutrient foods, patients will begin to lower their risk for AMD and other medical conditions. Eating more fish, supplementing DHA, and limiting the intake of vegetable oils will positively shift the dietary ratio of omega-6 to omega-3 and improve eye health and lower cardiovascular risk.

WHOLE FOODS IN THE PREVENTION OF NEOVASCULARIZATION AND ANGIOGENESIS

There is emerging information about the beneficial effects of the phytonutrients from whole foods on the prevention of angiogenesis. Angiogenesis from the choroidal vasculature leads to neovascularization of the macula and the extremely debilitating, exudative AMD. Recent research has found that certain phytonutrients suppress endothelial cell growth and prevent angiogenesis. EGCG from green tea has been shown to block vascular endothelial growth factor (VEGF) in vitro and prevent neovascularization in an embryonic membrane and mouse corneal tissue [174]. Pomegranate extract [175], an isoflavone from soy, a polyphenol from oranges, and a flavonoid from berries [161] have all been shown to inhibit angiogenesis and inhibit VEGF. Furthermore, resveratrol, another phytonutrient from red wine, can prevent angiogenesis when administered orally [176]. Another phytonutrient, procyanidin, found in cocoa, can inhibit vascular endothelium proliferation after oxidative stimulation [177].

While research still needs to address the long-term effect of these phytonutrients on AMD, encouraging patients to eat berries, soy products, oranges, pomegranates, and dark chocolate is not likely to cause harm. Furthermore, eating whole fruits and vegetables and drinking green tea and red wine (in moderation) may not only benefit AMD, but prevent cancer, since the growth of solid tumors is dependent on angiogenesis [178]. We are encouraged by the potential of phytonutrients to prevent and limit angiogenesis in exudative AMD.

CARBOHYDRATES AND AMD

While whole grains that are high in nutrients and fiber are an important tool in the nutritional management of AMD, refined carbohydrates should be avoided [179]. A 2007 study found that individuals who consumed a diet rich in refined carbohydrates with a high glycemic index had a higher risk of AMD progression when compared with individuals who consumed a diet with a low glycemic index [180]. Physicians should encourage AMD patients to limit refined carbohydrates.

VIII. NUTRITIONAL ISSUES IN AMD MANAGEMENT

Absorption and Availability of Dietary Carotenoids

The two main issues with regard to carotenoid bioavailability are release of carotenoids from the food source and digestive absorption. Since carotenoids are typically intracellular in fruits and vegetables, the cell wall must be compromised for the carotenoids to be available for micellization, the process of creating a micelle, which facilitates the absorption of fat and fat-soluble nutrients. Gentle cooking, processing by chopping or shredding, and thorough mastication are the best ways to increase the availability of carotenoids from plant sources, while gastric digestion is less efficient [181–183]. Furthermore, there does seem to be a difference in how effectively the xanthophylls and carotenes are released. Xanthophylls seem to be more readily freed from the food matrix and more effectively micellized than carotenes, but carotenes are more efficiently absorbed by enterocytes [184, 185].

Efficient micellization and absorption of carotenoids are also dependent on dietary fat intake because they are fat-soluble nutrients. While bile salts are important for forming micelles, fat from a meal helps the carotenoids to become soluble and allows for micelle formation and absorption [184, 186]. Consequently, carotenoid-rich fruits and vegetables should be eaten with a small amount of dietary fat to aid intestinal absorption. An excellent way to enhance carotenoid absorption from a salad or salsa is to add avocado or avocado oil [187]. Another important issue with regard to food preparation is cooking; while gentle cooking fractures cell walls and makes carotenoids more bioavailable, overcooking at high heats can destroy carotenoids [188, 189].

Cooking Oil Selection

In order to achieve optimal DHA from the diet, patients should evaluate their selection of cooking oils. They should avoid vegetable oils, like corn, safflower, sunflower, cottonseed, and soybean oil, which have very high relative ratios of omega-6 to omega-3 PUFAs [190, 191]. Additionally, these oils are often hydrogenated, which generates *trans* fats. Margarine should also be avoided, as should cooking with high heat and deep-frying, which damage oils. Instead patients should choose olive oil and canola oil, which contain a higher proportion of omega-3 fats. Nut oils such as hazelnut, almond, avocado, macadamia, coconut, pistachio, and red palm oils contain omega-9 and some short-chain saturated fats, which behave more favorably in the body than saturated animal fats. Regardless of which cooking oils are selected, the less processed the better. Extra virgin olive oil contains more antioxidants, which are the ingredients that confer the slightly green color to this oil. Some healthful oils, including walnut, flax, and pumpkinseed oil, are highly unsaturated and therefore very sensitive to heat when unprocessed. They should not be used for cooking, but can be stored in the refrigerator and added to cereal, salad, vegetables, and sauces.

Vitamin D in Older Adults

Older adults have a much higher risk for developing vitamin D deficiency. Elderly individuals typically have insufficient dietary vitamin D intake, inadequate sun exposure, and impaired renal conversion of provitamin D to calcitriol (Vitamin D3) [192, 193]. Additionally, sun exposure is not a reasonable way for older individuals to achieve appropriate vitamin D levels due to seasonal variation in the ultraviolet light levels that produce provitamin D and the risk for further macular damage from high-energy light exposure. Furthermore, ultraviolet damage to the skin from sunlight exposure is associated with an increased risk for skin cancer. Sun protection measures should be encouraged, and patients should be counseled to effectively achieve appropriate levels of vitamin D through diet and nutritional supplements [194].

Older individuals require more vitamin D than younger patients because of the aforementioned issues associated with achieving suitable vitamin D levels. The USDA recommends that men and women over 50 years of age get 10 μg (400 IU) of vitamin D each day, and that people over 70 get 15 μg (600 IU) daily. These recommendations are not recommended dietary allowances (RDAs), but suggestions of adequate intakes (AIs). The USDA lists the tolerable upper intake level for vitamin D as 50 μg (2000 IU) per day [143]. While the USDA advocates at least 600 IU/day, many nutritional experts recommend 800 to 1000 IU of calcitriol (vitamin D3), the preferred form of vitamin D, for adults [195, 196].

IX. SPECIAL CONSIDERATIONS FOR CAROTENOID INTAKE AND ABSORPTION

WARFARIN

Warfarin (Coumadin) is a common oral anticoagulant that inhibits vitamin K reductase. Warfarin affects the synthesis of the vitamin-K-dependent clotting factors by preventing the recycling of vitamin K. Many physicians and dieticians counsel patients on warfarin to completely avoid leafy vegetables, salads, or green vegetables due to their high vitamin K content, which can thus impair anticoagulation with warfarin. While this advice may reduce some forms of dietary vitamin K, it also prevents the dietary intake of carotenoids. Counseling and education should accompany any new prescription for warfarin. By explaining that changing dietary factors can affect warfarin's anticoagulant strength, a patient can be encouraged to maintain a diet that includes consistent amounts of carotenoid-rich vegetables. Warfarin dosage titration can be performed with the patient eating a steady and dependable amount of vegetables [197].

OBESITY

Obesity is a risk factor for the development of AMD, in part because adipose tissue sequesters fat-soluble vitamins such as vitamin D and carotenoids. Studies have shown lower plasma values of carotenoids in obese individuals [198, 199]. Basically, obesity is related to a relative carotenoid deficiency that may put patients at further risk for AMD [102]. It has also been established that MPOD levels are lower for obese individuals [97]. Consequently, obese patients will require a diet with higher levels of carotenoids and more fruits and vegetables.

GASTRIC BYPASS

It is well known that nutritional deficiencies are common in bariatric surgery patients. These nutritional deficiencies are related to both poor dietary intake and malabsorption [200, 201]. Fat-soluble nutrient deficiency is more likely for procedures that include biliopancreatic diversion due to impaired micelle formation and lipase activity [202]. A 1982 study found that carotenoid levels dropped rapidly and remained low in patients after jejunoileal bypass surgery [203]. To date, carotenoid level changes have not been studied for the now, more common Roux-en-Y gastric bypass. However, it is felt that overall malabsorption is less common for Roux-en-Y gastric bypass than previous procedures that diverted crucial absorptive gastrointestinal mucosa and the biliary and pancreatic digestive apparatus [204].

It is essential to understand the bypass procedure that a patient has undergone. Communication with the patient's surgeon may also be central to providing appropriate care. Furthermore, it is important to counsel gastric bypass patients to include vegetables in their diet. In addition to dietary counseling, it would be prudent to monitor carotenoid levels in bariatric surgery patients after gastric bypass to ensure patients are attaining healthy levels.

MALABSORPTION SYNDROMES

Malabsorption due to decreased gastrointestinal absorptive surface area can be caused by previous bowel resection, intestinal bypass, celiac sprue, Crohn's disease, AIDS enteropathy, chemotherapy, abdominal radiation therapy, amyloidosis, and intestinal lymphoma. Malabsorption can also be caused by poor micelle formation and fat solubilization, which occurs with parenchymal liver disease, cirrhosis, or biliary obstruction. Furthermore, pancreatic insufficiency from chronic pancreatitis, pancreatic resection, and cystic fibrosis can lead to malabsorption of fat-soluble nutrients due to impaired lipase activity [205, 206]. Deficiency of fat-soluble vitamins and nutrients must be considered in patients with malabsorption syndromes, and serum carotenoid testing is warranted to monitor nutritional status.

ORLISTAT

Orlistat, currently marketed under the brand names Xenical and Alli, is a reversible inhibitor of the lipase enzyme in the gut. By preventing lipase activity, dietary triglycerides cannot be hydrolyzed to absorbable monoglycerides and fatty acids. Undigested triglycerides pass unabsorbed into the stool. At the prescription dose of 120 mg, three times a day with meals, orlistat blocks the absorption of approximately 30% of dietary fat [207]. Fat-soluble vitamins and nutrients will also have a decreased absorption as they will pass with the undigested dietary fat [208]. Since an over-the-counter formulation of orlistat is now widely available, it is important to ask patients if they are using orlistat (Alli) and might be at risk for fat-soluble nutrient deficiency. Roche, the pharmaceutical company that produces orlistat, recommends that patients take a daily multivitamin supplement with the important fat-soluble vitamins at least two hours before taking orlistat. Furthermore, patients with malabsorption syndromes should not take orlistat because the drug will further aggravate gastrointestinal symptoms and nutrient deficiencies.

OLESTRA

Olestra (Olean) is a fat replacement created by Procter & Gamble. Olestra is a molecule created by linking fatty acids to a central sucrose molecule. This molecule is not digested and not absorbed. Olestra passes through the gastrointestinal tract unchanged into the stool. Since the molecule has multiple fatty acid groups, olestra can dissolve fat-soluble vitamins and carotenoids and prevent their absorption. In human studies of olestra, subjects who were fed up to 10 times the average serving amount on a daily basis had reduced absorption of carotenoids and vitamins A, D, E, and K. However, in typical amounts, the reduced absorption of fat-soluble nutrients is felt to be less than 10% [209]. While probably safe for healthy individuals, patients with malabsorption syndromes should avoid olestra to prevent exacerbating nutritional deficiencies.

X. SPECIAL CONSIDERATIONS FOR OMEGA-3 FATTY ACIDS

VEGETARIANS

Vegans and ovo-lacto vegetarians who do not eat fish are at risk for being deficient in DHA [210–212]. The major dietary omega-3 PUFA in strict vegetarians is the essential fatty acid alpha-linolenic acid (ALA) available from plant sources like flax and walnuts. ALA, a short-chain PUFA, must be lengthened. Studies have shown that healthy men can only convert 8% of dietary ALA to EPA and 0% to 4% to DHA. Due to the effects of estrogen, young women can convert about 21% of dietary ALA to EPA and 9% to DHA under optimal circumstances [213, 214]. Because vegetarians have a relatively high intake of LA, their high ratio of omega-6 to omega-3 PUFAs can reduce elongation of ALA to DHA by 40% to 50% [212, 215]. In summary, relying on the body to convert plant-derived ALA to DHA is not sufficient for optimum health [212, 215].

Vegetarians should be encouraged to eat fish, take fish oil supplements, or take marine algae oil supplements to achieve appropriate levels of DHA. For strict vegetarians, the best way to get DHA is to go to the source, or at least close to it. The source of most DHA and EPA on the planet is from marine algae. Ocean microalgae make DHA and EPA naturally. Since the aquatic food chain starts with these ocean algae, fish get their DHA and EPA from eating the algae or other organisms that have eaten the algae [216].

Eggs yolks are another potential source of DHA. Interestingly, eggs that are high in DHA and EPA come from chickens that have been fed marine algae, fish meal, or fish oil. Please note that some eggs come from chickens fed flax meal. These eggs will have omega-3 as ALA, but much less DHA and EPA. Educate patients to read the egg cartons and choose the eggs with the highest amount of DHA and EPA.

XI. SUNGLASSES FOR AMD

The perfect sunglasses not only block 100% of the UVA and UVB wavelengths, but also limit high-energy blue light. Sunglasses that block blue light tend to have an amber tint and can cause some minor color distortion. The amount of color distortion in amber lenses varies among different brands. The Neox lens that can be found in Callaway Golf Eyewear is a lens that blocks 100% of blue light up to 430 nm but allows the remainder of the visual spectrum to pass through, causing less color distortion. Most reputable optical shops have a machine that can test the ability of a pair of sunglasses to block the appropriate wavelengths.

XII. SUMMARY

The nutritional approach to lowering the risk factors for the development of AMD and slowing the progression of the disease includes the following:

- Minimize cardiovascular risk factors, including smoking, hypertension, and hyperlipidemia.
- Support and promote daily exercise.
- Encourage patients to protect their eyes from high-energy light through the use of hats and sunglasses. Appropriate sunglasses should block UV wavelengths and limit high-energy blue light.
- Counsel patients to eat more fish (at least two servings a week) and take 1 to 2 g of a fish oil supplement or marine algae supplement with DHA and EPA.
- Instruct high-risk patients to take an antioxidant supplement that includes vitamin C, mixed tocopherols (vitamin E), alpha-lipoic acid, zinc, copper, lutein, and zeaxanthin. Omega-3 PUFAs are also an important supplement for high-risk patients.
- Educate patients to eat whole foods that are high in lutein and zeaxanthin like spinach, kale, greens, and broccoli.
- Teach patients that whole fruits and vegetables have a mix of vitamins, minerals, and plant antioxidants that will promote eye health. Encourage patients to consume berries, citrus fruits, apples, nuts, legumes, and green tea.
- Recommend patients take 800 IU of vitamin D as calcitriol (vitamin D3) daily, since they are to avoid sunlight for AMD prevention. Another acceptable approach is to dose supplemental vitamin D to normalize blood levels.
- Educate patients to limit processed carbohydrates.
- Discourage high-fat diets and suggest patients limit their intake of fried foods and vegetable oils. Recommend patients choose lean red meats, poultry, and fish when eating meat. Encourage patients to cook with monounsaturated oils like olive oil and canola oil.

REFERENCES

1. Bressler, N.M., *Age-related macular degeneration is the leading cause of blindness.* JAMA, 2004. 291(15): p. 1900–1.
2. Klein, R., B.E. Klein, and K.L. Linton, *Prevalence of age-related maculopathy. The Beaver Dam Eye Study.* Ophthalmology, 1992. 99(6): p. 933–43.
3. *Population by Age, Sex, Race, and Hispanic Origin: 2006,* in *Current Population Survey, Annual Social and Economic Supplement,* U.S.C. Bureau, Editor. 2007.
4. David S. Friedman, M.D., M.P.H., *Vision Problems in the U.S.* 2002, Prevent Blindness America. p. 18–21.
5. Friedman, D.S., et al., *Prevalence of age-related macular degeneration in the United States.* Arch Ophthalmol, 2004. 122(4): p. 564–72.
6. Chopdar, A., U. Chakravarthy, and D. Verma, *Age related macular degeneration.* BMJ, 2003. 326(7387): p. 485–8.
7. Pratt, S., *Dietary prevention of age-related macular degeneration.* J Am Optom Assoc, 1999. 70(1): p. 39–47.
8. Zarbin, M.A., *Age-related macular degeneration: Review of pathogenesis.* Eur J Ophthalmol, 1998. 8(4): p. 199–206.
9. Pauleikhoff, D., *Neovascular age-related macular degeneration: Natural history and treatment outcomes.* Retina, 2005. 25(8): p. 1065–84.
10. Spaide, R.F., D. Armstrong, and R. Browne, *Continuing medical education review: Choroidal neovascularization in age-related macular degeneration—what is the cause?* Retina, 2003. 23(5): p. 595–614.
11. Anastasopoulos, E., F. Yu, and A.L. Coleman, *Age-related macular degeneration is associated with an increased risk of hip fractures in the Medicare database.* Am J Ophthalmol, 2006. 142(6): p. 1081–3.
12. Knudtson, M.D., et al., *Age-related eye disease, quality of life, and functional activity.* Arch Ophthalmol, 2005. 123(6): p. 807–14.
13. Buch, H., et al., *Age-related maculopathy: A risk indicator for poorer survival in women: The Copenhagen City Eye Study.* Ophthalmology, 2005. 112(2): p. 305–12.
14. Clemons, T.E., N. Kurinij, and R.D. Sperduto, *Associations of mortality with ocular disorders and an intervention of high-dose antioxidants and zinc in the Age-Related Eye Disease Study: AREDS Report No. 13.* Arch Ophthalmol, 2004. 122(5): p. 716–26.
15. Duan, Y., et al., *Age-related macular degeneration is associated with incident myocardial infarction among elderly Americans.* Ophthalmology, 2007. 114(4): p. 732–7.
16. Wong, T.Y., et al., *Age-related macular degeneration and risk for stroke.* Ann Intern Med, 2006. 145(2): p. 98–106.
17. *Amsler Grid Testing.* What is AMD?:www.amd.org/site/PageServer?pagename = Amsler-Grid.
18. Chakravarthy, U., et al., *Evolving European guidance on the medical management of neovascular age related macular degeneration.* Br J Ophthalmol, 2006. 90(9): p. 1188–96.
19. Moisseiev, J., et al., *The impact of the macular photocoagulation study results on the treatment of exudative age-related macular degeneration.* Arch Ophthalmol, 1995. 113(2): p. 185–9.
20. Hart, P.M., et al., *Visual outcomes in the subfoveal radiotherapy study: A randomized controlled trial of teletherapy for age-related macular degeneration.* Arch Ophthalmol, 2002. 120(8): p. 1029–38.
21. Epstein, P., *Trials that matter: Two faces of progress in the treatment of age-related macular degeneration.* Ann Intern Med, 2007. 146(7): p. 532–4.
22. Rasmussen, H., et al., *Clinical protocol. An open-label, phase I, single administration, dose-escalation study of ADGVPEDF.11D (ADPEDF) in neovascular age-related macular degeneration (AMD).* Hum Gene Ther, 2001. 12(16): p. 2029–32.
23. Lim, J.I., *Macular degeneration: The latest in current medical management.* Retina, 2006. 26(6 Suppl): p. S17–20.
24. Tomany, S.C., et al., *Risk factors for incident age-related macular degeneration: Pooled findings from 3 continents.* Ophthalmology, 2004. 111(7): p. 1280–7.
25. Kahn, H.A., et al., *The Framingham Eye Study. I. Outline and major prevalence findings.* Am J Epidemiol, 1977. 106(1): p. 17–32.
26. Bressler, S.B., et al., *Racial differences in the prevalence of age-related macular degeneration: The Salisbury Eye Evaluation (SEE) Project.* Arch Ophthalmol, 2008. 126(2): p. 241–5.
27. van Leeuwen, R., et al., *The risk and natural course of age-related maculopathy: Follow-up at 6 1/2 years in the Rotterdam study.* Arch Ophthalmol, 2003. 121(4): p. 519–26.

28. Mukesh, B.N., et al., *Five-year incidence of age-related maculopathy: The Visual Impairment Project.* Ophthalmology, 2004. 111(6): p. 1176–82.

29. Klaver, C.C., et al., *Genetic risk of age-related maculopathy. Population-based familial aggregation study.* Arch Ophthalmol, 1998. 116(12): p. 1646–51.

30. Smith, W., and P. Mitchell, *Family history and age-related maculopathy: The Blue Mountains Eye Study.* Aust N Z J Ophthalmol, 1998. 26(3): p. 203–6.

31. Klein, M.L., W.M. Mauldin, and V.D. Stoumbos, *Heredity and age-related macular degeneration. Observations in monozygotic twins.* Arch Ophthalmol, 1994. 112(7): p. 932–7.

32. Heiba, I.M., et al., *Sibling correlations and segregation analysis of age-related maculopathy: The Beaver Dam Eye Study.* Genet Epidemiol, 1994. 11(1): p. 51–67.

33. Meyers, S.M., T. Greene, and F.A. Gutman, *A twin study of age-related macular degeneration.* Am J Ophthalmol, 1995. 120(6): p. 757–66.

34. Allikmets, R., et al., *Mutation of the Stargardt disease gene (ABCR) in age-related macular degeneration.* Science, 1997. 277(5333): p. 1805–7.

35. Despriet, D.D., et al., *Complement factor H polymorphism, complement activators, and risk of age-related macular degeneration.* JAMA, 2006. 296(3): p. 301–9.

36. Yates, J.R., and A.T. Moore, *Genetic susceptibility to age-related macular degeneration.* J Med Genet, 2000. 37(2): p. 83–7.

37. Baird, P.N., et al., *Gene-environment interaction in progression of AMD—the CFH gene, smoking and exposure to chronic infection.* Hum Mol Genet, 2008.

38. Moshfeghi, D.M., and M.S. Blumenkranz, *Role of genetic factors and inflammation in age-related macular degeneration.* Retina, 2007. 27(3): p. 269–75.

39. Seddon, J.M., S. George, and B. Rosner, *Cigarette smoking, fish consumption, omega-3 fatty acid intake, and associations with age-related macular degeneration: The US Twin Study of Age-Related Macular Degeneration.* Arch Ophthalmol, 2006. 124(7): p. 995–1001.

40. Dandekar, S.S., et al., *Does smoking influence the type of age related macular degeneration causing visual impairment?* Br J Ophthalmol, 2006. 90(6): p. 724–7.

41. Thornton, J., et al., *Smoking and age-related macular degeneration: A review of association.* Eye, 2005. 19(9): p. 935–44.

42. Moeini, H.A., H. Masoudpour, and H. Ghanbari, *A study of the relation between body mass index and the incidence of age related macular degeneration.* Br J Ophthalmol, 2005. 89(8): p. 964–6.

43. Seddon, J.M., et al., *Progression of age-related macular degeneration: Association with body mass index, waist circumference, and waist-hip ratio.* Arch Ophthalmol, 2003. 121(6): p. 785–92.

44. Schaumberg, D.A., et al., *Body mass index and the incidence of visually significant age-related maculopathy in men.* Arch Ophthalmol, 2001. 119(9): p. 1259–65.

45. Knudtson, M.D., R. Klein, and B.E. Klein, *Physical activity and the 15-year cumulative incidence of age-related macular degeneration: The Beaver Dam Eye Study.* Br J Ophthalmol, 2006. 90(12): p. 1461–3.

46. Seddon, J.M., et al., *Progression of age-related macular degeneration: Prospective assessment of C-reactive protein, interleukin 6, and other cardiovascular biomarkers.* Arch Ophthalmol, 2005. 123(6): p. 774–82.

47. Zlateva, G.P., et al., *Comparison of comorbid conditions between neovascular age-related macular degeneration patients and a control cohort in the medicare population.* Retina, 2007. 27(9): p. 1292–9.

48. Hogg, R.E., et al., *Cardiovascular disease and hypertension are strong risk factors for choroidal neovascularization.* Ophthalmology, 2007.

49. Seddon, J.M., et al., *Association between C-reactive protein and age-related macular degeneration.* JAMA, 2004. 291(6): p. 704–10.

50. Boekhoorn, S.S., et al., *C-reactive protein level and risk of aging macula disorder: The Rotterdam Study.* Arch Ophthalmol, 2007. 125(10): p. 1396–401.

51. Vine, A.K., et al., *Biomarkers of cardiovascular disease as risk factors for age-related macular degeneration.* Ophthalmology, 2005. 112(12): p. 2076–80.

52. Tan, J.S., et al., *Cardiovascular risk factors and the long-term incidence of age-related macular degeneration: The Blue Mountains Eye Study.* Ophthalmology, 2007. 114(6): p. 1143–50.

53. Klein, R., et al., *Cardiovascular disease, its risk factors and treatment, and age-related macular degeneration: Women's Health Initiative Sight Exam ancillary study.* Am J Ophthalmol, 2007. 143(3): p. 473–83.

54. Kikuchi, M., et al., *Elevated C-reactive protein levels in patients with polypoidal choroidal vasculopathy and patients with neovascular age-related macular degeneration.* Ophthalmology, 2007. 114(9): p. 1722–7.

55. Totan, Y., et al., *Plasma malondialdehyde and nitric oxide levels in age related macular degeneration.* Br J Ophthalmol, 2001. 85(12): p. 1426–8.
56. Schaumberg, D.A., et al., *High-sensitivity C-reactive protein, other markers of inflammation, and the incidence of macular degeneration in women.* Arch Ophthalmol, 2007. 125(3): p. 300–5.
57. Braunstein, R.E., and J.R. Sparrow, *A blue-blocking intraocular lens should be used in cataract surgery.* Arch Ophthalmol, 2005. 123(4): p. 547–9.
58. Glazer-Hockstein, C., and J.L. Dunaief, *Could blue light-blocking lenses decrease the risk of age-related macular degeneration?* Retina, 2006. 26(1): p. 1–4.
59. Hawse, P., *Blocking the blue.* Br J Ophthalmol, 2006. 90(8): p. 939–40.
60. Sparrow, J.R., K. Nakanishi, and C.A. Parish, *The lipofuscin fluorophore A2E mediates blue light-induced damage to retinal pigmented epithelial cells.* Invest Ophthalmol Vis Sci, 2000. 41(7): p. 1981–9.
61. van Norren, D., and P. Schellekens, *Blue light hazard in rat.* Vision Res, 1990. 30(10): p. 1517–20.
62. Wu, J., et al., *Blue light induced apoptosis in rat retina.* Eye, 1999. 13(Pt 4): p. 577–83.
63. Borges, J., Z.Y. Li, and M.O. Tso, *Effects of repeated photic exposures on the monkey macula.* Arch Ophthalmol, 1990. 108(5): p. 727–33.
64. Ham, W.T., Jr., H.A. Mueller, and D.H. Sliney, *Retinal sensitivity to damage from short wavelength light.* Nature, 1976. 260(5547): p. 153–5.
65. Delcourt, C., et al., *Light exposure and the risk of age-related macular degeneration: The Pathologies Oculaires Liees a l'Age (POLA) study.* Arch Ophthalmol, 2001. 119(10): p. 1463–8.
66. Tomany, S.C., et al., *Sunlight and the 10-year incidence of age-related maculopathy: The Beaver Dam Eye Study.* Arch Ophthalmol, 2004. 122(5): p. 750–7.
67. Taylor, H.R., et al., *The long-term effects of visible light on the eye.* Arch Ophthalmol, 1992. 110(1): p. 99–104.
68. Snodderly, D.M., J.D. Auran, and F.C. Delori, *The macular pigment. II. Spatial distribution in primate retinas.* Invest Ophthalmol Vis Sci, 1984. 25(6): p. 674–85.
69. Bone, R.A., J.T. Landrum, and S.L. Tarsis, *Preliminary identification of the human macular pigment.* Vision Res, 1985. 25(11): p. 1531–5.
70. Handelman, G.J., et al., *Carotenoids in the human macula and whole retina.* Invest Ophthalmol Vis Sci, 1988. 29(6): p. 850–5.
71. Khachik, F., et al., *Separation and quantitation of carotenoids in foods.* Methods Enzymol, 1992. 213: p. 347–59.
72. Khachik, F., et al., *Separation and quantification of carotenoids in human plasma.* Methods Enzymol, 1992. 213: p. 205–19.
73. Khachik, F., et al., *Separation and identification of carotenoids and their oxidation products in the extracts of human plasma.* Anal Chem, 1992. 64(18): p. 2111–22.
74. Khachik, F., et al., *Identification, quantification, and relative concentrations of carotenoids and their metabolites in human milk and serum.* Anal Chem, 1997. 69(10): p. 1873–81.
75. Sommerburg, O., et al., *Fruits and vegetables that are sources for lutein and zeaxanthin: The macular pigment in human eyes.* Br J Ophthalmol, 1998. 82(8): p. 907–10.
76. Snodderly, D.M., G.J. Handelman, and A.J. Adler, *Distribution of individual macular pigment carotenoids in central retina of macaque and squirrel monkeys.* Invest Ophthalmol Vis Sci, 1991. 32(2): p. 268–79.
77. Hammond, B.R., Jr., B.R. Wooten, and D.M. Snodderly, *Individual variations in the spatial profile of human macular pigment.* J Opt Soc Am A Opt Image Sci Vis, 1997. 14(6): p. 1187–96.
78. Bone, R.A., et al., *Analysis of the macular pigment by HPLC: Retinal distribution and age study.* Invest Ophthalmol Vis Sci, 1988. 29(6): p. 843–9.
79. Nussbaum, J.J., R.C. Pruett, and F.C. Delori, *Historic perspectives. Macular yellow pigment. The first 200 years.* Retina, 1981. 1(4): p. 296–310.
80. Reading, V.M., and R.A. Weale, *Macular pigment and chromatic aberration.* J Opt Soc Am, 1974. 64(2): p. 231–4.
81. Kirschfeld, K., *Carotenoid pigments: Their possible role in protecting against photooxidation in eyes and photoreceptor cells.* Proc R Soc Lond B Biol Sci, 1982. 216(1202): p. 71–85.
82. Snodderly, D.M., *Evidence for protection against age-related macular degeneration by carotenoids and antioxidant vitamins.* Am J Clin Nutr, 1995. 62(6 Suppl): p. 1448S–61S.
83. Foote, C.S., Y.C. Chang, and R.W. Denny, *Chemistry of singlet oxygen. X. Carotenoid quenching parallels biological protection.* J Am Chem Soc, 1970. 92(17): p. 5216–8.
84. Landrum, J.T., R.A. Bone, and M.D. Kilburn, *The macular pigment: A possible role in protection from age-related macular degeneration.* Adv Pharmacol, 1997. 38: p. 537–56.

85. Beatty, S., et al., *Macular pigment and age related macular degeneration.* Br J Ophthalmol, 1999. 83(7): p. 867–77.
86. Stringham, J.M., and B.R. Hammond, Jr., *Dietary lutein and zeaxanthin: Possible effects on visual function.* Nutr Rev, 2005. 63(2): p. 59–64.
87. Obana, A., et al., *Macular carotenoid levels of normal subjects and age-related maculopathy patients in a Japanese population.* Ophthalmology, 2008. 115(1): p. 147–57.
88. Beatty, S., et al., *Macular pigment and risk for age-related macular degeneration in subjects from a Northern European population.* Invest Ophthalmol Vis Sci, 2001. 42(2): p. 439–46.
89. Haegerstrom-Portnoy, G., *Short-wavelength-sensitive-cone sensitivity loss with aging: A protective role for macular pigment?* J Opt Soc Am A, 1988. 5(12): p. 2140–4.
90. Hammond, B.R., Jr., B.R. Wooten, and D.M. Snodderly, *Preservation of visual sensitivity of older subjects: Association with macular pigment density.* Invest Ophthalmol Vis Sci, 1998. 39(2): p. 397–406.
91. SanGiovanni, J.P., et al., *The relationship of dietary carotenoid and vitamin A, E, and C intake with age-related macular degeneration in a case-control study: AREDS Report No. 22.* Arch Ophthalmol, 2007. 125(9): p. 1225–32.
92. Moeller, S.M., et al., *Associations between intermediate age-related macular degeneration and lutein and zeaxanthin in the Carotenoids in Age-related Eye Disease Study (CAREDS): Ancillary study of the Women's Health Initiative.* Arch Ophthalmol, 2006. 124(8): p. 1151–62.
93. *Antioxidant status and neovascular age-related macular degeneration. Eye Disease Case-Control Study Group.* Arch Ophthalmol, 1993. 111(1): p. 104–9.
94. Seddon, J.M., et al., *Dietary carotenoids, vitamins A, C, and E, and advanced age-related macular degeneration. Eye Disease Case-Control Study Group.* JAMA, 1994. 272(18): p. 1413–20.
95. Goldberg, J., et al., *Factors associated with age-related macular degeneration. An analysis of data from the first National Health and Nutrition Examination Survey.* Am J Epidemiol, 1988. 128(4): p. 700–10.
96. Ciulla, T.A., et al., *Macular pigment optical density in a midwestern sample.* Ophthalmology, 2001. 108(4): p. 730–7.
97. Hammond, B.R., Jr., T.A. Ciulla, and D.M. Snodderly, *Macular pigment density is reduced in obese subjects.* Invest Ophthalmol Vis Sci, 2002. 43(1): p. 47–50.
98. Bone, R.A., et al., *Lutein and zeaxanthin in the eyes, serum and diet of human subjects.* Exp Eye Res, 2000. 71(3): p. 239–45.
99. Hammond, B.R., Jr., et al., *Sex differences in macular pigment optical density: Relation to plasma carotenoid concentrations and dietary patterns.* Vision Res, 1996. 36(13): p. 2001–12.
100. Carroll, Y.L., B.M. Corridan, and P.A. Morrissey, *Carotenoids in young and elderly healthy humans: Dietary intakes, biochemical status and diet-plasma relationships.* Eur J Clin Nutr, 1999. 53(8): p. 644–53.
101. Rock, C.L., et al., *Diet and lifestyle correlates of lutein in the blood and diet.* J Nutr, 2002. 132(3): p. 525S–30S.
102. Mares, J.A., et al., *Predictors of optical density of lutein and zeaxanthin in retinas of older women in the Carotenoids in Age-Related Eye Disease Study, an ancillary study of the Women's Health Initiative.* Am J Clin Nutr, 2006. 84(5): p. 1107–22.
103. Bone, R.A., et al., *Lutein and zeaxanthin dietary supplements raise macular pigment density and serum concentrations of these carotenoids in humans.* J Nutr, 2003. 133(4): p. 992–8.
104. SanGiovanni, J.P., et al., *The relationship of dietary lipid intake and age-related macular degeneration in a case-control study: AREDS Report No. 20.* Arch Ophthalmol, 2007. 125(5): p. 671–9.
105. Hodge, W.G., et al., *Evidence for the effect of omega-3 fatty acids on progression of age-related macular degeneration: A systematic review.* Retina, 2007. 27(2): p. 216–21.
106. Vu, H.T., et al., *Does dietary lutein and zeaxanthin increase the risk of age related macular degeneration? The Melbourne Visual Impairment Project.* Br J Ophthalmol, 2006. 90(3): p. 389–90.
107. Salem, N., Jr., et al., *Mechanisms of action of docosahexaenoic acid in the nervous system.* Lipids, 2001. 36(9): p. 945–59.
108. Neuringer, M., et al., *Dietary omega-3 fatty acid deficiency and visual loss in infant rhesus monkeys.* J Clin Invest, 1984. 73(1): p. 272–6.
109. Neuringer, M., et al., *Biochemical and functional effects of prenatal and postnatal omega 3 fatty acid deficiency on retina and brain in rhesus monkeys.* Proc Natl Acad Sci USA, 1986. 83(11): p. 4021–5.
110. Jump, D.B., *The biochemistry of n-3 polyunsaturated fatty acids.* J Biol Chem, 2002. 277(11): p. 8755–8.

111. Simopoulos, A.P., *Omega-3 fatty acids in inflammation and autoimmune diseases.* J Am Coll Nutr, 2002. 21(6): p. 495–505.

112. Simopoulos, A.P., *The importance of the ratio of omega-6/omega-3 essential fatty acids.* Biomed Pharmacother, 2002. 56(8): p. 365–79.

113. Kris-Etherton, P.M., et al., *Polyunsaturated fatty acids in the food chain in the United States.* Am J Clin Nutr, 2000. 71(1 Suppl): p. 179S–88S.

114. Cordain, L., et al., *The paradoxical nature of hunter-gatherer diets: Meat-based, yet non-atherogenic.* Eur J Clin Nutr, 2002. 56(1 Suppl): p. S42–52.

115. Parekh, N., et al., *Association between vitamin D and age-related macular degeneration in the Third National Health and Nutrition Examination Survey, 1988 through 1994.* Arch Ophthalmol, 2007. 125(5): p. 661–9.

116. Crossland, M., and G. Rubin, *The Amsler chart: Absence of evidence is not evidence of absence.* Br J Ophthalmol, 2007. 91(3): p. 391–3.

117. Goldstein, M., et al., *Results of a multicenter clinical trial to evaluate the preferential hyperacuity perimeter for detection of age-related macular degeneration.* Retina, 2005. 25(3): p. 296–303.

118. Trustees, B.O., *Policy statement: Frequency of ocular examinations.* 2006, American Academy of Ophthalmology.

119. Olmedilla-Alonso, B., F. Granado-Lorencio, and I. Blanco-Navarro, *Carotenoids, retinol and tocopherols in blood: Comparability between serum and plasma (Li-heparin) values.* Clin Biochem, 2005. 38(5): p. 444–9.

120. Su, Q., et al., *Improved quantification of retinol, tocopherol and carotenoid in human plasma by HPLC using retinol acetate as internal standard.* Asia Pac J Clin Nutr, 2003. 12(Suppl): p. S63.

121. Lee, B.L., A.L. New, and C.N. Ong, *Simultaneous determination of tocotrienols, tocopherols, retinol, and major carotenoids in human plasma.* Clin Chem, 2003. 49(12): p. 2056–66.

122. *Carotene, Beta,* in *CPT 82380,* Lab Corporation of America: www.labcorp.com/datasets/labcorp/html/chapter/mono/sc004400.htm.

123. *Carotenes, fractionated, plasma or serum,* in *CPT 82380:* www.questdiagnostics.com.

124. *ARUP's Laboratory Test Directory (800) 522-2787,* in *0021021: Carotenes, Fractionated, Plasma or Serum:* www.aruplab.com/guides/ug/tests/0021021.jsp.

125. Berendschot, T.T., and D. van Norren, *Objective determination of the macular pigment optical density using fundus reflectance spectroscopy.* Arch Biochem Biophys, 2004. 430(2): p. 149–55.

126. Iannaccone, A., et al., *Macular pigment optical density in the elderly: Findings in a large biracial Midsouth population sample.* Invest Ophthalmol Vis Sci, 2007. 48(4): p. 1458–65.

127. Gallaher, K.T., et al., *Estimation of macular pigment optical density in the elderly: Test-retest variability and effect of optical blur in pseudophakic subjects.* Vision Res, 2007. 47(9): p. 1253–9.

128. Snellen, E.L., et al., *Neovascular age-related macular degeneration and its relationship to antioxidant intake.* Acta Ophthalmol Scand, 2002. 80(4): p. 368–71.

129. Tanumihardjo, S.A., J. Li, and M.P. Dosti, *Lutein absorption is facilitated with cosupplementation of ascorbic acid in young adults.* J Am Diet Assoc, 2005. 105(1): p. 114–8.

130. *National Institutes of Health state-of-the-science conference statement: Multivitamin/mineral supplements and chronic disease prevention.* Ann Intern Med, 2006. 145(5): p. 364–71.

131. Seddon, J.M., *Multivitamin-multimineral supplements and eye disease: Age-related macular degeneration and cataract.* Am J Clin Nutr, 2007. 85(1): p. 304S–7S.

132. Albanes, D., et al., *Alpha-tocopherol and beta-carotene supplements and lung cancer incidence in the alpha-tocopherol, beta-carotene cancer prevention study: Effects of base-line characteristics and study compliance.* J Natl Cancer Inst, 1996. 88(21): p. 1560–70.

133. Goodman, G.E., et al., *The Beta-Carotene and Retinol Efficacy Trial: Incidence of lung cancer and cardiovascular disease mortality during 6-year follow-up after stopping beta-carotene and retinol supplements.* J Natl Cancer Inst, 2004. 96(23): p. 1743–50.

134. Black, H.S., *Pro-carcinogenic activity of beta-carotene, a putative systemic photoprotectant.* Photochem Photobiol Sci, 2004. 3(8): p. 753–8.

135. Siems, W., et al., *Beta-carotene breakdown products may impair mitochondrial functions—potential side effects of high-dose beta-carotene supplementation.* J Nutr Biochem, 2005. 16(7): p. 385–97.

136. *A randomized, placebo-controlled, clinical trial of high-dose supplementation with vitamins C and E, beta carotene, and zinc for age-related macular degeneration and vision loss: AREDS report no. 8.* Arch Ophthalmol, 2001. 119(10): p. 1417–36.

137. Huang, H.Y., et al., *The efficacy and safety of multivitamin and mineral supplement use to prevent cancer and chronic disease in adults: A systematic review for a National Institutes of Health state-of-the-science conference.* Ann Intern Med, 2006. 145(5): p. 372–85.

138. Omenn, G.S., et al., *Effects of a combination of beta carotene and vitamin A on lung cancer and cardiovascular disease.* N Engl J Med, 1996. 334(18): p. 1150–5.

139. Berger, A., *What does zinc do?* BMJ, 2002. 325(7372): p. 1062.

140. Prasad, A.S., *Zinc: The biology and therapeutics of an ion.* Ann Intern Med, 1996. 125(2): p. 142–4.

141. Rowin, J., and S.L. Lewis, *Copper deficiency myeloneuropathy and pancytopenia secondary to overuse of zinc supplementation.* J Neurol Neurosurg Psychiatry, 2005. 76(5): p. 750–1.

142. *Dietary reference intakes for vitamin A, vitamin K, arsenic, boron, chromium, copper, iodine, iron, manganese, molybdenum, nickel, silicon, vanadium, and zinc.* 2001, National Academy Press: Washington, DC.

143. *Dietary Reference Intakes: Recommended Intakes for Individuals:*www.iom.edu/Object.File/Master/21/372/0.pdf.

144. Ellis, R., et al., *Phytate:zinc and phytate X calcium:zinc millimolar ratios in self-selected diets of Americans, Asian Indians, and Nepalese.* J Am Diet Assoc, 1987. 87(8): p. 1043–7.

145. Kelsay, J.L., R.A. Jacob, and E.S. Prather, *Effect of fiber from fruits and vegetables on metabolic responses of human subjects. III. Zinc, copper, and phosphorus balances.* Am J Clin Nutr, 1979. 32(11): p. 2307–11.

146. Menzano, E., and P.L. Carlen, *Zinc deficiency and corticosteroids in the pathogenesis of alcoholic brain dysfunction—a review.* Alcohol Clin Exp Res, 1994. 18(4): p. 895–901.

147. Naber, T.H., et al., *The value of methods to determine zinc deficiency in patients with Crohn's disease.* Scand J Gastroenterol, 1998. 33(5): p. 514–23.

148. Igic, P.G., et al., *Toxic effects associated with consumption of zinc.* Mayo Clin Proc, 2002. 77(7): p. 713–6.

149. Collins, N., *Zinc supplementation: Yea or nay?* Adv Skin Wound Care, 2003. 16(5): p. 226–30.

150. Hoffman, H.N., 2nd, R.L. Phyliky, and C.R. Fleming, *Zinc-induced copper deficiency.* Gastroenterology, 1988. 94(2): p. 508–12.

151. Tavani, A., et al., *Intake of selected micronutrients and the risk of surgically treated benign prostatic hyperplasia: A case-control study from Italy.* Eur Urol, 2006. 50(3): p. 549–54.

152. Cuajungco, M.P., and G.J. Lees, *Zinc and Alzheimer's disease: Is there a direct link?* Brain Res Brain Res Rev, 1997. 23(3): p. 219–36.

153. *The effect of five-year zinc supplementation on serum zinc, serum cholesterol and hematocrit in persons randomly assigned to treatment group in the age-related eye disease study: AREDS Report No. 7.* J Nutr, 2002. 132(4): p. 697–702.

154. Hooper, P.L., et al., *Zinc lowers high-density lipoprotein-cholesterol levels.* JAMA, 1980. 244(17): p. 1960–1.

155. Packer, L., K. Kraemer, and G. Rimbach, *Molecular aspects of lipoic acid in the prevention of diabetes complications.* Nutrition, 2001. 17(10): p. 888–95.

156. Kowluru, R.A., and S. Odenbach, *Effect of long-term administration of alpha-lipoic acid on retinal capillary cell death and the development of retinopathy in diabetic rats.* Diabetes, 2004. 53(12): p. 3233–8.

157. Biewenga, G.P., G.R. Haenen, and A. Bast, *The pharmacology of the antioxidant lipoic acid.* Gen Pharmacol, 1997. 29(3): p. 315–31.

158. Voloboueva, L.A., et al., *(R)-alpha-lipoic acid protects retinal pigment epithelial cells from oxidative damage.* Invest Ophthalmol Vis Sci, 2005. 46(11): p. 4302–10.

159. Tanito, M., et al., *Sulforaphane induces thioredoxin through the antioxidant-responsive element and attenuates retinal light damage in mice.* Invest Ophthalmol Vis Sci, 2005. 46(3): p. 979–87.

160. Hanneken, A., et al., *Flavonoids protect human retinal pigment epithelial cells from oxidative-stress-induced death.* Invest Ophthalmol Vis Sci, 2006. 47(7): p. 3164–77.

161. Joussen, A.M., et al., *Treatment of corneal neovascularization with dietary isoflavonoids and flavonoids.* Exp Eye Res, 2000. 71(5): p. 483–7.

162. Cremer, D.R., et al., *Safety evaluation of alpha-lipoic acid (ALA).* Regul Toxicol Pharmacol, 2006. 46(1): p. 29–41.

163. Cremer, D.R., et al., *Long-term safety of alpha-lipoic acid (ALA) consumption: A 2-year study.* Regul Toxicol Pharmacol, 2006. 46(3): p. 193–201.

164. Hammond, B.R., Jr., et al., *Dietary modification of human macular pigment density.* Invest Ophthalmol Vis Sci, 1997. 38(9): p. 1795–801.

165. Johnson, E.J., et al., *Relation among serum and tissue concentrations of lutein and zeaxanthin and macular pigment density.* Am J Clin Nutr, 2000. 71(6): p. 1555–62.

166. Berendschot, T.T., et al., *Influence of lutein supplementation on macular pigment, assessed with two objective techniques.* Invest Ophthalmol Vis Sci, 2000. 41(11): p. 3322–6.

167. Richer, S., et al., *Double-masked, placebo-controlled, randomized trial of lutein and antioxidant supplementation in the intervention of atrophic age-related macular degeneration: The Veterans LAST study (Lutein Antioxidant Supplementation Trial).* Optometry, 2004. 75(4): p. 216–30.

168. Richer, S., J. Devenport, and J.C. Lang, *LAST II: Differential temporal responses of macular pigment optical density in patients with atrophic age-related macular degeneration to dietary supplementation with xanthophylls.* Optometry, 2007. 78(5): p. 213–9.

169. Schalch, W., et al., *Xanthophyll accumulation in the human retina during supplementation with lutein or zeaxanthin—the LUXEA (LUtein Xanthophyll Eye Accumulation) study.* Arch Biochem Biophys, 2007. 458(2): p. 128–35.

170. Cangemi, F.E., *TOZAL Study: An open case control study of an oral antioxidant and omega-3 supplement for dry AMD.* BMC Ophthalmol, 2007. 7: p. 3.

171. Bartlett, H.E., and F. Eperjesi, *Effect of lutein and antioxidant dietary supplementation on contrast sensitivity in age-related macular disease: A randomized controlled trial.* Eur J Clin Nutr, 2007. 61(9): p. 1121–7.

172. Morris, M.S., et al., *Intake of zinc and antioxidant micronutrients and early age-related maculopathy lesions.* Ophthalmic Epidemiol, 2007. 14(5): p. 288–98.

173. Chung, H.Y., H.M. Rasmussen, and E.J. Johnson, *Lutein bioavailability is higher from lutein-enriched eggs than from supplements and spinach in men.* J Nutr, 2004. 134(8): p. 1887–93.

174. Cao, Y., and R. Cao, *Angiogenesis inhibited by drinking tea.* Nature, 1999. 398(6726): p. 381.

175. Toi, M., et al., *Preliminary studies on the anti-angiogenic potential of pomegranate fractions in vitro and in vivo.* Angiogenesis, 2003. 6(2): p. 121–8.

176. Cao, Y., R. Cao, and E. Brakenhielm, *Antiangiogenic mechanisms of diet-derived polyphenols.* J Nutr Biochem, 2002. 13(7): p. 380–90.

177. Kenny, T.P., et al., *Cocoa procyanidins inhibit proliferation and angiogenic signals in human dermal microvascular endothelial cells following stimulation by low-level H_2O_2.* Exp Biol Med (Maywood), 2004. 229(8): p. 765–71.

178. Folkman, J., *Angiogenesis in cancer, vascular, rheumatoid and other disease.* Nat Med, 1995. 1(1): p. 27–31.

179. Everitt, A.V., et al., *Dietary approaches that delay age-related diseases.* Clin Interv Aging, 2006. 1(1): p. 11–31.

180. Chiu, C.J., et al., *Dietary carbohydrate and the progression of age-related macular degeneration: A prospective study from the Age-Related Eye Disease Study.* Am J Clin Nutr, 2007. 86(4): p. 1210–8.

181. Faulks, R.M., and S. Southon, *Challenges to understanding and measuring carotenoid bioavailability.* Biochim Biophys Acta, 2005. 1740(2): p. 95–100.

182. Goni, I., J. Serrano, and F. Saura-Calixto, *Bioaccessibility of beta-carotene, lutein, and lycopene from fruits and vegetables.* J Agric Food Chem, 2006. 54(15): p. 5382–7.

183. Bernhardt, S.A.S., *Impact of different cooking methods on food quality: Retention of lipophilic vitamins in fresh and frozen vegetables.* J Food Eng, 2006. 77(2): p. 327–33.

184. Yonekura, L., and A. Nagao, *Intestinal absorption of dietary carotenoids.* Mol Nutr Food Res, 2007. 51(1): p. 107–15.

185. Novotny, J.A., et al., *Plasma appearance of labeled beta-carotene, lutein, and retinol in humans after consumption of isotopically labeled kale.* J Lipid Res, 2005. 46(9): p. 1896–903.

186. Roodenburg, A.J., et al., *Amount of fat in the diet affects bioavailability of lutein esters but not of alpha-carotene, beta-carotene, and vitamin E in humans.* Am J Clin Nutr, 2000. 71(5): p. 1187–93.

187. Unlu, N.Z., et al., *Carotenoid absorption from salad and salsa by humans is enhanced by the addition of avocado or avocado oil.* J Nutr, 2005. 135(3): p. 431–6.

188. Tyssandier, V., et al., *Processing of vegetable-borne carotenoids in the human stomach and duodenum.* Am J Physiol Gastrointest Liver Physiol, 2003. 284(6): p. G913–23.

189. Clevidence, B.H., D. Rao, and J. Dura-Novotny, *Effect of cooking method on xanthophyll content of yellow-fleshed potato.* United States Japan Natural Resources Protein Panel, 2005. 34: p. 280–84.

190. Johnson, G.H., D.R. Keast, and P.M. Kris-Etherton, *Dietary modeling shows that the substitution of canola oil for fats commonly used in the United States would increase compliance with dietary recommendations for fatty acids.* J Am Diet Assoc, 2007. 107(10): p. 1726–34.

191. Wijendran, V., and K.C. Hayes, *Dietary n-6 and n-3 fatty acid balance and cardiovascular health.* Annu Rev Nutr, 2004. 24: p. 597–615.

192. Kinyamu, H.K., et al., *Dietary calcium and vitamin D intake in elderly women: Effect on serum parathyroid hormone and vitamin D metabolites.* Am J Clin Nutr, 1998. 67(2): p. 342–8.

193. Cashman, K.D., *Calcium and vitamin D.* Novartis Found Symp, 2007. 282: p. 123–38; discussion 138–42, 212–8.

194. Gennari, C., *Calcium and vitamin D nutrition and bone disease of the elderly.* Public Health Nutr, 2001. 4(2B): p. 547–59.

195. Garland, C.F., et al., *The role of vitamin D in cancer prevention.* Am J Public Health, 2006. 96(2): p. 252–61.

196. Bischoff-Ferrari, H.A., et al., *Estimation of optimal serum concentrations of 25-hydroxyvitamin D for multiple health outcomes.* Am J Clin Nutr, 2006. 84(1): p. 18–28.

197. Marcason, W., *Vitamin K: What are the current dietary recommendations for patients taking coumadin?* J Am Diet Assoc, 2007. 107(11): p. 2022.

198. Wallstrom, P., et al., *Serum concentrations of beta-carotene and alpha-tocopherol are associated with diet, smoking, and general and central adiposity.* Am J Clin Nutr, 2001. 73(4): p. 777–85.

199. Vioque, J., et al., *Plasma concentrations of carotenoids and vitamin C are better correlated with dietary intake in normal weight than overweight and obese elderly subjects.* Br J Nutr, 2007. 97(5): p. 977–86.

200. Madan, A.K., et al., *Vitamin and trace mineral levels after laparoscopic gastric bypass.* Obes Surg, 2006. 16(5): p. 603–6.

201. Shuster, M.H., and J.A. Vazquez, *Nutritional concerns related to Roux-en-Y gastric bypass: What every clinician needs to know.* Crit Care Nurs Q, 2005. 28(3): p. 227–60; quiz 261–2.

202. Slater, G.H., et al., *Serum fat-soluble vitamin deficiency and abnormal calcium metabolism after malabsorptive bariatric surgery.* J Gastrointest Surg, 2004. 8(1): p. 48–55; discussion 54–5.

203. Vahlquist, A., et al., *Serum carotene, vitamin A, retinol-binding protein and lipoproteins before and after jejunoileal bypass surgery.* Int J Obes, 1982. 6(5): p. 491–7.

204. Alvarez-Leite, J.I., *Nutrient deficiencies secondary to bariatric surgery.* Curr Opin Clin Nutr Metab Care, 2004. 7(5): p. 569–75.

205. Bai, J.C., *Malabsorption syndromes.* Digestion, 1998. 59(5): p. 530–46.

206. Kastin, D.A., and A.L. Buchman, *Malnutrition and gastrointestinal disease.* Curr Opin Gastroenterol, 2002. 18(2): p. 221–8.

207. Davidson, M.H., et al., *Weight control and risk factor reduction in obese subjects treated for 2 years with orlistat: A randomized controlled trial.* JAMA, 1999. 281(3): p. 235–42.

208. Sundl, I., et al., *Effects of orlistat therapy on plasma concentrations of oxygenated and hydrocarbon carotenoids.* Lipids, 2006. 41(2): p. 113–8.

209. Peters, J.C., et al., *Assessment of the nutritional effects of olestra, a nonabsorbed fat replacement: Introduction and overview.* J Nutr, 1997. 127(8 Suppl): p. 1539S–1546S.

210. Fokkema, M.R., et al., *Short-term carnitine supplementation does not augment LCPω3 status of vegans and lacto-ovo-vegetarians.* J Am Coll Nutr, 2005. 24(1): p. 58–64.

211. Fokkema, M.R., et al., *Short-term supplementation of low-dose gamma-linolenic acid (GLA), alpha-linolenic acid (ALA), or GLA plus ALA does not augment LCP omega 3 status of Dutch vegans to an appreciable extent.* Prostaglandins Leukot Essent Fatty Acids, 2000. 63(5): p. 287–92.

212. Rosell, M.S., et al., *Long-chain n-3 polyunsaturated fatty acids in plasma in British meat-eating, vegetarian, and vegan men.* Am J Clin Nutr, 2005. 82(2): p. 327–34.

213. Plourde, M., and S.C. Cunnane, *Extremely limited synthesis of long chain polyunsaturates in adults: Implications for their dietary essentiality and use as supplements.* Appl Physiol Nutr Metab, 2007. 32(4): p. 619–34.

214. Williams, C.M., and G. Burdge, *Long-chain n-3 PUFA: Plant v. marine sources.* Proc Nutr Soc, 2006. 65(1): p. 42–50.

215. Gerster, H., *Can adults adequately convert alpha-linolenic acid (18:3n-3) to eicosapentaenoic acid (20:5n-3) and docosahexaenoic acid (22:6n-3)?* Int J Vitam Nutr Res, 1998. 68(3): p. 159–73.

216. Doughman, S.D., S. Krupanidhi, and C.B. Sanjeevi, *Omega-3 fatty acids for nutrition and medicine: Considering microalgae oil as a vegetarian source of EPA and DHA.* Curr Diabetes Rev, 2007. 3(3): p. 198–203.
217. Wang, J.J., et al., *Cataract surgery and the 5-year incidence of late-stage age-related maculopathy: Pooled findings from the Beaver Dam and Blue Mountains eye studies.* Ophthalmology, 2003. 110(10): p. 1960–7.
218. Klein, R., et al., *The relationship of ocular factors to the incidence and progression of age-related maculopathy.* Arch Ophthalmol, 1998. 116(4): p. 506–13.
219. Holden, J.E., et al., *Carotenoid Content of U.S. Foods: An update of the database.* J Food Comp Anal, 1999. 12: p. 169–96.

2 Rhinosinusitis

Food and Nutrient Approaches to Disease Management and Prevention

Mary L. Hardy, M.D., and Elizabeth R. Volkmann, M.D.

I. INTRODUCTION

Rhinosinusitis is a common clinical problem affecting one in seven adults, or 31 million individuals, in the United States each year [67]. Studies estimate a direct annual health care cost of $5.8 billion [2], which includes clinical encounters and 500,000 surgical procedures performed on the paranasal sinuses [63]. "I have a sinus problem" is one of the most common reasons for a patient visit to a physician in the United States and accounts for 25 million office visits each year [38]. The indirect costs of rhinosinusitis include 73 million days of restricted activity per year [2]. Despite the high incidence and health care burden of rhinosinusitis, treatment options vary considerably across medical disciplines [42]. This chapter emphasizes food and nutrient optimization for managing and preventing rhinosinusitis.

II. DEFINITION

Rhinosinusitis is defined as symptomatic inflammation of the paranasal sinuses and nasal cavity [74]. In recent years, *rhinosinusitis* has replaced the term *sinusitis* because the syndrome is often preceded by, and rarely occurs without, concurrent nasal airway inflammation [74]. Rhinosinusitis is classified as acute if less than 4 weeks, subacute if 4 to 8 weeks, or chronic if 8 weeks or longer. If three or more episodes of acute rhinosinusitis occur per year without persistent symptoms between episodes, the condition is termed *recurrent rhinosinusitis*. Rhinosinusitis can be further characterized by etiology such as acute bacterial rhinosinusitis or viral rhinosinusitis.

III. PRESENTATION

Signs and symptoms of rhinosinusitis differ according to the underlying cause of the inflammation, although there often is substantial crossover of symptoms. Acute bacterial rhinosinusitis typically manifests as purulent nasal drainage lasting 10 days or more accompanied by nasal obstruction, facial pain, pressure, or fullness [66]. Additional signs may include maxillary tooth discomfort, hyposmia or anosmia, cough, fever, and failure of transillumination of the maxillary sinuses [66].

Radiological imaging, such as computed tomography scanning, is no longer necessary for the diagnosis of rhinosinusitis, if the patient meets the clinical criteria and the provider does not suspect a complication or alternate diagnosis [74].

In viral rhinosinusitis, symptoms are similar to acute bacterial rhinosinusitis; however, they are present for less than 10 days and typically do not worsen over time [74]. The previous notion that purulent nasal drainage distinguishes bacterial from viral infections lacks sensitivity and is no longer used in clinical practice to discriminate between the two sources [74]. Approximately 0.5% to 2% of cases of viral rhinosinusitis develop into bacterial infection [31].

Chronic rhinosinusitis manifests with purulent nasal discharge, obstruction, facial pain, pressure, or fullness lasting for 8 weeks or longer [74]. Additional diagnostic criteria include documentation of inflammation via one or more of the following: radiographic imaging showing inflammation of the paranasal sinuses; polyps in the nasal cavity or middle meatus; and/or purulent mucus or edema in the middle meatus or ethmoid region [74].

IV. DIFFERENTIAL DIAGNOSIS

Differentiating rhinosinusitis from other possible diseases may be challenging during the initial evaluation. Table 2.1 presents a list of conditions that may present in a similar fashion to rhinosinusitis, and their distinguishing characteristics.

TABLE 2.1
Differential Diagnosis of Rhinosinusitis

Diagnosis	Distinguishing features
Cold or flu virus	Symptoms present less than 1 week
	Symptoms do not worsen with time
Allergies	Symptoms include itchy nose, eyes, or throat, and recurrent sneezing
	Symptoms appear to occur only during exposure to allergens
Migraine and other headaches	The headache is recurrent
	The headache has a significant impact on daily activities
	Symptoms do not include nasal congestion
Dental problems	Medical history may include recent dental work
Foreign object in nasal passage	Suggestive history
	Typically occurs in pediatric patients
Temporal arteritis	Headache is unilateral
	Symptoms include proximal muscle weakness
	Typically occurs in elderly patients
Temporomandibular joint disorders	History of teeth grinding
	Pain elicited upon palpation of the temporomandibular joint
Vasomotor rhinitis	Symptoms include nasal obstruction, rhinorrhea, and congestion
	Often occurs in pregnant women
	Typically a diagnosis of exclusion

Source: Adapted from [81].

V. PATHOPHYSIOLOGY

The major pathogens implicated in acute bacterial rhinosinusitis for adults and pediatric patients are *Streptococcus pneumoniae* and *Haemophilus influenza* [66]. In pediatric cases, *Moraxella catarrhalis* causes 25% of acute bacterial rhinosinusitis. Less frequent species known to cause rhinosinusitis in certain patient subgroups include β- and α-hemolytic streptococci, *Staphylococcus aureus*, and anaerobes [66]. In most cases, a preceding viral infection causes inflammation and congestion in the nasal passage, obstructing the sinuses and creating a hospitable environment for subsequent bacterial growth. Fungi, even though normal flora of the upper airway, can cause acute rhinosinusitis in immunocompromised or diabetic patients [20]. The most common cause of noninvasive fungal rhinosinusitis is *Aspergillus* [81].

While acute rhinosinusitis is typically infectious in nature, chronic rhinosinusitis may result from a combination of factors, including infection and allergic responses [29]. For example, allergic rhinitis is more often associated with chronic rhinosinusitis compared with isolated acute bacterial rhinosinusitis [19]. Moreover, patients with chronic rhinosinusitis demonstrate an exaggerated humoral and cellular immune response to airborne fungi [80]. In a study of patients with chronic rhinosinusitis, 57% had a positive in vitro or skin allergy test [30]. The edema and inflammation associated with allergic rhinitis may engender increased susceptibility of the sinuses to infection by blocking drainage and delaying mucociliary clearance [1].

VI. RISK FACTORS

MEDICAL CONDITIONS

Several factors may contribute to the occurrence, persistence, or recurrence of rhinosinusitis. The presence of an allergic diathesis predisposes to infections as described above. Atopic children, in general, have higher incidence of chronic rhinosinusitis [9]. Also, patients with asthma often suffer from concomitant chronic rhinosinusitis and exhibit increased asthma exacerbations until the rhinosinusitis is controlled [85]. Other medical risk factors include cystic fibrosis, immunocompromised states, ciliary dyskinesia, and anatomic variation, such as septal deviation [74].

ENVIRONMENTAL FACTORS

In a survey study of 66 million adults from 1988 to 1994, the prevalence of both acute and recurrent or chronic rhinosinusitis increased with direct exposure to cigarettes and other tobacco products [48]. Researchers suggest that cigarette smoke and other air pollutants can damage the cilia responsible for moving mucus through the sinuses [81]. Changes in atmospheric pressure, such as flying, climbing to high altitudes, or swimming, may predispose the individual to sinus blockage and subsequent infection [81]. Finally, anaerobic bacterial infections associated with dental procedures precipitate 10% of rhinosinusitis cases [81].

NUTRITIONAL FACTORS

Nutritional deficiencies have also been implicated as risk factors for the development of rhinosinusitis and other upper respiratory tract infections. In a study of children undergoing surgery for placement of tympanostomy tubes for frequent otitis media, patients had reduced levels of vitamin A and selenium [50]. Another prospective trial examined the blood levels of various vitamins and minerals in children with chronic rhinosinusitis and found significantly lower levels of vitamin C, vitamin E, copper, and zinc in chronic rhinosinusitis patients compared to age-matched controls [86].

TABLE 2.2
Complications of Rhinosinusitis

Complication	Clinical Characteristics
Osteomyelitis	Increased in adolescent males with frontal sinusitis
	Manifests as headache, fever, and soft swelling over the bone
Orbital infection	Develops in ethmoid sinusitis
	Pressure on optic nerve may lead to vision loss
Thrombosis	Develops in ethmoid or frontal sinuses
	Pupil may be fixed and dilated
Widespread or more	May result in abscesses or meningitis
severe infection	Infection spreads to brain, either through bones or blood vessels
	More likely in immunocompromised patients

Source: Adapted from [66].

VII.   COMPLICATIONS

Complications of rhinosinusitis include periorbital swelling, erythema, and facial pain [66]. In rare cases, rhinosinusitis can cause serious medical problems if left untreated (Table 2.2).

VIII.   TREATMENT

CONVENTIONAL MANAGEMENT

The primary objectives for treatment of both acute and chronic rhinosinusitis include the following: reduce swelling, eradicate infection, drain the sinuses, and ensure that the sinuses remain open. Conventional treatment involves using corticosteroids, antibiotics, decongestants and antihistamines to achieve these objectives. However, many patients may not require such an aggressive treatment approach [74]. For instance, several studies have demonstrated a lack of benefit of antibiotics for clinically diagnosed acute rhinosinusitis [57, 82]. In a large, randomized controlled trial of patients with acute rhinosinusitis, Williamson and colleagues [93] found that neither amoxicillin nor the corticosteroid budesonide nor both were superior to placebo for resolving symptoms. Another randomized controlled trial found that patients diagnosed with acute rhinosinusitis experience no advantage with antibiotic treatment (amoxicillin-clavulanate) compared with placebo and are, in fact, more likely to experience adverse effects [7]. Difficulty in distinguishing viral and bacterial rhinosinusitis in the general practice setting likely contributes to the lack of benefit of antibiotics among certain patients, and inappropriate use of antibiotics may lead to resistance of these medicines.

NASAL IRRIGATION AND HYDRATION

An important remedy for clearing the sinuses is nasal irrigation. Numerous studies suggest that daily irrigation of the nasal passages with a hypertonic solution (e.g., saline) relieves rhinosinusitis symptoms, reduces antibiotic use, and limits the occurrence of acute exacerbations [20, 33, 64, 71]. Saline irrigation is also helpful for patients who suffer from allergic rhinitis [22, 23]. Nasal irrigation floods the nasal cavity with warm saline solution, clearing out excess mucus and allergens while moisturizing the nasal cavity. Either a soft ear syringe, a *neti pot*, or a water pick with a special attachment may be used. A randomized controlled trial comparing the efficacy of saline and Dead Sea salt solution in nasal irrigation found that patients with chronic rhinosinusitis who used the Dead Sea salt solution had significantly better symptoms of relief than patients who used regular saline [21]. Extremely cost-effective, nasal irrigation is also safe to perform in children.

Maintenance of hydration is a key factor in the successful management of rhinosinusitis. Increased oral intake of fluids, such as teas and soups, may improve ciliary function and decrease congestion [20]. Use of a humidifier is also recommended [40]. Inhalation of the steam generated from hot liquids further moisturizes the nasal cavities [81], which are dry in patients who chronically use corticosteroid-based nasal sprays and decongestants. To deliver steam inhalation, the patient should boil a pot of water, form a tent over the pot by covering the head with a towel, and inhale the steam.

To enhance the benefits of steam inhalation, various herbal medicines can be added to the solution. Essential oils of eucalyptus (*Eucalyptus globules*), pine (*Pinus* spp.), and peppermint (*Mentha piperita*) act primarily as antimicrobials, but also possess anti-inflammatory and expectorant properties [12]. A small controlled study evaluating the effects of a mixture of eucalyptus, pine, peppermint, and nutmeg (*Ravensara aromatica*) on sinus infection symptoms had patients use three drops of the mixture in a steam inhalation for 10 minutes, three times a day for five days [52]. After five days of treatment, the essential oil group (eight subjects) had clear mucus and no congestion, while the control group (three subjects) had green mucus and persistent congestion. Synthetic forms of eucalyptus are used in cough medicines and ointments (e.g., Vicks VapoRub) as a decongestant and antiseptic [51].

Nutritional Strategies in Rhinosinusitis (Table 2.3)

Horseradish (*Armoracia rusticana*) exhibits congestion-clearing effects similar to other spicy foods such as cayenne (*Capsicum* spp.) pepper and curry (*Murraya koenigii*) [81]. In addition, horseradish acts as an antimicrobial [44]. In a prospective cohort study of 251 centers in Germany, patients with acute rhinosinusitis treated with an herbal drug containing *Nasturtium* and horseradish root demonstrated a reduction in symptoms similar to patients treated with conventional antibiotics [26]. Moreover, the patients treated with horseradish root had fewer adverse effects compared with the antibiotic group. When possible, patients should be encouraged to consume these substances directly from foods, as opposed to capsules, because the healing effects of these spices are thought to be due in part to their taste and smell.

The proteolytic enzyme bromelain, obtained from the pineapple stalk, has been used in rhinosinusitis as an anti-inflammatory and mucolytic. A study of children diagnosed with acute rhinosinusitis found that patients treated with a bromelain supplement had a shorter mean period of symptoms compared with patients treated with conventional therapy [5]. In another study, acute and chronic rhinosinusitis patients taking bromelain demonstrated improvements in nasal mucosal inflammation and in overall symptoms [83]. Bromelain oral dosage is typically 500 to 1000 mg/day [37] and the majority of studies provided the substance for 1 week in several divided doses per day [29]. Proteolytic enzymes from papaya and a few other fruits exert similar effects although perhaps not studied specifically in sinusitis.

Population-based survey studies in the United States have demonstrated that 24% to 32% of patients with chronic rhinosinusitis have used herbal therapy alone or as an adjuvant treatment for their condition [3, 46]. One such herbal preparation is Sinupret, which was developed in Germany for rhinosinusitis [29]. The formula, available in solution or tablet form, is comprised of five herbal extracts (*Gentiana lutea, Primula veris, Rumex sp., Sambucus nigra, Verbena officinalis*). A systematic review of 22 clinical studies with Sinupret in the treatment of rhinosinusitis demonstrated that combined with standard antibacterial therapy, Sinupret significantly reduced the acute signs and symptoms of rhinosinusitis [56]. Adjuvant treatment with Sinupret typically lasted 1 to 2 weeks in these studies. A randomized controlled trial of patients with acute rhinosinusitis found that patients who took Sinupret for 2 weeks (two tablets given three times per day) in addition to conventional antibiotics had fewer symptoms and better radiographical findings compared with patients who took antibiotics alone [61].

Nutritional Strategies for Allergic Rhinitis (Table 2.4)

Allergic rhinitis is a well-known risk factor for rhinosinusitis and can be ameliorated with nutritional interventions. Spirulina, a cyanobacteria with a high protein content, has been shown to be

TABLE 2.3
Nutrients for Rhinosinusitis*

Nutrient	Function	Top Sources
Vitamin A	Enhance function of white blood cells Increase antibody response to antigens Maintain function of mucosal tissues	Carrots, spinach, collard greens, kale, turnip greens, winter squash, Swiss chard, red bell pepper, sweet potato, peas, parsley, acorn squash, yellow corn, brussels sprouts, apricots, cantaloupe, mango, watermelon, peaches, papaya
Vitamin C	Anti-inflammatory	Papaya, red bell peppers, broccoli, brussels sprouts, strawberries, oranges, cantaloupe, kiwifruit, cauliflower, kale
Copper	Elimination of free radicals	Crimini mushrooms, turnips, spinach, kale, summer squash, asparagus, eggplant, tomato, cashews, ginger root, green beans, sesame seeds, mustard seeds, sunflower seeds, beans
Selenium	Protect cells from free radical damage	Crimini mushrooms, cod, shrimp, halibut, salmon, turkey, barley, chicken, sunflower seeds, asparagus, spinach
Zinc	Enhance function of white blood cells Decrease IgE-mediated release of antihistamine	Crimini mushrooms, summer squash, asparagus, collard greens, miso, broccoli, green peas, pumpkin seeds, sesame seeds, mustard seeds
Omega-3 fatty acids	Anti-inflammatory	Flaxseeds, walnuts, salmon, halibut, shrimp, tofu, scallops, winter squash, broccoli, cauliflower, brussels sprouts, soybeans, strawberries, miso
Bromelain	Mucolytic Anti-inflammatory	Pineapple
Hot spices (capsaicin)	Clear sinuses Promote drainage Relieve pain	Horseradish Cayenne (good source of vitamin A)
Probiotics	Enhance immune function	Yogurt, cottage cheese, aged cheese, miso, pickles, wine

Source: Adapted from [41, 53, 89].

* For chronic rhinosinusitis, patients may benefit from eliminating common food allergens including eggs, peanuts, milk and dairy products, wheat, corn, and concentrated sources of sugar.

an effective immune modulator and potential allergy remedy [54]. Containing phenolic acid, tocopherols, beta-carotenes, and gamma-linolenic acid, this alga has several anti-inflammatory properties, including inhibition of histamine release from mast cells [70], as well as cyclooxygenase-2 [72], and cytokines [54]. In a randomized crossover study, patients with allergic rhinitis who received spirulina for 12 weeks had significantly reduced interleukin (IL)-4 levels (32%) [54]. Another study found that dietary spirulina consumption increased immunoglobulin A (IgA) levels in human saliva [36]. Lower levels of secretory IgA are associated with increased susceptibility to upper respiratory tract infections (URTIs) [45, 91]. Furthermore, patients who have selective IgA deficiency experience recurrent, moderately severe URTIs [14], such as ear infections, sinusitis, bronchitis, and pneumonia [4].

In addition to its favorable effects on local immunity, spirulina has been shown to decrease allergic rhinitis symptoms, including nasal discharge, sneezing, nasal congestion, and itching [13]. In a double-blind, placebo-controlled study that evaluated the effectiveness and tolerability of spirulina for treating patients with allergic rhinitis, spirulina consumption significantly improved the symptoms and physical findings compared with placebo [13]. In this study, patients took five tablets each day, consuming either 2000 mg/day spirulina or placebo for 6 months. Patients were not permitted to take any anti-allergy or rhinitis medication during the study period.

Quercetin is a nutrient with anti-inflammatory activity of potential use in the management of allergic rhinitis [37]. Found in highest concentrations in apples and onions, quercetin inhibits

---

TABLE 2.4
Foods for Allergic Rhinitis

Foods to Consume	Foods to Avoid
Organic fruits and vegetables	Dairy products
-apples & onions (contain quercetin)	Yeast products (bread, refined sugars, alcohol)
Extra virgin olive oil	Artificial food additives
Flaxseeds	Salt
Rosemary	
Salmon, halibut	
Spirulina	

Source: Adapted from [41, 53].

---

histamine release [6], and decreases the gene expression of tumor necrosis factor alpha, IL-1β, IL-6, and IL-8 [58]. Subjects with nasal allergies treated with a nasal spray that included quercetin experienced significant relief of nasal symptoms that was comparable to oral antihistamine preparations [73]. Supplemental quercetin can be dosed at 400 to 500 mg orally three times per day [29].

Urtica dioica, also known as stinging nettles, has been used in the management of allergic rhinitis [84]. In one double-blind, controlled trial, patients with allergic rhinitis who took two 300-mg capsules of freeze-dried extracts of *Urtica dioica* at the onset of symptoms reported reductions in symptoms [59]. Nettle is one of the most nutrient-dense commonly used herbs, containing high amounts of vitamin A, potassium, calcium, and magnesium [65]. Interestingly, nettles also contain histamine, which is a pro-inflammatory molecule. However, histamine also acts as an autocoid (a local hormone) to modulate the immune response [55], and injections of histamine have been used effectively in the past to treat numerous allergic conditions including cluster headaches, penicillin reactions, and cold urticaria with associated anaphylaxis [39]. If taken in capsule form, dosage is 240 to 300 mg tablets given two to three times per day. Patients can also consume nettle in a tea by mixing two to three teaspoons of the herb in 16 ounces of hot water.

Butterbur (*Petasites hybridus*) is a herbaceous plant in the Asteraceae family whose leaves and roots contain eremophilan-type sesquiterpenes that may effectively manage symptoms of allergic rhinitis [43]. Butterbur inhibits the biosynthesis of leukotrienes associated with spasmolytic activity and type-I hypersensitivity [76, 77], and has been evaluated as a treatment for asthma and allergic rhinitis [76]. A prospective, randomized, double-blind, parallel group comparison study of a standardized formula of butterbur extract (Ze 339, 8 mg total petasine, one tablet given three times per day), fexofenadine (Telfast 180, one tablet, once daily) and placebo in 330 patients, demonstrated that butterbur Ze 339 and fexofenadine are equally effective relative to placebo [78].

IX. PREVENTION

PROBIOTICS

Primary preventative measures to reduce the risk of rhinosinusitis include avoidance of viral URTIs with probiotics. The goal of probiotics is to establish microbial colonies that support mucosal integrity [34]. Numerous studies have demonstrated that foods containing *Lactobacilli* reduce the incidence and severity of the common cold [16, 17, 25, 47, 94]. A randomized, double-blind, placebo-controlled intervention study found that adults who consumed a probiotic bacteria supplement for 3 months were less likely to develop URTIs and reported fewer symptoms during URTI episodes than controls [94]. Moreover, participants who consumed the probiotic supplement had significantly higher levels of T-lymphocytes, including CD4+ and CD8+ cells, and monocytes during the first

14 days of supplementations compared with the placebo group. By reducing the risk of URTIs, a well-established risk factor for rhinosinusitis, probiotic bacteria may decrease the incidence of rhinosinusitis. A double-blind, placebo-controlled multicenter study of patients with chronic recurrent rhinosinusitis demonstrated that participants receiving a probiotic for 6 months had fewer relapses, an increased interval to the first relapse, and less usage of antibiotics compared to the placebo group [32]. The findings were significant during the treatment period, as well as during the 8-month follow-up observation period.

Xylitol is another substance that may help preserve a microbial balance favorable for the oral mucosa. Randomized trials conducted in Finland have demonstrated that xylitol taken in a regimen of 1.67 g five times a day as a chewing gum or 2 g five times a day as a solution reduced the incidence of acute otitis media by 35% to 40% in young children [86, 87]. The main limitation of the use of sugar alcohols is a dose-dependent osmotic laxative effect. The Finnish studies of xylitol for acute otitis media prevention have also shown that 10 g of xylitol daily, given as 2 g five times a day, is well tolerated in children as young as 9 months of age.

Substances that may disrupt the natural microflora of the mucosa lining the upper respiratory and gastrointestinal tracts include antibiotics [24]. Antimicrobial agents active against both gram-positive and gram-negative organisms have a greater impact on the intestinal flora and may lead to overgrowth of unfavorable pathogens [24]. High sugar intake has also been implicated as a causative factor in intestinal dysbiosis [35]. While the mechanism for this alteration in microflora has yet to be fully elucidated, researchers postulate that high sugar intake increases bile output. Because certain species of intestinal bacteria utilize bile acids for energy, increased production of bile acids may result in a competitive advantage for this group of bacteria [60].

NUTRITIONAL STRATEGIES

Oral supplementation with essential fatty acids [90], zinc [75], selenium [49, 50], and cod liver oil [49, 50] can decrease the incidence of URTIs. Interestingly, from the 1920s to the 1940s, many children in the United States received cod liver oil, a rich source of vitamins A and D, as well as omega-3 fatty acids [79]. Due to an unpleasant taste and concern over vitamin A toxicity [8], cod liver oil largely fell out of favor. However, a recent randomized study of Latino children living in New York City found that daily supplementation of lemon-flavored cod liver oil and a children's multivitamin containing selenium significantly reduced the mean number of URTI physician visits over a 6-month period [49]. Supplemental nutrients were well tolerated by the children, and 70% of participants completed the full course of treatment.

One randomized controlled trial of elderly individuals observed that neither daily multivitamin-mineral supplementation, nor vitamin E (alpha-tocopherol) favorably affected the incidence and severity of URTIs [27]. These findings contrast with the results of previous studies that demonstrated a reduction in the incidence and duration of infections in elderly patients with multivitamin supplementation [10, 11]. The different results may reflect differences in the patient populations (institutionalized vs. noninstitutionalized patients) or supplementation regimens (synthetic vs. natural forms) under study. For instance, the earlier studies assessed institutionalized elderly patients who may be more likely to have nutrient deficiencies compared with the noninstitutionalized patients assessed in the study by Graat and colleagues [27]. Therefore, although studies do suggest a benefit from supplementation, the evidence is not uniformly positive.

Dietary alterations also help prevent symptoms of allergic rhinitis. Ivker [40] recommends that affected patients adopt a *Candida* control diet, avoiding foods containing yeast, such as bread, refined sugars, cheeses, peanuts, and alcoholic beverages, and instead eating fruits and vegetables, which are alkalinizing and rich in probiotics, although direct evidence for this intervention is lacking. Because allergic fungal rhinosinusitis has been implicated as a causative factor of chronic rhinosinusitis [68, 80], eating a yeast-free diet may decrease nutritional exposure to fungal antigens, which may divert the immune system from fighting rhinosinusitis-related pathogens. Dairy, wheat, and corn are reported to promote a more globular mucus, impair sinus drainage, and promote antigen exposure [37]. As such, the belief that consuming dairy products increases mucus production is an oversimplification of a more complex issue, which has not been tested in clinical trials.

COMPLEMENTARY THERAPIES

Acupuncture is effective in the prevention and treatment of both allergic and nonallergic rhinitis [15, 62, 95, 96]. A recent randomized controlled trial of children with persistent allergic rhinitis found that children who received acupuncture for 8 weeks reported fewer daily rhinitis symptoms and more symptom-free days compared with children who received sham acupuncture during both the treatment period and follow-up observation period [62]. There were no serious adverse effects of the acupuncture noted. Though less well-studied, acupuncture has also been successfully used to treat patients with chronic sinusitis [69].

A novel strategy for improving paranasal sinus ventilation is humming [28]. Humming has been shown to increase nasal levels of nitric oxide, which has antifungal and antibacterial activity [92]. A case report of a patient with chronic rhinosinusitis who hummed for 1 hour daily for 4 days demonstrated a significant reduction in sinus symptoms by day four of the study [18]. Future randomized, controlled studies are needed to assess the validity of the humming approach.

ENVIRONMENTAL FACTORS

Improving air quality reduces allergen exposure, and therefore reduces allergic predisposition. Decreased exposure to animal dander and dust mites through removal of carpeting and feather bedding is associated with improvement in rhinosinusitis symptoms [37]. Clinicians also suggest encasing pillows and bedding in allergy-reduction coverings or plastic and using a negative ion generator [40]. Avoidance of exogenous irritants, such as cigarette smoking, is also encouraged. An observational study of over 20,000 adults found that the prevalence of both acute and recurrent or chronic rhinosinusitis was increased with direct cigarette exposure [48].

X. SUMMARY

- Acute bacterial rhinosinusitis is suggested over viral infections when
  a. Symptoms or signs are present for 10 days or more
  b. Symptoms or signs worsen with time
- Chronic rhinosinusitis occurs when
  a. Symptoms or signs are present for 8 weeks or more
  b. There is documentation of sinus inflammation through imaging
- Recurrent rhinosinusitis occurs when there are three or more episodes of acute bacterial rhinosinusitis per year.
- Patients with chronic and recurrent rhinosinusitis should be assessed for factors that contribute to the pathogenesis of rhinosinusitis, such as allergic rhinitis and immunocompromised states.
- Risk factors for rhinosinusitis include atopic conditions, cigarette smoking, altitude changes, and nutritional deficiencies (vitamin A, vitamin C, vitamin E, copper, selenium, zinc).
- Management strategies for treating and preventing rhinosinusitis include
  a. Performing regular steam inhalation
  b. Drinking hot teas such as ginger and broth-based soups
  c. Consuming spicy foods (horseradish, hot pepper)
  d. Performing nasal washes with saline solution
  e. Using plant-derived remedies such as Sinupret (two to three capsules/day) and bromelain (500 to 1000 mg/day)
  f. Consuming a well-balanced diet rich in omega-3 fatty acids and vitamin A

- Management strategies for allergic rhinitis include:
  a. Using the phytonutrient quercetin (400 to 500 mg three times/day)
  b. Consuming spirulina (2000 mg/day), an alga rich in chlorophyll shown to increase secretory IgA
  c. Initiating environmental controls that may reduce the inflammatory response
  d. Identifying and avoiding known allergens including food allergens

REFERENCES

1. Alho OP, Karttunen R, Karttunen TJ. Nasal mucosa in natural colds: effects of allergic rhinitis and susceptibility to recurrent sinusitis. *Clin Exp Immunol.* Aug 2004;137(2):366–372.
2. Anand VK. Epidemiology and economic impact of rhinosinusitis. *Ann Otol Rhinol Laryngol Suppl.* May 2004;193:3–5.
3. Blanc PD, Trupin L, Earnest G. Alternative therapies among adults with a reported diagnosis of asthma or rhinosinusitis: data from a population-based survey. *Chest.* Nov 2001;120(5):1461–1467.
4. Braconier JH, Nilsson B, Oxelius VA, et al. Recurrent pneumococcal infections in a patient with lack of specific IgG and IgM pneumococcal antibodies and deficiency of serum IgA, IgG2 and IgG4. *Scand J Infect Dis.* 1984;16:407–410.
5. Braun JM, Schneider B, Beuth HJ. Therapeutic use, efficiency and safety of the proteolytic pineapple enzyme Bromelain-POS in children with acute sinusitis in Germany. *In Vivo.* Mar–Apr 2005;19(2):417–421.
6. Bronner C, Landry Y. Kinetics of the inhibitory effect of flavonoids on histamine secretion from mast cells. *Agents Act.* Apr 1985;16(3–4):147–151.
7. Bucher HC, Tschudi P, Young J, et al. Effect of amoxicillin-clavulanate in clinically diagnosed acute rhinosinusitis: a placebo-controlled, double-blind, randomized trial in general practice. *Arch Intern Med.* 2003;163(15):1793–1798.
8. Caffey J. Chronic poisoning due to excess of vitamin A: description of the clinical and roentgen manifestations in seven infants and young children. *Pediatrics.* Apr 1950;5(4):672–688.
9. Campbell JM, Graham M, Gray HC, Bower C, Blaiss MS, Jones SM. Allergic fungal sinusitis in children. *Ann Allergy Asthma Immunol.* Feb 2006;96(2):286–290.
10. Chandra RK. Nutrition and immunity in the elderly. *Nutr Rev.* Dec 1992;50(12):367–371.
11. Chavance M, Herbeth B, Lemoine A, Zhu BP. Does multivitamin supplementation prevent infections in healthy elderly subjects? A controlled trial. *Int J Vitam Nutr Res.* 1993;63(1):11–16.
12. Chester AC. Chronic sinusitis. *Am Fam Phys.* 1996;53:877–887.
13. Cingi C, Conk-Dalay M, Cakli H, et al. The effects of spirulina on allergic rhinitis. *Eur Arch Otorhinolaryngol.* 2008 Mar 15 [Epub ahead of print].
14. Daele J, Zicot AF. Humoral immunodeficiency in recurrent upper respiratory tract infections. Some basic, clinical and therapeutic features. *Acta Otorhinolaryngology Belg.* 2000;54:373–390.
15. Davies A, Lewith G, Goddard J, Howarth P. The effect of acupuncture on nonallergic rhinitis: a controlled pilot study. *Altern Ther Health Med.* Jan 1998;4(1):70–74.
16. de Vrese M, Winkler P, Rautenberg P, et al. Effect of Lactobacillus gasseri PA 16/8, Bifidobacterium longum SP 07/3, B. bifidum MF 20/5 on common cold episodes: a double blind, randomized, controlled trial. *Clin Nutr.* Aug 2005;24(4):481–491.
17. de Vrese M, Winkler P, Rautenberg P, et al. Probiotic bacteria reduced duration and severity but not the incidence of common cold episodes in a double blind, randomized, controlled trial. *Vaccine.* Nov 10 2006;24(44–46):6670–6674.
18. Eby GA. Strong humming for one hour daily to terminate chronic rhinosinusitis in four days: a case report and hypothesis for action by stimulation of endogenous nasal nitric oxide production. *Med Hypotheses.* 2006;66(4):851–854.
19. Emanuel IA, Shah SB. Chronic rhinosinusitis: allergy and sinus computed tomography relationships. *Otolaryngol Head Neck Surg.* Dec 2000;123(6):687–691.
20. Fagnan LJ. Acute sinusitis: a cost-effective approach to diagnosis and treatment. *Am Fam Physician.* Nov 15 1998;58(8):1795–1802, 1805–1896.
21. Friedman M, Vidyasagar R, Joseph N. A randomized, prospective, double-blind study on the efficacy of dead sea salt nasal irrigations. *Laryngoscope.* 2006;116(6):878–882.

22. Garavello W, Di Berardino F, Romagnoli M, Sambataro G, Gaini RM. Nasal rinsing with hypertonic solution: an adjunctive treatment for pediatric seasonal allergic rhinoconjunctivitis. *Int Arch Allergy Immunol.* Aug 2005;137(4):310–314.

23. Garavello W, Romagnoli M, Sordo L, Gaini RM, Di Berardino C, Angrisano A. Hypersaline nasal irrigation in children with symptomatic seasonal allergic rhinitis: a randomized study. *Pediatr Allergy Immunol.* Apr 2003;14(2):140–143.

24. Gismondo MR. Antibiotic impact on intestinal microflora. *Gastroenterol Int.* 1998;11:29–30.

25. Goldin BR, Gorbach SL. Clinical indications for probiotics: an overview. *Clin Infect Dis.* Feb 2008;46(2):S96–100.

26. Goos KH, Albrecht U, Schneider B. Efficacy and safety profile of a herbal drug containing nasturtium herb and horseradish root in acute sinusitis, acute bronchitis and acute urinary tract infection in comparison with other treatments in the daily practice/results of a prospective cohort study. *Arzneimittelforschung.* 2006;56(3):249–257.

27. Graat JM, Schouten EG, Kok FJ. Effect of daily vitamin E and multivitamin-mineral supplementation on acute respiratory tract infections in elderly persons: a randomized controlled trial. *Jama.* Aug 14 2002;288(6):715–721.

28. Granqvist S, Sundberg J, Lundberg JO. Paranasal sinus ventilation by humming. *J Acoust Soc Am.* May 2006;119(5):2611–2617.

29. Guo R, Canter PH, Ernst E. Herbal medicines for the treatment of rhinosinusitis: a systematic review. *Otolaryngol Head Neck Surg.* Oct 2006;135(4):496–506.

30. Gutman M, Torres A, Keen KJ, et al. Prevalence of allergy in patients with chronic rhinosinusitis. *Otolarygnol Head Neck Surg.* May 2004;130(5):545–552.

31. Gwaltney JM, Jr. Acute community-acquired sinusitis. *Clin Infect Dis.* Dec 1996;23(6):1209–1223; quiz 1224–1225.

32. Habermann W, Zimmermann K, Skarabis H, Kunze R, Rusch V. Reduction of acute recurrence in patients with chronic recurrent hypertrophic sinusitis by treatment with a bacterial immunostimulant (Enterococcus faecalis Bacteriae of human origin). *Arzneimittelforschung.* 2002;52(8):622–627.

33. Harvey R, Hannan SA, Badia L, Scadding G. Nasal saline irrigations for the symptoms of chronic rhinosinusitis. *Cochrane Database Syst Rev.* 2007(3):CD006394.

34. Hatakka K, Saxelin M. Probiotics in intestinal and nonintestinal infectious diseases—clinical evidence. *Curr Pharm Des.* 2008;14(14):135–1367.

35. Hawrelak JA, Myers SP. The causes of intestinal dysbiosis: a review. *Altern Med Rev.* Jun 2004;9(2):180–197.

36. Hayashi O, Hirahashi T, Katoh T, et al. Class specific influence of dietary spirulina platensis on antibody production in mice. *J Nutr Sci Vitaminol.* Dec 1998;44(6):841–851.

37. Helm S, Miller AL. Natural treatment of chronic rhinosinusitis. *Alter Med Rev.* 2006;11(3):196–207.

38. Hickner JM, Bartlett JG, Besser RE, Gonzales R, Hoffman JR, Sande MA. Principles of appropriate antibiotic use for acute rhinosinusitis in adults: background. *Ann Emerg Med.* Jun 2001;37(6):703–710.

39. Horton BT. The clinical use of histamine. *Postgrad Med.* 1951;9:1–11.

40. Ivker RS. Chronic sinusitis. 2007. In *Integrative Medicine* (2nd ed.), ed. D. Rakel. Philadelphia: Saunders Elsevier.

41. Jaber R. Respiratory and allergic diseases: from upper respiratory tract infections to asthma. *Prim Care.* Jun 2002;29(2):231–261.

42. Kaszuba SM, Stewart MG. Medical management and diagnosis of chronic rhinosinusitis: A survey of treatment patterns by United States otolaryngologists. *Am J Rhinol.* Mar–Apr 2006;20(2):186–190.

43. Käufeler R, Polasek W, Brattström A, et al. Efficacy and safety of butterbur herbal extract Ze 339 in seasonal allergic rhinitis: postmarketing surveillance study. *Adv Ther.* Mar–Apr 2006;23(2):373–384.

44. Kienholz VM, Kemkes B. The antibacterial action of ethereal oils obtained from horse radish root (*Cochlearia amoracia* L) [in German]. *Arzneim Forsch.* 1961;11:917–918.

45. Klentrou P, Cieslak T, MacNeil M, et al. Effect of moderate exercise on salivary immunoglobulin A and infection risk in humans. *Europ J Appl Physiol.* 2002;87:153–158.

46. Krouse HJ, Krouse JH. Complementary therapeutic practices in patients with chronic sinusitis. *Clin Excell Nurse Pract.* Nov 1999;3(6):346–352.

47. Lenoir-Wijnkoop I, Sanders ME, Cabana MD, et al. Probiotic and prebiotic influence beyond the intestinal tract. *Nutr Rev.* Nov 2007;5(11):469–489.

48. Lieu JE, Feinstein AR. Confirmations and surprises in the association of tobacco use with sinusitis. *Arch Otolaryngol Head Neck Surg.* Aug 2000;126(8):940–946.

49. Linday LA, Dolitsky JN, Shindledecker RD. Nutritional supplements as adjunctive therapy for children with chronic/recurrent sinusitis: pilot research. *Int J Pediatr Otorhinolaryngol.* Jun 2004;68(6):785–793.

50. Linday LA, Dolitsky JN, Shindledecker RD, Pippenger CE. Lemon-flavored cod liver oil and a multivitamin-mineral supplement for the secondary prevention of otitis media in young children: pilot research. *Ann Otol Rhinol Laryngol.* Jul 2002;111(7 Pt 1):642–652.

51. Lis Balchin M. *Aromatherapy science.* 2006. Grayslake, IL: Pharmaceutical Press.

52. Machon L. Use of four essential oils in the treatment of sinus infections. Unpublished dissertation. 2001. Hunder, NY: R J Buckle Associates.

53. Mateljan G. *The World's Healthiest Foods, Essential Guide for the Healthiest Way of Eating.* 2006. Seattle, WA: George Mateljan Foundation.

54. Mao TK, Van de Water J, Gershwin ME. Effects of a Spirulina-based dietary supplement on cytokine production from allergic rhinitis patients. *J Med Food.* Spring 2005;8(1):27–30.

55. Melmon KL, Rocklin RE, Rosenkranz RP. Autocoids as modulators of the inflammatory and immune response. *Am J Med.* Jul 1981;71:100–106.

56. Melzer J, Saller R, Schapowal A, Brignoli R. Systematic review of clinical data with BNO-101 (Sinupret) in the treatment of sinusitis. *Forsch Komplement Med (2006).* Apr 2006;13(2):78–87.

57. Merenstein D, Whittaker C, Chadwell T, et al. Are antibiotics beneficial for patients with sinusitis complaints? A randomized double-blind clinical trial. *J Fam Pract.* Feb 2005;54(2):152–153.

58. Min YD, Choi CH, Bark H, et al. Quercetin inhibits expression of inflammatory cytokines through attenuation of NF-kappaB and p38 MAPK in HMC-1 human mast cell line. *Inflamm Res.* May 2007;56(5):210–215.

59. Mittman P. Randomized, double blind study of freeze dried urtica dioica in the treatment of allergic rhinitis. *Planta Med.* 1990;56:44–47.

60. Moore WE, Cato EP, Holdeman LV. Some current concepts in intestinal bacteriology. *Am J Clin Nutr* 1978; 31:S33–S42.

61. Neubauer N, Marz RW. Placebo-controlled, randomized double-blind clinical trial with Sinupret sugar coated tablets on the basis of a therapy with antibiotics and decongestant nasal drops in acute sinusitis. *Phytomedicine.* 1994;45:96.

62. Ng DK, Chow PY, Ming SP, et al. A double-blind, randomized, placebo-controlled trial of acupuncture for the treatment of childhood persistent allergic rhinitis. *Pediatrics.* Nov 2004;114(5):1242–1247.

63. Owings MF, Kozak LJ. Ambulatory and inpatient procedures in the United States, 1996. *Vital Health Stat 13.* Nov 1998(139):1–119.

64. Papsin B, McTavish A. Saline nasal irrigation: its role as an adjunct treatment. *Can Fam Physician.* Feb 2003;49:168–173.

65. Pedersen M. *Nutritional herbology.* 1987. Boutiful, UT: Pedersen Publishing.

66. Piccirillo JF. Clinical practice. Acute bacterial sinusitis. *N Engl J Med.* Aug 26 2004;351(9):902–910.

67. Pleis JR, Lethbridge-Cejku M. Summary health statistics for U.S. adults: National Health Interview Survey, 2005. *Vital Health Stat 10.* Dec 2006;232:153.

68. Ponikau JU, Sherris DA, Kern EB, et al. The diagnosis and incidence of allergic fungal sinusitis. *Mayo Clin Proc.* Sep 1999;74(9):877–884.

69. Pothman R, Yeh HL. The effects of treatment with antibiotics, laser and acupuncture upon chronic maxillary sinusitis in children. *Am J Chin Med.* 1982;10(1–4):55–58.

70. Price JA, Sanny C, Shevlin D. Inhibition of mast cells by algae. *J Med Food.* Winter 2002;5(4):205–210.

71. Rabago D, Zgierska A, Mundt M, et al. Efficacy of daily hypertonic saline nasal irrigation among patients with sinusitis: a randomized controlled trial. *J Fam Pract.* Dec 2002;51(12):1049–1055.

72. Reddy CM, Bhat VB, Kiranmai G, Reddy MN, Reddanna P, Madyastha KM. Selective inhibition of cyclooxygenase-2 by C-phycocyanin, a biliprotein from Spirulina platensis. *Biochem Biophys Res Commun.* Nov 2 2000;277(3):599–603.

73. Remberg P, Björk L, Hedner T, Sterner O. Characteristics, clinical effect profile and tolerability of a nasal spray preparation of Artemisia abrotanum L. for allergic rhinitis. *Phytomedicine.* Jan 2004;11(1):36–42.

74. Rosenfeld RM, Andes D, Bhattacharyya N, et al. Clinical practice guideline: adult sinusitis. *Otolaryngol Head Neck Surg.* Sep 2007;137(3 Suppl):S1–31.

75. Sazawal S, Black RE, Jalla S, Mazumdar S, Sinha A, Bhan MK. Zinc supplementation reduces the incidence of acute lower respiratory infections in infants and preschool children: a double-blind, controlled trial. *Pediatrics.* Jul 1998;102(1 Pt 1):1–5.

76. Schapowal A (on behalf of Petasites Study Group). Randomised controlled trial of butterbur and cetirizine for treating seasonal allergic rhinitis. *Br Med J.* 2002;324:144–146.

77. Schapowal A (on behalf of Petasites Study Group). Butterbur Ze 339 for the treatment of intermittent allergic rhinitis: dose-dependent efficacy in a prospective, double-blind, placebo-controlled study. *Arch Otolaryngol Head Neck Surg.* 2004;130:1381–1386.

78. Schapowal A (on behalf of Petasite Study Group). Treating intermittent allergic rhinitis: a prospective, randomized, placebo and antihistamine-controlled study of Butterbur extract Ze 339. *Phytother Res.* Jun 2005;19(6):530–537.

79. Semba RD. Vitamin A as "anti-infective" therapy, 1920–1940. *J Nutr.* Apr 1999;129(4):783–791.

80. Shin SH, Ponikau JU, Sherris DA, et al. Chronic rhinosinusitis: an enhanced immune response to ubiquitous airborne fungi. *J Allergy Clin Immunol.* Dec 2004;114(6):1369–1375.

81. Simon H. In Depth Report on Sinusitis. *New York Times.* March 28, 2008 Available at http://health.nytimes.com/health/guides/disease/sinusitis/overview.html.

82. Stalman W, van Essen GA, van der Graaf Y, de Melker RA. The end of antibiotic treatment in adults with acute sinusitis-like complaints in general practice? A placebo-controlled double-blind randomized doxycycline trial. *Br J Gen Pract.* Dec 1997;47(425):794–799.

83. Taub SJ. The use of bromelains in sinusitis: a double-blind clinical evaluation. *Eye Ear Nose Throat Mon.* Mar 1967;46(3):361–362.

84. Thornhill SM, Kelly AM. Natural treatment of perennial allergic rhinitis. *Altern Med Rev.* Oct 2000;5(5):448–454.

85. Tosca MA, Cosentino C, Pallestrini E, et al. Medical treatment reverses cytokine pattern in allergic and nonallergic chronic rhinosinusitis in asthmatic children. *Pediatr Allergy Immunol.* Jun 2003;14(3):238–241.

86. Uhari T, Kontiokari M, Koskela M, Niemela, M. Xylitol chewing gum in prevention of acute otitis media: double blind randomised trial, *BMJ.* 1996;313:1180–1184.

87. Uhari M, Kontiokari T, and Niemela M. A novel use of xylitol sugar in preventing acute otitis media, *Pediatrics.* 1998;102:879–884.

88. Unal M, Tamer L, Pata YS, et al. Serum levels of antioxidant vitamins, copper, zinc and magnesium in children with chronic rhinosinusitis. *J Trace Elem Med Biol.* 2004;18(2):189–192.

89. United States Department of Agriculture. Nutrient Profiles. April 14 Available at http://www.ars.usda.gov/Services/docs.htm?docid=7783.

90. Venuta A, Spano C, Laudizi L, Bettelli F, Beverelli A, Turchetto E. Essential fatty acids: the effects of dietary supplementation among children with recurrent respiratory infections. *J Int Med Res.* Jul-Aug 1996;24(4):325–330.

91. Volkmann ER, Weekes NY. Basal SIgA and cortisol levels predict stress-related health outcomes. *Stress and Health.* 2006;22:11–23.

92. Weitzberg E, Lundberg JO. Humming greatly increases nasal nitric oxide. *Am J Respir Crit Care Med.* Jul 2002;166(2):131–132.

93. Williamson IG, Rumsby K, Benge S, et al. Antibiotics and topical nasal steroid for treatment of acute maxillary sinusitis: a randomized controlled trial. *Jama.* Dec 5 2007;298(21):2487–2496.

94. Winkler P, de Vrese M, Laue C, Schrezenmeir J. Effect of a dietary supplement containing probiotic bacteria plus vitamins and minerals on common cold infections and cellular immune parameters. *Int J Clin Pharmacol Ther.* Jul 2005;43(7):318–326.

95. Wolkenstein E, Horak F. Protective effect of acupuncture on allergen provoked rhinitis. *Wien Med Wochenschr.* 1998;148(19):450–453.

96. Xue CC, An X, Cheung TP, et al. Acupuncture for persistent allergic rhinitis: a randomised, sham-controlled trial. *Med J Aust.* Sep 17 2007;187(6):337–341.

97. Yarnell E, Abascal K, Hooper CG. *Clinical botanical medicine.* 2003. Larchmont, NY: Mary Ann Liebert, Inc.

3 Chemosensory Disorders

Alan R. Hirsch, M.D.

I. INTRODUCTION

Approximately 90% of taste or flavor is actually smell [1]. It is a nonpathological form of synesthesia, wherein orthonasal smell is perceived as aroma and retronasal smell, from the posterior of the mouth, through the oropharynx, is construed as taste [2, 3]. This chapter explores how diminution and alteration in taste and smell influence food selection and nutrient needs.

II. EPIDEMIOLOGY

Chemosensory dysfunction is endemic. Approximately 15 million Americans 55 or older have olfactory abnormalities, and more than 200,000 individuals seek the medical advice of general practitioners and specialists each year because of complaints regarding smell or taste [4]. Causes of chemosensory dysfunction are myriad, and the underlying disorders are often, in and of themselves, associated with nutritional dysfunction [5].

III. PATHOPHYSIOLOGY

Smell is the only sensation to reach the cortex before reaching the thalamus. Furthermore, it is the only sensory system that is primarily ipsilateral in its projection to the cortex. In the future, neuroimaging techniques will be able to expand the understanding of this evolutionarily, precortical limbic system sense that is intertwined with our daily nutrition.

ANATOMY OF SMELL

Dirhinous inhalation is olfactorily asymmetric due to the olfactory cycle, which alternates open nostrils every 4 to 8 hours. Parenthetically, olfaction demonstrates greatest sensitivity ipsilateral to the restricted nostril, as a result of eddy currents, which are created by the smaller aperture. These tumultuous gusts of odorant, like rhinal tornadoes, stochastically distribute the odorants, with greater concentration reaching the olfactory epithelium at the top of the nose, as opposed to bypassing this area in favor of the bronchi and lungs [6].

Once an odor passes through the olfactory epithelium, it must stimulate the olfactory nerve, which consists of unmyelinated olfactory fila. The olfactory nerve has the slowest conduction rate of any nerve in the body. The olfactory fila pass through the cribiform plate of the ethmoid bone and enter the olfactory bulb. During trauma, much damage occurs in this bulb [7]. Different odors localize in different areas of the olfactory bulb.

Inside the olfactory bulb is a conglomeration of neuropil called the glomeruli. Approximately 2000 glomeruli reside in the olfactory bulb. Four different cell types make up the glomeruli: processes of receptor cell axons, mitral cells, tufted cells, and second-order neurons that give off collaterals to the granule cells and to cells in the periglomerular and external plexiform layers. The mitral and tufted cells form the lateral olfactory tract and establish a reverberating circuit with the granule cells. The mitral cells stimulate firing of the granule cells, which in turn inhibit firing of the mitral cells [8].

A reciprocal inhibition exists between the mitral and tufted cells. This results in a sharpening of olfactory acuity. The olfactory bulb receives several efferent projections, including the primary olfactory fibers, the contralateral olfactory bulb and the anterior nucleus, the inhibitory prepiriform cortex, the diagonal band of Broca with neurotransmitters acetylcholine and gamma-aminobutyric acid (GABA), the locus coeruleus, the dorsal raphe, and the tuberomamillary nucleus of the hypothalamus.

The olfactory bulb's efferent fibers project into the olfactory tract, which divides at the olfactory trigona into the medial and lateral olfactory striae. These project to the anterior olfactory nucleus, the olfactory tubercle, the amygdaloid nucleus (which in turn projects to the ventral medial nucleus of the hypothalamus, a feeding center), the cortex of the piriform lobe, the septal nuclei, and the hypothalamus (in particular the anterolateral regions of the hypothalamus, which are involved in reproduction).

The anterior olfactory nucleus receives afferent fibers from the olfactory tract and projects efferent fibers, which decussate in the anterior commissure and synapse in the contralateral olfactory bulb. Some of the efferent projections from the anterior olfactory nucleus remain ipsilateral, and synapse on internal granular cells of the ipsilateral olfactory bulb.

The olfactory tubercle receives afferent fibers from the olfactory bulb and the anterior olfactory nucleus. Efferent fibers from the olfactory tubercle project to the nucleus accumbens as well as the striatum. Neurotransmitters of the olfactory tubercle include acetylcholine and dopamine.

The area on the cortex where olfaction is localized, that is, the primary olfactory cortex, includes the prepiriform area, the periamygdaloid area, and the entorhinal area. The piriform cortex and the amygdala are the primary olfactory cortex, while the insula and orbitofrontal cortex are secondary olfactory cortex association areas [9]. Afferent projections to the primary olfactory cortex include the mitral cells, which enter the lateral olfactory tract and synapse in the prepiriform cortex (lateral olfactory gyrus) and the corticomedial part of the amygdala. Efferent projections from the primary olfactory cortex extend to the entorhinal cortex, the basal and lateral amygdaloid nuclei, the lateral preoptic area of the hypothalamus, the nucleus of the diagonal band of Broca, the medial forebrain bundle, the dorsal medial nucleus and submedial nucleus of the thalamus, and the nucleus accumbens.

It should be noted that the entorhinal cortex is both a primary and a secondary olfactory cortical area. Efferent fibers project via the uncinate fasciculus to the hippocampus, the anterior insular cortex next to the gustatory cortical area, and the frontal cortex. This may explain why temporal lobe epilepsy that involves the uncinate often produces parageusias of burning rubber, uncinate fits [10].

Some of the efferent projections of the mitral and tufted cells decussate in the anterior commissure and form the medial olfactory tract. They then synapse in the contralateral parolfactory area and the contralateral subcallosal gyrus. The exact function of the medial olfactory stria and tract is not clear. The accessory olfactory bulb receives afferent fibers from the bed nucleus of the accessory olfactory tract and the medial and posterior corticoamygdaloid nuclei. Efferent fibers from the accessory olfactory bulb project through the accessory olfactory tract to the same afferent areas, for example, the bed nucleus of the accessory olfactory tract and the medial and posterior corticoamygdaloid nuclei. It should be noted that the medial and posterior corticoamygdaloid nuclei project secondary fibers to the anterior and medial hypothalamus, the areas associated with reproduction. Therefore the accessory olfactory bulb in humans may be the mediator for human pheromones [11].

Neurotransmitters That Mediate Smell

Neurotransmitters of the olfactory cortex are myriad, including glutamate, aspartate, cholecystokinin, luteinizing hormone-releasing hormone (LHRH), and somatostatin. Furthermore, perception of odors causes modulation of olfactory neurotransmitters within the olfactory bulb and the limbic system. Virtually all known neurotransmitters are present in the olfactory bulb. Thus odorant modulation of neurotransmitter levels in the olfactory bulb, tract, and limbic system intended for transmission of sensory information may have unintended secondary effects on a variety of different behaviors and disease states that are regulated by the same neurotransmitters. For instance, odorant modulation of dopamine in the olfactory bulb/limbic system may affect manifestations of Parkinson's disease. Mesolimbic override to many of the components of Parkinson's disease has been well documented, for example, motoric activation associated with emotional distress and fear of injury in a fire.

THE PHYSIOLOGY OF TASTE

Salt, sweet, sour, bitter, unami, and possibly lipids are mediated through taste receptors on taste buds located primarily in the fungiform, but also circumvallate papillae. The fungiform papillae have the lowest threshold to salt and sweet, whereas the circumvallate are more sensitive to sweet stimuli [12, 13]. Cranial nerve VII, IX, and X, mediating the gustatory stimuli, enter the pons and pontomedullary junction, ascending and descending through the tractus solitarius, finally terminating topographically on the ipsilateral nucleus of the tractus solitarius with cranial nerve VII chorda tympani fibers synapsing rostrally and glossopharyngeal fibers caudally. Second-order taste neurons progress through the parabrachial pontine nuclei where they diverge. One either bypasses or synapses in the thalamus with tertiary-order neurons progressing to the primary gustatory cortex in the insula. The other bypasses the thalamus and projects diffusely to the ventral forebrain with widespread limbic system connections.

ETIOLOGIES OF CHEMOSENSORY DISORDERS

Nasal Obstruction

Decreased ability to detect odors can occur secondary to nasal obstruction from adenoid hypertrophy. Adenoidectomy causes a recovery of the threshold of odor detection.

Steroid-dependent anosmia is a syndrome whose triad includes inhalant allergy, nasal polyps, and steroid reversal anosmia [14]. Its pathology is that of polyps, which cause a mechanical obstruction preventing odorants from reaching the olfactory epithelium.

Unknown Etiology

Acute viral hepatitis causes a reduction in olfactory sensitivity with dysgeusia and associated anorexia, which improve as the illness improves. Olfactory sensitivity in acute viral hepatitis is inversely proportional to the plasma bilirubin and directly proportional to the plasma retinal-binding protein level.

Endocrine Disorders

Several endocrine disorders are associated with anosmia. In hypothyroidism, 39% of afflicted individuals are aware of an alteration of sense of taste, 17% have dysosmia or distortion in sense of smell, and 39% have dysgeusia. Thyroid replacement reverses these problems. All individuals with both olfactory or gustatory problems and hypothyroidism have low parotid zinc levels.

Pseudohypoparathyroidism is a syndrome that includes short stature, rounded face, mental retardation, brachymetacarpia, brachymetatarsia, hypocalcemia, hyperphosphatemia, and resistance to parathyroid hormone. Hyposmias and hypogeusia are also seen in pseudohypoparathyroidism. Patients are usually unaware of their hyposmia and are unresponsive to hormones. The hyposmia has been well described as due to the X-linked dominant chromosome. Its onset is at birth.

Turner's syndrome, or chromatin-negative gonadal dysgenesis, is characterized by short stature, cubitus valgus, webbed neck, shield-like thorax, and XO-chromosome pattern. Though patients are unaware of olfactory defects, they are found to have both hyposmia and hypogeusia [15].

Olfactory sensitivity of patients with adrenal cortical insufficiency is increased approximately 100,000-fold over that of normal persons. Treatment with carbohydrate-active steroids (i.e., prednisone 20 mg q d) reduces it toward normal in 1 day. Since the olfactory response occurs prior to any change in electrolytes or body weight, one can postulate that endogeneous CNS carbohydrate-active steroids normally inhibit olfaction.

Congenital adrenal hyperplasia is a nonhypertensive virilizing illness, in which salt is not lost. Increases have been found in olfactory and gustatory sensitivity. Treatment with steroids reduces the hypersensitivity to normal in 8 to 14 days. Long before the reduction of olfactory and gustatory sensitivity, 17-ketosteroids and pregnanetriol return to normal, so it is unlikely that the reduction in olfactory sensitivity is due to carbohydrate-active steroids alone.

Kallmann's syndrome involves a deficiency of gonadotrophin-associated hypogonadism and impaired olfactory acuity. Clomiphene induces luteinizing hormone and follicle-stimulating hormone release, which causes an increase in both gonadotrophin and testosterone. The olfactory deficit does not respond to clomiphene.

Meningiomas

Olfactory meningiomas are classically described as causing loss of ability to detect odors. These meningiomas, which occur along the olfactory groove, account for less than 10% of all intracranial meningiomas. They usually develop in middle-aged patients, with hyposmia as the first, and for years, the only symptom. Eventually, however, the meningiomas enlarge, causing dementia and impaired vision.

Temporal Lobe Lesions

The temporal lobe also has an important influence on olfaction. One patient, after he had a bilateral resection of the medial temporal lobe that involved the amygdala, uncus, anterior two-thirds of the hippocampus and parahippocampal gyrus, was studied for his olfactory sensitivity. Although he could detect odors, he could not identify them, and when given two odors, he could not distinguish whether they were the same or different. This suggests that the medial temporal lobe is critical for perception of odor quality [16].

Further evidence for this can be seen in temporal lobectomy patients, who demonstrate a mild, bilateral reduction in absolute olfactory sensitivity. In the ipsilateral nostril, odor perception is reduced, as is odor identification. Patients with temporal lobe epilepsy who have had no surgery display a bilateral reduction in odor identification. Of patients with temporal lobe tumors, 20% have an olfactory disturbance [17].

Coronary artery bypass surgery can cause both dysosmia and cacosmia (whereby odors are distorted and previously hedonically pleasant aromas are now perceived as unpleasant). This may be secondary to temporal lobe infarction [18].

Thalamic and Hypothalamic Lesions

Estrogen-receptor-positive breast cancer patients are found to have hyposmia, possibly secondary to hypothalamic lesions [19]. Significantly, hypothalamic lesions produce an increase in incidence of spontaneous mammary tumors in female rats. This suggests that a hypothalamic lesion may be the primary defect in both estrogen receptor positive breast carcinoma and associated hyposmia.

Korsakoff's psychosis involves a lesion of the dorsal medial nucleus of the thalamus. Patients with Korsakoff's psychosis display an impaired ability to identify odors. The impairment is proportional to the reduction in their cerebral spinal fluid 3-methoxy-4-hydroxy-phenylethylene glycol (CSF MHPG), a norepinephrine metabolite [20]. CSF MHPG is reduced in Parkinson's disease and in senile dementia of the Alzheimer's type as well, and these patients also display an impaired ability to identify odors [21, 22]. It may be, therefore, that norepinephrine is important for olfaction, and that a drug to increase norepinephrine would increase olfactory ability.

One such drug is d-amphetamine. This d-2 dopamine receptor agonist increased olfactory detection in rats given 0.2 mg/kg body weight. With much higher doses (i.e., 1.6 mg/kg), the rats' ability to detect odors was reduced [23, 24]. The mechanism whereby it increases odor detection ability is unknown. D-amphetamine may act as a reticular-activity-system stimulator. It may also act by increasing catecholamine levels in the olfactory tubercle, anterior olfactory nucleus, amygdala, and entorhinal cortex. It may stimulate the locus coeruleus to release norephinephrine, which projects to the lateral olfactory tract. The lateral olfactory tract then would act to inhibit granule cell discharge, causing a reduction in the inhibition of mitral cell discharge. The mitral cells would thus be allowed to fire, causing an increase in olfactory acuity. The latter mechanism is probably not applicable to d-amphetamine, however, because in experiments with rats, norephinephrine depletion of the olfactory bulb had no effect on odor detection ability, implying that d-amphetamine operates on a central basis.

Parkinsonism

Parkinsonism is associated with a decrease in odor sensitivity in 75% of cases and a reduced ability to identify odors in 90% of cases. These olfactory deficits occur independently of age, gender, stage, and duration of the disease. Before they were tested, 72% of patients with Parkinson's disease were unaware of their deficits in olfaction, which tend to occur early in the disease process for those with dementia as well as without, and do not worsen with time [25]. In monozygotic twins with Parkinson's disease, olfactory impairment has a low concordance rate, indicating that this aspect of the disease is probably not inherited [26].

Many mechanisms have been postulated for the olfactory defects associated with Parkinson's disease. One is that the same environmental agent that caused the Parkinson's disease damaged the olfactory pathway. A second possible mechanism is that the olfactory receptor cells actively transport viruses, proteins, and environmental toxins upward, bypassing the blood-brain barrier and directly infiltrating the central nervous system. The substance so transported could damage both the olfactory epithelium and olfactory system before proceeding on to the substancia nigra to cause the Parkinson's disease. A third hypothesis is that the underlying Parkinson's disease could reduce the olfactory system's resistance to viral or environmental toxins, which then could destroy olfactory pathways. According to a fourth hypothesis, the degenerative process of Parkinson's disease may favor destruction of the olfactory pathways as it affects substancia nigra. A fifth hypothesis is that reduction in CNS neurotransmitters causes reduction in olfaction. The absence of effect of Sinemet on olfaction in Parkinson's disease argues against this hypothesis. In its favor is that d-2 dopamine-receptor agonist d-amphetamine increases olfaction in rats, as mentioned.

Aging

Olfactory deficit begins to be demonstrated at age 35 [27, 28]. Olfaction in aging individuals has been extensively studied [29]. Odor sensitivity, in regard to both absolute threshold and odor identification, is reduced with age. Over 50% of people between 65 and 80 years of age have major impairments in olfaction. For those over the age of 80 years, the proportion with major impairments rises to 75%. Over the age of 75 years, 25% are totally anosmic. These effects of aging parallel those found in other senses.

Many possible mechanisms have been postulated for age-induced olfactory defects. One theory holds that degenerative processes caused by toxins and viruses produce a cumulative effect on the olfactory epithelium. A second theory suggests that age-related immunocompromise predisposes people to upper respiratory infections (URIs), which may be followed by postviral URI-induced anosmia. A third hypothesis suggests that in the elderly, the central neural pathway degenerates, or that neurotransmitters, for instance norepinephrine, are reduced. A fourth theory postulates ossification of the foramina of the cribiform plate with secondary occlusion and compression of the olfactory filia. None of these theories exclude any of the others.

The implications of olfactory deficits among the older population are important, particularly regarding the detection of gas used for heating and cooking. Older persons succumb to accidental poisonings from leaking gas at a much higher rate than do younger people; 75% of such deaths were among persons over 60 years of age. Among persons over 65 years of age, 30% could not smell town gas in concentrations below 50 parts per 10,000, if they could smell it at all. Among those under age 65, in comparison, 95% could smell town gas in concentrations below 20 parts per 10,000. Half of the people over age 60 could not detect the odor of gas at the maximum concentration allowed by the Department of Transportation. One-seventh of persons 70 to 85 years of age could not detect the odor of gas at explosive concentrations.

In reference to ethyl mercaptan, the agent that is added to propane gas to give it a noxious odor, persons 70 to 85 years of age have a threshold 10 times higher than that of persons under age 70.

This impaired olfactory ability implies impaired gustatory abilities as well, since odor forms a large component of the sense of taste. This may account for the fact that the older population often consumes an unbalanced diet, such as one lacking in vegetables. Green peppers, for instance, have a bitter taste and a pleasant odor, but to this group, they merely taste bitter, making it unlikely that these foods will be eaten.

Also, retronasal odor perception, odor perceived while chewing and swallowing, is reduced. Despite this, older persons rarely complain of food lacking taste, possibly because of the slow, gradual loss of smell. Those who prepare food for this population should use higher concentrations of odorants compared with those preparing food for the young. Because of this population's deficits, foods with enhanced flavor are preferred.

Alzheimer's Disease (AD)

Patients with AD are usually unaware of their olfactory deficits [30]. Serby et al. postulated that the reduced odor threshold and identification ability found in this disorder are secondary to reduced acetylcholine in the olfactory system [31]. Acetylcholine has been found to be low in the olfactory tubercle in patients with AD. Arguing in favor of this hypothesis is that application of nasal acetylcholine produces an increase in olfactory sensitivity.

Koss et al. postulate that the decrease in olfactory sensitivity in Alzheimer's disease is secondary to temporal lobe dysfunction [32, 33]. As mentioned, olfactory defects are found in individuals with temporal lobectomies, and the same mechanism may operate in AD. Person et al. suggest that the olfactory pathway is the initial site of involvement both in AD and in Pick's disease [34].

In Alzheimer's disease, neuritic plaque and neurofibrillary tangles form in the olfactory bulb, olfactory tract, anterior olfactory nucleus, prepyriform cortex, uncus, and corticomedial part of the amygdaloid nucleus. Interestingly, the anterior olfactory nucleus, the uncus, and the corticomedial part of the amygdaloid nucleus all receive afferent input from the olfactory bulb. In the entorhinal cortex, layer II stellate cells, which are the end point for the lateral olfactory tract, are lost. Secondary connections of the olfactory cortex are involved with memory and cognition, including the amygdala, the dorsal medial nucleus of the thalamus, and the hippocampus.

A unified theory that could possibly explain the occurrence of both olfactory deficits and AD is a variant of that described for Parkinson's disease: Viruses may enter the olfactory pathway via the olfactory epithelium, thereby bypassing the blood-brain barrier [35]. Once inside the olfactory pathway, the viruses could spread into the secondary connections of the limbic system. This route of infection is known to operate in the case of St. Louis encephalitis and amebiasis.

Roberts' theory is that Alzheimer's disease begins in the nose and is caused by aluminosilicates [36]. Labeled glucose placed into the oropharynx is rapidly transported transneuronally to the glomeruli in the olfactory bulb. From there it spreads into the olfactory projections (i.e., the nucleus of Meynert, the locus ceruleus, and the brainstem raphe nuclei). Aluminum and silicon are found to increase in the brain with aging [37]. Widely dispersed in the environment, aluminosilicates can be found in diverse products, including talc, deionizers, antacids, underarm spray, dental powder, cat litter, cigar ash, and cigarette ash. Roberts strongly recommends reducing exposure to these aerosolized toxins.

Toxic Agents

In addition to aluminum and silicon mentioned above as possible causes of Alzheimer's disease, other, more classic toxic agents, notably lead and arsenic, are well known to affect olfaction.

Perfume workers, varnish workers, and those exposed to cadmium dust also experience a marked reduction in olfactory abilities.

In a Texas petrochemical plant, workers who smoked cigarettes showed reduced olfactory sensitivity; the diminished acuity directly correlated with the amount they smoked [38]. Another aspect of cigarette smoking concerns its effect on the trigeminally mediated reflex transitory apnea (the "took-my-breath-away" reflex). Cigarette smoking raised the threshold of the reflex by 67% [39]. The mechanism is probably secondary to smoke-induced ciliastasis, which causes a mucostasis that in turn induces a viscid static mucus. The viscid mucus impairs the transfer of odor molecules from the air to free nerve endings. Secondhand smoke may act through a similar mechanism to raise both olfactory and trigeminal thresholds.

Trauma

Subfrontal exploration of the anterior fossa can stretch or tear the olfactory nerves. Surgical repair of a dural tear with grafts covering the cribiform plate can block regenerating stem cells.

Head injury is a common cause of olfactory defects. Many possible mechanisms have been suggested. One is that acceleration injury produces shearing forces on the olfactory nerves as they pass through the cribiform plate of the ethmoid bone. Fracture of the cribiform plate may compress the olfactory nerves or a hematoma may compress them, thereby impairing olfaction. Another theory suggests that the primary insult in trauma is the destruction of pathways of central connection of olfaction [40].

Averaging the results of many studies of olfaction in head injury victims, we find that roughly 5% of victims have olfactory disorders. No correlation has been observed between the loss of olfaction and the age of the victim at the time of the accident, or the category of the accident.

The incidence of olfactory disorder is proportional to the severity of the injury, but even a trivial injury can induce anosmia. In trauma severe enough to induce amnesia, occipital trauma is 5 times as likely to produce anosmia as is trauma to the forehead.

Usually any olfactory loss occurs shortly after the trauma, but sometimes it may not occur until several months later. Recovery from olfactory defects usually begins during the first few weeks after head trauma, but it can be delayed until as long as 5 years later.

Half of the individuals with anosmia secondary to head trauma experience distorted smell in response to odorants. Costanzo reported on 77 persons with anosmia due to head injury: 33% recovered, 27% worsened, and 40% remained unchanged. Costanzo and Becker reported on a sample of 1167 patients: 50% recovered, except for cases where injury was so severe as to cause amnesia of more than 24 hours. In these cases, fewer than 10% recovered [41].

Temporary anosmia of short duration, often found after trauma, could be due to mechanical blockage of airways, nasal hemorrhaging, inflammation, CSF rhinorrhea, or an increase in intracranial pressure. Increased intracranial pressure may reduce circulation of the olfactory bulbs, causing secondary infarctions therein with associated anosmia.

Nutritional Deficiencies

Some primary nutritional deficiency states have also been associated with chemosensory pathology. Hypovitaminosis A induces both hyposmia and hypogeusia [42] that usually resolves within 2 months with vitamin A replacement. The mechanism of the deficit may be a result of epithelial proliferation and drying, which forms a physical barrier, preventing odorants and tastants from reaching their respective receptors [43].

Chemosensory dysfunction has also been reported in those deficient in B complex vitamins [44].

Wernicke-Korsakoff syndrome, with thiamine deficiency, demonstrates hyposmia [20].

Dysosmia and dysgeusia are seen in those with reduced B12 levels and pernicious anemia [44, 45].

Hypocupria causes a reversible hypogeusia and is responsive to both copper sulfate and zinc sulfate [46, 47].

Patients with anosmia induced by head trauma have been found to have reduced total serum zinc and increased total serum copper. This same chemical imbalance is found in the syndrome of idiopathic hypogeusia with dysgeusia, hyposmia, and dysosmia. The importance of zinc is further demonstrated in patients treated with L-histidine, which induces zincuria, causing a secondary hypozincemia and reduced total body zinc. This, in turn, causes hypogeusia, hyposmia, anorexia, dysgeusia, and dysosmia. All of these symptoms are corrected by treating the patient with zinc. Improvement occurs even when the patient is still receiving L-histidine.

The pathophysiology of hypozincemia may be like that of hypovitaminosis A, a structural barrier due to production of hyperkeratosis [48].

IV. PATIENT EVALUATION

When chemosensory disorders are associated with some of the underlying conditions mentioned above, it is important to diagnose the treatable medical conditions. This assessment is more relevant among hospitalized persons where the incidence of olfactory impairment is probably greater than among the general population [49, 50].

Standard medical [51] and neurological texts [52–54] indicate that assessment of the olfactory nerve, cranial nerve I (CNI), is an essential part of a complete neurological examination. Given the likelihood of olfactory dysfunction among hospitalized patients, particularly those with neurological disorders, olfactory testing should be routine.

Diagnoses Associated with Olfactory Impairment

Lack of olfactory data may impair diagnostic accuracy. For example, Post's pseudodementia, which does not involve olfactory impairment, is often misdiagnosed as Alzheimer's disease [55], which does involve olfactory impairment. In recent experiments, Solomon, Patrie et al. demonstrated that olfactory testing can aid in distinguishing these disorders [56]. Similarly, olfactory deficits are seen in idiopathic Parkinson's disease but not 1-methyl-4-phenyl-1,2,3,6-tetrahydropyridine (MPTP)-induced Parkinson's disease [57], progressive supranuclear palsy [58], or essential tremor [59]. Olfactory deficits are seen in a substantial proportion of those with sinusitis or migraines, but not in those with cluster headaches [60–62].

Olfactory deficits may be the first manifestation of an underlying disease state. Without olfactory data, B12 deficiency [5, 63] and olfactory groove meningiomas [64], which display olfactory dysfunction early on, may remain undetected until more serious neurological deficits occur. Psychiatric disorders, including general anxiety disorder [65] and sexual dysfunction [66], also are associated with olfactory dysfunction; thus, detection of olfactory deficits may signal the possibility of these conditions.

Assessment of CNI allows detection of hyposmia or anosmia regardless of its origin. Patients may then receive medications, vitamins, food supplements [67], or special treatment to correct the underlying pathology, for example, polypectomy for nasal polyps [68], steroids for allergic rhinitis [69]. Appropriate counseling emphasizes risks to personal safety such as spoiled or oversalted food, gas leaks, and smoke [70, 71]. Lifestyle changes, such as food tasters and gas detectors, can be advised.

Assessing Olfaction

Self-recognition of olfactory deficits is poor. Geriatric patients and those with neurogenitive disorders such as Alzheimer's disease doften are unaware of their olfactory losses [80]. Of those with Parkinson's disease, fewer than 15% recognize their olfactory deficits [25]. Younger people also lack insight into such problems. Half of anosmic workers exposed to cadmium [81], and 100% of hyposmic chefs [82], were unaware of any deficits. And, according to an unpublished study by this author, 87.5% of hyposmic or anosmic firefighters were unaware of their deficits. Thus, to limit testing to those who complain of problems would leave many cases of smell loss undetected.

Simple and easy ways to assess olfaction include the presentation of readily available fragrant substances such as coffee, almond, lemon, tobacco, anise, oil of clove, toothpaste, eucalyptus, vanilla, peppermint, camphor, rosewater, and soap [51–54]. In addition, formalized tests of olfaction are widely available, including the Chicago Smell Test [72, 73], the University of Pennsylvania Smell Identification Test (UPSIT) [74], the olfactory threshold test of Amoore [75], and the Alcohol Sniff Test [76–79].

Given the prevalence of olfactory disorder, the ease of testing it and the substantial evidence that identifying such impairment can enhance accuracy of diagnoses, it seems well worth physicians' time and effort to test olfaction. Moreover, patients suffering from hyposmia and anosmia can be treated and advised to take precautions to reduce such risks to their safety as spoiled food and leaking gas.

Yet anecdotal evidence and medical literature suggest that in clinical practice, CNI is rarely tested [54]. To evaluate, we reviewed histories and physical examinations in 90 patient charts at a Chicago teaching hospital. Charts were selected from all adult patients admitted to this hospital from April through September 1988 who met the following criteria: a neurologic diagnosis upon discharge; ability to follow directions and respond verbally; and not intubated, comatose, or admitted to an intensive care unit. None of the 94 physical exams performed by attending-level internists and neurologists indicated that CNI was tested. While four charts (4.2%) note "cranial nerves intact" or "neuro exam grossly normal," thereby implying that olfactory testing may have been performed, it appears to have been an overgeneralization.

A number of factors may account for this olfactory testing lacuna. Traditional tests lack standardization and those that are standardized are difficult to perform at the bedside. Traditional tests, such as holding vanilla, cloves, or coffee to the patient's nose, are not administered in a controlled manner [94], and there are only a few standardized tests of olfactory ability, including the Chicago Smell Test [72, 73], threshold tests of Amoore [75], the olfactory test of the Connecticut Chemosensory Clinical Research Center [95], and the most widely used test, the University of Pennsylvania Smell Identification Test (UPSIT) [96], a 40-question scratch-and-sniff test, adjusted for age and sex, the results of which have been validated in nearly 4000 normal controls [74].

Difficulties with these standardized tests prevent their widespread use. The Chicago Smell Test is not widely available. Individual odor olfactory threshold tests from Olfacto-Labs require several bulky bottles and so are not practical for the clinician [97]. The UPSIT requires the patient to provide 40 responses and so requires a substantial amount of time to administer, and patients with cognitive dysfunction may have difficulty completing it.

Alternatively, the Alcohol Sniff Test (AST) [76–78] can easily be performed at the bedside, even with children [98] and those with cognitive impairment [79]. The AST is rapid, cost-effective, and requires only a tape measure and an alcohol pad, and thus would seem ideal for use in a clinical setting. Olfactory ability is quantitatively determined by placing the 0 cm marker of the tape measure at the philtrum. With the patient's eyes closed, an alcohol pad, one-quarter exposed, is placed at the 40 cm marker and gradually moved inward on inhalation at 1 cm/s until detected. This is repeated four times, waiting 45 s between each test, and the results are averaged. If detection is greater than or equal to 17 cm, it indicates normosmia; detection between 8 and 17 cm indicates hyposmia; and detection at less than 8 cm suggests anosmia. The AST has been validated in comparison to threshold testing [76], and threshold testing correlates with the UPSIT [99].

A statistically significant correlation exists between the UPSIT and AST. UPSIT scores, in addition, are used to discriminate among anosmic, hyposmic, normosmic, and malingering patients.

At the risk of deblaterating, the AST can grossly be interpreted such that if alcohol can be detected beyond the chin, olfaction is normal. Using this method is both time efficient and validated as a screen for olfactory deficit. More detailed testing such as the UPSIT, functional MRI, and so on, can then be performed on those with an abnormal AST.

V. TREATMENT

Chemosensory disorders have been shown to be responsive to several nutritional approaches.

REPLETING NUTRIENTS

Phosphatidylcholine

Acetylcholine is important in olfaction as evidenced by the fact that a normal person's olfactory sense is impaired by taking scopolamine, which decreases the effect of acetylcholine. We cannot ascribe this impairment to drying of the nasal mucus since drying actually improves olfaction [100], so we ascribe it to a decrease in acetylcholine. As further evidence of the importance of acetylcholine in olfaction, patients with senile dementia of the Alzheimer's type lose their ability to detect and identify odors relatively early; in this disease, reduced choline acetyltransferase causes a reduction of acetylcholine in the basal nucleus of Meynert [101]. Phosphatidylcholine is converted via choline acetyltransferase into acetylcholine. Thus, choline provides the essential precursor [102]. The amount of choline circulating in the body affects its content in the brain and affects release of acetylcholine in the CNS. Insufficient choline impairs nerve cells' ability to transmit messages across synapses. By supplementing choline, therefore, we can amplify these messages in some forms of chemosensory disorders [103].

Phosphatidylcholine has been used to increase blood choline, brain choline, and brain acetylcholine levels in patients with brain diseases associated with impaired acetylcholine neurotransmission, such as tardive dyskinesia [104]. Due to its central role in the composition and function of neuronal membranes, phosphatidylcholine has also been used for patients with brain diseases associated with dissolution of neuronal membranes such as Alzheimer's disease [105]. By providing phosphatidylcholine to hyposmic patients, we may enhance their acetylcholine and improve olfaction.

In an open-label followed by a double-blind trial of phosphatidylcholine at 9 g/day for 3 months, mixed results were seen. A 40% improvement on the open-label study was followed by a negative result on the double-blind study. However, this could be due to a flaw in the study design. It may be suggestive that several experimental subjects dropped out of the double-blind trial with phosphatidylcholine, saying that they disliked the taste of licorice. Since none of the patients voiced this complaint initially, it seems possible that their sense of smell, and therefore of taste, improved during treatment, making them more aware of the licorice taste. None of the control subjects who dropped out mentioned the licorice taste as a reason [106]. Given the above, in those with idiopathic hyposmia or anosmia, we often start a 3-month trial of phosphatidylcholine (Phoschol) at 9 g/day in three divided doses.

Thiamine

While a pilot trial of thiamine 100 mg/day showed no effect, anecdotally some anosmic and hyposmic patients showed remarkable improvement with this treatment [107].

Vitamin A

Since vitamin A exists in the olfactory epithelium and could be involved in olfactory neuron regeneration, it theoretically could improve hyposmia or anosmia [108].

Of 56 anosmic patients studied, 89% who underwent intramuscular vitamin A injections regained full or partial olfactory ability. Oral retinoid treatment (Etretinate) has also been reported to be effective [109]. Patients with cirrhosis and hypovitaminosis A display improvement in both taste and smell thresholds in response to vitamin A treatment [110].

Caffeine

Caffeine inhibits adenosine receptors and thus may facilitate taste sensitivity. Although study results are mixed, there is a suggestion that topical caffeine enhances taste to sweet and bitter [111, 112].

Zinc

Zinc has undergone a peripetic course as the standard-bearer for treatment of smell and taste disorders. The zeitgeist of zinc was in the 1960s and 1970s when a series of articles suggested its efficacy in a wide range of chemosensory disorders [47, 113, 114]. Zinc was originally used during the polio epidemic in an attempt to prevent spread of the disease to victims' families. Family members were treated intranasally to destroy the receptor neuroepithelium. The stratagem was effective only for several months, since stem cells proliferated and underwent transformation into fully developed bipolar olfactory receptor cells, thus allowing the treated persons again to be exposed to the polio virus. This effect of zinc was the basis for the idea of using zinc on the stem cells of anosmics to stimulate the development of bipolar olfactory receptor cells.

The frequent association between olfactory impairment and exposure to trace metals suggests another rationale for using zinc. Mercury, lead, cadmium, and gold have been associated with olfactory dysfunction. Iron deficiency alters taste and food selection. Zinc metabolism is abnormal in such altered physiologic states, with hyposmia, as liver disease and first trimester pregnancy. Hypothyroid patients with hyposmia and hypogeusia have low parotid zinc levels. Treatment with Synthroid improves olfaction and taste as it returns parotid zinc levels to normal. Patients with postinfluenza hypogeusia and hyposmia have low parotid zinc and low serum zinc.

Clinical trials have not produced the results one might anticipate from the observations above. A study of 106 patients with hypogeusia following influenza revealed that although zinc treatment corrected their low serum levels, it did not improve hypogeusia and hyposmia. A double-blind, crossover trial did not demonstrate efficacy of zinc and treatment of hypogeusia [115]. Another paper, comparing zinc-treated versus non-zinc-treated patients, found no difference in taste ability [116]. Moreover, zinc is not necessarily benign; toxicity may occur. At 100 mg/day, a level at or below suggested therapeutic doses, inhibition of immune function, anemia, and neutropenia have been reported [117].

We have anecdotally found zinc to be remarkably effective in postcardiac transplantation dysosmia and hyposmia, despite the presence of normal zinc levels [118]. Zinc at concentrations beyond those in a multivitamin should be used with caution. I would consider only using zinc with laboratory evidence of hypozincemia or specific states where zinc has demonstrated efficacy including cirrhosis, dialysis, D-penicillimine treatment, and age-related macular degeneration.

INCREASING PATIENT AWARENESS OF ALTERED EATING HABITS

Chemosensory disorders in general are linked to changes in food selection. Most notably there is an aversion to foods that are bitter in taste and sweet in smell, as in dark chocolate, coffee, green peppers, and other green leafy vegetables. Also, a predilection develops toward more textured and trigeminally mediated foods, as sensory compensation for loss and in an attempt to recreate a sapid experience, with such foods as sushi or hot chili peppers.

Table 3.1 presents the different types of chemosensory impairment and the resulting impact on food selection and body weight:

- For congenital chemosensory dysfunction, no significant difference in weight, eating patterns, or food preferences compared to normosmics exists.
- People with acquired, noncongenital chemosensory dysfunction experience changes in food preferences and enhanced intake of salt and sugar.
- People with dysgeusia tend to ingest intense trigeminal stimuli, like mint, in an attempt to overcome the unpleasant sensation.
- In those with chemosensory loss, about 10% gain a substantial amount of weight, possibly increasing eating due to the narcissistic drive for the sensory experience or a lack of sensory specific satiety. An approximately equal number lose weight, possibly secondary to

TABLE 3.1
Change in Nutrition with Chemosensory Disorders [118–122]

Chemosensory Disorders	Food Complaints	Increased Appetite	Decreased Appetite	Decreased Enjoyment	Increased Use of Sugar, Salt, & Spices	% Who Gained 10% or More of Body WT after Chemosensory Dysfunction	% Who Lost 10% or More Body WT after Chemosensory Dysfunction
Anosmia (noncongential)	50% to 60%	20%	31%	88%	20% to 40% 4% decreased	14%	6.50%
Anosmia (congenital)	20%	No data	No data	No data	No data	No data	No data
Hyposmia	31% to 80%	30%	10% to 20%	50%	20% to 50% 20% decreased	1.50%	10.60%
Dysosmia & phantosmia	75% to 85%	No data	24%	83%	50%	No data	No data
Ageusia	100%	No data	100%	No data	No data	No data	No data
Hypogeusia	75%	No data	67%	33%	No data	No data	No data
Dysgeusia & phantageusia	72% to 85%	24%	30% to 67%	42% to 70%	40% to 60% 18% decreased	15% to 20%	15% to 20%

lack of interest in food or an associated depression, or due to the hedonically unpleasant distortion in the taste of foods.

- Dysguesia triggers most noted and avoided include meats, fresh fruits, coffee, eggs, carbonated beverages, and vegetables [119].
- Among patients with anorexia there is an elevation in sour and bitter recognition thresholds, but there is no abnormality in sweet or salt taste detection thresholds. Neither are there abnormal sweet superthreshold intensity judgments or detection threshold in anorexics or bulimics [120–122]. Furthermore, anorexics demonstrated an aversion to high-fat foods, but this may have been due to texture rather than taste [123].
- In those with obesity there are normal sweet taste thresholds and normal sweet superthreshold intensity judgments [124–127]. In regard to sweet hedonics, studies are inconclusive with results suggesting more, same, or less sweet preference [125, 126, 128, 129]. While high-fat, low-sugar mixtures appear to be preferred in the obese [130], not all studies confirm this preference [131, 132]. Diverse results from studies suggest that presently unidentified subgroups of taste response exist among those with obesity and chemosensory disorders.

Bringing awareness to the predispositions of food selection can help some patients moderate their food selection.

USE OF TASTANTS

Olfactory stimulation through intermittent odor presentation has previously been demonstrated to have efficacy in weight reduction [133]. Powdered crystallized tastants were demonstrated to induce weight loss in 108 people over 6 months [134]. We replicated the above study with a sample size of 1436 obese and overweight participants.

Nonnutritional, noncaloric, nonsalt flavors were crystallized and pulverized into a powdered form, each with a different basic flavor. Each participant was given sweet and savory tastants, presented as pairs in the order of cheddar cheese and cocoa, onion and spearmint, horseradish and banana, ranch dressing and strawberry, taco and raspberry, and parmesan and malt, and instructed to sprinkle these on whatever they ate—the savory flavors on salty foods, the sweet flavor on sweet foods—and otherwise not to change their eating or exercise routines.

Over a 6-month period, use of tastants was associated with a 30.5 pound weight loss or 14.7% of body mass. We hypothesized that this modality may be less effective in those who suffer from chemosensory dysfunction. This may particularly apply to those over the age of 35, the age at which olfactory ability starts to fade, and to men, whose baseline olfactory ability is worse than that of women [28, 135].

Several underlying mechanisms may contribute to weight loss. The tastants may enhance flavor. They may cause people to focus on eating and create mindful awareness of eating. The tastes themselves may increase the release of cholecystokinin (CCK) or cause CCK to be released earlier so satiety is reached before as many calories are consumed (sensory specific satiety augmenting alliesthesia). The tastants may make foods taste the same and remove the interest of food. The tastants might be socially awkward in some situations so the participants choose not to eat. The tastants may act to restore sensory perception of food. The tastants may influence food selection to more healthful foods. Tastants are new and novel and may add renewed interest to dieting. The tastants reinforce chronobiology and may therefore prevent dyssynchronosis, which is associated with weight gain.

The tastants we studied are commercially available.* In addition, patients can use their nose to help them lose weight by sniffing food before eating it, blowing bubbles in food, eating foods hot,

---

* The Sensa Weight Loss System can be accessed at www.scienceofsmell.com.

and chewing food throughly. These strategies enhance the olfactory chemosensory intensity of the food, and induce early satiety.

VI. SUMMARY

Compromised senses of smell and taste influence food selection, food preparation, and dietary patterns. Chemosensory impairments tend to have insidious onset and many patients are therefore unaware that these sensations are diminished or altered. Physicians can diagnose chemosensory disorders using a simple screening test. Familiarity with the medical conditions and iatrogenic factors can increase clinical suspicion of smell and taste impairment. Diagnosis can bring awareness to patients for altered food habits and issues pertaining to home safety. It can also assist clinicians in identifying underlying nutrient deficiencies that can be repleted. Tastants, spicy foods, and greater awareness in eating can help overcome some of the physiologic consequences of diminished taste. Unlike a chimera, an invisible universe at the tip of our nose is ripe for future exploration!

REFERENCES

1. Hirsch AR. Scentsation, olfactory demographic and abnormalities. *Intl J Aromatherap,* 1992; 4:1:16–17.
2. Bingham AF, Birch GG, deGraaf C, Behan JM, Perring KD. Sensory studies with sucrose maltol mixtures. *Chem Sen,* 1990; 15:447–456.
3. Murphy C, Cain WS. Taste and olfaction: Independence vs. interaction. *Physiol Behav,* 1980; 24:601–605.
4. Murphy C, Schubert CR, Cruickshanks KJ, Klein BEK, Klein R, Nondahl DM. Prevalence of olfactory impairment in older adults. *JAMA,* 2002; 288:2307–2312.
5. Estrem SA, Renner G. Disorders of smell and taste. *Otolaryngol Clin North Am,* 1987; 20(1)133–147.
6. Frye RE. Nasal patency and the aerodynamics of nasal airflow: Measurement by rhinomanometry and acoustic rhinometry, and the influence of pharmacological agents. In: Doty RL (Ed). *Handbook of Olfaction and Gustation,* Second Ed., Revised and Expanded. New York: Marcel Dekker, Inc., 2003, pp. 439–459.
7. Hirsch AR, Wyse JP. Posttraumatic dysosmia: Central vs peripheral. *J Neurol Orthop Med Surg,* 1993; 14:152–155.
8. Brodal A. *Neurological Anatomy in Relation to Clinical Medicine,* 3rd ed., Vol 10. New York: Oxford University Press, 1969.
9. Doty RL, Bromley SM, Moberg PJ, Hummel T. Laterality in human nasal chemoreception. In: Christman S (Ed). *Cerebral Asymmetries in Sensory and Perceptual Processing.* Amsterdam (the Netherlands): Elsevier, 1997, pp. 492–542.
10. Acharya V, Acharya J, Luders H. Olfactory epileptic auras. *Neurology,* 1996; 46:A446.
11. Hirsch AR. *Scentsational Sex.* Boston: Element Books, 1998.
12. Jeppson P. Studies on the structure and innervation of taste buds. *Acta Otolaryngol,* 1969; 259:1–95.
13. Smith DV. Taste, smell and psychophysical measurement. In: Meiselman HL, Rivlin RS (Eds). *Clinical Measurement of Taste and Smell.* New York: Macmillan, 1986, pp. 1–18.
14. Jefek BW, Moran DT, Eller PM. Steroid-dependent anosmia. *Arch Otolaryngol,* 1987; 113:547–549.
15. Heinkin R. Abnormalities of taste and olfaction in patients with chromatin negative gonadal dysgenesis. Taste and olfaction in Turner's syndrome. *J Clin Endocrin,* 1967;27:1437.
16. Eichenbaum H, Morton T, Potter H, Corkin S. Selective olfactory deficits in case H.M. *Brain,* 1983; 106(2):459–472.
17. Eskenazi B, Cain W, Novelly R, Mattson R. Odor perception in temporal lobe epilepsy patients with and without temporal lobectomy. *Neuropsychologia,* 1986; 24:553–562.
18. Mohr PD. Early neurological complications of coronary artery bypass surgery. *BMJ,* 1986; 292:60–61.
19. Lehrer S, Levine E, Bloomer W. Abnormally diminished sense of smell in women with estrogen receptor positive breast cancer. *Lancet,* 1985; 2:333.

20. Mair RG, Doty RL, Kelly KM, Wilson CS, Langlais PJ, McEntree WJ, Vollmecke TA. Multimodal sensory deficits in Korsakoff's psychosis. *Neuropsychologia,* 1986; 24:831–839.
21. Potter H, Butters N. An assessment of olfactory deficits in patients with damage to prefrontal cortex. *Neuropsychologia,* 1980; 18:621–628.
22. Ward CD, Hess WA, Calne DB. Olfactory impairment in Parkinson's disease. *Neurology,* 1983; 33:943–946.
23. Doty RL, Ferguson-Segall M. Odor detection performance of rats following d-amphetamine treatment: A signal detection analysis. *Psychopharmacology (Berl),* 1987; 93:87–93.
24. Doty RL, Ferguson-Segall M, Lucki I, Kreider M. Effects of intrabulbar injections of 6-hydroxydopamine on ethyl acetate odor detection in castrate and non-castrate male rats. *Brain Res,* 1988; 44:95–103.
25. Doty RL, Deems DA, Stellar S. Olfactory dysfunction in Parkinsonism: A general deficit unrelated to neurologic signs, disease stage, or disease duration. *Neurology,* 1988; 38:1237.
26. Doty RL, Riklan M, Deems D, Reynolds C, Stellar S. The olfactory and cognitive deficits of Parkinson's disease: Evidence for independence. *Ann Neurol,* 1989; 25:166–171.
27. Delahunty CM. Changing sensitivity of odour, taste, texture and mouth-feel with ageing. (Workshop summary). How do age-related changes in sensory physiology influence food liking and food intake? *Food Qual Pref,* 2004; 15:907–911.
28. Hawkes C, Fogo A, Shah M. Smell identification declines from age 36 years and mainly affects pleasant odors. *Chem Sen,* 2005; 30:A152–A153.
29. Stevens J, Cain W, Weinstein D. Aging impairs the ability to detect gas odors. *Fire Technol,* 1987; 23:198–204.
30. Doty R, Reys P, Gregor T. Presence of both odor identification and detection deficits in Alzheimer's disease. *Brain Res Bull,* 1987; 18:598.
31. Serby M, Corwin J, Novatt A, Conrad P, Rotrosen J. Olfaction in dementia. *Neurosurg Psychiat,* 1985; 14:848–849.
32. Koss E, Weiffenbach J, Haxby J, Friedland R. Olfactory detection and identification performance are dissociated in early Alzheimer's disease. *Neurology,* 1988; 38:1228.
33. Koss E, Weiffenbach J, Haxby J, Friedland R. Olfactory detection and identification performance are dissociated in early Alzheimer's disease. *Lancet,* 1987; 1:622.
34. Pearson R, Esiri M, Hiorns R, Wilcock G, Powell T. Anatomical correlates of the distribution of the pathological changes in the neocortex in Alzheimer's disease. *Proc Natl Acad Sci, USA,* 1985; 82:4531–4534.
35. Monath T, Cropp B, Harrison A. Mode of entry of a neurotropic arbovirus into the central nervous system. *Lab Invest,* 1983; 48:399.
36. Roberts R. Alzheimer's disease may begin in the nose and may be caused by aluminosilicates. *Neurbiol Aging,* 1986; 7:561–567.
37. Schwartz A, Frey J, Lukas R. Risk factors in Alzheimer's disease: Is aluminum hazardous to your health? *BNI Quarterly,* 1988; 4:2.
38. Frye R, Schwartz B, Doty R. Dose-related effects of cigarette smoking on olfactory function. *JAMA,* 1990; 263:1233.
39. Cain W, Cometto-Muniz JE. Perception of nasal pungency in smokers and nonsmokers. *Psychol Behav,* 1982; 29:727–732.
40. Levin H, High W, Eisenberg H. Impairment of olfactory recognition after closed head injury. *Brain,* 1985; 108:579–591.
41. Costanzo R, Becker D. Smell and taste disorders in head injury and neurosurgery patients. In: Meiselman HL, Rivlin RS (Eds). *Clinical Measurement of Taste and Smell.* New York: Macmillan, 1986, pp. 565–568.
42. Sauberlich HE. Vitamin metabolism and requirements. *S Afr Med J,* 1975; 49:2235–2244.
43. Friedman MI, Mattes RD. Chemical senses and nutrition. In: Getchell TV, et al., (Eds). *Smell and Taste in Health and Disease.* New York: Raven Press, 1991, p. 392.
44. Green RF. Subclinical pellagra and idiopathic hypogeusia. (Letter) *JAMA,* 1971; 218:8:1303.
45. Smith AD. Legaloblastic anemias. In: Williams WJ, Beutler E, Erslev AJ, Lichtman MA (Eds). *Hematology,* 3rd ed. New York: McGraw-Hill, 1983, pp. 434–465.
46. Smith DV, Seiden AM. Olfactory dysfunction. In: Laing DG, Doty RL, Briepohl W (Eds). *The Human Sense of Smell.* Chapter 14. New York: Springer-Verlag, 1995, pp. 298.

47. Schechter PJ, Friedewald WT, Bronzert DA, Raff MS, Henkin RI. Idiopathic hypogeusia: A description of the syndrome and a single blind study with zinc sulfate. *Int Rev Neurobiol Suppl,* 1972; 1:125–140.
48. Weismann K, Christensen E, Dreyer V. Zinc supplementation in alcoholic cirrhosis. *Acta Med Scand,* 1979; 205:361–366.
49. Public Health Service. *Report of the Panel on Communicative Disorders to the National Advisory Neurological and Communicative Disorders and Stroke Council.* (NIH Publication No. 79-1914). Washington, DC: National Institute of Health, 1979, p. 319.
50. Ackerman BH, Kasbekar N. Disturbances of taste and smell induced by drugs. *Pharmacotherapy,* 1997; 17:482–496.
51. Bates B. *Guide to Physical Examination.* Philadelphia: JB Lippincott, 1974, p. 272.
52. Haerer AF. *DeJong's The Neurological Examination.* 5th Ed. Philadelphia: Lippincott, 1992, p. 89.
53. Parsons M. *Color Atlas of Clinical Neurology.* Chicago: Year Book Medical, 1983, p. 18.
54. Fuller G. *Neurological Examination Made Easy.* Edinburgh, Scotland: Churchille Livingstone, 1993, p. 47.
55. Post F. Dementia, depression, and pseudodementia. In: Benson DV, Blumer D (Eds). *Psychiatric Aspects of Neurologic Disease.* New York: Grune and Stratton, 1975, pp. 99–120.
56. Solomon GS, Petrie WM, Hart JR, Brackin, Jr. HB. Olfactory dysfunction discriminates Alzheimer's dementia from major depression. *J Neuropsychiat Clin Neurosci,* 1998; 10:1:64–67.
57. Doty RL, Singh A, Tetrude J, Langston JW. Lack of olfactory dysfunction in MPTP-induced Parkinsonism. *Ann Neurol,* 1992; 32:97–100.
58. Sajjadian A, Doty RL, Gutnick DN, Chirurgi RJ, Sivak M, Perl D. Olfactory dysfunction in amyotrophic lateral sclerosis. *Neurodegeneracy,* 1994; 3:153–157.
59. Busenbark KL, Huber ST, Greer G, Pahwa R, Koller WC. Olfactory function in essential tremor. *Neurology,* 1992; 42:1631–1632.
60. Hirsch AR. Olfaction in migraineurs. *Headache,* 1992; 32:233–236.
61. Loury MC, Kennedy DN. Chronic sinusitis and nasal polyposis. In: Getchell TV, et al (Eds). *Smell and Taste in Health and Disease.* New York: Raven, 1991, pp. 517–528.
62. Hirsch AR, Thakkar N. Olfaction in a patient with unclassifiable cluster headache-like disorder. *Headache Quart,* 1995; 6:113–122.
63. Hirsch AR. Neurotoxicity as a result of ambient chemicals: Denham Springs, La. *International Congress on Hazardous Waste: Impact on Human and Ecological Health.* U.S. Department of Health and Human Services. Atlanta: Public Health Agency for Toxic Substances and Disease Registry, 1995, p. 229.
64. Jafek BW, Hill DP. Surgical management of chemosensory disorders. *ENTJ,* 1989; 66:398–404.
65. Hirsch AR, Trannel TH. Chemosensory disorders and psychiatric diagnoses. *J Neurol Ortho Med Surg,* 1996; 17:25–30.
66. Hirsch AR. Concurrence of chemosensory and sexual dysfunction. *Bio Psychiat,* 1998; 43:52S.
67. Davidson TM, Jalowayski A, Murphy C, Jacobs RJ. Evaluation and treatment of smell dysfunction. *West J Med,* 1987; 146:434–438.
68. Scott AE, Cain WS, Leonard G. Nasal/sinus disease and olfactory loss at the Connecticut Chemosensory Clinical Research Center. *Chem Senses,* 1989; 14:745.
69. Scott AE, Cain WS, Clavet G. Topical corticosteroids can alleviate olfactory dysfunction. *Chem Senses,* 1988; 13:735.
70. Chalke HD, Dewhurst JR. Accidental coal-gas poisoning. *Brit Med J,* 1957; 2:915–917.
71. Costanzo RM, Zasler ND. Head trauma. In: Getchell TV, et al. (Eds). *Smell and Taste in Health and Disease.* New York: Raven, 1991, pp. 711–730.
72. Hirsch AR, Gotway MB. Validation of the Chicago Smell Test (CST) in subjective normosmic neurologic patients. *Chem Senses,* 1993; 18:570–571.
73. Hirsch AR, Gotway MB, Harris AT. Validation of the Chicago Smell Test (CST) in patients with subjective olfactory loss. *Chem Senses,* 1993; 18:571.
74. Doty RL. *Smell Identification Test Administration Manual.* Hadden Heights, NY: Sensonics, 1995.
75. Amoore JE, Ollman BG. Practical test kits for quantitatively evaluating sense of smell. *Rhinol,* 1983; 21:49–54.
76. Davidson TM, Murphy C. Rapid clinical evaluation of anosmia: The alcohol sniff test. *Arch Otolaryngol Head Neck Surg,* 1997; 123:591–594.
77. Schlotfeld CR, Geisler MW, Davidson TM, Murphy C. Clinical application of the alcohol sniff test on HIV positive and HIV negative patients with nasal sinus disease. *Chem Senses,* 1998; 23:610.

78. Middleton CB, Geisler MW, Davidson TM, Murphy C. Relationship between the alcohol sniff test and sensory olfactory event-related potentials: Validation of a psychophysical test. *Chem Senses*, 1998; 23:610.

79. Freed CL, Dalve-Endres AM, Davidson TM, Murphy C. Rapid screening of olfactory function in Down's syndrome. *Chem Senses,* 1998; 23:610.

80. Nordin S, Monsoh AU, Murphy C. Unawareness of smell loss in normal aging and Alzheimer's disease: Discrepancy between self-reporting and diagnosed smell sensitivity. *J Gerentol,* 1995; 50:187–192.

81. Adams RG, Crabtree N. Anosmia in alkaline battery workers. *Br J Industr Med,* 1961; 18:216–221.

82. Hirsch AR. Smell and taste: How the culinary experts compare to the rest of us. *Food Technol,* 1987; 23:198–204.

83. Venstrom D, Amoore JE. Olfactory threshold in relation to age, sex, or smoking. *J Food Sci,* 1968; 33:264–265.

84. Vital Durand M. Recurrent anosmia under beta-blockers. *Presse Med,* 1985; 14:2064.

85. Levinsons JL, Kennedy K. Dysosmia, dysgeusia, and nifedipine. [Letter] *Ann Intern Med,* 1985; 102:135–136.

86. Solomon GS. Anosmia in Alzheimer's disease. *Percept Mot Skills,* 1994; 79:1249–1250.

87. Hirsch AR. Olfactory dysfunction as a symptom in various conditions. *J Neurol Orthop Med Surg,* 1992; 13:298–302.

88. Hirsch AR, Cleveland LB. Olfaction and chronic spinal cord injury. *J Neuro Rehab,* 1998; 12:101–104.

89. Van Damme PA, Freihofer HP. Disturbances of smell and taste after high central midface fractures. *J Craniomaxillofac Surg,* 1992; 20:248–250.

90. Duncan HJ, Seiden AM. Long-term follow-up of olfactory loss secondary to head trauma and upper respiratory tract infection. *Arch Otolaryngol Head Neck Surg,* 1995; 121:1183–1187.

91. Hawkes CM. Diagnosis and treatment of Parkinson's disease: Anosmia is a common finding. *BMJ,* 1995; 310:447–452.

92. Pearce RK, Hawkes CH, Daniel SE. Anterior olfactory nucleus in Parkinson's disease. *Mov Disord,* 1995; 10:283–287.

93. Doty RL, Li C, Mannon L, Yousem DG. Olfactory dysfunction in multiple sclerosis. *N Eng J Med,* 1997; 336;1918–1919.

94. Adams R, Victor M. *Principles of Neurology.* New York: McGraw-Hill, 1989, pp. 482–496.

95. Gent JP, Cain WS, Bartoshuk LM. Taste and smell management in a clinical setting. In: Meiselman HL, Rivlin RS (Eds). *Clinical Measurement of Taste and Smell.* New York: Macmillan, 1986, pp. 107–111.

96. Doty RL, Newhouse MG, Azzalina JD. Internal consistency and short-term test-retest reliability of the University of Pennsylvania Smell Identification Test. *Chem Sen,* 1985; 10:297–300.

97. Bakay L, Cares HL. Olfactory meningiomas. *Acta Neurochirurgia Fasc,* 1973; 26:1–12.

98. Davidson TM, Freed C, Healy MP, Murphy C. Rapid clinical evaluation of anosmia in children: The Alcohol Sniff Test. *Ann NY Acad Sci,* 1998; 855:787–792.

99. Doty RL, Shaman P, Applebaum SL, Gilberson R, Sikorsky L, Rosenberg L. Smell identification ability: Changes with age. *Science,* 1984; 226:1441–1443.

100. Serby M. Olfaction and neuropsychiatry [Abstr.]. Distributed at Dr. Serby's lecture at the Institute for Research and Behavioral Neurosciences, New York, December 12, 1987.

101. Adams RB. *Principles of Neurology.* New York: McGraw-Hill, 1989, p. 927.

102. Wurtman RJ. Sources of choline and lecithin in the diet. In: Barbeau JH, Growden JH, Wurtman RJ (Eds). *Nutrition and the Brain, Vol. 5.* New York: Raven Press, 1979, pp. 73–81.

103. Wurtman RJ, Hefti F, Melamed E. Precusor control of neurotransmitter synthesis. *Pharmacol Rev,* 1981; 32:315–335.

104. Jackson IV, Nuttal EA, Ibe IO, et al. Treatment of tardive dyskinesia with lecithin. *Am J Psychiat,* 1979; 136:1458–1460.

105. Little A, Levy R, Chuaqui-Kidd P, et al. Double blind placebo control trial of high dose lecithin in Alzheimer's disease. *J Neurol Nursury Psychiat,* 1985; 48:736–742.

106. Hirsch AR, Dougherty DD, Aranda JG, Vanderbilt JG, Weclaw GC. Medications for olfactory loss: Pilot studies. *J Neurol Orthop Med Surg,* 1996; 17:108–114.

107. Hirsch AR, Baker J. Lack of efficacy of thiamine treatment for chemosensory disorder. *J Psychiat Clin Neurosci,* 2001; 13:1:151.

108. Duncan RB, Briggs M. Treatment of uncomplicated anosmia by vitamin A. *Arch Otolaryngol,* 1962; 75:116–124.

109. Roydhouse N. Retinoid therapy and anosmia. *New Zealand Med J,* 1988; 101:465.

110. Garrett-Laster M, Russell RM, Jacques PF. Impairment of taste and olfaction in patients with cirrhosis: The role of vitamin A. *Human Nutr,* 1984; 38C:203–214.

111. Schiffman SS, Diaz C, Beeker TG. Caffeine intensifies taste of certain sweeteners: Role of adenosine receptor. *Pharm Biochem Behav*, 1986; 24:429–432.

112. DeMet E, Stein MK, Tran C, Chicz-DeMet A, Sangdahl C, Nelson J. Caffeine taste test for panic disorder: Adenosine receptor supersensitivity. *Psychiatr Res,* 1989; 30:231–242.

113. Henkin RI, Keiser HR, Jaffee IA, Sternlieb I, Scheinberg IH. Decreased taste sensitivity after D-penicillamine reversed by copper administration. *Lancet,* 1967; 2:1268–1271.

114. Henkin RI, Bradley DF. Regulation of taste acuity by thiols and metal ions. *Proc Natl Acad Sci, USA,* 1969; 62:30–37.

115. Henkin RI, Schechter PJ, Friedewald WT, Demets DL, Raff M. A double blind study of the effects of zinc sulfate on taste and smell dysfunction. *Am J Med Sci,* 1976; 272:285–299.

116. Deems DA, Doty RL, Settle RG, Moore-Gillon V, Shaman P, Mester AF, Kimmelman CP, Brightman VJ, Snow Jr., JB. Smell and taste disorders. A study of 750 patients from the University of Pennsylvania Smell and Taste Center. *Arch Otolaryngol Head Neck Surg,* 1991; 117:519–528.

117. Fosmire GJ. Zinc toxicity. *Am J Clin Nutr,* 1990; 51:225–227.

118. Hirsch AR. Unpublished.

119. Markley EJ, Mattes-Kulig DA, Henkin RI. A classification of dysgeusia. *J Am Dietet Assoc,* 1983; 83:578–580.

120. Casper RC, Kirschner B, Sandstead HH, Jacob RA, Davis JM. An evaluation of trace metals, vitamins, and taste function in anorexia nervosa. *Am J Clin Nutr,* 1980; 33:1801–1808.

121. Lacey JH, Stanley PA, Crutchfield SM. Sucrose sensitivity in anorexia nervosa. *J Psychosom Res,* 1977; 21:17–21.

122. Sunday SR, Halmi KA. Taste perceptions and hedonics in eating disorders. *Psychol Behav,* 1990; 48:587–594.

123. Mela DJ. Sensory assessment of fat content in fluid dairy products. *Appetite,* 1988; 10:37–44.

124. Grinker J. Obesity and sweet taste. *Am J Clin Nutr,* 1978; 31:1078–1087.

125. Drewnowski A. Sweetness and obesity. In: Dobbing J (Ed). *Sweetness.* New York: Springer-Verlag, 1987, pp. 177–201.

126. Fritjers JER, Rasmussen-Conrad EL. Sensory discrimination, intensity perception, affective judgment of sucrose-sweetness in the overweight. *J Gen Psychol,* 1982; 107:233–247.

127. Witherly SA, Pangborn RM, Stern JS. Gustatory responses and eating duration of obese and lean adults. *Appetite,* 1980; 1:53–63.

128. Rodin J, Moskowitz HR, Bray GA. Relationship between obesity, weight loss, and taste responsiveness. *Physiol Behav,* 1976; 17:591–597.

129. Spitzer L, Rodin J. Human eating behavior: A critical review of studies in normal weight and overweight individuals. *Appetite,* 1981; 2:293–329.

130. Drewnowski A. Fat and sugar: Sensory and hedonic aspects of sweet, high-fat foods. In Friedman MI, Tordoff MG, Kare MR (Eds). *Chemical Senses: Appetite and Nutrition.* New York: Marcel Dekker, 1991, pp. 69–83.

131. Pangborn RM, Bos KEO, Stern J. Dietary fat intake and taste responses to fat in milk by under-, normal, and overweight women. *Appetite,* 1985; 6:25–40.

132. Warwick ZS, Schiffman SS, Anderson JJB. Relationship of dietary fat content to preferences in young rats. *Physiol Behav,* 1990; 48:581–586.

133. Hirsch AR, Gomez R. Weight reduction through inhalation of odorants. *J Neurol Orthop Med Surg,* 1995; 16:28–31.

134. Hirsch AR, Gallant-Shean M. Use of tastants to facilitate weight loss. *Chem Sen,* 2003; 28:A124.

135. Doty RJ, Applebaum SL, Zusho H, et al. A cross-cultural study of sex differences in odor identification ability. *Neurophysiological,* 1985; 8:667–672.

Section II

Cardiovascular and Pulmonary Diseases

4 Dyslipidemia and Atherosclerosis

Douglas W. Triffon, M.D., and Erminia M. Guarneri, M.D.

I. INTRODUCTION

The prevention of cardiovascular disease requires a global approach to risk factor reduction. The benefit of targeting multiple risk factors has been reported in several recent trials [1, 2]. A 50% reduction in cardiovascular events can be achieved in diabetic patients with concomitant treatment of hypertension, hyperlipidemia, elevated glucose, smoking, excess weight, poor diet, and lack of exercise [2]. The additive effects of nutrient supplementation on top of standard therapy have been the focus of several recent trials [3, 4]. Omega-3 oils can decrease cardiovascular events when added to usual therapy post–myocardial infarction. A meta-analysis of folate therapy trials reveals a significant reduction of stroke by 18% [5]. Vitamin D deficiency may increase cardiovascular risk factors and cardiac disease. Nutrient supplementation should be considered as part of a global strategy to lower cardiovascular risk.

II. EPIDEMIOLOGY

Atherosclerosis has become one of the major progressive lifelong diseases in the modern era, affecting the lives of one out of two men, and one out of three women. In the United States, 13 million people have a history of coronary heart disease. Each year, 1.2 million new cases of myocardial infarction or fatal coronary heart disease occur. Coronary heart disease is the leading cause of death in the United States, accounting for 37% of deaths in men and 41% of deaths in women. The disease starts silently in adolescence and slowly progresses throughout life. It results in clinical events usually after 55 years of age in men and after 65 years of age in women. Events occur earlier in life in those with clustering of multiple risk factors such as cigarette smoking, diabetes, low high density lipoprotein (HDL), elevated lipoprotein(a), small dense low density lipoprotein (LDL), and recently recognized genetic polymorphisms.

III. PATIENT EVALUATION

OVERALL RISK ASSESSMENT

Modern lifestyles contribute to the development of vascular disease through job stress, lack of time to exercise, and diets high in fat and refined carbohydrates and low in fruits and vegetables. The Interheart Study defined the relative risks for acute myocardial infarction of various cardiovascular risk factors in a population of 29,972 subjects from 52 different countries [6]. Nine risk factors were found to account for 90% of the population's attributable risk in men and 94% of the risk in women (see Table 4.1).

TABLE 4.1
Results of the Interheart Study

Cardiovascular Risk Factor	Relative Risk	Percent Attributable Risk
Smoking	2.87	35.7%
Elevated Apolipoprotein B/Apolipoprotein A1	3.25	49.2%
Hypertension	1.91	17.9%
Diabetes	2.37	9.9%
Abdominal obesity	1.12	20.1%
Psychosocial factors	2.67	32.5%
Daily consumption of fruit and vegetables	0.7	13.7%
Regular alcohol consumption (>=3/week)	0.91	6.7%
Regular physical activity	0.86	12.2%

Smoking and raised Apolipoprotein B to Apolipoprotein A1 ratio were the strongest risk factors for acute myocardial infarction. Avoiding smoking, and eating a diet low in fat and high in fruits and vegetables, together with regular physical exercise, would reduce the risk of myocardial infarction by 75%.

The results of the Interheart Study revealed that hyperlipidemia was the most important risk factor overall in terms of population attributable risk of 49.2%. Results underscore the importance of controlling the risk of elevated lipids in clinical practice. Our current guideline framework for cholesterol treatment is based on estimated short-term risk of cardiovascular disease, which could have an undesirable consequence. It may encourage the delay in treatment of a lifelong disease and may not make the practitioner truly aware of the high lifetime risk of many of the patients in his or her practice. One-third of patients who sustain a heart attack each year are in the low-risk group, according to the Framingham 10-year risk. A second third of heart attacks each year occur in the intermediate risk group. The risk of the heart attacks was missed by the traditional Framingham risk score and the opportunity to prevent the cardiovascular event was also missed. Lifetime risk of cardiovascular disease is another time frame to assess and enter into treatment decisions. The lifetime risk of cardiovascular disease has been studied in 7926 subjects from the Framingham Heart Study who were 50 years of age and were free of cardiac disease [7]. The results indicate that more than 50% of men and 40% of women will develop cardiovascular disease during their life. The presence of diabetes confers the highest lifetime risk of heart disease of 67%, which underscores its place in the Adult Treatment Panel (ATP) III guidelines as a coronary equivalent risk factor (see Table 4.2). Cholesterol of more than 240 mg/dL at age 50 years confers in men a 65% lifetime risk of cardiovascular disease. The same total cholesterol of greater than 240 mg/dL confers a lifetime risk of cardiovascular disease of 48% in a woman. An elevated blood pressure between 140 to 159 mmHg systolic and 90 to 99 mmHg diastolic confers a lifetime risk of cardiovascular disease of 62% in men and 52% in women. The total cholesterol and blood pressure elevations studied are common in clinical practice and carry a higher long-term risk that the physician or patient often

TABLE 4.2
Lifetime Risk of Cardiovascular Disease

Risk Factor	Lifetime Risk Men	Lifetime Risk Women
Total cholesterol > 240 mg/dL	64.6%	48.3%
Blood pressure >140–159/90–99	61.6%	52.3%
Diabetes	67.1%	57.3%
Smoking	51.5%	39%
Obesity (BMI>30 kg/m^2)	58%	43%

does not appreciate. Optimizing risk factors can reduce the long-term risks to 5% in men and 8% in women and extend survival by 11 years in a man and by 8 years in a woman. The physician can assess the 10-year Framingham risk and the lifetime risk and treat any patient with a lifetime risk of greater than 40% as high risk.

LDL CHOLESTEROL

LDL cholesterol has been the main target of therapy in reducing the risks of hyperlipidemia. Multiple trials have substantiated the success of lowering LDL cholesterol in reducing cardiac events. A meta-analysis of 14 randomized trials including 90,056 participants reported a 12% relative reduction in total mortality over 5 years for every 40 mg/dL decrease in LDL cholesterol [8]. Yet, residual cardiovascular risk remains after treating to goal LDL cholesterol as revealed by multiple studies such as the 4S Trial, Lipid Trial, Care, Heart Protection Trial, West of Scotland Trial, and Afcaps/TEXcaps Trial. Seventy-five percent of cardiovascular events still are occurring in these trials of LDL reduction. More intensive LDL cholesterol lowering to 70 mg/dL leads to a further 16% relative reduction in events as seen in a pooled analysis of the Prove-IT, Ideal, and TNT Trials, but residual risk still remains. Possible causes of this residual risk appear in Table 4.3.

Residual risk may remain once LDL cholesterol is lowered if triglycerides remain elevated. A report from an analysis of 4849 middle-aged men followed for 8 years indicated that triglycerides were an independent risk factor for coronary heart disease at any level of LDL cholesterol [9]. A recent meta-analysis of 29 prospective studies, which assessed the independent risk of triglycerides in 262,525 participants, reported an adjusted odds ratio of 1.72 for the highest tertile of triglycerides versus the lowest tertile [10]. The Prove-IT Trial reported a lower composite endpoint of death, myocardial infarction (MI), and recurrent acute coronary syndrome with a triglyceride of less than 150 mg/dL independent of LDL [11]. Each 10 mg/dL lowering of triglycerides resulted in a 1.6% lower incidence of the composite endpoint. The lowest incidence of events occurred in the subgroup with an LDL less than 70 mg/dL, triglyceride less than 150 mg/dL, and an hsCRP less than 2 mg/L. Results underscore the need to treat beyond LDL in order to maximize risk reduction.

TABLE 4.3
Possible Causes of Residual Cardiovascular Risk at Goal LDL-C

Low HDL cholesterol
Lp(a)
Small dense LDL cholesterol
Elevated apo B or particle number LDL-P
Elevated trigylcerides
Remnant particles
Impaired fasting glucose
Hypertension
Inflammation
Elevated thrombotic risk factors
Metabolic syndrome
Phytosterol absorption
Genetic polymorphisms
Smoking
Postprandial lipemia
Lack of exercise
High fat diet
Diet low in fruit and vegetables
Stress
Chronic renal disease

TABLE 4.4
LDL and Non-HDL Cholesterol Treatment Goals

Risk Category	LDL-C Goal	Non-HDL-C Goal
High risk (CHD or CHD risk equivalent)	100 mg/dL optional goal 70 mg/dL	130 mg/dL optional goal 100 mg/dL
Moderate risk (10 yr risk < 20%)	130 mg/dL	160 mg/dL
Low risk (0–1 risk factors)	160 mg/dL	190 mg/dL

NON-HDL CHOLESTEROL

Non-HDL cholesterol is a helpful way to assess the combined risk of LDL cholesterol and triglycerides. Non-HDL cholesterol can be computed by subtracting the HDL from the total cholesterol and is more predictive of risk than LDL. The relative merits of LDL versus non-HDL cholesterol were compared in an analysis of 5794 subjects from the Framingham Study followed for 15 years [12]. An elevated non-HDL cholesterol increased the risk at any level of LDL, but LDL did not add to the risk prediction of non-HDL cholesterol. The superior risk prediction of non-HDL cholesterol was found in subjects with triglycerides under 200 mg/dL as well. The targets for non-HDL cholesterol are 30 mg/dL higher than the target for LDL. Both LDL and non-HDL cholesterol goals should be achieved to reduce residual risk (see Table 4.4).

APO B

Apo B has also been reported to be a better predictor of cardiac risk than LDL cholesterol and is an alternative to non-HDL cholesterol as a more comprehensive molecule to measure in clinical practice [12]. Apo B reflects the number of atherogenic particles in VLDL and LDL, while non-HDL represents the concentration of cholesterol carried in these particles. The Health Professionals Follow-up Study assessed the relative risk of apo B versus non-HDL in predicting nonfatal MI or coronary heart disease death in 6 years of follow-up [12]. The relative risk for apo B was 3.01 versus 2.76 for non-HDL and 1.81 for LDL. Both apo B and non-HDL cholesterol were stronger predictors of risk than LDL, though particle number, as reflected in apo B, was more predictive than the cholesterol content carried in these particles. Whether apo B should be incorporated into the guidelines remains controversial. It would add cost, but can be measured nonfasting. Non-HDL would not increase costs and also can be measured nonfasting.

Residual cardiovascular risk is also associated with low HDL even on statin treatment. Thirty-five percent of adult men have HDL less than 40 mg/dL, and 39% of adult women have an HDL less than 50 mg/dl. For every decrease in HDL of 1 mg/dL, the risk of coronary heart disease increases 2% to 3% [13]. The TNT Trial reported the predictive value of HDL in 9770 patients with coronary heart disease [14]. HDL was found to be predictive of cardiovascular events in these statin-treated patients, even in patients with LDL less than 70 mg/dL. Similar data have been reported from the 4S, Care, and Lipid trials [13]. Low HDL continues to predict increased risk despite statin treatment and very low LDL levels. Whether raising HDL in statin-treated patients decreases clinical events is the subject of the ongoing AIM-HIGH Trial. This trial will test the effect of extended release niacin and simvastatin versus simvastatin alone on cardiovascular outcomes.

LP(A)

Another risk factor that may increase risks beyond LDL is Lp(a). Lp(a) was reported to be an independent predictor of cardiovascular risk in the Procam Study. A total of 4849 men were followed for 8 years and the primary endpoint was nonfatal MI and cardiovascular death. The relative risk for Lp(a) was found to be 5.3 versus 4.3 for LDL. The Framingham Offspring Study reported the risk of coronary heart disease from Lp(a) in 2919 men followed for 15.4 years [17]. Elevated Lp(a) was an independent risk factor for coronary heart disease and was similar in magnitude to a total cholesterol of 240 mg/dL or an HDL below 35 mg/dL.

Lp(a) may carry the majority of oxidized phospholipids found on apo B. Tsimikas et al. reported from a 10-year analysis of the Bruneck Study that there was no difference in the risk prediction of cardiovascular disease between plasma levels of oxidized phospholipids on apo B and Lp(a) levels [19]. Both predicted future events independent of traditional risk factors. The risk of Lp(a) was increased by higher levels of Lp-PLA2 activity. Lp-PLA2 further oxidizes phospholipids on Lp(a) and hence may amplify its risk. An elevated Lp(a) in the presence of an elevated Lp-PLA2 can increase risk up to 3.5-fold. Patients who have elevation of both factors may be at much higher risk than the LDL itself might predict because of this synergistic effect on oxidized phospholipids. Lp-PLA2 is a lipoprotein-bound phospholipase that is secreted by monocytes and macrophages. Eighty percent is bound to LDL and 20% is bound to HDL and VLDL. Lp-PLA2 binds to apo B on LDL and preferentially binds to small dense LDL. Lp-PLA2 generates two proinflammatory lipid mediators, lysophosphatidylcholine and oxidized nonesterified fatty acids. A meta-analysis of 14 studies of Lp-PLA2 involving 20,549 subjects revealed that Lp-PLA2 was an independent predictor of cardiovascular disease with a relative risk of 1.6 [20]. Lp-PLA2 is additive to the risk prediction of high-sensitivity CRP (hsCRP) in patients with LDL less than 130 mg/dL [18]. Lp-PLA2 levels do not correlate with levels of hsCRP.

HsCRP

HsCRP is an acute phase reactant and has a higher variability than other lipid risk factors. Two separate measurements of hsCRP averaged, and optimally 2 weeks apart, are adequate to determine a person's risk. If a value of hsCRP of over 10 mg/L is found, then a search for intercurrent infection or inflammation should occur and the value should be disregarded and repeated in 2 weeks. Low-risk hsCRP is 1.0 mg/L; average risk is 1.0 to 3.0 mg/L; and high risk is greater than 3.0 mg/L. The high-risk hsCRP has a two-fold increase in relative risk. Clinical events are reduced more effectively when both LDL and hsCRP are lowered. The effects of statins on lowering hsCRP are independent of their effects on lowering LDL. Data from the Prove-IT Trial revealed that the lowest risk of recurrent myocardial infarction or death from coronary causes among 3745 patients with acute coronary syndromes occurred when both an LDL level of less than 70 mg/dL and an hsCRP of less than 2 mg/L were achieved [22]. The risk of recurrent events of an hsCRP of greater than 2 mg/L was similar to the risk of LDL cholesterol of greater than 70 mg/dL. Similar data have been reported from the Afcaps/TEXcaps Trial.

Lipid Ratios

In general, lipid ratios are more predictive of cardiovascular risk than individual lipid values [23]. Whether apo B/apo A-1 ratios are superior to TC/HDL ratios is controversial in the literature. Both the Interheart Study and Afcaps/TEXcaps Trial reported that the apo B/apo A-1 ratio was the best lipid predictor of risk. The EPIC-Norfolk Study did not find any improvement in the risk prediction of cardiovascular events in a primary prevention population of apo B/apo A-1 versus TC/HDL ratio [24]. The EPIC-Norfolk Study included very few diabetics and excluded statin-treated subjects. Both of these groups have less risk prediction by cholesterol content versus particle number. Nevertheless, a more global assessment of risk would incorporate one of these ratios along with a measure of inflammation. Ridker showed that adding hsCRP to TC/HDL ratios does significantly improve risk prediction [23]. Lp(a) may independently predict risk and may be especially useful when there is a strong family history of premature heart disease. Apo B/apo A-1 ratio combined with hsCRP and Lp(a) may comprise a global lipid target that may help to better assess the residual risk in patients that is missed by lowering only LDL.

HOMOCYSTEINE

McCully first described homocysteine as a vascular disease risk factor in 1969 [25]. He reported the autopsy findings from children who died of homocysteinuria and hypothesized that elevated homocysteine levels may be linked to atherosclerosis. Homocysteine is an intermediate metabolite in the metabolism of the amino acid methionine to cysteine. There are two enzyme systems that are important in this conversion, methylenetetrahydrofolate reductase and cystathionine beta-synthase. Folate, B6, and B12 are cofactors that are needed for proper function of these enzymes. Homocysteine increases thrombogenicity of the blood, damages the endothelium, and increases oxidation.

Several epidemiologic studies have established a correlation between homocysteine levels and cardiovascular mortality [26, 27]. A meta-analysis of 30 studies confirmed an independent relationship between homocysteine and ischemic heart disease and stroke [28]. Two prospective treatment trials of homocysteine have had mixed results. The NORVIT Study investigated the effect of homocysteine lowering in 3749 men with recent MI. Subjects were randomized to one of four treatments: the combination of 800 μg of folic acid, 400 μg of B12, and 40 mg of B6; or 800 μg of folic acid with 400 μg of B12; or 40 mg of B6 alone; or placebo. Homocysteine levels were lowered by 27% in both groups that were treated with combinations that contained folic acid and B12. Folate levels increased by five- to six-fold, and B12 levels increased 60% in the combination therapy groups. There was no decrease in homocysteine in the group treated with B6 alone. The primary endpoint of the trial was a composite of fatal and nonfatal MI, fatal and nonfatal stroke, and sudden cardiac death. There was no benefit of any of the treatment regimens on the incidence of the primary outcome. There was a trend toward an increase of events in the combination therapy group that contained folic acid, B12, and B6 (relative risk, 1.22; 95% confidence interval, 1.00 to 1.50; P = 0.05).

The HOPE 2 Trial studied 5522 patients with cardiovascular disease or diabetes. Treatment was randomized between a combination of 2.5 mg folic acid, 1 mg of B12, and 50 mg of B6, or placebo. There was no significant difference in the combined endpoint of death from cardiovascular causes, MI, and stroke between the folic acid, B12, and B6 vitamin group and the placebo group. There was a 25% reduction of stroke in the vitamin-treated group. A meta-analysis of eight homocysteine treatment trials reported that folic acid supplementation reduced the risk of stroke by 18%. A beneficial effect was more likely with treatment for more than 36 months, a homocysteine lowering of more than 20%, and no prior history of stroke. Homocysteine lowering may have a greater effect on the reduction of stroke than of coronary disease. A 3 μmol/L reduction of homocysteine is associated with an 11% reduction in coronary disease and a 19% reduction in stroke.

Present evidence does not support using folic acid, B12, and B6 vitamin supplementation post-MI, or post-stent, or in patients with known cardiovascular disease. The major vascular outcome to show benefit from supplementation with folate, B vitamins in general, and lowering homocysteine is the primary prevention of stroke. Elevated homocysteine levels have been associated with an increased risk for the development of dementia and Alzheimer disease. To date, no placebo-controlled treatment trials have been completed to determine the value of folic acid, B12, and B6 vitamin supplementation to prevent dementia and Alzheimer's disease.

VITAMIN D

Vitamin D may be an important nutrient in the prevention of cardiovascular disease. It affects inflammation, vascular calcification, renin activity, and blood pressure; prevents proliferation of vascular smooth muscle cells; and increases anti-inflammatory cytokines. Vitamin D receptors are found in cardiac tissues such as blood vessels and cardiac muscle cells. Vitamin D deficiency stimulates the release of parathyroid hormone, which leads to myocardial hypertrophy and also increases inflammation via release of cytokines from vascular smooth muscle cells. Vitamin D levels have been found to vary inversely with the amount of vascular calcification [29]. An increase in vascular calcification, as determined by a coronary calcium score, has been shown to be an independent predictor of cardiovascular risk [30].

The majority of vitamin D is cutaneously synthesized, with only a few good food sources such as eel, herring, and salmon. Vitamin D deficiency results from inadequate sun exposure, pigmented skin, or low dietary intake. The best measure of vitamin D status is a 25-hydroxyvitamin D level. 1,25-dihydroxyvitamin D levels are not the best measure of vitamin D status since they have a short half life in the blood, and often are increased in early stage vitamin D deficiency to compensate for a drop in 25-hydroxyvitamin D levels. Vitamin D deficiency is present in one-third to one-half of middle-aged or older adults worldwide. Data from the Framingham Offspring Study report a 28% incidence of low 25-hydroxyvitamin D levels, defined as below 15 ng/mL [31]. The low vitamin D level was associated with a 63% increase in cardiovascular events over a 5.4 year follow-up period.

A meta-analysis of 18 randomized controlled trials of vitamin D supplementation in 57,311 subjects revealed a 7% reduction in total mortality [32]. The average dose of vitamin D used in these trials was 528 IU. It appears that the administration of very common doses of vitamin D can reduce total mortality. Prospective, randomized trials of vitamin D supplementation are needed to assess the long-term effects of vitamin D on cardiovascular morbidity and mortality. One should consider measuring a vitamin D level as part of a yearly physical since a low level is also associated with increased incidence of colon cancer, prostate cancer, multiple sclerosis, rheumatoid arthritis, and type 1 diabetes mellitus.

Omega-3 Fats

Omega-3 oils may have cardioprotective properties by decreasing atherosclerosis, inflammation, thrombosis, and arrhythmias. Fish oil supplementation has been studied in 11,324 survivors of MI in the GISSI Prevenzione Study [33]. One gram of fish oil was found to reduce the primary endpoint of death, MI, or stroke by 10%. There was a 14% reduction in death and a 17% reduction in cardiovascular death. There was a 54% reduction in sudden death. This benefit was on top of standard post-MI care including beta-blockers, statins, aspirin, and ACE-inhibitors. The JELIS Study also reported a 19% reduction in major coronary events in 18,645 subjects randomized to eicosapentaenoic acid plus statin versus statin alone [34]. Fish oil can reduce cardiovascular events in addition to that achieved by statin therapy.

Vitamin E

The Nurses Health Study, which was observational in design, concluded a 34% reduction in cardiovascular events in subjects taking vitamin E supplementation [35]. Since that initial observation, multiple studies have attempted to evaluate vitamin E in the primary and secondary prevention of cardiovascular disease. In the primary prevention project, 4495 patients were followed for 3.6 years on 300 IU of vitamin E supplementation without demonstrating improvement in cardiovascular morbidity [36]. Multiple secondary prevention studies including HOPE [37] and GISSI-P [33] failed to demonstrate benefit from vitamin E supplementation. The HDL-Atherosclerosis Treatment Study (HATS) compared treatment regimens of lipid-modifying therapy and antioxidant-vitamin therapy, alone and together [38]. The 3-year, double-blind trial included 160 patients with coronary disease, low levels of HDL cholesterol, and normal levels of LDL cholesterol. Patients were assigned to one of four treatment regimens: simvastatin (10 to 20 mg/day) plus niacin (2 to 4 g/day); antioxidants; simvastatin (10 to 20 mg/day) plus niacin (2 to 4 g/day) plus antioxidants; or placebo. The primary endpoints were arteriographic evidence of change in coronary stenosis and the occurrence of a first cardiovascular event (fatal/nonfatal MI, stroke, or revascularization). The average stenosis progressed with placebo (3.9%), antioxidants (1.8%), and simvastatin plus niacin plus antioxidants (0.7%). There was a 0.4% regression with simvastatin plus niacin alone (p < 0.001). In conclusion, the combination of simvastatin plus niacin greatly reduced the rate of major coronary events (60% to 90%) and substantially slowed progression of coronary atherosclerosis in patients with low HDL cholesterol. While HATS further supported the use of niacin for raising HDL and reducing plaque formation in combination with statin therapy, no further advantage was seen in the group receiving antioxidants and combination statin-niacin therapy. These studies did not attempt to assess the inflammatory and oxidative state of subjects prior to initiation and following therapy.

In a randomized, double-blind placebo control trial, subjects were given 1600 IU of RRR-alpha-tocopherol versus placebo and followed for 6 months [39]. Subjects taking the vitamin E had a statistically significant reduction in hsCRP and urinary F2 isoprostanes and monocyte superoxide anion and tumor necrosis factor release compared with baseline and placebo. Despite this reduction in oxidative and inflammatory markers, no change was seen in carotid intima medial thickness. Multiple trial design concerns have been raised to explain the inconsistency of the observational and randomized study data [40]. These include (1) not using the right type of supplement formulation, (2) not using the correct dosage, (3) not using a complex antioxidant mixture, (4) not choosing the right study population, and (5) not looking at functional biomarkers. One of the important variables missing from all of these studies is nutritional status. Until biomarkers and nutritional status are included with these research variables, it is premature to conclude that antioxidants offer no benefit in cardiovascular disease prevention.

IV. DRUG–NUTRIENT INTERACTIONS

The treatment of hyperlipidemia with statins may decrease mitochondrial levels of coenzyme Q10 and increase the incidence of myalgias. Coenzyme Q10 is an important nutrient for proper mitochondrial function. The benefits of coenzyme Q10 administration in statin-treated patients are controversial. A small randomized trial of supplementation with coenzyme Q10 in statin-treated patients did not reveal any benefit in the prevention of myalgia symptoms [41]. Another small trial reported that supplementation with coenzyme Q10 did reduce myalgia symptoms by 40% [42]. Larger trials are needed to clarify the benefit of coenzyme Q10 in the prevention or treatment of statin-induced myalgias.

Both niacin (also known as vitamin B3) and fibrates can increase homocysteine levels by up to 50% [43]. The mechanism of the elevation of homocysteine is an interference with the metabolism of folate and homocysteine by niacin and fibrates. The elevation in homocysteine can be prevented by folate, B12, and B6 supplementation. The benefit of B vitamin supplementation beyond doses to normalize serum levels to improve cardiovascular outcomes needs further study. Physical exam findings, laboratory evidence, and known risk factors such as gastric hypochlorhydria and gastric bypass surgery can suggest that folate, B12, or B6 should be supplemented for reasons apart from cardiovascular health.

V. COMORBID CONDITIONS

Although genetics account for approximately 20% of cardiovascular risk, 70% to 90% of chronic disease is related to an individual's lifestyle and environment. CDC data from 2006 reported that 29 states in America have greater than 25% of their population meeting the definition of obesity defined as body mass index (BMI) greater than or equal to 30. This epidemic of obesity is associated with diabetes mellitus, hypertension, low HDL cholesterol, elevated LDL cholesterol, and inflammation. The CDC predicts that one out of three children born in the year 2000 will develop diabetes in their lifetime and it is estimated that approximately 50% of American adults between the ages of 60 and 69 already have the metabolic syndrome [44]. The causes of cardiovascular disease are multifactorial and treatment frequently requires lifestyle change. Almost all cardiac risk factors are dependent on lifestyle and environment. As medicine has become increasingly dependent on the pharmaceutical industry, the focus has shifted from treating the whole person to a disease-driven model focused mainly on the presenting problem. Prevention is the best intervention for cardiovascular disease, yet in a recent survey of primary care physicians and cardiologists, discussions of lifestyle including nutrition, exercise, and psychosocial stressors continues to be poorly addressed [45]. Poor nutrition and physical inactivity are identified as probably the true leading underlying causes of death in the United States [46]. Increasing BMI has been linked to diabetes mellitus, hyperlipidemia, and hypertension in a linear fashion. Inversely, as the BMI is lowered, improvement is appreciated in all risk factors in the same linear fashion. Multiple avenues of research have shown lifestyle intervention alone can alter the course of disease. For example, in the Diabetes Prevention Study, type 2 diabetes was prevented in high-risk individuals who underwent individualized counseling on weight loss and physical activity alone when compared to appropriately matched controls and patients taking metformin alone [47].

VI. DIET CONSIDERATIONS

An initial approach to a patient's nutrition should simply start with total caloric consumption, which is a crucial variable affecting obesity. The Department of Agriculture reports an 8% increase in food consumption from 1990 to 2000, and the CDC reports that the doubling of the prevalence of obesity between 1971 and 2000 correlated with a 22% increase in calorie consumption for women and a 9% increase for men [48]. Interestingly, despite indications that the percentage of calories consumed as fat is decreasing, surveys indicate that we are consuming more calories overall [49]. Reduction in total caloric intake should be emphasized as a first-line approach to weight loss.

Fats and carbohydrates are the major macronutrients affecting cardiovascular health. Fats are broken down into saturated, monounsaturated, and polyunsaturated fatty acids. Saturated fatty acids contain no double bonds in their fatty acid chains and they are typically solid at room temperature. They are the predominant fats in dairy products, red meat, and tropical oils, such as coconut oil. Saturated fats increase total and LDL cholesterol as well as inflammation. Overall, the intake of saturated fat is associated with an increase in the incidence of cardiovascular disease [50]. However, the Nurse's Health Study showed that when you simply replace saturated fat intake with carbohydrate intake there is a very small reduction in cardiovascular risk. In contrast, replacement of saturated fat with monounsaturated or polyunsaturated fats was associated with an almost 10-fold greater decrease in risk [51].

Monounsaturated fats have been associated with lower cardiovascular disease (CVD) risk. Foods rich in monounsaturated fat include olive oil, canola oil, many types of nuts, and avocados. The Mediterranean diet is high in monounsaturated fats, namely olive oil. The largest prospective study to look at the benefits of monounsaturated fats and a modified Mediterranean diet is the Lyon Diet Heart Study [52]. This study randomized patients with known CVD to a modified Mediterranean diet or the American Heart Association step 1 diet. The modified Mediterranean diet includes a high consumption of fresh fruits and vegetables; the use of whole-grain rather than refined carbohydrates; low to moderate amounts of dairy, fish, and poultry; low amounts of red meat; minimal amounts of processed foods; and a low to moderate consumption of wine. The primary monounsaturated fat is alpha-linolenic acid (ALA) enriched canola oil. The experimental group experienced 60% fewer cardiovascular events and 80% fewer late diagnoses of cancer. This was further supported in the Indo-Mediterranean Diet Heart Study, where the Indo-Mediterranean diet group experienced 49% fewer cardiovascular events, 62% fewer sudden deaths, and 51% fewer nonfatal MIs in comparison to the National Cholesterol Education Program diet group [53]. Both the Lyon and Indo-Mediterranean diets are high in omega-3 content and are anti-inflammatory. High-fat and diets high in refined sugar reduce endothelium-dependent relaxation and increase inflammatory markers such as interleukin-18 and tumor necrosis factor. Hu and Willet reviewed 147 epidemiological and dietary intervention studies and concluded these nutrition principles for prevention of cardiovascular disease [54]:

1. Increase consumption of omega-3 fatty acids from fish, fish oil supplements, and plant sources.
2. Substitute nonhydrogenated unsaturated fats for saturated and *trans* fats.
3. Consume a diet high in fruits, vegetables, nuts, and whole grains, and low in sugar and refined grain products.
4. Avoid processed foods.
5. Choose foods, food combinations, and preparation methods that are low on the glycemic index.

VII. CONCLUSIONS

Global cardiovascular risk reduction requires a comprehensive assessment and treatment of vascular risk factors. Better targets than LDL cholesterol are needed. Either apo B/apo A-1 or TC/HDL plus hsCRP may represent a more comprehensive lipid target for the assessment and treatment of cardiovascular risk.

Strategies to more adequately reduce cardiovascular events include

- Optimizing control of hypertension, obesity, and diabetes
- Replacing diets high in saturated fats and refined carbohydrates with fiber, fruit and vegetables, nuts, and legumes
- Optimal nutrient supplementation with omega-3 oils, vitamin D, and possibly B vitamins

With a global approach to cardiovascular risk, events can be reduced by 50% to 75% compared to the 25% to 35% reductions seen with statin treatment alone [2, 6].

ACKNOWLEDGMENT

The authors thank DOW Chemical for their professional development support.

REFERENCES

1. Peter SS, Björn D, Neil RP, et al. Prevention of coronary and stroke events with atorvastatin in hypertensive patients who have average or lower-than-average cholesterol concentrations, in the Anglo-Scandinavian Cardiac Outcomes Trial—Lipid Lowering Arm (ASCOT-LLA): a multicentre randomised controlled trial. *Lancet*, April 5, 2003; 361(9364): 1149–1158.
2. Gæde P, Vedel P, et al. Multifactorial intervention and cardiovascular disease in patients with type 2 diabetes. *NEJM*, 2003; 348(5): 383–393.
3. Yokoyama M, et al. Effects of eicosapentaenoic acid on major coronary events in hypercholesterolaemic patients (JELIS): a randomised open-label, blinded endpoint analysis. *Lancet*, Mar 31, 2007; 369(9567): 1090–1098.
4. Dietary supplementation with n-3 polyunsaturated fatty acids and vitamin E after myocardial infarction: results of the GISSI-Prevenzione trial. *Lancet*, 1999; 354: 447–455.
5. Wang X, et al. Efficacy of folic acid supplementation in stroke prevention: a meta-analysis. *Lancet*, 2007; 369: 1876–1882.
6. Effect of potentially modifiable risk factors associated with myocardial infarction in 52 countries (The INTERHEART study): case control study. *Lancet*, September 11, 2004; 364: 937–952.
7. Prediction of lifetime risk for cardiovascular disease by risk factor burden at 50 years of age. *Circulation*, 2006; 113: 791–798.
8. Efficacy and Safety of Cholesterol-Lowering Treatment: Prospective Meta-analysis of Data from 90056 Participants in 14 Randomized Trials of Statins. *Lancet*, October 8, 2005; 366: 1267–1278.

9. Assman G, et al. The emergence of triglycerides as a significant risk factor in coronary artery disease. *Europ Heart J*, 1998; 19(suppl M): M8–M14.

10. Sarwar N, et al. Triglycerides and the risk of coronary heart disease; 10,158 incident cases among 262,525 participants in 29 Western prospective studies. *Circulation*, 2007; 115: 450–458.

11. The impact of triglyceride level beyond low density cholesterol after acute coronary syndrome in the PROVE IT-TIMI 22 Trial. *JACC*, Feb 19, 2008; 51(7): 724–730.

12. Liu J, et al. Non-high-density lipoprotein and very-low-density lipoprotein cholesterol and their risk predictive values in coronary heart disease. *Am J Cardiol*, 2006; 98: 1363–1368.

13. Gordon DJ, Probstfield JL, Garrison RJ, et al. High-density lipoprotein cholesterol and cardiovascular disease: four prospective American studies. *Circulation*, 1989; 79: 8–15.

14. Barter P, et al. HDL Cholesterol, very low levels of LDL cholesterol, and cardiovascular events. *NEJM*, 2007; 357: 1301–1310.

15. Sacks F. The role of high-density lipoprotein (HDL) cholesterol in the prevention and treatment of coronary heart disease: expert group recommendations. *Am J Cardiol*, July 15, 2002; 139–143.

16. Pischon T, Girman C, et al. Non-high-density lipoprotein cholesterol and Apoliprotein B in the prediction of coronary heart disease in men. *Circulation*, 2005; 112: 3375–3383.

17. Assmann G, Schulte H, et al. Hypertriglyceridemia and elevated lipoprotein (a) are risk factors for major coronary events in middle-aged men. *Am J Cardiol*, 1996; 77(14): 1179–1184.

18. Bostom AG, Cupples LA, et al. Elevated plasma lipoprotein(a) and coronary heart disease in men aged 55 years and younger. A prospective study. *JAMA*, 1996; 7(276): 544–548.

19. Kiechl S, Willeit J, et al. Oxidized phospholipids, lipoprotein(a), lipoprotein-associated phospholipase A2 activity, and 10-year cardiovascular outcomes. *ATVB*, 2007; 27: 1788.

20. Garza C, Montori VM, et al. Association between lipoprotein-associated phospholipase A2 and cardiovascular disease: A systematic review. *Mayo Clinic Proceedings*, 2007; 82(2): 159–165.

21. Ballantyne CM, et al. Lipoprotein-associated phospholipase A2, high-sensitivity C-reactive protein, and risk for incident coronary heart disease in middle-aged men and women in the Atherosclerosis Risk in Communities (ARIC) Study. *Circulation*, 2004; 109: 837–842.

22. Ridker PM, et al. C-reactive protein levels and outcomes after statin therapy. *NEJM*, 2005; 352: 20–28.

23. Ridker PM, Stampfer MJ, Rifai N. Novel risk factors for systemic atherosclerosis: a comparison of C-reactive protein, fibrinogen, homocysteine, lipoprotein(a), and standard cholesterol screening as predictors of peripheral arterial disease. *JAMA*, May 16, 2001; 285(19): 2481–2485.

24. Role of the Apolipoprotein B–Apolipoprotein A-I ratio in cardiovascular risk assessment: A case–control analysis in EPIC-Norfolk. *Ann Intern Med*, 2007; 146: 640–648.

25. McCully KS. Vascular pathology of homocysteinemia: implications for the pathogenesis of arteriosclerosis. *Am J Pathol*, 1969; 56: 111–128.

26. Bostom AG, Rosenberg IH, et al. Nonfasting plasma total homocysteine levels and all-cause and cardiovascular disease mortality in elderly Framingham men and women. *Arch Int Med*, May 24, 1999; 159(10): 1077–1080.

27. Nygard O, Nordrehaug JE, Refsum H, Ueland PM, Farstad M, Vollset SE. Plasma homocysteine levels and mortality in patients with coronary artery disease. *N Engl J Med*, 1997; 337: 230–236.

28. Homocysteine and risk of ischemic heart disease and stroke. A meta-analysis. The Homocysteine Studies Collaboration. *JAMA*, 2002; 288: 2015–2022.

29. Watson KE, Abroiat ML, Malone LL, Hoed JM, Doherty T, Detrano R, Demer LL. Active serum vitamin D levels are inversely correlated with coronary calcification. *Circulation*, 1997; 96: 1755–1760.

30. Park R, Detrano R, Xiang M, Fu P, Ibrahim Y, LaBree L, Azen S. Combined use of computed tomography coronary calcium scores and C-reactive protein levels in predicting cardiovascular events in nondiabetic individuals. *Circulation*, Oct 2002; 106: 2073–2077.

31. Wang TJ, Pencina MJ, Booth SL, Jacques PF, Ingelsson E, Lanier K, Benjamin EJ, D'Agostino RB, Wolf M, Vasan RS. Vitamin D deficiency and risk of cardiovascular disease. *Circulation*, Jan 2008; 117: 503–511.

32. Autier P, Gandini S. Vitamin D supplementation and total mortality: A meta-analysis of randomized controlled trials. *Arch Intern Med*, 2007; 167: 1730–1737.

33. GISSI-Prevenzione Investigators. Dietary supplementation with n-3 polyunsaturated fatty acids and vitamin E after myocardial infarction: results of the GISSI-Prevenzione trial. *Lancet*, 1999; 354: 447–455.

34. Yokoyama M, Origasa H, et al. Effects of eicosapentaenoic acid on major coronary events in hypercholesterolaemic patients (JELIS): a randomised open-label, blinded endpoint analysis. *Lancet*, Mar 31, 2007; 369(9567): 1090–1098.

35. Lopez-Garcia E, Schulze MB, et al. Consumption of (n-3) fatty acids is related to plasma biomarkers of inflammation and endothelial activation in women. *J Nutrition*, Jul 2004; 134(7): 1806–1811.

36. Sacco M, Pellegrini F, et al. Primary prevention of cardiovascular events with low-dose aspirin and vitamin E in type 2 diabetic patients: results of the Primary Prevention Project (PPP) trial. *Diabet Care*, Dec 2003; 26(12): 3264–3272.

37. Yusuf S, Sleight P, et al. Effects of an angiotensin-converting inhibitor, raqmipril, on cardiovascular events in high-risk patients. The Heart Outcomes Prevention Evaluation Study Investigators. *NEJM*, Jan 20, 2000; 342(3): 145–153.

38. Brown BG, Zhao XQ, et al. Simvastatin and niacin, antioxidant vitamins, or the combination for the prevention of coronary disease. *NEJM*, Nov 29, 2001; 345(22): 1583–1592.

39. Devaraj D, Tang R, et al. Effect of high-dose alpha-tocopherol supplementation on biomarkers of oxidative stress and inflammation and carotid atherosclerosis in patients with coronary disease. *Am J Clin Nutr*, Nov 2007; 86: 1392–1398.

40. Blumberg J, Frei B. Why clinical trials of vitamin E and cardiovascular diseases may be fatally flawed. Commentary on "The relationship between dose of vitamin E and suppression of oxidative stress in humans." *Free Radical Biology and Medicine*, 2007; 43: 1374–1376.

41. Young JM, et al. Effect of coenzyme Q(10) supplementation on simvastatin-induced myalgia. *Am J Cardiol*, Nov 1, 2007; 100(9): 1400–1403.

42. Caso G, Kelly P, et al. Effect of coenzyme q10 on myopathic symptoms in patients treated with statins. *Am J Cardiol*, May 15, 2007; 99(10): 1409–1412.

43. Dierkes J, Westphal S. Effect of drugs on homocysteine concentrations. *Semin Vasc Med*, May 2005; 5(2): 124–139.

44. Narayaan KM, Boyle JP, Thompson TJ, Sorenson SW, Williamson DF. Lifetime risk for diabetes mellitus in the United States. *JAMA*, 2003; 290: 1884–1890.

45. Mosca L, Linfante AH, Benjamin EJ, Berra K, Hayes SN, Walsh BW, Fabunmi RP, Kwan J, Mills T, Simpson SL. National study of physician awareness and adherence to cardiovascular disease prevention guidelines. *Circulation*, 2005; 111: 499–510.

46. Mokdad AH, Marks JS, Stroup DF, Gerberding JL. Actual causes of death in the United States, 2000. *JAMA*, 2004; 291: 1238–1245.

47. Tuomilehto et al. Prevention of type 2 diabetes mellitus by changes in lifestyle among subjects with impaired glucose tolerance. *NEJM*, May 2003; 344(18): 1343–1350.

48. Ogden CL, Carroll MD, Curtin LR, McDowell MA, Tabak CJ, Flegal KM. Prevalence of overweight and obesity in the United States 1999-2004. *JAMA*, 2006; 295: 1549–1555.

49. Eckle RH, Krauss, RM. American Heart Association Call t7:1491: Obesity as a Major Risk Factor for Coronary Heart Disease. *Circulation*, 1998; 97: 2099–2100.

50. Ascherio A. Epidemiologic studies on dietary fats and coronary heart disease. *Am J Med*, 2002; 113 Suppl 9B: 9S–12S.

51. Hu FB, Stampfer MJ, Manson JE, et al. Dietary fat intake and the risk of coronary heart disease in women. *NEJM*, 1997; 33.

52. de Lorgeril M, Salen P, Martin JL, et al. Mediterranean diet, traditional risk factors, and the rate of cardiovascular complications after myocardial infarction: final report of the Lyon Diet Heart Study. *Circulation*, 1999; 99: 779–785.

53. Singh RB, Dubnov G, Niaz MA, et al. Effect of an Indo-Mediterranean diet on progression of coronary artery disease in high risk patients (Indo-Mediterranean Diet Heart Study): a randomized single-blind trial. *Lancet*, 2002; 360: 1455–1461.

54. Hu FB, Wilett WC. Optimal diets for prevention of coronary heart disease. *JAMA*, 2002; 288: 2569–2578.

5 Hypertension

Utilizing Nutrition in Treatment

Mark C. Houston, M.D., M.S.

I. INTRODUCTION

Short-term reduction in blood pressure (BP) utilizing nutrition results in intermediate and long-term improvements in morbidity and mortality, including cerebrovascular accidents (CVA), coronary heart disease (CHD), and myocardial infarction (MI) [1, 2]. In the Health Professionals Follow-up Study [1], diets rich in potassium reduced CVA by 41% in hypertensive subjects. In the Lyon Diet Heart Study [2], a Mediterranean type diet reduced the incidence of a second MI by 76%. These studies and others reveal the importance of micronutrients, macronutrients, and nutraceuticals for preventing and treating hypertension and the cardiovascular complications of this disease.

Many national and global organizations and policy directives on nutrition and hypertension such as JNC-7 [3], the Nutrition Committee of the AHA [4], the World Health Organization (WHO), Canadian Hypertension Society, the Institute of Medicine report to Congress on the Nutritional Needs of the Elderly [5], INTERSALT [6], the European Society of Hypertension (ESH)–European Society of Cardiology (ESC), International Society of Hypertension (ISH) [7], and the British Hypertension Society(BHS) recognize the positive impact of nutrition on hypertension, CHD, atherosclerosis, and CVA.

The best means to reduce BP and target organ damage (TOD) in hypertensive patients is an integrative approach that uses nutrition, vitamins, antioxidants, minerals, functional foods, nutraceutical supplements, weight loss, exercise, judicious alcohol use, and complete cessation of tobacco and caffeine combined with optimal pharmacologic therapy. Reducing BP requires a combination of lifestyle modifications and drug therapy, especially for those patients [3] with multiple CHD risk factors, TOD, or clinical cardiovascular disease (CCD). Tables 5.1 and 5.2 can help guide patient-specific treatments. Lifestyle changes may prevent or delay the onset of hypertension, reduce BP levels, slow disease progression, and potentiate the effects of antihypertensive drugs, thereby allowing for fewer drugs and/or lower doses. Finally, there may be additive or synergistic improvements in cardiovascular risk factors, vascular function, structure, and health [8, 9]. Patients with BP below 140/90 mm Hg who have no risk factors, TOD, or cardiovascular disease (CCD) may be initially and successfully treated with lifestyle modifications [3].

A large percentage of essential hypertensive patients are appropriate candidates for preliminary and prolonged lifestyle modifications as long as the BP is frequently evaluated and clinical TOD, CCD, DM, or significant risk factors are not present at that time and do not develop later. As many as 50% to 60% of essential hypertensive patients are included in this classification [9–11]. Optimal nutrition, antioxidants, vitamins, minerals, functional foods, and nutraceutical supplements are effective therapies in these patients and provide excellent adjunctive treatment in patients taking antihypertensive drugs. The patient's nutritional analysis should be evaluated at baseline. All nutrients that are deficient must be repleted to normal levels. The lifestyle modifications mentioned above should always be continued following initiation of drug therapy [8–11].

This paper will review the basic science and clinical studies of nutraceutical supplements, vitamins, antioxidants, minerals, macronutrients, and micronutrients and their impact on the prevention and treatment of hypertension. Correlations and mechanisms of action based on vascular biology will provide a unique framework for understanding the clinical use of these therapeutic interventions. Pharmacologic therapy with antihypertensive drugs is beyond the scope of this paper, but some general discussion is provided to emphasize the importance of balance when treating essential hypertension. Integrating nutrition with pharmacologic therapy reduces BP and TOD and improves the worldwide dismal statistics of BP control [3, 12–15].

II. PATHOPHYSIOLOGY

Oxidative stress with an imbalance between reactive oxygen species (ROS) and the antioxidant defense mechanisms contributes to the etiology of human hypertension [16–21]. Oxidative stress

TABLE 5.1
JNC-7 Classification of Blood Pressure (BP) for Adults
Aged 18 Years and Older

| | | | | Management* | |
| | | | | Initial Drug Therapy | |
BP Classification	Systolic BP, mmHg*	Diastolic BP, mmHg*	Lifestyle Modification	Without Compelling Indication	With Compelling Indications
Normal	<120 and	<80	Encourage	No antihypertensive drug indicated	
Prehypertension	120–139 or	80–89	Yes	Thiazide-type diuretics for most; may consider ACE inhibitor,	Drug(s) for the compelling indications‡
Stage 1 Hypertension	140–159 or	90–99	Yes	ARB, β-blocker, CCB, or combination	Drug(s) for the compelling indications Other antihypertensive drugs (diuretics, ACE inhibitor, ARB, β-blocker, CCB) as needed
Stage 2 Hypertension	≥ 160 or	≥ 100	Yes	Two-drug combination for most (usually thiazide-type diuretic and ACE inhibitor or ARB or and ACE inhibitor or ARB or β-blocker or CCB)§	Drug(s) for the compelling indications Other antihypertensive drugs (diuretics, ACE inhibitor, ARB, β-blocker, CCB) as needed

Source: [3].
Abbreviations: ACE, angiotensin-converting enzyme; ARB, angiotensin-receptor blocker; CCB, calcium channel blocker
* Treatment determined by highest BP category.
‡ Treat patients with chronic kidney disease or diabetes to BP goal of less than 130/80 mmHg.
§ Initial combined therapy should be used cautiously in those at risk for orthostatic hypertension.

TABLE 5.2
Hypertension Treatment JNC-7

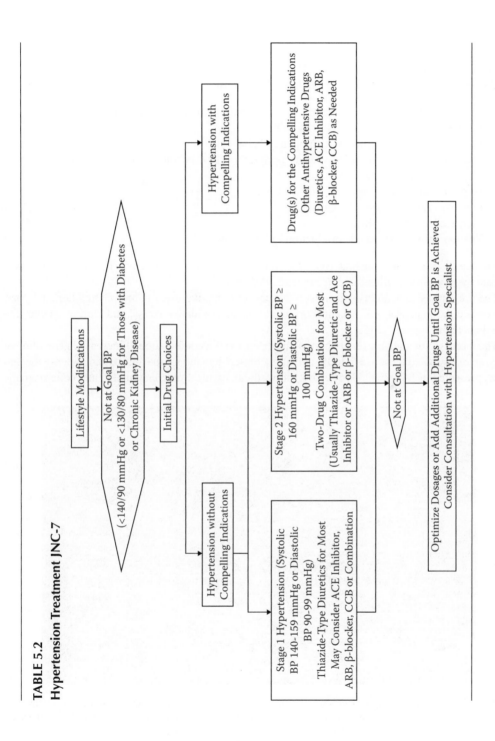

has been implicated in many hypertensive disorders including lead-induced [18, 22–24], uremic, cyclosporine-induced [25–28], salt-sensitive [29, 30], preeclampsia, essential hypertension [31–35], diabetes mellitus [36, 37] and in hypertension induced by high-fat and high-refined-carbohydrate diets [38–41].

Hypertensive patients have an impaired endogenous and exogenous antioxidant defense mechanism [42–49]. In addition, hypertensive patients have more oxidative stress and a greater than normal response to oxidative stress [16, 17, 19, 20, 43, 44, 47, 50, 51].

The proposed mechanisms of ROS-induced hypertension in humans are as follows [52–54]:

- Structural and functional damage from direct action on endothelial cells
- Degradation of nitric oxide (NO) by ROS
- Effects on eicosanoid metabolism in endothelial cells
- Oxidative modification of low density lipoprotein (LDL) cholesterol
- Hyperglycemia
- Hyperinsulinemia
- Increased fatty acid mobilization
- Increased catecholamines
- The increase of superoxide production by angiotensin II

Imbalance of vasodilators such as NO, vasoconstrictors such as angiotensin II, and ROS can perpetuate hypertension as illustrated in Figure 5.1 [55–58].

The present research and conclusions of the role of oxidative stress in animal and human hypertension are the interrelations of neurohormonal systems, oxidative stress, and cardiovascular disease depicted in Figure 5.2 [59].

The increased oxidative stress in human hypertension is a combination of increased generation of ROS, an exacerbated response to ROS, and an increased demand for the antioxidant defense mechanisms presented in Table 5.3 [59–61]. Low intracellular, extracellular, enzymatic, and nonenzymatic

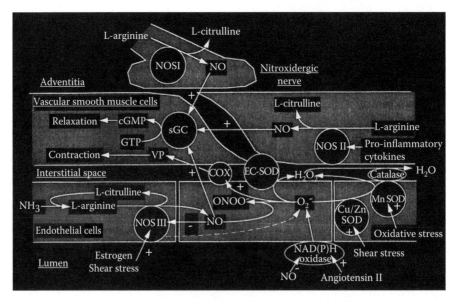

FIGURE 5.1   Reactive oxygen species and nitric oxide [77]. Some of the complex interactions involved in regulating the balance of nitric oxide (NO) and superoxide (O_2^-) within the vasculature. NOS I indicates neuronal NOS; NOS II, inducible NOS; NOS III, endothelial NOS; EC-SOD, extracellular superoxide dismutase; Mn SOD, manganese SOD; Cu/Zn SOD, copper/zinc SOD; sGC, soluble guanylate cyclase; ONOO$^-$, peroxynitrite; H_2O_2, hydrogen peroxide; GTP, guanosine 5'-triphosphate; COX, cyclooxygenase; and VP, vasoconstrictor prostanoids. (From [77].)

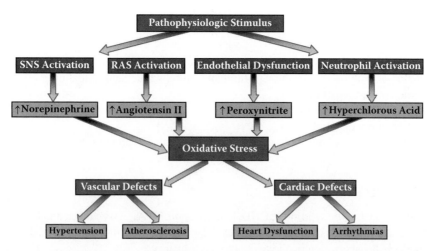

FIGURE 5.2 Role of different extra-cardiac and extra-vascular systems in the genesis of oxidative stress and development of cardiovascular abnormalities [59]. SNS, sympathetic nervous system; RAS, renin-angiotensin system.

TABLE 5.3
The Cytotoxic Reactive Oxygen Species and the Natural Defense Mechanisms

Reactive Oxygen Species		Antioxidant Defense Mechanisms	
Free Radicals		*Enzymatic Scavengers*	
$O_2 \bullet^-$	Superoxide anion radical	SOD	Superoxide dismutase
$OH \bullet$	Hydroxyl radical		$2O_2 \bullet^- + 2H+ \rightarrow H_2O_2 + O_2$
$ROO \bullet$	Lipid peroxide (peroxyl)	CAT	Catalase (peroxisomal-bound)
$RO \bullet$	Alkoxyl		$2H_2O_2 \rightarrow O_2 + H_2O$
$RS \bullet$	Thiyl	GTP	Glutathione peroxidase
$NO \bullet$	Nitric oxide		$2GSH + H_2O_2 \rightarrow GSSG + 2H_2O$
$NO_2 \bullet$	Nitrogen dioxide		$2GSH + ROOH \rightarrow GSSG + ROH + 2H_2O$
$ONOO^-$	Peroxynitrite		
$CCl_3 \bullet$	Trichloromethyl		
		Nonenzymatic scavengers	
		Vitamin A	
Non-radicals		Vitamin C (ascorbic acid)	
H_2O_2	Hydrogen peroxide	Vitamin E (α-tocopherol)	
HOCl	Hypochlorous acid	β-carotene	
$ONOO^-$	Peroxynitrite	Cysteine	
$^1O_2$	Singlet oxygen	Coenzyme Q	
		Uric acid	
		Flavonoids	
		Sulfhydryl group	
		Thioether compounds	

The superscripted bold dot indicates an unpaired electron and the negative charge indicates a gained electron. GSH, reduced glutathione; GSSG, oxidized glutathione; R, lipid chain. Singlet oxygen is an unstable molecule due to the two electrons present in its outer orbit spinning in opposite directions.
Source: [59].

antioxidants result in a net reduction in antioxidant reserves [59]. The cardiovascular effects of excess ROS are as follows:

- Peroxidation of polyunsaturated fatty acids in membrane lipid bilayers
- Oxidation of proteins by induction of lipid and carbohydrate auto-oxidation proteolysis
- Oxidation of carbohydrates
- Oxidation of DNA and subsequent damage
- Oxidation of organic molecules
- Up-regulation of and damage to genetic machinery, gene expression transcription factors, and DNA synthesis

III. EPIDEMIOLOGY

Diabetes mellitus, metabolic syndrome, CHD, hypertension, CVA, CHF, cancer, and hyperlipidemia have reached epidemic levels in the United States [62, 63]. These nutritionally related diseases result from the modern-day aberration in a long evolutionary history.

Humans have evolved from a pre-agricultural, hunter-gatherer society to a commercial agriculture with highly processed foods that has imposed unnatural and unhealthy nutrition. The human genetic makeup is 99.9% that of our Paleolithic ancestors for the past 35,000 years, yet our nutrition is vastly different (Table 5.4) [64]. The macronutrient and micronutrient variations contribute to the higher incidence of hypertension and other cardiovascular diseases through a complex nutrient-gene interaction [62–65]. Poor nutrition, coupled with obesity and a sedentary lifestyle, have resulted in an exponential increase in nutritionally related diseases [62]. In particular, the high Na^+/K^+ ratio and low omega-3 to omega-6 fatty acid ratio and increased intake of saturated and *trans* fats of modern diets have contributed to hypertension, stroke, CHD, CHF, diabetes, dyslipidemia, and renal disease [66–73].

Humans are genetically geared to a pre-agricultural, hunter-gatherer nutritional and exercise lifestyle. Table 5.4 contrasts modern-day intake of potassium, sodium, fiber, protein, carbohydrate, and fat with that of hunter-gatherers from the Paleolithic era [62, 67–74]. The genes of Paleolithic humans and modern humans differ much less than the nutrient intake.

Nutrients and ROS are powerful, influential factors to which the human genome is exposed. These nutrients and ROS determine the amount and activity of specific proteins by functioning as regulators of gene transcription [62, 63, 75, 76], nuclear RNA processing [62, 63, 77], and messenger

---

TABLE 5.4
Evolutionary Nutritional Impositions

	Paleolithic Intakes[*]	Modern Intakes[*]
K+	> 10,000 mEq/day (256 g)	150 mEq/day (6 g)
Na+	< 50 mmol /day (1.2 g)	175 mmol/day (4 g)
Na+ / K+ ratio	< 0.13 /day	> 0.67/day
Fiber	> 100 g/day	9 g/day
Protein	37%	20%
Carbohydrate	41%	40%–50%
Fat	22%	30%–40%
P/S Ratio	1.4	0.4

Source: [64, 130].

P/S Ratio = Polyunsaturated to saturated fats ratio

[*]Evolution from pre-agricultural, hunter-gatherer milieu to an agricultural, refrigeration society has imposed an unnatural and unhealthful nutritional selection process.

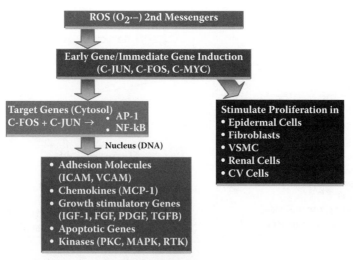

Redox-Sensitive Transcriptional Factors

FIGURE 5.3 ROS are intracellular signal transduction systems and modulators of transcriptional pathways. (From [61].)

RNA stability and degradation [62, 63, 78] (Figure 5.3). These factors, in turn, determine and influence energy metabolism, cell differentiation, and cell growth [62] (Figure 5.4). The clinical outcomes of nutrient regulation of gene expression may be beneficial or detrimental in their effects on cardiovascular disease, BP, glucose, and lipids [63] (Figure 5.5).

IV. TREATMENT APPROACHES

ELECTROLYTES

Sodium (Na+)

The average sodium intake in the United States is 5000 mg/day with some areas of the country consuming 15,000 to 20,000 mg/day [12]. However, the minimal requirement for sodium is probably about 500 mg/day [12]. Epidemiologic, observational, and controlled clinical trials demonstrate that an increased sodium intake is associated with higher blood pressure [79]. A reduction in sodium

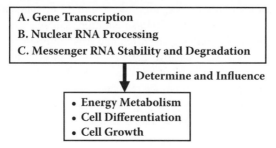

FIGURE 5.4 Nutrient–gene interactions and gene expression: "The interaction of nature and nurture." (From [62, 63, 65, 75, 76, 77, 78].)

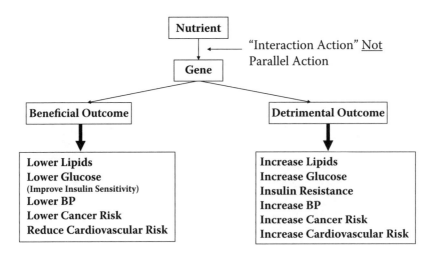

FIGURE 5.5   Nutrient regulation of gene expression.

intake in hypertensive patients, especially the salt-sensitive patients, will significantly lower blood pressure by 4–6/2–3 mm Hg [68, 80–82]. The blood pressure reduction is proportional to the severity of sodium restriction [68, 83, 84].

The effect of dietary sodium on BP is modulated by other components of the diet [85–88]. Sodium-chloride-induced hypertension is augmented by diets low in potassium [85, 86], calcium, and magnesium [85, 87, 89] and attenuated by high potassium, magnesium, and calcium (especially Na⁺ sensitive). The DASH-II diet is particularly instructive in this regard [68]. Gradual reductions in sodium from 150 to 100 to 50 mmol/day in association with a high fruit, vegetable, and low-fat dairy intake with adequate potassium, calcium, magnesium, and fiber intake was the most effective in reducing BP.

Despite the enormous body of literature on salt and hypertension, debate still exists as to a true causal relationship [87, 88]. Nevertheless, sodium does have a major impact on cardiovascular, cerebrovascular, and renal disease [88–103]. Studies have documented a direct relationship between sodium intake and increased platelet reactivity [89], stroke (independent of BP) [90, 91], left ventricular hypertrophy [92], MI [92], CHF [92], sudden death [92], and left ventricular filling [93]. The renal plasma flow falls and glomerular filtration rate and glomerular filtration increase leading to an increase in intraglomerular capillary pressure, microalbuminuria, proteinuria, glomerular injury, and renal insufficiency [92, 94–97]. Sodium also reduces arterial compliance independent of BP changes [98, 99].

Salt sensitivity (> 10% increase in mean arterial pressure [MAP] with salt loading) is a key factor in determining the cardiovascular, cerebrovascular, renal and blood pressure response to dietary salt intake [100–103]. Cardiovascular events are more common in salt-sensitive patients than in salt-resistant ones, independent of BP [102, 103]. In addition, salt sensitivity is most pronounced in elderly patients with isolated systolic hypertension and it is modified by polymorphisms of the angiotensinogen gene [104–106]. Salt-sensitive patients do not inhibit their sympathetic nervous system activity [106] or increase NO production with salt loading [107]. Sodium interacts at the vascular level with other minerals, calcium, trace elements, and fatty acids [108–110].

The evidence is very suggestive that reduction of dietary salt intake reduces target organ damage (brain, heart, kidney, and vasculature) that is both dependent on the small BP reduction, but also independent of the decreased BP.

Potassium (K⁺)

The average U.S. dietary intake of potassium (K⁺) is 45 mEq/day with a potassium to sodium (K⁺/Na⁺) ratio of less than 1:2 [12]. The recommended intake of K⁺ is 650 mEq/day with a K⁺/Na⁺

ratio of over 5:1 [12]. Numerous epidemiologic, observational, and clinical trials have demonstrated a significant reduction in BP with increased dietary K^+ intake [12, 111, 112]. The magnitude of BP reduction with a K^+ supplementation of 60 to 120 mEq/day is 4.4/2.5 mm Hg in hypertensive patients and 1.8/1.0 mm Hg in normotensive patients [113, 114]. Alteration of the K^+/Na^+ ratio to a higher level is important for both antihypertensive as well as cardiovascular and cerebrovascular effects [89, 115]. High potassium intake reduces the incidence of cardiovascular and cerebrovascular accidents independent of the BP reduction [48, 66, 114].

Gu et al. [115] recently demonstrated for the first time that potassium supplementation at 60 mmol of KCl per day for 12 weeks significantly reduced systolic blood pressure (SBP) –5.0 mm Hg (range –2.13 to –7.88 mm Hg) (p < 0.001). This study confirmed that the higher the initial BP, the greater the response and that the urinary sodium-potassium ratio correlates best with BP reduction as does the dietary sodium-potassium ratio [89] compared to either urinary sodium or potassium individually [115].

Magnesium (Mg^{++})

A high dietary intake of magnesium of at least 500 to 1000 mg/day reduces BP in most of the reported epidemiologic, observational, and clinical trials, but the results are less consistent than those seen with Na^+ and K^+ [12, 79, 114, 116–122]. In most epidemiologic studies, there is an inverse relationship between dietary magnesium intake and BP [109, 114, 118, 119, 122–127]. A study of 60 essential hypertensive subjects given magnesium supplements showed a significant reduction in BP over an 8 week period documented by 24 hour ambulatory BP, home, and office blood BP [117]. The intake of multiple minerals in a natural form such as Mg^{++}, K^+, and Ca^{++} is more effective than Mg^{++} alone in reducing BP.

Magnesium competes with Na^+ for binding sites on vascular smooth muscle and acts like a calcium channel blocker (CCB), increases PGE, binds in a necessary-cooperative manner with potassium, inducing endothelial vasodilation (EDV) and BP reduction [12, 79, 109, 127–129]. Magnesium regulates both SBP, diastolic blood pressure (DBP), intracellular Ca^{++}, Na^+, K^+, and pH as well as left ventricular mass, insulin sensitivity, and arterial compliance [126, 127].

Calcium (Ca^{++})

Population studies show a link between hypertension and calcium [12, 114, 130], but clinical trials that administer calcium supplements to patients have shown inconsistent effects on BP [131, 132]. Higher dietary calcium is not only associated with a lower BP, but also with a decreased risk of developing hypertension [114, 133]. A 23% reduction in the risk of developing hypertension was noted in those individuals on greater than 800 mg/day compared to those on less than 400 mg/day [114, 134].

A recent meta-analysis of the effect of Ca^{++} supplementation in hypertensive patients found a reduction in systolic BP of 4.3/1.5 mm Hg [110, 135, 136]. Foods containing Ca^{++} were more effective than supplements in reducing BP [110, 136]. Karanja et al. [137] assessed the effects of $CaCO_3$ (calcium carbonate) versus calcium contained in the diet and found significant increases in magnesium, riboflavin, and vitamin D in the dietary group that correlated with Ca^{++} intake. There is an additive or synergistic effect on BP reduction with a combination of minerals and vitamins as compared to Ca^{++} alone [68, 74].

MACRONUTRIENTS

Protein

Observational and epidemiologic studies demonstrate a consistent association between a high protein intake and a reduction in BP [138–141]. The protein source is an important factor in the BP effect; animal protein being less effective than nonanimal protein [142]. However, lean or wild animal protein with less saturated fat and more essential omega-3 and reduced omega-6 fatty acids may reduce BP, lipids, and CHD risk [141–143]. The Intermap Study showed an inverse correlation of BP with total protein intake, especially with protein intake from nonanimal sources [142].

The Intersalt Study [139] supported the hypothesis that higher dietary protein intake has favorable influences on BP in 10,020 men and women in 32 countries worldwide. The average SBP and DBP were 3.0 and 2.5 mm Hg lower respectively for those whose dietary protein was 30% above the overall mean than for those 30% below the overall mean (81 vs. 44 g/day).

Fermented milk supplemented with whey protein concentrate significantly reduces BP in animal models (rats) and human studies [144]. Kawase et al. studied 20 healthy men given 200 mL of fermented milk/whey protein twice daily for 8 weeks. The SBP was reduced significantly ($p < 0.05$) in the treatment group compared to the control group [144]. Natural bioactive substances in milk and colostrum including minerals, vitamins, and peptides have been demonstrated to reduce BP [145, 146]. These findings are consistent with the combined diet of fruits, vegetables, grains, and low-fat dairy in DASH-I and DASH-II studies in reducing BP [68, 74].

Soy protein at intakes of 25 to 30 g/day lowers BP and increases arterial compliance [147, 148]. Soy contains many active compounds that produce these antihypertensive effects, including isoflavones, amino acids, saponins, phytic acid, trypsin inhibitors, fiber, and globulins [147, 148].

In two unpublished studies by Pitre et al. [149] in spontaneously hypertensive rats, hydrolyzed ion-exchange whey protein isolate (BioZate-1™, Davisco, Eden Prairie, Minnesota) demonstrated significant reductions in mean arterial pressure and heart rate compared to an ion-exchange whey protein isolate. BioZate-1™ at an oral dose of 30, 75, and 150 mg/kg reduced mean arterial pressure by 10% to 18% and heart rate (HR) 10% that was sustained for 24 hours ($p < 0.05$ for both). The maximum effect occurred 1 to 6 hours after dosing. Pins and Keenan [150] administered 20 g of hydrolyzed whey protein to 30 hypertensive subjects and noted a BP reduction of 11/7 mm Hg compared to controls that is mediated by an angiotensin converting enzyme inhibitor (ACEI) mechanism. Whey protein must be hydrolyzed in order to exhibit the dose-related antihypertensive effect.

Bovine-casein-derived peptides and whey-protein-derived peptides exhibit ACEI activity [144, 145, 150, 151]. The enzymatic hydrolysis of whey protein isolates releases ACEI peptides [149]. The relative in vitro ACEI activity (IC50 – the amount of the substance that causes a 50% inhibition of ACE activity is 0.45 mg/mL for BioZate-1™, 376 mg/mL for whey protein isolate compared to 1.3×10^{-6} for captopril).

Sardine muscle protein, which contains Valyl-Tyrosine (VAL-TYR), significantly lowers BP in hypertensive patients [152]. Kawasaki et al. treated 29 hypertensive patients with 3 mg of Valyl-Tyrosine sardine muscle concentrated extract for 4 weeks and lowered BP 9.7 mm Hg/5.3 mm Hg ($p < 0.05$) [152]. Valyl-Tyrosine is a natural ACEI. In addition to ACEI effects, protein intake may also reduce catecholamine responses and induce natriuresis [153]. The optimal protein intake, depending on level of activity, renal function, stress and other factors, is about 1.0 to 1.5 g/kg/day [154, 155].

Fats

Observational, epidemiologic, biochemical, cross-sectional studies, and clinical trials of the effect of fats on BP have been disappointing and inconsistent [156–160]. An exhaustive meta-analysis and review of these studies is reported by Morris [156]. Research suggests that rather than the ratio of fat to carbohydrates and proteins, the type of dietary fat, total daily intake, and relative ratios of specific types of fats may be more important in determining the BP effect in patients.

The amount and ratio of the polyunsaturated fats (PUFA) and monounsaturated fats (MUFA), which include omega-3 fatty acids (ω-3 FA), omega-6 fatty acids (ω-6 FA), and omega-9 fatty acids (ω-9 FA) may be particularly influential in blood pressure. The ω-3 FA and ω-6 FA are essential fatty acid families, whereas ω-9 FA (oleic acid) can be manufactured by the body from the dietary precursor stearic acid. The omega-3 PUFA are strong determinants of cell growth, energy metabolism, energy balance, and insulin sensitivity [62, 161, 162]. A ratio of omega-3 to omega-6 PUFA of between 1:2 to 1:1 is considered beneficial to cardiovascular health and approaches that of our Paleolithic ancestors and the Inuit Eskimos [64].

TABLE 5.5
Metabolic Pathways of the Omega-3 and Omega-6 Fatty Acids

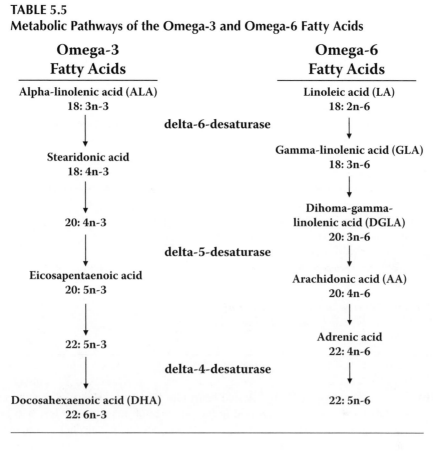

Omega-3 Fatty Acids		Omega-6 Fatty Acids
Alpha-linolenic acid (ALA) 18: 3n-3		Linoleic acid (LA) 18: 2n-6
	delta-6-desaturase	
Stearidonic acid 18: 4n-3		Gamma-linolenic acid (GLA) 18: 3n-6
20: 4n-3		Dihoma-gamma-linolenic acid (DGLA) 20: 3n-6
	delta-5-desaturase	
Eicosapentaenoic acid 20: 5n-3		Arachidonic acid (AA) 20: 4n-6
22: 5n-3		Adrenic acid 22: 4n-6
	delta-4-desaturase	
Docosahexaenoic acid (DHA) 22: 6n-3		22: 5n-6

Omega-3 PUFA

Alpha-linolenic acid (ALA), eicosapentaenoic acid (EPA), and docosahexaenoic acid (DHA) comprise the primary members of the omega-3 PUFA family (Table 5.5). Omega-3 fatty acids are found in coldwater fish such as herring, haddock, salmon, trout, tuna, cod, and mackerel; fish oils; flax, flax seed, and flax oil; and nuts [12, 163]. Omega-3 PUFA significantly lower BP in observational, epidemiologic, and in some small prospective clinical trials through a variety of mechanisms (Table 5.6) [12, 156, 164–170]. A meta-analysis of 31 studies on the effects of fish oil on BP have shown a dose-related response in hypertension as well as a relationship to the specific concomitant diseases associated with hypertension [109, 171–177]. At fish oil doses of < 4 g/day, there was no change in BP in the mildly hypertensive subjects. At 4 to 7 g/day, BP fell 1.6 to 2.9 mm Hg, and at over 15 g/day, BP decreased 5.8 to 8.1 mm Hg [109, 171–177].

A study of 399 healthy males showed that a 1% increase in adipose tissue alpha-linolenic acid content was associated with a 5 mm Hg decrease in SBP, DBP, and MAP [117].

Knapp et al. [169] demonstrated a significant reduction in BP (p < 0.01) in a group of hypertensive subjects given 15 g/day of fish oil. Bao et al. [163] studied 69 obese, hypertensive subjects for 16 weeks treated with fish oil (3.65 grams omega-3 FA per day), evaluated by 24 hour ambulatory BP monitoring (24 hour ABM). The best BP results were seen in subjects on combined fish oil and weight loss. BP fell 13.0/9.3 mm Hg and heart rate fell 6 beats per minute on average.

Mori et al. [161] studied 63 hypertensive, hyperlipidemic patients treated with omega-3 fatty acids (3.65 g/day for 16 weeks) and found significant reductions in BP (P < 0.01). Studies indicate

TABLE 5.6
Omega-3 and PUFA: Mechanisms of Action

- Stimulates nitric oxide (NO) and PGI but decreases TxA_2 and leukotrienes (168)
- Improves insulin sensitivity and lowers BP
  - N-3 skeletal muscle phospholipid content
  - Membrane fluidity, membrane phospholipid content (167) regulate gene expression
  - Mitochondrial up-coupling protein and FA oxidation in liver and skeletal muscle
  - Thermogenesis gene induction (Reduces body fat) (increases heat production) energy balance improves
  - Mitochondrial and peroxisomal oxidation in skeletal muscle (131)
  - ↓ TG droplets, ↑ Glucose uptake, Glycogen storage
  - Improved glucose tolerance (134)
- Intracellular and inter organ fuel partitioners directing FA away from storage to oxidation (131)
  - PPARα ligand activators (lipid oxidation) (131)
  - SREBP-1 suppression (↓ lipogenic genes)
- Improved cardiac function
- Improved endothelial dysfunction (213)
- Reduced plasma norepinephrine
- Change calcium flux

PPAR = Peroxisome-proliferator-activated receptor
SREBP-1 = Sterol-response-element-binding protein
Source: [65, 161, 162].

---

that DHA is very effective in reducing BP and heart rate [164, 165]. However, formation of EPA and ultimately DHA from ALA is decreased in the presence of increased linoleic acid in the diet (omega-6 FA), increased dietary saturated fats and *trans* fatty acids, alcohol and aging through inhibitory effects or reduced activity of delta-6-desaturase, and to a lesser extent delta-5-desaturase and delta-4-desaturase [164, 165]. The omega-3 and omega-6 metabolic pathways are presented in Table 5.5. Eating coldwater fish three times per week is as effective as high-dose fish oil in reducing BP in hypertensive patients, and the protein in the fish may also have antihypertensive effects [12, 170].

Omega-6 Fatty Acids

The omega-6 FA family, which includes linoleic acid (LA), gamma-linolenic acid (GLA), dihomo-gamma-linolenic acid (DGLA), and arachidonic acid (AA), does not usually lower BP significantly [156] (Table 5.5), but may prevent increases in BP induced by saturated fats [108, 178]. The omega-6 FA are found in flax, flax seed, flax seed oil, conjugated linoleic acid (CLA), canola oil, nuts, evening primrose oil, borage oil, and black current oil.

GLA and DGLA will enhance synthesis of vasodilating prostaglandins PGE_1 and PGI_2 preventing the increase in BP by feeding saturated fats [109, 178]. GLA also completely blocks stress-induced hypertension [179, 180] due to increased PGE_1 [181], decreased plasma aldosterone, and reduced adrenal angiotensin II receptor density and affinity [180].

Omega-9 Fatty Acids (omega-9 FA)

Olive oil is rich in monounsaturated fats (MUFA) (omega-9 FA) (oleic acid), which have been associated with BP and lipid reduction in Mediterranean and other diets [12, 182]. Ferrara et al. studied 23 hypertensive subjects in a double-blind, randomized, crossover study for 6 months comparing MUFA with PUFA [182]. Extra virgin olive oil (MUFA) was compared to sunflower oil (PUFA), rich in linoleic acid (W-6 FA). The SBP fell 8 mm Hg ($p < 0.05$) and the DBP fell 6 mm Hg ($p < 0.01$)

in the MUFA-treated subjects compared to the PUFA-treated subjects. In addition, the need for antihypertensive medications was reduced by 48% in the MUFA group versus 4% in the PUFA (omega-6 FA) group (p < 0.005).

Olive oil is rich in oleic acid (omega-9 FA). Extra virgin oil has 5 mg of phenols in 10 g of olive oil, a rich polyphenol antioxidant [182, 183]. About 4 tablespoons of extra virgin olive oil is equal to 40 g. The combined antioxidant and antilipid effect of MUFA probably accounts for the BP effects by improved NO bioavailability, reduced ROS, improved endothelial function, vasodilation, and inhibition of the oxLDL stimulation of the angiotensin II receptor (A-II R) [43, 44, 55, 56, 59, 60, 184, 185].

Fiber

The clinical trials with various types of fiber to reduce BP have been generally favorable, but inconsistent [186]. Soluble fiber, guar gum, guava, psyllium, and oat bran reduce BP and reduce the need for antihypertensive medications in hypertensive, diabetic, and hypertensive-diabetic patients [187–190]. Vuksan et al. [188] reduced SBP 9.4 mm Hg in hypertensive subjects with the fiber Glucomannan. Keenan gave oat bran as beta-glucan to hypertensive patients and reduced BP 7.5 mm Hg/5.5 mm Hg. The doses required to achieve these BP reductions are approximately 60 g of oatmeal per day, 40 g dry weight of oat bran per day, 3 g of beta-glucan per day, or 7 g of psyllium per day [147].

Vitamins

Vitamin C

Vitamin C is a potent water-soluble antioxidant that recycles vitamin E, improves endothelial dysfunction, and produces a diuresis (Table 5.7) [165, 191–195]. The dietary intake of vitamin C or plasma ascorbate concentration in humans is inversely correlated to SBP, DBP, and heart rate [56–58, 196–214]. However, controlled intervention trials have been somewhat less consistent or inconclusive as to the relationship of vitamin C administration and BP [57, 199, 206–208, 209, 215, 216].

Ness et al. [57] published a systematic review on hypertension and vitamin C and concluded that if vitamin C has any effect on BP, it is small. However, in the 18 studies that were reviewed worldwide, 10 of 14 showed a significant BP reduction with increased plasma ascorbate levels and

---

TABLE 5.7
Vitamin C: Mechanisms of Action

- Reduces ED and improves EDVD and lowers BP and SVR in HBP, HLP, CHD, smokers
- Diuresis
- Increase NO and PGI_2
- Decrease adrenal steroid production
- Improve sympathovagal balance
- Decrease cystosolic Ca^{++}
- Antioxidant
- Recycles vitamin E, glutathione, uric acid
- Reduces neuroendocrine peptides
- Reduces thrombosis and decreases TxA_2
- Reduces lipids ($\downarrow$TC, $\downarrow$LDL, $\downarrow$TG, $\uparrow$HDL)
- Reduces leukotrienes
- Improves aortic collagen, elasticity, and aortic compliance
- Increase cGMP and activate VSM K^+ channels

Source: [196–213].

3 of 5 demonstrated a decreased BP with increased dietary vitamin C [57]. In four small, randomized clinical trials of 20 to 57 subjects, one had significant BP reduction, one had no significant BP reduction, and two were not interpretable [57]. In two uncontrolled trials, there was a significant reduction in BP [57].

Duffy et al. [199] evaluated 39 hypertensive subjects (DBP 90 to 110 mm Hg) in a placebo-controlled 4 week study. A 2000 mg loading dose of vitamin C was given initially followed by 500 mg/day. The SBP was reduced 11 mm Hg ($p = 0.03$), DBP decreased by 6 mm Hg ($p = 0.24$), and MAP fell 10 mm Hg ($p < 0.02$).

Fotherby et al. [210] studied 40 mild hypertensive and normotensive patients in a double-blind, randomized, placebo-controlled, crossover study for 6 months. Men and women ages 60 to 80 years (mean age 72 ± 4 years) were given vitamin C 250 mg twice daily for 3 months, and then crossed over after a 1-week washout period. The 24-hour ABM showed a decrease in SBP 2.0 + 5.2 mm Hg ($p < 0.05$), but there was no significant change in DBP. However, the higher the BP was, the greater the response to vitamin C. The conclusion from this study was that vitamin C reduced primarily daytime SBP as measured by 24 hour ABM in hypertensive, but not normotensive patients. In the hypertensive patients, SBP was reduced by 3.7 + 4.2 mm Hg ($p < 0.05$) and DBP fell 1.2 + 3.7 mm Hg (NS).

Block et al. [217] in an elegant depletion-repletion study of vitamin C demonstrated an inverse correlation of plasma ascorbate levels, SBP and DBP. During this 17-week controlled diet study of 68 normotensive men aged 39 to 59 years with mean DBP of 73.4 mm Hg and mean SBP of 122.2 mm Hg, vitamin C depletion at 9 mg/day for 1 month was followed by vitamin C repletion at 117 mg/day repeated twice. Plasma ascorbate was inversely related to DBP ($p < 0.0001$, correlation -0.48) and to SBP in logistic regression. People in the bottom quartile of plasma ascorbate had a DBP 7 mm Hg higher than those in the top quartile. One-fourth of the DBP variance was accounted for by plasma ascorbate alone. Of the other plasma nutrients examined, only ascorbate was significantly and inversely correlated with DBP ($p < 0.0001$, $r = -0.48$) for the 5 week plasma ascorbate levels. Each increase at week five in the plasma ascorbate level was associated with a 2.4 mm Hg lower DBP at week nine.

TABLE 5.8
Vitamin C: Conclusions

1. BP is inversely correlated with vitamin C intake and plasma ascorbate levels in humans and animals in epidemiologic, observational, cross-sectional, and controlled prospective clinical trials.

2. A dose-response relationship between lower BP and higher plasma ascorbate levels is suggested.

   A. DBP fell about 2.4 mm Hg per plasma ascorbate quartile in a depletion repletion study.

   B. SBP fell 3.6 to 17.8 mm Hg for each 50 μmol/L increase in plasma ascorbate level.

   C. BP may be inversely correlated to tissue levels of ascorbate.

   D. Doses of 100 to 1000 mg/day are needed.

3. SBP is reduced proportionately more than DBP, but both are decreased. 24-hour ABM indicates a predominate daytime SBP reduction and lower HR. Office BP shows a reduction in SBP and DBP as well.

4. The greater the initial BP, the greater the BP reduction.

5. BP is reduced in hypertensives, normotensives, hyperlipidemics, diabetics, and in patients with a combination of these diseases.

6. Improves ED in HBP, HLP, PAD, DM, CHD, CHF, smokers, and in conduit arteries, epicardial coronary arteries, and forearm resistance arteries.

7. Long-term epidemiological studies indicate an inverse correlation of vitamin C intake and ascorbate levels with RVR of CVD, CHD, and CVA.

8. The lipid profile seems to be beneficial with small reductions in TC, TG, and LDL and oxLDL and with increases in HDL (women).

9. Combinations of vitamin C with other antioxidants such as vitamin E, beta-carotene, or selenium provide synergistic anti-hypertensive effects.

Most epidemiologic studies demonstrate an inverse relationship between plasma ascorbate levels, dietary intake, and BP, with a reduction in SBP of 3.6 to 17.8 mm Hg for each 50 umol/liter increase in plasma ascorbate [57, 196, 197, 201–205, 218, 219].

The present conclusions correlating vitamin C and BP are shown in Table 5.8. The observational, epidemiologic, and prospective clinical trials point strongly to a role of vitamin C in reducing BP in hypertensive patients and normotensive patients as well as those in other disease categories.

Vitamin D

Epidemiological, clinical, and experimental investigations all demonstrate a relationship between the plasma levels of 1,25-dihydroxycholecalciferol (1,25 $(OH)_2$ D_3), the active form of vitamin D and BP [220–226], including a vitamin-D-mediated reduction in BP in hypertensive patients.

Vitamin D may have an independent and direct role in the regulation of BP [220–222] and insulin metabolism [221, 222]. A study of 34 middle-aged men demonstrated that serum levels of 1,25 (OH_2) D_3 were inversely correlated to BP ($p < 0.02$).

Vascular tissue contains a receptor or receptors for both the calcium-regulating parathyroid hormone and 1,25 $(OH)_2$ D_3 [227]. MacCarthy demonstrated that 1,25 $(OH)_2$ D_3 antagonizes the mitogenic effect of epidermal growth factor on proliferation of vascular smooth muscle cells [228].

Lind, in double-blind, placebo-controlled studies, found that BP was lowered with vitamin D during long-term treatment of patients with intermittent hypercalcemia [223, 224]. In another study, Lind et al. demonstrated that total and ionized calcium levels were increased, but DBP was significantly decreased, and the hypotensive effect of vitamin D was inversely related to the pretreatment serum levels of 1,25 $(OH)_2$ D_3 and additive to antihypertensive medications [225]. In a group of 148 women with low 25 $(OH)_2$ D_3 levels, the administration of 1200 mg calcium plus 800 IU of vitamin D_3 reduced SBP 9.3% more ($p < 0.02$) compared to 1200 mg of calcium alone. The HR fell 5.4% ($p = 0.02$), but DBP was not changed [226].

Vitamin B6 (Pyridoxine)

Vitamin B6 is a readily metabolized and excreted water-soluble vitamin [229]. Six different B6 vitamins exist, but pyridoxal 5′ phosphate (PLP) is the primary and most potent active form. Much of vitamin B6's antihypertensive effects are due to its participation in neurotransmitter and hormone biosynthesis, amino acid reactions with kynureninase, cystathionine synthetase, cystathionase, and membrane L-type calcium channels [229, 230].

One human study by Aybak et al. [231] proved that high-dose vitamin B6 significantly lowered BP. This study compared nine normotensive men and women with 20 hypertensive subjects, all of whom had significantly higher BP, plasma norepinephrine and HR compared to control normotensive patients. Patients received 5 mg/kg/day of vitamin B6 for 4 weeks. The SBP fell from 167 + 13 to 153 + 15 mm Hg, an 8.4% reduction ($p < 0.01$) and the DBP fell from 108 + 8.2 to 98 + 8.8 mm Hg, a 9.3% reduction ($p < 0.005$).

In summary, vitamin B6 has multiple antihypertensive effects that resemble those of central alpha agonists such as clonidine, calcium channel blockers, and diuretics. Finally, changes in insulin sensitivity and carbohydrate metabolism may lower BP in selected hypertensive individuals with the metabolic syndrome of insulin resistance. Chronic intake of vitamin B6 at 200 mg/day is safe and has no adverse effects. Even doses up to 500 mg/day are probably safe [229].

Lycopene (Carotenoid)

Lycopene is a non-provitamin-A carotenoid, a potent antioxidant found in tomatoes and tomato products, guava, pink grapefruit, watermelon, apricots, and papaya in high concentrations [232]. Lycopene has recently been shown to produce a significant reduction in BP, serum lipids, and oxidative stress markers [233, 234]. Paran et al. [234] evaluated 30 patients with Grade I hypertension, ages 40 to 65, taking no antihypertensive or antilipid medications, treated with a tomato lycopene extract for 8 weeks. The SBP was reduced from 144 to 135 mm Hg (9 mm Hg reduction, $p < 0.01$)

and DBP fell from 91 to 84 mm Hg (7 mm Hg reduction, $p < 0.01$). A similar study of 35 subjects with Grade I hypertension showed similar results on SBP, but not DBP [233]. Serum lipids were significantly improved in both studies without change in serum homocysteine.

CoQ10 (Ubiquinone)

Coenzyme Q-10 (CoQ10) is a potent lipid phase antioxidant, free radical scavenger, cofactor and coenzyme in mitochondrial energy production and oxidative phosphorylation that lowers SVR and BP [12, 205, 218, 235–243].

Serum levels of CoQ10 decrease with age and are lower in patients with diseases characterized by oxidative stress such as hypertension, CHD, hyperlipidemia, diabetes mellitus, and atherosclerosis. Enzymatic assays showed a deficiency of CoQ10 in 39% of 59 patients with essential hypertension versus only 6% deficiency in controls ($p < 0.01$) [238]. There is a high correlation of CoQ10 deficiency and hypertension. Supplements are needed to maintain normal serum levels in many of these disease states and in some patients taking statin drugs for hyperlipidemia [205].

Human studies have also demonstrated significant and consistent reductions in BP in hypertensive subjects following oral administration of 100 to 225 mg/day of CoQ10 [219, 235, 237, 238, 242].

Burke et al. [243] conducted a 12-week, randomized, double-blind, placebo-controlled trial with 60 mg of oral CoQ10 in 76 subjects with isolated systolic hypertension (ISH). The mean reduction in SBP in the treated group was 17.8 + 7.3 mm Hg ($p < 0.01$), but DBP did not change. Only 55% of the subjects were responders achieving a reduction in SBP > 4 mm Hg, but in this group the SBP fell 25.9 + 6.4 mm Hg. There was a trend between SBP reduction and increase in CoQ10 levels. Adverse effects were virtually nonexistent.

CoQ10 has consistent and significant antihypertensive effects in patients with essential hypertension. The major conclusions from in vitro, animal and human clinical trials indicate the following:

1. Compared to normotensive patients, essential hypertensive patients have a high incidence of CoQ10 deficiency documented by serum levels.
2. Doses of 120 to 225 mg/day of CoQ10, depending on the delivery method and concomitant ingestion with a fatty meal, are necessary to achieve a therapeutic level of over 2 µg/mL. This dose is usually 1 to 2 mg/kg/day of CoQ10. Use of a special delivery system allows better absorption and lower oral doses.
3. Patients with the lowest CoQ10 serum levels may have the best antihypertensive response to supplementation.
4. The average reduction in BP is about 15/10 mm Hg based on reported studies.
5. The antihypertensive effect takes time to reach its peak level, usually at about 4 weeks, then BP remains stable. The antihypertensive effect is gone within 2 weeks after discontinuation of CoQ10.
6. Approximately 50% of patients on antihypertensive drugs may be able to stop between one and three agents. Both total dose and frequency of administration may be reduced.
7. Even high doses of CoQ10 have no acute or chronic adverse effects.

Alpha-Lipoic Acid

Alpha-lipoic acid is a potent and unique thiol compound-antioxidant that is both water and lipid soluble [165]. Alpha-lipoic acid helps to recirculate tissue and blood levels of vitamins and antioxidants in both lipid and water compartments such as vitamin C and vitamin E, glutathione and cysteine [165, 244, 245]. Alpha-lipoic acid binds excess aldehydes, reduces aldehyde production, and increases aldehyde excretion. The reduction in aldehydes leads to closure of L-type calcium channels, which decreases cystosolic calcium. Lower cystosolic calcium levels reduce systemic vascular resistance and blood pressure [244, 245]. Mechanisms of action are summarized in Table 5.9 and depicted in Figure 5.6. R-alpha-lipoic acid lowers BP in humans in doses of about 200 mg/day.

TABLE 5.9
Alpha-Lipoic Acid Mechanisms of Action

1. Increases levels of glutathione, cysteine, vitamin C and E.

2. Binds endogenous aldehydes, reduces production, and increases excretion.

3. Normalizes membrane calcium channels by providing sulfhydryl groups (-SH) which reduces cytosolic free calcium, SVR, vascular tone, and BP. DHLA is redox partner of alpha lipoic acid.

4. Improves insulin sensitivity and glucose metabolism, reduces advanced glycosylation and products (AGEs) and thus aldehydes.

5. Increases NO levels, stability, and duration of action via increase nitrosothiols such as S-nitrosocysteine and S-nitroglutathione which carry NO.

6. Reduces cytokine-induced generation of NO (iNOS).

7. Inhibits release and translocation of NFκB from cytoplasm into nucleus of cell which decreases controlled gene transcription and regulation of endothelin-I, tissue factor, VCAM-1.

8. Improves ED through beneficial effects on NO, AGEs, vitamin C and E, glutathione, cysteine, endothelin, tissue factor, VCAM-1, linoleic and myristic acid.

9. Reduces monocyte binding to endothelium (VCAM-1).

10. Increases linoleic acid and reduces myristic acid.

Source: [244–245].

L-Arginine

L-arginine is an amino acid that is the primary precursor for the production of nitric oxide (NO) [246, 247], which has numerous cardiovascular effects [219, 247], mediated through conversion of L-arginine to NO by endothelial NOS to increase cyclic GMP levels in vascular smooth muscle,

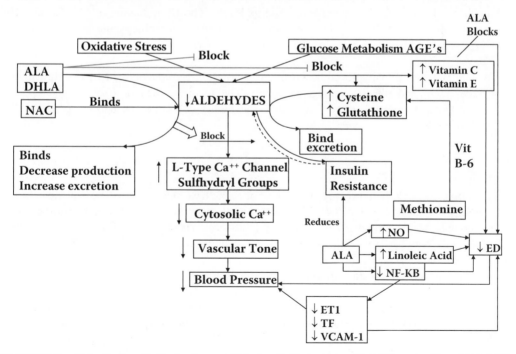

FIGURE 5.6 Alpha-lipoic acid: Mechanism—Aldehydes, Oxidative Stress, Ca++ Channels. (From [244, 245].) ALA = Alpha-lipoic acid, DHLA = Dihydrolipoic acid, NAC = N-acetyl cysteine, ED = Endothelial dysfunction, ET1 = Endothelin, TF = Tissue factor, VCAM-1 = Vascular cell adhesion molecule-1

improve ED, and reduce vascular tone and BP [248]. Patients with hypertension, hyperlipidemia, and atherosclerosis have elevated serum levels of asymmetric dimethylarginine, which inactivates NO [219, 249].

Human studies in hypertensive and normotensive subjects of parenteral and oral administrations of L-arginine demonstrate an antihypertensive effect [248, 250–252]. Siani et al. [248] evaluated six healthy [253], normotensive volunteers. Diet one was the control diet containing 3.5 to 4 g of L-arginine per day. Diet two contained natural-arginine-enriched foods at 10 g of L-arginine per day. Diet three consisted of diet one plus an L-arginine supplement of 10 g/day. The BP decreased significantly in both diets two and three. In diet two, the BP fell 6.2/5.0 mm Hg (p < 0.03 for SBP and p < 0.002 for DBP). In diet three, the BP fell 6.2/6.8 mm Hg (p < 0.01 for SBP and p < 0.006 for DBP).

L-arginine is not normally the rate-limiting step in NO synthesis [254, 255]. Alternative mechanisms may exist whereby l-arginine lowers BP through direct effects of the amino acid on the vasculature or endothelium, as well as release of hormones, vasodilating prostaglandins, improved renal NO or endothelial NO bioavailability [248].

Taurine

Taurine is a sulfonic beta-amino acid that has been used to treat hypertension [256–258], hypercholesterolemia, arrhythmias, atherosclerosis, CHF, and other cardiovascular conditions [256, 257, 259–261].

Human studies have noted that essential hypertensive subjects have reduced urinary taurine as well as other sulfur amino acids [262, 263]. Taurine lowers BP [258–261, 264, 265] and HR [260]; decreases arrhythmias [260], CHF symptoms [260], and SNS activity [258, 260]; increases urinary sodium [264, 266]; and decreases PRA, aldosterone [266], plasma norepinephrine [265], and plasma and urinary epinephrine [258, 267]. A study of 31 Japanese males with essential hypertension placed on an exercise program for 10 weeks showed a 26% increase in taurine levels and a 287% increase in cysteine levels. The BP reduction of 14.8/6.6 mm Hg was proportional to both taurine level elevations and plasma norepinephrine reduction. Fujita et al. [258] reduced BP 9/4.1 mm Hg (p < 0.05) in 19 hypertension subjects given 6 g of taurine for 7 days.

Concomitant use of enalapril with taurine provides additive reductions in BP, LVH, arrhythmias [268, 269], and platelet aggregation [269]. The recommended dose of taurine is 2 to 3 g/day at which no adverse effects are noted, but higher doses may be needed to reduce BP significantly [258].

Specific Foods

Garlic

Clinical trials utilizing the correct type and dose of garlic have shown consistent reductions in BP in hypertensive patients [12, 165, 270–279]. Not all garlic preparations are processed similarly and are not comparable in antihypertensive potency [280–290]. There is a consistent dose-dependent reduction in BP with garlic mediated through the renin angiotensin aldosterone system and the NO system (see Table 5.10) [281].

Approximately 10,000 µg of allicin per day, the amount contained in four cloves or 4 g of garlic, is required to achieve a significant BP-lowering effect [12, 270, 271]. In humans the average reduction in SBP is 5 to 8 mm Hg [291]. Garlic is probably a natural ACEI and CCB that increases bradykinin and NO-inducing vasodilation, reducing systemic vascular resistance (SVR) and BP and improving vascular compliance. Studies supporting the various mechanisms of action are presented in Table 5.10.

Approximately 30 hypertensive clinical trials have been completed to date, and 23 reported results with placebo control, four used nonplacebo controls, and three did not report results [291].

TABLE 5.10
Garlic: Mechanism of Action

- ACEi (Gamma-glutamyl peptides, flavonolic compounds)
- Increase NO [228]
- Decrease sensitivity to NE [228]
- Increase adenosine [228, 229, 230, 231]
- Vasodilation and reduced SVR [277]
- Inhibit AA metabolites (TxA$_2$) [277]
- Reduced aortic stiffness [277]
- Magnesium (natural CCB vasodilator)
- Decreased ROS

Source: [117, 273, 280–290].

These trials studied BP as the primary outcome, and seven excluded concomitant antihypertensive medications. Significant reductions in DBP of 2% to 7% were noted in three trials and reductions in SBP of 3% in one trial when compared to placebo. Other trials reported BP reductions in the garlic-treated subjects (within-group comparisons).

Seaweed

Wakame (*Undaria Pinnatifida*) is the most popular, edible seaweed in Japan [292]. In humans, 3.3 g of dried Wakame for 4 weeks significantly reduced both the SBP 14 + 3 mm Hg and the DBP 5 + 2 mm Hg (p < 0.01) [293]. A study of 62 middle-aged, male patients with mild hypertension given a potassium-loaded, ion-exchanging sodium-adsorbing potassium-releasing seaweed preparation showed significant BP reductions at 4 weeks on 12 and 24 g/day of the seaweed (p < 0.01) [294]. The MAP fell 11.2 mm Hg (p < 0.001) in the sodium-sensitive patients and 5.7 mm Hg (p < 0.05) in the sodium-insensitive patients, which correlated with plasma rennin activity (PRA).

The primary effect of Wakame appears to be through its ACEI activity from at least four parent tetrapeptides and possibly their dipeptide and tripeptide metabolites, especially those containing the amino acid sequence tyrosine-lysine in some combination [292]. Its long-term use in Japan has demonstrated its safety. Many other foods have demonstrated ACEI activity in vitro, but whether they are active after oral ingestion in vivo remains to be proven in human studies [282, 285, 289, 290, 292, 295–311] (Table 5.11).

Celery

Animal studies have demonstrated a significant reduction in BP using a component of celery oil, 3-N-butyl phthalide [312, 313]. Celery, celery extract, and celery oil contain apigenin, which relaxes vascular smooth muscle. CCB-like substances and components that inhibit tyrosine hydroxylase, which reduces plasma catecholamine levels, lower SVR and BP [312, 313]. Consuming four stalks of celery per day, 8 teaspoons of celery juice three times daily, or its equivalent in extract form of celery seed (1000 mg twice a day) or oil (one-half to 1 teaspoon three times daily in tincture form) seems to provide an antihypertensive effect in human essential hypertension [255, 313–315]. In a Chinese study of 16 hypertensive subjects, 14 had significant reductions in BP [313–315]. Celery also has diuretic effects that may reduce BP [313–315].

Pycnogenol

Pycnogenol, a bark extract from the French maritime pine, at doses of 200 mg/day resulted in a significant reduction in systolic BP from 139.9 to 132.7 mm Hg (p < 0.05) in 11 patients with mild

TABLE 5.11

Natural Antihypertensive Compounds Categorized by Antihypertensive Class

Diuretics

1. Hawthorne berry
2. Vitamin B6 (pyridoxine)
3. Taurine
4. Celery
5. GLA
6. Vitamin C (ascorbic acid)
7. K^+
8. Mg^{++}
9. Ca^{++}
10. Protein
11. Fiber
12. CoQ10
13. L-Carnitine

Beta Blockers

1. Hawthorne berry

Central Alpha Agonists (reduce sympathetic nervous system activity)

1. Taurine
2. K^+
3. Zinc
4. Na^+ restriction
5. Protein
6. Fiber
7. Vitamin C
8. Vitamin B6
9. CoQ10
10. Celery
11. Gamma linolenic acid/dihomo gamma linolenic acid (GLA/DGLA)
12. Garlic

Direct Vasodilators

1. Omega-3 FA
2. MUFA (omega-9 fatty acid)
3. K^+
4. Mg^{++}
5. Ca^{++}
6. Soy
7. Fiber
8. Garlic
9. Flavonoids
10. Vitamin C
11. Vitamin E
12. CoQ10
13. L-Arginine
14. Taurine
15. Celery
16. Alpha linolenic acid

Calcium Channel Blockers (CCB)

1. Alpha lipoic acid
2. Vitamin C (ascorbic acid)
3. Vitamin B6 (pyridoxine)
4. Magnesium (Mg^{++})
5. N-acetylcysteine
6. Vitamin E
7. Hawthorne berry
8. Celery
9. Omega-3 fatty acids (EPA and DHA)
10. Calcium
11. Garlic

Angiotensin Converting Enzyme Inhibitors (ACEI)

1. Garlic
2. Seaweed–various (Wakame, etc.)
3. Tuna protein/muscle
4. Sardine protein/muscle
5. Hawthorne berry
6. Bonito fish (dried)
7. Pycnogenol
8. Casein
9. Hydrolyzed whey protein
10. Sour milk
11. Gelatin
12. Sake
13. Essential fatty acids (omega-3 fatty acids)
14. Chicken egg yolks
15. Zein
16. Dried salted fish
17. Fish sauce
18. Zinc
19. Hydrolyzed wheat germ isolate

Angiotensin Receptor Blockers (ARBs)

1. Potassium (K^+)
2. Fiber
3. Garlic
4. Vitamin C
5. Vitamin B6 (pyridoxine)
6. CoQ10
7. Celery
8. Gamma linolenic acid/dihomo gamma linolenic acid (GLA/DGLA)

hypertension over 8 weeks. Diastolic BP fell from 93.8 to 92.0 mm Hg (NS). Serum thromboxane concentrations were significantly reduced ($p < 0.05$) [316].

V. PHARMACOLOGY

Many of the natural compounds in food, certain nutraceutical supplements, vitamins, antioxidants, or minerals function in a similar fashion to a specific class of antihypertensive drugs. Although the potency of these natural compounds may be less than the antihypertensive drug, when used in combination with other nutrients and nutraceuticals, the antihypertensive effect is magnified. Many of these nutrients have varied, additive, and synergistic mechanisms of action in lowering BP. Table 5.11 summarizes these natural compounds into the major antihypertensive drug classes such as diuretics, beta blockers, central alpha agonists, calcium channel blockers, angiotensin-converting enzyme inhibitors, and angiotensin receptor blockers.

VI. SUMMARY AND RECOMMENDATIONS

1. Endothelial dysfunction and vascular smooth muscle dysfunction play a primary role in the initiation and perpetuation of hypertension, CVD, and TOD.
2. Nutrient-gene interactions are a predominant factor in promoting beneficial or detrimental effects in cardiovascular health and hypertension.
3. Natural whole foods and supplemental nutrients can prevent, control, and treat hypertension through numerous vascular biology mechanisms.
4. Oxidative stress initiates and propagates hypertension and cardiovascular disease.
5. Antioxidants can prevent and treat hypertension.
6. Whole-food and phytonutrient concentrates of fruits, vegetables, and fiber with natural combinations of balanced phytochemicals, nutrients, antioxidants, vitamins, minerals, and appropriate macronutrients and micronutrients are generally superior to single component or isolated artificial or single component natural substances for the prevention and treatment of hypertension and CVD.
7. There is a role for the selected use of single and component nutraceuticals, vitamins, antioxidants, and minerals in the treatment of hypertension based on scientifically controlled studies as a complement to optimal nutritional, dietary intake from food and other lifestyle modifications.
8. Exercise, weight reduction, smoking cessation, alcohol and caffeine restriction, as well as other changes in lifestyle must be incorporated.

The clinical approach we use in our clinic is as follows:

Nutrition	Daily Intake
1. DASH I, DASH II-Na$^+$ and PREMIER diets	—
2. Sodium restriction	50–100 mmol
3. Potassium	100 mEq
4. Potassium/sodium ratio	> 5:1
5. Magnesium	1000 mg
6. Zinc	25–50 mg
7. Protein: total intake (30% total calories)	1.0–1.8 g/kg
A. Nonanimal sources preferred but lean or wild animal protein in moderation is acceptable	
B. Hydrolyzed whey protein	30 g
C. Soy protein (fermented is best)	30 g
D. Sardine muscle concentrate extract	3 mg
E. Coldwater fish	3x/week
F. Fowl, poultry	3–4/week

8. Fats: 30% total calories
    - A. Omega-3 fatty acids PUFA   2–3 g
        (DHA, EPA, coldwater fish)
    - B. Omega-6 fatty acids PUFA   1 g
        (canola oil, nuts)
    - C. Omega-9 fatty acids MUFA   4 tablespoons or
        (extra virgin olive oil) (olives)   5–10 olives
    - D. Saturated FA (lean, wild animal meat) (30%)   <10% total calories
    - E. P/S ratio (polyunsaturated/saturated) fats   > 2.0
    - F. Omega-3/Omega-6 PUFA ratio   1:1–1:2
    - G. No *trans* fatty acids   (0%)
        (hydrogenated margarines, vegetable oils)
    - H. Nuts: almonds, walnuts, hazelnuts, etc.
10. Carbohydrates (30% to 40% total calories)
    - A. Reduce or eliminate refined sugars and simple
        carbohydrates
    - B. Increase complex carbohydrates and fiber
        whole grains (oat, barley, wheat)
        vegetables, beans, legumes,
        i.e., oatmeal or   60 g
        oatbran (dry) or   40 g
        beta-glucan or   3 g
        psyllium   7 g
11. Garlic   4 cloves/d
12. Wakame seaweed (dried)   3.0–3.5 g
13. Celery
    Celery stalks or   4 stalks
    Celery juice or   8 teaspoons TID
    Celery seed extract or   1000 mg BID
    Celery oil (tincture)   ½–1 teaspoon TID
14. Lycopene   10 mg
    Tomatoes and tomato products,
    guava, watermelon, apricots, pink grapefruit, papaya

Exercise   **Recommendation**
- Aerobically   7 days/weeks
                              60 minutes day
                              4200 KJ/week
- Resistance training   3x/week to daily

Weight Loss   **Recommendation**
- To ideal body weight (IBW)
- Lose 1–2 pounds/week
- Body mass index (BMI)   < 25
- Waist circumference   < 35 inches in female
                              < 40 inches in male
- Total body fat   < 16% in males
                              < 22% in females
- Increase lean muscle mass

Alcohol Restriction   **Recommendation < 20 g/day**
  Wine   < 10 ounces (preferred – red wine)
  Beer   < 24 ounces
  Liquor   < 2 ounces (100 proof whiskey)

Caffeine Elimination	NONE
Tobacco and Smoking	STOP

Avoid Drugs and Interactions That Increase BP

Vitamins, Antioxidants, and Nutraceutical Supplements	Daily Intake
1. Vitamin C	250 to 500 mg BID
2. Vitamin B6	100 mg QD to BID
3. CoQ10	60 mg QD to BID
4. Lipoic acid (with biotin)	100 to 200 mg BID
5. Taurine	1.0 to 1.5 grams BID
6. L-arginine (food and supplements)	5 grams BID

REFERENCES

1. Ascherio A, Rimm EB, Hernan MA, et al. Intake of potassium, magnesium, calcium and fiber and risk of stroke among US men. *Circulation* 1998; 98:1198–1204.
2. De Lorgeril M, Salen P, Martin JL, Monjaud I, Delaye J, Mamelle N. Mediterranean diet, traditional risk factors and the rate of cardiovascular complications after myocardial infarction: final report of the Lyon diet heart study. *Circulation* 1999; 99:779–785.
3. The Seventh Report of the Joint National Committee on Prevention, Detection, Evaluation, and Treatment of High Blood Pressure (JNC-7). *JAMA* 2003; 289:2560–2572.
4. Krauss R, Deckelbaum R, Ernst N, et al. Dietary guidelines for healthy American adults: a statement for health professionals from the nutrition committee, American Heart Association. *AHA Medical/Scientific Statement* 1996; 94:1795–1800.
5. Institute of Medicine. The role of nutrition in maintaining health in the nation's elderly: evaluating coverage of nutrition services for the medicare population. Washington, DC: National Academy Press, 2000.
6. INTERSALT Cooperative Research Group. INTERSALT: an international study of electrolyte excretion and blood pressure: results for 24-hour urinary sodium and potassium excretion. *BMJ* 1988; 297:319–328.
7. 2003 European Society of Hypertension – European Society of Cardiology Guidelines for the Management of Arterial Hypertension Guidelines Committee. *J Hypertens* 2003; 21:1011–1053.
8. Houston MC, Meador BP, Schipani LM. *Handbook of Antihypertensive Therapy.* 10th Edition. Philadelphia: Hanley and Belfus, Inc., 2000, pp. 1–176.
9. Houston MC. New insights and approaches to reduce end organ damage in the treatment of hypertension: subsets of hypertension approach. *Am Heart J* 1992; 123:1337–1367.
10. Houston MC. New insights and new approaches for the treatment of essential hypertension: selections of therapy based on coronary heart disease risk factor analysis, hemodynamic profiles, quality of life, and subsets of hypertension. *Am Heart J* 1989; 117:911–951.
11. Houston, MC. Hypertension strategies for therapeutic intervention and prevention of end-organ damage. *Primary Care Clin North Am* 1991; 18:713–753.
12. Warner MG. Complementary and alternative therapies for hypertension. *Compl Health Pract Rev* 2000; 6:11–19.
13. Burt VL, Whelton P, Roccella EJ, et al. Prevalence of hypertension in the US adult population: results from the Third National Health and Nutrition Examination Survey, 1988-1991 (comments). *Hypertension* 1995; 25:305–313.
14. Sheps SG, Roccella EJ. Reflections on the sixth report of the Joint National Committee on Prevention, Detection, Evaluation, and Treatment of High Blood Pressure. *Curr Hypertens Rep* 1999; 1: 342–345.
15. Wolf-Maier K, Cooper RS, Banegas JR, et al. Hypertension prevalence and blood pressure levels in six European countries, Canada and the United States. *JAMA* 2003; 289:2363–2369.
16. Akpaffiong MJ, Taylor AA. Antihypertensive and vasodilator actions of antioxidants in spontaneously hypertensive rats. *Hypertension* 1998; 11:1450–1460.
17. Kitiyakara C, Wilcox CS. Antioxidants for hypertension. *Opin Nephrol Hypertens* 1998; 7:531–538.

18. Vaziri ND, Liang K, Ding Y. Increased nitric oxide inactivation by reactive oxygen species in lead-induced hypertension. *Kidney Int* 1999; 56:1492–1498.
19. Griendling KK, Minieri CA, Ollerenshaw JD, Alexander RW. Angiotensin II stimulates NADH and NADDH oxidase activity in cultured vascular endothelial smooth muscle cells. *Circ Res* 1994; 74:1141–1148.
20. Sagar S, et al. Oxygen free radicals in essential hypertension. *Mol Cell Biochem* 1992; 110:103–108.
21. Nayak DU, Karmen C, Frishman WH, Vakili BA. Antioxidant vitamins and enzymatic and synthetic oxygen-derived free radical scavengers in the prevention and treatment of cardiovascular disease. *Heart Dis* 2001; 3:28–45.
22. Gonick HC, Ding Y, Bondy SC, Ni Z, Vaziri ND. Lead-induced hypertension: interplay of nitric oxide and reactive oxygen species. *Hypertension* 1997; 30:1487–1492.
23. Vaziri ND, Ding Y, Ni Z, Gonick HC. Altered nitric oxide metabolism and increased oxygen free radical activity in lead-induced hypertension: effect of lazaroid therapy. *Kidney Int* 1997; 52:1042–1046.
24. Ding Y, Vaziri ND, Gonick HC. Lead-induced hypertension, II: response to sequential infusions of L-arginine, superoxide dismutase, and nitroprusside. *Environ Res* 1998; 76:107–113.
25. Vaziri ND, Ni Z, Zhang YP, Ruzicks EP, Maleki P, Ding Y. Depressed renal and vascular nitric oxide synthase expression in cyclosporine-induced hypertension. *Kidney Int* 1998; 54:482–491.
26. Navarro-Antolin J, Hernandez-Perera O, Lopez-Ongil S, Rodriguez-Puyol M, Rodriguez-Puyol D, Lamas S. CsA and FK506 up-regulate eNOS expression: role of reactive oxygen species and AP-1. *Kidney Int Suppl* 1998; 68:S20–S24.
27. Lopez-Ongil S, Hernandez-Perera O, Navarro-Antolin J, Perez de Lema G, Rodriguez-Puyol M, Lamas S, Rodriguez-Puyol D. Role of reactive oxygen species in the signaling cascade of cyclosporine A-mediated up-regulation of eNOS in vascular endothelial cells. *Br J Pharmacol* 1998; 124:447–454.
28. Vaziri ND, Oveisi F, Ding Y. Role of increased oxygen free radical activity in the pathogenesis of uremic hypertension. *Kidney Int* 1998; 53:1748–1754.
29. Atarashi K, Ishiyama A, Takagi M, Minami M, Kimura K, Goto A, Omata M. Vitamin E ameliorates the renal injury of Dahl salt-sensitive rats. *Am J Hypertens* 1997; 10:116S–119S.
30. Swei A, Lacy F, DeLano FA, Schmid-Schonbein GW. Oxidative stress in the Dahl hypertensive rat. *Hypertension* 1997; 30:1628–1633.
31. Kitiyakara C, Wilcox C. Antioxidants for hypertension. *Curr Opin Nephrol Hypertens* 1998; 7:531–538.
32. Lacy F, O'Conner DT, Schmid-Schonbein GW. Plasma hydrogen peroxide production in hypertensives and normotensive subjects at genetic risk of hypertension. *J Hypertens* 1998; 16:291–303.
33. Tse WY, Maxwell SR, Thomason H, Blann A, Thorpe GH, Waite M, Holder R. Antioxidant status in controlled and uncontrolled hypertension and its relationship to endothelial damage. *J Hum Hypertens* 1994; 89:843–849.
34. Romero-Alvira D, Roche E. High blood pressure, oxygen radicals and antioxidants: etiological relationships. *Med Hypotheses* 1996; 46:414–420.
35. Roggensack AM, Zhang Y, Davidge ST. Evidence for peroxynitrite formation in the vasculature of women with preeclampsia. *Hypertension* 1999; 33:83–89.
36. Giugliano D, Ceriello A, Paolisso G. Diabetes mellitus, hypertension, and cardiovascular disease: which role for oxidative stress? *Metabolism* 1995; 44:363–368.
37. Orie NN, Zidek W, Tepel M. Reactive oxygen species in essential hypertension and non-insulin dependent diabetes mellitus. *Am J Hypertens* 1999; 12:1169–1174.
38. Faure P, Rossini E, Lafond JL, Richard MJ, Favier A, Halimi S. Vitamin E improves the free radical defense system potential and insulin sensitivity of rats fed high fructose diets. *J Nutr* 1997; 127:103–107.
39. Aliev G, Bodin P, Burnstock G. Free radical generators cause changes in endothelial and inducible nitric oxide synthases and endothelin-1 immuno-reactivity in endothelial cells from hyperlipidemic rabbits. *Mol Genet Metab* 1998; 63:191–197.
40. Roberts CK, Vaziri ND, Wang XQ, Barnard RJ. Enhanced NO inactivation and hypertension induced by a high-fat, refined carbohydrate diet. *Hypertension* 2000; 36:423–429.
41. Barnard RJ, Roberts CK, Varon SM, Berger JJ. Diet-induced insulin resistance precedes other aspects of metabolic syndrome. *J Appl Physiol* 1999; 84:1311–1315.
42. Wen Z, Killalea S, McGettigan P, Feely J. Lipid peroxidation and antioxidant vitamins C and E in hypertensive patients. *Ir J Med Sci* 1996; 165:210–212.
43. Kumar KV, Das UN. Are free radicals involved in the pathology of human essential hypertension? *Free Radic Res Commun* 1993; 19:59–66.

44. Russo C, Olivieri O, Girelli D, Faccini G, Zenari ML, Lombardi S, Corrocher R. Antioxidant status and lipid peroxidation in patients with essential hypertension. *J Hypertens* 1998; 16:1267–1271.

45. Laursen JB, Rajagopalan S, Galis Z, Tarpey M, Freeman BA, Harrison DG. Role of superoxide in angiontensin II-induced but not catecholamine-induced hypertension. *Circulation* 1997; 95:588–593.

46. Loverro G, Greco P, Capuano F, Carone D, Cormio G, Selvaggi L. Lipoperoxidation and antioxidant enzymes activity in pregnancy complicated with hypertension. *Eur J Obstet Gynecol Reprod Biol* 1996; 70:123–127.

47. Tse WY, Maxwell SR, Thomason H, Blann A, Thorpe GH, Waite M, Holder R. Antioxidant status in controlled and uncontrolled hypertension and its relationship to endothelial damage. *J Hum Hypertens* 1994; 8:843–849.

48. Villar J, Montilla C, Muniz-Grijalvo O, Muriana FG, Stiefel P, Ruiz-Gutierrez V, et al. Erythrocyte Na^+-Li^+ countertransport in essential hypertension: correlation with membrane lipid levels. *J Hypertens* 1996; 14:969–973.

49. Mihailovic MB, Avramovic DM, Jovanovic IB, Pesut OJ, Matic DP, Stojanov VJ. Blood and plasma selenium levels and GSH-Px activities in patients with arterial hypertension and chronic heart disease. *J Environ Pathol Toxicol Oncol* 1998; 17:285–289.

50. Lacy F, O'Connor DT, Schmid-Schonbein GW. Plasma hydrogen peroxide production in hypertensives and normotensive subjects at genetic risk of hypertension. *J Hypertens* 1998; 16:291–303.

51. Huang A, Sun D, Kaley G, Koller A. Superoxide released to high intra-arteriolar pressure reduces nitric oxide-mediated shear stress- and agonist-induced dilations. *Circ Res* 198; 83:960–965.

52. DeFronzo R, Ferrannini E. Insulin resistance: a multifaceted syndrome responsible for NIDDM, obesity, hypertension, and atherosclerotic cardiovascular disease. *Diabet Care* 1991; 14:173–194.

53. Singal PK, Beamish RE, Dhalla NS. Potential oxidative pathways of catecholamines in the formation of lipid peroxides and genesis of heart disease. *Adv Exp Med Biol* 1983; 161:391–401.

54. Paolisso G, Giugliano D. Oxidative stress and insulin action: is there a relationship? *Diabetolog* 1996; 39:357–363.

55. McIntyre M, Bohr DF, Dominiczak AF. Endothelial function in hypertension. The role of superoxide anion. *Hypertension* 1999; 34:539–545.

56. Ceriello A, Giugliano D, Quatraro A, et al. Anti-oxidants show an anti-hypertensive effect in diabetic and hypertensive subjects. *Clin Sci* 1991; 81:739–742.

57. Ness AR, Chee D, Elliot P. Vitamin C and blood pressure—an overview. *J Hum Hypertens* 1997; 11:343–350.

58. Galley HF, Thornton J, Howdle PD, Walker BE, Webster NR. Combination oral antioxidant supplementation reduces blood pressure. *Clin Sci* 1997; 92:361–365.

59. Dhalla NS, Temsah RM, Netticadam T. The role of oxidative stress in cardiovascular diseases. *J Hypertens* 2000; 18:655–673.

60. Koska J, Syrova D, Blazicek P, et al. Malondialdehyde, lipofuscin and activity of antioxidant enzymes during physical exercise in patients with essential hypertension. *J Hypertens* 1999; 17:529–535.

61. Wolf G. Free radical production and angiotensin. *Curr Hypertens Rep* 2000; 2:167–173.

62. Price PT, Nelson CM, Clarke SD. Omega-3 polyunsaturated fatty acid regulation of gene expression. *Curr Opin Lipidol* 2000; 11:3–7.

63. Talmud PJ, Waterworth DM. In-vivo and in-vitro nutrient-gene interactions. *Curr Opin Lipidol* 2000; 11:31–36.

64. Eaton SB, Eaton SB III, Konner MJ. Paleolithic nutrition revisited: a twelve-year retrospective on its nature and implications. *Eur J Clin Nutr* 1997; 51:207–216.

65. Berdanier CD. Nutrient-gene interactions. In: Ziegler EE, Filer LJ Jr, eds. *Present Knowledge in Nutrition.* 7th Ed. Washington, DC: ILSI Press, 1996, pp. 574–580.

66. Khaw K-T, Barrett-Connor E. Dietary potassium and stroke-associated mortality: a 12-year prospective population study. *N Engl J Med* 1987; 316:235–240.

67. He J, Ogden LG, Vupputuri S, et al. Dietary sodium intake and subsequent risk of cardiovascular disease in overweight adults. *JAMA* 1999; 282:2027–2034.

68. Sacks FM, Svetkey LP, Vollmer WM, Appel LJ, Bray GA, et al. Effects on blood pressure of reduced dietary sodium and the dietary approaches to stop hypertension (DASH) diet. *N Engl J Med* 2001; 344:3–10.

69. Broadhurst CL. Balanced intakes of natural triglycerides for optimum nutrition: an evolutionary and phytochemical perspective. *Med Hypotheses* 1997; 49:247–261.

70. Ravnskov U. The questionable role of saturated and polyunsaturated fatty acids in cardiovascular disease. *J Clin Epidemiol* 1998; 51:443–460.

71. Gillman MW, Cupples A, Millen BE. Inverse association of dietary fats with development of ischemic stroke in men. *JAMA* 1997; 278:2145–2150.

72. Ascherio A, Willett WC. Health effects of *trans* fatty acids. *Am J Clin Nutr* 1997; 66:1006S–1010S.

73. Tavani A, Negri E, D'Avanzo B, et al. Margarine intake and risk of nonfatal acute myocardial infarction on Italian women. *Eur J Clin Nutr* 1997; 51:30–32.

74. Appel LJ, Moore TJ, Obarzanek E, et al. A clinical trial of the effects of dietary patterns on blood pressure. *N Engl J Med* 1997; 336:1117–1124.

75. Desvergne B, Wahli W. Peroxisome proliferator-activated receptors: nuclear control of metabolism. *Endocr Rev* 1999; 20:649–688.

76. Jump DB, Clarke SD. Regulation of gene expression by dietary fat. *Annu Rev Nutr* 1999; 19:63–90.

77. Stabile LP, Klautky SA, Minor SM, Salati LM. Polyunsaturated fatty acids inhibit the expression of the glucose-6-phosphate dehydrogenase gene in primary rat hepatocytes by a nuclear posttranscriptional mechanism. *J Lipid Res* 1998; 39:1951–1963.

78. Weiss SL, Sunde RA. Selenium regulation of classical glutathione peroxidase expression requires the $3'$ untranslated region in Chinese hamster ovary cells. *J Nutr* 1997; 127:1304–1310.

79. Kotchen TA, McCarron DA. AHA Science Advisory. Dietary electrolytes and blood pressure. *Circulation* 1998; 98:613–617.

80. Midgley JP, Matthew AG, Greenwood CM, Logan AG. Effect of reduced dietary sodium on blood pressure: a meta-analysis of randomized controlled trials [comments]. *JAMA* 1996; 275:1590–1597.

81. Cutler JA, Follmann, Allender PS. Randomized trials of sodium reduction: an overview. *Am J Clin Nutr* 1997; 65:643S–651S.

82. Graudal NA, Galloe AM, Garred P. Effects of sodium restriction on blood pressure, renin, aldosterone, catecholamines, cholesterols, and triglyceride: a meta-analysis. *JAMA* 1998; 279:1383–1391.

83. Svetkey LP, Sacks FM, Obarzanek E, et al. The DASH diet, sodium intake and blood pressure (the DASH-Sodium Study): rationale and design. *JADA* 1999; 99:S96–S104.

84. Egan BM, Lackland DT. Biochemical and metabolic effects of very-low-salt diets. *Am J Med Sci* 2000; 320:233–239.

85. Hamet P, Daignault-Gelinas M, Lambert J, Ledoux M, Whissell-Cambiotti L, Bellavance F, Mongean E. Epidemiological evidence of an interaction between calcium and sodium intake impacting on blood pressure: a Montreal study. *Am J Hypertens* 1992; 5:378–385.

86. Liu ZQ, Yang JJ, Mu YM, Liang YX, Wang DJ, Zhu CF, Sun TY. Adding potassium and calcium to the dietary salt as a hypertension-preventive approach in adolescents with higher blood pressure and their family members: a single blind randomized-controlled trial. *Am J Hypertens* 2001; 14:145A. Abstract P-345.

87. Kotchen TA, Kotchen JM. Dietary sodium and blood pressure: interactions with other nutrients. *Am J Clin Nutr* 1997; 65:708S–711S.

88. Morris CD. Effect of dietary sodium restriction on overall nutrient intake. *Am J Clin Nutr* 1997; 65:687S–691S.

89. Hu G, Tian H. A comparison of dietary and non-dietary factors of hypertension and normal blood pressure in a Chinese population. *J Hum Hypertens* 2001; 15:487–493.

90. Perry IJ, Beevers DG. Salt intake and stroke: a possible direct effect. *J Hum Hypertens* 1992; 6:23–25.

91. Reid R, Lindop G, Brown W, Lever AF, Lucie N, Webb D. Similar blood pressure but different outcome in rats with DOC and post-DOC hypertension. *J Hypertens* 1983; 1:303–310.

92. Messerli FH, Schmieder RE, Weir MR. Salt: a perpetrator of hypertensive target organ disease? *Arch Intern Med* 1997; 157:2449–2452.

93. Langenfeld MRW, Schmieder RE, Schobel HP, Friedrich A. Dietary salt intake and left ventricular diastolic function in early essential hypertension. In: Program and Abstracts of the XVI Scientific Meeting of the International Society of Hypertension; June 26, 1996; Glasgow, Scotland. Abstract 128.2.

94. Gu J-W, Anand V, Shek EW, et al. Sodium induces hypertrophy of cultured myocardial myoblasts and vascular smooth muscle cells. *Hypertension* 1998; 31:1083–1087.

95. Yu HCM, Burrell LM, Black MJ, et al. Salt induces myocardial and renal fibrosis in normotensive and hypertensive rats. *Circulation* 1998; 98:2621–2628.

96. Heeg JE, de Jong PE, van der Hem GK, de Zeeuw D. Efficacy and variability of the antiproteinuric effect of ACE inhibition by lisinopril. *Kidney Int* 1989; 36:272–279.

97. Bakris GL, Smith A. Effects of sodium intake on albumin excretion in patients with diabetic nephropathy treated with long-acting calcium antagonists. *Ann Intern Med* 1996; 125:201–204.

98. Safar ME, Asmar RG, Benetos A, London GM, Levy BI. Sodium, large arteries and diuretic compounds in hypertension. *J Hypertens Suppl* 1992; 10:S133–S136.

99. Draaijer P, Kool MJ, Maessen JM, et al. Vascular distensibility and compliance in salt-sensitive and salt-resistant borderline hypertension. *J Hypertens* 1993; 11:1199–1207.

100. Kawasaki T, Delea CS, Bartter FC, Smith H. The effect of high-sodium and low-sodium intakes on blood pressure and other related variables in human subjects with idiopathic hypertension. *Am J Med* 1978; 64:193–198.

101. Weinberger MH. Salt sensitivity of blood pressure in humans. *Hypertension* 1996; 27:481–490.

102. Morimoto A, Usu T, Fujii T, et al. Sodium sensitivity and cardiovascular events in patients with essential hypertension. *Lancet* 1997; 350:1734–1737.

103. Weinberger MH, Fineberg NS, Fineberg SE, Weinberger M. Salt sensitivity, pulse pressure and death in normal and hypertensive humans. *Hypertens* 2001; 37:429–432.

104. Weinberger MH, Miller JZ, Luft FC, Grim CE, Fineberg NS. Definitions and characteristics of sodium sensitivity and blood pressure resistance. *Hypertens* 1986; 8:127–134.

105. Johnson AG, Nguyen TV, Davis D. Blood pressure is linked to salt intake and modulated by the angiotensinogen gene in normotensive and hypertensive elderly subjects. *J Hypertens* 2001; 19: 1053–1060.

106. Miyajima E, Yamada Y. Reduced sympathetic inhibition in salt-sensitive Japanese young adults. *Am J Hypertens* 1999; 12:1195–1200.

107. Cubeddu LX, Alfieri AB, Hoffmann IS, Jimenez E, Roa CM, et al. Nitric oxide and salt sensitivity. *Am J Hypertens* 2000; 13:973–979.

108. McCarron DA. Diet and blood pressure--the paradigm shift. *Science* 1998; 281:933–934.

109. Das UN. Minerals, trace elements, and vitamins interact with essential fatty acids and prostaglandins to prevent hypertension, thrombosis, hypercholesterolaemia and atherosclerosis and their attendant complications. *IRCS Med Sci* 1985; 13:684.

110. Birkett NJ. Comments on a meta-analysis of the relation between dietary calcium intake and blood pressure. *Am J Epidemiol* 1998; 148:223–228.

111. Whelton PK, He J. Potassium in preventing and treating high blood pressure. *Semin Nephrol* 1999; 19:494–499.

112. Siani A, Strazzullo P, Giacco A, Pacioni D, Celentano E, Mancini M. Increasing the dietary potassium intake reduces the need for antihypertensive medication. *Ann Intern Med* 1991; 115:753–759.

113. Whelton PK, He J, Cutler JA, et al. Effects of oral potassium on blood pressure: meta-analysis of randomized controlled clinical trials. *JAMA* 1997; 227:1624–1632.

114. McCarron DA, Reusser ME. Nonpharmacologic therapy in hypertension: from single components to overall dietary management. *Prog Cardiovasc Dis* 1999; 41:451–460.

115. Gu D, He J, Xigui W, Duan X, Whelton PK. Effect of potassium supplementation on blood pressure in Chinese: a randomized, placebo-controlled trial. *J Hypertens* 2001; 19:1325–1331.

116. Ahsan SK. Magnesium in health and disease. *J Pak Med Assoc* 1998; 48:246–250.

117. Weiss D. Cardiovascular disease: risk factors and fundamental nutrition. *Int J Integrative Med* 2000; 2:6–12.

118. Widman L, Wester PO, Stegmayr BG, Wirell MP. The dose dependent reduction in blood pressure through administration of magnesium: a double blind placebo controlled cross-over trial. *Am J Hypertens* 1993; 6:41–45.

119. Paolisso G, Gambardella A, Balbi V, Galzerano D, Verza M, Varricchio M, D'Onofrio F. Effects of magnesium and nifedipine on insulin action, substrate oxidation and blood pressure in aged subjects. *Am J Hypertens* 1993; 6:920–926.

120. Kisters K, Krefting ER, Barenbrock M, Spieker C, Rahn KH. Na$^+$ and Mg2$^+$ contents in smooth muscle cells in spontaneously hypertensive rats. *Am J Hypertens* 1999; 12:648–652.

121. Sanders GM, Sim KM. Is it feasible to use magnesium sulfate as a hypotensive agent in oral and maxillofacial surgery? *Ann Acad Med Singapore* 1998; 27:780–785.

122. Altura BM, Altura BT, Carella A. Magnesium deficiency-induced spasms of umbilical vessels: relation to preeclampsia, hypertension, growth retardation. *Science* 1983; 221:376–378.

123. Saris NE, Mervaala E, Karppanen H, Khawaja JA, Lewenstam A. Magnesium. An update on physiological, clinical and analytical aspects. *Clin Chim Acta* 2000; 294:1–26.

124. Sudhakar K, Sujatha M, Rao VB, Jyothy A, Reddy PP. Serum and erythrocyte magnesium levels in hypertensives and their first degree relatives. *J Indian Med Assoc* 1999; 97:211–213.

125. Corica F, Corsonello A, Buemi M, De Gregorio T, Malara A, Mauro VN, Macaione S, Ientile R. Platelet magnesium depletion in normotensive and hypertensive obese subjects: the role of salt-regulating hormones and catecholamines. *Magnes Res* 1999; 12:287–296.

126. Resnick LM. Magnesium in the pathophysiology and treatment of hypertension and diabetes mellitus: where are we in 1997? *Am J Hypertens* 1997; 10:368–370.

127. Laurant P, Touyz RM. Physiological and pathophysiological role of magnesium in the cardiovascular system: implications in hypertension. *J Hypertens* 2000; 18:1177–1191.

128. Haenni A, Johansson K, Lind L, Lithell H. Magnesium improves endothelium-dependent vasodilation in the human forearm. *Am J Hypertens* 2001; 14:68A. Abstract P-116.

129. Siegel G, Walter A, Gustavsson H, Lindman B. Magnesium and membrane function in vascular smooth muscle. *Artery* 1981; 9:232–252.

130. McCarron DA. Role of adequate dietary calcium intake in the prevention and management of salt sensitive hypertensive. *Am J Clin Nutr* 1997; 65:712S–716S.

131. Cappuccio FP, Elliott P, Allender PS, et al. Epidemiologic association between dietary calcium intake and blood pressure: a meta-analysis of published data. *Am J Epidemiol* 1995; 142:935–945.

132. Allender PS, Cutler JA, Follmann D, et al. Dietary calcium and blood pressure: a meta-analysis of randomized clinical trials. *Ann Intern Med* 1996; 124:825–831.

133. McCarron DA. Calcium metabolism in hypertension. *Keio J Med* 1995; 44:105–114.

134. Witteman JCM, Willett WC, Stampfer MJ, et al. A prospective study of nutritional factors and hypertension among US women. *Circulation* 1989; 80:1320–1327.

135. Bucher HC, Cook RJ, Guyatt GH, et al. Effects of dietary calcium supplementation on blood pressure. A meta-analysis of randomized controlled trials. *JAMA* 1996; 275:1016–1022.

136. Griffith L, Guyatt GH, Cook RJ, et al. The influence of dietary and nondietary calcium supplementation on blood pressure: an updated meta-analysis of randomized clinical trials. *Am J Hypertens* 1999; 12:84–92.

137. Karanja N, Morris CD, Rufolo P, et al. The impact of increasing dietary calcium intake on nutrient consumption, plasma lipids and lipoproteins in humans. *Am J Hypertens* 1994; 59:900–907.

138. Obarzanek E, Velletri PA, Cutler JA. Dietary protein and blood pressure. *JAMA* 1996; 274:1598–1603.

139. Stamler J, Elliott P, Kesteloot H, Nichols R, Claeys G, Dyer AR, Stamler R. Inverse relation of dietary protein markers with blood pressure. Findings for 10,020 men and women in the Intersalt Study. Intersalt Cooperative Research Group. International study of salt and blood pressure. *Circulation* 1996; 94:1629–1634.

140. He J, Welton PK. Effect of dietary fiber and protein intake on blood pressure: a review of epidemiologic evidence. *Clin Exp Hypertens* 1999; 21:785–796.

141. Zhou B. The relationship of dietary animal protein and electrolytes to blood pressure. A study on three Chinese populations. *Int J Epidemiol* 1994; 23:716–722.

142. Elliott P, Dennis B, Dyer AR, et al. Relation of dietary protein (total, vegetable, animal) to blood pressure: INTERMAP epidemiologic study. Presented at the 18th Scientific Meeting of the International Society of Hypertension, Chicago, IL, August 20-24, 2000.

143. Wolfe BM. Potential role of raising dietary protein intake for reducing risk of atherosclerosis. *Can J Cardiol* 1995; 11:127G–131G.

144. Kawase M, Hashimoto H, Hosoda M, Morita H, Hosono A. Effect of administration of fermented milk containing whey protein concentrate to rats and healthy men on serum lipids and blood pressure. *J Dairy Sci* 2000; 83:255–263.

145. Groziak SM, Miller GD. Natural bioactive substances in milk and colostrum: effects on the arterial blood pressure system. *Br J Nutr* 2000; 84:S119–S125.

146. Barr SI, McCarron DA, Heaney RP, Dawson-Hughes B, Berga SL, Stern JS, Oparil S. Effects of increased consumption of fluid milk on energy and nutrient intake, body weight, and cardiovascular risk factors in healthy older adults. *J Am Diet Assoc* 2000; 100:810–817.

147. Hasler CM, Kundrat S, Wool D. Functional foods and cardiovascular disease. *Curr Atheroscler Rep* 2000; 2:467–475.

148. Tikkanen MJ, Adlercreutz H. Dietary soy-derived isoflavone phytoestrogens: could they have a role in coronary heart disease prevention? *Biochem Pharmacol* 2000; 60:1–5.

149. Pitre M, Santure M, Bachelard H. Antihypertensive effects of whey protein hydrolysates in conscious, unrestrained spontaneously hypertensive rats. Hypertension Research Unit, Pavillon CHUL Research Center, Laval University, Ste-Foy, Quebec, Canada. (Unpublished data by permission.)

150. Pins J, Keenan J. The antihypertensive effects of a hydrolyzed whey protein supplement. *Cardiovasc Drugs Ther* 2002; 16(Suppl):68.

151. Yamamoto N, Akino A, Takano T. Antihypertensive effect of different kinds of fermented milk in spontaneously hypertensive rats. *Biosci Biotechnol Biochem* 1994; 58:776–778.

152. Kawasaki T, Seki E, Osajima K, Yoshida M, Asada K, Matsui T, Osajima Y. Antihypertensive effect of valyl-tyrosine, a short chain peptide derived from sardine muscle hydrolyzate, on mild hypertensive subjects. *J Hum Hypertens* 2000; 14:519–523.

153. Kuchel O. Differential catecholamine responses to protein intake in healthy and hypertensive patients. *Am J Physiol* 1998; 275:R1164–R1173.
154. Millward DJ. Optimal intakes of protein in the human diet. *Proc Nutr Soc* 1999; 58:403–413.
155. Lemon PWR. Is increased dietary protein necessary or beneficial for individuals with a physically active lifestyle? *Nutr Rev* 1996; 54:S169–S175.
156. Morris MC. Dietary fats and blood pressure. *J Cardiovasc Risk* 1994; 1:21–30.
157. National Diet Heart Study Research Group. The National Diet Heart Study final report. *Circulation* 1968; 37–38:1228–1230.
158. Chee D, Stamler J. Relationship of dietary linolenic acid and omega-3 PUFA to BP: results from the MRFIT #2. AHA 40th Annual Conference on Cardiovascular Disease Epidemiology and Prevention. March 1-4, 2000. San Diego.
159. Witteman J, Willett W, Stampfer M, Golditz G, Sacks F, Speizer F, et al. A prospective study of nutritional factors and hypertension among US women. *Circulation* 1989; 80:1320–1327.
160. Ascherio A, Rimm EB, Giovannucci EL, Colditz GA, Rosner B, Willett WC, Sacks F, Stampfer MJ. A prospective study of nutritional factors and hypertension among US men. *Circulation* 1992; 86:1475–1484.
161. Mori TA, Bao DQ, Burke V, Puddey IB, Watts GF, Beilin LJ. Dietary fish as a major component of a weight-loss diet: effect on serum lipids, glucose and insulin metabolism in overweight hypertensive subjects. *Am J Clin Nutr* 1999; 70:817–825.
162. Baur LA, O'Connor J, Pan DA, Kriketos AD, Storlien LH. The fatty acid composition of skeletal muscle membrane phospholipid: its relationship with the type of feeding and plasma glucose levels in young children. *Metabolism* 1998; 47:106–112.
163. Bao DQ, Mori TA, Burke V, et al. Effects of dietary fish and weight reduction on ambulatory blood pressure in overweight hypertensives. *Hypertension* 1998; 32:710–717.
164. Mori TA, Bao DQ, Burke V, Puddey IB, Beilin LJ. Docosahexaenoic acid but not eicosapentaenoic acid lowers ambulatory blood pressure and heart rate in humans. *Hypertension* 1999; 34:253–260.
165. DeBusk RM. Dietary supplements and cardiovascular disease. *Curr Atheroscler Rep* 2000; 2:508–514.
166. Alexander JW. Immunonutrition: the role of omega-3 fatty acids. *Nutrition* 1998; 14:627–633.
167. Toft I, Bønaa KH, Ingebretsen OC, Nordøy A, Jenssen T. Effects of ω-3 polyunsaturated fatty acids on glucose homeostasis and blood pressure in essential hypertension: a randomized, controlled trial. *Ann Intern Med* 1995; 123:911–918.
168. Bønaa KH, Bjerve KS, Straume B, Gram IT, Thelle D. Effect of eicosapentaenoic and docosahexaenoic acids on blood pressure in hypertension: a population-based intervention trial from the Tromso study. *N Engl J Med* 1990; 322:795–801.
169. Knapp HR, FitzGerald GA. The antihypertensive effects of fish oil: a controlled study of polyunsaturated fatty acid supplements in essential hypertension. *N Engl J Med* 1989; 320:1037–1043.
170. Appel LJ, Miller ER, Seidler AJ, Whelton PK. Does supplementation of diet with 'fish oil' reduce blood pressure? A meta-analysis of controlled clinical trials. *Arch Intern Med* 1993; 153:1429–1438.
171. Engler MM, Engler MB, Goodfriend TL, Ball DL, Yu Z, Su P, Koretz DL. Docosahexaenoic acid is an anti-hypertensive nutrient that affects aldosterone production in SHR. *Proc Soc Exp Biol Med* 1999; 221:32–38.
172. Prisco D, Paniccia R, Bandinelli B, Filippini M, Francalanci I, Giusti B, Giurlani L, Gensini GF, Abbate R, Neri Serner GG. Effect of medium-term supplementation with a moderate dose of n-3 polyunsaturated fatty acids on blood pressure in mild hypertensive patients. *Thromb Res* 1998; 91:105–112.
173. Rousseau D, Moreau D, Raederstorff D, Sergiel JP, Rupp H, Muggli R, Grynberg A. Is a dietary n-3 fatty acid supplement able to influence the cardiac effect of the psychological stress? *Mol Cell Biochem.* 1998; 178:353–366.
174. Health effects of omega 3 polyunsaturated fatty acids in seafoods. In: Simopoulos AP, Kifer RR, Martin RE, Barlow SM, eds. *World Rev Nutr Dietet.* Vol. 66. Basel: Karger, 1991, pp. 1–592.
175. Woodcock BE, Smith E, Lambert WH, Jones WM, Galloway JH, Greaves M, Preston FE. Beneficial effect of fish oil on blood viscosity in peripheral vascular disease. *BMJ* 1984; 288:592–594.
176. Morris M, Sacks F, Rosner B. Does fish oil lower blood pressure? A meta-analysis of controlled trials. *Circulation* 1993; 88:523–533.
177. Engler MB, Ma YH, Engler MM. Calcium-mediated mechanisms of eicosapentaenoic acid-induced relaxation in hypertension rat aorta. *Am J Hypertens* 1999; 12:1225–1235.
178. Hassall CH, Kirtland SJ. Dihomo-gamma-linolenic acid reverses hypertension induced in rats by diets rich in saturated fat. *Lipids* 1984; 19:699–703.
179. Mills DE, Ward R. Attenuation of psychosocial stress-induced hypertension by gamma-linolenic acid (GLA) administration in rats. *Proc Soc Exp Biol Med* 1984; 176:32–37.

180. Engler MM, Schambelan M, Engler MB, Ball DL, Goodfriend TL. Effects of gamma-linolenic acid on blood pressure and adrenal angiotensin receptors in hypertensive rats. *Proc Soc Exp Biol Med* 1998; 218:234–237.

181. Mamalakis G, Kafatos A, Tornaritis M, Alevizos B. Anxiety and adipose essential fatty acid precursors for prostaglandin E1 and E2. *J Am Coll Nutr* 1998; 17:239–243.

182. Ferrara LA, Raimondi S, d'Episcopa I, et al. Olive oil and reduced need for antihypertensive medications. *Arch Intern Med* 2000; 160:837–842.

183. Papadopoulos G, Boskou D. Antioxidant effect of natural phenols in olive oil. *J Am Oil Chem Soc* 1991; 68:669–671.

184. Mensink RP, Katan MB. Effect of dietary fatty acids on serum lipids and lipoproteins: a meta-analysis of 27 trials. *Arterioscler Thromb* 1992; 12:911–919.

185. Reaven P, Parthasarathy S, Grasse BJ, Miller E, Steinberg D, Witzum JL. Effects of oleate-rich and linoleate-rich diets on the susceptibility of low density lipoprotein to oxidative modification in mildly hypercholesterolemic subjects. *J Clin Invest* 1993; 91:668–676.

186. He J, Whelton PK. Effect of dietary fiber and protein intake on blood pressure: a review of epidemiologic evidence. *Clin Exp Hypertens* 1999; 21:785–796.

187. Pereira MA, Pins JJ. Dietary fiber and cardiovascular disease: experimental and epidemiologic advances. *Curr Atheroscler Rep* 2000; 2:494–502.

188. Vuksan V, Jenkins DJA, Spadafora P, et al. Konjac-Mannan (Glucomannan) improves glycemia and other associated risk factors for coronary heart disease in type 2 diabetes. *Diabet Care* 1999; 22:913–919.

189. Keenan JM, Pins JJ, Frazel C, et al. Oat ingestion reduces systolic and diastolic blood pressure among moderate hypertensives: a pilot trial. *J Fam Pract* 2000 (In Press).

190. Pins JJ, Geleva D, Keenan JM, et al. Whole grain cereals reduce antihypertensive medication need, blood lipid and plasma glucose levels. *J Am Coll Nutr* 1999; 18:529. Abstract.

191. Sherman DL, Keaney JF, Biegelsen ES, et al. Pharmacological concentrations of ascorbic acid are required for the beneficial effect on endothelial vasomotor function in hypertension. *Hypertension* 2000; 35:936–941.

192. Ting HH, Creager MA, Ganz P, Roddy MA, Haley EA, Timimi FK. Vitamin C improves endothelium-dependent vasodilation in forearm resistance vessels of humans with hypercholesterolemia. *Circulation* 1997; 95:2617–2622.

193. Taddei S, Virdis A, Ghiadoni L, Magagna A, Salvetti A. Vitamin C improves endothelium-dependent vasodilation by restoring nitric oxide activity in essential hypertension. *Circulation* 1998; 97:2222–2229.

194. Levine GN, Frei B, Koulouris SN, Gerhard MD, Keaney JF, Vita JA. Ascorbic acid reverses endothelial vasomotor dysfunction in patients with coronary artery disease. *Circulation* 1996; 93:1107–1113.

195. Heitzer T, Just H, Münzel T. Antioxidant vitamin C improves endothelial dysfunction in chronic smokers. *Circulation* 1996; 94:6–9.

196. Bates CJ, Walmsley CM, Prentice A, Finch S. Does vitamin C reduce blood pressure? Results of a large study of people aged 65 or older. *J Hypertens* 1998; 16:925–932.

197. Ness AR, Khaw K-T, Bingham S, Day NE. Vitamin C status and blood pressure. *J Hypertens* 1996; 14:503–508.

198. Moran JP, Cohen L, Green JM, Xu G, Feldman EB, Hames CG, Feldman DS. Plasma ascorbic acid concentrations relate inversely to blood pressure in human subjects. *Am J Clin Nutr* 1993; 57:213–217.

199. Duffy SJ, Gokce N, Holbrook M, et al. Treatment of hypertension with ascorbic acid. *Lancet* 1999; 354:2048–2049.

200. Schilling J, Holzer P, Guggenbach M, Gyurech D, Marathia K, Geroulanos S. Reduced endogenous nitric oxide in the exhaled air of smokers and hypertensives. *Eur Respir J* 1994; 7:467–471.

201. Hemila H. Vitamin C and lowering of blood pressure: need for intervention trials? *J Hypertens* 1991; 9:1076–1077.

202. Feldman EB. The role of vitamin C and antioxidants in hypertension. *Nutr M.D.* 1998; 24:1–4.

203. Trout DL. Vitamin C and cardiovascular risk factors. *Am J Clin Nutr* 1991; 53:322–325.

204. Salonen JT, Salonen R, Ihanainen M, et al. Blood pressure, dietary fats, and antioxidants. *Am J Clin Nutr* 1988; 48:1226–1232.

205. Enster L, Dallner G. Biochemical, physiological and medical aspects of ubiquinone function. *Biochim Biophys Acta* 1995; 1271:195–204.

206. Simon JA. Vitamin C and cardiovascular disease: a review. *J Am Coll Nutr* 1992; 11:107–125.

207. Osilesi O, Trout DL, Ogunwole J. Glover EE. Blood pressure and plasma lipids during ascorbic acid supplementation in borderline hypertensive and normotensive adults. *Nutr Res* 1991; 11:405–412.

208. Lovat LB, Lu Y, Palmer AJ, Edwards R, Fletcher AE, Bulpitt CJ. Double blind trial of vitamin C in elderly hypertensives. *J Hum Hypertens* 1993; 7:403–405.

209. Ghosh SK, Ekpo EB, Shah IU, Girling AJ, Jenkins C, Sinclair AJ. A double-blind placebo controlled parallel trial of vitamin C treatment in elderly patients with hypertension. *Gerontology* 1994; 40: 268–272.

210. Fotherby MD, Williams JC, Forster LA, Craner P, Ferns GA. Effect of vitamin C on ambulatory blood pressure and plasma lipids in older persons. *J Hypertens* 2000; 18:411–415.

211. Koh ET. Effect of vitamin C on blood parameters of hypertensive subjects. *J Okla State Med Assoc* 1984; 77:177–182.

212. Block G, Mangels AR, Patterson BH, Levander OA, Norkus E, Taylor PR. Body weight and prior depletion affect plasma ascorbate levels attained on identical vitamin C intake: a controlled-diet study. *J Am Coll Nutr* 1999; 18:628–637.

213. Grossman M, Dobrev D, Himmel HM, Ravens U, Kirsh W. Ascorbic acid-induced modulation of venous tone in humans. *Hypertension* 2001; 37:949–954.

214. Yoshioka M, Aoyama K, Matsoshita T. Effects of ascorbic acid on blood pressure and ascorbic acid metabolism in spontaneously hypertensive rats. *Int J Vitam Nutr Res* 1985; 55:301–307.

215. Gale CR, Martyn CN, Winter PD, Cooper C. Vitamin C and risk of death from stroke and coronary heart disease in cohort of elderly people. *BMJ* 1995; 310:1563–1566.

216. Egan DA, Garg R, Wilt TJ, et al. Rationale and design of the arterial disease multiple intervention trial (ADMIT) pilot study. *Am J Cardiol* 1999; 83:569–575.

217. Block G, Mangels AR, Norkus EP, Patterson BH, Levander OA, Taylor PR. Ascorbic acid status and subsequent diastolic and systolic blood pressure. *Hypertension* 2001; 37:261–267.

218. Cooke JP. Nutraceuticals for cardiovascular health. *Am J Cardiol* 1998: 82:43S–45S.

219. Kendler BS. Nutritional strategies in cardiovascular disease control: an update on vitamins and conditionally essential nutrients. *Prog Cardiovasc Nurs* 1999; 14:124–129.

220. Dakshinamurti K, Lal KJ. Vitamins and hypertension from Simopoulos AP (ed): Nutrients in the control of metabolic diseases. *World Rev Nutr Diet*. Basal, Karger, 1996; 69:40–73.

221. Hanni LL, Huarfner LH, Sorensen OH, Ljunghall S. Vitamin D is related to blood pressure and other cardiovascular risk factors in middle-aged men. *Am J Hypertens* 1995; 8:894–901.

222. Boucher BJ. Inadequate vitamin D status: does it contribute to the disorders comprising syndrome 'X'? *Br J Nutr* 1998; 79:315–327.

223. Lind L, Wengle BO, Junghall S. Blood pressure is lowered by vitamin D (alphacalcidol) during long term treatment of patients with intermittent hypercalcemia. *Acta Med Scand* 1987; 222:423–427.

224. Lind L, Lithell H, Skarfos E, et al. Reduction of blood pressure by treatment with alphacalcidol. *Acta Med Scand* 1988; 223:211–217.

225. Lind L, Wengle BO, Wide L, Sorensen OH, Ljunghall S. Hypertension in primary hyperparathyroidism—reduction of blood pressure by long-term treatment with vitamin D (alphacalcidol). A double-blind, placebo-controlled study. *Am J Hypertens* 1988; 1:397–402.

226. Pfeifer M, Begerow B, Minne HW, Nachtigall D, Hansen C. Effects of a short-term vitamin D(3) and calcium supplementation on blood pressure and parathyroid hormone levels in elderly women. *J Clin Endocrinol Metab* 2001; 86:1633–1637.

227. Bukoski RD, McCarron DA. Altered aortic reactivity and lowered blood pressure associated with high Ca^{++} intake in the SHR. *Am J Physiol* 1986; 251:H976–H983.

228. MacCarthy EP, Yamashita W, Hsu A, et al. 1,25 dihydroxy vitamin D3 and rat vascular smooth muscle cell growth. *Hypertension* 1989; 13:954–959.

229. Bender DA. Non-nutritional uses of vitamin B-6. *Br J Nutr* 1999; 81:7–20.

230. Dakshinamurti K, Paulose CS, Viswanathan M. Vitamin B6 and hypertension. *Ann N Y Acad Sci* 1990; 575:241–249.

231. Aybak M, Sermet A, Ayyildiz MO, Karakilcik AZ. Effect of oral pyridoxine hydrochloride supplementation on arterial blood pressure in patients with essential hypertension. *Arzneimittelforschung* 1995; 45:1271–1273.

232. Katz DL. *Nutrition in Clinical Practice*. Philadelphia: Lippincott Williams and Wilkins, 2001, pp. 370–371.

233. Paran E, Engelhard YN. Effect of lycopene, an oral natural antioxidant on blood pressure. *J Hypertens* 2001; 19:S74. Abstract P 1.204.

234. Paran E, Engelhard Y. Effect of tomato's lycopene on blood pressure, serum lipoproteins, plasma homocysteine and oxidative stress markers in grade I hypertensive patients. *Am J Hypertens* 2001; 14:141A. Abstract P-333.

235. Digiesi V, Cantini F, Oradei A, Bisi G, Guarino GC, Brocchi A, Bellandi F, Mancini M, Littarru GP. Coenzyme Q-10 in essential hypertension. *Mol Aspects Med* 1994; 15:S257–S263.
236. Langsjoen PH, Langsjoen AM. Overview of the use of Co Q 10 in cardiovascular disease. *Biofactors* 1999; 9:273–284.
237. Singh RB, Niaz MA, Rastogi SS, Shukla PK, Thakur AS. Effect of hydrosoluble coenzyme Q10 on blood pressure and insulin resistance in hypertensive patients with coronary heart disease. *J Hum Hypertens* 1999; 13:203–208.
238. Digiesi V, Cantini F, Brodbeck B. Effect of coenzyme Q10 on essential hypertension. *Curr Ther Res* 1990; 47:841–845.
239. Morisco C, Trimarco B, Condorelli M. Effect of coenzyme Q10 therapy in patients with congestive heart failure: a long-term multicenter randomized trial. *Clin Investig* 1993; 71:S134–S136.
240. Kontush A, et al. Plasma ubiquinol is decreased in patients with hyperlipidemia. *Atherosclerosis* 1997; 129:119–126.
241. Yokoyama H, et al. Coenzyme Q10 protects coronary endothelial function from ischemia reperfusion injury via an antioxidant effect. *Surgery* 1996; 120:189–196.
242. Digiesi V, et al. Mechanism of action of coenzyme Q10 in essential hypertension. *Curr Ther Res* 1992; 51:668–672.
243. Burke BE, Neustenschwander R, Olson RD. Randomized, double-blind, placebo-controlled trial of coenzyme Q10 in isolated systolic hypertension. *South Med J* 2001; 94:1112–1117.
244. Vasdev S, Ford CA, Parai S, et al. Dietary alpha-lipoic acid supplementation lowers blood pressure in spontaneously hypertensive rats. *J Hypertens* 2000; 18:567–573.
245. Bierhaus A, Chevion S, Chevion M, Hoffman M, Quehenberger P, Illmer T, Luther T, Berentshtein E, Tritschler H, Muller M, Wahl P, Ziegler R, Nawroth PP. Advanced glycation end product-induced activation of NF-kappa B is suppressed by alpha lipoic acid in cultured endothelial cells. *Diabetes* 1997; 46:1481–1490.
246. Cooke JP, Dzau VJ. Nitric oxide synthase: role in the genesis of vascular disease. *Annu Rev Med* 1997; 48:489–509.
247. Cooke JP, Tsao PS. Endothelial alterations in atherosclerosis: the role of nitric oxide. In: Webb D, Vallance P, eds. *Endothelial Function in Hypertension*. Heidelberg: Springer-Verlag, 1997, pp. 29–38.
248. Siani A, Pagano E, Iacone R, Iacoviell L, Scopacasa F, Strazzullo P. Blood pressure and metabolic changes during dietary L-arginine supplementation in humans. *Am J Hypertens* 2000; 13:547–551.
249. Vallance P, Leone A, Calver A, Collier J, Moncada S. Endogenous dimethyl-arginine as an inhibitor of nitric oxide synthesis. *J Cardiovasc Pharmacol* 1992; 20:S60–S62.
250. Higashi Y, Oshima T, Ozono R, Watanabe M, Matsuura H, Kajiyama G. Effects of L-arginine infusion on renal hemodynamics in patients with mild essential hypertension. *Hypertension* 1995; 25:898–902.
251. Higashi Y, Oshima T, Watanabe M, Matsuura H, Kajiyama G. Renal response to L-arginine in salt-sensitive patients with essential hypertension. *Hypertension* 1996; 27:643–648.
252. Campese VM, Amar M, Anjali C, Medhat T, Wurgaft A. Effect of L-arginine on systemic and renal haemodynamics in salt-sensitive patients with essential hypertension. *J Hum Hypertens* 1997; 11:527–532.
253. Kelly JJ, Williamson P, Martin A, Whitworth JA. Effects of oral L-arginine on plasma nitrate and blood pressure in cortisol-treated humans. *J Hypertens* 2001; 19:263–268.
254. MacAllister RJ, Calver AL, Collier J, Edwards CMB, Herreros B, Nussey SS, Vallance P. Vascular and hormonal responses to arginine: provision of substrate for nitric oxide or non-specific effect? *Clin Sci* 1995; 89:183–189.
255. Duke JA. *The Green Pharmacy: Herbs, Foods and Natural Formulas to Keep You Young. Anti-Aging Prescriptions*. Pennsylvania: Rodale Publishers St. Martin's Press, 2001, pp. 1–546.
256. Huxtable RJ. Physiologic actions of taurine. *Physiol Rev* 1992; 72:101–163.
257. Ciehanowska B. Taurine as a regulator of fluid-electrolyte balance and arterial pressure. *Ann Acad Med Stetin* 1997; 43:129–142.
258. Fujita T, Ando K, Noda H, Ito Y, Sato Y. Effects of increased adrenomedullary activity and taurine in young patients with borderline hypertension. *Circulation* 1987; 75:525–532.
259. Birdsall TC. Therapeutic applications of taurine. *Altern Med Rev* 1998; 3:128–136.
260. Huxtable RJ, Sebring LA. Cardiovascular actions of taurine. *Prog Clin Biol Res* 1983; 125:5–37.
261. Nakagawa M, Takeda K, Yoshitomi T, Itoh H, Nakata T, Sasaki S. Antihypertensive effect of taurine on salt-induced hypertension. *Adv Exp Med Biol* 1994; 359:197–206.
262. Kohashi N, Okabayashi T, Hama J, Katori R. Decreased urinary taurine in essential hypertension. *Prog Clin Biol Res* 1983; 125:73–87.

263. Ando K, Fujita T. Etiological and physiopathological significance of taurine in hypertension. *Nippon Rinsho* 1992; 50:374–381.

264. Meldrum MJ, Tu R, Patterson T, Dawson R, Petty T. The effect of taurine on blood pressure and urinary sodium, potassium and calcium excretion. *Adv Exp Med Biol* 1994; 359:207–215.

265. Tanabe Y, Urata H, Kiyonaga A, Ikede M, Tanake H, Shindo M, Arakawa K. Changes in serum concentrations of taurine and other amino acids in clinical antihypertensive exercise therapy. *Clin Exp Hypertens* 1989; 11:149–165.

266. Gentile S, Bologna E, Terracina D, Angelico M. Taurine-induced diuresis and natriuresis in cirrhotic patients with ascites. *Life Sci* 1994; 54:1585–1593.

267. Mizushima S, Nara Y, Sawamura M, Yamori Y. Effects of oral taurine supplementation on lipids and sympathetic nerve tone. *Adv Exp Med Biol* 1996; 403:615–622.

268. Tao L, Rao MR. Effects of enalapril and taurine on left ventricular hypertrophy and arrhythmia in renovascular hypertensive rat. *Yao Xue Xue Bao* 1996; 31:891–896.

269. Ji Y, Tao L, Rao MR. Effects of taurine and enalapril on blood pressure, platelet aggregation and the regression of left ventricular hypertrophy in two-kidney-one-clip renovascular hypertensive rats. *Yao Xue Xue Bao* 1995; 30:886–890.

270. Auer W, Eiber A, Hertkorn E, Hoehfeld E, Koehrle U, Lorenz A, Mader F, Marx W, Otto G, Schmid-Otto B. Hypertension and hyperlipidaemia: garlic helps in mild cases. *Br J Clin Pract* 1990; 69:3–6.

271. McMahon FG, Vargas R. Can garlic lower blood pressure? A pilot study. *Pharmacotherapy* 1993; 13:406–407.

272. Lawson LD. Garlic: a review of its medical effects and indicated active compounds. In: Lawson LD, Bauer R, eds. *Phytomedicines of Europe: Chemistry and Biological Activity.* Washington, DC: American Chemical Society, 1998, pp. 76–209.

273. Pedraza-Chaverri J, Tapia E, Medina-Campos ON, de los Angeles Granados M, Franco M. Garlic prevents hypertension induced by chronic inhibition of nitric oxide synthesis. *Life Sci* 1998; 62:71–77.

274. Orekhov AN, Grunwald J. Effects of garlic on atherosclerosis. *Nutrition* 1997; 13:656–663.

275. Ernst E. Cardiovascular effects of garlic (Allium savitum): a review. *Pharmatherapeutica* 1987; 5:83–89.

276. Silagy CA, Neil AW. A meta-analysis of the effect of garlic on blood pressure. *J Hypertens* 1994; 12:463–468.

277. Silagy C, Neil A. Garlic as a lipid lowering agent: a meta analysis. *J R Coll Physicians Lond* 1994; 28:39–45.

278. Ojewole JAO, Adewunmi CO. Possible mechanisms of antihypertensive effect of garlic: evidence from mammalian experimental models. *Am J Hypertens* 2001; 14:29A. Abstract.

279. Kleinjnen J, Knipschild P, Ter Riet G. Garlic, onions and cardiovascular risk factors: a review of the evidence from human experiments with emphasis on commercially available preparations. *Br J Clin Pharmacol* 1989; 28:535–544.

280. Reuter HD, Sendl A. Allium sativum and Allium ursinum: chemistry, pharmacology and medicinal applications. *Econ Med Plant Res* 1994; 6:55–113.

281. Mohamadi A, Jarrell ST, Shi SJ, Andrawis NS, Myers A, Clouatre D, Preuss HG. Effects of wild versus cultivated garlic on blood pressure and other parameters in hypertensive rats. *Heart Dis* 2000; 2:3–9.

282. Clouatre D. *European Wild Garlic: The Better Garlic.* San Francisco: Pax Publishing, 1995.

283. Sendl A, Elbl G, Steinke B, Redl K, Breu W, Wagner H. Comparative pharmacological investigations of Allium ursinum and Allium sativum. *Planta Med* 1992; 58:1–116.

284. Sendl A, Schliack M, Losu R, Stanislaus F, Wagner H. Inhibition of cholesterol synthesis in vitro by extracts and isolated compounds prepared from garlic and wild garlic. *Atherosclerosis* 1992; 94:79–85.

285. Wagner H, Elbl G, Lotter H, Guinea M. Evaluation of natural products as inhibitors of angiotensin I converting enzyme (ACE). *Pharmacol Lett* 1991; 15–18.

286. Das I, Khan NS, Sooranna SSR. Potent activation of nitric oxide synthase by garlic: a basis for its therapeutic application. *Curr Med Res Opin.* 1994; 13:257–263.

287. Torok B, Belagyi J, Rietz B, Jacob R. Effectiveness of garlic on the radical activity radical generating sytems. *Arzneimittelforschung* 1994; 44:608–611.

288. Jarrell ST, Bushehri N, Shi S-J, Andrawis N, Clouatre D, Preuss HG. Effects of Wild Garlic (*Allium ursinum*) on blood pressure in SHR. *J Am Coll Nutr* 1996; 15:532. Abstract.

289. Mutsch-Eckner M, Meier B, Wright AD, Sticher O. Gamma-glutamyl peptides from *Allium sativum* bulbs. *Phytochemistry* 1992; 31:2389–2391.

290. Meunier MT, Villie F, Jonadet M, Bastide J, Bastide P. Inhibition of angiotensin I converting enzyme by flavonolic compounds: in vitro and in vivo studies. *Planta Med* 1987; 53:12–15.
291. Ackermann RT, Mulrow CD, Ramirez G, Gardner CD, Morbidoni L, Lawrence VA. Garlic shows promise for improving some cardiovascular risk factors. *Arch Intern Med* 2001; 161:813–824.
292. Suetsuna K, Nakano T. Identification of an antihypertensive peptide from peptic digest of wakame (undaria pinnatifida). *J Nutr Biochem* 2000; 11:450–454.
293. Nakano T, Hidaka H, Uchida J, Nakajima K, Hata Y. Hypotensive effects of wakame. *J Jpn Soc Clin Nutr* 1998; 20:92.
294. Krotkiewski M, Aurell M, Holm G, Grimby G, Szckepanik J. Effects of a sodium-potassium ion-exchanging seaweed preparation in mild hypertension. *Am J Hypertens* 1991; 4:483–488.
295. Hata Y, Yamamoto M, Ohni M, Nakajima K, Nakamura Y, Takano T. A placebo-controlled study of the effect of sour milk on blood pressure in hypertensive subjects. *Am J Clin Nutr* 1996; 64:767–771.
296. Maruyama S, Mitachi H, Awaya J, Kurono M, Tomizuka N, Suzuki H. Angiotensin I-converting enzyme inhibitory activity of the c-terminal hexapeptide of as1-casein. *Agric Biol Chem* 1987; 51:2557–2561.
297. Kohmura M, Nio N, Kubo K, Monoshima Y, Munekata E, Ariyoshi Y. Inhibition of angiotensin-converting enzyme by synthetic peptides of human β-casein. *Agric Biol Chem* 1989; 53:2107–2114.
298. Miyoshi S, Ishikawa I, Kaneko T, Fukui F, Tanaka M, Maruyama S. Structures and activity of angiotensin-converting enzyme inhibitors in an α-zein hydrolysate. *Agric Biol Chem* 1991; 55: 1313–1318.
299. Yano S, Suzuki K, Funatsu G. Isolation from α-zein of thermolysin peptides with angiotensin I-converting enzyme inhibitory activity. *Biosci Biotechnol Biochem* 1996; 60:661–663.
300. Ohshima G, Shimabukuro H, Nagasama K. Peptide inhibitors of angiotensin-converting enzyme in digests of gelatin by bacterial collagenase. *Biochim Biophys Acta* 1979; 566:128–137.
301. Saito S, Wanezaki (Nakamura) K, Kawato A, Imayasu S. Structure and activity of angiotensin I converting enzyme inhibitory peptides from sake and sake lees. *Biosci Biotechnol Biochem* 1994; 58: 1767–1771.
302. Nakamura Y, Yamamoto N, Sakai K, Okubo A, Yamazaki S, Takano T. Purification and characterization of angiotensin I-converting enzyme inhibitors from sour milk. *J Dairy Sci* 1995; 78:777–783.
303. Suetsuna K. Study on the inhibitory activities against angiotensin I-converting enzyme of the peptides derived from sardine muscle. Doctoral Thesis, Tohoku University, Miyagi, Sendai, Japan, 1992.
304. Matsufuji H, Matsui T, Ohshige S, Kawasaki T, Osajima K, Osajima Y. Antihypertensive effects of angiotensin fragments in SHR. *Biosci Biotechnol Biochem* 1995; 59:1398–1401.
305. Kohama Y, Oka H, Kayamori Y, Tsujikawa K, Mimura T, Nagase Y, Satake M. Potent synthetic analogues of angiotensin-converting enzyme inhibitor derived from tuna muscle. *Agric Biol Chem* 1991; 55:2169–2170.
306. Astawan M, Wahyuni M, Yasuhara T, Yamada K, Tadokoro T, Maekawa A. Effects of angiotensin I-converting enzyme inhibitory substances derived from Indonesian dried-salted fish on blood pressure of rats. *Biosci Biotechnol Biochem* 1995; 59:425–429.
307. Yokoyama K, Chiba H, Yoshikawa M. Peptide inhibitors for angiotensin I-converting enzyme from thermolysin digest of dried bonito. *Biosci Biotechnol Biochem* 1992; 56:1541–1545.
308. Okamoto (Kaimura) A, Matsumoto E, Iwashita A, Yasuhara T, Kawamura Y, Koizumi Y, Yanagida F. Angiotensin I-converting enzyme inhibitory action of fish sauce. *Food Sci Technol Int* 1995; 1:101–106.
309. Suetsuna K. Purification and identification of angiotensin I-converting enzyme inhibitors from the red algae Porphyra yezoensis. *J Mar Biotechnol* 1998; 6:163–167.
310. Suetsuna K. Separation and identification of angiotensin I-converting enzyme inhibitors from peptic digest of Hizikia fusiformis protein. *Nippon Suisan Gakkaishi* 1998; 64:862–866.
311. Blaszó G, Gáspár R, Rüve HJ, Rohdewald P. ACE inhibition and hypotensive effect of a procyanidins containing extract from the baric of pinus pinaster sol. *Pharm Pharmacol Lett* 1996; 1:8–11.
312. Le OT, Elliot WJ. Dose response relationship of blood pressure and serum cholesterol to 3-N-butyl phthalide, a component of celery oil. *Clin Res* 1991; 39:750A. Abstract.
313. Duke JA. *The Green Pharmacy Herbal Handbook.* Emmaus, PA: Rodale Press, 2000, pp. 68–69.
314. Castleman M. *The Healing Herbs: The Ultimate Guide to the Curative Power of Nature's Medicines.* Emmaus, PA: Rodale Press, 1991, pp. 105–107.
315. Heinerman J. *Heinerman's New Encyclopedia of Fruits and Vegetables.* Paramus, NJ: Prentice Hall, 1995, pp. 93–95.
316. Hosseini S, Lee J, Sepulveda RT, et al. A randomized, double-blind, placebo-controlled, prospective 16 week crossover study to determine the role of pycnogenol in modifying blood pressure in mildly hypertensive patients. Nutr Res 2001; 21:1251–1260.

6 Congestive Heart Failure and Cardiomyopathy

The Metabolic Cardiology Solution

Stephen T. Sinatra, M.D.

I. INTRODUCTION

The consensus opinion is that failing hearts are energy starved. Disruption in the metabolic processes controlling myocardial energy metabolism is characteristic in failing hearts, and this loss of energetic balance directly impacts heart function. Treatment options that include metabolic intervention with therapies shown to preserve energy substrates or accelerate energy turnover are indicated for at-risk populations or patients at any stage of disease.

II. EPIDEMIOLOGY

More than 5 million Americans suffer from chronic congestive heart failure (CHF) and 550,000 new cases are diagnosed annually, making CHF the most costly diagnosis in the Medicare population and the most common cause of hospitalization in patients over age 65. With an aging population, the number of CHF cases continues to grow annually, as evidenced by the growth in hospital discharges, which increased from 400,000 in 1979 to more than 1.08 million in 2005, or 171%.

Approximately 28% of men and women over the age of 45 have mild to moderate diastolic dysfunction with preserved ejection fraction.[1] Decline in diastolic heart function marks an early stage of disease that can progress in the absence of clinical and metabolic intervention.

The same study presented additional data that CHF is a growing medical concern, with the lifetime risk of developing CHF for those over the age of 40 years now at 20%, a level well in excess of many conditions commonly monitored with age.[1]

III. PATHOPHYSIOLOGY

CHF is a clinical syndrome characterized by well-established symptoms, clinical findings, and standard of care pharmaceutical interventions. CHF occurs when the heart muscle weakens or the myocardial wall becomes stiff, resulting in an inability to meet the metabolic demands of the peripheral tissues. This chronic condition is predisposed by hypertension, cardiac insult such as myocardial infarction, ischemic heart disease, valvular disease, chronic alcohol abuse, or infection of the heart muscle, to mention a few. They all contribute to dysfunction or permanent loss of myocytes and decrease in contractility, cardiac output, and perfusion to vital organs of the body. Frequently, excess fluid accumulates in the liver, lungs, lining of the intestines, and the lower extremities.

Many cardiovascular diseases such as hypertension, coronary artery disease, and cardiomyopathies can lead to the progressive onset of CHF that is accompanied by systolic and/or diastolic dysfunction. Most patients with systolic cardiac dysfunction exhibit some degree of diastolic involvement, but approximately half of patients with CHF show marked impairment of diastolic function with well-preserved ejection fraction. Deficits in both systolic and diastolic dysfunction frequently go undiagnosed until onset of overt heart failure.

BASICS OF CARDIAC ENERGY METABOLISM

It is now widely accepted that one characteristic of the failing heart is the persistent and progressive loss of energy. The requirement for energy to support the systolic and diastolic work of the heart is absolute. Therefore, a disruption in cardiac energy metabolism, and the energy supply–demand mismatch that results, can be identified as the pivotal factor contributing to the inability of failing hearts to meet the hemodynamic requirements of the body. In her landmark book, *ATP and the Heart*, Joanne Ingwall[2] describes the metabolic maelstrom associated with the progression of CHF, and identifies the mechanisms that lead to a persistent loss of cardiac energy reserves as the disease process unfolds.

The heart contains approximately 700 milligrams of ATP, enough to fuel about 10 heartbeats. At a rate of 60 beats per minute, the heart will beat 86,400 times in the average day, forcing the heart to produce and consume an amazing 6000 g of ATP daily, and causing it to recycle its ATP pool 10,000 times every day. This process of energy recycling occurs primarily in the mitochondria of the myocyte. These organelles produce more than 90% of the energy consumed in the healthy heart, and in the heart cell, the approximately 3500 mitochondria fill about 35% of the cell volume. Disruption in mitochondrial function significantly restricts the energy-producing processes of the heart, causing a clinically relevant impact on heart function that translates to peripheral tissue involvement.

The heart consumes more energy per gram than any other organ, and the chemical energy that fuels the heart comes primarily from adenosine triphosphate, or ATP (Figure 6.1). The chemical energy held in ATP is resident in the phosphoryl bonds, with the greatest amount of energy residing in the outermost bond holding the ultimate phosphoryl group to the penultimate group. When energy is required to provide the chemical driving force to a cell, this ultimate phosphoryl bond is broken and chemical energy is released. The cell then converts this chemical energy to mechanical energy to do work. In the case of the heart, this energy is used to sustain contraction, drive ion pump function, synthesize large and small molecules, and perform other necessary activities of the cell.

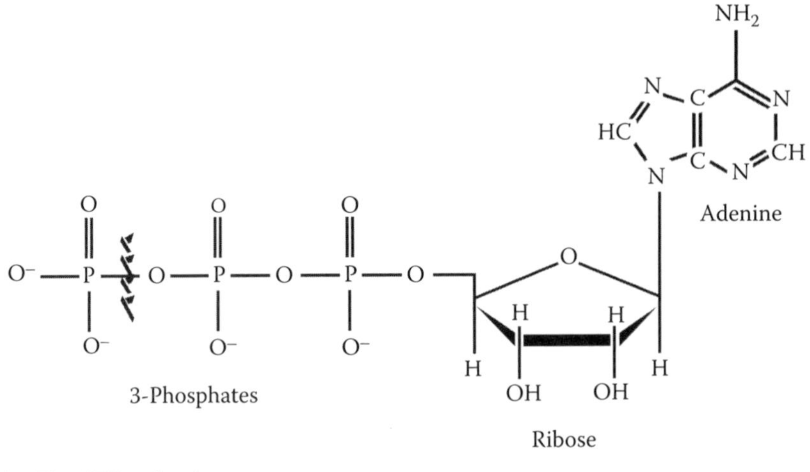

FIGURE 6.1   The ATP molecule.

The consumption of ATP in the supply of cellular energy yields the metabolic byproducts adenosine diphosphate (ADP) and inorganic phosphate (Pi). A variety of metabolic mechanisms have evolved within the cell to provide rapid rephosphorylation of ADP to restore ATP levels and maintain the cellular energy pool. In significant ways, these metabolic mechanisms are disrupted in CHF, tipping the balance in a manner that creates a chronic energy supply–demand mismatch.

The normal nonischemic heart is capable of maintaining a stable ATP concentration despite large fluctuations in workload and energy demand. In a normal heart, the rate of ATP synthesis via rephosphorylation of ADP closely matches ATP utilization. The primary site of ATP rephosphorylation is the mitochondria, where fatty acid and carbohydrate metabolic products flux down the oxidative phosphorylation pathways. ATP recycling can also occur in the cytosol via the glycolytic pathway of glucose metabolism, but in normal hearts this pathway accounts for only about 10% of ATP turnover. ATP levels are also maintained through the action of creatine kinase in a reaction that transfers a high-energy phosphate creatine phosphate (PCr) to ADP to yield ATP and free creatine. Because the creatine kinase reaction is approximately 10-fold faster than ATP synthesis via oxidative phosphorylation, creatine phosphate acts as a buffer to assure a consistent availability of ATP in times of acute high metabolic demand. Although there is approximately twice as much creatine phosphate in the cell as ATP, there is still only enough to supply energy to drive about 10 heartbeats, making the maintenance of high levels of ATP availability critical to cardiac function.

The content of ATP in heart cells progressively falls in CHF, frequently reaching and then stabilizing at levels that are 25% to 30% lower than normal.[3,4] The fact that ATP falls in the failing heart means that the metabolic network responsible for maintaining the balance between energy supply and demand is no longer functioning normally in these hearts. It is well established that oxygen deprivation in ischemic hearts contributes to the depletion of myocardial energy pools,[2,4] but the loss of energy substrates in the failing heart is a unique example of chronic metabolic failure in the well-oxygenated myocardium. The mechanism explaining energy depletion in heart failure is the loss of energy substrates and the delay in their re-synthesis. In conditions where energy demand outstrips supply, ATP is consumed at a rate that is faster than it can be restored via oxidative phosphorylation or the alternative pathways of ADP rephosphorylation. The net result of this energy overconsumption is the loss of ATP catabolic products that leave the cell by passing across the cell membrane into the bloodstream. This loss of catabolic byproducts lowers the cellular concentration of energy substrates and depletes energy reserves. In diseased hearts the energy pool depletion via this mechanism can be significant, reaching levels that exceed 40% in ischemic heart disease and 30% in heart failure.

Under high workload conditions, even normal hearts display a minimal loss of energy substrates. These substrates must be restored via the *de novo* pathway of ATP synthesis. This pathway is slow and energy costly, requiring consumption of six high-energy phosphates to yield one newly synthesized ATP molecule. The slow speed and high-energy cost of *de novo* synthesis highlights the importance of cellular mechanisms designed to preserve energy pools. In normal hearts the salvage pathways are the predominant means by which the ATP pool is maintained. While *de novo* synthesis of ATP proceeds at a rate of approximately 0.02 nM/min/g in the heart, the salvage pathways operate at a 10-fold higher rate.[5] The function of both the *de novo* and salvage pathways of ATP synthesis is limited by the cellular availability of 5-phosphoribosyl-1-pyrophosphate, or PRPP (Figure 6.2). PRPP initiates these synthetic reactions, and is the sole compound capable of donating the D-ribose-5-phosphate moiety required to re-form ATP and preserve the energy pool. In muscle tissue, including that of the heart, formation of PRPP is slow and rate limited, impacting the rate of ATP restoration via the *de novo* and salvage pathways.

ENERGY STARVATION IN THE FAILING HEART

The long-term mechanism explaining the loss of ATP in CHF is decreased capacity for ATP synthesis relative to ATP demand. In part, the disparity between energy supply and demand in hypertrophied

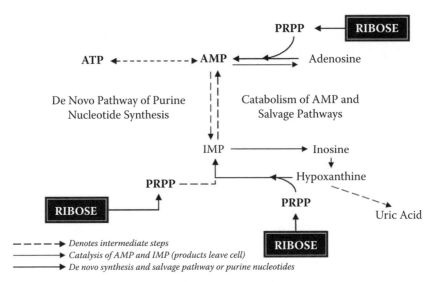

FIGURE 6.2 *De novo* synthesis and salvage of energy compounds.

and failing hearts is associated with a shift in relative contribution of fatty acid versus glucose oxidation to ATP synthesis. The major consequence of the complex readjustment toward carbohydrate metabolism is that the total capacity for ATP synthesis decreases, while the demand for ATP continually increases as hearts work harder to circulate blood in the face of increased filling pressures associated with CHF and hypertrophy. The net result of this energy supply–demand mismatch is a decrease in the absolute concentration of ATP in the failing heart; this decrease in absolute ATP level is reflected in lower energy reserve in the failing and hypertrophied heart. A declining energy reserve is directly related to heart function, with diastolic function being first affected, followed by systolic function, and finally global performance (Figure 6.3).

LaPlace's law confirms that pressure overload increases energy consumption in the face of abnormalities in energy supply. In failing hearts these energetic changes become more profound as left

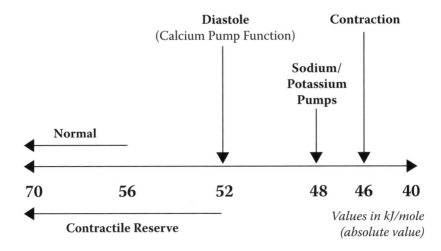

FIGURE 6.3   Free energy of hydrolysis of ATP required to fuel certain cell functions.

ventricle remodeling proceeds,[6-8] but they are also evident in the early development of the disease.[9] It has also been found that similar adaptations occur in the atrium, with energetic abnormalities constituting a component of the substrate for atrial fibrillation in CHF.[10] Left ventricular hypertrophy is initially an adaptive response to chronic pressure overload, but it is ultimately associated with a 10-fold greater likelihood of subsequent chronic CHF. While metabolic abnormalities are persistent in CHF and left ventricular hypertrophy, at least half of all patients with left ventricular hypertrophy–associated heart failure have preserved systolic function, a condition referred to as diastolic heart failure.

Oxidative phosphorylation is directly related to oxygen consumption, which is not decreased in patients with pressure-overload left ventricular hypertrophy.[11] Metabolic energy defects, instead, relate to the absolute size of the energy pool and the kinetics of ATP turnover through oxidative phosphorylation and creatine kinase. The deficit in ATP kinetics is similar in both systolic and diastolic heart failure and may be both an initiating event and a consequence. Inadequate ATP availability would be expected to initiate and accentuate the adverse consequences of abnormalities in energy-dependent pathways. Factors that increase energy demand, such as adrenergic stimulation and biochemical remodeling, exaggerate the energetic deficit. Consequently, the hypertrophied heart is more metabolically susceptible to stressors such as increased chronotropic and inotropic demand, and ischemia.

In humans, this metabolic deficit is shown to be greater in compensated left ventricular hypertrophy (with or without concomitant CHF) than in dilated cardiomyopathy.[12,13] Hypertensive heart disease alone was not shown to contribute to alterations in high-energy phosphate metabolism, but it can contribute to left ventricular hypertrophy and diastolic dysfunction that can later alter cardiac energetics.[14,15] Further, for a similar clinical degree of heart failure, volume overload hypertrophy does not, but pressure overload does, induce significant high-energy phosphate impairment.[16] Type 2 diabetes has also been shown to contribute to altering myocardial energy metabolism early in the onset of diabetes, and these alterations in cardiac energetics may contribute to left ventricular functional changes.[17] The effect of age on progression of energetic altering has also been reviewed, with results of both human[18] and animal[19] studies suggesting that increasing age plays a moderate role in the progressive changes in cardiac energy metabolism that correlates to diastolic dysfunction, left ventricular mass, and ejection fraction.

Cardiac energetics also provide important prognostic information in patients with heart failure, and determining the myocardial contractile reserve has been suggested as a method of differentiating which patients would most likely respond to cardiac resynchronization therapy (CRT) seeking to reverse LV remodeling.[20] Patients with a positive contractile reserve are more likely to respond to CRT and reverse remodeling of the left ventricle. Nonresponders show a negative contractile reserve, suggesting increased abnormality in cardiac energetics.

Studies confirm that energy metabolism in CHF and left ventricular hypertrophy is of vital clinical importance impacting both the heart and peripheral tissue. Loss of diastolic function associated with energy depletion can directly affect diastolic filling and stroke volume, limiting the delivery of oxygen-rich blood to the periphery. This chronic oxygen deprivation forces peripheral tissue, especially muscle, to adjust and down-regulate energy turnover mechanisms, a contributing cause of peripheral tissue involvement in CHF and a factor in the symptoms of fatigue, dyspnea, and muscle pain associated with the disease.

IV. PATIENT EVALUATION

While the symptoms of CHF are well known and diagnostic procedures are defined, early diastolic dysfunction may be more difficult to diagnose. Clinical suspicion can be raised by the symptoms of shortness of breath and fatigue. While CHF can generally be determined by a careful physical examination and chest x-ray, more complex cases may require further assessment, such as that uncovered by increases in B-type natriuretic peptide (BNP) or by right heart catheterization. An echocardiogram with careful assessment of the mitral valve velocity and function will assist the clinician in making the diagnosis.

It should be noted that a presumption of energy deficiency in all patients presenting with CHF symptoms is warranted. While the absolute energy requirement for diastolic filling exceeds that of systolic emptying, patients with systolic heart failure frequently present with diastolic and peripheral tissue involvement. Therefore, energy deficiency should be a paramount consideration.

Blood levels of certain of the nutrients involved in energy production can be assayed and have been shown to correlate with cardiomyocyte energy needs. Assays for free L-carnitine and CoQ10 are not routinely done by hospitals with the exception of the Mayo Clinic, but testing is routinely available and blood levels of CoQ10 and L-carnitine can be determined by qualified medical diagnostic laboratories, such as Quest Diagnostics or Metametrix Clinical Laboratory. The normal ranges show considerable variation. In my own clinical experience after testing hundreds of patients, I feel that the normal baseline levels of CoQ10 and L-carnitine approximate the plasma baseline levels of the Mayo Clinic, which are 0.43–1.53 µg/mL and 25–54 µmol/L for CoQ10 and free L-carnitine, respectively.

Although the medical literature generally supports the use of CoQ10 in CHF, the evaluated dose-response relationships for the nutrient have been confined to a narrow dose range, with the majority of clinical studies having been conducted in doses ranging from 90 to 200 mg daily. At such doses, some patients have responded, while others have not. In my patients with moderate to severe CHF or dilated cardiomyopathy, I generally use higher doses of CoQ10 in ranges of 300 to 600 mg in order to get a biosensitive result frequently requiring a blood level greater than 2.5 µg/mL and preferably up to 3.5 µg/mL.[21,22] Blood levels are particularly important and should be ordered, especially in patients who do not respond clinically when higher doses of CoQ10 and carnitine are utilized.

Some specialty laboratories provide both normal and optimal ranges. The slightly higher optimal range is clinically meaningful and more reflective of the range needed for patients with CHF. Since L-carnitine is predominantly made in the liver and kidney, additional consideration should be given to patients with renal failure or insufficiency because low levels of L-carnitine may adversely affect multiple organ systems. I suggest testing these patients more frequently to monitor L-carnitine levels in an attempt to move them into the optimum range. To maintain a blood level of L-carnitine sufficient to impact cardiac energy metabolism in CHF, I recommend 2000 to 2500 mg/day. Since L-carnitine is not well absorbed, smaller doses given multiple times a day on an empty stomach appear to be most effective. Most preparations of L-carnitine are offered in capsules. Patients on the medications listed in Table 6.1 are also at risk for low serum levels and priority should be placed on diagnostic testing in these patients.

D-ribose is produced by each cell individually and is not transported from one tissue to another. Therefore, a minimal blood level has not been established. In all energy-depleted patients, a lack of adequate D-ribose should be presumed, since the natural synthesis of D-ribose in tissue is generally inadequate to preserve or restore tissue energy levels in conditions of chronic energy deficiency. Blood levels of D-ribose range from 0.0 to 3.0 mg/dL and can be evaluated by laboratory evaluation, but results are of limited diagnostic value.

TABLE 6.1
Nutrient-Drug Interactions for Energy Nutrients

Nutrient	Drugs Depleting Tissue Levels
D-Ribose	There are no known nutrient-drug interactions
CoQ10	Statins, beta blockers, oral hypoglycemic agents, certain antidepressants
L-Carnitine	Dilantin

V. PHARMACOLOGIC TREATMENT

In large part, the objective of drug therapy is to inhibit certain of the compensatory mechanisms that may contribute to progression of CHF.

First-line pharmaceutical therapies for CHF include angiotensin-converting enzyme (ACE) inhibitors, diuretics, and digoxin. Angiotensin receptor blockers (ARBs) are also used as alternatives to ACE inhibitors in patients who are unable to tolerate the side effects of ACE inhibitors—cough being the most common and annoying symptom. Beta blockers have shown promising results in clinical trials designed to evaluate improvement in quality of life, exercise tolerance, and functional classification. Various types of diuretics are often utilized when fluid retention interferes with quality-of-life issues such as dyspnea and/or peripheral edema.

Digoxin, a natural constituent of the foxglove flowering plant, exerts a mild positive inotropic effect on cardiac contractility by inhibiting sodium-potassium pump function. Inhibiting this pump leads to accumulation of calcium within the cell, making it available to myosin to promote contraction. In general, however, while inotropic agents relieve symptoms in CHF patients, there is no evidence they prolong life and, in fact, may worsen the mortality rate. Inotropic agents such as Dobutamine increase contractility and cardiac output, but may force the heart to work beyond its energetic reserve, further reducing the cardiac energy pool. Inotropic agents may increase the frequency of cardiac arrhythmias and the potential for sudden cardiac death, effects that may be exacerbated by depletion of the cardiac energy pool.

Although the pharmacological treatment of CHF improves symptoms, the options are often limited. An integrative approach with positive lifestyle considerations and nutraceutical support will improve quality of life and reduce human suffering. Nutraceutical support with energy-enhancing nutraceuticals has improved quality-of-life issues in patients awaiting heart transplant. In my personal experience I've had several patients taken off transplant lists who improved so much while waiting for a transplant that they decided not to undergo the surgery.

VI. FOOD AND NUTRIENT TREATMENT

One of the major issues associated with heart failure is fluid retention. Compensatory mechanisms in heart failure lead to fluid and sodium retention to maintain blood pressure. Processed foods further increase fluid retention, an effect that may lead to increased blood pressure that could aggravate the energy-depleted condition.

Conversely, CHF patients are frequently deficient in magnesium and potassium, which are depleted in heart failure often by the use of diuretic medications. Low potassium can increase blood pressure, while depleted magnesium can lead to a number of factors, including poor energy metabolism and insulin resistance. Similarly, thiamin levels can be low in CHF, and this can further sodium retention and disease progression. Finally, patients with CHF should limit fluid consumption to two quarts per day. Fluids are broadly defined as foods that are liquid at room temperature, and therefore include water, milk, juices, Jell-O or gelatins, popsicles, and ice cream (see Table 6.2).

Because the failing heart shows a shift in metabolism from fatty acids to carbohydrates, and since ischemic disease contributes to CHF progression by depleting ATP substrates, dyslipidemia resulting from consumption of fatty foods is problematic. Patients should be instructed to choose lower fat dairy products, lean meats and fish, and to prepare foods with no added fat (see Table 6.3). This is a dilemma with diet alone because vegetarians generally have lower serum levels of CoQ10 and L-carnitine. Supplemental dosing can help avoid a diet high in saturated fats.

Energy metabolic deficit is additionally related to depletion of cellular compounds that contribute to energy metabolism, notably the pentose D-ribose, CoQ10, and L-carnitine. These nutrients are provided by foods that are metabolically active, such as red meat, heart, and liver. The normal diet is generally not adequate to provide sufficient levels of these nutrients and supplemental consumption is strongly recommended. Although one 6-ounce portion of wild Alaskan salmon may well provide 10–15 mg of CoQ10, it would take the equivalent of 10 pounds of salmon to give the

TABLE 6.2
Nutrient Recommendations for Congestive Heart Failure

Nutrient	Recommendation
Salt	Avoid: Processed salt in fast food, canned soups and sauces, lunch meats, frozen dinners, snack foods.
Magnesium	Increase: Wheat germ, navy beans, oatmeal, nuts, seeds, figs, tofu, low-fat dairy items, seafood.
Potassium	Increase: Fresh fruits and vegetables, beans, whole grains, low-fat dairy items, fish, potatoes.
Thiamin	Increase: Beans, peas, peanuts, whole grains, eggs, fish, poultry.
Fats	Avoid: All *trans* fats. Restrict: Saturated fats
Processed sugars	Avoid all.
Fluids	Restrict to 2 quarts per day or less. Alternatives: hard candies or gum to stimulate saliva, ice chips to lessen thirst.

additional CoQ10 required to help make a difference in the compromised patient with CHF. This dietary scenario is not possible or practical.

D-ribose is a pentose carbohydrate that is found in every living tissue. Natural synthesis is via the oxidative pentose phosphate pathway of glucose metabolism, but the poor expression of gatekeeper enzymes glucose-6-phosphate dehydrogenase and 6-phosphogluconate dehydrogenase limit its natural production in heart and muscle tissue. The primary metabolic fate of D-ribose is the formation of 5-phosphoribosyl-1-pyrophosphate (PRPP) required for energy synthesis and salvage. The concentration of PRPP in tissue defines the rate of flux down the energy synthetic pathway and, in this way, ribose is rate limiting for preservation of the cellular energy pool. As a pentose, D-ribose is not consumed by cells as a primary energy fuel. Instead, ribose is preserved for the metabolic task of stimulating *de novo* energy synthesis and salvage.

CoQ10 resides in the electron transport chain of the mitochondria and is vital for progression of oxidative phosphorylation. In CHF, oxidative phosphorylation slows due to a loss of mitochondrial protein and lack of expression of key enzymes involved in the cycle. Disruption of mitochondrial activity may lead to a loss of CoQ10 that can further depress oxidative phosphorylation. In patients taking statin-like drugs, the mitochondrial loss of CoQ10 may be exacerbated by restricted CoQ10 synthesis resulting from HGM-CoA reductase inhibition. Such a decrease in CoQ10 occurring after years of statin therapy may be a major factor in the increase in CHF over the last decades. A small study reported in the *American Journal of Cardiology* demonstrates that diastolic dysfunction occurs in approximately two-thirds of previously normal patients given low-dose statin therapy. Supplemental CoQ10 helps to resurrect the previous vulnerable myocardium.[23]

Carnitine is derived naturally in the body from the amino acids lysine and methionine. Its principal role is to facilitate the transport of fatty acids across the inner mitochondrial membrane to initiate beta-oxidation and to remove metabolic waste products from the inner mitochondria for disposal. Carnitine also exhibits antioxidant and free radical scavenger properties. Carnitine, like CoQ10, is found predominantly in animal flesh, and deficiencies in both of these nutrients are realized in those on vegetarian diets. The relationship between carnitine availability in heart tissue, carnitine metabolism in the heart, and left ventricular function is elucidated in Table 6.4.

TABLE 6.3
Foods High in Energy Nutrients

Energy Nutrient	Food Sources (descending order of importance)
D-Ribose	Veal, beef
CoQ10	Beef heart, wild salmon, chicken liver
L-Carnitine	Mutton, lamb, beef, pork, poultry

TABLE 6.4
Clinical and Laboratory Evaluation of D-Ribose, CoQ10, and L-Carnitine in Congestive Heart Failure

Nutrient	Research Result	Reference
D-Ribose	NYHA Class II/III CHF; Administration resulted in significant improvement in all indices of diastolic heart function and led to significant improvement in patient quality of life score and exercise tolerance. No tested parameters were improved with glucose (placebo) treatment.	25
	NYHA Class II-IV CHF; Ribose improved ventilation efficiency, oxygen uptake efficiency, stroke volume, Doppler Tei Myocardial Performance Index (MPI) and ventilatory efficiency while preserving VO_{2max}. All are powerful predictors of heart failure survival. Ribose stimulates energy metabolism along the cardiopulmonary axis, thereby improving gas exchange.	25–27
	Lewis rat model; Remote myocardium exhibits a decrease in function within four weeks following myocardial infarction. To a significant degree, ribose administration prevents the dysfunction. Increased workload on the remote myocardium impacts cardiac energy metabolism resulting in lower myocardial energy levels. Elevating cardiac energy level improves function and may delay chronic changes in a variety of CHF conditions.	28
CoQ10	CHF with dilated cardiomyopathy and/or hypertensive heart disease; Therapy maintained blood levels of CoQ10 above 2.0 µg/mL, and allowed 43% of the participants to discontinue one to three conventional drugs over the course of the study.	29
	Hypertensive heart disease with isolated diastolic dysfunction; Supplementation resulted in clinical improvement, lowered elevated blood pressure, enhanced diastolic cardiac function, and decreased myocardial wall thickness in 53% of study patients.	30
	Idiopathic dilated cardiomyopathy; Significant therapeutic effect of CoQ10. Affirmed the use of SPET-imaging as a way to measure the clinical impact of CoQ10 in hearts. Results are significant in that they show even small doses of coenzyme Q10 can have significant implications for some patients with dilated cardiomyopathy.	31
	End-stage CHF and cardiomyopathy; Designed to determine if CoQ10 could improve the pharmacological bridge to transplantation. Significant findings: (1) Following 6 weeks of therapy the study group showed elevated blood levels of CoQ10 (0.22 mg/dL to 0.83 mg/dL, increase of 277%). Placebo group showed no increase (0.18 mg/dL to 0.178 mg/dL). (2) Study group showed improvement in 6-minute walk test distance, shortness of breath, NYHA functional classification, fatigue, and episodes of waking for nocturnal urination with no changes in the placebo group. Results show that therapy may augment pharmaceutical treatment of patients with end-stage CHF and cardiomyopathy.	32
L-Carnitine	End-stage CHF and transplant; Compared to controls, concentration of carnitine in the heart muscle was significantly lower in patients; the level of carnitine in the tissue was directly related to ejection fraction. Study concluded that carnitine deficiency in heart tissue might be directly related to heart function.	33
	CHF and cardiomyopathy; Patients with CHF had higher plasma and urinary levels of carnitine, suggesting that carnitine was being released from the heart. Results showed that the level of plasma and urinary carnitine was related to the degree of left ventricular systolic dysfunction and ejection fraction, showing that plasma and urinary carnitine levels could serve as markers for myocardial damage and impaired left ventricular function.	34
	MI survivors; All-cause mortality significantly lower in the carnitine group than the placebo group (1.2% and 12.5%, respectively).	35
	MI survivors; Patients taking carnitine showed improvement in arrhythmia, angina, onset of heart failure, mean infarct size; reduction in total cardiac events. Significant reduction in cardiac death and nonfatal infarction versus placebo (15.6% vs. 26.0%, respectively).	36
	CHF; Improvement in ejection fraction and a reduction in left ventricular size in carnitine-treated patients. Combined incidence of CHF death after discharge was lower in the carnitine group than the placebo group (6.0% vs. 9.6%, respectively), a reduction of more than 30%.	37

The therapeutic advantage ribose provides in CHF suggests its value as an adjunct to traditional therapy for CHF.[24] Researchers and practitioners using ribose in cardiology practice recommend a dose range of 10 to 15 g/day as metabolic support for CHF or other heart disease. In my practice, patients are placed on the higher dose following a regimen of 5 g/dose three times per day. If patients respond favorably, the dose is adjusted to 5 g/dose two times per day. Individual doses of greater than 10 g are not recommended because high single doses of hygroscopic (water-retaining) carbohydrate may cause mild gastrointestinal discomfort or transient lightheadedness.

It is suggested that ribose be administered with meals or mixed in beverages containing a secondary carbohydrate source. In diabetic patients prone to hypoglycemia, I frequently recommend ribose in fruit juices. Ribose does have a negative glycemic impact and in diabetic patients taking insulin I've realized that bouts of hypoglycemia have occurred. This is why I've started with smaller doses and used a fruit juice to compensate for the reductions in blood sugar that I've clinically seen. Ribose has 20 calories per serving and doesn't necessarily have to be placed in a liquid. My patients have used a teaspoon of ribose in yogurt, protein shakes, as well as in oatmeal. Ribose can also be added to hot tea and is especially tasty in a green tea beverage. Ribose is a sugar and it tastes sweet.

VII. SUMMARY

The complexity of cardiac energy metabolism is often misunderstood, but is of vital clinical importance. One characteristic of the failing heart is a persistent and progressive loss of cellular energy substrates and abnormalities in cardiac bioenergetics that directly compromise diastolic performance, which has the capacity to impact global cardiac function. It took me 35 years of cardiology practice to learn that the heart is all about ATP, and the bottom line in the treatment of any form of cardiovascular disease, especially CHF and cardiomyopathy, is restoration of the heart's energy reserve. I've coined the term "Metabolic Cardiology"[38] to describe the biochemical interventions that can be employed to directly improve energy metabolism in heart cells. In simple terms, sick hearts leak out and lose vital ATP and when ATP levels drop, diastolic function deteriorates. The endogenous restoration of ATP cannot keep pace with this insidious deficit and relentless depletion. Treatment options that include metabolic intervention with therapies shown to preserve energy substrates or accelerate ATP turnover are indicated for at-risk populations or patients at any stage of disease.

In treating patients with mild CHF, I specifically recommend the following metabolic therapy (all per day):

- Multivitamin/mineral combination
- Fish oil: 1 g
- D-ribose: 10 to 15 g (two or three 5 g doses)
- CoQ10: 300 to 360 mg
- L-carnitine: 1500 to 2500 mg
- Magnesium: 400 to 800 mg

For severe CHF, dilated cardiomyopathy, and patients awaiting heart transplantation, I recommend (all per day):

- Multivitamin/mineral combination
- Fish oil: 1 g
- D-ribose: 15 g (three 5 g doses)
- CoQ10: 360 to 600 mg
- L-carnitine: 2500 to 3500 mg
- Magnesium: 400 to 800 mg

REFERENCES

1. Redfield MM, SJ Jacobson, JC Burnett, DW Mahoney, KR Bailey, RJ Rodenheffer. Burden of systolic and diastolic ventricular dysfunction in the community. Appreciating the scope of the heart failure epidemic. *JAMA*, 2003;289(2):194–202.
2. Ingwall JS. *ATP and the Heart*. Kluwer Academic Publishers, Boston, Massachusetts. 2002.
3. Ingwall JS. On the hypothesis that the failing heart is energy starved: Lessons learned from the metabolism of ATP and creatine. *Cur Hypertens Rep*, 2006;8:457–464.
4. Ingwall JS, RG Weiss. Is the failing heart energy starved? On using chemical energy to support cardiac function. *Circ Res*, 2004;95:135–145.
5. Manfredi JP, EW Holmes. Purine salvage pathways in myocardium. *Ann Rev Physiol*, 1985;47:691–705.
6. Gourine AV, Q Hu, PR Sander, AI Kuzmin, N Hanafy, SA Davydova, DV Zaretsky, J Zhang. Interstitial purine metabolites in hearts with LV remodeling. *Am J Physiol Heart Circ Physiol*, 2004;286:H677–H684.
7. Hu Q, Q Wang, J Lee, A Mansoor, J Liu, L Zeng, C Swingen, G Zhang, J Feygin, K Ochiai, TL Bransford, AH From, RJ Bache, J Zhang. Profound bioenergetic abnormalities in peri-infarct myocardial regions. *Am J Physiol Heart Circ Physiol*, 2006;291:H648–H657.
8. Ye Y, G Gong, K Ochiai, J Liu, J Zhang. High-energy phosphate metabolism and creatine kinase in failing hearts: A new porcine model. *Circulation*, 2001;103:1570–1576.
9. Maslov MY, VP Chacko, M Stuber, AL Moens, DA Kass, HC Champion, RG Weiss. Altered high-energy phosphate metabolism predicts contractile dysfunction and subsequent ventricular remodeling in pressure-overload hypertrophy mice. *Am J Physiol Heart Circ Physiol*, 2007;292:H387–H391.
10. Cha Y-M, PP Dzeja, WK Shen, A Jahangir, CYT Hart, A Terzic, MM Redfield. Failing atrial myocardium: Energetic deficits accompany structural remodeling and electrical instability. *Am J Physiol Heart Circ Physiol*, 2003;284:H1313–H1320.
11. Bache RJ, J Zhang, Y Murakami, Y Zhang, YK Cho, H Merkle, G Gong, AH From, K Ugurbil. Myocardial oxygenation at high workstates in hearts with left ventricular hypertrophy. *Cardiovasc Res*, 1999;42(3):567–570.
12. Smith CS, PA Bottomley, SP Schulman, G Gerstenblith, RG Weiss. Altered creatine kinase adenosine triphosphate kinetics in failing hypertrophied human myocardium. *Circulation*, 2006;114:1151–1158.
13. Weiss RG, G Gerstenblith, PA Bottomley. ATP flux through creatine kinase in the normal, stressed, and failing human heart. *Proc Nat Acad Sci*, 2005;102(3):808–813.
14. Beer M, T Seyfarth, J Sandstede, W Landschutz, C Lipke, H Kostler, M von Kienlin, K Harre, D Hahn, S Neubauer. Absolute concentrations of high-energy phosphate metabolites in normal, hypertrophied, and failing human myocardium measured noninvasively with (31)P-SLOOP magnetic resonance spectroscopy. *J Am Coll Cardiol*, 2002;40(7):1267–1274.
15. Lamb HJ, HP Beyerbacht, A van der Laarse, BC Stoel, J Doornbos, EE van der Wall, A de Roos. Diastolic dysfunction in hypertensive heart disease is associated with altered myocardial metabolism. *Circulation*, 1999;99(17):2261–2267.
16. Neubauer S, M Horn, T Pabst, K Harre, H Stromer, G Bertsch, J Sandstede, G Ertl, D Hahn, K Kochsiek. Cardiac high-energy phosphate metabolism in patients with aortic valve disease assessed by 31P-magnetic resonance spectroscopy. *J Investig Med*, 1997;45(8):453–462.
17. Diamant M, HJ Lamb, Y Groeneveld, EL Endert, JW Smith, JJ Bax, JA Romijm, A de Roos, JK Radder. Diastolic dysfunction is associated with altered myocardial metabolism in asymptomatic normotensive patients with well-controlled type 2 diabetes mellitus. *J Am Coll Cardiol*, 2003;41(2):328–335.
18. Schocke MF, B Metzler, C Wolf, P Steinboeck, C Kremser, O Pachinger, W Jaschike, P Lukas. Impact of aging on cardiac high-energy phosphate metabolism determined by phosphorous-31 2-dimensional chemical shift imaging (31P 2D CSI). *Magn Reson Imaging*, 2003;21(5):553–559.
19. Perings SM, K Schulze, U Decking, M Kelm, BE Strauer. Age-related decline of PCr/ATP-ratio in progressively hypertrophied hearts of spontaneously hypertensives rats. *Heart Vessels*, 2000;15(4):197–202.
20. Ypenburg C, A Sieders, GB Bleeker, ER Holman, EE van der Wall, MJ Schalij, JJ Bax. Myocardial contractile reserve predicts improvement in left ventricular function after cardiac resynchronization therapy. *Am Heart J*, 2007;154(6):1160–1165.
21. Sinatra ST. Coenzyme Q10 and congestive heart failure. Letter to the Editor, *Annals of Int Med*, 2000;133(9).
22. Sinatra ST. Refractory congestive heart failure successfully managed with high doses of coenzyme Q10 administration. *Molec Aspects Med*, 1997;18:299–305.

23. Silver MA, PH Langsjoen, S Szabo, H Patil, A Zelinger. Effect of atorvastatin on left ventricular diastolic function and ability of coenzyme Q10 to reverse that dysfunction. *Am J Cardiol,* 2004;94(10):1306–1310.

24. Omran H, S Illien, D MacCarter, JA St. Cyr, B Luderitz. D-Ribose improves diastolic function and quality of life in congestive heart failure patients: A prospective feasibility study. *Eur J Heart Failure,* 2003;5:615–619.

25. Vijay N, D MacCarter, M Washam, J St. Cyr. Ventilatory efficiency improves with d-ribose in congestive heart failure patients. *J Mol Cell Cardiol,* 2005;38(5):820.

26. Carter O, D MacCarter, S Mannebach, J Biskupiak, G Stoddard, EM Gilbert, MA Munger. D-Ribose improves peak exercise capacity and ventilatory efficiency in heart failure patients. *JACC,* 2005; 45(3 Suppl A):185A.

27. Sharma R, M Munger, S Litwin, O Vardeny, D MacCarter, JA St. Cyr. D-Ribose improves Doppler TEI myocardial performance index and maximal exercise capacity in stage C heart failure. *J Mol Cell Cardiol,* 2005;38(5):853.

28. Befera N, A Rivard, G Gatlin, S Black, J Zhang, JE Foker. Ribose treatment helps preserve function of the remote myocardium after myocardial infarction. *J Surg Res,* 2007;137(2):156.

29. Langsjoen PH, P Langsjoen, R Willis, et al. Usefulness of coenzyme Q10 in clinical cardiology: A long-term study. *Mol Aspects Med,* 1994;15:S165–175.

30. Burke BE, R Neuenschwander, RD Olson. Randomized, double-blind, placebo-controlled trial of coenzyme Q10 in isolated hypertension. *So Med J,* 2001;94(11):1112–1117.

31. Kim Y, et al. Therapeutic effect of coenzyme Q10 on idiopathic dilated cardiomyopathy: Assessment by iodine-123 labelled 150(p-iodophenyl)-3(R,S)-methyl-pentadecanoic acid myocardial single-photon emission tomography. *Eur J Nuc Med,* 1997;24:629–634.

32. Berman M, A Erman, T Ben-Gal, et al. Coenzyme Q10 in patients with end-stage heart failure awaiting cardiac transplantation: A randomized, placebo-controlled study. *Clin Cardiol,* 2004;27:295–299.

33. El-Aroussy W, A Rizk, G Mayhoub, et al. Plasma carnitine levels as a marker of impaired left ventricular functions. *Mol Cell Biochem,* 2000;213(1–2):37–41.

34. Narin F, N Narin, H Andac, et al. Carnitine levels in patients with chronic rheumatic heart disease. *Clin Biochem,* 1997;30(8):643–645.

35. Davini P, A Bigalli, F Lamanna, A Boem. Controlled study on L-carnitine therapeutic efficacy in post-infarction. *Drugs Exp Clin Res,* 1992;18:355–365.

36. Singh RB, MA Niaz, P Agarwal, et al. A randomized, double-blind, placebo-controlled trial of L-carnitine in suspected acute myocardial infarction. *Postgrad Med,* 1996;72:45–50.

37. Iliceto S, D Scrutinio, P Bruzzi, et al. Effects of L-carnitine administration on left ventricular remodeling after acute anterior myocardial infarction: The L-Carnitine Ecocardiografia Digitalizzata Infarto Miocardioco (CEDIM) trial. *J Am Coll Cardiol,* 1995;26(2):380–387.

38. Sinatra ST. *The Sinatra Solution/Metabolic Cardiology.* Laguna Beach, CA: Basic Health Publications, 2005.

7 Cardiac Arrhythmias

Fish Oil and Omega-3 Fatty Acids in Management

Stephen Olmstead, M.D., and Dennis Meiss, Ph.D.

I. INTRODUCTION

The accumulated evidence suggests that fish oil has heterogeneous antiarrhythmic properties. Its effects vary according to the type of arrhythmia, the underlying cardiac disorder, the amount and type of dietary fish consumption, and other factors. This chapter reviews the basic biochemistry of polyunsaturated fatty acids (PUFA) and electrophysiologic effects of omega-3 long-chain polyunsaturated fatty acids (LCPUFA), examines the antiarrhythmic properties of fish oil, and critically evaluates the available clinical evidence as to which patients may benefit and who may not benefit from fish oil supplementation.

II. EPIDEMIOLOGY

In 1976, Bang and coworkers insightfully proposed that the low mortality from coronary heart disease (CHD) observed in Greenland Inuit people despite a high dietary fat intake was due to the consumption of abundant amounts of omega-3 LCPUFA from fish and other seafoods.[1] The Greenland Inuit hypothesis came concurrently with publication of research by Gudbjarnason and his group showing that increased dietary availability of omega-3 LCPUFA supplied by cod liver oil lowered isoproterenol stress tolerance in rats leading to greater cardiac necrosis and death.[2] Over the ensuing decades, a considerable body of evidence from tissue culture and animal model studies has been developed showing that omega-3 LCPUFA favorably alter myocardial excitability and reduce the risk of ventricular arrhythmias.[3–10] Observational studies have disclosed that one to two fatty fish meals weekly and higher omega-3 LCPUFA blood levels are associated with a lower risk of sudden cardiac death (SCD).[11–14] Three randomized, controlled trials have demonstrated that fish consumption and fish oil supplementation decrease total and cardiovascular mortalities primarily by reducing the risk of SCD.[15–17] However, one large study found that men with angina pectoris and no prior myocardial infarction (MI) who regularly consumed fish or fish oil experienced an excess incidence of SCD.[18] Studies of fish oil in patients with implantable cardiac defibrillators (ICD) at high-risk for recurrent ventricular arrhythmias have yielded conflicting results ranging from protective benefit to proarrhythmic adverse effects.[19–21]

III. PATHOPHYSIOLOGY

POLYUNSATURATED FATTY ACID BIOCHEMISTRY

PUFA are carboxylic acids with hydrocarbon (acyl) tails of varying length containing two or more C=C double bonds. There are two families of PUFA: omega-3 and omega-6 (see Figure 7.1).[22] In omega-3 PUFA, the first C=C double bond is located at carbon 3 counting from the terminal or omega methyl group of the acyl tail. In omega-6 PUFA, the first C=C double bond is located at carbon 6 from the omega methyl group. Omega-3 and omega-6 PUFA are also called n-3 and n-6 fatty acids. Eukaryotes normally make and metabolize *cis* fatty acids; the C=C double bonds in both monounsaturated and PUFA are in the *cis* conformation, meaning the substituent groups are oriented in the same direction. Both PUFA families are essential for human health. Following intake, omega-3 and omega-6 PUFA are both ubiquitously disseminated throughout the body and mediate or regulate a host of physiological processes that include cardiovascular, immunological, hormonal, metabolic, neural, and visual functions. At the cellular level, these effects are brought about by changes in membrane lipid structure, alterations of membrane physical properties, interactions with membrane receptors and ion channels, modulation of eicosanoid signaling, and control of gene transcription.[23]

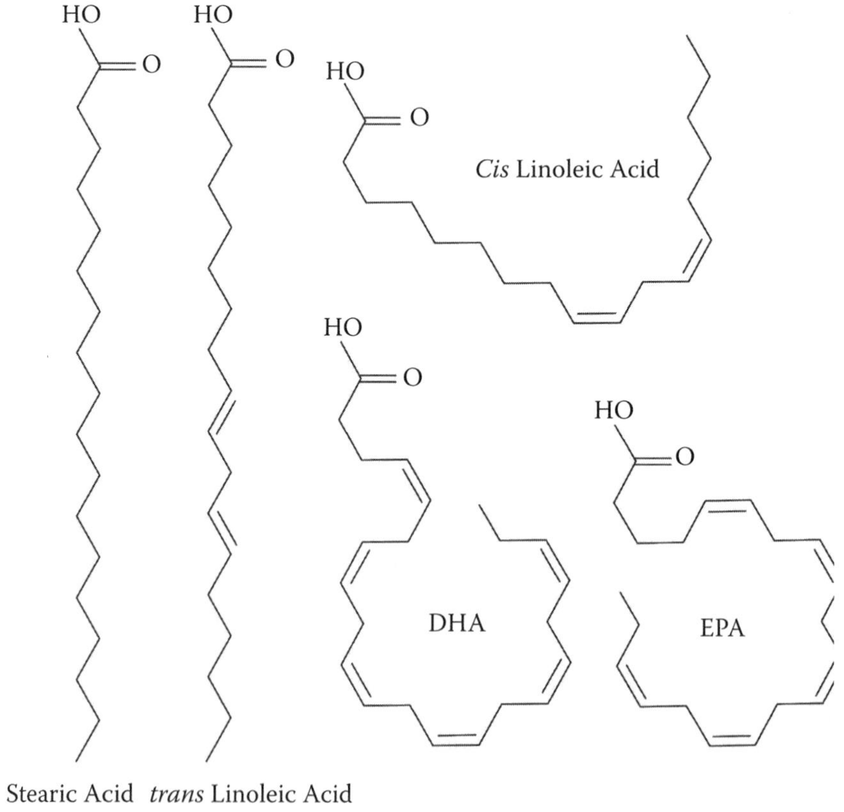

FIGURE 7.1 Fatty acid structures. The structures of the long-chain polyunsaturated fatty acids EPA and DHA are compared to the *cis* isomer of the omega-6 polyunsaturated fatty acid linoleic acid, the *trans* isomer of linoleic acid, and stearic acid, a common dietary saturated fatty acid. Note how the acyl tail of the *cis* isomers folds back on itself. This results in less dense lipid packing within cell membranes. The *cis* conformation makes a polyunsaturated fatty acid structurally equivalent to a saturated fatty acid leading to greater lipid packing and reduced cell membrane fluidity. (From ProThera, Inc. With permission.)

Polyunsaturated Fatty Acid Metabolism

Although omega-3 and omega-6 PUFA are necessary for normal cellular function, humans and other mammals lack the ability to insert a C=C double bond at the omega-3 and omega-6 positions, making dietary intake of these fatty acids essential. The omega-3 alpha-linolenic acid (18: 3n-3) and the omega-6 linoleic acid (18: 3n-6) are the primary essential fatty acids because they cannot be synthesized by mammalian cells. These essential fatty acids may be transformed in the liver into longer chain PUFA (see Figure 7.2). Alpha-linolenic acid is the precursor of the omega-3 LCPUFA eicosapentaenoic acid (EPA; 20: 5n-3) and docosahexaenoic acid (DHA; 22: 6n-3). Linoleic acid is the precursor of the omega-6 arachidonic acid (AA; 20: 4n-6). The conversion of alpha-linolenic acid to EPA and DHA is very inefficient.[24,25] EPA and DHA synthesis is further compromised by high dietary intake of omega-6 PUFA because alpha-linolenic acid and linoleic acid compete for entry into metabolic pathways.[25] Excessive consumption of omega-6 PUFA relative to omega-3 PUFA predisposes to a proinflammatory, prothrombotic, and vasoconstrictive physiology.[23] This makes dietary intake of EPA and DHA, commonly found in oily fish and other marine sources, vital to meet the body's need for omega-3 LCPUFA.

Polyunsaturated Fatty Acid Membrane Physiology

Omega-3 LCPUFA have profound effects on cell membrane physiology. These effects are believed to be due to the multiple *cis* C=C double bonds that cause the acyl tail to fold back upon itself[26] (see Figure 7.1). This highly flexible three-dimensional conformation results in significantly less lipid packing within the membrane than is permitted by saturated or *trans* unsaturated fatty acids. In general, cell membranes with excessive concentrations of saturated or *trans* unsaturated fatty acids are stiff and inflexible while membranes containing higher amounts of *cis* LCPUFA are more fluid and dynamic.[27] DHA in particular has profound effects on membrane function.[28] These include increased membrane permeability,[29] enhanced membrane fusion,[30] more efficient vesicle formation,[31] greater membrane inplane plasticity,[32] increased phospholipid "flip-flops,"[33] and promotion of intramembrane lipid domain formation.[34] It is also becoming increasingly clear that membrane physical properties significantly influence the function of membrane proteins such as cell signaling receptors and ion channels.[35,36]

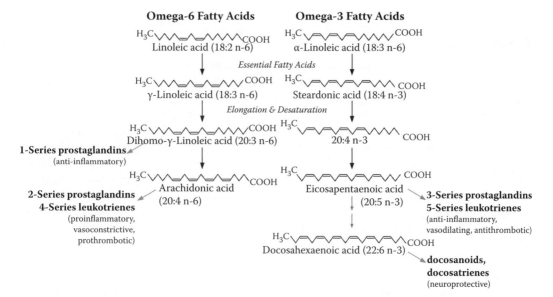

FIGURE 7.2 Metabolic pathways for essential fatty acids. The essential omega-6 linoleic and omega-3 α-linolenic polyunsaturated fatty acids compete for the same desaturation and elongation enzymes. An imbalance of dietary intake of omega-6 to omega-3 polyunsaturated fatty acids, common in modern diets, results in excessive production and membrane content of the omega-6 arachidonic acid, a precursor of proinflammatory, prothrombotic, and vasoconstrictive 2-series prostaglandins and 4-series leukotrienes. (From ProThera, Inc. With permission.)

Omega-3 Long-Chain Polyunsaturated Fatty Acid Electrophysiology

A series of in vitro and animal experiments have elucidated the basic electrophysiology of omega-3 LCPUFA. In a perfused isolated rabbit heart, LCPUFA antagonize hypoxia-mediated ventricular arrhythmias.[3] In rats, dietary LCPUFA reduced the risk of ventricular fibrillation (VF) during coronary occlusion and reperfusion.[4] In marmoset monkeys, dietary LCPUFA reduced vulnerability to ventricular arrhythmias during coronary occlusion and reperfusion.[6] Omega-3 LCPUFA have been found to be more effective than omega-6 LCPUFA at increasing the VF threshold.[37] Exercise studies of dogs have shown that intravenous infusions of fish oil can prevent ischemia-induced VF.[7] In the dog model, EPA, DHA, and alpha-linolenic acid possessed similar anti-arrhythmic effects.[38] Elegant experiments involving cultured neonatal rat cardiomyocytes have provided extensive insights into the antiarrhythmic mechanisms of omega-3 LCPUFA at the transmembrane ion channel level.[9,39,41,42] The electrophysiologic effects of omega-3 LCPUFA are summarized below:

- Increase action potential duration (QT interval)[8]
- Increase atrioventricular conduction (PR interval)[8]
- Decrease rate of contraction[39]
- Maintain steady myocyte resting potential[40]
- Increase effective refractory period[40]
- Inhibit the fast-voltage-dependent sodium current (I_{NA})[9,41,42]
- Accelerate I_{NA} channel transition from resting to inactive state[9,41,42]
- Stabilize the I_{NA} channel inactive state[9,41,42]
- Inhibit voltage-gated L-type calcium current[9,41,42]
- Inhibit sarcoplasmic reticulum calcium release[9,41,42]
- Inhibit repolarizing outward potassium current (I_{tol})[9,41,42]
- Inhibit fast outward potassium current (I_{Kr})[9,41,42]
- Inhibit delayed-rectifier potassium current (I_{Ks})[9,41,42]
- Activate inward potassium current (I_{ir})[9,41,42]

Current Hypothesis

Experimental data primarily by Leaf and coworkers show that free omega-3 LCPUFA must partition into or enter the lipophilic acyl chains of membrane phospholipids to exert antiarrhythmic effects.[41–43] Only the free omega-3 LCPUFA are antiarrhythmic. They do not become incorporated into membrane phospholipids or form other covalent bonds to exert their antiarrhythmic effects, because when the free omega-3 LCPUFA are extracted from myocytes, the antiarrhythmic effects cease. Free LCPUFA concentrations in the nM to mcM range have been found to be antiarrhythmic. These molar concentrations and resultant free omega-3 LCPUFA to phospholipid ratios are considered too low for omega-3 LCPUFA to cause a generalized increase in membrane fluidity due to reduced lipid packing. Current thinking hypothesizes that free omega-3 LCPUFA enhance the fluidity of membrane microdomains surrounding channel proteins. Theoretically, small localized increases in free omega-3 LCPUFA concentrations in perichannel microdomains could correct membrane protein hydrophobic mismatches in which the size of the hydrophobic portion of the transmembrane portion of the channel protein is less than the hydrophobic portion of the lipid bilayer. Omega-3 LCPUFA, by virtue of the folding of their double-bonded acyl tails, will reduce the size of the hydrophobic portion of the lipid bilayer.[36] This may alter the resting conformation of the ion channels and alter their conductance. Further research remains to be done to test this hypothesis for the antiarrhythmic mechanism of action of omega-3 LCPUFA.

IV. TREATMENT CONSIDERATIONS

Prevention of Arrhythmias after MI

At least three prospective studies have shown an inverse relation between fish intake and CHD mortality.[44–46] These studies appeared to confirm the Greenland Inuit hypothesis that regular consumption of foods rich in omega-3 LCPUFA confers protection against CHD.

1. The Diet and Reinfarction Trial (DART).[15] DART randomized 2033 Welsh men under age 70 who had suffered an acute MI into four groups to receive no dietary advice or dietary advice on reduced fat intake, increased fish intake, or increased fiber intake. Patients who received dietary advice to increase fish intake and could not tolerate fish were asked to take three MaxEPA® capsules delivering 500 mg daily of EPA. The portion of fish intake advised was relatively small, providing around 300 g of fatty fish, or about 2.5 g of EPA, per week. Follow-up was obtained at 6 months and 2 years.

The risk of death at 2 years was reduced by 29% in subjects advised to increase fish intake or consume EPA supplements compared to those given no dietary fish advice ($p < 0.05$). The absolute risk reduction was 3.5%. The reduction in total mortality was due almost entirely to a 32.5% decrease in the risk of death from CHD ($p < 0.01$). The absolute reduction in ischemic heart disease death rate was 3.7%. There was no significant difference in the incidence of nonfatal MI between patients randomized to receive advice to increase fish consumption and those receiving no such advice. Dietary advice on reduced fat and increased fiber consumption also had no significant effect on mortality and reinfarction. The reduction in total mortality and ischemic heart disease mortality without an effect on the rate of recurrent MI was interpreted to mean fish oil reduces mortality by decreasing the incidence of arrhythmia-mediated SCD.

2. The Indian Experiment of Infarct Survival–4 (IEIS–4) Study randomized 360 patients admitted with suspicion of acute MI to receive fish oil containing 1.08 g of EPA and 0.72 g of DHA daily, 20 g daily of mustard oil containing 2.9 g of alpha-linolenic acid, or placebo.[16] The trial was double-blind. Over 90% of subjects received aspirin and approximately 30% were on beta-blockers. No information was provided on the use of lipid-lowering agents. Follow-up of all outcomes took place over 12 months.

The total of cardiac events after 1 year was significantly less in patients randomized to fish oil and mustard oil compared to the placebo group (24.5% and 28% vs. 34.7%). Relative to placebo, patients receiving fish oil had a 48.2% reduction in cardiac mortality (10.6% absolute risk reduction) while mustard oil reduced cardiac mortality by 40% (6.7% absolute risk reduction). Both fish oil and mustard oil significantly reduced the incidence of nonfatal reinfarction (13% and 15% vs. 25.4%). Fish oil was also found to reduce the incidence of left ventricular dilatation and ventricular arrhythmias.

3. The Gruppo Italiano per lo Studio della Sopravvivenza nell'Infarto Miocardico Prevenzione (GISSI-Prevenzione) is the largest trial to date on the effect of omega-3 LCPUFA on outcomes following acute MI.[17] This open-label trial randomized 11,324 recently discharged patients to 1 g fish oil, 300 mg vitamin E (synthetic dl-alpha-tocopherol), both, or neither. The fish oil contained 570 to 588 mg of DHA and 280 to 294 mg of EPA as ethyl esters. All subjects consumed a Mediterranean-type diet that included moderate fish consumption. Most patients were on a secondary CHD risk reduction program consisting of an antiplatelet agent (82.8%), a lipid-lowering agent (45.5%), an ACE inhibitor (39%), and/or a beta-blocker (38.5%).

After 3.5 years of follow-up, four-way analysis found patients randomized to fish oil had a significant 15% reduction in the relative risk of the aggregate endpoint of cardiovascular death, recurrent nonfatal MI, and stroke. The relative risk reduction in incidence of the aggregate endpoint was due to a decrease in death and nonfatal MI. Fish oil had no effect on the incidence of fatal or nonfatal stroke. All-cause mortality was reduced by 20.2% (2.1% absolute risk reduction). Cardiovascular death was reduced by 30% (2% absolute risk reduction). SCD was decreased by 45% (1.6% absolute risk reduction). Fish oil supplementation had no effect on the incidence of nonfatal cardiovascular events such as recurrent MI. Vitamin E supplementation alone had no effect on the aggregate endpoint, but in four-way analysis reduced cardiovascular deaths by 20% and sudden death by 35%. There was no increased benefit to combining fish oil with synthetic vitamin E. Of interest is that neither fish oil nor vitamin E was associated with any reported increased bleeding risk to revascularization procedures, calling into question the often repeated advice to discontinue these agents prior to surgery. This advice has no basis in clinical studies.

A time-course reanalysis of the original data reaffirmed the GISSI-Prevenzione trial results.[49] The survival curves of patients randomized to fish oil significantly diverged early from those of patients randomized to vitamin E or no treatment. Total mortality was 41% lower by 3 months. The risk of SCD was reduced by 53% by 4 months. Significant reductions in other cardiovascular deaths were observed 6 to 8 months after randomization. As with the DART findings, the early improvements in total mortality rate and reduced incidence of SCD provide support for the hypothesis that the omega-3 LCPUFA in fish oil exert their benefit through antiarrhythmic effects.

4. The Danish High-Dose n-3 Fatty Acid versus Corn Oil after Myocardial Infarction Study included 300 patients recruited following acute MI. The double-blind trial was designed to assess the effect of high-dose fish oil on serum lipid levels and outcomes.[50] Patients were randomized to receive 4 g daily of fish oil (2.28 to 2.36 g daily DHA and 1.12 to 1.16 g daily EPA) or corn oil. Approximately 85% of subjects received aspirin, about 60% were on beta-blockers, about 10% were using ACE inhibitors, and 68% were prescribed statins. Prior to study entry, 30% of those randomized to fish oil and 25% of subjects randomized to corn oil were regularly consuming fish oil. The median follow-up period was 18 months.

The cardiac death rate was identical in both groups (5.3%) as was total mortality (7.3%). Recurrent nonfatal MI occurred more frequently in patients receiving fish oil (14%) than in patients receiving corn oil (10%), but the difference was not significant. Patients receiving high-dose fish oil had significant reductions in serum triacylglycerol levels, especially in conjunction with statin therapy.

While the Danish study failed to find that fish oil reduced adverse outcomes following MI, a number of factors must be considered when evaluating the results of this trial. The first is the low rate of mortality and recurrent infarction. The observed mortality rate is about half that seen in DART and the GISSI-Prevenzione study. This means the study lacked the statistical power to observe a real benefit for fish oil. The low adverse events rate may have been related to a high rate of revascularization. In the GISSI-Prevenzione study, 24% of subjects had undergone revascularization after 42 months. In contrast, in the Danish trial, 31% of patients had undergone revascularization after a median time of 18 months. Recurrent adverse events were uncommon in revascularized patients. Another factor biasing this study against finding a benefit for fish oil is the high number of patients using fish oil prior to study entry. Patients already consuming and benefiting from fish oil would be unlikely to accrue significant additional benefits from recommended fish oil intake. The low mortality in both groups may have been related to the high consumption of fish oil and fish in the Danish population.

To summarize the effect of fish and fish oil following MI, four interventional trials have assessed the effect on adverse outcomes in patients following acute MI. Two relatively small trials yielded conflicting results. The Danish trial failed to show a reduction in mortality or nonfatal myocardial infarction rates. However, the high number of patients consuming fish oil prior to study entry, the high revascularization rate, and the low adverse event rate bias this study against finding a benefit for fish oil. IEIS–4 found that fish oil substantially reduced cardiac mortality and nonfatal reinfarction. However, the mortality and nonfatal reinfarction rates in the placebo group were approximately twice the rate reported by DART as well as by the GISSI-Prevenzione Trial. While the benefit of fish oil is apparent, the magnitude of any benefit may have been exaggerated. A more unfortunate and troubling worry is that the validity of a prior study by the IEIS–4 leading author has been questioned and fabrication of data has been alleged.[47,48] While the validity or integrity of the IEIS–4 data has not been questioned, the results of IEIS–4 are regrettably tainted by this unrelated allegation.

The two larger trials found significant benefit for fish oil. These studies unequivocally show that fish oil or fish reduce total and cardiovascular mortality following MI. The magnitude of the reduction of mortality rate post-MI is comparable to that obtained with statins, aspirin, ACE inhibitors, and beta-blockers.[51] Fish oil supplementation following MI offers additive benefits to those provided by standard therapies. Both studies demonstrate a reduction in the incidence of sudden death, but no significant effect on recurrent MI. An antiarrhythmic mechanism appears to be the likely means by which the risk of death is reduced in this population. Based on the available clinical evidence of concordant, large, randomized, controlled trials, the recommendation of 1 g of fish oil daily in patients following acute MI is warranted.

MORTALITY IN PATIENTS WITH ANGINA PECTORIS

A single study conducted by the DART principal investigator and coworkers assessed the long-term effect of increased dietary fish or fish oil intake on outcomes in men with chronic stable angina pectoris.[18] After 3 to 9 years of follow-up, mortality was 26% greater in people assigned to increased fish intake. The risk of SCD was increased by 54%. The excess risk was largely among patients given fish oil. The increase in mortality was confined to the second phase of the trial. An analysis of the data to evaluate the possibility of an interaction between fish oil and medications found that fish oil interacted favorably with beta-blockers to reduce the risk of SD. No adverse fish oil–medication interactions were apparent. The authors speculate that fish oil intake may have been associated with an increase in risk-taking behavior although the reasons for the observed increase in mortality with fish oil in this population are entirely unclear. The results provide a caveat against blanket recommendations for fish oil consumption and highlight the fact that patients with CHD are a heterogeneous population.

RISK OF SCD

Siscovik and coworkers in Seattle first reported that dietary intake and blood levels of omega-3 LCPUFA were inversely associated with the risk of SCD.[11] In a population-based, case-control study, they compared 334 patients with primary cardiac arrest attended by paramedics and 493 randomly identified, population-based community controls, matched for age and sex. All cases and controls had no history of clinical heart disease or fish oil supplement use. The spouses of case patients and controls were interviewed to determine dietary omega-3 LCPUFA intake from seafood during the preceding month. Blood specimens from 82 cases and 108 controls were analyzed to determine red blood cell membrane fatty acid composition. The investigators found that compared with no consumption of EPA and DHA, an intake of 5.5 g of omega-3 LCPUFA per month, approximately one fatty-fish meal per week and the mean of the third quartile, was associated with a 50%

reduction in the risk of primary cardiac arrest. A red blood cell omega-3 LCPUFA level of 5.0% of total fatty acids, the third quartile mean, was associated with a 70% reduction in the risk of primary cardiac arrest compared with a red blood cell membrane omega-3 LCPUFA level of 3.3% of total fatty acids, the lowest quartile mean.

These convincing data were subsequently confirmed by two prospective cohort studies among health care professionals. In the Physicians' Health Study, which followed apparently healthy male physicians for up to 17 years, the incidence of SCD was related to fish consumption.[12] The risk of SCD was significantly reduced by 52% in men consuming fish at least once a week compared with the risk in men who ate fish less than once a month. The authors went on to explore the relation between baseline blood levels of omega-3 LCPUFA and the incidence of SCD in a nested, case-control study within the Physicians' Health Study.[13] Higher baseline blood omega-3 LCPUFA levels were significantly associated with a reduction in the risk of SCD. After adjusting for confounding factors, compared to the lowest quartile blood levels, omega-3 LCPUFA levels in the third quartile were associated with a 72% reduction, and levels in the fourth quartile were associated with an 81% reduction in SCD risk (p for trend = 0.007). Red blood cell fatty acid analyses are not routinely available as clinical tests, but plasma fatty acid panels are available from integrative medicine clinical laboratories. Such testing may assist clinicians in risk assessment and assessment of dietary or supplemental fish oil interventions.

In the second prospective cohort study, the Health Professional Follow-Up Study, involving 45,722 men free of apparent heart disease, the relation of dietary intake of omega-6 PUFA and omega-3 PUFA from both seafood and plant sources to CHD risk was assessed.[52] Intake of both long-chain and intermediate-chain omega-3 PUFA was associated with lower CHD risk without any modification by omega-6 PUFA intake. Men with a median omega-3 LCPUFA intake of 250 mg/day or more had a reduced risk of SCD regardless of the amount of daily omega-6 PUFA intake. Plant-based intermediate-chain omega-3 PUFA appeared to reduce CHD risk when omega-6 LCPUFA intake from seafood is low, which has health implications for populations with low availability or consumption of fatty fish.

In another study, 5201 men and women over 65 were selected in four U.S. communities from Medicare rolls.[14] The consumption of tuna and other broiled or baked fish was associated with higher plasma EPA and DHA phospholipid levels, while intake of fried fish and fish sandwiches was not. The clinical correlates of this association were that tuna and other broiled or baked fish intake were related to a lower rate of ischemic heart disease (IHD) death and arrhythmias, but not nonfatal MI. Consumption of fried fish and fish sandwiches had no protective effect. This study highlights the importance of the type of fish, rich in omega-3 LCPUFA, and the method of preparation, baked or broiled, in conferring protection from SCD. These observational studies provide strong support for advising apparently healthy people to consume modest amounts of baked or broiled fatty fish one to two times per week or to consume fish oil supplements in a dose of 250 mg/day.

A growing body of evidence implicates dietary *trans* fatty acids (TFA) in an increased risk of SCD. TFA are unsaturated fatty acids in which at least one C=C double bond is in the *trans* configuration with the substituent groups oriented in the opposite directions.[53] In nature, TFA have only been found in a few bacteria and are not normally made by eukaryotic cells.[54] TFA are produced in large amounts when PUFA in vegetable oils are partially hydrogenated for use in commercial food production and cooking.[55] TFA are also found in beef and dairy products due to the metabolic activities of gut bacteria in ruminants.[56] Dietary TFA consist chiefly of *trans* oleic acid with one C=C double bond, *trans* linoleic acid with two C=C double bonds, and *trans* palmitoleic acid with one C=C double bond.[57] The *trans* configuration causes the acyl tail of TFA to resemble the linear structure of saturated fatty acids and facilitates greater lipid packing both within foodstuffs and within cell membranes (see Figure 7.1). Diets rich in saturated fats are known to increase the risk of VF and SCD in primates.[6,58] In a case-control study from investigators in Seattle, increased levels of red cell TFA were associated with a moderate increase in the risk of primary cardiac arrest.[56] Levels of *trans* isomers of oleic acid with its single C=C double bond were not associated with an increased risk, but levels of the *trans* isomer of linoleic acid with its two C=C double bonds were linked to a three-fold increase in the risk of SCD. It is conceivable that production of TFA during high-heat frying contributed to the lack of protective effect of fried fish on IHD death and arrhythmias observed in the previously described trial on Medicare recipients.[14] While further research is clearly warranted, dietary restrictions of TFA coupled with increased intakes of omega-3 LCPUFA seem prudent.

HIGH-RISK PATIENTS WITH IMPLANTABLE CARDIAC DEFIBRILLATORS

SCD is almost always caused by ventricular arrhythmias. SCD is the leading cause of death in Western countries and its incidence may be increasing.[59] Patients who have survived SCD are generally treated by placement of an implantable cardiac defibrillator (ICD). These patients are at high risk of recurrent arrhythmias and the ICD makes it possible to determine the nature and frequency of such arrhythmias and treat them by electrical shock or antitachycardia pacing.

Christensen and coworkers in Denmark evaluated the relation between serum omega-3 LCPUFA levels and the incidence of recurrent ventricular arrhythmias over a 12-month period in patients with an ICD.[60] They found that patients with more than one recurrent arrhythmic event had significantly lower serum omega-3 LCPUFA levels compared to patients without arrhythmias. When patients were divided into quintiles based on serum omega-3 LCPUFA levels, those in the lowest quintile had significantly more ventricular arrhythmic events than did those in the highest quintile (mean 1.3 event vs. 0.2 event, $p<0.05$).

The Fatty Acid Antiarrhythmia Trial (FAAT) randomized 402 patients with ICDs to either 4 g daily of fish oil (2.6 g EPA plus DHA) or olive oil.[19] The primary endpoint was time to first ICD event for ventricular tachycardia or fibrillation (VT or VF). As would be expected in patients with serious ventricular arrhythmias, 79% had coronary artery disease (CAD) and approximately half had severe left ventricular dysfunction with ejection fractions less than 0.30. Fish oil prolonged the time to first ICD event by 28%, but this failed to reach significance ($p=0.057$). When probable episodes of VT and VF were included in the analysis, the beneficial effect of fish oil became statistically significant. A high proportion (35%) of subjects did not comply with consuming either the fish oil or olive oil. When on-treatment analysis was confined to patients compliant for at least 11 months, fish oil significantly prolonged the time to first ICD event by 38%. Multivariate analysis found that fish oil reduced the risk of an ICD event for VT or VF by a highly significant 48%. The study authors suggest that regular consumption of fish oil may reduce the risk of potentially fatal ventricular arrhythmias in a high-risk population with a high proportion of patients suffering from CAD and severe left ventricular systolic dysfunction.

In contrast, a trial by Raitt and collaborators from Oregon found that omega-3 LCPUFA in fish oil may be proarrhythmic in certain patients with an ICD.[20] These investigators randomized 200 patients (73% with CAD) to either 1.8 g daily of fish oil or olive oil. The primary endpoint was time to first ICD treatment for VT or VF. At 6, 12, and 24 months, more patients receiving fish oil had ICD therapy for VT or VF than did patients randomized to olive oil. The difference was not statistically significant. Multivariate analysis revealed that VT as the ICD qualifying arrhythmia and low ejection fraction were independent predictors of time to ICD treatment for VT or VF, suggesting that omega-3 LCPUFA may have proarrhythmic properties in these patients, especially the subset of patients with VT as the qualifying arrhythmia.

The Study on Omega-3 Fatty Acids and Ventricular Arrhythmia (SOFA) was a double-blind, placebo-controlled trial carried out by Brouwer and colleagues at cardiology clinics across Europe.[21] The study enrolled 546 subjects with an ICD and a history of VT or VF. Patients were randomized to 2 g/day of fish oil (containing 464 mg EPA/335 mg DHA) or 2 g/day of high-oleic sunflower oil. The primary endpoint was appropriate ICD treatment (shock or antitachycardia pacing) for VT or VF or death. Fish oil did not improve event-free survival. Among subjects receiving fish oil, 27% received appropriate ICD therapy compared to 30% of patients receiving placebo. In the fish oil group, eight patients (3%) died, six (2%) from cardiac causes, compared to 14 (5%) deaths, 13 (5%) from cardiac causes, in the placebo group. The differences were not significant. Overall, fish oil conferred no survival or event-free benefit in these patients, but was also not associated with any proarrhythmic effects. In the subset of patients with a prior MI, there was a nonsignificant trend toward longer event-free survival (28% reaching the primary endpoint in the fish oil group versus 35% in the sunflower oil group; p = 0.13).

A meta-analysis of the three trials of fish oil in people with an ICD has been performed.[61] The analysis confirmed what is readily apparent in any close reading of the three studies: There is considerable heterogeneity in the response of this patient population to fish oil. Heterogeneity was particularly high between the Raitt study and the Leaf study (p = 0.01). In contrast, no significant heterogeneity was found between the Leaf study and the Brouwer study (p = 0.30) or between the Raitt study and the Brouwer study (p = 0.10). When the Leaf and Brouwer studies are analyzed together using a fixed-effects model, fish oil significantly reduced ICD discharge for recurrent ventricular arrhythmias. The current data prompt caution in the use of fish oil in patients with an ICD and suggest that high dose (>1 g/d) fish oil should be avoided in patients with primary VT especially in the absence of CHD.

ATRIAL DYSRHYTHMIAS

Atrial fibrillation (AF) is an increasingly common and complex atrial dysrhythmia.[62] AF is characterized by a process of electrical remodeling that perpetuates the arrhythmia and may be facilitated by inflammation and oxidative stress.[63] Omega-3 LCPUFA have been hypothesized to have benefit in the prevention of AF through antiarrhythmic and anti-inflammatory mechanisms of action.[64,65] Limited animal studies suggest that fish oil may reduce susceptibility to AF. In a rabbit model of increased vulnerability to rapid pacing-induced AF due to left atrial stretch, dietary supplementation with tuna oil significantly reduced the pressure and pacing thresholds for stretch-induced AF.[66] In a dog model, fish oil limited heart-failure-induced structural remodeling and prevented associated AF, but had no effect on atrial pacing remodeling and associated AF.[67] The benefit was thought to be related to omega-3 LCPUFA-mediated reductions in protein kinase activation.

Prospective cohort studies have yielded conflicting data. A population-based study of 4815 elderly people by Mozaffarian and colleagues found that consumption of tuna or other broiled or baked fish was associated with a reduced risk of AF.[68] The much larger Danish Diet, Cancer, and Health Study involving 47,949 people found that consumption of fish was not associated with a lower risk of AF.[69] However, this study was not designed to assess the effect of fish intake on risk of atrial arrhythmias and did not elicit any information on the use of fish oil supplements, an important potential confounding factor. Patients with heart disease were excluded from the study, and this may be the population that benefits most.

Clinical trials of fish oil and atrial dysrhythmias are sparse. In a small Italian study of 40 patients with dual-chamber pacemakers, omega-3 LCPUFA supplements (1 g/day) significantly reduced the incidence of atrial tachycardias.[70] When fish oil supplements were withdrawn, the incidence of recurrent atrial tachycardias reverted to baseline levels. While this study is suggestive, the number of subjects was small and the population highly selected. In a study of fish oil supplements in 160 patients undergoing coronary bypass surgery, significantly fewer subjects randomized to 2 g/day of fish oil experienced postoperative AF compared to patients receiving placebo (15.2% vs. 33.3%; p=0.013).[71] Fish oil in conjunction with cardiac surgery was not associated with any increase in bleeding risk. In all of these clinical studies, fish oil was not associated with significant adverse effects. Preliminary clinical data on fish oil and atrial arrhythmias are intriguing and certainly justify larger prospective clinical trials. Clinicians may wish to consider the use of fish oil in the prevention and treatment of atrial dysrhythmias.

V. SUMMARY

- Omega-3 LCPUFA are antiarrhythmic.
- Omega-3 LCPUFA reduce lipid packing in cell membranes affecting ion channels.
- *trans* fatty acids with two or more double bonds are proarrhythmic.
- 1 g/day of fish oil lowers mortality following MI.
- Doses in excess of 1 g/day of fish oil may increase risk of arrhythmia in patients with primary VT and idiopathic dilated cardiomyopathy.
- Fish oil may be used empirically to prevent atrial arrhythmias.
- No data support discontinuing fish oil prior to surgeries.

REFERENCES

1. Bang HO, Dyeberg J, Hjorne N. The composition of food consumed by Greenland Eskimos. *Acta Med Scand* 1976;200:69–73.
2. Gudbjarnason S, Óskarsdóttir G, Hallgrímsson J, Doell B. Role of myocardial lipids in development of cardiac necrosis. *Recent Adv Stud Cardiac Struct Metab* 1976;11:571–82.
3. Murnaghan MF. Effect of fatty acids on the ventricular arrhythmia threshold in the isolated heart of the rabbit. *Br J Pharmacol* 1981;73:909–15.
4. McLennan PL, Abeywardena MY, Charnock JS. Dietary fish oil prevents ventricular fibrillation following coronary artery occlusion and reperfusion. *Am Heart J* 1988;116:709–17.
5. McLennan PL. Relative effects of dietary saturated, monounsaturated, and polyunsaturated fatty acids on cardiac arrhythmias in rats. *Am J Clin Nutr* 1993;57:207–12.
6. McLennan PL, Bridle TM, Abeywardena MY, Charnock JS. Dietary lipid modulation of ventricular fibrillation threshold in the marmoset monkey. *Am Heart J* 1992;123:1555–61.
7. Billman GE, Hallaq H, Leaf A. Prevention of ischemia-induced ventricular fibrillation by omega 3 fatty acids. *Proc Natl Acad Sci USA* 1994;91:4427–30.
8. Billman GE, Kang JX, Leaf A. Prevention of ischemia-induced cardiac sudden death by n-3 polyunsaturated fatty acids in dogs. *Lipids* 1997;32:1161–8.
9. Leaf A, Xiao YF. The modulation of ionic currents in excitable tissues by n-3 polyunsaturated fatty acids. *J Membr Biol* 2001;184:263–71.
10. Leaf A, Xiao YF, Kang JX, Billman GE. Membrane effects of the n-3 fish oil fatty acids, which prevent fatal ventricular arrhythmias. *J Membr Biol* 2005;206:129–39.
11. Siscovick DS, Raghunathan TE, King I, et al. Dietary intake and cell membrane levels of long-chain n-3 polyunsaturated fatty acids and the risk of primary cardiac arrest. *JAMA* 1995;274:1363–7.
12. Albert CM, Hennekens CH, O'Donnell CJ, et al. Fish consumption and decreased risk of sudden cardiac death. *JAMA* 1998;279:23–8.
13. Albert CM, Campos H, Stampfer MJ, et al. Blood long-chain n-3 fatty acids and risk of sudden death. *N Engl J Med* 2002;346:1113–8.
14. Mozaffarian D, Lemaitre RN, Kuller LH, et al. Cardiac benefits of fish consumption may depend on the type of fish meal consumed. The Cardiovascular Health Study. *Circulation* 2003;107:1372–7.
15. Burr ML, Fehily AM, Gilbert JF, et al. Effects of changes in fat, fish, and fibre intakes on death and myocardial reinfarction: Diet And Reinfarction Trial (DART). *Lancet* 1989;2:757–61.
16. Singh RB, Niaz MA, Sharma JP, et al. Randomized, double-blind, placebo-controlled trial of fish oil and mustard oil in patients with suspected acute myocardial infarction: The Indian Experiment of Infarct Survival—4. *Cardiovasc Drugs Ther* 1997;11:485–91.
17. GISSI-Prevenzione Investigators. Dietary supplementation with n-3 polyunsaturated fatty acids and vitamin E after myocardial infarction: results of the GISSI-Prevenzione trial. *Lancet* 1999;354:447–55.
18. Burr ML, Ashfield-Watt PA, Dunstan FD, et al. Lack of benefit of dietary advice to men with angina: results of a controlled trial. *Eur J Clin Nutr* 2003;57:193–200.
19. Leaf A, Albert CM, Josephson M, et al. Prevention of fatal arrhythmias in high-risk subjects by fish oil n-3 fatty acid intake. *Circulation* 2005;112:2762–8.
20. Raitt MH, Conner WE, Morris C, et al. Fish oil supplementation and risk of ventricular tachycardia and ventricular fibrillation in patients with implantable defibrillators. A randomized controlled trial. *JAMA* 2005;293:2884–91.

21. Brouwer IA, Zock PL, Camm AJ, et al. Effect of fish oil on ventricular tachyarrhythmia and death in patients with implantable cardioverter defibrillators: the Study on Omega-3 Fatty Acids and Ventricular Arrhythmia (SOFA) randomized trial. *JAMA* 2006;295:2613–9.
22. Jump DB. The biochemistry of n-3 polyunsaturated fatty acids. *J Biol Chem* 2002;277:8755–8.
23. Colussi G, Catena C, Baroselli S, et al. Omega-3 fatty acids: from biochemistry to their clinical use in the prevention of cardiovascular disease. *Recent Patents Cardiovasc Drug Discov* 2007;2:13–21.
24. Burdge GC. Metabolism of alpha-linolenic acid in humans. *Prostaglandins Leukot Essent Fatty Acids* 2006;75:161–8.
25. Burdge GC, Calder PC. Conversion of alpha-linolenic acid to longer-chain polyunsaturated fatty acids in human adults. *Reprod Nutr Dev* 2005;45:581–97.
26. Onuki Y, Morishita M, Chiba Y, Tokiwa S, Takayama K. Docosahexaenoic acid and eicosapentaenoic acid induce changes in the physical properties of a lipid bilayer model membrane. *Chem Pharm Bull* 2006;54:68–71.
27. Valentine RC, Valentine DL. Omega-3 fatty acids in cellular membranes: a unified concept. *Prog Lipid Res* 2004;43:383–402.
28. Wassall SR, Brzustowicz MR, Shaikh SR, Cherezov V, Caffrey M, Stillwell W. Order from disorder, corralling cholesterol with chaotic lipids The role of polyunsaturated lipids in membrane raft formation. *Chem Phys Lipids* 2004;132:79–88.
29. Huster D, Albert JJ, Arnold K, Gawrisch K. Water permeability of polyunsaturated lipid membranes measured by ^{17}O NMR. *Biophys J* 1997;73:855–64.
30. Kafrawy O, Zerouga M, Stillwell W, Jenski LJ. Docosahexaenoic acid in phosphatidylcholine mediates cytotoxicity more effectively than other omega-3 and omega-6 fatty acids. *Cancer Lett* 1998;132:23–9.
31. Williams EE, Jenski LJ, Stillwell W. Docosahexaenoic acid (DHA) alters the structure and composition of membranous vesicles exfoliated from the surface of a murine leukemia cell line. *Biochem Biophys Acta* 1998;1371:351–62.
32. Smaby JM, Momsen MM, Brockman HL, Brown RE. Phosphatidylcholine acyl unsaturation modulates the decrease in interfacial elasticity induced by cholesterol. *Biophys J* 1997;73:1492–1505.
33. Armstrong VT, Brzustowicz MR, Wassall SR, Jenski LJ, Stillwell W. Rapid flip-flop in polyunsaturated (docosahexaenoate) phospholipid membranes. *Arch Biochem Biophys* 2003;414:74–82.
34. Stillwell W, Wassall SR. Docosahexaenoic acid: membrane properties of a unique fatty acid. *Chem Phys Lipids* 2003;126:1–27.
35. Lundbaek JA, Birn P, Hansen AJ, et al. Regulation of sodium channel function by bilayer elasticity: the importance of hydrophobic coupling. Effects of Micelle-forming amphiphiles and cholesterol. *J Gen Physiol* 2004;123:599–621.
36. Bruno MJ, Koeppe RE 2nd, Andersen OS. Docosahexaenoic acid alters bilayer elastic properties. *Proc Natl Acad Sci USA* 2007;104:9638–43.
37. McLennan PL, Bridle TM, Abeywardena MY, Charnock JS. Comparative efficacy of n-3 and n-6 poly-unsaturated fatty acids in modulating ventricular fibrillation threshold in marmoset monkeys. *Am J Clin Nutr* 1993;58:666–9.
38. Billman GE, Kang JX, Leaf A. Prevention of sudden cardiac death by dietary pure omega-3 polyunsatu-rated fatty acids in dogs. *Circulation* 1999;99:2452–7.
39. Kang JX, Leaf A. Effects of long-chain polyunsaturated fatty acids on the contraction of neonatal rat cardiac myocytes. *Proc Natl Acad Sci USA* 1994;91:9886–90.
40. Kang JX, Xiao YF, Leaf A. Free long-chain polyunsaturated fatty acids reduce membrane electrical excit-ability in neonatal rat cardiac myocytes. *Proc Natl Acad Sci USA* 1995;92:3997–4001.
41. Leaf A. The electrophysiologic basis for the antiarrhythmic and anticonvulsant effects of n-3 polyunsatu-rated fatty acids: heart and brain. *Lipids* 2001;36 Suppl:S107–10.
42. Leaf A, Kang JX, Xiao YF. Fish oil fatty acids as cardiovascular drugs. *Curr Vasc Pharmacol* 2008;6:1–12.
43. Leaf A. Electrophysiologic basis for the antiarrhythmic and anticonvulsant effects of omega 3 polyun-saturated fatty acids. *World Rev Nutr Diet* 2001;88:72–8.
44. Kromhout D, Bosschieter EB, de Lezenne Coulander C. The inverse relation between fish consumption and 20-year mortality from coronary heart disease. *N Engl J Med* 1985;312:1205–9.
45. Shekelle RB, Missell LV, Oglesby P, Shryock AM, Stamler J. Fish consumption and mortality from coro-nary heart disease. *N Engl J Med* 1985;313:820.
46. Norrell SE, Ahlbom A, Feychting M, Pedersen NL. Fish consumption and mortality from coronary heart disease. *Br Med J* 1986;293:426.

47. Expression of concern. *BMJ* 2005;331:266.
48. Al-Marzouki S, Evens S, Marshall T, Roberts I. Are these data real? Statistical methods for the detection of data fabrication in clinical trials. *BMJ* 2005;331:267–70.
49. Marchioli R, Barzi F, Bomba E, et al. Early protection against sudden death by n-3 polyunsaturated fatty acids after myocardial infarction. Time-course analysis of the results of the Gruppo Italiano per lo Studio della Sopravvivenza nell'Infarto Miocardico (GISSI)-Prevenzione. *Circulation* 2002;105:1897–1903.
50. Nilsen DW, Albrektsen G, Landmark K, et al. Effects of high-dose concentrate of n-3 fatty acids or corn oil introduced early after acute myocardial infarction on serum triacylglycerol and HDL cholesterol. *Am J Clin Nutr* 2001;74:50–6.
51. Lee KW, Lip GYH. The role of omega-3 fatty acids in the secondary prevention of cardiovascular disease. *Q J Med* 2003;96:465–80.
52. Mozaffarian D, Ascherio A, Hu FB, et al. Interplay between different polyunsaturated fatty acids and risk of coronary heart disease in men. *Circulation* 2005;111:157–64.
53. Emken EA. Nutrition and biochemistry of *trans* and positional fatty acid isomers in hydrogenated oils. *Annu Rev Nutr* 1984;4:339–76.
54. Ferreri C, Panagiotaki M, Chatgilialoglu C. *Trans* fatty acids in membranes: the free radical path. *Mol Biotechnol* 2007;37:19–25.
55. Mozaffarian D. *Trans* fatty acids—effects on systemic inflammation and endothelial function. *Atheroscler Suppl* 2006;7:29–32.
56. Lemaitre RN, King IB, Raghunathan TE, et al. Cell membrane trans-fatty acids and the risk of primary cardiac arrest. *Circulation* 2002;105:697–701.
57. Lemaitre RN, King IB, Mozaffarian D, Sootodehnia N, Siscovick DS. Trans-fatty acids and sudden cardiac death. *Atheroscler Suppl* 2006;7:13–5.
58. Charnock JS. Dietary fats and cardiac arrhythmia in primates. *Nutrition* 1994;10:161–9.
59. Zheng ZJ, Croft JB, Giles WH, et al. Sudden cardiac death in the United States, 1989 to 1998. *Circulation* 2001;104:2158–63.
60. Christensen JH, Riahi S, Schmidt EB, et al. n-3 Fatty acids and ventricular arrhythmias in patients with ischaemic heart disease and implantable cardioverter debrillators. *Europace* 2005;7:338–44.
61. Jenkins DJ, Josse AR, Beyene J, et al. Fish-oil supplementation in patients with implantable cardioverter defibrillators: a meta-analysis. *CMAJ* 2008;178:157–64.
62. Gersh BJ, Tsang TS, Seward BJ. The changing epidemiology and natural history of nonvalvular atrial fibrillation: clinical implications. *Trans Am Clin Climatol Assoc* 2004;115:149–60.
63. Korantzopoulos P, Kolettis T, Siogas K, Goudevenos J. Atrial fibrillation and electrical remodeling: the potential role of inflammation and oxidative stress. *Med Sci Monit* 2003;9:RA225–9.
64. Harrison RA, Elton PJ. Is there a role for long-chain omega3 or oil-rich fish in the treatment of atrial fibrillation? *Med Hypotheses* 2005;64:59–63.
65. Liu T, Li G. Anti-inflammatory effects of long-chain omega 3 fatty acids: potential benefits for atrial fibrillation. *Med Hypotheses* 2005;65:200–1.
66. Ninio DM, Murphy KJ, Howe PR, Saint DA. Dietary fish oil protects against stretch-induced vulnerability to atrial fibrillation in a rabbit model. *J Cardiovasc Electrophysiol* 2005;16:1189–94.
67. Sakabe M, Shiroshita-Takeshita A, Maguy A, et al. Omega-3 polyunsaturated fatty acids prevent atrial fibrillation associated with heart failure but not atrial tachycardia remodeling. *Circulation* 2007;116:2101–9.
68. Mozaffarian D, Psaty BM, Rimm EB, et al. Fish intake and risk of incident atrial fibrillation. *Circulation* 2004;110:368–73.
69. Frost L, Vestergaard P. n-3 Fatty acids consumed from fish and risk of atrial fibrillation or flutter: the Danish Diet, Cancer, and Health Study. *Am J Clin Nutr* 2005;81:50–4.
70. Biscione F, Totteri A, De Vita A, Lo Bianco F, Altamura G. Effect of omega-3 fatty acids on the prevention of atrial arrhythmias. *Ital Heart J Suppl* 2005;6:53–9. (Article in Italian)
71. Calò L, Bianconi L, Colivicchi F, et al. n-3 Fatty acids for the prevention of atrial fibrillation after coronary artery bypass surgery: a randomized, controlled trial. *J Am Coll Cardiol* 2005;45:1723–8.

8 Asthma

Nutrient Strategies in Improving Management

Kenneth Bock, M.D., and Michael Compain, M.D.

I. INTRODUCTION

Asthma is a well-characterized immune response that targets the lung. Our understanding of the condition has evolved from the simple manifestations of airway reactivity with cough, wheezing, and shortness of breath to the present awareness of asthma as one of a growing number of inflammatory conditions that are at the interface of genetics and environmental influences.

Although primary care physicians have a full array of pharmacological therapies available in a classic step-care structure, these treatments of course have their attendant side effects. Fortunately, there is now a good body of basic and clinical research showing how nutritional and environmental factors can either trigger asthma or be used to modify and treat it. This offers the opportunity for nonpharmacological interventions that can be both preventive and therapeutic.

II. EPIDEMIOLOGY

There are an estimated 300 million people with asthma, and the geographic distribution is not uniform.[1] As with other immune and allergic disorders, asthma is on the rise. Between 1981 and 2002, asthma prevalence in U.S. children increased from 3% to approximately 6%.[2] Over the past several decades, an association has been found between the increase in allergy and asthma and the spread of a Western lifestyle.[3] This has often been attributed to environmental pollution, but there may be other factors involved, such as the degradation of nutritional quality in the food supply of industrialized nations,[4] or diminished vitamin D levels due to decreased sun exposure. Furthermore, there are questions being raised about the effect of early life environmental influences such as exposure to microorganisms on immune development in industrialized societies.

Air quality is a major contributing factor. In addition to the known inhalant allergens such as dust mites, mold, and cockroach antigens, there are well-established associations with indoor pollutants such as cigarette smoke.[5-7] Although there is not clear evidence that outdoor pollution is causing an increase in prevalence, it is documented that compounds such as sulfur dioxide,[8] ozone[9] and particulates exacerbate asthma. This certainly suggests that these pollutants are at least partly responsible for the increased prevalence in urban areas.[10,11] The effect of pollutants also raises the issue of oxidative stress in genetically susceptible individuals, which may have therapeutic implications.[12] Investigation is also taking place regarding other genetic factors that may play a role in the way people with asthma respond to pollutants.[13] Furthermore, there is speculation as to whether environmental immunotoxins such as heavy metals might contribute to the increased prevalence of atopic disease.[14]

III. PATHOPHYSIOLOGY

The rapid expansion of our understanding of immunology has revealed insights into the genesis of allergic phenomena in general and asthma in particular. This is particularly relevant to issues regarding immune tolerance.

The pathophysiology of airway inflammation has been known for many years, with the role of IgE, eosinophils, and mast cells established. These effectors are in turn known to be directed by proinflammatory cytokines such as IL-4, IL-5, IL-9, and IL-13, which are elaborated by TH_2 lymphocytes.

Until recently it was felt that the TH_2 lymphocytes were involved in a dance of mutual regulation/inhibition with TH_1 lymphocytes.[15] It now appears more likely that some other group of T cells, called regulatory T (Treg) cells, elaborate cytokines such as IL-10 and Transforming Growth Factor Beta (TGFB) to modulate the activity of effector T cells. Regulatory T cells themselves are subject to many influences. Vitamin D, for example, has been shown to promote Treg cells,[16,17] and vitamin D deficiency has been proposed as one of the causes of the increased prevalence of asthma.[18] Allergy and asthma appear to represent situations where Treg control of TH_2 cells is loosened.[19,20]

But what messages do the regulatory T cells receive that cause them to direct a response of immune tolerance versus one of reactivity? This is the central question that underpins the development of allergic responses such as asthma.

The Hygiene Hypothesis was proposed to explain a body of epidemiologic evidence[3] that indicates that atopic and autoimmune conditions are more common in industrialized societies. It was found that the presence of older siblings and early daycare were associated with reduced incidence of later wheezing and atopy.[21,22] Furthermore, there are studies showing that children who live on farms or have early exposure to animals have reduced risk of developing allergy.[23] The increased exposure to antibiotics in industrialized societies, both therapeutically and in the food supply, has a negative effect on intestinal flora. In fact, a variety of studies have demonstrated that childhood use of antibiotics is indeed associated with increased risk of later development of asthma and allergy.[24–26] These data are consistent with our growing appreciation of how early exposure to commensal organisms is essential for developing immune tolerance.

Species of healthful bacteria that inoculate the intestinal tract early in life secrete lipopolysaccharides, which interact with toll-like receptors on dendritic and epithelial cells at the GI mucosa. This leads to cell signaling, which stimulates regulatory T cells to elaborate IL-10 and TGFB, keeping the effector T cells (TH_1 and TH_2) in check. The result is an immune response of either tolerance or appropriate inflammation when the gut-associated lymphoid tissue (GALT) is exposed to other antigens. The GALT is estimated to represent 65% of our immune tissue and therefore holds sway over immune responses throughout the body. In sum, the intestinal immune system not only tolerates healthful bacteria, but requires them for its early education and long-term immune regulation. There is even evidence that gastric presence of *Helicobacter pylori* is associated with a 30% to 50% reduction of asthma incidence.[27,28] Therefore, when these toll receptor ligands are absent or depleted by antibiotics early in life, the result is immune dysregulation and inflammatory disorders such as asthma and allergy. Recent evidence suggests an increased incidence of genetic polymorphisms involving the function of toll receptors themselves in individuals with asthma.[29]

The gut flora has a significant effect on intestinal permeability. Increased intestinal permeability is commonly present in atopic diseases[30] and may cause sensitization to a larger number of antigens that then have access to the GALT. Therapeutic agents such as steroids can increase permeability further,[31] so that short-term benefit may come at the price of further sensitization. NSAIDs also increase intestinal permeability. The use of probiotics has been shown to reduce permeability in atopic individuals.[32]

Oxidative stress is another aspect of the inflammatory process that may offer therapeutic opportunities in asthma. In addition to environmental oxidants, which may trigger lung injury, the inflammatory process itself generates free radicals. A number of studies have shown that people with asthma have a higher incidence of genetic polymorphisms for glutathione S-transferase activity, which would make them more susceptible to oxidative stress.[33,34] Levels of antioxidants such as vitamin C, carotenoids, and selenium have also been found to be lower in people with asthma than in controls.[35–37]

IV. NUTRITIONAL THERAPIES

There have been numerous epidemiological and interventional studies to explore the use of diet and nutrients in the treatment of asthma, although the studies are generally smaller and have less statistical power than those in the literature supporting conventional pharmacological therapies.

One area of investigation has been the role of foods as triggers. Although the incidence of classic IgE food allergy is relatively low,[38] there is evidence of IgG-mediated food sensitivity and food intolerances leading to increased airway reactivity in a higher percentage of patients.[39–41] Given the fact that food allergies are poorly understood and frequently undiagnosed, an elimination diet can be used for both diagnosis and treatment. (Chapter 15, "Food Reactivities," elaborates on diagnosis and treatment options.)[38,42,43] Food allergies may be especially important in asthma that flares randomly and seems unrelated to inhaled triggers.

Another potential source of dietary impact on asthma is that of food additives.[44–46] This has been reviewed extensively in the case of wine reactions in asthma. Although it was formerly felt that sulfites were largely responsible, there is now more controversy regarding the incidence as well as the cause of this phenomenon.[47,48] In either case, wine sensitivity is frequently reported by people with asthma. A diet trial without additives may be of benefit in some patients, and commercially available food and wine products are now offered sulfite-free.

There is evidence that increased fish consumption has been associated with lowered risk,[49,50] which may be due to the anti-inflammatory effect of omega-3 oils or a relative decrease in the intake of proinflammatory arachidonic acid from meat and poultry. Increased seafood consumption might also provide more vitamin D or micronutrients such as selenium or iodine. Due to their high mercury content, however, large fish such as tuna, shark, and swordfish should generally be avoided. Although mercury has not been directly tied to asthma, it promotes oxidative stress and TH_2 skewing of immune function, which one would expect to be deleterious in those with asthma.

There is also an association between asthma and obesity. Obese individuals and asthmatics seem to have polymorphisms for receptors that are significant in both inflammation and asthma.[51] Leptin has been shown to increase airway reactivity in animal studies,[52] and adipokines from fat cells are known to foster inflammation. Obesity has an obvious restrictive effect on lung function, and conversely, asthma can often impede an exercise and conditioning program. Furthermore, the frequent use of corticosteroids will promote obesity. Together, these factors can generate a number of vicious cycles in those with severe asthma.

The role of micronutrients in the diet has been studied more extensively. As noted above, there is strong epidemiologic literature showing the inverse association between antioxidant levels and asthma activity.[53–55] This has led to the proposition that the decline in antioxidant content in the highly processed Western diet is partly responsible for the prevalence trends. Given the fact that a large prospective diet intervention trial is unlikely to happen, it would seem reasonable to recommend that asthmatics increase their intake of colored fruits and vegetables in order to raise antioxidant capacity.

Other micronutrient and trace elements such as selenium[56] and manganese[57] have also been found to be at reduced levels in people with asthma. The data on magnesium are mixed. In addition to the extensive literature on the therapeutic use of magnesium, there remains the question of whether there is an actual magnesium deficiency in patients with asthma, and the studies point in both directions.[58–62] A diet high in nuts, seeds, and leafy green vegetables to provide magnesium seems prudent.

Magnesium has been shown to be a bronchodilator in vitro[63] and in vivo.[64] Interventional studies with magnesium deal extensively with the use of intravenous magnesium in the acute setting and they have shown it to be effective.[65,66] There is less clarity about the use of oral magnesium in the treatment of chronic asthma, with some studies supporting its use[67,68] and others not.[69] Since this cation is very safe in those with adequate renal function, one practical approach might be to check a red blood cell magnesium level and supplement those who are deficient or low normal. Measuring serum selenium levels and supplementing in doses up to 200 μg might also be considered. Zinc is another nutrient found to be at reduced levels in asthmatics, and there is evidence that zinc deficiency creates a cytokine environment conducive to asthma.[70] Zinc deficiency may decrease the activity of delta-6-desaturase, which is an important enzyme in the metabolism of essential fatty acids.

Vitamin B6 has been shown to have an inhibitory effect on inflammatory mediators such as thromboxanes and leukotrienes.[71] Among its many physiologic functions, B6 is important in trytophan metabolism, which may be abnormal in asthmatics,[72] and B6 levels have been found to be low in asthmatics.[73] Small studies have shown clinical improvement with B6 supplementation in the dosage range of 100 to 200 mg/day.[74]

Vitamin E has been less well studied as a therapeutic agent, but there has been an association noted between reduced intake history and increased presence of asthma.[75] In addition, one prospective diet study showed reduced asthma incidence with higher dietary vitamin E consumption.[76] Vitamin E obtained from the diet is a mixture of alpha-, beta-, delta-, and gamma-tocopherols and the corresponding tocotrienols. Vitamin E from supplements tends to be only alpha-tocopherol. Clinical trials should be evaluated for the type of vitamin E used. Presently there are select vitamin E supplements that contain the full spectrum of tocopherols and tocotrienols, similar to the vitamin E obtained from diet. Additionally, antioxidant nutrients work well in groups, so using vitamin E in conjunction with vitamin C, selenium, carotenoids, and flavonoids might offer further benefit. Vitamin C alone has been studied with some positive results.[77]

Diverse dietary polyphenolic compounds can mediate antioxidant reactions. One recently studied compound is an extract of pine bark called pycnogenol. Two controlled trials[78,79] of this agent have shown significant benefit with a dose of about 2 mg/kg body weight per day up to 200 mg. Lycopene, an antioxidant that confers the red color to tomatoes, guava, and pink grapefruit, has also been found beneficial.[80] Another class of nutrients that has been used in supplemental form is flavonoids such as quercetin.[81] This compound has been shown to down-regulate the inflammatory contribution of mast cells,[82,83] as well as the expression of cytokines in bronchial epithelium.[84] It has also been shown in vitro to induce gene expression of TH_1 cytokines in monocytes and to inhibit the TH_2 cytokine IL-4.[85] Quercetin has been employed therapeutically in a dose range of 1 to 2 g/day, but well-controlled studies have not been performed. The herb *Euphorbia stenoclada* has been used traditionally in the treatment of asthma, and it appears that quercetin may be the major active ingredient.[86,87]

The role of prostanoids and leukotrienes in the inflammatory response of asthma is well documented,[88,89] and was exploited in the development of drugs such as the montelukasts. Because essential fatty acids are integral in the genesis of leukotrienes, they present logical therapeutic options. Eicosapentaenoic acid (EPA), an omega-3 fatty acid from fish oil, produces the anti-inflammatory series 3 prostanoids (PGE3), and gamma linoleic acid (GLA) from borage and primrose oil generates the anti-inflammatory series 1 prostanoids (PGE1). Although GLA is an omega-6 EFA, the anti-inflammatory series 1 compounds are distinct from the proinflammatory series 2 (PGE2) that arise from arachadonic acid. The literature in the therapeutic use of supplemental EFAs is not as rich or convincing in asthma as it is in other inflammatory conditions such as rheumatoid arthritis and inflammatory bowel disease. Epidemiologic dietary exposure studies have been positive,[90–92] and a number of supplementation trials with EPA have been positive as well[93–96] but negative results have also been obtained.[97–99] It is important to note that compared to the micronutrients and antioxidants discussed above, EFAs have to be supplemented with some caution. In the dose range of 1 to 3 g, which was used in the clinical trials, one must consider the mild negative effect on coagulation as well as occasional gastrointestinal tolerability issues. Clinical benefit has also been shown in a small study using 10 to 20 g/day of perilla seed oil, which is high in the precursor compound alpha-linolenic acid.[100]

Adequate hydration is essential in asthma management. Water intake is important as is the adequacy of intracellular cations.

Propolis from bees has been studied in asthma.[101] In addition to the herbal extract of *Euphorbia stenoclada*, *Gnaphalium liebmannii*,[102] gingko,[103] and *Tylopohera indica* have also been studied as potential adjunct treatments for asthma.[104]

Results of nutritional therapies can be augmented with relaxation techniques shown to improve lung function and reduce medication use.[105,106] Studies of acupuncture have shown some improvement, but not in measures of lung function.[107–109]

V. PATIENT EVALUATION

The concept of asthma as a completely reversible condition has long been supplanted by the knowledge that active airway inflammation leads to tissue damage and chronic changes. Early and aggressive treatment is therefore essential.

The diagnosis of asthma is usually straightforward and easily established by the primary care physician on clinical grounds and pulmonary function testing. One caveat is that the contribution of factors such as GERD may be more difficult to determine. Findings on history and physical exam may also, however, indicate the presence of coexisting nutritional factors that may influence the development and severity of a patient's asthma. The elements of a medical history suggesting common inhalant triggers such as dust, mold, and pollens should of course be obtained, but the discussion here focuses on the nutritional aspects.

A dietary history can be very revealing and can be obtained with a food diary. Foods that are eaten most frequently may in fact cause sensitization and are usually removed in elimination diets. In our clinical experience, removal of food triggers can be every bit as effective in treatment as environmental controls for dust and mold. In addition, a dietary history can reveal the degree of additives, preservatives, and sulfites consumed as well as the sufficiency of micronutrients discussed above.

Certain symptoms are often considered by nutritionally oriented practitioners to reflect possible food sensitivity. This especially includes postprandial symptoms such as dermal or oral pruritis, fatigue, gas, or bloating. Urticaria and recurrent apthous ulcers may raise the suspicion of food triggers. Certainly any symptom that the patient connects to a particular food should be considered.

Regarding micronutrients, one may also get clues from the history. Magnesium deficiency should be suspected in those with symptoms such as muscle cramps or twitches, or a tendency toward constipation. Poor wound healing and frequent infections might suggest zinc deficiency.

Physical examination may reveal infra-orbital darkening sometimes referred to as allergic shiners. Oral thrush may indicate an imbalance of gastrointestinal flora and apthous ulcers may be present. Eczema in an atopic distribution of antecubital and popliteal regions might cause one to suspect food triggers. Dry skin or follicular hyperkeratosis identified as roughness over the triceps region can represent an imbalance of essential fatty acids.

Laboratory evaluation may be helpful as well. Most commercial labs can run assays for erythrocyte magnesium, serum selenium, and plasma zinc. Measuring 25-hydroxyvitamin D is becoming common practice for a variety of reasons and should be checked in those with asthma. Several diagnostic techniques are available to assay food reactivities and they can buttress diagnostic use of an elimination diet.

VI. DRUG–NUTRIENT INTERACTIONS

The nutritional agents used in asthma therapy do not seem to adversely impact pharmacologic agents, outside of the concern that imbalances from higher dosing of essential fatty acids can influence coagulation. Nutritional agents can have a medication-sparing effect. Asthma medications as well as medications for other conditions discussed in this text may need to be adjusted downward.

There are certain classes of medications that are not used in asthma per se, but negatively impact some of the nutrient levels discussed above:

* Diuretics: magnesium depletion, dehydration
* Oral contraceptives: diminished vitamin B6
* Steroids: obesity, increased intestinal permeability
* NSAIDs: increased intestinal permeability
* Antibiotics: disturb gut flora (dysbiosis)

VII. SPECIAL CONSIDERATIONS

In light of the discussion under pathophysiology above, a word should be said about the concept of asthma prevention. Since primary care physicians are obviously caring for women of child-bearing age as well as for young children, they might consider the implications of the Hygiene Hypothesis, especially when treating individuals with a family history of atopy.

The use of antibiotics should be minimized in order to maintain normal intestinal flora. Consuming antibiotic-free meat and poultry products may also be helpful, as well as the regular consumption of probiotic supplements. In the perinatal period, one should weigh the theoretically beneficial effects of vaginal delivery and breastfeeding on the establishment of intestinal flora as well. Given the results of some of the prospective studies[110,111] and the extreme safety of these agents, it might be reasonable to consider probiotic supplementation in infants with a family history of allergy. There is even some evidence that the nutritional factors such as flavonoids used therapeutically may have a role in prevention as well.[112]

VIII. SUMMARY

There are many patients in whom nutritional interventions can effectively treat asthma, requiring either no other treatment or only occasional beta-agonist use instead of the chronic anti-inflammatory agents that they would otherwise require. For others, one can achieve a significant medication-sparing effect with decreased costs and side effects. Especially in children, one can create a more normal life and possibly avoid some of the vicious cycles that medications can create around obesity, intestinal permeability, and gut flora disturbances.

These are the major diagnostic and therapeutic points to consider in using a nutritional approach to asthma treatment:

* Investigate for food triggers by diet history, elimination diet, and if necessary, additional food allergy testing.
* Avoid preservatives and sulfites, which may function as triggers.
* Consider measurement of RBC magnesium, serum selenium, and plasma zinc.
* Increase flavonoids and micronutrients in diet by enhanced consumption of colored fruits and vegetables, whole grains, nuts, and seeds, as well as weekly fish consumption, avoiding large fish that may be high in mercury.
* Maintain ideal body weight.
* Consider supplementing the following minerals: magnesium 250 to 500 mg, selenium 200 µg, zinc 20 to 40 mg. Daily dosage refers to amount of elemental mineral, which can be bound to a variety of salts or amino acid chelates.

- Consider supplementing the following antioxidants: vitamin C at least 500 to 1000 mg, vitamin E 100 to 400 IU (high gamma-tocopherol), pycnogenol 2 mg/kg body weight/day up to 200 mg, lycopene 30 mg for exercise-induced asthma, and quercetin 1 to 2 g/day in divided doses.
- Balance essential fatty acids, which can frequently be achieved with supplemental dosing of fish oil 1 to 3 g/day (use caution due to coagulation effect in patients on anticoagulants, NSAIDS, etc.) and gamma-linolenic acid 240 to 960 mg.
- Supplement vitamin B6 at 100 to 200 mg/day.
- Dose vitamin D to normalize blood levels.
- Use relaxation techniques and yoga training as an adjunct to dietary recommendations.
- Practice primary prevention strategies for pregnant women and infants by encouraging breastfeeding, minimizing antibiotics, and using supplemental probiotics.

REFERENCES

1. Masoli M, Fabian D, et al. The global burden of asthma: executive summary of the GINA Dissemination Committee Report. *Allergy*, 2004; 59: 469–478.
2. National Health Interview Survey 1981–2004, National Center for Health Statistics. US Dept. of Health and Human Services
3. Asher M, Innes I. Worldwide time trends in the prevalence of asthma, allergic rhinoconjunctivitis, and eczema in childhood: ISAAC phase one and three report multicountry cross-sectional surveys. *Lancet*, 368: 733–743.
4. Magkos F, Arvaniti F, Zampelas A. Organic food: nutritious food or food for thought? A review of the evidence. *Int J Food Sci Nutr*, 2003 Sep; 54(5): 357–371.
5. Guidelines for the Diagnosis and Management of Asthma, NAEP Expert Panel Report II. *NIH Publ* 97-4051, Bethesda MD, National Heart, Lung and Blood Inst, 1997.
6. Evans R, Mellins R, et al. Improving care for minority children with asthma: professional education in public health clinics. *Pediatrics*, 1997; 99: 157–164.
7. Sarnat JA, Asthma and air quality. *Curr Opin Pulm Med*, 2007 Jan; 13(1): 63–66.
8. Sole D, Camelo-Nunes IC, et al. Prevalence of asthma, rhinitis and atopic eczema in Brazilian adolescents related to exposure to gaseous air pollutants and socioeconomic status. *J Investig Allergol Clin Immunol*, 2007; 17(1): 6–13.
9. Villeneuve PJ, Chen L, et al. Outdoor pollution and emergency department visits for asthma among children and adults: a case-crossover study in northern Alberta, Canada. *Eviron Health*, 2007 Dec 24; 6(1): 40.
10. Hock G, Brunekreef B. Effect of photochemical air pollution on acute respiratory symptoms in children. *Am J Respir Crit Care Med*, 1995; 151: 27–32.
11. Byrd RS, Joad JP. Urban asthma. *Curr Opin Pulm Med*, 2006; 12(1): 68–74.
12. Imboden M, Downs S, et al. Glutathione S-transferase genotypes modify lung function decline in the general population: SAPALDIA cohort study. *Resp Res*, 2007; 8: 2.
13. London SJ. Gene-air pollution interactions in asthma. *Proc Am Ther Soc*, 2007 Jul; 4(3): 217–220.
14. Gurrie MJ. Exogenous Type I cytokines modulate mercury-induced hyper-IgE in the rat. *Clin Exp Immunol*, 2000; 121: 17–22.
15. Massarella G, Bianco A, et al. The Th_1/Th_2 lymphocyte polarization in asthma. *Allergy*, 2000; 55: suppl. 61: 6–9.
16. Gregori S, Giarratana N, et al. A 1 alpha, 25-dihydroxyD(3) analog enhances regulatory T-cells and arrests autoimmune diabetes in NOD mice. *Diabetes*, 2002; 51: 1367–1374.
17. Xystrakis E, Kusumakar S, et al. Reversing the defective induction of IL-10-secreting regulatory T-cells in glucocorticosteroid-resistant asthma patients. *J Clin Invest*, 2006; 116: 146–155.
18. Litonjua A, Weiss S. Is Vitamin D deficiency to blame for asthma epidemic? *J Allerg Clin Immunol*, 2007 Nov; 120(5):1031–1035.
19. Umetsu D, Akbar O, DeKruyff. Regulatory T Cells control the development of allergic disease and asthma. *J Allerg Clin Immunol*, 112(3): 480–487.
20. Romagna S. Regulatory T Cells: which role in the pathogenesis and treatment of allergic disorders? *Allergy*, 2006; 61: 3–14.
21. von Mutius E. The influence of birth order on the expression of atopy in families: a gene-environment interaction? *Clin Exp Allergy*, 1998; 28: 1454–1456.

22. Ball T, Castro-Rodriguez J, et al. Siblings, day-care attendance, and the risk of asthma and wheezing during childhood. *N Engl J Med*, 2000; 343: 538–543.

23. Braun-Fahrlander C, Riedler J, et al. Environmental exposures to endotoxin and its relation to asthma in school age children. *NEJM*, 2002; 347: 869–877.

24. Wickens K, Pearce N, et al. Antibiotic use in early childhood and the development of asthma. *Clin Exp Aller*, 1999; 29: 766–771.

25. Yan F, Polk DB. Commensal bacteria in the gut: learning who our friends are. *Curr Opin Gastroenterol*, 2004; 20: 565–571.

26. Kozyrskyj A, Ernst P, Becker A. Increased risk of childhood asthma from antibiotic use in early life. *Chest*, 2007; 31: 1753–1759.

27. Matysiak-Budnik T, Heyman M. Food allergy and H. Pylori. *J Ped Gastro Nutr*, 2002; 34: 5–12.

28. H. Pylori may protect against asthma, other respiratory conditions. *Int Med World Report*, 2007; (1): 15.

29. Yang IA, et al. The role of TLR's and.... *Curr Opin Allerg Clin Immunol*, 2006 Feb; 6(1): 23–28.

30. Bernard A. Increased intestinal permeability in bronchial asthma. *J Allerg Clin Immunol*, 1996; 97: 1173–1178.

31. Kiziltas S, Imeryuz N, et al. Corticosteroid therapy augments gastroduodenol permeability to sucrose. *Am J Gastroenterol*, 1998 Dec; 93(12): 2420–2425.

32. Rosenfeldt V, Benfeldt B. Effect of probiotics on gastrointestinal symptoms and small intestinal permeability in children with atop dermatitis. *J Pediatrics*, 2004: 612–616.

33. Romieu, GSTM1 and GSTP1 and respiratory health. *Eur Resp J*, 2006 Nov; 28(5): 953–959.

34. Tamer L, et al. GST gene polymorphisms. *Respirology*, 2004 Nov; 9(4): 493–498.

35. Suguira H, Ichinose M, et al. Oxidative and nitrative stress in bronchila asthma. *Antiox Redox Signal*, 2008 April; 10(4): 785–798.

36. Misso NL, et al. Plasma concentration of dietary and non-dietary antioxidants....*Eur Respir J*, 2005 Aug; 9(4): 493–498.

37. Ford ES, et al. Serum antioxidant concentrations among U.S. adults with self-reported asthma. *J Asthma*, 2004; 41(2): 179–187.

38. Bousquet J, Michel F. Food allergy and asthma. *Ann Allerg*, 1998 Dec; Part II; 61: 70–74.

39. Anthony HM et al. Food intolerance. *Lancet*, 1994 July 9; 344: 136–137.

40. Watson W, et al. Food hypersensitivity and changes in airway function. *J Allerg and Clin Immunol*, 1992; (I/Part II): 184/159.

41. Wilson N, et al. Bronchial hyperactivity in food and drink intolerance. *Ann Allerg*, 1988 Dec; 61: 75–79.

42. Hoj L, et al. A double blind controlled trial of elemental diet in severe, perennial asthma. *Allergy* 1981; 36: 257–262.

43. Borok G, et al. Childhood asthma—food the trigger? *South Afr Med Journ*, 1990 March 3; 77: 269.

44. Weber R, Col MC, et al. Food additives and allergy. *Ann Allerg*, 70: 183–191.

45. Lessof MH, et al. Reactions to food additives. *Clin and Exp Allergy*, 1995; 25 (suppl): 27–28.

46. Hodge L, Yank Y, et al. Assessment of food chemical intolerance in adult asthmatic subjects. *Thorax*, 1996 Aug; 51(8): 805–809.

47. Valley H, et al. Changes in hyperresponsiveness following high- and low-sulfite wine challenge in wine-sensitive asthma patients. *Clin Exp Allerg*, 2007 July; 37(7): 1062–1066.

48. Vally H, Thompson PJ. Role of sulfite additives in wine-induced asthma: single dose and cumulative dose studies. *Thorax*, 2001 Oct; 56(10): 763–769.

49. Hodge L. Consumption of oily fish and asthma risk. *Med J Australia*, 1996; 164: 137–140.

50. Thien F, et al. Oily fish and asthma—a fish story? *Med J Australia*, 1996 Feb 5; 164: 135–136.

51. Beuther DA. Obesity and asthma. *Am J Resp Crit Care Med*, 2006 Jul 15; 174(2): 112–119.

52. Lu FL, Johnston RA, et al. Increased pulmonary responses to ozone exposure in obese db/db mice. *Am J Physiol Cell Mol Physiol*, 2006 May; 290(5): L856–65.

53. Kelly J, et al. Altered lung antioxidant status in patients with mild asthma. *Lancet*, 1999; 354: 482–483.

54. Ochs-Balcom HM, Grant BJ, et al. Antioxidants, oxidative stress and pulmonary function in individuals diagnosed with asthma or COPD. *Eur J Clin Nutr*, 2006 Aug; 60(8): 991–999.

55. Misso NL, Brooks-Wildhaber J, et al. Plasma concentration of dietary and nondietary antioxidants are low in severe asthma. *Eur Resp J*, 2005 Aug; 26(2): 257–264.

56. Kadrabova J, et al. Selenium status is decreased in patients with intrinsic asthma. *Biol Trace Elem Res*, 1996; 52: 241–248.

57. Kocyigit A, Armutcu F, et al. Alterations in plasma essential trace elements.....and the possible role of these elements on oxidative status in patients with childhood asthma. *Biol Trac Elem Res*, 2004 Jan; 97(1): 31–41.

58. Panaszek K, Barg W, Obojski A. The use of magnesium in bronchial asthma: a new approach to an old problem. *Arch Immunol Ther Exp*, 2007 Feb 5; 5(1): 354.

59. Sedighi M, Pourpak Z, et al. Low magnesium concentrations in erthrocytes of children with acute asthma. *Iran J Aller*, 2006 Dec; 5(4): 183–186.

60. Kazaks AG, Uriu-Adams JY, et al. Multiple measures of magnesium status are comparable in mild asthma and control subjects. *J Asthma*, 2006 Dec; 43(10): 783–788.

61. Zerras E, Papatherdorou G, et al. Reduced intracellular magnesium concentration in patients with acute asthma. *Chest*, 2003 Jan; 123(1): 113–118.

62. Sinert R, Spektor M, et al. Ionized magnesium levels and the ratio of ionized calcium to magnesium in asthma patients before and after treatment with magnesium. *Scand J Clin Lab Invest*, 2005; 65(8): 659–670.

63. Spivy WH, Skobellof EM, Levin RM. Effect of magnesiuim chloride on rabbit bronchial smooth muscle. *Ann Emerg Med*, 1990; 19: 1107–1112.

64. Nuppen M, Vanmaele L, et al. Bronchodilating effect of intravenous magnesium sulfate in acute severe bronchial asthma. *Chest*, 1990; 97: 373–377.

65. Skobelloff EM, Spivy WH, McNamara RM, et al. Intravenous magnesium sulfate for treatment of acute severe asthma in the emergency department. *JAMA*, 1989; 262: 1210–1213.

66. Ciarallo J, Sauer A, Shannon MW. Intravenous magnesium for moderate to severe asthma: results of a randomized, placebo-controlled trial. *J Pediatr*, 1996; 129: 809–814.

67. Gantijo-Amaral E, Ribeiro MA, et al. Oral magnesium supplementation in asthmatic children: a double blind placebo-controlled trial. *Eur J Clin Nutr*, 2007 Jan; 61(1): 54–60.

68. Bede D, Suranyi A, et al. Urinary magnesium excretion in asthmatic children receiving magnesium supplementation: a randomized, placebo-controlled double blind study. *Manges Res*, 2003 Dec; 16(4): 1262–1270.

69. Fogarty A, Lewis SA, et al. Oral magnesium and vitamin C supplementation in asthma: a parallel group randomized placebo-controlled trial. *Clin Exp Allerg*, 2003 Oct; 33(10): 1355–1359.

70. Tudor R, Zalewski PD, et al. Zinc in health and chronic disease. *J Nutr Health Aging*, 2005; 9(1): 45–51.

71. Saaereks V, Ylatilo P, et al. Opposite effects of nicotinic acid and pyridoxine on systemic prostacycline, thromboxane and leukotriene production in man. *Pharmacol Toxicol*, 2002 June; 90(6): 338–342.

72. Collip PJ, Chen SY, et al. Tryptophan metabolism in bronchial asthma. *Ann Allerg*, 1975 Sep; 35(3): 153–158.

73. Reynolds RD, Natta CL. Depressed plasma pyridoxal phosphate concentration in adult asthmatics. *J Clin Nutr*, 1985 Apr; 41(4): 684–688.

74. Collipp PJ, Goldzier S 3rd, et al. Pyridoxine treatment of childhood bronchial asthma. *Annal Allerg*, 1975 Aug; 35(2): 93–97.

75. Fogarty A, Lewis S, et al. Dietary vitamin E, IgE concentration and atopy. *Lancet* 2000; 356: 1573–1574.

76. Troisi RJ, Willet WC, et al. A prospective study of diet and adult onset asthma. *Am J Resp Crit Care Med*, 1995; 151: 1401–1408.

77. Bielory L, Gandhi R. Asthma and vitamin C. *Ann Allerg*, 1994 Aug; 73(2): 89–96.

78. Lau BH, Riesen SK, et al. Pycnogenol as an adjunct in the management of childhood asthma. *J Asthma*, 2004; 41(8): 825–832.

79. Hosseini S, Pishnamazi S, et al. Pycnogenol in the management of asthma. *J Med Food*, 2001 Winter; 4(4): 201–209.

80. Neuman I, Nahum H. Reduction of exercise-induced asthma oxidative stress by lycopene, a natural antioxidant. *Allergy*, 2000; 55: 1184–1189.

81. Tanaka T, Higa S, et al. Flavanoids as potential anti-allergy substances. *Curr Med Chem – Antiinflamm and Anti-Allerg Ag*, 2003 (2): 57–65.

82. Min YD, Choi CH, et al. Quercetin inhibits expression of inflammatory cytokines through attenuation of NFkB and p38MAPk in the HMC-1 human mast cell line. *Inflamm Res*, 2007 May; 56(5): 210–215.

83. Kandere-Grzybowska K, Kempuraj D, et al. Regulation of IL1-induced selective IL6 release from human mast cells and inhibition by quercetin. *Br J Pharmacol*, 2006 May; 148(2): 208–215.

84. Nanua S, Zick SM, et al. Quercetin blocks airway epithelial cell chemokine expression. *Am J Resp Cell Mol Biol*, 2006 Nov; 35(5): 602–610.

85. Nair MP, Kandaswami C, et al. The flavonoid, quercetin, differentially regulates Th-1 (IFNgamma) and Th-2 (IL4) cytokine gene expression by normal peripheral blood mononuclear cells. *Biochem Biophys Acta*, 2002 Dec 16; 1593(1): 29–36.

86. Ekpo OE, Pretorius E. Asthma, Euphorbia hirta and its anti-inflammatory properties. *South Afr J Science*, 2007 May/June; 103: 201–203.

87. Chaabi M, Freund-Michel V, et al. Anti-proliferative effect of Euphorbia stenoclada in human airway smooth muscle cells in culture. *J Ethnopharm*, 2007; 109: 134–139.

88. Carey MA, Germolec DR, et al. Cyclogenase enzymes in allergic inflammation and asthma. *Leukot Essent Fatty Acids*, 2003; 69(2–3): 157–162.

89. Calabrses C, Triggliano M, et al. Arachadonic acid metabolism in inflammatory cells of patients with bronchial asthma. *Allergy*, 2000; 55(suppl 61): 27–30.

90. Oddy WH, deKler NH, et al. Ratio of omega 6 to omega 3 fatty acids and childhood asthma. *J Asthma*, 2004; 41(3): 319–326.

91. Schwarz J, Weiss ST. The relationship of dietary fish intake to level of pulmonary function in the first National Health and Nutrition Survey. *Eur Respir J*, 1994; 7: 1821–1824.

92. Hodge L, Salmoc CM, et al. Effect of dietary intake of omega 3 and omega 6 fatty acids on severity of asthma in children. *Eur Respir J*, 2008; 11: 361–365.

93. Mihrshahi S, Peat JK, et al. Effect of omega 3 fatty acid concentration in plasma on symptoms of asthma at 18 months of age. *Ped Allerg Immunol*, 2004 Dec; 15(6): 517–522.

94. Nagakkura T, Matsuda S, et al. Dietary supplementation with fish oil rich in omega 3 polyunsaturated fatty acids in children with bronchial asthma. *Eur Respir J*, 2000 Nov; 16(5): 861–865.

95. Peat J, Mihrsahi S, et al. Three year outcomes of dietary fatty acid modification and house dust mite reduction in the Childhood Asthma Prevention Study. *J Allerg Clin Immunol*, 114(4): 807–813.

96. Dry J, Vincent D. Effect of a fish oil diet on asthma: results of a one year double blind trial. *Int Arch Allerg Appl Immunol*, 1991; 85: 156–157.

97. Reisman J, Schachter HM, et al. Treating asthma with omega 3 fatty acids: where is the evidence? *BMC Compl Altern Med*, 2006 Jul 19; 6: 26.

98. Thien, et al. Dietary fish oil effects on seasonal hay fever and asthma in pollen-sensitive subjects. *Am J Resp Dis*, 1993; 147: 1138–1143.

99. Arm J, et al. The effect of dietary supplementation with fish oil lipids on the airway response to inhalant allergy and bronchial asthma. *Am Rev Resp Dis*, 1989; 139: 1395–1400.

100. Markham A, Wilkinson J. Complementary and alternative medicine in the management of asthma. An examination of the evidence. *J Asthma*, 2004; 41(2): 131–139.

101. Khayyall MT, El-Ghazaly MA, et al. A clinical study of the potential beneficial effects of a propolis food product as an adjuvant in asthmatic patients.

102. Sanchez-Mendoza ME, Torres G, et al. Mechanisms of relaxant of a crude hexane extract of Gnaphalium liebmannii in guinea pig tracheal smooth muscle. *J Ethnopoharmocol*, 2007; 111: 142–147.

103. Wilkins JH, et al. Effects of a platelet activating factor-antagonist (BN52063) on bronchoconstriction and platelet activation during exercise-induced asthma. *Br J Clin Pharmacol*, 1990; 29: 85–91.

104. Shivpuri DN, et al. Treatment of asthma with an alcoholic extract of Tylophora Indica: a crossover, double blind study. *Ann Allerg*, 1972 July; 30: 407–412.

105. Lowe TH. Efficacy of 'functional relaxation' in comparison to terbutaline and a 'placebo relaxant' method in patients with acute asthma. *Psychother Psychosom*, 2001; 70: 151–157.

106. Jain SC, Rai L, et al. Effect of yoga training on exercise tolerance in adolescents with childhood asthma. *J Asthma*, 1991; 28: 437–442.

107. Shapiro MY, Berkman N, et al. Short term acupuncture treatment is of no benefit in patients with moderate persistent asthma. *Chest*, 2002; 121(5): 1396–1400.

108. Biernacki W, Peake MD, Acupuncture in the treatment of stable asthma. *Respir Med*, 1998; 92: 1143–1145.

109. Joo S, Schott C, et al. Immunological effects of acupuncture in the treatment of allergic asthma: a randomized, controlled trial. *J Altern Compl Med*, 2000; 6(6): 519–525.

110. Bjorksten B. Evidence of probiotics in prevention of allergy and asthma. *Curr Drug Targ – Inflam Allerg*, 2005; 4: 599–604.

111. Kalliomaki M, Salminen S, et al. Probiotics in primary prevention of atopic disease: a randomized, placebo-controlled trial. *Lancet*, 2001; 357: 1076–1079.

112. Willers SM, Devereux G, Craig LCA, et al. Maternal food consumption during pregnancy and asthma, respiratory and atopic symptoms in 5-year-old children. *Thorax*, 2007; 62: 773–779.

9 Chronic Obstructive Pulmonary Disease

A Nutrition Review

David R. Thomas, M.D.

I. INTRODUCTION

An understanding of the role of nutrition in chronic obstructive pulmonary disease (COPD) must begin with recent advances in the understanding of the pathophysiology of COPD. COPD is a genetic, particle-associated, cytokine-mediated inflammatory disease of the pulmonary airways.[1] The underlying prerequisite for the development of COPD is a complex genetic abnormality where products of certain genes interact with environmental stimuli to produce an excessive response that results in clinical expression of the disease. This genetic variation in the host response to the toxic gases and particles present in the environment contributes to our understanding of why only a fraction of smokers of the same age and gender who have smoked equivalent amounts develop COPD.[2]

II. EPIDEMIOLOGY

Only a fraction of smokers of the same age and gender who have smoked equivalent amounts develop COPD.[3] Epidemiologic tools have helped delineate several predisposing host factors, including alpha-1 antitrypsin deficiency, genetically induced airway hyperresponsiveness, exposure to tobacco smoke, air pollution, occupational exposure, lung maturity at birth, and socioeconomic status. Several aspects of nutrition, including diet, genetic variation in nutrient needs, metabolic response to toxicants, and obesity, can be predisposing factors.

III. PATHOPHYSIOLOGY

The molecular basis of COPD is becoming increasingly understood. The inhalation of toxic particulate matter from the environment, especially in the form of cigarette smoke, leads to activation of proinflammatory cytokines, including interleukin-8, tumor necrosis factor alpha, and leucotriene B4, that have a direct effect on destruction of pulmonary tissues. In addition, oxidative stress and an imbalance between protease and anti-protease production contribute to the inflammation.

The diagnosis of COPD includes heterogeneous pathological conditions that result in limitations of airflow. COPD includes both chronic bronchitis, characterized by fibrosis and obstruction of small airways, and emphysema, characterized by enlargement of airspaces, destruction of lung parenchyma, loss of lung elasticity, and closure of small airways. Chronic bronchitis is defined by a productive cough lasting for more than 3 months in each of two successive years. This reflects mucous hypersecretion and may not necessarily be associated with airflow limitation. Most patients with COPD have overlap of both pathological mechanisms, but may differ in the relative proportion of emphysema and obstructive bronchiolitis.[4] COPD is distinct from asthma where there is variable airflow obstruction that is spontaneously reversible or reversible with treatment. COPD is characterized by slowly progressive development of airflow limitation that is poorly reversible. However, some people may have coexistent syndromes of asthma and COPD.

Clear phenotypes can be clinically distinguished in people with COPD. Historically, clinicians have observed a "blue bloater" phenotype, characterized by chronic bronchitis symptoms. Those with predominantly chronic bronchitis are often obese. A "pink puffer" phenotype is characterized by low body weight and symptoms predominantly of emphysema. Despite the fact that these clinical phenotypes are not always clearly defined, this clinical observation has driven research into the relationship of body weight and COPD.

Compared to those with a reference body mass index (BMI) between 18.5 to 24.9, people with a BMI greater than 28 are more likely to develop asthma or chronic bronchitis [odds ratio (OR) 2.10, 95% confidence intervals (CI) 1.31 to 3.36, and 1.80, 95% CI 1.32 to 2.46, respectively]. People who develop emphysema are more likely to have a BMI less than 18.5 (OR 2.97, 95% CI 1.33 to 6.68).[5] Data from this longitudinal study show that obesity precedes the diagnosis of COPD and is not the result of a reduction of physical activity due to the respiratory impairment. These data also confirm the clinical observation that people with emphysema are more likely to have a low BMI.

IV. TREATMENT APPROACHES

There is no cure for COPD. The only intervention that has been shown to slow the progressive decline in the clinical measurement of progression of COPD (FEV_1, the lung forced vital capacity in 1 second) is cessation of inhalation of particulate matter in the form of cigarette smoking.[6] Although smoking is the major causal mechanism in COPD, quitting smoking does not result in resolution of the inflammatory response in the airways.[7] All other interventions in the management of COPD must be considered palliative.[8]

V. RELATIONSHIP OF COPD AND NUTRITIONAL STATUS

Between 25% to 33% of people with moderate to severe COPD are reported to be malnourished.[9] The definitions of malnutrition vary considerably, but frequently include weight loss or low body weight. Low body weight in those with COPD is associated with impaired pulmonary status, reduced diaphragmatic mass, and lower exercise capacity, and it independently predicts a higher mortality rate.[10,11]

Various mechanisms have been proposed for the weight loss occurring with COPD. Failure to consume adequate calories or inability to eat large meals due to dyspnea (starvation), an elevated cost of ventilation and an elevated resting energy expenditure (inadequate nutrition),[12,13] muscle loss due to dyspnea-related inactivity (sarcopenia), the effects of inflammation (cachexia), or use of corticosteroids[14] may contribute to weight loss.

In 412 subjects with moderate to severe COPD, BMI and bioelectrical impedance were used to form four categories of nutritional depletion: (1) Cachexia was defined as a BMI less than 21 and a low fat-free mass. (2) Semi-starvation was defined as a BMI less than 21 and a normal sex-adjusted fat-free mass. (3) Muscle atrophy was defined as a BMI greater than or equal to 21 and a low sex-adjusted fat-free mass. (4) No nutritional depletion was considered to be a BMI greater than or equal to 21 and a normal fat-free mass. Subjects were followed for 2 to 5 years and mortality was assessed at the end of the study. The subjects with a low fat-free mass (either cachexia or muscle atrophy) were at highest risk of death (relative risk 1.91, 95% CI 1.37 to 2.67 and 1.96, 95% CI 1.21 to 3.17, respectively), compared with the no depletion group. A low BMI without a low fat-free mass was not associated with a higher mortality.[15] These data suggest that the classical parameters of inadequate nutrient intake are not associated with a higher mortality.

VI. ETIOLOGY OF WEIGHT LOSS IN COPD

The association of lower body weight, increased caloric need, and poor outcome has focused clinical research on the hypothesis that inadequate intake of protein and calories results in clinical deterioration in people with COPD. By this reasoning, replenishment of nutrients should produce weight gain and improve clinical outcome. However, the results from individual clinical trials of nutritional support in people with COPD have been variable. Little effect has been seen in trials with less than 2 weeks duration.

A recent meta-analysis combined 14 randomized clinical trials involving 487 people with COPD who had nutritional support for more than 2 weeks. The majority of the individual trials have been small and of short duration. Even when the analysis is limited to studies longer than 2 weeks, very little support is found for the hypothesis that simple nutritional supplementation is beneficial. Nutritional support had no significant effect on weight gain, anthropometric measures, lung function, or exercise capacity in patients with stable COPD, even when nutritional supplementation was combined with a multidisciplinary rehabilitation program and exercise therapy. Tables 9.1 and 9.2 present the study parameters and results.[16] Few studies have evaluated health-related quality of life,

---

TABLE 9.1
Randomized Controlled Trials with Greater Than 2 Weeks Duration of Nutritional Supplements in COPD Patients

Study Author	Number	Intervention
Lewis MJ, et al., 1987	10 intervention vs. 11 controls, undernourished	500–100 Kcal standard (Isocal HCN) vs. usual diet for 8 weeks
Efthimiou J, 1988	7 intervention, undernourished vs. 7 well nourished	640–1280 Kcal/d standard (build-up) vs. none for 12 weeks
Knowles JB, et al., 1988	13 intervention vs. 12 controls, mixed nutritional status	Increased intake 18%–26% standard (Sustacal) vs. usual diet for 8 weeks
Otte KE, et al., 1989	13 intervention vs. 15 controls, undernourished	400 Kcal/d supplement vs. diluted supplement for 13 weeks
Whittaker JS, et al., 1990	6 intervention vs. 4 controls, malnourished	1000 Kcal/d, standard (Isocal) vs. diluted control for 16 days
Fuenzalida CE, et al., 1990	5 subjects with weight loss vs. 4 controls	1080 Kcal/d, standard (Sustacal HC) vs. usual diet for 21 days
Rogers RM, et al., 1992	15 intervention vs. 13 controls, malnourished	1.7 times REE, 1.5 g/kg/day protein vs. none
DeLetter, 1994	18 intervention vs. 17 controls, undernourished	355 Kcal/d standard formula (Pulmocare) vs. none for 8 weeks
Schols AMWJ, et al., 1995	33 intervention vs. 38 controls, nourished	420 Kcal, 14% protein supplement vs. none for 8 weeks
Schols AMWJ, et al., 1995	39 intervention vs. 25 controls, undernourished	420 Kcal/d, 14% protein supplement vs. none for 8 weeks
Goris AHC, et al., 2003	11 intervention vs. 9 controls, undernourished	Standard (Respifor) vs. none for 12 weeks
Steiner MC, et al., 2003	42 intervention vs. 43 controls, mixed nutritional status	570 Kcal/d, standard (Respifor) vs. none for 7 weeks
Teramoto S, et al., 2004	20 intervention vs. 20 controls, undernourished	20% fat, 18% protein, low carbohydrate vs. none for 4 weeks
Weekes CE, et al., 2004	20 intervention vs. 17 controls, undernourished or at risk	Fortified milk vs. none for 6 months

Source: Compiled from [16].

TABLE 9.2
Meta-Analysis of Outcome Measures for Nutritional Support in COPD Patients

Outcome	Number of Trials	Number of Patients/Controls	Effect Size	95% Confidence Interval
Weight	12	214/215	1.15 kg	–0.85 to 3.14
Arm muscle circumference	8	111/103	0.03 cm	–0.77 to 0.83
Tricep skinfold thickness	6	63/61	1.36 mm	–0.14 to 2.86
6-minute walk	3	38/39	3.4 m	–46.1 to 52.9
FEV_1	6	80/70	–0.12	–0.44 to 0.20
PI_{max}	6	81/71	3.55 cm water	–1.9 to 9.0
PE_{max}	6	81/73	8.21 cm water	–0.48 to 16.9
HRQOL (SF-36)	1			
Vitality	1	31/28	4.70	0.40 to 9.00
Health change	1	31/28	11.00	4.40 to 17.52
HRQOL (CRQ) dyspnea	1	25/35	–0.39	–1.10 to 0.50
Hospital admissions	1	31/28	0.40	0.14 to 1.18

Key: FEV_1=forced expiratory volume in 1 second; PI_{max}=maximum inspiratory pressure; PE_{max}=maximum expiratory
pressure; HRQOL=Health related quality of life; SF-36=Short form 36 quality of life instrument; CRQ=Clinical
respiratory quality instrument.
Source: Compiled from [16].

but in those that did, little overall effect is seen. While larger and better studies are needed, the current data suggest that provision of supplemental calories or protein has had little effect on people with COPD. In addition, those with COPD who receive enteral feedings have been prospectively observed to have a decreased survival rate compared to untreated patients.[17]

The weight loss in people with COPD has also been attributed to an increased oxygen cost of ventilation (O_2 cost). In small numbers of malnourished patients with COPD, the O_2 cost of ventilation was higher (4.28 +/– 0.98 mL, n=9), relative to the normally nourished COPD group (2.61 +/– 1.07, n=10), and normal control subjects (1.23 +/– 0.51, n=7).[18]

The measured Resting Energy Equivalent (REE) has been shown to be significantly higher in people with COPD who were undernourished (1.15 +/– 0.02), compared to an adequately nourished COPD group (0.99 +/– 0.03) and normal controls (0.93 +/– 0.02).[19] These findings suggest that those with COPD may require additional protein and calories to overcome the increased work of breathing. However, the finding of an elevated REE in people with COPD is not consistent across all studies. In 172 people in a rehabilitation setting, only 26% of those with COPD had an REE greater than 110%. The subjects with an elevated REE were older and had lower total lung capacities, suggesting worse disease.[20] The depletion in fat-free mass was not different between hypermetabolic and normometabolic patients. REE alone may not explain the weight loss in people with COPD as it may be offset by a decrease in daily activities.[21] The total energy expenditure in these patients may not be different from healthy control patients.[22]

The dismal results from nutritional intervention trials have redirected the assessment of the etiology of weight loss in people with COPD. Weight loss due to inadequate nutrition or increased protein-energy requirement should respond to the provision of adequate calories. Because clinical trials of supplemental calories or protein have shown little effect, the weight loss in those with COPD may be caused by factors intrinsic to the disease itself.

Reduced food intake alone does not seem to be the primary cause of weight loss in people with COPD. The weight loss with COPD involves depletion in both fat mass and fat-free mass. The loss of fat-free mass is more important and appears to be due to a depression of protein synthesis.

Although weight-losing COPD patients are not catabolic, nutritional supplementation alone does not appear to reverse the loss of fat-free mass.[23]

Recent advances in understanding the pathogenesis of COPD suggest that the disease is a result of proinflammatory cytokine activation. This suggests that the weight loss in people with COPD is related to this inflammatory state.

The syndrome of cachexia, which is widely recognized in a number of disease states,[24] has been linked to weight loss in COPD.[25,26] Patients with severe emphysema have increased levels of tumor necrosis factor-alpha, soluble tumor necrosis receptors R55 and R75, interleukin-6, and lipopoly-saccharide binding protein.[27] In addition, C-reactive protein, a marker for inflammation, is elevated in those with COPD who have a decreased fat-free mass. In a study of 102 patients with clinically stable COPD, C-reactive protein levels were elevated in 48 patients. In these patients, REE and interleukin-6 levels were higher compared to other patients, and inversely correlated with exercise capacity and 6-minute walking distance. C-reactive protein correlated with both body mass index and fat mass index.[28]

Cytokines have a direct negative effect on muscle mass, and an increase in concentration of inflammatory markers has been associated with a reduced lean mass.[29-31] Patients with cachexia experience severe progressive loss of skeletal muscle. The loss of skeletal muscle mass is due to a combination of reduced protein synthesis and increased protein degradation. While reduced protein synthesis plays a role, protein degradation is the major cause of loss of skeletal muscle mass in cachexia.

Both fat and fat-free mass are depleted in cachexia syndromes, a similar picture to the weight loss observed in COPD patients. Low-grade systemic inflammation is significantly elevated in patients with COPD compared to healthy control patients. Inflammation was highest in COPD patients with muscle wasting defined by a low fat-free mass.[32]

In addition to the effect of cytokines on skeletal muscle, cytokines act in the hypothalamus to cause an imbalance between the orexigenic and anorexigenic regulatory pathways. Cytokines directly result in feeding suppression, and lower intake of nutrients and cachexia is nearly always accompanied by anorexia. Interleukin-1 beta and tumor necrosis factor act on the glucose-sensitive neurons in the ventromedial hypothalamic nucleus (a "satiety" site) and the lateral hypothalamic area (a "hunger" site).[33] In the anorexia-cachexia syndrome, the peripheral signals for an energy deficit reaching the hypothalamus fail to produce a response, which propagates the cachectic process.[34] By this mechanism, proinflammatory cytokines lead to a decrease in nutrient intake. The decrease in intake appears to contribute to, but not directly cause, the loss of body mass.

This decreased subjective desire to eat has been observed in cachectic COPD patients. Cachexia, defined as weight loss greater than 7.5% of body weight and BMI less than 24.1 kg/m^2, was diagnosed in 33% (34/103) subjects with COPD.[35] The levels of interleukin-6 and the interleukin-6 to interleukin-10 ratio were significantly higher in the cachectic COPD patients, along with a decreased appetite.

In those with COPD who participated in 8 weeks of 500 to 750 Kcal/d nutritional supplementation, the 14 patients who did not gain weight were compared with 10 who gained 10% or more of their body weight. The nonresponders were older, had an elevated systemic inflammatory response, and had anorexia, suggesting that cachexia may be the mediator of nonresponse.[36]

VII.   MANAGEMENT OF CACHEXIA IN COPD

In contrast to starvation, cachexia is remarkably resistant to hypercaloric feeding. Both enteral and parenteral feeding in cancer cachexia have consistently failed to show any benefit in terms of weight gain, nutritional status, quality of life, or survival.[37] These findings in cancer cachexia are similar to the results in nutritional supplementation studies in COPD, where enteral feeding has been associated with higher mortality. For this reason, attention has been directed to other adjunctive measures.

Pharmacological treatment of anorexia with agents that modulate cytokine production has produced weight gain in the cachexia syndrome.[38] Steroids and hormonal agents such as megesterol acetate are currently widely used in the treatment of cancer and HIV cachexia and anorexia.[39] Megestrol acetate has also been shown to increase appetite and body weight in underweight COPD patients.[40] Both steroids and hormonal agents act through multiple pathways, such as increasing neuropeptide-Y levels to increase appetite, and down-regulating proinflammatory cytokines. As with the studies in nutritional supplementation, the weight gain has been predominantly in the fat mass compartment.

Thalidomide significantly attenuated both total weight loss and loss of lean body mass in patients with cancer and acquired immunodeficiency syndrome.[41] The action is linked to inhibition and degradation of tumor necrosis factor-alpha. Eicosapentaenoic acid, an omega-3 fatty acid, can halt weight loss in cancer cachexia and may increase lean body mass at high doses.[42] The effect is postulated to result from its ability to down-regulate proinflammatory cytokines and proteolysis-inducing factor. In 64 patients with COPD, 32 were randomized to receive a 400 Kcal/d nutritional supplement containing 0.6 g of omega-3 fatty acids, and 32 patients received a 400 Kcal/d nutritional supplement containing 0.07 g of omega-3 fatty acids. The intervention group supplementation contained 0.40 g of omega-6 fatty acids, while the control group received 0.93 g of omega-6 fatty acids.[43a] After 2 years of supplementation, the BMI, serum protein levels, and serum albumin levels significantly increased in both groups but there was no difference between groups. No significant difference was observed in resting blood gas analysis, in pulmonary function tests, or St. George Respiratory Questionnaire scores between groups. The percent of predicted 6-minute walk test distance improved by 6% in the omega-3 supplement group, the Borg dyspnea scale score improved in both groups (but less in the omega-3 supplemented group), and there was less decrease in arterial oxygen saturation measured by pulse oximetry in the intervention group (1.9% vs. 0.5%) compared to the control group. Serum levels of leukotriene-B4 decreased in the 0.6g omega-3 supplemented group, but interleukin-8 and tumor necrosis factor-alpha levels did not change in either group. These data suggest that the clinical improvement in people with COPD supplemented with omega-3 fatty acids for 2 years is marginal. However, the observed decrease in serum cytokine levels is provocative and deserves further research.

These results of pharmacologic interventions suggest that improvement in cachexia may result from a common suppressive effect of these agents on proinflammatory cytokines. While improved appetite and weight gain have been observed, whether these pharmacological agents improve functional outcome is not clear.

Although it is clear that systemic inflammation plays a role in weight loss in patients with COPD, other factors may be involved. People with COPD also show a higher prevalence of low plasma levels of testosterone and insulin-like growth factor-I compared with healthy subjects of the same age.[43b,44] Therefore, the use of anabolic agents to correct hypogonadism or as an adjunct to increase lean body mass has been investigated in controlled studies.

Treatment with oxandrolone for 16 weeks produced gains in body weight, body cell mass, and fat-free mass in 7 of 11 subjects with COPD. Furthermore, levels of interleukin-1, leptin, interleukin-6, and tumor necrosis factor-alpha decreased in the subjects with weight gain, suggesting that the effect was associated with a reduction in inflammation.[45]

Nandrolone decanoate, another anabolic steroid, plus a nutritional supplement (420 Kcal/d) plus exercise was compared to the nutritional supplement and exercise alone for 8 weeks. All patients gained weight, but greater gain in lean body mass occurred in the group receiving the anabolic steroid.[46] Stanozolol, another anabolic steroid, was evaluated in a small study of 17 undernourished (BMI less than 20) COPD patients for 9 weeks. Both groups received exercise interventions. Nine of 10 patients in the stanozol group gained weight (mean 1.8 kg) and increased their lean body mass, while all control patients lost weight and did not increase their lean body mass.[47] There was no improvement in inspiratory muscle mass and no effect on endurance exercise capacity. The results of adding an anabolic steroid to other interventions have been promising, but only small treatment effects have been observed to date.

Creatine supplementation in subjects with COPD led to an increase in fat-free mass by a mean of 1.09 kg. Creatine supplementation increased peripheral muscle strength and endurance, and improved health status. However, it did not improve exercise capacity.[48]

Recombinant human growth hormone (rhGH) has been shown to induce protein anabolism and muscle growth in a number of different disease states. In the only placebo-controlled trial done to date, no improvement in muscle function or exercise tolerance was noted.[49] More concerning is that an increase in REE was noted, suggesting that rhGH treatment might actually worsen pulmonary status by increasing respiratory demand.

VIII. COMORBIDITIES

As many as 35% to 72% of patients with COPD have been reported to be osteopenic, and 36% to 60% of patients with COPD have osteoporosis.[50–52] Patients requiring oral glucocorticoid therapy have lower T-scores and more fractures than those treated with bronchodilators only. Glucocorticoid-induced osteoporosis is well-documented in the literature.[53–55] Patients placed on high-dose glucocorticoid therapy exhibit a rapid loss of bone mineral density within the first 6 months.[56] Patients receiving oral glucocorticoid therapy (average dose 20 mg) have a 1.8-fold (95% CI 1.08 to 3.07) increased incidence of vertebral fractures.[57] For these reasons, people with COPD should be screened for bone mineral density; those who require glucocorticoid treatment are at particularly high risk.

The standard treatment for people at risk for osteoporosis should include 400 to 800 IU vitamin D and 1000 to 1500 mg elemental calcium per day.[58] There are some data to suggest that doses in the range of 800 IU of vitamin D may improve muscle function, including respiratory function.[59]

1,25-hydroxyvitamin D, the active vitamin D metabolite, binds to a highly specific nuclear receptor in muscle tissue, leading to improved muscle function and reduced risk of falling.[60] Higher plasma concentrations of 1,14-dihydrocholecalciferol are associated with increased muscle strength, physical activity, and ability to climb stairs, and lower concentrations are associated with higher frequency of falls among elderly people.[61,62] The effects of vitamin D on muscle may also be mediated by de novo protein synthesis,[63] affecting muscle cell growth through the highly specific nuclear vitamin D receptor expressed in human muscle.[64] In one study, treatment with 1,25-hydroxyvitamin D increased the relative number and size of type II muscle fibers of older women within 3 months of treatment.[65]

Calcium and vitamin D supplementation have been shown in some, but not all, studies to be beneficial in patients receiving long-term corticosteroid therapy. In general, calcium and vitamin D alone are insufficient to completely prevent the bone loss associated with high-dose glucocorticoid treatment, and additional therapy is required.

Drugs that specifically act on bone by decreasing resorption are bisphosphonates, calcitonin, selective estrogen receptor modulators, and estrogen. In large randomized controlled trials, alendronate reduced both vertebral and nonvertebral fractures.[66] It is most beneficial in those at highest risk—women with at least one vertebral fracture or documented osteoporosis. Symptomatic vertebral fractures were decreased by 28% to 36% over 4 years of treatment, and the risk of hip fracture was reduced 50%.[67] A similar reduction in vertebral fracture incidence has been observed with risedronate.

Bisphosphonates may be useful in corticosteroid-induced osteoporosis and in men with osteoporosis.[68] Bisphosphonates may be poorly absorbed and may cause gastric side effects. To maximize uptake, tablets must be taken after an overnight fast, with a full glass of water, and food avoided for half an hour. Dosing must be adjusted for renal function.

Calcitonin, combined with vitamin D and calcium, does not reduce bone loss to a greater degree than calcium and vitamin D used alone. Thus, calcitonin may not produce added benefit in preventing or treating glucocorticoid-induced osteoporosis.[69]

Hypogonadism is associated with development of osteoporosis in both men and women, and occurs more commonly in people with COPD. Sex hormone replacement therapy can reduce bone loss in these patients.[70] There is a reduction in hip and vertebral fractures of 34%, and total reduction in fracture risk by 24%.[71] However, long-term side effects, particularly breast cancer and cardiovascular events, limit the indications for use of sex hormone replacement therapy.

Patients should be encouraged to participate in physical therapy programs to increase exercise endurance and to maintain muscle strength.[72]

IX. SUMMARY AND CONCLUSIONS

People with moderate to severe COPD frequently have a low BMI and commonly lose weight. This weight loss is associated with impaired pulmonary status, reduced diaphragmatic mass, and lower exercise capacity, and it independently predicts a higher mortality rate.

Adequate nutrition is essential to maintaining health and functional status, and should be addressed early in the course of COPD. Although adequate nutrition is important in the management of all COPD patients, hypercaloric feeding is not helpful and may be harmful.

Clinical trials of supplemental protein and energy to reverse weight loss and improve functional status have been disappointing. The etiology of this weight loss does not appear to be related to nutrient intake and increasingly appears to be related to the syndrome of cachexia.

Interventions for reversing cachexia have shown modest increases in body weight and functional status. Current therapy is empirically directed at improving appetite and body weight. The data suggest that a component of this response is related to suppression of proinflammatory cytokines. Future research into reversing the cachexia syndrome in people with COPD must focus on improving reduced protein synthesis and increased protein degradation.

REFERENCES

1. Petty TL. COPD in perspective. *Chest* 2002;121(5 Suppl):116S–120S.
2. Vestbo J, Hogg JC. Convergence of the epidemiology and pathology of COPD. *Thorax* 2006;61(1):86–88.
3. Vestbo J, Hogg JC. Convergence of the epidemiology and pathology of COPD. *Thorax* 2006;61(1):86–88.
4. Barnes PJ. Chronic obstructive pulmonary disease. *New Engl J Med* 2000;343:269–280.
5. Guerra S, Sherrill DL, Bobadilla A, Martinez FD, Barbee RA. The relation of body mass index to asthma, chronic bronchitis, and emphysema. *Chest* 2002;122(4):1256–1263.
6. Anthonisen NR, Connett JE, Murray RP. Smoking and lung function of Lung Health Study participants after 11 years. *Am J Respir Crit Care Med* 2002;166:675–679.
7. Rutgers SR, Postma DS, ten Hacken NH, et al. Ongoing airway inflammation in patients with COPD who do not currently smoke. *Thorax* 2000;55:12–18.
8. Rabe KF, Hurd S, Anzueto A, Barnes PJ, Buist SA, Calverley P, Fukuchi Y, Jenkins C, Rodriguez-Roisin R, van Weel C, Zielinski J. Global strategy for the diagnosis, management, and prevention of chronic obstructive pulmonary disease. *Am J of Resp Crit Care Med* 2007;176:532–555.
9. Schols A. Nutritional modulation as part of the integrated management of chronic obstructive pulmonary disease. *Proc Nutr Soc* 1999;58:321.
10. Sahebjami H, Doers JT, Render MC, et al. Anthropometric and pulmonary function test profile of outpatients with stable chronic obstructive pulmonary disease. *Am J M* 1993;94(5):469–474.
11. Wilson DO, Rogers RM, Wright E, et al. Body weight in chronic obstructive pulmonary disease—The National Institutes of Health Intermittent Positive-Pressure Breathing Trial. *Am Rev Resp Dis* 1989;139(6):1435–1438.
12. Mannix ET, Manfredi F, Farber MO. Elevated O_2 cost of ventilation contributes to tissue wasting in COPD. *Chest* 1999;115(3):708–713.
13. Jounieaux V, Mayeux I. Oxygen cost of breathing in patients with emphysema or chronic bronchitis in acute respiratory failure. *Am J Resp Crit Care Med* 1995;152(6 pt 1):2181–2184.
14. Decramer M, de Bock V, Dom R. Functional and histologic picture of steroid-induced myopathy chronic obstructive pulmonary disease. *Am J Resp Crit Care Med* 1996;153:1958–1964.
15. Schols AMWJ, Broekhuizen R, Weling-Scheepers CA, Wouters EF. Body composition and mortality in chronic obstructive pulmonary disease. *Am J Clin Nutr* 2005;82:53–59.

16. Ferreira IM, Brooks D, Lacasse Y, Goldstein RS, White J. Nutritional supplementation for stable chronic obstructive pulmonary disease. *Cochr Dat System Rev* 2007;4.
17. Freeborne N, Lynn J, Desbiens NA. Insights about dying from the SUPPORT project: the Study to Understand Prognoses and Preferences for Outcomes and Risks of Treatments. *J Am Geriatr Soc* 2000;48:S33–S38.
18. Donahoe M, Rogers RM, Wilson DO, Pennock BE. Oxygen consumption of the respiratory muscles in normal and in malnourished patients with chronic obstructive pulmonary disease. *Am Rev Resp Dis* 1989;140(2):385–391.
19. Wilson DO, Donahoe M, Rogers RM, Pennock BE. Metabolic rate and weight loss in chronic obstructive lung disease. *JPEN* 1990;14(1):7–11.
20. Creutzberg EC, Schols AM, Bothmer-Quaedvlieg FC, Wouters EF. Prevalence of an elevated resting energy expenditure in patients with chronic obstructive pulmonary disease in relation to body composition and lung function. *Euro J Clin Nutr* 1998;52(6):396–401.
21. Baarends EM, Schols AMWJ, Westerterp KR, Wouters EF. Total daily energy expenditure relative to resting energy expenditure in clinically stable patients with COPD. *Thorax* 1997;52:780–785.
22. Hugli O, Schutz Y, Fitting JW. The daily energy expenditure in stable chronic obstructive pulmonary disease. *Am J Resp Crit Care Med* 1996;153:294–300.
23. Congleton J. The pulmonary cachexia syndrome: aspects of energy balance. *Proc Nutr Soc* 1999;58(2):321–328.
24. Thomas DR. Loss of skeletal muscle mass in aging: examining the relationship of starvation, sarcopenia and cachexia. *Clin Nutr* 2007;26(4):389–399.
25. De Francia MD, Barbier D, Mege JL, Orehek J. Tumor necrosis factor-alpha levels and weight loss in chronic obstructive pulmonary disease. *Am J Resp Crit Care Med* 1994;150:1453–1455.
26. Aguilaniu B, Goldstein-Shapses S, Pajon A, et al. Muscle protein degradation in severely malnourished patients with chronic obstructive pulmonary disease subject to short-term total parenteral nutrition. *JPEN* 1992;16:248–254.
27. Schols MWJ, Buurman WA, Staal van den Brekel A, Dentener MA, Wouters EFM. Evidence for a relation between metabolic derangements and increased levels of inflammatory mediators in a subgroup of patients with chronic obstructive pulmonary disease. *Thorax* 1996;51:819–824.
28. Broekhuizen R, Wouters EF, Creutzberg EC, Schols AM. Raised CRP levels mark metabolic and functional impairment in advanced COPD. *Thorax* 2006;61(1):17–22.
29. Visser M, Pahor M, Taaffe DR, et al. Relationship of interleukin-6 and tumor necrosis factor-alpha with muscle mass and muscle strength in elderly men and women: the Health ABC Study. *J Gerontol A* 2002;57(5):M326–32.
30. Schols AM, Buurman WA, Staal van den Brekel AJ, Dentener MA, Wouters EF. Evidence for a relation between metabolic derangements and increased levels of inflammatory mediators in a subgroup of patients with chronic obstructive pulmonary disease. *Thorax* 1996;51:819–824.
31. Anker SD, Ponikowski PP, Clark AL, et al. Cytokines and neurohormones relating to body composition alterations in the wasting syndrome of chronic heart failure. *Eur Heart J* 1999;20:683–693.
32. Van Helvoort HA, Heijdra YF, Thijs HM, Vina J, Wanten GJ, Dekhuijzen PN. Exercise-induced systemic effects in muscle-wasted patients with COPD. *Med Sci Sport Exer* 2006;38(9):1543–1552.
33. Espat NJ, Moldawer LL, Copeland III EM. Cytokine-mediated alterations in host metabolism prevent nutritional repletion in cachectic cancer patients. *J Surg Oncol* 1995;58:77–82.
34. Morley JE, Thomas DR, Wilson MM. Cachexia: pathophysiology and clinical relevance. *Am J Clin Nutr* 2006;83(4):735–743.
35. Koehler F, Doehner W, Hoernig S, Witt C, Anker SD, John M. Anorexia in chronic obstructive pulmonary disease–association to cachexia and hormonal derangement. *Inter J Card* 2007;119(1):83–89.
36. Creutzberg EC, Schols AMWJ, Weling-Scheepers CAPM, Buurman WA, Wouters EFM. Characterization of nonresponse to high caloric oral nutritional therapy in depleted patients with chronic obstructive pulmonary disease. *Am J Resp Crit Care Med* 2000;161:745–752.
37. Gordon JN, Green SR, Goggin PM. Cancer cachexia. *Quart J Med* 2005;98(11):779–788.
38. Thomas DR. Guidelines for the use of orexigenic drugs in long-term care. *Nutr Clin Pract* 2006;21(1):82–87.
39. Deans C, Wigmore SJ. Systemic inflammation, cachexia and prognosis in patients with cancer. *Curr Opin Clin Nutr Metabol Care* 2005;8:265–269.
40. Weisberg J, Wanger J, Olson J, et al. Megestrol acetate stimulates weight gain and ventilation in underweight COPD patients. *Chest* 2002;121:1070–1078.

41. Gordon JN, Trebble TM, Ellis RD, Duncan HD, Johns T, Goggin PM. Thalidomide in the treatment of cancer cachexia: a randomised placebo controlled trial. *Gut* 2005;54:540–545.

42. Fearon KC, Von Meyenfeldt MF, Moses AG, et al. Effect of a protein and energy dense N-3 fatty acid enriched oral supplement on loss of weight and lean tissue in cancer cachexia: a randomised double blind trial. *Gut* 2003;52:1479–1486.

43a. Matsuyama W, Mitsuyama H, Watanabe M, Oonakahara K, Higashimoto I, Osame M, Arimura K. Effects of omega-3 polyunsaturated fatty acids on inflammatory markers in COPD. *Chest* 2005;128(6):3817–3827.

43b. Kamischke A, Kemper DE, Castel MA, Lüthke M, Rolf C, Behre HM, Magnussen H, Nieschlag E. Testosterone levels in men with chronic obstructive pulmonary disease with or without glucocorticoid therapy. *Eur Respir J* 1998;11:41–45.

44. Casaburi R, Goren S, Bhasin S. Substantial prevalence of low anabolic hormone levels in COPD patients undergoing rehabilitation. *Am J Resp Crit Care Med* 1996;153:A128.

45. Yeh SS, Hafner A, Mantovani G, Levine DM, Parker TS. Relationship between body composition and cytokines in cachectic patients with chronic obstructive pulmonary disease. *J Amer Geri Soc* 2003;51:890.

46. Schols AMWJ, Soeters PN, Mostert R, Pluymers RJ, Wouters EFM. Physiologic effects of nutritional support and anabolic steroids in patients with chronic obstructive pulmonary disease. *Am J Resp Crit Care Med* 1995;153:1268–1274.

47. Ferreira IM, Verreschi IT, Nery LE, et al. The influence of 6 months of oral anabolic steroids on body mass and respiratory muscles in undernourished COPD patients. *Chest* 1998;114:19–28.

48. Fuld JP, Kilduff LP, Neder JA, Pitsiladis Y, Lean ME, Ward SA, Cotton MM. Creatine supplementation during pulmonary rehabilitation in chronic obstructive pulmonary disease. *Thorax* 2005;60(7):531–537.

49. Burdet L, de Muralt B, Schutz Y, Pichard C, Fitting JW. Administration of growth hormone to underweight patients with chronic obstructive pulmonary disease: a prospective, randomized, controlled study. *Am J Resp Crit Care Med* 1997;156:1800–1806.

50. Shane E, Silverberg SJ, Donovan D, et al. Osteoporosis in lung transplantation candidates with end-stage pulmonary disease. *Am J Med* 1996;101:262–269.

51. Iqbal F, Michaelson J, Thaler L, et al. Declining bone mass in men with chronic pulmonary disease: contribution of glucocorticoid treatment, body mass index, and gonadal function. *Chest* 1999;116:1616–1624.

52. Incalzi RA, Caradonna P, Ranieri P, et al. Correlates of osteoporosis in chronic obstructive pulmonary disease. *Respir Med* 2000;94:1079–1084.

53. Adinoff AD, Hollister JR. Steroid-induced fractures and bone loss in patients with asthma. *N Engl J Med* 1983;309:265–268.

54. Adler RA, Rosen CJ. Glucocorticoids and osteoporosis. *Endocrinol Metab Clin North Am* 1994;23:641–654.

55. Goldstein MF, Fallon JJ, Harning R. Chronic glucocorticoid therapy-induced osteoporosis in patients with obstructive lung disease. *Chest* 1999;116:1733–1749.

56. Pearce G, Tabensky DA, Delmas PD, et al. Corticosteroid-induced bone loss in men. *J Clin Endocrinol Metab* 1998;83:801–806.

57. McEvoy C, Ensrud K, Bender E, et al. Association between corticosteroid use and vertebral fractures in older men with chronic obstructive pulmonary disease. *Am J Resp Crit Care Med* 1998;157:704–709.

58. Reid IR. Therapy of osteoporosis: calcium, vitamin D, and exercise. *Am J Med Sci* 1996;312:278–286.

59. Bischoff HA, Stahelin HB, Dick W, Akos R, Knecht M, Salis C, et al. Effects of vitamin D and calcium supplementation on falls: a randomized controlled trial. *J Bone Miner Res* 2003;18:343–351.

60. Bischoff HA, Borchers M, Gudat F, et al. In situ detection of 1,25-dihydroxyvitamin D3 receptor in human skeletal muscle tissue. *Histochem J* 2001;33:19–24.

61. Mowe M, Haug E, Bohmer T. Low serum calcidiol concentration in older adults with reduced muscular function. *J Am Geriatr Soc* 1999;47:220–226.

62. Dhesi JK, Bearne LM, Moniz C, Hurley MV, Jackson SH, Swift CG, et al. Neuromuscular and psychomotor function in elderly subjects who fall and the relationship with vitamin D status. *J Bone Miner Res* 2002;17:891–897.

63. Boland R. Role of vitamin D in skeletal muscle function. *Endocr Rev* 1986;7:434–447.

64. Bischoff HA, Borchers M, Gudat F, et al. In situ detection of 1,25-dihydroxyvitamin D3 receptor in human skeletal muscle tissue. *Histochem J* 2001;33:19–24.

65. Sorensen OH, Lund B, Saltin B, et al. Myopathy in bone loss of ageing: improvement by treatment with 1 alpha-hydroxycholecalciferol and calcium. *Clin Sci (Colch)* 1979;56:157–161.

66. Cummings SR, Black DM, Thompson DE, Applegate WB, Barrett-Connor E, Musliner TA, et al. Effect of alendronate on risk of fracture in women with low bone density but without vertebral fractures: results from the Fracture Intervention Trial. *JAMA* 1998;280:2077–2082.

67. Black DM, Cummings SR, Karpf DB, Cauley JA, Thompson DE, Nevitt MC, et al. Randomised trial of effect of alendronate on risk of fracture in women with existing vertebral fractures. Fracture Intervention Trial Research Group. *Lancet* 1996;348:1535–1541.

68. Adachi JD, Cranney A, Goldsmith CH, et al. Intermittent cyclic therapy with etidronate in the prevention of corticosteroid-induced bone loss. *J Rheumatol* 1994;21:1922–1926.

69. Sambrook P, Birmingham J, Kelly P, et al. Prevention of corticosteroid osteoporosis: a comparison of calcium, calcitriol, and calcitonin. *N Engl J Med* 1993;328:1747–1752.

70. Lane NE, Lukert BP. The science and therapy of glucocorticoid-induced bone loss. *Endocrinol Metab Clin North Am* 1998;27:465–483.

71. Rossouw JE, Anderson GL, Prentice RL, LaCroix AZ, Kooperberg C, Stefanick ML, et al. Risks and benefits of estrogen plus progestin in healthy postmenopausal women: principal results from the Women's Health Initiative randomized controlled trial. *JAMA* 2002;288:321–333.

72. Henderson NK, White CP, Eisman JA. The roles of exercise and fall risk reduction in the prevention of osteoporosis. *Endocrinol Metab Clin North Am*, 1998 Jun;27:369–387.

Section III

Gastrointestinal Diseases

10 Gastroesophageal Reflux Disease

Mark Hyman, M.D.

I. INTRODUCTION

Although humans have suffered from heartburn for millennia, gastroesophageal reflux disease, or GERD, has only been recently recognized as a disease. GERD is defined as chronic symptoms or mucosal damage resulting from the abnormal reflux of gastric or duodenal contents into the esophagus. The disease and its treatment have been the target of aggressive pharmaceutical marketing to both professionals and consumers. Proton pump inhibitors (PPIs) as a class of medications are the third best-selling pharmaceutical drug worldwide.

Symptoms related to GERD are among the most common presenting complaint to the primary care physician. GERD has been recently recognized to increase the risk for erosive esophagitis, strictures, and Barrett's esophagus, a metaplastic change of the esophageal epithelium associated with an increased risk of adenocarcinoma. Significant questions remain about true risk of reflux and adenocarcinoma. Mounting evidence documents harm from long-term pharmacologic acid suppression, including osteoporosis, depression, B12 and mineral deficiencies, small intestinal bacterial overgrowth, irritable bowel syndrome, pneumonia, and *Clostridium difficile* infectious diarrhea.

Clearly a new approach is needed that addresses the underlying causes of GERD and uses pharmacologic agents only to mitigate causative factors, while relying on dietary, nutritional, and other lifestyle therapies that are targeted toward the underlying causes and restoring normal intestinal function.

Conventional approaches to GERD include limiting dietary triggers, elevating the head of the bed, and pharmacologic treatments. Pharmacologic treatments that include antacids, H2 blockers, proton pump inhibitors, and motility agents are highly effective immediately upon use. However, their cessation can lead to rebounding symptoms and often results in long-term use. Novel approaches are needed to treat the underlying cause of GERD and offer resolution. This chapter probes two questions: Why has the normal physiological function been disrupted, and how can normal function be restored? Several roles for food and nutrients emerge.

II. EPIDEMIOLOGY

One in 10 American adults has daily episodes of heartburn, 10% to 20% have weekly symptoms, and 44% have occassional symptoms. GERD is a medical condition experienced by 25% to 35% of the U.S. population. When does heartburn became pathologic, leading to erosive esophagitis? Labeling everyone who experiences occasional heartburn as having GERD has led to significant overmedication. There is considerable overlap in symptoms between patients with severe erosive esophagitis leading to strictures and Barrett's esophagus, and those with nonerosive disease, making clinical decisions difficult.[1]

A concern of clinicians who are presented with patients with chronic GERD is how to measure their risk of adenocarcinoma. While the overall incidence of GERD has increased 300% to 500% over the last 30 to 40 years in developed countries, the number of individuals with adenocarcinoma of the esophagus remains low, but it is the fastest rising cancer and the third most common digestive cancer. In 2002, only half of the 13,100 esophageal cancers were adenocarcinomas. The number needed to treat is quite large to prevent each case of esophageal adenocarcinoma. In fact, because the cancer is rare there are few prospective cohort studies of patients with reflux to assess risk of cancer. Only 50% of patients with GERD have esophagitis. A recent review of the evidence does not support the use of endoscopy to screen patients with GERD for Barrett's esophagus.[2] There are no randomized trials to support this widespread practice and serious questions remain about the benefits and cost-effectiveness of the procedure. Obesity and nighttime symptoms are the two risk factors for progression to esophageal adenocarcinoma.

III. PATHOPHYSIOLOGY AND ETIOLOGY

The pathophysiology of GERD is clear, while the etiology remains controversial. Symptoms may or may not occur upon reflux of gastric contents and occasionally bile and pancreatic secretions into the esophagus. The degree of symptoms does not correlate with the severity of the disease. Severe symptoms may be associated with nonerosive disease, while Barrett's esophagus and adenocarcinoma may develop in asymptomatic patients.

In addition to the typical symptoms of GERD, which are heartburn, regurgitation, and dysphagia, atypical symptoms may include coughing, chest pain, and wheezing. Other consequences may result from abnormal reflux, including damage to the lungs (e.g., pneumonia, asthma, idiopathic pulmonary fibrosis), vocal cords (e.g., laryngitis, globus, cancer), ear (e.g., otitis media), and teeth (e.g., enamel decay).

A number of dietary and lifestyle factors have been demonstrated to trigger reflux, including portion size, late-night eating, fried foods, spicy foods, citrus, tomato-based foods, caffeine, alcohol, chocolate, mint, and smoking. These trigger reflux for a variety of reasons. Mint relaxes the lower esophageal sphincter tone, spicy foods increase parietal cell activity, deep-fried foods delay gastric emptying, and late-night eating leads to being horizontal on a full stomach.

Physiologically, GERD is caused by lower esophageal sphincter (LES) relaxation not related to swallowing and due to stimulation of mechanoreceptors programmed in the brainstem. Gastric distension is a major trigger for this stimulation, so how one eats may be as important as what one eats.

Obesity and pregnancy also increase the risk of reflux through direct compression of stomach contents and other mechanisms.[3] Pregnancy increases reflux because of multiple alterations in physiology and function, including elevation of progesterone, morning sickness, need for increased volume of food, and worsening of hiatal hernias; going to bed earlier and eating later makes lying down on a full stomach inevitable. Also, acidic foods are often selected during pregnancy partly because of the body's cues to absorb more minerals. Certain medications, including NSAIDs, aspirin, and steroids, increase the risk of gastritis and GERD. Calcium channel blockers, beta-blockers, nitrates, tricyclic antidepressants, anti-cholinergics, and progesterone all reduce lower esophageal sphincter tone leading to reflux. Bisphosphonates such as alendronate can cause esophagitis.

The role of *Helicobacter pylori* infection in reflux is controversial. Studies on eradication of *H. pylori* infection in GERD have been mixed, with some showing benefit and others not. There is evidence that long-term acid suppression with PPIs in patients with *H. pylori* infection increases the risk of gastric carcinoma.[4] *H. pylori* may proliferate if PPIs are used long term. A diagnostic evaluation for and treatment of *H. pylori* is reasonable; however, it may make GERD worse before it makes it better.

H. pylori infection has been linked to food allergy,[5] rosacea, atherosclerosis, B12 deficiency, Raynaud's, and Sjögren's and other autoimmune diseases.[6]

Dysfunction of the enteric nervous system from altered autonomic tone between the sympathetic and parasympathetic systems is implicated in reflux.[7] Physical or psychological stress increases sympathetic tone, increasing contraction of the pylorus and gastric outlet while relaxing the lower esophageal sphincter (LES), and sets the conditions for reflux. Autonomic dysfunction promotes an acquired gastroparesis leading to postprandial dyspepsia and bloating. Activation of the parasympathetic nervous system through the relaxation response or deep breathing relaxes the pylorus and increases LES tone, preventing reflux.[8]

Zinc deficiency may lead to altered intestinal permeability, triggering inflammation, food allergies, and increased sympathetic tone.[9] Zinc is necessary for proenzyme activation in the stomach. Zinc deficiency alters normal stomach physiology. Magnesium deficiency may also contribute to altered intestinal motility contributing to reflux.[10] Use of proton pump inhibitors inhibits mineral absorption, further exacerbating the effects of magnesium and zinc deficiency.

Gluten intolerance and celiac disease have also been linked to reflux, and a gluten-free diet frequently results in resolution of reflux.[11] This should prompt more research investigating the link between food allergies, sensitivities, and intolerances and GERD. A recent study suggests this is the case.[12] More controversial are the role of IgG and non-IgE-mediated food allergies and GERD. While little data exist, clinical experience with elimination diets supports a trial for treatment.

While data are limited,[13] clinical experience suggests that dysbiosis, or the alteration of normal gut flora,[14] small intestinal bacterial overgrowth (SIBO),[15] leads to increased intestinal inflammation, disruption of the normal epithelial barrier function, and stimulation of the enteric nervous system. It is commonly experienced as postprandial bloating, and may also manifest as reflux. Small bowel yeast overgrowth secondary to the use of antibiotics, steroids, hormones, or a diet high in refined sugars and carbohydrates also may trigger upper intestinal symptoms. Alteration in the gut pH alters the microbial environment and results in bacterial and yeast overgrowth.[16,17] Bile reflux often goes undiagnosed. Gastric pH is rarely measured, and patients are often empirically placed on PPIs for alkaline reflux. This leads to further small intestinal bacterial overgrowth and irritable bowel syndrome (IBS).

There is an overlap in prevalence of GERD and IBS. They form a continuous spectrum of functional gastrointestinal motility disorders. Most (>50%) patients with GERD have delayed gastric emptying, which sets the stage not only for GERD but also bacterial overgrowth and IBS.

Food quality has been shown to play a role in altered gastric and intestinal function. Calorie-dense, high-fat[18] foods contribute to reflux. High-glycemic-load foods with highly processed sugar content can also adversely influence gastric emptying and result in worsening reflux.

IV. PATIENT EVALUATION

Esophagogastroduodenoscopy (EGD), radiography (upper GI series), ambulatory pH monitoring, and motility studies document the dysfunction but do little to uncover the etiology of reflux other than hiatal hernia. Their benefit and cost-effectiveness as diagnostic or screening tools for Barrett's esophagus or adenocarcinoma is not supported by existing research.

Testing for *H. pylori* should be performed. Serology or antibody testing, stool antigen, and urea breath testing can all document infection. Breath testing and stool antigen testing should be used to confirm eradication 8 weeks after treatment to reduce false negatives.

DIAGNOSTICS OF PHYSIOLOGY AND FUNCTION

Novel functional tests can help direct therapy to underlying causes of reflux. They are typically not used by conventional physicians or gastroenterologists, but provide useful lenses for looking at the etiology and patterns of gut dysfunction, which may contribute to GERD.

Though problematic due to a high rate of false positives and some false negatives, IgG food reactivity testing can help identify trigger foods linked not only to intestinal dysfunction such as irritable bowel syndrome,[19] but obesity[20] and systemic inflammatory diseases.

Testing for celiac disease is essential for any patient with chronic intestinal symptoms, reflux[21] or any inflammatory or chronic disease. Testing should include IgA and IgG antigliadin antibodies;

total IgA (to check for IgA deficiency); IgA tissue transglutaminase antibodies; and anti-endomesial antibodies. Assessing HLA DQ2 and D8 genotypes can help further clarify the diagnosis; however, these are present in approximately 30% of the general population.[22]

Assessment of body weight and central obesity contributes to understanding the etiology of reflux.

Urinary organic acid analysis identifies markers of overgrowth of intestinal flora including small bowel overgrowth[23] and yeast overgrowth.[24] These nonhuman microbial metabolites are absorbed through the intestinal epithelium and excreted in the urine.

Digestive stool analysis provides a broad picture of intestinal health, including information about digestion, absorption, immune function, metabolic markers of dysbiotic intestinal flora, and microbiology such as assessment of beneficial flora, pathogenic bacteria, yeast, and parasites.

Nutritional analysis should include plasma or red blood cell (RBC) zinc, RBC magnesium (also can become deficient from competitive absorption with calcium for those taking Tums and even prescription medications for GERD, not only by decreased stomach acid), vitamin D, serum iron, ferritin, and methylmalonic acid (B12 assessment).

Amino acid analysis can be helpful in assessing deficiencies that are caused by or result from reflux or intestinal imbalances.

V. PATIENT TREATMENT

PHARMACOLOGIC INTERVENTIONS AND RISKS

Heartburn had been traditionally treated with sodium bicarbonate and antacids such as calcium carbonate. H2 blockers followed by proton pump inhibitors (PPIs) have become the main treatment modalities and among the mostly widely used and profitable pharmaceuticals. After Lipitor and Plavix, drugs for cholesterol and heart disease, proton pump inhibitors are currently the third top-selling drugs in America in a $252 billion drug market. Nexium and Prevacid are in the top 10 best-selling drugs and account for $5.7 and $4.0 billion in sales annually. Over-the-counter antacids including Tums, Rolaids, and Maalox account for $1 billion in annual sales.

Conventional reflux medications include:

- Calcium carbonate
- Antacid-alginic acid combinations
- H2 blockers (cimetidine, famotidine, nizatidine, ranitidine)
- Proton pump inhibitors (esomeprazole, lansoprazole, omeprazole, pantoprazole, rabeprazole)

Prolonged and aggressive pharmacological suppression of gastric acid production with proton pump inhibitors or H2 blockers has become common practice for treating a mostly benign lifestyle condition. Mounting evidence documents the risks of long-term suppression of the normal physiological acid required for the initiation of protein digestion in the stomach, mineral absorption, normal intrinsic factor function, and the activation of pancreatic enzymes.

DRUG–FOOD INTERACTIONS AND DRUG–NUTRIENT INTERACTIONS

1. Medication is permissive. Instead of losing weight, eating less, or eating fewer fatty "rich" foods, people use a pill.
2. Medication reduces stomach acid. However, foods such as vinegar, spices, and decaffeinated coffee, which raise stomach acid, improve diabetes. The mechanisms of these foods are not established, but are certainly cause for concern that pharmacologically suppressing stomach acid may have the converse effect on diabetes.

3. Suppression of parietal cell acid function also impairs intrinsic factor function and B12 absorption.[25] Long-term used of PPIs is associated with B12 deficiency and all its associated complications including depression, neuropathy, fatigue, and dementia. Measuring serum B12 levels is an inadequate measure of functional B12 status. Serum methylmalonic acid is a more sensitive indicator of B12 deficiency.

4. Stomach acid is required for protein absorption. When proteins are inadequately broken down to their constituent amino acids, they travel further down the GI tract where they are exposed to gut-associated lymphoid tissue (GALT). These partially digested proteins can trigger food intolerances and immune up-regulation. PPIs may contribute to the development of IgG or non-IgE mediated food sensitivities.

5. Adequate gastric acid is necessary for proper mineral absorption. PPIs have been linked to calcium, magnesium,[26] zinc,[27] and iron[28] deficiency.

6. Inadequate mineral status leads to greater uptake of heavy metal toxicants because zinc, for example, is a necessary cofactor for metallothionein, which complexes and removes intracellular metals, and selenium is a cofactor for glutathione peroxidase, necessary for detoxification and as part of our antioxidant system.

7. Chronic use of acid-blocking drugs leads to an increase in the development of osteoporosis and increase in hip fracture because blocking acid prevents absorption of calcium and other minerals necessary for bone health.[29]

8. *H. pylori* can shift from cohabitation status to disease-causing concentrations.

Protein and food maldigestion are common side effects of pharmacological acid suppression, and may cause bloating, abdominal pain, and diarrhea. Small bowel bacterial overgrowth is common. Studies link PPIs to community-acquired *Clostridium difficile* infection.[30]

Immune Dysregulation and Acid Blockade: Cancer and Allergies

PPIs may also increase the risk of gastric cancer.[31] Other consequences of long-term PPI use include an increase in gastric polyps,[32] community-acquired pneumonia, and pediatric pneumonia and gastroenteritis.[33]

In developing countries, allergic diseases such as asthma (30 million cases), environmental allergies (50 million cases) and, particularly IgE type 1 hypersensitivity food allergy (9 million cases) are increasing at an alarming rate.[34] Adding autoimmunity (24 million cases), we are facing an epidemic of inflammatory and allergic disease. The prevailing hypothesis is that increased hygiene and reduced exposure to infection agents in early childhood impedes normal development of tolerance and immunity.[35]

However, another hypothesis merits consideration and is supported by the literature.[36] Food reactivities including intolerances, allergies, and hyperreactivities can result from reduced gastric digestion of protein induced by acid-suppressing therapies, including PPIs and H2 blockers. In 152 patients medicated with acid-blocking medication, 25% developed IgE antibodies to regular food constituents as confirmed by oral provocation and skin testing. Allergenicity of potential food allergens is reduced 10,000-fold by gastric digestion. Though not yet adequately investigated, impaired or partial digestion of dietary proteins may also induce delayed hypersensitivity or IgG antibody formation to dietary constituents. This may be compounded by bacterial overgrowth in the small intestine induced by PPIs, which alters intestinal permeability leading to activation of the GALT and both local and systemic inflammation.

A vicious cycle of inflammation, altered motility, autonomic dysfunction, nutrient malabsorption, maldigestion, altered intestinal flora, and dysbiosis can be triggered by the collective influence of our processed, low-fiber, high-sugar, nutrient-deficient, low-phytonutrient-content diet; stress; and the overuse of antibiotics, acid-suppressing medication, NSAIDs, aspirin, steroids, and anti-hypertensives.

In sum, long-term use of powerful acid-suppression medication can alter normal digestion, lead to nutrient malabsorption, disrupt normal intestinal flora and immunity, increase the risk of cancer and allergic disease, induce nutrient deficiency, and cause pneumonia, colitis, and osteoporosis. These medications should be used with caution only as a last resort for a relatively benign condition. Considering the fact that therapy with PPIs does not affect progression of Barrett's esophagus to esophageal adenocarcinoma, the rationale for long-term treatment is questionable.

SURGICAL INTERVENTIONS AND RISKS

Surgical treatments for reflux are controversial and include laparoscopic Nissen fundoplication, radiofrequency heating of the gastroesophageal junction known as the Stretta procedure, and endo-scopic gastroplasty known as the EndoCinch procedure. Treatment benefits from 50% to 75% of properly selected patients but postsurgical complications including dysphagia and bloating occur in 20% of patients. Within 3 to 5 years of the procedure, 52% of patients are taking reflux medication again.[37] After being highly touted, Stretta was removed from the market due to an alarmingly high incidence of severe complications including death.

FOOD AND NUTRIENT TREATMENTS

Clinical tools can be useful in improving gut function and addressing GERD and nonulcer dyspep-sia. A starting point is to remove what harms and provide what heals. The details may be different from person to person, but the concept will guide diagnosis and therapy. This is an area of medicine where the practical art has exceeded the clinical science; however, the positive clinical outcomes from this low-risk approach warrant its application because conventional approaches routinely fail.

A careful dietary history and response to common triggers is essential. Assessing and modifying triggering factors or behaviors such as stress levels, use of medications that alter intestinal function and lead to altered motility or dysbiosis, smoking, late-night eating, poor sleep quality, and abdomi-nal obesity are important.

TREATMENT OF POTENTIAL CAUSES

Elimination of Dietary Triggers

Elimination of typical dietary triggers can often be helpful, including caffeine, alcohol, chocolate, garlic, onions, and peppermint; and spicy, fried or fatty, citrus- or tomato-based, and processed or junk foods. A whole-food, low-glycemic-load, phytonutrient-rich, plant-based, high-fiber diet often resolves the symptoms of reflux.

Modification of Medications

Medicine begets medicine. Nutrient interventions described throughout this text can reduce the dose or eliminate the need for several of the medications known to worsen GERD. A careful medi-cation history and cessation or substitution of medications that alter motility, such as calcium chan-nel blockers, beta-blockers, alpha-adrenergic agonists, theophylline, nitrates, and progesterone, are important. Also important to consider are medications that alter intestinal permeability, such as steroids, aspirin, and NSAIDs, leading to increasing intestinal inflammation, which in turn increases sympathetic tone in the enteric nervous system.

Food Allergy Elimination Diet

Though largely based on empirical observation and clinical experience, a food allergy elimina-tion diet based on common food allergens or IgG testing may improve symptoms and is a benign intervention. A 2- to 3-week elimination diet of the most common food allergens with careful food reintroduction of each food class every 3 days may identify trigger foods. The most common food allergens include gluten, dairy, eggs, yeast, corn, soy, citrus, nightshades, and nuts. Gluten elimination in celiac patients relieves reflux.

The purpose of eliminating common food sensitivities is to reduce the total antigenic load on the GALT, to reduce altered motility that results from immunologic irritation of the enteric nervous system increasing sympathetic tone, and to allow the repair of the gut mucosa and restoration of normal intestinal permeability.

The goal of the elimination diet is to reduce the overall antigenic load, repair the gut mucosa, and reintroduce foods slowly to identify any GI or systemic symptoms. Depending on the severity of dysbiosis and altered intestinal permeability, this process can take anywhere from 4 to 12 weeks. Careful food reintroduction to identify trigger foods is an essential component of the elimination/ challenge process. Diagnosis and treatment of food reactivities is discussed in Chapter 15. A comprehensive gut repair program is necessary for optimal treatment of altered gut function, normalization of intestinal flora, enzyme function, and the enteric nervous system.

Treatment of *Helicobacter Pylori*

Controversy remains because *H. pylori* have colonized human stomachs since Paleolithic times, and its eradication in the population as a whole has been linked to increases in asthma and allergic diseases via the Hygiene Hypothesis. Whether this is an epiphenomenon of increased "hygiene" or a causal relationship still remains to be proven.[38]

While no consensus exists, and some experts propose that certain strains of *H. pylori* may protect against GERD,[39] it is reasonable to attempt to eradicate *H. pylori* in GERD with one course of treatment, which can often relieve symptoms, while reducing the risk of peptic ulcer disease and gastric cancer. However, it is important to note that eradication of *H. pylori* increases risk of gastric cancer, but reduces risk of adenocarcinoma of the esophagus.

Certain foods inhibit or reduce *H. pylori* populations, including cruciferous vegetables and licorice, as does maintaining an appropriate pH.

This bacterium has come into prominence over the last few years as the cause of stomach ulcers but also may be linked to reflux. It is found in 90% to 100% of people with duodenal ulcers, 70% of people with gastric ulcers, and about 50% of people over the age of 50. Benign cohabitation with *H. pylori* is common but may progress to symptomatic infection. It may be associated with stomach cancer as well as inflammation throughout the body, and may even be linked to heart disease. It is often acquired in childhood and is the cause of lifelong gastritis or stomach inflammation. Large-population studies may miss unique subgroups with susceptibility because genetic and nutritional differences between individuals can determine whether or not *H. pylori* causes gut symptoms or cancer. For those with elevated C-reactive protein, inflammatory diseases, chronic digestive symptoms, or a family history of gastric cancer, treatment is recommended. Currently most physicians only treat documented ulcers. However, this may neglect many people who could benefit from treatment. A trial of a single course of treatment may be helpful in some patients with GERD.

Low stomach acid predisposes to the growth of *H. pylori* as do low antioxidant defense systems. Low levels of vitamin C and E in gastric fluids promote the growth of *H. pylori*.[40] Natural therapies can sometimes be effective, but pharmacological triple therapy, two antibiotics and a proton pump inhibitor, is often necessary for eradication of *H. pylori*.[41]

Food and Nutrient Treatment of Dysbiosis

Again, largely based on clinical experience and empirical observation, normalizing intestinal function through a comprehensive approach can resolve reflux symptoms. Restoring normal intestinal function takes 2 to 3 months and requires a methodical approach often referred to as the 4R program. Alterations of gut flora may be the cause of reflux. However, treatment with antibiotics for *H. pylori* and the long-term use of PPIs that disrupt further digestion by altering pH may lead to dysbiosis. In either case, to treat the cause of reflux or the side effects of medication, a gut repair protocol often results in significant clinical improvement.

4R: Remove, Replace, Reinoculate, and Repair

Remove

The first step is removing any triggers for altered intestinal function, including food allergens and pathogens. The most common microbial influences on the gut include small bowel bacterial overgrowth, yeast overgrowth, *H. pylori* infection, and parasites. It may also require treatment for environmental toxins including heavy metals.

Targeted antimicrobial therapies are often necessary. Successful treatment of small bowel bacterial overgrowth with rifiaxmin (Xifaxin) has been well documented.[42] Common antifungal therapies include both herbal and pharmacological treatments. Medications used include fluconazole, itraconazole, nystatin, terbinafine, and ketoconazole. Herbal and natural therapies include caprylic acid, undecylenic acid, oregano, and berberine. Pharmacologic treatments for parasites include metronidazole, iodoquinole (Yodoxin), paramomycin (Humatin), trimethoprim/sulfamethoxazole, and nitazoxanide (Alinia). Herbal therapies for parasites include artemesia,[43] oregano, and berberine. Treatment of *H. pylori* can be accomplished with triple therapy[44] and may respond to herbal therapies.[45]

Replace

Removing of triggers is followed by replacing insufficient digestive enzymes, hydrochloric acid, and prebiotics.

Broad-spectrum digestive enzyme support can improve intestinal function and reduce symptoms of GERD and bloating. Plant- or animal-based enzymes may be used. Enzymes that may need to be replaced include proteases, lipases, cellulases, and saccharidases, which are normally secreted by the pancreas or intestinal mucosa.

Two to three enzymes are taken with meals. Dyspeptic symptoms may also result from hypochlorhydria and be clinically indistinguishable from acid reflux. It is more common in those over 60 years old. Zinc is necessary for HCl production.

A trial of hydrochloric acid (betaine HCl) with meals may be diagnostic. A starting dose of 500 to 600 mg per tablet or capsule is taken at the start of the meal and titrated up to five tablets or capsules until a warm feeling occurs in the stomach area. The warm feeling indicates excess acid and that the dose should be reduced at the next meal. Generally after a few months of gut repair, treatment with HCl and enzymes is no longer necessary.

Reinoculate

The next step, done concurrently, is reinoculating the gut with beneficial bacteria or probiotics.[46]

Mounting evidence links altered intestinal flora or dysbiosis to many chronic diseases of the 21st century, including obesity, allergy, atopy, irritable bowel syndrome, and inflammatory diseases, as well as cancer. For therapeutic effect anywhere from 10 billion to 450 billion probiotic organisms have been used. Cultured and fermented traditional foods such as sauerkraut, tempeh, and miso contain live bacteria. Probiotic supplementation is usually necessary for therapeutic reinoculation of intestinal flora. Live or freeze-dried bacteria packaged in powders, tablets, or capsules are available and contain a variety of *Lactobacillus* species, *Bifidobacteria, Streptococcus,* and *Saccharomyces boulardii*. Prebiotics such as fructans, inulin, arabinogalactans, and fructooliosaccharides provide substrates for colonization and growth of normal commensal flora in probiotics.

Repair

Reinoculation is followed by repairing a damaged intestinal epithelium with zinc, glutamine, omega-3 fatty acids, gamma oryzanol, herbal anti-inflammatories such as turmeric and ginger, and a whole-food, high-fiber, phytonutrient-rich diet.[47]

The last step in normalization of digestive and intestinal function is to repair through providing nutritional support for regeneration and healing of the intestinal mucosa. Key nutrients that are involved in intestinal mucosal differentiation, growth, functioning, and repair include glutamine, zinc, pantothenic acid and essential fatty acids such as eicosapentaenoic acid, docosahexaenoic acid, and gamma linolenic acid.

Colonocytes use glutamine as their energy substrate. PPIs reduce glutamine availability, creating an iatrogenic glutamine insufficiency. Stress also reduces glutamine availability. The amino acid glutamine,[48] which provides both a source of fuel and precursors for growth to the rapidly dividing cells of the intestinal lining, can aid in repair and healing of gut mucosal injury. Glutamine improves gut and systemic immune function, especially in patients on long-term parenteral nutrition. Glutamines improve repair of gut mucosa after damage from radiation or chemotherapy, and reduce episodes of bacterial translocation and clinical sepsis in critically ill patients.

Zinc carnosine reduces NSAID-induced epithelial injury, induces mucosal repair, and reduces intestinal permeability.[49] Chewable or powdered deglycyrrhizinated licorice root is an herbal anti-inflammatory, which may reduce heartburn, reflux, and gastritis.[50] It provides a protective coating to the esophagus and the gastric mucosa. Aloe vera reduces mucosal inflammation, reduces reflux, and improves gut healing.[51] Dosing of these and many other nutrient and herbal treatments are outlined in Chapter 11. The ultimate repair of the gut results from removing insults such as toxic foods, allergens, and infections while replacing enzymes and hydrochloric acid, adding fiber and prebiotics, reinoculating with beneficial flora, and finally the use of healing nutrients.

Special Considerations

Patients with peptic ulcer disease should be tested and aggressively treated for *H. pylori*. Pregnant women can undertake a 4R program but should be careful to ensure adequate caloric intake and follow conventional precautions regarding use of medications and herbs.

Additional Benefits of the 4R Approach

Many chronic and inflammatory diseases of the 21st century, including obesity, are related to gut dysfunction. The 4R approach can ameliorate or cure many other chronic health problems and should be used as a first step in approaching most patients with chronic complex illnesses. It is a low-risk, high-yield therapeutic modality that merits more aggressive clinical use and further study.

SUMMARY

GERD is a common, annoying, but mostly benign condition. Acid-suppressive therapies may be effective in reducing symptoms but lead to unnecessary and potentially life-threatening complications. Addressing underappreciated underlying etiologies including food sensitivities, celiac disease, *Helicobacter pylori* infection, small bowel bacterial and yeast overgrowth, and normalizing gut function through a 4R program, as well as addressing more commonly recognized lifestyle factors and dietary habits, leads to the relief of symptoms in the majority of patients. It is necessary to highlight for patients the long-term negative consequences of short-term symptom suppression. This awareness helps them to take the time necessary to use these tools of functional medicine to support long-term health and well-being. A therapeutic approach to GERD is summarized in Table 10.1.

TABLE 10.1
Therapeutic Options for Gastroesophageal Reflux Disease (GERD)

I. Lifestyle and Dietary Recommendations for Treatment of GERD

A. *Dietary Triggers*
- Caffeine, alcohol, chocolate, garlic, onions, and peppermint; and spicy, fried or fatty, citrus- or tomato-based, and processed or junk foods

B. *Lifestyle and Behavioral Factors*
- Avoid large meals
- Finish eating within 3 hours of bedtime
- Practice active relaxation to increase parasympathetic tone
- Eat slowly
- Chew food completely
- Ensure adequate quality sleep
- Stop smoking
- Raise the head of the bed 6–8 inches
- Lose weight

C. *Medications That May Induce Reflux*
- Calcium channel blockers
- Beta-blockers
- Alpha-adrenergic agonists
- Theophylline
- Nitrates
- Progesterone
- Aspirin
- NSAIDs

D. *Food Allergy Elimination Diet*
- A 2-week trial of an oligo-antigenic diet followed by food challenge
  - Gluten, dairy, eggs, yeast, corn, soy, citrus, nightshades, and nuts

II. Treatment of Microbial Imbalances or Infections

A. *Helicobacter pylori Treatment*

Select Natural Therapies
- Bismuth subcitrate 240 mg twice daily before meals for 2 weeks. It can cause a temporary harmless blackening of the tongue and stool.
- DGL or deglycyrrhizinated licorice can both help eradicate the organism and relieve symptoms.
- Myrrh gum resin.

Medications
- Amoxicillin 1 g twice a day, clarithromycin 500 mg twice a day, omeprazole 20 mg twice a day for 10 days
- Prevpac: Lansoprazole/amoxicillin/clarithromycin combination twice a day for 14 days
- Helidac (bismuth/metronidazole/tetracycline) four times a day with meals for 2 weeks
- Tritec (ranitidine bismuth citrate) 400 mg twice a day for 28 days

B. *Treatment of Small Bowel Bacterial Overgrowth*

Nonprescription Preparations
- Oregano, citrus seed extract, *Isatis*, or berberine compounds.
- Special spices for the gut include garlic, onions, turmeric, ginger, cinnamon, sage, rosemary, oregano, and thyme. All of these can be added to the diet to support healthy digestive functioning.

Medications
Occasionally prescription medication may be needed. Some of the useful compounds include:
- Rifamixin 200–400 mg three times a day (the preferred treatment and a nonabsorbed antibiotic)
- Metronidazole 250 mg three times a day for 7 days (for anaerobes such as Bacteroides or Clostridia species)

TABLE 10.1   *(continued)*

- Tetracycline 500 mg twice a day for 7 days (also for anaerobes)
- Ciprofloxacin 500 mg twice a day for 3 days (for aerobes)

C. *Treatment of Yeast Overgrowth*

- Address predisposing factors (such as chronic use of antibiotics, steroids, hormones)
- Trial of yeast control diet: elimination of refined carbohydrates, sugar and fermented foods
- Testing for yeast overgrowth
- Nonprescription antifungals (oregano, garlic, citrus seed extract, berberine, tannins, undecylenate, *Isatis tinctoria*, Caprylic acid)
- Antifungal medications (nystatin, fluconazole, itraconazole, terbinafine, ketoconazole)
- Immunotherapy
- Identify potential environmental toxic fungi (Stachybotrys, strains of Aspergillus, Chaetomium, and Penicillium)
- 4R program
- Stress reduction

D. *Treatment of Parasites*

Nonprescription parasite treatments

- Take digestive enzymes for a few months—parasites often cause malabsorption and maldigestion
- Avoid vitamins during treatment because vitamins help the parasites flourish
- Use herbal therapies *Artemesia annua,* oregano, and berberine-containing plants (*Hydrastis Canadensis, Berberis vulgaris, Berberis aquifolium and Coptis chinesis*)

Prescription Medication for Parasites

- Humatin (paramomycin) in adult doses of 250 mg three times daily for 14 days and Bactrim DS or Septra DS (trimethoprim and sulfamethoxazole) every 12 hours for 14 days.
- Yodoxin (iodoquinole) 650 mg three times daily for 14 days. Yodoxin is antifungal as well as antiparasitic.
- Flagyl (metronidazole) 500 mg three times a day for 10 days with meals.
- Alinia (nitazoxanid) 500 mg three times a day for 10 days.

III. Use of Digestive Enzymes and Hydrochloric Acid

Enhance digestion by replacing missing digestive enzymes and HCl and recommending consumption of soluble fiber (vegetables, fruits, beans, most grains—except those containing gluten).

Most effective enzymes are from animals and are also available by prescription. Use 2-3 just before or at the beginning of a meal. They are generally well tolerated and without side effects. Look for a formula containing at least:

- Protease 100,000 USP units
- Lipase 20,000 USP units
- Amylase 100,000 USP units

Vegetarians can take a mixed plant-based form of digestive enzymes. Use 2–3 just before or at the beginning of a meal. These are grown from Aspergillus fungus so be careful if the patient has mold or yeast sensitivities.

Optimal formulas contain about 500 mg of enzymes per tablet or capsule and also contain:

- Amylase 100,000 USP units
- Protease 100,000 USP units
- Lipase 10,000 USP units
- Lactase 1600 units

Digestive bitters may also aid digestion. Swedish bitters or other aperitifs stimulate digestion function including enzymes and HCl. Herbal bitters that include gentian and artichoke, cardamom, fennel, ginger, and dandelion are also available in more concentrated forms that can be added to water.

IV. Probiotics and Prebiotics

In addition to supplementing with the healthy bacteria, studies have shown that providing food for the flora can improve outcomes. The food for probiotics is called prebiotics and includes mostly nondigestible plant components that are used by

continued

TABLE 10.1   *(continued)*

the flora for their nourishment. Some common foods that fulfill these criteria include fructose-containing oligosaccharides, which occur naturally in a variety of plants such as onion, asparagus, chicory, banana, and artichoke.

Follow These Guidelines When Selecting Probiotics and Prebiotics:

- Use a 12-week course of a probiotic to restore normal symbiosis or ecological balance. Often long-term therapy is needed.
- Take 5–10 billion organisms a day on an empty stomach in divided doses (twice a day).
  Preparations include freeze-dried bacteria packaged in powders, tablet, or capsule form.
- Higher doses may be necessary with preparations containing 50–450 billion organisms.
- Look for reputable, refrigerated brands of mixed flora including *Lactobacillus acidophilus, Lactobacillus rhamnosis* or GG and *B. bifidum.*
- Some products contain no live flora because they are very susceptible to damage from heat or processing or improper storage.
- Some strains do not colonize the gut well.
- Try some strains backed by research such as *Lactobacillus* GG (Culturelle), and the DDS-1 strain of *Lactobacillus acidophilus*, or VSL #3.
- Eat prebiotic sources of fiber including onion, asparagus, burdock root, Jerusalem artichoke chicory, and banana or consider supplements of fructose-containing oligosaccharides such as inulin or chicory root.

V. Nutrients for Gut Repair

Specialized gut support products and nutrients provide the necessary support for gut healing and repair. These are the final tools for correcting digestive problems, healing a leaky gut, and reducing relapse and recurrence of digestive and immune problems. These should be taken for 1–3 months depending on the severity of symptoms and response to treatment. These compounds needed for gut repair can be divided into four main categories:

A. *Gut Food*

- Glutamine 1000–10,000 mg/day

This is a nonessential amino acid that is the preferred fuel for the lining of the small intestine and can greatly facilitate healing. It can be taken for 1 to 2 months. It generally comes in powder form and is often combined with other compounds that facilitate gut repair.

B. *Nutrients and Antioxidants*

- Zinc carnosine 75–150 mg twice a day between meals
- Zinc 20–50 mg
- Vitamin A 5000–10,000 U/day
- Vitamin B5 pantothenic acid 100–500 mg/day
- Vitamin E 400 to 800 IU/day in the form of mixed tocopherols

These can be taken separately, or as part of a good high-potency multivitamin.

C. *Essential Fats and Oils*

- GLA (gamma linolenic acid) 2–6 g/day
- Gamma-oryzanol (rice brain or rice brain oil) 100 mg three times a day
- Omega 3 fatty acids 3 to 6 g/day of EPA/DHA

D. *Anti-inflammatories and Gut Detoxifiers*

- N-acetylcysteine 500 mg twice a day
- Reduced glutathione 300 mg twice a day
- Quercitin 500 mg twice a day and other bioflavonoids

ACKNOWLEDGMENTS

Leo Galland, M.D., Patrick Hanaway, M.D., and Gerard Mullin, M.D. contributed research and input in the preparation of the manuscript.

REFERENCES

1. Scott M, Gelhot AR. Gastroesophageal reflux disease: diagnosis and management. *Am Fam Physician.* 1999 Mar 1; 59(5):1161–9, 1199. Review.
2. Shaheen N, Ransohoff DF. Gastroesophageal reflux, Barrett esophagus, and esophageal cancer: scientific review. *JAMA.* 2002 Apr 17; 287(15):1972–81. Review.
3. El-Serag HB, Graham DY, Satia JA, Rabeneck L. Obesity is an independent risk factor for GERD symptoms and erosive esophagitis. *Am J Gastroenterol.* 2005 Jun; 100(6):1243–50.
4. Suerbaum S, Michetti P. Helicobacter pylori infection. *N Engl J Med.* 2002 Oct 10; 347(15):1175–86. Review.
5. Matysiak-Budnik T, Heyman M. Food allergy and Helicobacter pylori. *J Pediatr Gastroenterol Nutr.* 2002 Jan; 34(1):5–12. Review.
6. Gasbarrini A, Franceschi F. Does H. pylori infection play a role in idiopathic thrombocytopenic purpura and in other autoimmune diseases? *Am J Gastroenterol.* 2005 Jun; 100(6):1271–3.
7. Bhatia V, Tandon RK. Stress and the gastrointestinal tract. *J Gastroenterol Hepatol.* 2005 Mar; 20(3):332–9. Review.
8. Keohane J, Quigley EM. Functional dyspepsia: the role of visceral hypersensitivity in its pathogenesis. *World J Gastroenterol.* 2006 May 7; 12(17):2672–6. Review.
9. Davidson G, Kritas S, Butler R. Stressed mucosa. *Nestle Nutr Workshop Ser Pediatr Program.* 2007; 59:133–42; discussion 143–6. Review.
10. Landin WE, Kendall FM, Tansy MF. Metabolic performance and GI function in magnesium-deficient rats. *J Pharm Sci.* 1979 Aug; 68(8):978–83.
11. Cuomo A, Romano M, Rocco A, Budillon G, Del Vecchio Blanco C, Nardone G. Reflux oesophagitis in adult coeliac disease: beneficial effect of a gluten free diet. *Gut.* 2003 Apr; 52(4):514–7.
12. Semeniuk J, Kaczmarski M. Gastroesophageal reflux (GER) in children and adolescents with regard to food intolerance. *Adv Med Sci.* 2006; 51:321–6.
13. Waldron B, Cullen PT, Kumar R, Smith D, Jankowski J, Hopwood D, Sutton D, Kennedy N, Campbell FC. Evidence for hypomotility in non-ulcer dyspepsia: a prospective multifactorial study. *Gut.* 1991 Mar; 32(3):246–51.
14. Othman M, Agüero R, Lin HC. Alterations in intestinal microbial flora and human disease. *Curr Opin Gastroenterol.* 2008 Jan; 24(1):11–6. Review.
15. Lin HC. Small intestinal bacterial overgrowth: a framework for understanding irritable bowel syndrome. *JAMA.* 2004 Aug 18; 292(7):852–8. Review.
16. O'May GA, Reynolds N, Macfarlane GT. Effect of pH on an in vitro model of gastric microbiota in enteral nutrition patients. *Appl Environ Microbiol.* 2005 Aug; 71(8):4777–83.
17. Gościmski A, Matras J, Wallner G. Microflora of gastric juice in patients after eradication of Helicobacter pylori and treatment with a proton pump inhibitor. *Wiad Lek.* 2002; 55(1–2):19–28. Polish.
18. Fox M, Barr C, Nolan S, Lomer M, Anggiansah A, Wong T. The effects of dietary fat and calorie density on esophageal acid exposure and reflux symptoms. *Clin Gastroenterol Hepatol.* 2007 Apr; 5(4):439–44.
19. Atkinson W, Sheldon TA, Shaath N, Whorwell PJ. Food elimination based on IgG antibodies in irritable bowel syndrome: a randomised controlled trial. *Gut.* 2004 Oct; 53(10):1459–64.
20. Wilders-Truschnig M, Mangge H, Lieners C, Gruber HJ, Mayer C, März W. IgG antibodies against food antigens are correlated with inflammation and intima media thickness in obese juveniles. *Exp Clin Endocrinol Diabetes.* 2008, Apr; 16(4):241–245.
21. Lee SK, Green PH. Celiac sprue (the great modern-day imposter). *Curr Opin Rheumatol.* 2006 Jan; 18(1):101–7. Review.
22. Alaedini A, Green PH. Narrative review: celiac disease: understanding a complex autoimmune disorder. *Ann Intern Med.* 2005 Feb 15; 142(4):289–98. Review.
23. Elsden SR, Hilton MG, Waller JM. The end products of the metabolism of aromatic amino acids by Clostridia. *Arch Microbiol.* 1976 Apr 1; 107(3):283–8.
24. Shaw W, Kassen E, Chaves E. Increased urinary excretion of analogs of Krebs cycle metabolites and arabinose in two brothers with autistic features. *Clin Chem.* 1995 Aug; 41(8 Pt 1):1094–104.
25. Ruscin JM, Page RL 2nd, Valuck RJ. Vitamin B(12) deficiency associated with histamine(2)-receptor antagonists and a proton-pump inhibitor. *Ann Pharmacother.* 2002 May; 36(5):812–816.
26. Epstein M, McGrath S, Law F. Proton-pump inhibitors and hypomagnesemic hypoparathyroidism. *N Engl J Med.* 2006 Oct 26; 355(17):1834–6.

27. Ozutemiz AO, Aydin HH, Isler M, Celik HA, Batur Y. Effect of omeprazole on plasma zinc levels after oral zinc administration. *Indian J Gastroenterol*. 2002 Nov-Dec; 21(6):216–8.

28. Hutchinson C, Geissler CA, Powell JJ, Bomford A. Proton pump inhibitors suppress absorption of dietary non-haem iron in hereditary haemochromatosis. *Gut*. 2007 Sep; 56(9):1291–5. Epub 2007 Mar 7.

29. Yang YX, Lewis JD, Epstein S, Metz DC. Long-term proton pump inhibitor therapy and risk of hip fracture. *JAMA*. 2006 Dec 27; 296(24):2947–53.

30. Dial S, Delaney JAC, Barkun AN, Suissa S. Use of gastric acid-suppressive agents and the risk of community acquired Clostrium difficile-associated disease. *JAMA*. 2005; 294(23): 2989–95.

31. Waldum HL, Gustafsson B, Fossmark R, Qvigstad G. Antiulcer drugs and gastric cancer. *Dig Dis Sci*. 2005 Oct; 50 Suppl 1:S39–44. Review.

32. Jalving M, Koornstra JJ, Wesseling J, Boezen HM, DE Jong S, Kleibeuker JH. Increased risk of fundic gland polyps during long-term proton pump inhibitor therapy. *Aliment Pharmacol Ther*. 2006 Nov 1; 24(9):1341–8.

33. Hauben M, Horn S, Reich L, Younus M. Association between gastric acid suppressants and Clostridium difficile colitis and community-acquired pneumonia: analysis using pharmacovigilance tools. *Int J Infect Dis*. 2007 Sep; 11(5):417–22.

34. Leonardi S, Miraglia del Giudice M, La Rosa M, Bellanti JA. Atopic disease, immune system, and the environment. *Allergy Asthma Proc*. 2007 Jul-Aug; 28(4):410–7. Review.

35. Guarner F. Hygiene, microbial diversity and immune regulation. *Curr Opin Gastroenterol*. 2007 Nov; 23(6):667–72. Review.

36. Untersmayr E, Jensen-Jarolim E. The effect of gastric digestion on food allergy. *Curr Opin Allergy Clin Immunol*. 2006 Jun; 6(3):214–9.

37. Lundell L, Miettinen P, Myrvold HE, Hatlebakk JG, Wallin L, Malm A, Sutherland I, Walan A. Nordic GORD Study Group. Seven-year follow-up of a randomized clinical trial comparing proton-pump inhibition with surgical therapy for reflux oesophagitis. *Br J Surg*. 2007 Feb; 94(2):198–203.

38. Blaser MJ, Chen Y, Reibman J. Does Helicobacter pylori protect against asthma and allergy? *Gut*. 2008 Jan 14.

39. Loffeld RJ, Werdmuller BF, Kuster JG, Pérez-Pérez GI, Blaser MJ, Kuipers EJ. Colonization with cagA-positive Helicobacter pylori strains inversely associated with reflux esophagitis and Barrett's esophagus. *Digestion*. 2000; 62(2–3):95–9.

40. Kim HJ, Kim MK, Chang WK, Choi HS, Choi BY, Lee SS. Effect of nutrient intake and Helicobacter pylori infection on gastric cancer in Korea: a case-control study. *Nutr Cancer*. 2005; 52(2):138–46.

41. Wolle K, Malfertheiner P. Treatment of Helicobacter pylori. *Best Pract Res Clin Gastroenterol*. 2007; 21(2):315–24. Review.

42. Majewski M, McCallum RW. Results of small intestinal bacterial overgrowth testing in irritable bowel syndrome patients: clinical profiles and effects of antibiotic trial. *Adv Med Sci*. 2007; 52:139–42.

43. Karunajeewa HA, Manning L, Mueller I, Ilett KF, Davis TM. Rectal administration of artemisinin derivatives for the treatment of malaria. *JAMA*. 2007 Jun 6; 297(21):2381–90. Review.

44. Bergamaschi A, Magrini A, Pietroiusti A. Recent advances in the treatment of Helicobacter pylori infection. *Recent Patents Anti-Infect Drug Disc*. 2007 Nov; 2(3):197–205. Review.

45. Paraschos S, Magiatis P, Mitakou S, Petraki K, Kalliaropoulos A, Maragkoudakis P, Mentis A, Sgouras D, Skaltsounis AL. In vitro and in vivo activities of Chios mastic gum extracts and constituents against Helicobacter pylori. *Antimicrob Agents Chemother*. 2007 Feb; 51(2):551–9.

46. Isolauri E. Probiotics in human disease. *Am J Clin Nutr*. 2001 Jun; 73(6):1142S–6S. Review.

47. Duggan C, Gannon J, Walker WA. Protective nutrients and functional foods for the gastrointestinal tract. *Am J Clin Nutr*. 2002 May; 75(5):789–808. Review.

48. Vicario M, Amat C, Rivero M, Moretó M, Pelegrí C. Dietary glutamine affects mucosal functions in rats with mild DSS-induced colitis. *J Nutr*. 2007 Aug; 137(8):1931–7.

49. Mahmood A, FitzGerald AJ, Marchbank T, Ntatsaki E, Murray D, Ghosh S, Playford RJ. Zinc carnosine, a health food supplement that stabilises small bowel integrity and stimulates gut repair processes. *Gut*. 2007 Feb; 56(2):168–75.

50. Tarnawski A, Hollander D, Cergely H. Cytoprotective drugs. Focus on essential fatty acids and sucralfate. *Scand J Gastroenterol Suppl*. 1987; 127:39–43. Review.

51. Effects of aloe vera and sucralfate on gastric microcirculatory changes, cytokine levels and gastric ulcer healing in rats. *World J Gastroenterol*. 2006 Apr 7; 12(13):2034–9.

11 Peptic Ulcer Disease and *Helicobacter pylori*

Georges M. Halpern, M.D., Ph.D.

I. INTRODUCTION

Here are some facts and numbers [1]:

- 10% of Americans feel heartburn every day.
- 44% of Americans have heartburn monthly.
- 20 million Americans will suffer from an ulcer in their lifetime.
- The major cause of ulcer is *Helicobacter pylori* (*H.pylori*).
- The second leading cause is NSAIDs.
- Over-the-counter (OTC) antacids account for $1 billion sales every year.
- >60 million Americans experience acid indigestion once a month.
- >15 million experience it daily.
- >10 million are hospitalized each year for gastric problems, at a cost of $40 billion.
- 6000 Americans die each year from ulcer-related complications.
- >40,000 have surgery (persistent symptoms, complications of ulcers).

Should the primary care provider be actively involved to change this course? Obviously, "yes." Can foods or natural substances help? The answer is "yes," but not necessarily what one may think and the choice may prove difficult. This chapter will help you select the appropriate strategy best suited for your specific patient.

II. EPIDEMIOLOGY

Peptic ulcer disease is common worldwide. The overall lifetime prevalence is about 12% for men and 9% for women. The lifetime risk of peptic ulcer disease is about 10%. At any given time, about 2% of the general population of the United States has symptomatic peptic ulcer disease, which translates into about 4 million people who have active peptic ulcers; about 350,000 new cases are diagnosed each year. Four times as many duodenal ulcers as gastric ulcers are diagnosed. Approximately 3000 deaths per year in the United States are due to duodenal ulcer and 3000 to gastric ulcer. There has been a marked decrease in reported hospitalization and mortality rates for peptic ulcer in the United States, but changes in criteria for selecting the underlying cause of death might account for some of the apparent decrease in ulcer mortality rates. Hospitalization rates for duodenal ulcers decreased nearly 50% from 1970 to 1978, but hospitalization rates for gastric ulcers did not decrease [2]. Physician office visits for peptic ulcer disease have decreased in the last few decades. The hospitalization rate is approximately 30 patients per 100,000 cases. Although this decrease in hospitalization rates may reflect a decrease in duodenal ulcer disease incidence, it appears that changes in coding practices, hospitalization criteria, and diagnostic procedures have contributed to the reported declines in peptic ulcer hospitalization and mortality rates; the mortality rate has decreased modestly in the last few decades and is approximately 1 death per 100,000 cases. In Peru, the prevalence of gastric ulcer and duodenal ulcer decreased from 3.15% and 5.05% respectively in 1985, to 1.62% and 2.00% respectively in 2002 [3]. There is no good evidence to support the popular belief that peptic ulcer is most common in the spring and autumn; the most consistent pattern appears to be low ulcer rates in the summer. There is strong evidence that cigarette smoking, regular use of aspirin or nonsteroidal anti-inflammatory drugs (NSAIDs, including coxibs), and prolonged use of steroids are associated with the development of peptic ulcer. There is some evidence that coffee may affect ulcers, but most studies do not implicate alcohol, food, or psychological stress as causes of ulcer disease. Genetic factors play a role in both duodenal and gastric ulcer; the first-degree relatives of patients with duodenal ulcer have a 2- to 3-fold increase in risk of getting duodenal ulcer and relatives of gastric ulcer patients have a similarly increased risk of getting a gastric ulcer. About half of the patients with duodenal ulcer have elevated plasma pepsinogen I; a small increase in risk of duodenal ulcer is found in persons with blood group O and in subjects who fail to secrete blood group antigens into the saliva. In most Western countries, morbidity from duodenal ulcer is more common than from gastric ulcer, even though deaths from gastric ulcer exceed or equal those from duodenal ulcer, while in Japan, both morbidity and mortality are higher for gastric ulcer than for duodenal ulcer [2].

H. pylori is associated with peptic ulcers in adults (<60, mostly males); while NSAIDs are the major cause of peptic ulcers in the elderly (mostly women). The currently accepted knowledge is that *H. pylori* is transmitted by the fecal-oral route, which may or may not be water- or food-borne.

H. pylori is so common as to seem ubiquitous in many areas of the world. In developing nations, four of five persons are infected by age 20 [4]. However, in the United States, infection is unusual in children, and the likelihood of being infected is roughly correlated with age and ethnic background [4]. Today the prevalence of *H. pylori* infection in the United States is about 30%, which represents a 50% decline from 30 years ago. Persons born before 1950 are much more likely to have the infection than those born after 1950. Twice as many Black and Hispanic people are infected as White people [5]. This difference is not racial but reflects socioeconomic and educational factors, especially socioeconomic status during childhood. Although the prevalence of *H. pylori* infection is relatively low in the United States and other countries in which the standard of living is high, the prevalence exceeds 50% in industrialized areas of Asia and Europe. The EUROGAST Study Group [6] found that among asymptomatic persons 25 to 34 years of age, the prevalence of infection in Minneapolis–St. Paul (MN) was 15%, compared with 62% in Yokote, Japan, and 70% in parts of Poland. Because infection is typically acquired in childhood and is almost ubiquitous in Russia, Asia, Latin America, South America, and parts of Europe, patient age and country of origin may be important for detection. Mortality data (1971–2004) from eight different countries, including Argentina, Australia, Chile, Hong Kong, Japan, Mexico, Singapore, and Taiwan, were characterized by a decline in gastric and duodenal ulcer mortality [7]. Gastritis is almost always associated with *H. pylori* infection, but peptic ulcer disease develops in only about one in six infected persons. A number of studies [8] have shown that more than 90% of patients with duodenal ulcer and more than 70% of those who have gastric ulcer are infected with *H. pylori*. However, recent reports [9] describe ulcer disease that is *H. pylori*-negative and apparently not associated with use of NSAIDs, suggesting there may be other rare causative factors.

III. PATHOPHYSIOLOGY

Peptic ulcers are defects in the gastric or duodenal mucosa that extend through the *muscularis mucosa*. *H. pylori* infection and NSAID use are the most common etiologic factors. *H. pylori* can elevate acid secretion in people who develop duodenal ulcers, decrease acid through gastric atrophy in those who develop gastric ulcers or cancer, and leave acid secretion largely unchanged in those who do not develop these diseases. Duodenal ulcers did not occur in achlorhydric people or in those secreting <15 mmol/h of acid; duodenal ulcers can be healed, but not cured, by pharmacological suppression of acid secretion below this threshold. Areas of gastric metaplasia in the duodenum can be colonized by *H. pylori*, causing inflammation (duodenitis) and leading to further damage of the mucosa. The extent of gastric metaplasia is related to the amount of acid entering the duodenum— lowest in patients with pernicious anemia who secrete no acid and highest in patients with acid hypersecretion due to gastrin-secreting tumors (Zollinger-Ellison syndrome). Acid hypersecretion in duodenal ulcer disease is virtually always due to *H. pylori* infection because secretion returns to normal after the infection is eradicated. The predominantly antral gastritis in duodenal ulcer disease leads to acid hypersecretion by suppressing somatostatin cells and increasing gastrin release from the G cells in the gastric antrum. Other less common causes are mastocytosis, and basophilic leukemias. Under normal conditions, a physiologic balance exists between peptic acid secretion and gastroduodenal mucosal defense. Mucosal injury and, thus, peptic ulcer occur when the balance between the aggressive factors and the defensive mechanisms is disrupted. Aggressive factors, such as NSAIDs, *H. pylori*, alcohol (liquor), bile salts, acid, and pepsin, can alter the mucosal defense by allowing back diffusion of hydrogen ions and subsequent epithelial cell injury. The defensive mechanisms include tight intercellular junctions, mucus, mucosal blood flow, cellular restitution, and epithelial renewal. *H. pylori* infection predisposes to distal gastric cancer, but patients who develop this complication have diminished acid secretion. Low acid secretion in gastric cancer was, until recently, thought to be predominantly due to gastric corpus gastritis, the associated gastric atrophy leading to loss of parietal cells. However, *H. pylori*-associated acid hyposecretion can in part be reversed by eradicating *H. pylori*, suggesting that hyposecretion is due to inflammation rather than to permanent loss of cells.

Most strains of *H. pylori* can be divided into two distinct phenotypes based on the presence or absence of a vacuolating toxin (Vac A toxin) and the products of the cag pathogenicity island (cagPI), a large chromosomal region that encodes virulence genes and is similar to that found in other enteric pathogens such as *Escherichia coli* and *Salmonella typhi*. People infected with strains of *H. pylori* with the cagPI have more severe mucosal damage and are more likely to have duodenal ulcers or gastric cancer. However, research has not yet identified *H. pylori* genes that predispose to either duodenal ulcer or gastric cancer. Furthermore, in developing countries, where *H. pylori* infects most of the population, cagPI strains of *H. pylori* are present in almost all infected people but only a few develop clinical disease [10].

IV. TREATMENT RECOMMENDATIONS

FOOD

Since *H. pylori* infection is the leading cause of PUD and it is transmitted through gastrointestinal exposure, some patients and their practitioners are focused on risk of reinfection. Food and nutrient selection should instead be focused on what improves gastrointestinal linings and immune resistance.

A diet imposed by a physician or a dietician creates stress and will not be followed for more than a few days. Some remedies, such as the recommendation of large amounts of milk, can exacerbate symptoms. Furthermore, most people are wired to like or dislike foods, dishes, textures, and smells, or carry prejudices they were infected with at a young age. A clinically measurable example is the "Supertasters" who find cruciferous vegetables intensely (and therefore avoidably) bitter. Therefore rather than imposing a diet, certain foods should be recommended over others.

Broccoli sprouts, brussels sprouts, and other leafy vegetables of the large "cabbage" family must be cooked (microwave is okay) to prevent infection due to ubiquitous *E. coli*. Lactic fermentation of cabbage, for example, sauerkraut, is safe, and provides the added benefits of a probiotic.

Yogurt, kefir, and other lactic-fermented foods do help, and could cure a peptic ulcer (see Table 11.1) [11–52]. Conversely, large amounts of live probiotics, even 10^{10} live lactic bacteria, pale when compared to the $>10^{14}$ bacteria that form our usual intestinal flora. Somewhere between 300 and 1000 different species live in the gut, with most estimates at about 500 [53]. Probiotics alone do not seem to make much difference; if absorbed during a treatment with antibiotics, they will be wiped out.

TABLE 11.1
Brief Review of Natural Products Proposed to Control/Eradicate *H. pylori*, or Cure Peptic Ulcers

Nutrient/Food/Herb	Proposed Mechanism of Action	Dosing and Precautions
Aloe vera [11] gel *Aloe barbadensis*	Reduction of leukocyte adherence in postcapillary venule. Increased level of IL-10; decreased level of TNF-α. Reduction of gastric inflammation. Elongated gastric glands. Healing of gastric ulcers.	1 teaspoon (5 g) of gel after meals. *Caveat*: Use only the translucent gel without alloin, a cathartic purgative.
Astragaloside IV [12] *Astragalus zahlbruckneri*	Participation of NO (nitric oxide), prostaglandins, and sulfhydryls.	100 mg t.i.d.
Broccoli sprouts, brussels sprouts [13–15] (sulforaphanes)	Antioxidant. Stimulate nrf-2 gene-dependent antioxidant enzyme activities. Protect and repair gastric mucosa during *H. pylori* infection Bacteriostatic against 3 reference strains and 45 clinical isolates of *H. pylori* irrespective of their resistance to conventional antibiotics. Brief exposure to sulforaphane was bactericidal. Consumption of broccoli sprouts twice daily for 7 days resulted in normal urea breath tests, which remained normal at day 35. 78% of patients became stool antigen-negative and 60% remained negative at day 35.	50 g of cooked broccoli/brussels sprouts b.i.d. for 7 days.
Cat's Claw/Uña de Gato [16] *Uncaria tomentosa, Uncaria guianensis* (3% alkaloids [rhynchophylline]; 15% polyphenols)	Carboxyl-alkyl esters; pentacyclic oxindole alkaloids (POA). Proanthocyanidins. Antioxidants, anti-inflammatory. Cytoprotection with inhibition of TNF-α production (>70%).	Inner bark of stems and leaves. 1 g of vine powder capsules t.i.d. (and up to 5 g daily) with lemon juice (½ teaspoon/cup of water). *Caveat*: Potentiates Coumadin/ warfarin.
Centella asiatica, Gotu kola [17]	Brahmi, bacosides A and B. Bacoside assists in release of NO. Asiaticosides are immuno-stimulants. Extract and asiaticosides reduced size of ulcers at day 3 and 7 with concomitant attenuation of myeloperoxidase activity in ulcer tissue. Epithelial cell proliferation and angiogenesis were promoted, as well as expression of basic fibroblast growth factor in the ulcer tissues.	Eaten raw as salad leaf (Sri Lanka). Boil ½ teaspoon dry leaves/ cup of water; drink 3 cups daily. *Caveat*: Potentiates sedative effects of diphenhydramine, barbiturates, tricyclic antidepressants, zolpidem, anticonvulsants. Interferes with oral anti-diabetics and insulin.

TABLE 11.1   *(continued)*

Nutrient/Food/Herb	Proposed Mechanism of Action	Dosing and Precautions
Cranberry [18] *Vaccinium oxycoccus palustris*	Polyphenol antioxidants with antibacterial activity. Anti-adhesion against *H. pylori*. [13]C urea breath test was negative after 1 week of treatment. Eradication was 82.5%; better in female patients (95.2%).	250 mL of juice b.i.d.
Dangshen [19] *Conopsis pilosula*	Reduces gastric acid secretion, and gastrointestinal movements and propulsion.	Roots: 10–15 g daily in decoction.
Dragon's Blood [20] *Dracaena cochinchinensis*	New flavonoids derivatives 6 and 7 and (2S)-4',7-dihydroxy-8-methylflavan were very active against *H. pylori* (ATC c45504) with MIC values of 29.5, 29.5 and 31.3 microM respectively.	10 grains q.d., preferably in liquor. *Caveat*: Cathartic (risk of diarrhea).
Ginger [21] *Zigimber officinale* rhizome	Sesquiterpenoids. Phenylpropanoloids (gingerols, shogaols). Zingerone (during cooking). Sialagogue (stimulates production of saliva). Gastrokinetic. Ginger rhizome extract containing the gingerols inhibit the growth of *H. pylori* Cag+ strains *in vitro*.	1–5 g of fresh ginger daily. *Caveat*: Interacts with warfarin. Cholecystokinetic contraindicated if gallstones. Can cause heartburn if taken in large amounts or as powder.
Guarana [22] *Paullinia cupana*	Tannins and other polyphenols. Pretreatment with guarana (50 & 100 mg/kg orally) provides gastroprotection against pure ethanol, similar to caffeine (2–30mg/kg orally). But guarana protected against indomethacin-induced gastric ulceration while caffeine was ineffective.	Guarana extract: 500 mg q.d. with food. *Caveat*: Risk of seizures at high doses (cf. caffeine). Do not mix with ephedrine!
DGL [23] Deglycyrrhizinated licorice, Caved-S®	Equal to cimetidine. 44% healing vs. 6% with placebo	>760 mg chewed before each meal. Daily dosage: 4.5 g.
Marigold [24, 25] *Calendula officinalis*	Methanolic extract and its 1-butanol-soluble fraction show gastroprotective effects. The active constituents are saponin glycosides A, B, C, D and F against indomethacin-induced lesions in rats. In 90% of patients, spontaneous pain disappeared. Gastric acidity was statistically decreased posttreatment.	Calendula extract (45% water): 1–5 mL b.i.d.
Mastic gum [26–28] Resin from *Pistacia lenticus,* from the island of Chios, Greece	Decreases free acidity in 6-hour pylorus-ligated rats and cytoprotective against 50% ethanol in rats. Acid fraction of total mastic extract was very active (MBC=0.139mg/mL), as well as isomasticadienolic acid (MBC=0.202mg/mL). A double-blind study on 38 patients	1 g daily.

continued

TABLE 11.1   *(continued)*

Nutrient/Food/Herb	Proposed Mechanism of Action	Dosing and Precautions
	with 1 g daily for 2 weeks provided symptomatic relief in 80% of mastic patients (vs. 50% in the placebo group); endoscopically proven healing occurred in 70% mastic patients vs. 22% with placebo (p < 0.01). No side effects were reported.	
Optiberry® [29] Blend of wild blueberry, strawberry, cranberry, wild bilberry, elderberry, and raspberry seed extracts, with standardized levels of malvidin, cyanidin, delphinidin and petunidin.	Anthocyanins: better bioavailability with antioxidant activity. *H. pylori* strain 49503 suspension in PBS was exposed for 18 h to Optiberry 0.25–1% concentration that significantly inhibited (p < 0.05) *H. pylori* and increased its susceptibility to clarithromycin.	30 mg b.i.d. with meals.
Parsley [30] *Petroselinum crispum* Tannins, flavonoids, sterols, triterpenes.	Inhibits gastric secretion, protects gastric mucosa against injuries caused by pyloric ligation, indomethacin, and cytodestructive agents at 1–2 g/kg in rats.	6g daily. *Caveat*: Emmenagogue and abortifaciens (apiol). Photosensitizer (furanocoumarins and psoralens). Rich in oxalic acid (urolithiasis).
Plantain [31–33] *Musa spp.* Extract from unripe plantain bananas. Effects may vary according to variety; *Hom* seems to be more active.	Stimulates growth of gastric mucosa. Antiulcer caused by aspirin, indomethacin, phenylbutazone, prednisolone, and cysteamine in rats; caused by histamine in guinea pigs. Increased staining of alcian blue in apical cells with staining in deeper layers of mucosal glands. Extract of *Hom* variety is both gastroprotective (vs. indomethacin) and ulcer healing.	5–10 g of powder daily, with food. *N.B.* Ripe fruit plantain and dessert bananas are inactive.
Evening Primrose [34, 35] *Oenothera biennis* The seeds contain 7–10% of gamma-linolenic acid (GLA), an omega-6 PUFA. The oil (EPO) is used in medicine (anti-inflammatory).	EPO (5–10 mg/kg) inhibits damage induced by pylorus ligation and NSAIDs; it demonstrates anti-secretory and anti-ulcerogenic effects in rats. EPO inhibited growth of *H. pylori*, suppressed acid production, healed the ulcer, and protected gastric mucosa from aspirin- and steroid-induced damage in humans.	4–8 g of EPO daily, divided in small doses to be taken throughout the day. *Caveat*: Seizures in some patients, notably if taking antipsychotic phenothiazines.
Polyunsaturated Fatty Acids, PUFAs [36] Commonly found in seed and marine oils. GLA (omega-6), docosahexaenoic (DHA) and EPA (omega-3 C20:5) acids are most effective.	Linolenic acid is associated with membrane function [^{14}C studies].	Diets rich in PUFAs protect against duodenal ulcers by inhibiting growth of *H. pylori*. Doses of 10^{-3}M or 2.5×10^{-4}M are effective in killing most *H. pylori*.
Probiotics, Yogurt/Yoghurt [37, 38] Live microorganisms which when administered in adequate amounts confer a health benefit on the host; mostly lactic bacteria.	Lactic bacteria inhibit growth of *H. pylori*. Regular intake of yogurt containing Bb12 and La5 (AB yogurt) decreased the urease activity (^{13}C breath test) after 6 w of therapy	2–4 6 oz. or 8 oz. yogurts with live active cultures/day. Brands associating *bifidobacteria* claim more efficacy.

TABLE 11.1   *(continued)*

Nutrient/Food/Herb	Proposed Mechanism of Action	Dosing and Precautions
	(p < 0.0001), and *H. pylori* infection in 59 adults vs. 11 in milk (placebo) control group. Pretreatment with AB yogurt for 4 w improved the efficacy of quadruple 1 w treatment of *H. pylori* infection despite microbial resistance.	
Propolis [39] A resinous substance that bees collect from tree buds or other botanical sources. The composition of propolis is variable, depending on season, bee species and geographic location.	The composition of propolis will vary from hive to hive, district to district, and season to season. Even propolis samples taken from within a single colony can vary, making controlled clinical tests virtually impossible. Propolis has been shown to target *H. pylori*, and is anti-inflammatory and antioxidant. Combination of propolis and clarithromycin improved inhibition of *H. pylori* synergistically.	Two 250 mg capsules t.i.d. for 1 w. *Caveat*: Propolis may cause severe allergic reactions if the user is sensitive to bees or bee products.
Quercetin [40] 3,3',4',5,7-pentahydroxy-2-phenylchromen-4-one. The aglycone form of a number of other flavonoid glycosides, such as rutin and quercetin.	Quercetin is the most active of the flavonoids with significant anti-inflammatory activity; it inhibits both the manufacture and release of histamine; it exerts potent antioxidant activity and vitamin C-sparing action. Pretreatment (120') with 200 mg/kg quercetin prevented gastric necrosis due to ethanol; all animals treated with quercetin showed increased gastric mucus production.	Foods rich in quercetin include capers (1800 mg/kg), lovage (1700 mg/kg), apples (440 mg/kg), tea (*Camellia sinensis*), onions (higher concentrations of quercetin occur in the outermost rings), red grapes (higher concentration in red wine), citrus fruits, broccoli, and other leafy green vegetables. Organic tomatoes have 79% more quercetin than conventionally grown ones. FRS soft chews is a commercial supplement: 2 soft chews t.i.d. *Caveat*: Quercetin is contraindicated with antibiotics; it may interact with fluoroquinolones. It is also a potent inhibitor of CYP3A4 (drug interaction).
Reishi, Lingzhi [41] *Ganoderma lucidum*	Reishi polysaccharide (GLPS) 250 and 500 mg/kg by intragastric administration healed ulcers in rats, with suppression of TNF-α gene expression and ornithine decarboxylase (ODC) activity. GLPS at 0.25–1 mg/mL increased mucus synthesis. Besides suppression of TNF-α, GLPS induced c-Myc and ODC gene expression.	1–2 capsules of 500 mg (with spores) of ReishiMax® b.i.d with vitamin C supplement (250mg) or fruit juice.
Sanogastril® [42] Extract of *glycine maximus* with *Lactobacillus bulgaricus* LB51.	Active against gastric hyperacidity; 80% of gastric and duodenal ulcers improved after 10 days of treatment.	Chew 1–3 1.5 g tablet(s) each day. Active within 5 minutes in 70% of cases.

continued

TABLE 11.1 *(continued)*

Nutrient/Food/Herb	Proposed Mechanism of Action	Dosing and Precautions
Sea-Buckthorn [43] *Hippophae rhamnoides*	Constituents of sea-buckthorn berries, particularly oils, have exceptional properties as antioxidants. In rats, oral administration of CO_2-extracted oil from seeds and pulp at dosage of 7 mL/kg/day significantly reduced ulcer formation by water immersion or reserpine in rats. At 3.5 mL/kg/day it also reduced gastric ulcer by pylorus ligation and sped up healing of acetic acid-induced gastric ulcer ($P < 0.01$).	Fresh juice, syrup, and berry or seed oils are used for stomach ulcers. The recommended dosage for esophagus and stomach disorders is ½ teaspoon 2–3 times a day of sea-buckthorn oil.
Swallowroot, Sariva [44] *Decalepis hamiltonii* Bioactive polysaccharide (SRPP)	Prevented (80–85%) stress-induced gastric ulcers in animal models. Normalized gastric mucin, antioxidants, and upregulated X 3 H(+),K(+)-ATPase. Protected gastric mucosa and epithelial glands. Inhibited *H. pylori* growth at 77mg/mL. SRPP is nontoxic.	Decoction of root (India, Ayurvedic) t.i.d.
Green Tea [45] *Camellia sinensis*	Inhibition of *H. pylori* urease with IC(50) of 13 µg/mL. Active components are catechins. In Mongolian gerbils infected with *H. pylori*, 500, 1000, and 2000 ppm of green tea extract in water suppressed gastritis and *H. pylori* in 6 w, in dose-dependent manner.	4–8 cups (2.25 g of tea per 6 oz of water) daily. Decaffeinated green tea is available.
Turmeric, Curcumin [46] *Curcuma longa* Its rhizomes are boiled for several hours and then dried in hot ovens, after which they are ground into a deep orange-yellow powder. Turmeric contains up to 5% essential oils and up to 3% curcumin, a polyphenol. It can exist in at least two tautomeric forms, keto and enol. The keto form is preferred in solid phase and the enol form in solution.	Anti-H_2 histamine receptor. In pylorus-ligated rat stomachs, it reduced gastric secretion and prevented lesions. Pretreatment with *Curcuma longa* extract reduced Dimaprit® (H_2 agonist)-induced cAMP production in a concentration-dependent manner. The ethanol and ethylacetate extracts are both active as H_2 receptor competitive blockers.	Two 500 mg curcumin 95% capsules b.i.d.
Vitamin C [47, 48] Ascorbic acid	Adding vitamin C (ascorbic acid) for 1 w to the triple treatment (omeprazole 20 mg q.d. + clarithromuycin 500 mg q.d. + amoxicillin 1 g q.d.) can reduce the dosage of clarithromycin from 500 to 250 mg and help eradicate *H. pylori* [37]. However, administration of 5 g q.d. vitamin C during 28 days had no effect on *H. pylori* infection [38].	250 mg b.i.d.

TABLE 11.1   *(continued)*

Nutrient/Food/Herb	Proposed Mechanism of Action	Dosing and Precautions
Water hyssop, Brahmi [49] *Bacopa monniera* Contains 2 saponins (bacopaside I and II), betulinic acid, wogonin, oxeoxindin, apigenin, and luteolin.	In both normal and diabetic (NIDDM) rats, *B. monniera* extract (BME, 20–100mg/kg) did not influence blood glucose levels. BME (50mg/kg) showed significant anti-ulcer and ulcer-healing activities. The ulcer-protective effects of BME were more pronounced in nondiabetic rats; BME affects various mucosal offensive and defensive factors.	1–2 225 mg tablet(s) b.i.d. Antioxidant. Treats epilepsy. Nootropic (enhances cognition); protects against memory deterioration due to phenytoin.
Bolivian Medicinals [50] *Phoradendron crassifolium* and *Franseria artemisioides* Tanins, saponins, flavonoids, and coumarins.	Cytoprotective against ethanol-induced ulcer in rats. Cytoprotective activity is comparable to atropine.	As decoction, several times daily. *Caveat*: *Phoradendron* is a mistletoe, with poorly defined toxicity. *Franseria artemisioides* is a ragweed, with cross-allergenicity with all *Ambrosiae*.
Zinc-Carnosine [51] Chelate of elemental zinc and carnosine in a 1:1 ratio.	Carnosine is a free radical scavenger that prevents lipid peroxidation. Zinc-carnosine blocks the effects of TNF-α or IL-1β in MKN28 human gastric cells, and reduces IL-8 in supernatant. It prevents reduction of mucus production caused by ethanol, and inhibits proliferation of *H. pylori* by inactivating urease. Many studies confirm 100% control of symptoms and >80% endoscopic cure after 8 w of treatment. Zinc-carnosine improved efficacy and shortens duration of treatment with antibiotics.	75 mg q.d. or b.i.d., preferably chewable, for 8 weeks.
Traditional Chinese Medicine (TCM) [52] 30 Chinese herbals divided into the groups below	*In vitro* assessment of ethanol extracts against *H. pylori*. Extracts of group #1 were active at a concentration of 40 µg/mL while extracts of groups #2 and #3 were active at 60 µg/mL. These 30 well-known plants require more studies for identification of active components and standardization, but offer great hope for eradication of *H. pylori*, possibly in combination.	As "tea" (decoction) t.i.d. *Caveat*: sourcing, toxicology, standardization—and even proper identification—are poor, unknown, or ignored. Contamination with heavy metals, pathogens, pesticides, etc. is common.

TCM Treatment of Peptic Ulcer

Insufficiency-Cold Type: Modified Decoction of Astragalus
Astragalus root
Cinnamon twig bark
White peony root
Cuttlefish bone
Dahurian angelica root
Prepared licorice root

continued

TABLE 11.1 *(continued)*

Nutrient/Food/Herb	Proposed Mechanism of Action	Dosing and Precautions

Stagnated-Heat Type: Modified Two-Old Herbs Decoction + Eliminating Pathogenic Heat from Liver

Coptis rhizome

Cape jasmine fruit

Scutellaria root

Anemarrhema rhizome

White peony root

Tangerine peel

Piniella tuber

Poria

Finger citron

Dendrobium

Prepared licorice root

N.B. If presence of hematemesis or melena, add 6 g of natoginseng powder to be taken after decoction.

Advanced Stomach Support Formula, Standardized

Corydalis tuber

Astragalus root

San-qi root

Chekiang fritillary bulb

Chinese licorice root

Gambir leaf & stem

Bletilla striata (Thumb.) root

Sepia esculenta (Hoyle) shell

Qi-Stagnation Type: Modified Powder Against Cold Limbs + Sichuan Chinaberry Powder

Bupleurum root

Cyperus tuber

White peony root

Bitter orange

Tangerine peel

Sichuan chinaberry

Corydalis tuber

Aucklandia root

Perilla stem

Ark shell

Finger citron

Prepared licorice root

Foods rich in quercetin should be part of the diet: Apples, tea, and red wine are the most acceptable. A regular consumption of onions and capers is recommended. Regular, moderate consumption of red wine (even de-alcoholized) during meals will control *H. pylori* proliferation [54] and toxicity [55].

To provide a supplemental, absorbable iron supply, a diet rich in red meat, liver, and other innards is recommended in patients with confirmed blood loss due to a bleeding ulcer. The only iron we can readily absorb comes from animal sources. These same foods are rich in vitamin B12, which can be absorbed less readily in a hypochlorhydric environment of acid-suppressing medication.

Beverages can increase stomach acid production. Patients must be aware of the acid-inducing properties of some beverages (presented in Figure 11.1). Of particular note is that milk but not fermented dairy products induce acid production.

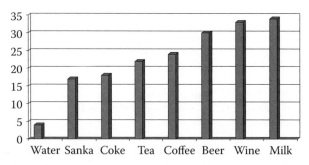

FIGURE 11.1   Stomach acid output 3.5 hours after consumption of beverage. The volume of each beverage consumed was 360 mL except for wine, which was 240 mL. The acid output was measured in mmol/3.5 hours.

Nutrient and Herbal Supplements

The marketing of "natural cures" is an exponentially growing business on the Internet, in magazines, health food stores, supermarkets, or large outlets (e.g., Costco, Wal-Mart). Most claims are unsubstantiated, and most products are unreliable if not toxic.

Table 11.1 summarizes current acceptable knowledge based on extensive research on Medline/PubMed in early 2008. Most products have not been submitted to the test of controlled clinical studies and base their claims on limited animal or lab results. Here, more than ever, caution is required.

Treatment of peptic ulcer disease can involve nutrient-drug interactions. Specifically, if proton pump inhibitors have been used for a long period of time, the patient's vitamin B12 status must be checked, and oral supplementation or injection considered.

V.   SUMMARY

I can recommend the following, for a good record on safety and efficacy. Most foods can be consumed regularly; supplements' activity should be checked after 8 weeks.

- Cooked broccoli sprouts: 50 g daily
- Cranberry juice (pure): 250 mL twice daily
- Deglycyrrhizinated licorice: 760 mg t.i.d.
- Mastic gum: 1 g daily
- Unripe plantain powder: 5 to 10 g daily
- Yogurt, natural, low fat, with live cultures (possibly *Bifidobacteria*): 2 to 4 6-ounce servings daily
- Diet high in vegetables rich in quercetin, and moderate amounts of red wine (even de-alcoholized) with meals
- Sanogastril®: 1 to 3 tablets daily
- Green tea (eventually decaffeinated): *ad libitum*
- Zinc-carnosine: 75 mg q.d. or b.i.d. (preferably chewable)

REFERENCES

1. Yamada T, Alpers DH, Kaplowitz N, Laine L, Owyang C, Powell DW. *Textbook of gastroenterology,* 4th ed. Philadelphia: Lippincott, Williams & Wilkins, 2003.
2. Kurata GH, Haile BM. Epidemiology of peptic ulcer disease. *Clin Gastroenterol* 1984;13:289–307.

3. Ramírez-Ramos A, Watanabe-Yamamoto J, Takano-Morón J, Gilman RH, Recavarren Arce S, Arias-Stella J, Yoshiwara-Wakabayashi E, Rodríguez-Ulloa C, Miyagui-Maeda J, Chinga-Alayo E, Mendoza-Requena D, Leey-Casella J, Rosas-Aguirre A, Velapatiño-Cochachi B, Guerra Valencia D. Decrease in prevalence of peptic ulcer and gastric adenocarcinoma at the Policlínico Peruano Japones, Lima, Peru, between the years 1985 and 2002. Analysis of 31,446 patients. *Acta Gastroenterol Latinoam* 2006;36:139–146.

4. Breuer T, Malaty HM, Graham DY. The epidemiology of H pylori-associated gastroduodenal diseases. In: Ernst PB, Michetti P, Smith PD, eds. *The immunobiology of* H pylori: *from pathogenesis to prevention.* Philadelphia: Lippincott-Raven, 1997:1–14.

5. Graham DY, Malaty HM, Evans DG, et al. Epidemiology of *Helicobacter pylori* in an asymptomatic population in the United States: effect of age, race, and socioeconomic status. *Gastroenterology* 1991;100(6):1495–1501.

6. The EUROGAST Study Group. Epidemiology of, and risk factors for, *Helicobacter pylori* infection among 3194 asymptomatic subjects in 17 populations. *Gut* 1993;34(12):1672–1676.

7. Sonnenberg A. Time trends of ulcer mortality in non-European countries. *Am J Gastroenterol* 2007;102:1101–1107.

8. Isenberg JI, Soll AH. Epidemiology, clinical manifestations, and diagnosis of peptic ulcer. In: Bennett JC, Plum F, eds. *Cecil textbook of medicine,* 20th ed. Philadelphia: Saunders, 1996:664–666.

9. Sprung DJ, Apter MN. What is the role of *Helicobacter pylori* in peptic ulcer and gastric cancer outside the big cities? *J Clin Gastroenterol* 1998;26(1):60–63.

10. Calam J, Baron JH. ABC of the upper gastrointestinal tract. *BMJ* 2001;323:980–982.

11. Eamlamnam K, Patumraj S, Visedopas N, Thong-Ngam D. Effects of aloe vera and sucralfate on gastric microcirculatory changes, cytokine levels and gastric ulcer healing in rats. *World J Gastroenterol* 2006;12(13):2034–2039.

12. Navarrete A, Arrieta J, Terrones L, Abou-Gazar H, Calis I. Gastroprotective effect of Astragaloside IV: role of prostaglandins, sulfhydryls and nitric oxide. *J Pharm Pharmacol* 2005;57(8):1059–1064.

13. Yanaka A, Zhang S, Tauchi M, Suzuki H, Shibahara T, Matsui H, Nakahara A, Tanaka N, Yamamoto M. Role of nrf-2 gene in protection and repair of gastric mucosa against oxidative stress. *Inflammopharmacology* 2005;13(1–3):83–90.

14. Fahey JW, Haristoy X, Dolan PM, Kensler TW, Scholtus I, Stephenson KK, Talalay P, Lozniewski A. Sulforaphane inhibits extracellular, intracellular, and antibiotic-resistant strains of *Helicobacter pylori* and prevents benzo[a]pyrene-induced stomach tumors. *Proc Natl Acad Sci USA* 2002; 99(11):7810–7815.

15. Galan MV, Kishan AA, Silverman AL. Oral broccoli sprouts for the treatment of *Helicobacter pylori* infection: a preliminary report. *Dig Dis Sci* 2004;49(7–8):1088–1090.

16. Gattuso M, Di Sapio O, Gattuso S, Pereyra EL. Morphoanatomical studies of *Uncaria tomentosa* and *Uncaria guianensis* bark and leaves. *Phytomedicine* 2004;11(2–3):213–223.

17. Cheng CL, Guo JS, Luk J, Koo MW. The healing effects of *Centella* extract and asiaticoside on acetic acid induced gastric ulcers in rats. *Life Sci* 2004;74(18):2237–2349.

18. Shmuely H, Yahav J, Samra Z, Chodick G, Koren R, Niv Y, Ofek I. Effect of cranberry juice on eradication of *Helicobacter pylori* in patients treated with antibiotics and a proton pump inhibitor. *Mol Nutr Food Res* 2007;51(6):746–751.

19. Wang ZT, Du Q, Xu GJ, Wang RJ, Fu DZ, Ng TB. Investigations on the protective action of *Condonopsis pilosula* (Dangshen) extract on experimentally-induced gastric ulcer in rats. *Gen Pharmacol* 1997; 28(3):469–473.

20. Zhu Y, Zhang P, Yu H, Li J, Wang MW, Zhao W. Anti-*Helicobacter pylori* and thrombin inhibitory components from Chinese Dragon's Blood, *Dracaena cochinchinensis*. *J Nat Prod* 2007;70(10): 1570–1577.

21. Mahady GB, Pendland SL, Yun GS, Lu ZZ, Stoia A. Ginger (*Zinzinber officinalis* Roscoe) and the gingerols inhibit the growth of Cag A+ strains of *Helicobacter pylori*. *Anticancer Res* 2003;23(SA): 3699–3702.

22. Campos AR, Barros AI, Santos FA, Rao VS. Guarana (*Paullinia cupana* Mart.) offers protection against gastric lesions induced by ethanol and indomethacin in rats. *Phytother Res* 203;17(10):1199–1202.

23. Glick L. Deglycyrrhizinated liquorice for peptic ulcer. *Lancet* 1982;2(8302):817.

24. Yoshikawa M, Murakami T, Kishi A, Kageura T, Matsuda H. Medicinal flowers. III. Marigold.(1): hypoglycemic, gastric emptying inhibitory, and gastroprotective principles and new oleanane-type triterpene oligoglycosides, calendasaponins A, B, C, and D, from Egyptian *Calendula officinalis*. *Chem Pharm Bull* (Tokyo) 2001;49(7):863–870.

25. Chakürski I, Matev M, Stefanov G, Koïchev A, Angelova I. Treatment of duodenal ulcers and gastroduodenitis with a herbal combination of *Symphitum officinalis* and *Calendula officinalis* with and without antacids. *Vutr Boles* 1981;20(6):44–47.

26. Al-Said MS, Ageel AM, Parmar NS, Tariq M. Evaluation of mastic, a crude drug obtained from *Pistacia lentiscus* for gastric and duodenal anti-ulcer activity. *Ethnopharmacol* 1986;15(3):271–278.

27. Paraschos S, Magiatis P, Mitakou S, Petraki K, Kalliaropoulos A, Maragkoudakis P, Mentis A, Sgouras D, Skaltsounis AL. *In vitro* and *in vivo* activities of Chios mastic gum extracts and constituents against *Helicobacter pylori*. *Antimicrob Agents Chemother* 2007;51(2):551–559.

28. Al-Habbal MJ, Al-Habbal Z, Huwez FU. A double-blind controlled clinical trial of mastic and placebo in the treatment of duodenal ulcer. *Clin Exp Pharmacol Physiol* 1984;11(5):541–544.

29. Chatterjee A, Yasmin T, Bagchi D, Stohs SJ. Inhibition of *Helicobacter pylori in vitro* by various berry extracts, with enhanced susceptibility to clarithromycin. *Mol Cell Biochem* 2004;265(1–2):19–26.

30. Al-Howiriny T, Al-Sohaibani M, El-Tahir K, Rafatullah S. Prevention of experimentally-induced gastric ulcers in rats by an ethanolic extract of Parsley *Petroselinum crispum*. *Am J Chin Med* 2003;31(5):699–711.

31. Best R, Lewis DA, Nasser N. The anti-ulcerogenic activity of the unripe plantain banana (*Musa* species). *Br J Pharmacol* 1984;82(1):107–116.

32. Goel RK, Gupta S, Shankar R, Sanyal AK. Anti-ulcerogenic effect of banana powder (*Musa sapientum* var. *paradisiaca*) and its effect of mucosal resistance. *J Ethnopharmacol* 1986;18(1):33–44.

33. Pannangpetch P, Vuttivirojana A, Kularbkaew C, Tesana S, Kongyingyoes B, Kukongviriyapan V. The antiulcerative effect of Thai *Musa* species in rats. *Phytother Res* 2001;15(5):407–410.

34. al-Shabanah OA. Effect of evening primrose oil on gastric ulceration and secretion induced by various ulcerogens and necrotizing agents in rats. *Food Chem Toxicol* 1997;35(8):769–775.

35. Das UN. Hypothesis: *cis*-unsaturated fatty acids as potential anti-peptic ulcer drugs. *Prostaglandins Leukot Essent Fatty Acids* 1998;58(5):377–380.

36. Thompson L, Cockayne A, Spiller RC. Inhibitory effect of polyunsaturated fatty acids on the growth of *Helicobacter pylori*: a possible explanation of the effect of diet on peptic ulceration. *Gut* 1994;35(11):1557–1561.

37. Wang KY, Li SN, Liu CS, Perng DS, Su YC, Wu DC, Lai CH, Wang TN, Wang WM. Effects of ingesting Lactobacillus- and Bifidobacterium-containing yogurt in subjects with colonized *Helicobacter pylori*. *Am J Clin Nutr* 2004;80(3):737–741.

38. Sheu BS, Cheng HC, Kao AW, Wang ST, Yang YJ, Yang HB, Wu JJ. Pretreatment with Lactobacillus- and Bifidobacterium-containing yogurt can improve the efficacy of quadruple therapy in eradicating residual *Helicobacter pylori* infection after failed triple therapy. *Am J Clin Nutr* 2006;83(4):864–869.

39. Nostro A, Cellini L, Di Bartolomeo S, Canatelli MA, Di Campli E, Procopio F, Grande R, Marzio L, Alonzo V. Effects of combining extracts from propolis or *Zigiber officinalis* with clarithromycin on *Helicobacter pylori*. *Phytother Res* 2006;20(3):187–190.

40. Alarcon de la Lastra C, Martin MJ, Motilva V. Antiulcer and Gastroprotective effects of quercetin: a gross and histologic study. *Pharmacology* 1994;48(1):56–62.

41. Gao Y, Zhou S, Wen J, Huang M, Xu A. Mechanism of the antiulcerogenic effect of *Ganoderma lucidum* polysaccharides on indomethacin-induced lesions in the rat. *Life Sci* 2002;72(6):731–745.

42. www.yalacta.com/US/sanogastril/sanoga.htm.

43. Xing J, Yang B, Dong Y, Wang B, Wang J, Kallio HP. Effects of sea buckthorn (*Hippophae rhamnoides* L.) seed and pulp oil on experimental models of gastric ulcer in rats. *Fitoterapia* 2002;73(7–8):644–650.

44. Srikanta BM, Siddaraju MN, Dharmesh SM. A novel phenol-bound pectic polysaccharide from *Decalepis hamiltonii* with multi-step ulcer preventive activity. *World J Gastroenterol* 2007;13(39):5196–207.

45. Matsubara S, Shibata H, Ishikawa F, Yokokura T, Takahashi M, Sugimura T, Wakabayashi K. Suppression of *Helicobacter pylori*-induced gastritis by green tea extract in Mongoian gerbils. *Biochem Biophys Res Commun* 2003;310(3):715–719.

46. Kim DC, Kim SH, Choi BH, Baek NI, Kim D, Kim MJ, Kim KT. Curcuma longa extract protects against gastric ulcers by blocking H_2 histamine receptors. *Biol Pharm Bull* 2005;28(12):2220–2224.

47. Chuang CH, Sheu BS, Kao AW, Cheng HC, Huang AH, Yang HB, Wu JJ. Adjuvant effect of vitamin C on omeprazole-amoxicillin-clarithromycin triple therapy for *Helicobacter pylori* eradication. *Hepatogastroenterology* 2007;54(73):320–326.

48. Kamiji MM, Oliveira RB. Effect of vitamin C administration on gastric colonization by *Helicobacter pylori*. *Arch Gastroenterol* 2005;42(3):167–172.

49. Darababu M, Prabha T, Pryambada S, Agrawal VK, Aryya NC, Goel RK. Effect of *Bacopa monnieri* and *Azadirachta indica* on gastric ulceration and healing in NIDDM rats. *Indian J Exp Biol* 2004;42(4):389–397.

50. Gonzales E, Iglesias I, Carretero E, Villar A. Gastric cytoprotection of Bolivian medicinal plants. J *Ethnopharmacol* 2000;70(3):329–333.
51. Halpern GM. *Zinc-carnosine: Nature's safe and effective remedy for ulcers.* Garden City Park, NY: SquareOne Publishers, 2005, 42p.
52. Li Y, Xu C, Zhang Q, Liu JY, Tan RX. *In vitro* anti-*Helicobacter pylori* action of 30 Chinese medicines used to treat ulcer diseases. *J Ethnopharmacol* 2005;98(3):329–333.
53. Steinhoff U. Who controls the crowd? New findings and old questions about the intestinal microflora. *Immunol Lett* 2005;99(1):12–16.
54. Daroch F, Hoeneisen M, Gonzalez CL, et al. *In vitro* antibacterial activity of Chilean red wines against *Helicobacter pylori. Microbios* 2001;104:79–85.
55. Tombola F, Campello S, De Luca L, Ruggiero P et al. Plant polyphenols inhibit VacA, a toxin secreted by the gastric pathogen *Helicobacter pylori. FEBS Lett* 2003;543:184–189.

12 Viral Hepatitis, Nonalcoholic Steatohepatitis, and Postcholecystectomy Syndrome

Trent William Nichols, Jr., M.D.

I. INTRODUCTION

The liver detoxifies potentially harmful foreign substances and endogenous metabolic byproducts. Failure to detoxify harms the liver, gallbladder, and human host. Historically, the focus on liver disease management has been reducing the toxic burden where possible. More recent research points to biochemical individuality in response to the same toxin burden.

Hepatitis and cholecystitis can be thought of as genetotrophic diseases, those for which genetic uniqueness creates demands for specific nutrients beyond the average and for which unmet nutrient demands are associated with disease [1]. This chapter focuses on dietary patterns, food, and nutrients that can augment the liver's detoxifying system in the face of liver and gallbladder disease.

II. EPIDEMIOLOGY

Viral hepatitis is also changing with immigrants and adoptees from areas where hepatitis B virus (HBV) is endemic and where hepatitis B is often acquired transplacentally with a chronic carriage rate of 90% without medical intervention. Due to improved viral testing, blood transfusions have decreased as a cause of transferring hepatitis B and C. Intravenous drug use, unsafe sex and tattoos are now the leading means of acquiring hepatitis B and C. There are 1.4 million deaths annually in the United States from hepatocellular carcinoma and cirrhosis as a complication of hepatitis B [2]. Hepatitis C infects an estimated 3 to 4 million people in the United States and is only self-limiting in 15%. Of the 85% who have chronic hepatitis C, the majority will have elevated or fluctuating serum alanine aminotransferase (ALT) and one-third will have persistently normal ALT. The latter group is presently not eligible for peg interferon and ribavirin therapy despite their continued liver injury and detectable viremia [3].

Nonalcoholic steatohepatitis (NASH) has recently become the third cause for liver transplantation and is projected to be the leading cause sometime in the future as obesity and diabetes prevalence increases. The spectrum of fatty liver ranges from NAFLD (nonalcoholic fatty liver disease) with normal enzymes to NASH as the leading cause of transaminasemia. NAFLD is now present in 17% to 33% of Americans [4].

Also partly due to the epidemic of obesity and diabetes, gallstone disease has a population prevalence of 5% to 25%. Prevalence varies significantly among different ethnic groups. Northern Europeans have a much higher incidence than African Americans. Seventy percent of Pima Indians in Arizona and California have gallstones because of hereditary factors and a diet high in saturated fat and starches. In Mexico, Pima Indians eating a more traditional diet have a much lower rate. Women are disproportionately affected across races [5].

In summary, inheritance, gender, lifestyle habits, nutrition, and health status influence the activities of various detoxification enzymes. Polymorphism of liver detoxification enzymes has been associated with increased prevalence of many degenerative diseases [6].

III.   PATHOPHYSIOLOGY

Liver detoxification is a two-phase process, where each phase requires nutrients. If those nutrients are inadequately present, the liver's ability to manage the oxidative byproducts is compromised. Phase I detoxification is conducted by the specialized members of the cytochrome P450 mixed-function oxidase family of enzymes, resulting in production of a new class of compounds called biotransformed intermediates. These are converted into a form that can be easily excreted. Many toxins are fat soluble and tend to accumulate into fatty tissues. Phase II detoxification involves the combination of these newly biotransformed intermediates with substances in the liver to make them water-soluble for excretion as nontoxic substances in the urine and bile [7].

For phase I and the eight separate phase II processes to function properly, specific nutrients are required: Vitamins C, E, and B complex; bioflavinoids; glutathione; and the sulfur-containing amino acid cysteine [8]. The amino acids glycine, taurine, and methionine and vitamins and minerals are additionally needed to activate the conjugation phase II pathways [9].

Viral hepatitis and NASH both exert inflammatory stress on the liver. The liver in turn requires more detoxifying nutrients to manage inflammation, mitochrondrial stress, and other processes occurring at the molecular and cellular levels. When the molecular insults are not fully neutralized, inflammation results. Free radicals overwhelm the antioxidant reserve of the mitochondria of the cell. Repeated and ongoing inflammation results in liver damage visible at the tissue level, when fibrosis from the stellate cells overzealously attempts to wall off the inflammation to keep it from spreading. This process may result in altered architecture of the liver lobule reducing access to the arterial and portal blood flow and bile removal leading to cirrhosis and portal hypertension [10]. When the liver is inflamed, insulin resistance and abdominal fat increase the steatosis in the liver and predispose the gallbladder to stone formations.

In chronic hepatitis, hepatic hypoxia and oxidative stress may occur during the inflammatory and fibrotic processes that characterize these chronic liver diseases of viral origin. As a consequence, new vascular structures are formed to provide oxygen and nutrients and prevent cellular damage from oxidative stress. Angiogenesis with growth factors and molecules involved in matrix remodeling, cell migration, and vessel maturation-related factors are involved with liver disease and liver regeneration [11].

A study published in the *Journal of Hepatology* confirmed the above hypothesis on the pathophysiology of hepatitis C. This study investigated the relationship between oxidative stress, insulin resistance, steatosis, and fibrosis in patients with chronic hepatitis C (CHC). IgG against malondialdehyde-albumin adducts and HOMA-IR (homeostasis model assessment derived from fasting plasma glucose and insulin level) were measured as markers of oxidative stress and insulin resistance in 107 consecutive CHC patients. Oxidative stress was present in 61% of the patients, irrespective of age, gender, viral load, BMI, aminotransferase level, histology activity index (HAI), and hepatitis C virus (HCV) genotype. Insulin resistance and steatosis were demonstrated in 80% and 70% of patients respectively. In patients infected by HCV genotype non-3, but not in those with genotype 3 infection, HOMA-IR ($p < 0.03$), steatosis ($p = 0.02$) and fibrosis ($p < 0.05$) were higher in those with oxidative stress than in those without. The researchers concluded that oxidative stress and insulin resistance contribute to steatosis in patients infected with HCV genotype non-3, thereby accelerating the progression of fibrosis [12].

IV. CLINICAL DIAGNOSIS

The majority of patients with NASH and NAFLD are asymptomatic. The diagnosis tends to be suspected only when chemical abnormalities are noted or fatty liver is seen on ultrasound or CT scan of abdomen. Some patients may come to medical attention because of fatigue, malaise, and vague right-upper quadrant abdominal discomfort. Physical examination has demonstrated hepatomegaly in three-fourths of patients in several studies. Fulminate liver failure has been reported in patients treated with certain nucleoside analogs, antimiotic agents, and tetracycline. In other patients with inborn errors of metabolism, such as tyrosinemia, fatty liver or steatosis appears to progress rapidly to cirrhosis and commonly leads to death from various liver-related complications, including hepatocellular carcinoma. Liver biopsy is seldom necessary to diagnose NAFLD and is currently made to exclude other causes of chronic hepatitis [13].

However, many patients with chronic illnesses have some impairment of liver detoxification of which they and many of their doctors are unaware. They don't have elevated AST, ALT, or GGT, but are often on a number of pharmaceuticals and often have drug interactions and sensitivities. Symptoms include sensitivities to perfumes, car exhaust, fumes from gasoline or paint, and common household cleansing agents and chemicals. Physical examination often reveals palmar erythema, which hepatologists would say indicates that the patients have cirrhosis, but they don't. These patients are experiencing liver disease at the molecular and cellular level, which is not yet visible on a tissue level. Primary care doctors aware of the molecular process by which liver disease develops can monitor these patients, reduce toxicant exposures, and increase nutrients required for liver detoxification pathways. Proactive interventions may stall liver disease and may also treat the other chronic illnesses for which the patients are being treated in the primary care setting.

Hypertriglyceridemia is associated with fatty liver (NASH and NAFLD). A ratio of the triglycerides divided by the HDL of 3.0 or greater and triglycerides of 130 mg/dL or greater can be used in the absence of standardized insulin assays to screen patients for insulin resistance [14]. However, this ratio is not a reliable marker of insulin resistance in African Americans or Hispanics [15].

Also available are specialized laboratory tests to screen for impaired liver detoxification. One such test is called the functional liver detox challenge test to acetaminophen, benzoate, salicylic acid, and caffeine, which can be obtained from Genova Diagnostic Laboratory. This test evaluates specific aspects of the cytochrome p450 detoxification, measuring the clearance of challenge substances in two salivary specimens; the products of detoxifying reactions are also assessed in an overnight urine specimen.

Since insulin resistance is a risk factor for gallbladder disease, hypertriglyceridemia is also associated with gallbladder disease. Gallbladder disease, which is predominantly gallstone disease, is manifested right-upper quadrant abdominal pain that can radiate to the back and is usually associated with fatty food ingestion. Ultrasound of the gallbladder is the gold standard. Lab testing of biliary obstruction with transient elevated transaminasemia, bilirubinemia, alkaline phosphates, and elevated GGT are noted.

V. VIRAL HEPATITIS

Antioxidants protect the liver from oxidative damage to the mitochondria. Antioxidants are also highly protective of angiogenesis and fibrosis [16].

Researchers at Shandong University China investigated the impacts of interferon alpha-2b (IFN alpha-2b) on the oxidative stress states in the treatment of chronic hepatitis B (CHB) with different genotypes. Thirty-five patients with chronic hepatitis B and 18 healthy volunteers as a control were enrolled in the study. In control and patient groups, the serum ALT and aspartate aminotransferase (AST), serum malondialdehyde (MDA) levels, and serum total antioxidative stress capacity (TAC) were measured spectrophotometrically. After the therapy with interferon alpha-2b via intramuscular injection three times a week for 12 weeks, these parameters were measured again in the patient group. The serum levels of MDA after the treatment with IFN alpha-2b were significantly lower than the pretreatment levels ($P < 0.05$), which even returned to the normal concentration ($P > 0.05$) in the responsive group. There were also significant increases in the TAC after the IFN alpha-2b therapy in this group. However, the significant differences in the TAC levels before and after the INF alpha-2b treatment were not observed in the nonresponsive group. The researchers concluded that oxidative stress could be improved with IFN alpha-2b treatment of chronic hepatitis B patients. The results suggested that antioxidant treatment for chronic hepatitis B patients may help improve the effect of anti-virus therapy [17].

The aim of another study was to determine oxidant/antioxidant status of patients with chronic hepatitis C (CHC), and the effect of pegylated interferon alpha-2b plus ribavirin combination therapy on oxidative stress. Nineteen patients with chronic HCV infection and 28 healthy controls were included in the research. In control and patient groups, serum alanine aminotransferase (ALT) and aspartate aminotransferase (AST) levels, erythrocyte malondialdehyde (MDA) levels, erythrocyte CuZn-superoxide dismutase (SOD), and erythrocyte glutathione peroxidase (GSH-Px) activities were measured. After pegylated interferon alpha-2b and ribavirin combination therapy for 48 weeks, these parameters were measured again in the patient group. The results were that serum MDA levels increased significantly in CHC patients (n: 19) before the treatment when compared with healthy subjects (n: 28) 9.28 +/– 1.61, 4.20 +/– 1.47 nmol/mL, p < 0.001 respectively). MDA concentration decreased significantly (p < 0.001) after the treatment as well as ALT and AST activity in erythrocytes of these patients. Superoxide dismutase and glutathione peroxidase were significantly lower in erythrocytes of patients with CHC before treatment compared with the control group (both p < 0.001). These results show that patients with chronic HCV infection are under the influence of oxidative stress associated with lower levels of antioxidant enzymes. These impairments return to the level of healthy controls after pegylated interferon alpha-2b plus ribavirin combination therapy of CHC patients. They concluded that although interferon and ribavirin are not antioxidants, their antiviral capacity might reduce viral load and inflammation, and perhaps through this mechanism might reduce virus-induced oxidative stress [18].

In another study, 100 patients with chronic HCV infection who failed interferon treatment were enrolled and randomly assigned to receive combined intravenous and oral antioxidants or placebo, or oral treatment alone. Primary endpoints were liver enzymes, HCV-RNA levels, and histology. The investigators found that combined oral and intravenous antioxidant therapy was associated with a significant decline in ALT levels in 52% of patients who received antioxidant therapy versus 20% of patients who received placebo (P = 0.05). Histology activity index (HAI) score at the end of treatment was reduced in 48% of patients who received antioxidant therapy versus 26% of patients who received placebo (P = 0.21). HCV-RNA levels decreased by 1-log or more in 28% of patients who received antioxidant therapy versus 12% who received placebo (P = NS). In part II of the trial, oral administration of antioxidants was not associated with significant alterations in any of the endpoints. The authors concluded that antioxidant therapy has a mild beneficial effect on the inflammatory response of chronic HCV infection patients who are nonresponders to interferon. Combined antiviral and antioxidant therapy may be beneficial for these patients [19].

Burt Berkson, a medical doctor at the Integrative Medical Center of New Mexico, New Mexico State University, described a low-cost and efficacious treatment program in three patients with cirrhosis, portal hypertension, and esophageal varices secondary to chronic hepatitis C infection. This regimen combined three potent antioxidants (alpha-lipoic acid [thioctic acid], silymarin, and selenium) that possess antiviral, free radical quenching, and immune boosting qualities. The triple antioxidant combination of alpha-lipoic acid 300 mg twice daily, silymarin 300 mg daily, and selenium 200 mcg twice a day was chosen for a conservative treatment of hepatitis C because these substances protect the liver from free radical damage, increase the levels of other fundamental antioxidants, and interfere with viral proliferation. The three patients presented in this study followed the triple antioxidant program and recovered quickly and their laboratory values remarkably improved. Furthermore, liver transplantation was avoided and the patients were back at work, carrying out their normal activities, and feeling healthy. The author offered a more conservative approach to the treatment of hepatitis C that is exceedingly less expensive.

One year of this triple antioxidant therapy costs less than $2,000, as compared to more than $300,000 a year for liver transplant surgery. The author concluded that the conservative triple antioxidant treatment approach should be considered prior to liver transplant surgery evaluation, or during the transplant evaluation process. If there is a significant improvement in the patient's condition, liver transplant surgery may be avoided [20]. Because alpha-lipoic acid increases the liver cells' ability to make glutathione, it has been used to treat other forms of hepatitis [21, 22].

VI. STEATOHEPATITIS

More than 20% of Americans have nonalcoholic fatty liver disease (NAFLD), and it is the leading cause of abnormal liver enzymes in the United States. Nonalcoholic steatohepatitis (NASH), a more serious form of NAFLD, can proceed to cirrhosis and even hepatocellular carcinoma. These liver diseases represent the hepatic component of the metabolic syndrome, and this spectrum of liver disease represents a major health problem both in the United States and worldwide, with NASH projected to be the leading reason for liver transplantation in the near future.

Unfortunately, from a strictly clinical medicine perspective, NASH is a disease in search of an effective therapy. Most of the current regimens have been tested in open label, uncontrolled trials that have been carried out over a relatively short period of time and most of these studies did not adhere to a strict histologic endpoint [23]. None have been convincingly effective. However, understanding how liver disease at the tissue level is the result of aberrant molecular and cellular processes that began generally years beforehand presents broader possibilities for treatment interventions and is therefore a reason to diagnose disease early.

Diet and Weight Reduction

Hepatic steatosis is closely linked to diet. Lifestyle choices and altered genetic signaling are intertwined in a vicious cycle that produces abnormalities in lipid and glucose metabolism. Joseph L. Goldstein, M.D., Nobel laureate and professor of medicine and genetics at Southwestern School of Medicine, University of Texas, said that although many assume the process requires years of poor diet, inadequate exercise, and less than optimal lifestyle, it could be accelerated enormously. He cited the 2004 documentary *Super Size Me* in which Morgan Spurlock monitored his metabolic function while consuming all his meals at a fast-food restaurant over a 30-day period. "Morgan Spurlock was able to develop metabolic syndrome in less than a month and it took him six months to reverse it." Goldstein stated the major physiological change in Spurlock as well as others with metabolic syndrome is a fatty liver. "One of the most important mediators of metabolic function in the liver is sterol regulatory element binding protein (SREBP). A high glucose intake in the diet triggers the pancreas to produce increased amounts of insulin. The liver continues to produce glucose despite the high glucose intake. Ultimately, the downstream effects of sustained hyperglycemia lead to type 2 diabetes mellitus and the abnormally elevated SREPB-1c activity leads to increased synthesis of fatty acids and triglyceride in the liver, resulting in a fatty liver [24]."

Refined carbohydrates can increase inflammation and triglyceride levels. A study of 74 obese patients undergoing bariatric surgery at Johns Hopkins was conducted by Steve Solga, M.D., and Anna Mae Diehl, M.D. All patients underwent a preoperative dietary evaluation using a standardized 24-hour food recall. Food intake was evaluated for total calories and macronutrients and compared to liver histopathology from biopsies routinely obtained during surgery. The authors found there were no significant associations between either total caloric intake or protein intake and either steatosis, fibrosis, or inflammation. However, higher carbohydrate intake was associated with significantly higher odds of inflammation, while higher fat intake was associated with significantly lower odds of inflammation [25]. This contradicted previous recommendation of fat restriction and the increase therefore of carbohydrates.

It has also been demonstrated that rapid weight loss may actually elevate liver enzymes. It can also cause spasm of the gall bladder and theoretically cause more oxidative stress by release of toxins that have been stored in fat. Therefore, most experts recommend that the reduction of weight in obese patients with NAFLD should be gradual (< 1.6 kg per week) [26].

Sibutramine (Meridia) and orlistat (Xenical) used in weight reduction have shown improved results of liver function tests and decreased sonographic evidence of steatosis in NASH patients [27].

Bariatric surgery has also been studied in NASH. Roux-en-Y gastric bypass surgery was retrospectively studied in 29 patients undergoing surgery. At that time, patients had achieved a mean weight loss of 116.9 lb, with a significant decrease in body mass index (28.9 ± 5.8 kg/m^2 vs. 47.8 ± 6.6 kg/m^2), relative to presurgery baseline. Mean scores revealed that liver histology other than portal fibrosis improved after gastric bypass. The author concluded that fibrosis or scarring may be permanent. "Liver function tests showed some improvement in test results after gastric bypass, but even at baseline the values were within the normal range," noted Dr. R.H. Clements, emphasizing the role of biopsy in diagnosing NASH [28].

Toxin Avoidance

The most studied toxin that can be avoided is smoking tobacco products. Smoking has now also been demonstrated to increase the fibrosis and progression to cirrhosis in both chronic viral hepatitis and NASH. Cigarette smoking induces three major adverse effects on the liver: direct or indirect toxic effects, immunological effects, and oncogenic effects. Smoking yields chemical substances with cytotoxic potential that increase necro-inflammation and fibrosis. In addition, smoking increases the production of pro-inflammatory cytokines (IL-1, IL-6, and TNF-α) that would be involved in liver cell injury. Smoking affects both cell-mediated and humoral immune responses by blocking lymphocyte proliferation and inducing apoptosis of lymphocytes. Smoking also increases serum and hepatic iron, which induce oxidative stress and lipid peroxidation that lead to activation of stellate cells and development of fibrosis. Smoking yields oncogenic chemicals that increase the risk of hepatocellular carcinoma in patients with viral hepatitis and are independent of viral infection as well. Tobacco smoking has been associated with suppression of p53 (tumor suppressor gene). Heavy smoking affects the sustained virological response to interferon therapy in hepatitis C patients, which can be improved by repeated phlebotomy to alleviate the secondary polycythemia caused by it [29].

In certain underdeveloped countries, it appears likely that industrial toxins in food and water exposure play a role in NASH. There is increasing interest in the potential interaction of toxins and liver detoxification and their interactions with nutrients [30].

The majority of research studies of NASH exclude any patients who consume alcohol as the pathology is virtually identical with steatosis, including Mallory bodies (alcoholic hyaline) in both entities. Alcohol consumption is considered a risk factor in NAFLD progressing to NASH [31].

Specific Foods

Sulfur-containing cruciferous vegetables are broccoli, brussels sprouts, and cauliflower. Sulfation couples toxins with a sulfur-containing compound, important in detoxifying drugs, food additives, environmental toxins, and toxins from gut bacteria. This is also the main pathway for detoxifying steroid and thyroid hormones.

Citrus fruits contain glucuronic acid, which provides the process of glucuronidation with toxins. This detoxification is important because many commonly used over-the-counter medications are handled through this pathway, including aspirin, as are food additives such as benzoates and menthol.

NUTRIENTS

A number of nutrients or natural occurring substances have also been tried for NASH. These have included betaine, ursodeoxycholic acid, vitamin E, N-acetylcysteine, S-adenosylmethionine (SAMe), phosphatidylcholine, silymarin (milk thistle), probiotics, carnitine, and glutathione.

Betaine

Betaine is N-trimethylglycine, a methyl donor initially found in sugar beets, and has been used in a number of clinical trials along with folate and vitamin B12 to reduce homocysteine, a toxic amino acid implicated in cardiovascular and neurodegenerative disease. A small clinical trial conducted at the Mayo Clinic and published in the *American Journal of Gastroenterology* in 2001 demonstrated that betaine, a naturally occurring metabolite of choline which had been shown to raise S-adenosylmethionine (SAMe) levels, may decrease hepatic steatosis. Ten adult patients with NASH were enrolled and received betaine in two daily doses for 12 months. A significant improvement in serum levels of AST ($p = 0.002$) and ALT ($p = 0.007$) occurred during treatment. Aminotransferase normalized in three of seven patients that completed the year-long trial. Similarly, a marked improvement in the degree of steatosis, necroinflammatory grade, and stage of fibrosis was also noted at one year [32].

The effect of betaine on steatohepatitis has been elucidated. In this study, the effects of betaine on fat accumulation in the liver induced by high-sucrose diet and mechanisms by which betaine could attenuate or prevent hepatic steatosis was examined. Male C57BL/6 mice were divided into four groups (eight mice per group) and started on one of four treatments: standard diet (SD), SD + betaine, high-sucrose diet (HS), and HS + betaine. Betaine was supplemented in the drinking water at a concentration of 1% (anhydrous). Long-term feeding of high-sucrose diet to mice caused significant hepatic steatosis accompanied by markedly increased lipogenic activity. Betaine significantly attenuated hepatic steatosis in this animal model, and this change was associated with increased activation of hepatic AMP-activated protein kinase (AMPK) and attenuated lipogenic capability (enzyme activities and gene expression) in the liver [33].

Ursodeoxycholic Acid

Ursodeoxycholic acid, a bile salt that has been approved by the FDA for primary biliary cirrhosis (PBC), is marketed as URSO Forte™ and URSO 250. URSO has in more than 10 years of clinical studies proven its effectiveness and safety to delay the progression of PBC, normalize liver function tests, and decrease the incidence of esophageal varices by 60%.

In pilot studies it was found by itself not to be effective in NASH, and therefore was used in combination with antioxidants and other agents.

Patients with elevated aminotransferase levels with biopsy-proven NASH were randomly assigned to receive UDCA 12 to 15 mg/kg a day with vitamin E 400 IU twice a day (UDCA/Vit E), UDCA with placebo (UDCA/P), or placebo/placebo (P/P). After 2 years, they underwent a second liver biopsy. Forty-eight patients were included, 15 in the UDCA/Vit E group, 18 in the UDCA/P group, and 15 in the P/P group; 8 patients dropped out, none because of side effects. Baseline parameters were not significantly different between the three groups. BMI remained unchanged during the study. AST and ALT levels diminished significantly in the UDCA/Vit E group. Neither the AST nor the ALT levels improved in the P/P group and only the ALT levels improved in the UDCA/P group. Histologically, the activity index was unchanged at the end of the study in the P/P and UDCA/P groups, but it was significantly better in the UDCA/Vit E group, mostly as a result of regression of steatosis. The authors concluded that 2 years of treatment with UDCA in combination with vitamin E improved laboratory values and hepatic steatosis of patients with NASH. Larger trials are warranted [33].

Ursodeoxycholic acid and previously chenodeoxycholic acid have been used in gallstone disease for about two decades. The standard treatment is laparoscopic cholecystectomy, making gallstone disease the second most costly digestive disorder in most Western countries. Despite a rapid convalescence, the procedure is not devoid of morbidity or even mortality, with bile duct injury occurring in 0.1% to 0.5% of cases in even the most experienced hands. Moreover, postoperatively some 20% of patients continue to suffer from pain (the main indication for treatment). In patients with mild symptoms, surgical treatment has been associated with a higher morbidity than the natural course of the disease. Medical dissolution therapy with bile acids is an alternative for patients with mild-to-moderate symptoms due to cholesterol gallstones. Chenodeoxycholic acid (CDCA, chenodiol) has now been largely replaced by the safer and more efficient ursodeoxycholic acid (UDCA) marketed as Actigall and Urso. The main drawbacks of UDCA treatment are its low efficacy (approximately 40%), slowness in action, and the possibility of stone recurrence. However, this treatment is extremely safe, and the efficacy and slowness can be somewhat improved by better patient selection. According to the author, patient symptoms may respond to this therapy even without complete stone dissolution [34].

N-acetylcysteine

N-acetylcysteine has been used to increase glutathione in the liver, which is one of the detoxifying enzymes used for liver conjugation of toxins. Its use in NASH follows this logic that abnormalities in liver detoxification may be in part important in pathogenesis of fatty liver and transaminasemia. N-acetylcysteine (NAC) was studied in a model of NASH in a research project with male Sprague-Dawley rats with three groups of diets. Group 1 (control, n = 8) was free accessed to regular dry rat chow (RC) for 6 wk. Group 2 (NASH, n = 8) was fed with 100% fat diet for 6 wk. Group 3 (NASH+NAC (20), n = 9) was fed with 100% fat diet plus 20 mg/kg per day of NAC orally for 6 wk. All rats were sacrificed to collect blood and liver samples at the end of the study. Researchers found the levels of total glutathione (GSH) and hepatic malondialdehyde (MDA) were increased significantly in the NASH group as compared with the control group (P < 0.05). Livers from group 2 showed moderate to severe macrovesicular steatosis, hepatocyte ballooning, and necroinflammation. NAC treatment improved the level of GSH (P < 0.05), and led to a decrease in fat deposition and necroinflammation. The authors concluded that NAC treatment could attenuate oxidative stress and improve liver histology in rats with NASH [35].

S-adenosylmethionine

In another model, rats were fed a methionine-choline deficient (MCD) diet and given S-adenosylmethionine (SAMe), or 2(RS)-n-propylthiazolidine-4(R)-carboxylic acid (PTCA), two agents that stimulate glutathione (GSH) biosynthesis on the development of experimental steatohepatitis. These two agents suppressed abnormal enzyme activities in the treated rats whereas the control rats developed elevated transaminasemia. MCD rats developed severe liver pathology manifested by fatty degeneration, inflammation, and necrosis, which significantly improved with therapy. Blood levels of GSH were significantly depleted in MCD rats but normalized in the treated groups. The researchers found a significant up-regulation of genes involved in tissue remodeling and fibrosis (matrix metalloproteinases, collagen-alpha1), suppression of cytokines signaling, and the inflammatory cytokines in the livers of rats fed MCD. The authors concluded that GSH-enhancing therapies significantly attenuated the expression of deleterious proinflammatory and fibrogenic genes in this dietary model [36].

Phosphatidylcholine

Phosphatidylcholine (PC), an essential fatty acid found in cell walls, was demonstrated to be reduced in a mouse model of starvation-induced hepatic steatosis. After 24 hours of fasting it appears that starvation reduced the phospholipids (PL). Phosphatidylcholine was used in another animal model of NASH. Rats were fed orotic acid (OA) containing triglyceride (TG) or PC (20% of dietary lipid, PC + OA group) for 10 days. Rats fed the TG diet without OA supplementation served as the control group. Administering OA significantly increased the weights and TG accumulation in livers of the TG + OA group compared with the control group. The researchers found that the PC + OA group did not show TG accumulation and OA-induced increases of these enzyme activities, and a significant increase in the activity of carnitine palmityl transferase, a rate-limiting enzyme of fatty acid beta-oxidation, was found in the PC + OA group. They concluded that dietary PC appears to alleviate the OA-induced hepatic steatosis and hepatomegaly, mainly through the attenuation of hepatic TG synthesis and enhancement of fatty acid beta-oxidation in Sprague-Dawley rats [37].

Silymarin

Silymarin or milk thistle has been used in a number of clinical trials of NASH. Silybin is the main component of silymarin that is absorbed when linked with a phytosome. This substance reduces in rats the lipid-peroxidation and the activation of hepatic stellate cells. In humans, some noncontrolled studies show that silybin is able to reduce insulin resistance, liver steatosis, and plasma markers of liver fibrosis [38].

Silybin in combination with vitamin E and phospholipids to improve its antioxidant activity was used in the following study. Eighty-five patients were divided into two groups: those affected by NAFLD (group A) and those with HCV-related chronic hepatitis associated with NAFLD (group B). After treatment, group A showed a significant reduction in ultrasonographic scores for liver steatosis. Liver enzyme levels, hyperinsulinemia, and indexes of liver fibrosis showed an improvement in treated individuals. A significant correlation among indexes of fibrosis, BMI, insulinemia, plasma levels of cytokines, degree of steatosis, and gamma-glutamyl transpeptidase was observed. The author's data suggest that silybin conjugated with vitamin E and phospholipids could be used as a complementary approach to the treatment of patients with chronic liver damage [39].

Probiotics

Beneficial bacteria have been demonstrated to have protective effects exerted directly by specific bacterial species, control of epithelial cell proliferation and differentiation, production of essential mucosal nutrients, such as SCFAs and amino acids, prevention of overgrowth of pathogenic organisms, and stimulation of intestinal immunity. Oral probiotics are living microorganisms that upon ingestion in specific numbers exert health benefits beyond those of inherent basic nutrition [40]. The accumulation of fat in hepatocytes with a necroinflammatory component—steatohepatitis—that may or may not have associated fibrosis is becoming a frequent lesion, as discussed earlier. Probiotics have therefore attracted attention for their inclusion in the therapeutics for NASH after being used in inflammatory bowel disease and irritable bowel syndrome. Although steatohepatitis is currently recognized to be a leading cause of cryptogenic cirrhosis, the pathogenesis has not been fully elucidated. Among the various factors implicated, intestinal bacterial overgrowth may play a role. In fact, various rat models of intestinal bacterial overgrowth have been associated with liver lesions similar to NASH, and bacterial overgrowth has been observed significantly more often in patients with NASH compared with control subjects. The authors discuss the relationship among intestinal bacterial overgrowth, steatohepatitis development, and probiotic treatment [41].

Carnitine

The lipid-lowering effect of carnitine and its precursors, lysine and methionine, were studied in an animal model of alcoholic steatosis where Sprague-Dawley rats were fed ethanol as 36% of total calories. The ethanol caused hepatic steatosis. Supplementation of the ethanol diet with 1%

DL carnitine, 0.5% L-lysine, and 0.2% L-methionine significantly lowered ethanol-induced lipid fractions. It was concluded that dietary carnitine more effectively prevented alcohol-induced hyperlipidemia and accumulation of fat in livers. A deficiency of functional carnitine may indeed exist in chronic alcoholic cases [42]. A deficiency in nutrients such as carnitine, choline, and other amino acids may result from total parental nutrition (TPN) due to formulation, poor delivery, and degradation of TPN. Carnitine deficiency has been documented on long-term TPN resulting in fatty liver. Mobilization of long-chain fatty acids into the mitochondria cannot occur without fatty acid shuttling, resulting with an increase in free fatty acids and the development of hepatic steatosis. However, human studies with carnitine supplementation have failed to confirm previously mentioned effects on fatty liver [43] [44]. In an experimental model of insulin resistance using fructose-fed rats, L-carnitine reduced skeletal muscle lipid, including triglycerides, and reduced oxidative stress [45].

Glutathione

Glutathione in the form of glutathione-sulfate transferase (GSH) helps to process a large number of xenobiotics. The availability of GSH depends upon the sufficient amounts of its amino acid precursors (cysteine, glycine and glutamic acid). Magnesium is an essential cofactor in GSH synthesis and B vitamins for methionine recycling and reducing agent. S-adenosylmethionine (SAMe) is a methyl donor and precursor of GSH. Low SAMe levels have been seen in experimental liver injury, and impaired methylation is associated with elevated homocysteine, vitamins B2, B6, B12, folic acid, and serine. B6 and magnesium support amino acid coupling, which is another process in which nutrients combine with drug toxins and detoxify them [46]. Hyperhomocysteinemia causes steatosis and the methylenetetrahydrofolate reductase (MTHFR) gene polymorphism (A1298) has been described in 57 well-diagnosed NASH patients and thus is a risk factor for this disease [47]. Vitamins B6, B12, folic acid, and a methyl donor all exist at critical biochemical interactions in the methionine cycle between SAMe and high levels of homocysteine, signaling a breakdown of this vital process [48].

VII.   POSTCHOLECYSTECTOMY SYNDROME

The history of medical therapy for gallstone disease as a major alternative to surgery was rather short and confined to the 1970s and 1980s before the development of laparoscopic cholecystectomy. The discovery that long-term therapy with ursodiol or chenodiol bile salts could slowly dissolve cholesterol gallstones or the impact of stone dissolution via extracorporeal shockwave lithotripsy was the impetus for nonsurgical treatment of gallstone disease. Additionally there was the development of methyl tert-butyl ether that is instilled via percutaneous transhepatic catheter or endoscopic route, dissolving the stones rapidly without major side effects. However, after laparoscopic cholecystectomy was perfected and the problem resolved with intraductal stones that were initially missed, the enthusiasm for nonsurgical therapy rapidly diminished to a therapy only considered when the patient is not a candidate for surgery or steadily refuses surgery [49].

After the gallbladder is removed, a number of patients (10% to 15%) complain of symptoms. These symptoms can represent either the continuation of symptoms thought to be caused by the gallbladder or the development of new symptoms normally attributed to the gallbladder. Postcholecystectomy syndrome (PCS) also includes the development of symptoms caused by removal of the gallbladder with diarrhea or even abdominal pain following cholecystectomy. This is termed the postcholecystectomy syndrome and is often limited to 6 months postcholecystectomy. Bile is thought to be the cause of PCS in patients with mild gastroduodenal symptoms or diarrhea. Removal of the reservoir function of the gallbladder alters bile flow and the enterohepatic circulation of bile by dumping bile into the small intestine after a meal.

One investigator found gastritis to be more frequent postoperatively (30% vs. 50%). Preoperatively, no cases of peptic ulcer disease (PUD) occurred, but three cases developed postoperatively in this study. It was also shown that fasting gastric bile acid concentration increased after cholecystectomy, and the increase was greater in patients with PCS [50].

Choline supplementation has been recommended by some for postcholecystectomy patients. Consider the following research article: In patients with sustained PCS, the content of the basic bile components (cholesterol, cholic acid, and total phosphorus) was measured. The cholate-cholesterol coefficient, which to a degree helps evaluate the lithogenic state of the bile, was calculated. The cholesterol concentration in the serum and bile was contrasted. A total of 104 patients were examined at different postoperative periods and it was found that in 70% of them the bile was not oversaturated with cholesterol. Two varients of the diet, differing in the ratio of fat and carbohydrate, were used. Under the effect of the fat-sparing, a reduced serum cholesterol concentration was noted along with a rise of the cholic acid content in the bile with a rise of the cholesterol level that led to an increase of the cholate-cholesterol coefficient. Against the background of the fat-sparing diet treatment, there was a diminution of the serum cholesterol content, and in the cholesterol and cholic acid concentration in the bile with a high cholate-cholesterol coefficient. The authors suggest choline supplementation may be helpful [51].

In a short-term follow-up study on nine female patients the researchers found no alterations in cholic acid (CA) or deoxycholic acid (DCA) pools after cholecystectomy. However, in the long term (greater than 6 months), cholecystectomy could promote changes of the intestinal bacterial flora and thereby lead to enhanced conversion of CA to DCA, causing an expansion of the DCA pool size and a reduction of the CA pool size. To test this hypothesis, pool sizes, fractional turnover rates (FTR), and synthesis or input rates of CA, chenodeoxycholic acid (CDCA) and DCA were determined in 12 female patients before and again 5 to 8 years after cholecystectomy. In the long term, pool size and synthesis rate of CA had not changed and DCA pool size had expanded by only 7.5% (not significant [NS]). DCA input increased by 32% (NS) but was balanced by an increase in FTR of 36%. In conclusion, cholecystectomy causes no changes in bile acid pool composition after 6 months and thus has no adverse effects on bile acid metabolism in the long term [52].

VIII. SUMMARY

Patients in my practice have established illnesses. This generally means that the nutrients involved in liver detoxification are in high demand, perhaps more than patients could easily obtain by select foods and diet alone. For this reason I have expanded on my dietary, food, and lifestyle interventions to optimize the nutrients needed for liver detoxification. In my gastroenterology and nutritional practice I presently have many patients on nutrient powders that can be consumed as foods or beverages at usually 2 scoops daily [10]. Table 12.1 provides details for clinical use.

In addition, viral hepatitis patients nutritionally are advised to reduce saturated fats in their diets and cease any alcohol ingestion. They are also encouraged to use one of the above-mentioned medical food liver detoxification products, and in many cases to add silymarin, standardized extract 300 mg twice daily. A trial at the NIH is now undergoing in patients with hepatitis C with silymarin at this concentration. If my patients decline medications or are not a candidate for them, then I strongly encourage them to follow the Berkson protocol of alpha-lipoic acid, selenium, and silymarin.

In addition to nutrient powders, I advise NAFLD patients to lose weight, to exercise with weight resistance training, and to do daily liver detoxification with one of the above-mentioned medical food detoxification products. NASH patients are advised the same plus silymarin standardized extract of silybin 300 mg twice daily. If no transaminases reduction is seen, then medical therapy with metformin is started before trying any other additional nutritional therapy.

TABLE 12.1
Nutrient Powders Formulated to Supplement Liver Detoxification

Ultra Clear™ supplies low-allergy-potential rice protein concentrate with added essential amino acids L-lysine and L-threonine to increase the biological value of the protein.

- Rich in the antioxidant vitamins A, C, E, and beta-carotene, which help protect against oxygen free radicals generated during the hepatic detoxification process.
- Provides high-molecular-weight rice dextrins as the carbohydrate source and medium-chain triglycerides as a source of readily absorbed and metabolized lipids.

Medi-Clear™ in addition to the minerals and vitamins has:

- L-Glutathione 25 mg, Lactobacillus Sporogenes 50 mg, N-Acetyl Cysteine 50 mg, Glycine 1.65 mg, Taurine 110 mg, Green Tea Extract (Catechin) 25 mg, MSM 100 mg, Quercetin Chalcone 250 mg, L-Glutamine 500 mg, Betaine (trimethlyglycine) 50 mg, Borage Oil 300 mg, Medium Chain Triglycerides 1.5 g, Olive Oil 1 g.
- Amino Acids : % of total amino acids: alanine 5.6, arginine 9.4, aspartic acid 9.0, cystine/2 2.2, glutamic acid 17.1, glycine 4.7, histidine 2.4, isoleucine 4.2, leucine 8.6, lysine 3.5, methionine 2.4, phenyalanine 5.2, proline 5.2, serine 5.6, threonine 3.6, tryptophan 1.3, tyrosine 5.3, valine 4.7.

Clear Detox™ rice protein provides a full complement of essential and nonessential amino acids, including the sulfur-containing amino acids cysteine and methionine.

- Reduced glutathione is involved in phase II detoxification of xenobiotic compounds. N-acetylcysteine also functions as an antioxidant and helps maintain tissue glutathione levels.
- In addition, it also has the potential to bind heavy metals such as mercury and cadmium. Methylsulfonylmethane (MSM) is an excellent source of bioavailable sulfur, an essential micronutrient vital for healthy tissues. As a critical component of the Krebs cycle, alpha-lipoic acid supports aerobic energy production.
- In addition, it supports healthy liver function by scavenging free radicals and regenerating other antioxidants such as vitamins C and E.
- This formula provides a synergistic combination of standardized milk thistle, artichoke, turmeric, greater celandine, and barberry extracts to support hepatic function by increasing bile flow, preserving glutathione concentrations, and promoting healthy turnover of liver tissue.

Note: Powders are Ultra Clear™, Clear Detox™, and Medi-Clear™ from Metagenics, Pure Encapsulation, and Thorne, respectively.

Postcholecystectomy patients are usually treated for IBS with probiotics. I have not used choline, but may suggest this in the future after doing the research on the topic.

REFERENCES

1. Williams, R., *Biochemical Individuality*. 1956, New York: John Wiley and Sons.
2. McMahon, B., *Issues in HBV*. Audio-Digest Gastroenterology, 2007; 21(7).
3. Berenguer, M. and T. Wright, *Sleisinger and Fordtran's Gastrointestinal and Liver Disease*, ed. M. Feldman, L.S. Friedman, and M.H. Sleisenger. Vol. 2. 2002, Philadelphia: Saunders. 2385.
4. Farrell, G. and C. Larter, *Nonalcoholic Fatty Liver Disease: From Steatosis to Cirrhosis*. Hepatology, 2006. 43(S1): p. S99–112.
5. Huang, C.S. and D.R. Lichtenstein, *Therapy of Digestive Disorders*. 2nd ed, ed. M.M. Wolfe. 2006, Philadelphia: WB Saunders. 1051.
6. Hyman, M., S.M. Baker, and D.S. Jones, *Textbook of Functional Medicine*, ed. D. Jones. 2006, Gig Harbor, WA: Institute of Functional Medicine. 820.
7. *Cassert & Doull's Toxicology—The Basic Science of Poison*. 6th ed, ed. K. CD. 2004, New York: McGraw-Hill.
8. Beutler, E., *Nutritional and Metabolic Aspects of Glutathione*. Annual Review of Nutrition, 1989. 9: p. 287–302.
9. Bland, J.S. and S. Benum, *The 20-Day Rejuvenation Diet Program*. 1997, New Canaan: Keats Publishing.

10. Nichols, T.W., *Optimal Digestive Health*. 2nd ed. 2005, Rochester, VT: Healing Arts Press. 598.
11. Chaparro, M. et al., *Angiogenesis in Chronic Inflammatory Liver Disease*. Hepatology, 2004. 39(5): p. 1185–1195.
12. Vidali, M. et al., *Interplay between Oxidative Stress and Hepatic Steatosis in the Progression of Chronic Hepatitis C*. J Hepatol, 2007.
13. Diehl, A.M., and F. Poordad, *Nonalcoholic Fatty Liver Disease*. 7th ed. Sleisenger & Fordtran's Gastrointestinal and Liver Disease, ed. M. Feldman, L.S. Friedman, and M.H. Sleisenger. Vol. II. 2002, Philadelphia: Saunders. 1393–1401.
14. McLaughlin, T. et al., *Use of Metabolic Markers to Identify Overweight Individuals Who Are Insulin Resistant*. Ann Int Med 2003. 139(10): p. 802–809.
15. Sumner, A. et al., *Fasting Triglyceride and the Trigylceride-HDL Cholesterol Ratio Are Not Markers of Insulin Resistance in African Americans*. Arch Intern Med 2005. 165(12): p. 1395–1400.
16. Yang, C. et al., *Lymphocytic Microparticles Inhibit Angiogenesis by Stimulating Oxidative Stress and Negatively Regulating VEGF-Induced Pathways*. Am J Physiol Regul Integr Comp Physiol, 2008. 294(2): p. R467–476.
17. Fan, Y., K. Wang, et al., *Oxidative Stress in Patients with Chronic Hepatitis B before and after Interferon alpha-2b Treatment*. Zhonghua Shi Yan He Lin Chuang Bing Du Xue Za Zhi 2007. 21(1): p. 23–25.
18. Levent, G., et al., *Oxidative Stress and Antioxidant Defense in Patients with Chronic Hepatitis C Patients before and after Pegylated Interferon alfa-2b Plus Ribavirin Therapy*. J Transl Med., 2006. 4: p. 25.
19. Gabbay, E., et al., *Antioxidant Therapy for Chronic Hepatitis C After Failure of Interferon: Results of Phase II Randomized, Double-Blind Placebo Controlled Clinical Trial*. World J Gastroenterol, 2007. 13(40): p. 5317–5323.
20. Berkson, B., *A Conservative Triple Antioxidant Approach to the Treatment of Hepatitis C. Combination of Alpha Lipoic Acid (Thioctic Acid), Silymarin, and Selenium: Three Case Histories*. Med Klin (Munich, 1999. 94. Suppl 3): p. 84–89.
21. Berkson, B., *Thiotic Acid in Treatment of Hepatotoxic Mushroom (Phalloides) Poisoning*. N Engl J Med, 1979. 300(7): p. 371.
22. Nichols, T.W., *Alpha Lipoic Acid: Biological Effect and Clinical Implications*. Altern Med Rev, 1997. 2(3): p. 177–183.
23. Nugent, C., and Z.M. Younossi, *Evaluation and Management of Obesity-Related Nonalcoholic Fatty Liver Disease*. Nat Clin Pract Gastroenterol Hepatol, 2007. 4(8): p. 432–441.
24. Bosworth, T., *Targetting the Trigger of Metabolic Syndrome*, in *Gatroenterology & Endiscopy News*. 2007, New York: McMahon Publishing. p. 1, 24–25.
25. *Dietary Composition and Nonalcoholic Fatty Liver Disease*. Dig Dis Sci, 2004. 49(10): p. 1578–1583.
26. Luyckx, F. et al., *Non-alcoholic Steatohepatitis: Association with Obesity and Insulin Resistance, and Influence of Weight Loss*. Diabetes Metab, 2000. 26(2): p. 98–106.
27. Sabuncu, T. et al., *The Effects of Sibutramine and Orlistat on the Ultrasonographic Findings, Insulin Resistance and Liver Enzyme Levels in Obese Patients with Non-alcoholic Steatohepatitis*. Rom J Gastroenterol, 2003. 12(3): p. 189–192.
28. Clements, R.H., *Gastric Bypass Surgery Significantly Improves NASH*, in *Medscape Gastroenterology*. 2005, Medscape: 22nd Annual Meeting of American Society of Bariatric Surgery.
29. El-Zayadi, A., *Heavy Smoking and Liver*. World J Gastroenterol, 2006. 12(38): p. 6098–6101.
30. Cave, M. et al., *Nonalcoholic Fatty Liver Disease: Predisposing Factors and the Role of Nutrition*. J Nutr Biochem, 2007. 18(3): p. 184–195.
31. Poullis et al., *Alcohol, Obesity and TNF- α*. Gut, 2001. 49: p. 313–314.
32. Duseja, A., *Metformin Is Effective in Achieving Biochemical Response in Patients with Nonalcoholic Fatty Liver Disease (NAFLD) Not Responding to Lifestyle Interventions*. Ann Hepatol, 2007. 6(4): p. 222–226.
33. Song, Z. et al., *Involvement of AMP-activated Protein Kinase in Beneficial Effects of Betaine on High-Sucrose Diet-Induced Hepatic Steatosis*. Am J Physiol Gastrointest Liver Physiol, 2007. 294(4): p. G894–902.
34. Konikoff, F., *Gallstones—Approach to Medical Management*. Med Gen Med, 2003. 5(4): p. 8.
35. Thong-Ngam, D. et al., *N-acetylcysteine Attenuates Oxidative Stress and Liver Pathology in Rats with Non-alcoholic Steatohepatitis*. World J Gastroenterol, 2007. 13(38): p. 5127–5132.
36. Oz, H. et al., *Glutathione-enhancing Agents Protect against Steatohepatitis in a Dietary Model*. J Biochem Mol Toxicol, 2006. 20: p. 2714–2724.
37. Buang, Y. et al., *Dietary Phosphatidylcholine Alleviates Fatty Liver Induced by Orotic Acid*. Nutrition, 2005. 21(7–8): p. 867–873.
38. Agrawal, S. et al., *Management of Nonalcoholic Steatohepatitis: An Analytic Review*. J Clin Gastroenterol, 2002. 35(3): p. 253–261.

39. Loguercio, C., *The Effect of a Silybin-vitamin e-phospholipid Complex on Nonalcoholic Fatty Liver Disease: A Pilot Study.* Dig Dis Sci, 2007. 52(9): p. 2387–2395.

40. Tappenden, K. et al., *The Physiological Relevance of the Intestinal Microbiota—Contributions to Human Health.* J Am Coll Nutr, 2007. 26(6): p. 679S–83S.

41. Nardone, G. et al., *Probiotics: A Potential Target for the Prevention and Treatment of Steatohepatitis.* J Clin Gastroenterol, 2004. 38(6 Suppl): p. S121–122.

42. Sachan, D. et al., *Ameliorating Effects of Carnitine and Its Precursors on Alcohol-induced Fatty Liver.* Am J Clin Nutr, 1984. 39(5): p. 738–744.

43. Leuschner, U., O. James, and H. Dancygier, *Steatohepatitis (NASH and ASH).* Falk Symposium No 121. 2001, Dordrecht Netherland: Kluwer Academic Publishers.

44. Farrell, G., et al., *Fatty Liver Disease: NASH and Related Disorders.* 2005, Boston: Blackwell Publishing. 337.

45. Rajasekar, P. et al., *Effect of L-carnitine on Skeletal Muscle Lipids and Oxidative Stress in Rats Fed High-Fructose Diet.* Exp Diabetes Res, 2007. 2007(72741).

46. Lyon, M. *Textbook of Functional Medicine*, ed. D. Jones. 2006, Gig Harbor, WA: Institute of Functional Medicine. 275–299.

47. Sazci, A. et al., *Methyenetetrahydrofolate Gene Polymorphisms in Patients with Nonalcholic Steatohepatitis (NASH).* Cell Biochem Funct, 2007. 26(3): p. 291–296.

48. Miller, A., *The Methionine-homocysteine Cycle and Its Effects on Cognitive Disease.* Altern Med Rev, 2003. 1: p. 7–19.

49. Health, M. *Gallstoned-Treatment in Adults.* GPAC—Guidelines and Protocols Advisory Committee 2007.

50. Abu Farsakh, N., *The Postcholecystectomy Syndrome. A Role for Duodenogastric Reflux.* Clin Gastroenterol Hepatol, 1996. 22(3): p. 197–201.

51. Pokrovskaia, G. et al., *Change in the Exocrine Function of the Liver after Cholecystectomy under the Influence of Diet Therapy.* Vopr Pitan, 1979. 1: p. 44–49.

52. Kullak-Ublick, G. et al., *Long-term Effects of Cholecystectomy on Bile Acid Metabolism.* Hepatology, 1995. 21(1): p. 41–45.

13 Irritable Bowel Syndrome

Linda A. Lee, M.D., and Octavia Pickett-Blakely, M.D.

I. INTRODUCTION

Irritable bowel syndrome (IBS) is a complex, chronic disorder characterized by abdominal pain or discomfort and altered bowel habits. IBS is symptom defined and is thought to arise from a perturbance in the brain-gut axis. The diagnosis of IBS, which is classified as a functional gastrointestinal (GI) disorder, rests on fulfillment of the Rome III criteria established by a multinational consensus group and is not associated with anatomical abnormalities. The diagnosis requires recurrent abdominal pain or discomfort of at least 6 months duration relieved by defecation and associated with changes in stool consistency or frequency (Table 13.1). Often patients are subgrouped into different categories based on their primary symptoms: constipation predominant (IBS-C), diarrhea predominant (IBS-D), or mixed. IBS-C is distinct from functional constipation, which is defined by its unique set of Rome III criteria. The diagnosis of IBS is further supported by the age of symptom onset, which typically is prior to the fifth decade of life, the lack of nocturnal symptoms, and the absence of weight loss or rectal bleeding. IBS is characterized by the absence of clinically measurable diagnostic tests. Therapy for IBS is thus directed toward addressing individual dietary patterns, food and nutrient intake, psychological factors, and comorbidities.

II. EPIDEMIOLOGY

IBS is the most commonly diagnosed GI condition with an estimated U.S. prevalence of 10% to 15% [1]. Symptoms of IBS frequently lead to office visits with primary care physicians and specialists. In 2002, over 2 million clinic visits were made for IBS [2]. Symptoms can be mild or severe, and can fluctuate in frequency and intensity. Studies have repeatedly demonstrated that functional GI disorders perturb quality of life more significantly than organic GI disorders and other chronic diseases such as rheumatoid arthritis [3, 4].

IBS occurs worldwide, but is less prevalent in Asia compared to the United States [5]. Women are affected three times more often than men. In the United States, Caucasians are 2.5 times more likely than African Americans to have IBS [6]. However, IBS has the same impact on health-related quality of life across ethnic groups [6, 7]. The impact of socioeconomic status on IBS prevalence is less clearly defined. Some studies associate IBS with affluence while others implicate poverty as a risk factor [8–11].

The economic impact of IBS is astonishing. IBS-related costs rose to $1.35 billion in the United States in 2003 [12–14]. The predicted costs are likely an underestimation because expenditures for prescription or over-the-counter medications were not included. Quality of life and work productivity are also adversely impacted by IBS symptoms. Consequently, IBS continues to be the second most common reason for work absenteeism [15]. For example, a survey of over 5,000 persons from U.S. households found that IBS patients missed an average of 13.4 days per year from work or school due to illness, whereas the average subject without a GI disorder missed only 4.9 days [16].

TABLE 13.1
Rome III Criteria for Irritable Bowel Syndrome
At least 3 months, with onset at least 6 months previously of recurrent abdominal pain or
discomfort* associated with two or more of the following:
- Improvement with defecation; *and/or*
- Onset associated with a change in frequency of stool; *and/or*
- Onset associated with a change in form (appearance) of stool

*Discomfort means an uncomfortable sensation not described as pain.

Risk factors for IBS may include environmental as well as genetic ones. A family aggregation study, which surveyed relatives of individuals with IBS, demonstrated a prevalence of 17%
in patients' relatives versus 7% in spouses' relatives [17]. Other studies have also shown a familial aggregation of IBS, but this could be complicated by environmental factors, such as sharing
acquired responses to abdominal symptoms or as some investigators believe, nutrition in fetal life
[18]. Studies of twins are conflicting, with some demonstrating concordance of IBS twice as great
in monozygotic compared to dizygotic twins [19, 20].

III.   PATHOPHYSIOLOGY

The pathophysiology of IBS is complex and still poorly understood. However, visceral hypersensitivity, disordered cortical pain processing, small bowel bacterial overgrowth, and increased intestinal permeability have been implicated and will be discussed below.

Visceral Hypersensitivity

Visceral hypersensitivity is defined as having a low threshold to painful stimuli arising from the
GI tract. In research settings, this has traditionally been assessed by measuring the pain response
to inflation of a balloon within the digestive tract. IBS patients tend to experience more pain compared to controls for a given volume inflated. This was first documented in 1973 when inflation of
a sigmoid balloon to 60 mL caused pain in 6% of controls but in 55% of patients with IBS [21].
Luminal distention, triggered postprandially and exacerbated by gas-producing foods, may lead to
the enhanced perception of bloating and abdominal pain in those with IBS.

Increased pain perception could be mediated at the level of extrinsic gut afferent nerves
responsible for sensory perception as well as by cortical processing that affects pain inhibition.
Visceral hypersensitivity is thought to arise from a disruption in normal serotonin (also known as
5-hydroxytriptamine or 5HT) signaling. Ninety-five percent of the serotonin in the human body
is found in the GI tract, mostly produced by enterochromaffin cells in the GI epithelium [22].
Enterochromaffin cells act as sensory transducers that release 5HT after meals. 5HT binds 5HT4
receptors present on visceral motor afferent nerves, which control GI reflexes that govern intestinal motility and secretion. 5HT also regulates visceral sensation by binding 5HT3 receptors
present on extrinsic gut afferent neurons, responsible for transmitting sensory signals from gut
to cortical regions [22]. The amount of 5HT that is functionally active at any one time is determined by the rate of production by enterochromaffin cells and the rate of reuptake into mucosal
enterocytes via serotonin reuptake transporters (SERT), where it is then catabolized. It has been
postulated that defects in 5HT production, SERT reuptake, or metabolism can affect the pool of
5HT available and lead to alterations in visceral motility, secretion, and sensation. Increased 5HT
bioavailability has been implicated in IBS-D, whereas reduced 5HT bioavailability is associated
with IBS-C [23, 24].

Data supporting a critical role of intestinal serotonin signaling in the pathogenesis of IBS have emerged from both animal and human studies. Postprandial plasma 5HT levels are lower in individuals with IBS-C and higher in IBS-D patients compared to controls [23, 24]. A transgenic, SERT gene knockout mouse demonstrates increased rectal transit time resulting in wetter stools [25]. A recent study of IBS-D and IBS-C patients revealed no differences in expression of SERT in colonic mucosa. Instead, expression of p11, a molecule that increases serotonergic receptor function (5HT1B), was increased in IBS [26]. Identification of additional factors regulating 5HT signaling may lead to the development of novel therapeutic agents.

Studies on post-infectious IBS (PI-IBS) also support the role of serotonin in IBS. Up to 17% of individuals with IBS report the first onset of IBS symptoms following a bout of infectious colitis [27]. Predictors of developing PI-IBS include female gender, prolonged diarrhea (greater than 15 days), psychological factors, and severity of initial illness [28]. PI-IBS has been reported following outbreaks of giardiasis [29], salmonellosis [28], shigellosis [30–32], and *Campylobacter jejuni* infection [33]. In a rodent model of 2,4,6-trinitrobenzene sulfonic acid (TNBS) induced colitis, 5HT gut mucosal content, the number of 5HT-immunoreactive cells, and the proportion of epithelial cells that were 5HT-immunoreactive was two-fold higher than in control animals [34]. Increased levels of enterochromaffin cells and 5HT levels have been identified in the rectal mucosa of individuals suffering from PI-IBS [27, 33].

In addition to abnormalities in serotonin processing and function, alterations in central processing of pain signaling have now been demonstrated using positron emission tomography (PET) and cortical functional magnetic resonance imaging (fMRI). Cortical fMRI indirectly measures cognitive activity and neuronal activation by assessing changes in oxyhemoglobin that occur as a result of fluctuations in cerebral blood flow [35]. fMRI has demonstrated that a painful rectal stimulus activates the anterior cingulate cortex (ACC), the central nervous system pain center, to a greater degree in IBS patients than controls [36]. A concern raised about interpretation of IBS fMRI studies is that anticipation of pain and somatization may contribute to the patterns of neuronal activation seen, so that alterations in cognitive response rather than visceral hypersensitivity may contribute to the difference in fMRI results [37, 38].

Small Intestinal Bacterial Overgrowth

Most studies have demonstrated about 10% of IBS patients have small intestinal bacterial overgrowth (SIBO). Antibiotic therapy may improve IBS symptoms in a subset of IBS patients with SIBO [39, 40]. Although the mechanism of SIBO development is not entirely clear, SIBO can cause symptoms of bloating, cramping, and diarrhea, which in the setting of visceral hyperalgesia can lead to significant distress. These symptoms arise from malabsorption of ingested fat, protein, carbohydrates, and vitamins as a result of bacterial utilization of these macro- and micronutrients. Impaired intestinal motility or diminished gastric acid secretion is a risk factor for the development of SIBO. Pimentel et al. demonstrated that patients with IBS and SIBO have reduced phase III of the migrating motor complex, the component of fasting gut motility responsible for clearing the small intestinal lumen of contents from the last meal [41]. These data implicate impaired motility as a possible etiology of SIBO, and thus, IBS symptoms in some patients. Furthermore, treatment of IBS symptoms with antibiotics and/or probiotics in an effort to restore the equilibrium of enteric flora has yielded promising results [39, 42, 43].

Increased Intestinal Permeability

Post-infectious IBS (PI-IBS) may result from an increase in intestinal permeability as a result of inflammation triggered by infection. Intestinal permeability is detected noninvasively by measuring urinary excretion of orally consumed probe molecules, such as mannitol and lactulose [44, 45]. Increased intestinal permeability is more frequently encountered among patients with IBS-D and PI-IBS, particularly in those with a history of atopy [46]. Although IBS has been classified as a functional disorder not typically associated with anatomic defects, an inflammatory component among those with PI-IBS or IBS-D has been reported. An increased number of activated T lymphocytes and mast cells have been noted in the colonic [47] and jejunal mucosa [48] of patients with IBS-D, and the presence of these mast cells near enteric nerves may account for visceral pain or sensitivity. Increased intestinal permeability may also be related to elevated proinflammatory cytokine production noted in peripheral blood monocytes of IBS-D patients [49].

IV. PHARMACOLOGY

A paucity of therapies exists with documented efficacy in the treatment of IBS. Interpretation of efficacy in clinical trials is hampered by the large placebo effect among IBS patients [50]. Some commonly used therapies are directed toward symptom management of abdominal cramping, constipation, diarrhea, and/or bloating. Others specifically target serotonin metabolism, which is now thought to be responsible for visceral hyperalgesia or cortical pain processing. Given the broad range in symptom severity and frequency, treatment of IBS must be individualized.

CONSTIPATION

A first-line therapy for both functional constipation and IBS-C is a high-fiber diet, although this strategy may backfire in those with IBS-C. Increasing fiber intake to 25 to 30 g/day is thought to increase GI transit, although data in this area are conflicting. A typical serving of a given fruit or vegetable may contain anywhere from 2 to 5 grams of fiber. Fiber is also available as a dietary supplement in both soluble and insoluble forms. Soluble fiber such as psyllium and partially hydrolyzed guar gum derived from plants is extensively fermented by colonic bacteria, leading to the production of substantial amounts of gas and volatile fatty acids. As a consequence, stool content is heavy in bacterial mass and low in fiber residue. Conversely, insoluble fiber, such as wheat bran or whole-wheat grains, is minimally metabolized by colonic flora, and thus produces less gas. However, in an IBS-C patient with visceral hypersensitivity, even minimal amounts of gas accumulation in the setting of altered motility may be perceived as significant abdominal cramping and bloating. Some IBS-C patients cannot tolerate excessive amounts of fiber in the diet, and in fact, report improvement with respect to bloating and gassiness when consuming less fiber. Despite bulking agents being widely prescribed, a recent meta-analysis found that they were no better than placebo in improving IBS symptoms [51]. Little data exist as to the efficacy of other laxatives in the treatment of IBS-C. Lubiprostone, a locally acting chloride channel activator currently FDA approved for the treatment of constipation, is now being investigated for use in IBS-C [52].

Tegaserod is a 5HT4 receptor agonist that was shown in clinical trials to be more effective than placebo in improving IBS symptoms in women with predominantly constipation [53]. Tegaserod stimulated intestinal and colonic transit and reduced abdominal discomfort while improving constipation. Its manufacturer withdrew Tegaserod from the U.S. market in 2007 because of safety concerns. Renzapride is a 5HT4 receptor full agonist/5HT3 receptor antagonist currently being investigated for efficacy in the treatment of constipation predominant IBS. Despite being shown to accelerate colonic transit in an early trial [54], in a more recent phase II clinical trial, no significant difference in relief from abdominal pain occurred between renzapride and placebo [55].

Increased recognition that IBS may arise from perturbances in serotonin metabolism have spurred anecdotal use of 5-hydroxytryptophan (5-HTP), the precursor to serotonin. 5-HTP is often used with vitamin B6, which is a cofactor needed for conversion of 5-HTP to 5HT. Although 5-HTP may be useful in the treatment of depression [56], there are no published clinical trials in the medical literature regarding its efficacy in IBS.

ABDOMINAL CRAMPING

Anticholinergic agents, such as dicyclomine or hyoscyamine, are often prescribed to reduce smooth muscle spasm, although well-designed clinical trials that have proven their efficacy in reducing global IBS symptoms are lacking [57]. Nevertheless, some patients report symptomatic improvement when taking them before triggering events or before ingestion of meals. In addition to its use in foods and fragrances, peppermint oil extract derived from the peppermint leaf has long been thought to have medicinal properties. Particular to the GI tract, it has been shown to result in smooth muscle relaxation, possibly via a calcium channel antagonist mechanism [58]. The effect of peppermint oil on GI motility has not been completely elucidated. There are data showing decreased small intestinal transit time as well as increased gastric emptying time [58]. Colonic spasm relief has also been demonstrated with peppermint oil [59]. The literature is sparse, however, on clinical trials examining the effect of peppermint oil on IBS symptoms. A small study in the pediatric literature showed dramatic symptom improvement after a 14-day trial of peppermint oil [60]. However, moderate symptom improvement was observed in the placebo group to a greater extent than the treatment group. A large placebo effect hampers the interpretation of data in many IBS clinical trials. In the adult population peppermint oil was effective in improving overall IBS scores in another trial [61]. Side effects reported in clinical trials with peppermint oil are heartburn and anal/perianal burning [62]. Heartburn may be reduced if an enteric-coated preparation is used [60].

DIARRHEA

Anti-motility agents are often used in those patients with diarrhea-predominant IBS. Loperamide can be a helpful adjunct by reducing peristalsis and intestinal secretion and delaying GI transit, allowing increased colonic water absorption. Alosetron, a 5HT3 receptor antagonist, has been shown to improve symptoms of IBS-D [63, 64]. Alosetron decreases stool frequency and abdominal discomfort. Reports of ischemic colitis and severe constipation requiring bowel resection have led to its availability only on a restricted basis. Among IBS patients, specific polymorphisms have been identified more frequently in the serotonin transporter gene SLC6A4, whose gene product is responsible for reuptake of serotonin from the synaptic cleft. Some polymorphisms are associated with increased colonic transit time in response to alosetron [65]. The SERT deletion/deletion promoter polymorphism is more common among those with diarrhea-predominant IBS in Koreans [66] and Caucasians [67], suggesting the possibility of identifying individuals who might respond more readily to pharmacologic agents that modify serotonin signaling. Newer agents that work via 5HT3 are under investigation.

ABDOMINAL PAIN AND BLOATING

Because visceral hypersensitivity is central to IBS pathophysiology, there is increased interest in the use of antidepressants, which may be effective in dampening visceral pain signaling and perception. Typically, antidepressant doses used for IBS are lower than those used for the treatment of depression. Tricyclic antidepressants may help to improve abdominal pain, but may not improve IBS [57, 68]. A disadvantage is that some patients cannot tolerate side effects associated with some of these agents. In a small study of IBS patients without depression, the selective serotonin reuptake inhibitor citalopram improved abdominal pain, bloating, impact of symptoms on daily life, and overall well-being [69].

As a role for mucosal inflammation has emerged in IBS, and with increased recognition that intestinal microflora can modulate the host immune response, probiotics have been pursued as a possible treatment strategy for managing IBS symptoms. Probiotics consist of live microorganisms that are ingested to confer health benefits. Support for the use of probiotics comes from several randomized placebo-controlled trials using highly specific bacterial strains in which some individual symptoms of IBS, such as abdominal pain or bloating, improved after 4 or 8 weeks of therapy [43, 70–72]. In a randomized placebo-controlled study using *B. infantis* 35624 in 77 IBS patients, symptomatic improvement was associated with normalization of the ratio of anti-inflammatory to proinflammatory cytokines [73], suggesting that certain bacterial strains may indeed modulate cytokine production. Highly specific bacterial strains are used in clinical trials, and a response to one strain does not mean that the same response will be achieved with any commercially available probiotic. Probiotic preparations abound and manufacturing of these compounds is not subject to regulation by the Food and Drug Administration, making the selection of an appropriate preparation difficult.

V. COMORBID CONDITIONS

Patients with IBS are more likely to have other functional GI disorders, such as dyspepsia, which has some overlapping symptoms [74, 75]. Patients with IBS are likely to have comorbid disorders that affect a variety of organ systems, such as cystitis, pelvic pain, fibromyalgia, and chronic fatigue syndrome [76, 77]. There is a high prevalence of IBS among patients with psychiatric illness [78], with up to 94% of IBS patients who present for medical care being affected [77]. A history of sexual or physical abuse can be elicited in many patients with functional GI disorders [79].

Food Intolerance and Allergies

In patients with IBS, even normal physiologic responses of the GI tract to the ingestion of food may trigger the gastrocolonic reflex and provoke symptoms in some individuals with visceral hypersensitivity [80]. High fat content may provoke colonic motility and GI symptoms in an IBS patient. Caffeine also stimulates colonic motility and exacerbates IBS symptoms.

Food intolerance is not equivalent to food allergy, which generates an immune response. Food allergy has an estimated prevalence up to 4% in adults and up to 8% in children [81] and is discussed in more detail in Chapter 15, "Food Reactivities." The most common food allergens in U.S. adults are tree nuts, peanuts, shellfish, and fish, and in children, they are egg, wheat, and soybean. Food allergies can be mediated by immunoglobulin E, which leads to an immediate reaction, or can be triggered by cell-mediated mechanisms that account for delayed responses. Negative skin prick testing in adults has a negative predictive value >95%, but a positive response unfortunately has only a positive predictive value of 30% to 40% [82], leaving food withdrawal and challenge still the most common way of diagnosing food allergy. Some studies have attempted to use the increased presence of IgG antibodies over baseline to food allergens to guide food withdrawal with some improvement in a subset of IBS patients [83–85]. However, tests that measure IgE or IgG antibodies to specific foods are of questionable utility, especially when IgG antibodies against various food substances are prevalent even among the non-IBS population [86, 87].

Food elimination diets still remain the primary tool for evaluating food allergy. However, interpretation of elimination diet results are complicated in IBS [83–85, 88, 89]. An elimination diet that is devoid of wheat byproducts, milk, soy, and eggs often means shifting from a diet rich in processed foods to one comprised of whole foods. The elimination of processed foods could reduce food allergen exposure, but also decreases the intake of poorly absorbed carbohydrates, such as fructose and sorbitol. Symptomatic improvement with food elimination may reflect a response to reduced dietary intake of carbohydrate rather than exclusion of a food allergen.

Celiac Disease

There is overlap between the symptoms of IBS and celiac disease (CD). Bloating, abdominal pain, and diarrhea can be seen in patients with either of these disorders. This overlap has been reported in the literature, with one report finding up to 5% of newly diagnosed IBS patients having CD, while another report found 20% of patients with CD meeting Rome I criteria for IBS [90, 91]. Furthermore, CD serologies and HLA DQ2 positivity in IBS-D patients are predictors of gluten-free diet responsiveness [92]. It is not entirely clear if these observations reflect increasing diagnostic yield of serologic tests, increased clinical suspicion, or IBS-"type" symptoms in CD patients due to the enteropathy. Nonetheless, given this association, it is quite reasonable and cost effective to screen patients with IBS for CD in populations where the prevalence is above 1% [93]. Current guidelines recommend screening by serologic testing for tissue transglutaminase IgA, which has a specificity greater than 95% and a sensitivity in the range of 90% to 96% [94].

VI. PATIENT EVALUATION

The patient history is the most important component in making the diagnosis of IBS as no physical exam findings are diagnostic of IBS. Rather, it is the absence of significant physical exam findings that is most consistent with IBS. A clinical presentation that fulfills the Rome III criteria may alone be diagnostic in the absence of alarm symptoms. The criteria for IBS are distinct from that of functional constipation, namely that the latter is not associated with abdominal pain or discomfort. A history of weight loss, nocturnal awakening for diarrhea or abdominal pain, anemia, or rectal bleeding should prompt a search for an alternative diagnosis. Similarly, if the onset of symptoms occurs after age 50, the diagnosis of IBS should be questioned. Screening questionnaires for IBS primarily exist to measure symptom severity and impact on quality of life once the diagnosis of IBS is made. Such questionnaires, such as the IBSQOL, are used primarily for research purposes. The IBS Severity Scale is the tool recommended to assess responsiveness to an intervention in clinical trials [95].

Serum laboratory tests in IBS typically are normal. Laboratory testing is done to help exclude the possibility of other underlying disorders, such as thyroid disease or celiac disease. Stool tests should be considered to rule out active intestinal infection in those with diarrhea. Testing for visceral hypersensitivity with balloon manometry and functional MRI or PET scanning are only done primarily for research purposes; no role for these tests as yet has been established in clinical practice. In a 2002 position statement, the American College of Gastroenterology Functional Gastrointestinal Disorders Task Force stated that because IBS patients do not have an increased incidence of organic disease, "available data do not support the performance of diagnostic tests amongst patients with IBS" in the absence of alarm symptoms such as rectal bleeding or weight loss.

VII. TREATMENT RECOMMENDATIONS

After the diagnosis of IBS is made, treatment begins by obtaining a thorough dietary history, in part to identify symptom aggravators and especially because most patients with IBS will describe intolerance to specific foods [96]. Particular attention should be paid to medications and supplements, as many agents are known to precipitate or aggravate constipation or diarrhea even in those without IBS. Common medications and supplements that cause altered bowel habits are listed in Table 13.2. It is important to obtain a food diary to understand what components in the diet could be responsible for symptom aggravation in IBS [88]. The diet should be reviewed for dietary intake of specific carbohydrates, which could easily aggravate symptoms in an individual with visceral hypersensitivity. Carbohydrates that could be problematic include lactose, fructose, and the sugar alcohols. Caffeine intake and a high-fat diet should be monitored as both are known to stimulate colonic motility.

Lactose

Lactose intolerance is a common cause of milk-related symptoms. Lactose is hydrolyzed in the small intestine by the enzyme lactase, expressed by the enterocytes found in intestinal villi. Lactase activity is highest during infancy. Down-regulation of lactase enzyme activity within the small

TABLE 13.2
Common Causative Agents of Constipation and Diarrhea

Agent	Constipation	Diarrhea
Supplements	Calcium	Magnesium
	Iron	Vitamin C
		Niacin
Herbals	St. John's Wort (*Hypericum perforatum*)	Goldenseal (*Hydrastasis canadenis*)
		Aloe vera
Prescription Drugs	Anti-cholinergics (oxybutynin)	Cholinesterase inhibitors (pyridostigmine)
	Opiods analgesics (morphine)	Biguanides (metformin)
	Calcium channel blockers (diltiazem)	Calcinuerin inhibitors (tacrolimus)
	Non-opiod analgesics (tramadol)	Immunosuppressants (mycophenolate mofetil)
	Psychotrophics (lithium)	Colchicine
	Antidepressants (sertraline)	Stimulants (amphetamine)
	Beta blockers (atenolol)	Proton pump inhibitors (pantoprazole)
	Stimulants (dextroamphetamine)	Antibiotics (flouroquinolones)
	Anticonvulsants (phenytoin)	Laxative agents (lactulose)
	Bile acid binders (cholestyramine)	HAART therapy
		Chemotherapy agents (flourouracil)
		Anti-Parkinson's (Tolcapone)

Source: [126–128].

intestine is a normal occurrence in the vast majority of adults, but the rate of loss is dependent on race and ethnicity [97]. Because milk is pervasive in the Western diet, many individuals are unaware that undigested lactose is the source of their GI symptoms. Undigested lactose delivered to the colon increases the osmotic load, producing a more watery stool. In addition, undigested lactose is fermented by luminal bacteria to produce diarrhea and gas. Systemic symptoms of lactose intolerance may also include headache, fatigue, and myalgias.

Lactose intolerance is measurable by lactose hydrogen breath testing and has a specificity between 89% and 100% and sensitivity 69% to 100% [98]. Although many IBS patients self-report lactose intolerance, lactose breath hydrogen testing has demonstrated no increased prevalence of lactose malabsorption in IBS patients compared to controls in various geographic populations [99, 100]. Whether adherence to a lactose-free diet improves IBS symptoms in those who are lactose intolerant has been debated. Differences in response to a lactose-free diet reflects regional prevalence of lactose malabsorption and dietary compliance; regions with high prevalence of lactose malabsorption report clinical improvement in response to a low-lactose diet [101–103]. This may explain why fermented foods, a widespread practice among traditional cultures to preserve food using the action of microorganisms, are widely held to be more easily digestible [104]. Foods such as yogurt or kefir, fermented with lactic-acid-producing organisms, may be better tolerated in individuals with lactose intolerance because these bacteria hydrolyze lactose.

FRUCTOSE

Fructose malabsorption may also aggravate IBS symptoms, particularly in combination with ingested sorbitol [105, 106]. Fructose is a monosaccharide absorbed by carrier-mediated facilitated diffusion, with an absorption capacity of about 50 g/day [107]. Fructose absorption is enhanced when ingested with glucose [107]. When not absorbed in the small intestine, fructose exerts an osmotic effect and is fermented by colonic bacteria to produce hydrogen, carbon dioxide, and short-chain fatty acids

[108]. In a small study of normal volunteers, 50% of individuals were found to malabsorb fructose after ingesting only 25 g, and two-thirds malabsorbed fructose after ingesting 50 g, as measured by fructose hydrogen breath testing [109]. GI symptoms from fructose malabsorption may be more prevalent among both the normal and IBS populations when one considers fructose ingestion has increased more than 1000% in the United States over the past 20 years with the addition of high fructose corn syrup to sweeten soft drinks and fruit juices, candy, cereals, and many processed foods [110]. Quantities of 25 to 50 g of fructose are equivalent to >500 mL (16.91 U.S. ounces) of a high-fructose-corn-syrup-sweetened soft drink [111]. Fructose malabsorption may not be more common among the IBS population [112] and does not have an etiologic role in IBS, but fructose malabsorption may indeed aggravate IBS symptoms. In a small study of IBS patients with documented fructose intolerance, improvement in pain, belching, bloating, fullness, indigestion, and diarrhea was reported in response to dietary avoidance of fructose [113]. Dietary guidelines to reduce symptoms of fructose malabsorption have been proposed and may be effective in managing patients with IBS [108]. At the very least, patients should read labels to eliminate soft drinks containing high fructose corn syrup. Fruit juice also contains significant fructose and so excessive intake should be monitored.

ARTIFICIAL SWEETENERS

In an effort to reduce caloric intake, patients may resort to consuming "sugar-free" products, which contain sorbitol, maltitol, or xylitol. Such artificial sweeteners may add to bloating and diarrhea symptoms in patients with IBS simply because they are poorly absorbed in the small intestine and ultimately fermented by colonic bacteria. Thus, patients are well-advised to avoid these artificial sweeteners, which are pervasive in chewing gum and soft drinks in particular.

Sucralose is a synthetic, non-nutritive sweetener found in a variety of foods. Although some GI complaints have been attributed to sucralose ingestion, it is unclear as to how it causes these symptoms. Most ingested sucralose is excreted intact in the feces [114], so colonic bacterial fermentation cannot account for symptoms. Aspartame (N-l-α-aspartyl-phenylalanine-1-methyl ester) is another artificial sweetener that is broken down and absorbed at the small intestinal brush border into aspartic acid and phenylalanine dipeptide [115]. Although aspartame is not known to perturb GI physiology itself [116], 26% of consumer complaints involved GI side effects after ingestion of aspartame-sweetened foods [117].

VIII.   OTHER THERAPIES

Recognition that IBS represents a disorder of the brain-gut axis has raised a possible role for psychological therapies in the management of IBS. Cognitive behavior therapy (CBT), a form of psychotherapy used to modify maladaptive thinking, has been successfully used for the treatment of several psychiatric disorders, such as anxiety and depression. CBT has been studied in multiple clinical trials and is now recommended as an IBS treatment option by the United Kingdom Department of Health [118]. Although a Cochrane review to evaluate the efficacy of hypnotherapy in the treatment of IBS identified few studies of sufficient quality or size for meta-analysis [119], there are some studies demonstrating hypnotherapy may also help to improve abdominal pain and global IBS symptoms in those who have failed medical therapy [120–123].

Relaxation therapies have also been studied in clinical trials as adjunctive therapy to medical therapy with promising results [124]. Despite multiple studies showing their efficacy, psychological therapies in IBS management are still underutilized.

IX.   SUMMARY

The treatment of IBS begins with the recognition that there is tremendous variability in symptom severity, frequency, and triggering events. Thus, successful management of IBS requires an effective physician-patient relationship and an individualized biopsychosocial approach [125]. Dietary counseling is essential as is attention to the role of psychological therapy in management of symptoms. Among the standard pharmacologic therapies currently used in the management of IBS, only alosetron and tegaserod have been shown to improve global IBS symptoms, but some therapies listed below have been shown to be helpful in improving a specific symptom for which they are listed. Some listed therapies still lack proven efficacy in clinical trials but are often used in clinical practice given their low side effect profiles.

APPROACH TO IBS

History and Physical Exam
- History: Note absence of alarm symptoms (rectal bleeding, anemia, weight loss).
- Note presence of comorbid illnesses, such as fibromyalgia, chronic pelvic pain, cystitis, chronic fatigue.
- Note history of sexual or physical abuse.
- Physical exam—normal.
- Laboratory tests—usually normal, including thyroid function tests; serum tissue transglutaminase IgA (celiac disease screen) and stool studies.

Management
IBS-C
- Dietary and medication history.
  - Increase dietary fiber to 25 to 30 g/day, which improves stool bulk, but may worsen bloating and gassiness.
  - Add a bulk laxative, such as insoluble or soluble fiber, which improves stool bulk, but may worsen bloating.
  - Increase daily water intake and physical exercise.
- Consider an osmotic laxative (PEG 3350), although it may worsen bloating.
- Consider lubiprostone, which is currently under investigation for IBS-C.
- Consider a stimulant laxative, although it may worsen cramping.

IBS-D
- Dietary history.
  - Consider lactose intolerance.
  - Consider fructose malabsorption.
  - Reduce caffeine.
  - Reduce dietary fat intake.
  - Do not skip meals.
- Antidiarrheal agents (e.g., loperamide) to decrease stool frequency and improve consistency.
- Anti-spasmodics taken prior to triggering events such as job stress, social events, and certain foods.
- Alosetron improves abdominal discomfort and diarrhea.

Bloating, abdominal cramping/pain
- Dietary recommendations.
  - Avoid carbonated beverages, chewing gum, artificial sweeteners, fructose consumption > 25 to 50 g/day, and a high-fat diet.
- Consider testing for lactose intolerance with the lactose hydrogen breath test.
- Consider testing for small intestine bacterial overgrowth with the lactulose hydrogen breath test.

- If the lactulose hydrogen breath test is positive, begin a trial of antibiotic therapy (e.g., rifaximin, norfloxacin, amoxicillin-clavulinic acid).
- Antispasmodics (hyoscyamine, dicyclomine, or peppermint oil) preferably taken prior to triggering events or foods, up to three or four times a day.
- Tricyclic antidepressants, SSRIs (selective serotonin reuptake inhibitors), or SNRIs (selective norepinephrine reuptake inhibitors).
- Cognitive behavior therapy, gut-directed hypnotherapy, relaxation therapy.

REFERENCES

1. Thompson, W.G. *A strategy for management of the irritable bowel.* Am J Gastroenterol, 1986. 81(2): p. 95–100.
2. Shaheen, N.J., et al. *The burden of gastrointestinal and liver diseases, 2006.* Am J Gastroenterol, 2006. 101(9): p. 2128–38.
3. Simren, M., et al. *Health-related quality of life in patients attending a gastroenterology outpatient clinic: functional disorders versus organic diseases.* Clin Gastroenterol Hepatol, 2006. 4(2): p. 187–95.
4. Frank, L., et al. *Health-related quality of life associated with irritable bowel syndrome: comparison with other chronic diseases.* Clin Ther, 2002. 24(4): p. 675–89; discussion, p. 674.
5. Cremonini, F., and N.J. Talley. *Irritable bowel syndrome: epidemiology, natural history, health care seeking and emerging risk factors.* Gastroenterol Clin North Am, 2005. 34(2): p. 189–204.
6. Wigington, W.C., W.D. Johnson, and A. Minocha. *Epidemiology of irritable bowel syndrome among African Americans as compared with whites: a population-based study.* Clin Gastroenterol Hepatol, 2005. 3(7): p. 647–53.
7. Gralnek, I.M., et al. *Racial differences in the impact of irritable bowel syndrome on health-related quality of life.* J Clin Gastroenterol, 2004. 38(9): p. 782–89.
8. Minocha, A., et al. *Prevalence, sociodemography, and quality of life of older versus younger patients with irritable bowel syndrome: a population-based study.* Dig Dis Sci, 2006. 51(3): p. 446–53.
9. Icks, A., et al. *Prevalence of functional bowel disorders and related health care seeking: a population-based study.* Z Gastroenterol, 2002. 40(3): p. 177–83.
10. Howell, S., et al. *The irritable bowel syndrome has origins in the childhood socioeconomic environment.* Am J Gastroenterol, 2004. 99(8): p. 1572–78.
11. Olafsdottir, L.B., H. Gudjonsson, and B. Thjodleifsson. *Epidemiological study of functional bowel disorders in Iceland.* Laeknabladid, 2005. 91(4): p. 329–33.
12. Leong, S.A., et al. *The economic consequences of irritable bowel syndrome: a US employer perspective.* Arch Intern Med, 2003. 163(8): p. 929–35.
13. Inadomi, J.M., M.B. Fennerty, and D. Bjorkman. *Systematic review: the economic impact of irritable bowel syndrome.* Aliment Pharmacol Ther, 2003. 18(7): p. 671–82.
14. Hulisz, D. *The burden of illness of irritable bowel syndrome: current challenges and hope for the future.* J Manag Care Pharm, 2004. 10(4): p. 299–309.
15. Quigley, E.M. *Changing face of irritable bowel syndrome.* World J Gastroenterol, 2006. 12(1): p. 1–5.
16. Drossman, D.A., et al. *U.S. householder survey of functional gastrointestinal disorders. Prevalence, sociodemography, and health impact.* Dig Dis Sci, 1993. 38(9): p. 1569–80.
17. Kalantar, J.S., et al. *Familial aggregation of irritable bowel syndrome: a prospective study.* Gut, 2003. 52(12): p. 1703–7.
18. Bengtson, M.B., et al. *Irritable bowel syndrome in twins: genes and environment.* Gut, 2006. 55(12): p. 1754–59.
19. Park, M.I., and M. Camilleri. *Genetics and genotypes in irritable bowel syndrome: implications for diagnosis and treatment.* Gastroenterol Clin North Am, 2005. 34(2): p. 305–17.
20. Wojczynski, M.K., et al. *Irritable bowel syndrome: a co-twin control analysis.* Am J Gastroenterol, 2007. 102(10): p. 2220–29.
21. Ritchie, J. *Pain from distension of the pelvic colon by inflating a balloon in the irritable colon syndrome.* Gut, 1973. 14(2): p. 125–32.
22. Gershon, M.D. *Review article: serotonin receptors and transporters—roles in normal and abnormal gastrointestinal motility.* Aliment Pharmacol Ther, 2004. 20 Suppl 7: p. 3–14.
23. Atkinson, W., et al. *Altered 5-hydroxytryptamine signaling in patients with constipation- and diarrhea-predominant irritable bowel syndrome.* Gastroenterology, 2006. 130(1): p. 34–43.

24. Dunlop, S.P., et al. *Abnormalities of 5-hydroxytryptamine metabolism in irritable bowel syndrome.* Clin Gastroenterol Hepatol, 2005. 3(4): p. 349–57.

25. Chen, J.J., et al. *Maintenance of serotonin in the intestinal mucosa and ganglia of mice that lack the high-affinity serotonin transporter: abnormal intestinal motility and the expression of cation transporters.* J Neurosci, 2001. 21(16): p. 6348–61.

26. Camilleri, M., et al. *Alterations in expression of p11 and SERT in mucosal biopsy specimens of patients with irritable bowel syndrome.* Gastroenterology, 2007. 132(1): p. 17–25.

27. Spiller, R.C. *Role of infection in irritable bowel syndrome.* J Gastroenterol, 2007. 42 Suppl 17: p. 41–47.

28. Mearin, F., et al. *Dyspepsia and irritable bowel syndrome after a Salmonella gastroenteritis outbreak: one-year follow-up cohort study.* Gastroenterology, 2005. 129(1): p. 98–104.

29. Dizdar, V., O.H. Gilja, and T. Hausken. *Increased visceral sensitivity in giardia-induced postinfectious irritable bowel syndrome and functional dyspepsia. Effect of the 5HT3-antagonist ondansetron.* Neurogastroenterol Motil, 2007. 19(12): p. 977–82.

30. Ji, S., et al. *Post-infectious irritable bowel syndrome in patients with Shigella infection.* J Gastroenterol Hepatol, 2005. 20(3): p. 381–86.

31. Kim, H.S., et al. *The development of irritable bowel syndrome after Shigella infection: 3 year follow-up study.* Korean J Gastroenterol, 2006. 47(4): p. 300–305.

32. Wang, L.H., X.C. Fang, and G.Z. Pan. *Bacillary dysentery as a causative factor of irritable bowel syndrome and its pathogenesis.* Gut, 2004. 53(8): p. 1096–1101.

33. Dunlop, S.P., et al. *Relative importance of enterochromaffin cell hyperplasia, anxiety, and depression in postinfectious IBS.* Gastroenterology, 2003. 125(6): p. 1651–59.

34. Linden, D.R., et al. *Serotonin availability is increased in mucosa of guinea pigs with TNBS-induced colitis.* Am J Physiol Gastrointest Liver Physiol, 2003. 285(1): p. G207–G216.

35. Amaro, E., Jr., and G.J. Barker. *Study design in fMRI: basic principles.* Brain Cogn, 2006. 60(3): p. 220–32.

36. Mertz, H., et al. *Regional cerebral activation in irritable bowel syndrome and control subjects with painful and nonpainful rectal distention.* Gastroenterology, 2000. 118(5): p. 842–48.

37. Lawal, A., et al. *Novel evidence for hypersensitivity of visceral sensory neural circuitry in irritable bowel syndrome patients.* Gastroenterology, 2006. 130(1): p. 26–33.

38. Naliboff, B.D., and E.A. Mayer. *Brain imaging in IBS: drawing the line between cognitive and non-cognitive processes.* Gastroenterology, 2006. 130(1): p. 267–70.

39. Pimentel, M., et al. *The effect of a nonabsorbed oral antibiotic (rifaximin) on the symptoms of the irritable bowel syndrome: a randomized trial.* Ann Intern Med, 2006. 145(8): p. 557–63.

40. Yang, J., et al. *Rifaximin versus other antibiotics in the primary treatment and retreatment of bacterial overgrowth in IBS.* Dig Dis Sci, 2008. 53(1): p. 169–74.

41. Pimentel, M., et al. *Lower frequency of MMC is found in IBS subjects with abnormal lactulose breath test, suggesting bacterial overgrowth.* Dig Dis Sci, 2002. 47(12): p. 2639–43.

42. Sharara, A.I., et al. *A randomized double-blind placebo-controlled trial of rifaximin in patients with abdominal bloating and flatulence.* Am J Gastroenterol, 2006. 101(2): p. 326–33.

43. Whorwell, P.J., et al. *Efficacy of an encapsulated probiotic Bifidobacterium infantis 35624 in women with irritable bowel syndrome.* Am J Gastroenterol, 2006. 101(7): p. 1581–90.

44. Camilleri, M., and H. Gorman. *Intestinal permeability and irritable bowel syndrome.* Neurogastroenterol Motil, 2007. 19(7): p. 545–52.

45. Bjarnason, I., A. MacPherson, and D. Hollander. *Intestinal permeability: an overview.* Gastroenterology, 1995. 108(5): p. 1566–81.

46. Dunlop, S.P., et al. *Abnormal intestinal permeability in subgroups of diarrhea-predominant irritable bowel syndromes.* Am J Gastroenterol, 2006. 101(6): p. 1288–94.

47. Barbara, G., et al. *Activated mast cells in proximity to colonic nerves correlate with abdominal pain in irritable bowel syndrome.* Gastroenterology, 2004. 126(3): p. 693–702.

48. Guilarte, M., et al. *Diarrhoea-predominant IBS patients show mast cell activation and hyperplasia in the jejunum.* Gut, 2007. 56(2): p. 203–9.

49. Liebregts, T., et al. *Immune activation in patients with irritable bowel syndrome.* Gastroenterology, 2007. 132(3): p. 913–20.

50. Patel, S.M., et al. *The placebo effect in irritable bowel syndrome trials: a meta-analysis.* Neurogastroenterol Motil, 2005. 17(3): p. 332–40.

51. Schoenfeld, P. *Efficacy of current drug therapies in irritable bowel syndrome: what works and does not work.* Gastroenterol Clin North Am, 2005. 34(2): p. 319–35, viii.
52. Johanson, J.F., et al. *Clinical trial: phase 2 trial of lubiprostone for irritable bowel syndrome with constipation.* Aliment Pharmacol Ther, 2008.
53. Evans, B.W., et al. *Tegaserod for the treatment of irritable bowel syndrome and chronic constipation.* Cochrane Database Syst Rev, 2007(4):CD003960.
54. Camilleri, M., et al. *Effect of renzapride on transit in constipation-predominant irritable bowel syndrome.* Clin Gastroenterol Hepatol, 2004. 2(10): p. 895–904.
55. George, A.M., N.L. Meyers, and R.I. Hickling. *Clinical trial: renzapride therapy for constipation-predominant irritable bowel syndrome—a multicentre, randomised, placebo-controlled, double-blind study in the primary healthcare setting.* Aliment Pharmacol Ther, 2008.
56. Shaw, K., J. Turner, and C. Del Mar. *Tryptophan and 5-hydroxytryptophan for depression.* Cochrane Database Syst Rev, 2002(1):CD003198.
57. *Evidence-based position statement on the management of irritable bowel syndrome in North America.* Am J Gastroenterol, 2002. 97(11 Suppl): p. S1–S5.
58. McKay, D.L., and J.B. Blumberg. *A review of the bioactivity and potential health benefits of peppermint tea (Mentha piperita L.).* Phytother Res, 2006. 20(8): p. 619–33.
59. Leicester, R.J., and R.H. Hunt. *Peppermint oil to reduce colonic spasm during endoscopy.* Lancet, 1982. 2(8305): p. 989.
60. Kline, R.M., et al. *Enteric-coated, pH-dependent peppermint oil capsules for the treatment of irritable bowel syndrome in children.* J Pediatr, 2001. 138(1): p. 125–28.
61. Cappello, G., et al. *Peppermint oil (Mintoil) in the treatment of irritable bowel syndrome: a prospective double blind placebo-controlled randomized trial.* Dig Liver Dis, 2007. 39(6): p. 530–36.
62. Grigoleit, H.G., and P. Grigoleit. *Peppermint oil in irritable bowel syndrome.* Phytomedicine, 2005. 12(8): p. 601–6.
63. Andresen, V., et al. *Effects of 5-hydroxytryptamine (serotonin) type 3 antagonists on symptom relief and constipation in nonconstipated irritable bowel syndrome: a systematic review and meta-analysis of randomized controlled trials.* Clin Gastroenterol Hepatol, 2008.
64. Krause, R., et al. *A randomized, double-blind, placebo-controlled study to assess efficacy and safety of 0. 5 mg and 1 mg alosetron in women with severe diarrhea-predominant IBS.* Am J Gastroenterol, 2007. 102(8): p. 1709–19.
65. Camilleri, M., et al. *Serotonin-transporter polymorphism pharmacogenetics in diarrhea-predominant irritable bowel syndrome.* Gastroenterology, 2002. 123(2): p. 425–32.
66. Park, J.M., et al. *Serotonin transporter gene polymorphism and irritable bowel syndrome.* Neurogastroenterol Motil, 2006. 18(11): p. 995–1000.
67. Yeo, A., et al. *Association between a functional polymorphism in the serotonin transporter gene and diarrhoea predominant irritable bowel syndrome in women.* Gut, 2004. 53(10): p. 1452–58.
68. Drossman, D.A., et al. *Further validation of the IBS-QOL: a disease-specific quality-of-life questionnaire.* Am J Gastroenterol, 2000. 95(4): p. 999–1007.
69. Tack, J., et al. *A controlled crossover study of the selective serotonin reuptake inhibitor citalopram in irritable bowel syndrome.* Gut, 2006. 55(8): p. 1095–1103.
70. Kim, H.J., et al. *A randomized controlled trial of a probiotic combination VSL# 3 and placebo in irritable bowel syndrome with bloating.* Neurogastroenterol Motil, 2005. 17(5): p. 687–96.
71. Niedzielin, K., H. Kordecki, and B. Birkenfeld. *A controlled, double-blind, randomized study on the efficacy of Lactobacillus plantarum 299V in patients with irritable bowel syndrome.* Eur J Gastroenterol Hepatol, 2001. 13(10): p. 1143–47.
72. Nobaek, S., et al. *Alteration of intestinal microflora is associated with reduction in abdominal bloating and pain in patients with irritable bowel syndrome.* Am J Gastroenterol, 2000. 95(5): p. 1231–38.
73. O'Mahony, L., et al. *Lactobacillus and bifidobacterium in irritable bowel syndrome: symptom responses and relationship to cytokine profiles.* Gastroenterology, 2005. 128(3): p. 541–51.
74. Talley, N.J., et al. *Overlapping upper and lower gastrointestinal symptoms in irritable bowel syndrome patients with constipation or diarrhea.* Am J Gastroenterol, 2003. 98(11): p. 2454–59.
75. Whitehead, W.E., et al. *Is functional dyspepsia just a subset of the irritable bowel syndrome?* Baillieres Clin Gastroenterol, 1998. 12(3): p. 443–61.
76. Whitehead, W.E., et al. *Comorbidity in irritable bowel syndrome.* Am J Gastroenterol, 2007. 102(12): p. 2767–76.

77. Whitehead, W.E., O. Palsson, and K.R. Jones. *Systematic review of the comorbidity of irritable bowel syndrome with other disorders: what are the causes and implications?* Gastroenterology, 2002. 122(4): p. 1140–56.

78. Garakani, A., et al. *Comorbidity of irritable bowel syndrome in psychiatric patients: a review.* Am J Ther, 2003. 10(1): p. 61–67.

79. Drossman, D.A., et al. *Sexual and physical abuse in women with functional or organic gastrointestinal disorders.* Ann Intern Med, 1990. 113(11): p. 828–33.

80. Whorwell, P., and R. Lea. *Dietary treatment of the irritable bowel syndrome.* Curr Treat Options Gastroenterol, 2004. 7(4): p. 307–16.

81. Sampson, H.A. *Update on food allergy.* J Allergy Clin Immunol, 2004. 113(5): p. 805–19; quiz, p. 820.

82. Nowak-Wegrzyn, A., and H.A. Sampson. *Adverse reactions to foods.* Med Clin North Am, 2006. 90(1): p. 97–127.

83. Zar, S., et al. *Food-specific IgG4 antibody-guided exclusion diet improves symptoms and rectal compliance in irritable bowel syndrome.* Scand J Gastroenterol, 2005. 40(7): p. 800–807.

84. Zar, S., M.J. Benson, and D. Kumar. *Food-specific serum IgG4 and IgE titers to common food antigens in irritable bowel syndrome.* Am J Gastroenterol, 2005. 100(7): p. 1550–57.

85. Atkinson, W., et al. *Food elimination based on IgG antibodies in irritable bowel syndrome: a randomised controlled trial.* Gut, 2004. 53(10): p. 1459–64.

86. Zar, S., D. Kumar, and M.J. Benson. *Food hypersensitivity and irritable bowel syndrome.* Aliment Pharmacol Ther, 2001. 15(4): p. 439–49.

87. Shanahan, F., and P.J. Whorwell. *IgG-mediated food intolerance in irritable bowel syndrome: a real phenomenon or an epiphenomenon?* Am J Gastroenterol, 2005. 100(7): p. 1558–59.

88. Drisko, J., et al. *Treating irritable bowel syndrome with a food elimination diet followed by food challenge and probiotics.* J Am Coll Nutr, 2006. 25(6): p. 514–22.

89. Zuo, X.L., et al. *Alterations of food antigen-specific serum immunoglobulins G and E antibodies in patients with irritable bowel syndrome and functional dyspepsia.* Clin Exp Allergy, 2007. 37(6): p. 823–30.

90. O'Leary, C., et al. *Celiac disease and irritable bowel-type symptoms.* Am J Gastroenterol, 2002. 97(6): p. 1463–67.

91. Sanders, D.S. *Celiac disease and IBS-type symptoms: the relationship exists in both directions.* Am J Gastroenterol, 2003. 98(3): p. 707–8.

92. Wahnschaffe, U., et al. *Predictors of clinical response to gluten-free diet in patients diagnosed with diarrhea-predominant irritable bowel syndrome.* Clin Gastroenterol Hepatol, 2007. 5(7): p. 844–50; quiz, p. 769.

93. Spiegel, B.M., et al. *Testing for celiac sprue in irritable bowel syndrome with predominant diarrhea: a cost-effectiveness analysis.* Gastroenterology, 2004. 126(7): p. 1721–32.

94. *AGA Institute medical position statement on the diagnosis and management of celiac disease.* Gastroenterology, 2006. 131(6): p. 1977–80.

95. Camilleri, M., et al. *Primary endpoints for irritable bowel syndrome trials: a review of performance of endpoints.* Clin Gastroenterol Hepatol, 2007. 5(5): p. 534–40.

96. Monsbakken, K.W., P.O. Vandvik, and P.G. Farup. *Perceived food intolerance in subjects with irritable bowel syndrome—etiology, prevalence and consequences.* Eur J Clin Nutr, 2006. 60(5): p. 667–72.

97. Jarvela, I.E. *Molecular genetics of adult-type hypolactasia.* Ann Med, 2005. 37(3): p. 179–85.

98. Arola, H., and A. Tamm. *Metabolism of lactose in the human body.* Scand J Gastroenterol Suppl, 1994. 202: p. 21–25.

99. Farup, P.G., K.W. Monsbakken, and P.O. Vandvik. *Lactose malabsorption in a population with irritable bowel syndrome: prevalence and symptoms. A case-control study.* Scand J Gastroenterol, 2004. 39(7): p. 645–49.

100. Vernia, P., et al. *Self-reported milk intolerance in irritable bowel syndrome: what should we believe?* Clin Nutr, 2004. 23(5): p. 996–1000.

101. Parker, T.J., et al. *Irritable bowel syndrome: is the search for lactose intolerance justified?* Eur J Gastroenterol Hepatol, 2001. 13(3): p. 219–25.

102. Vernia, P., et al. *Lactose malabsorption and irritable bowel syndrome. Effect of a long-term lactose-free diet.* Ital J Gastroenterol, 1995. 27(3): p. 117–21.

103. Bohmer, C.J., and H.A. Tuynman. *The effect of a lactose-restricted diet in patients with a positive lactose tolerance test, earlier diagnosed as irritable bowel syndrome: a 5-year follow-up study.* Eur J Gastroenterol Hepatol, 2001. 13(8): p. 941–44.

104. Caplice, E., and G.F. Fitzgerald. *Food fermentations: role of microorganisms in food production and preservation.* Int J Food Microbiol, 1999. 50(1–2): p. 131–49.

105. Rumessen, J.J., and E. Gudmand-Hoyer. *Functional bowel disease: malabsorption and abdominal distress after ingestion of fructose, sorbitol, and fructose-sorbitol mixtures.* Gastroenterology, 1988. 95(3): p. 694–700.

106. Rumessen, J.J., and E. Gudmand-Hoyer. *Functional bowel disease: the role of fructose and sorbitol.* Gastroenterology, 1991. 101(5): p. 1452–53.

107. Rumessen, J.J., and E. Gudmand-Hoyer. *Absorption capacity of fructose in healthy adults. Comparison with sucrose and its constituent monosaccharides.* Gut, 1986. 27(10): p. 1161–68.

108. Shepherd, S.J., and P.R. Gibson. *Fructose malabsorption and symptoms of irritable bowel syndrome: guidelines for effective dietary management.* J Am Diet Assoc, 2006. 106(10): p. 1631–39.

109. Beyer, P.L., E.M. Caviar, and R.W. McCallum. *Fructose intake at current levels in the United States may cause gastrointestinal distress in normal adults.* J Am Diet Assoc, 2005. 105(10): p. 1559–66.

110. Bray, G.A., S.J. Nielsen, and B.M. Popkin. *Consumption of high-fructose corn syrup in beverages may play a role in the epidemic of obesity.* Am J Clin Nutr, 2004. 79(4): p. 537–43.

111. Gibson, P.R., et al. *Review article: fructose malabsorption and the bigger picture.* Aliment Pharmacol Ther, 2007. 25(4): p. 349–63.

112. Nelis, G.F., M.A. Vermeeren, and W. Jansen. *Role of fructose-sorbitol malabsorption in the irritable bowel syndrome.* Gastroenterology, 1990. 99(4): p. 1016–20.

113. Choi, Y.K., et al. *Fructose intolerance in IBS and utility of fructose-restricted diet.* J Clin Gastroenterol, 2008. 42(3): p.233–238.

114. Roberts, A., et al. *Sucralose metabolism and pharmacokinetics in man.* Food Chem Toxicol, 2000. 38 Suppl 2: p. S31–S41.

115. Hooper, N.M., R.J. Hesp, and S. Tieku. *Metabolism of aspartame by human and pig intestinal microvillar peptidases.* Biochem J, 1994. 298 Pt 3: p. 635–39.

116. Bianchi, R.G., et al. *The biological properties of aspartame. II. Actions involving the gastrointestinal system.* J Environ Pathol Toxicol, 1980. 3(5–6): p. 355–62.

117. Bradstock, M.K., et al. *Evaluation of reactions to food additives: the aspartame experience.* Am J Clin Nutr, 1986. 43(3): p. 464–69.

118. Health, D.O. *Treatment choice in psychological therapies and counselling: evidence based clinical practice guidelines.* In *NHS Executive.* 2001: London.

119. Webb, A.N., et al. *Hypnotherapy for treatment of irritable bowel syndrome.* Cochrane Database Syst Rev, 2007(4):CD005110.

120. Palsson, O.S., et al. *Hypnosis treatment for severe irritable bowel syndrome: investigation of mechanism and effects on symptoms.* Dig Dis Sci, 2002. 47(11): p. 2605–14.

121. Whorwell, P.J., A. Prior, and E.B. Faragher. *Controlled trial of hypnotherapy in the treatment of severe refractory irritable-bowel syndrome.* Lancet, 1984. 2(8414): p. 1232–34.

122. Galovski, T.E., and E.B. Blanchard. *The treatment of irritable bowel syndrome with hypnotherapy.* Appl Psychophysiol Biofeedback, 1998. 23(4): p. 219–32.

123. Roberts, L., et al. *Gut-directed hypnotherapy for irritable bowel syndrome: piloting a primary care-based randomised controlled trial.* Br J Gen Pract, 2006. 56(523): p. 115–21.

124. van der Veek, P.P., Y.R. van Rood, and A.A. Masclee. *Clinical trial: short- and long-term benefit of relaxation training for irritable bowel syndrome.* Aliment Pharmacol Ther, 2007. 26(6): p. 943–52.

125. Drossman, D.A. *The functional gastrointestinal disorders and the Rome III process.* Gastroenterology, 2006. 130(5): p. 1377–90.

126. Fernandez-Banares, F. *Nutritional care of the patient with constipation.* Best Pract Res Clin Gastroenterol, 2006. 20(3): p. 575–87.

127. Boudreau, M.D., and F.A. Beland. *An evaluation of the biological and toxicological properties of Aloe barbadensis (miller), Aloe vera.* J Environ Sci Health C Environ Carcinog Ecotoxicol Rev, 2006. 24(1): p. 103–54.

128. Sellin, J.H. *A practical approach to treating patients with chronic diarrhea.* Rev Gastroenterol Disord, 2007. 7 Suppl 3: p. S19–S26.

14 Inflammatory Bowel Disease

Food and Nutrient Approaches

Melissa A. Munsell, M.D., and Gerard E. Mullin, M.D.

I. INTRODUCTION

Inflammatory bowel disease (IBD) is a chronic illness that is characterized by unremitting intestinal inflammation with tissue injury caused by increased oxidative and metabolic stress. Increased energy, macronutrient, micronutrient, and electrolyte requirements result from thermodynamic demands of inflammation and tissue losses from intestinal injury. Consequent protein-calorie malnutrition and micronutrient deficiencies are common among these patients and require close supervision and corrective supplementation[1] (Table 14.1). Along these lines, food harbors nutrients that are vital for optimal cellular function (i.e., antioxidants, polyphenols, omega-3 fatty acids, etc.) and regulate key components of the inflammatory cascade. Diet plays an important role in down-regulating the unresolved inflammation of IBD while optimizing healing and immunity. Thus, dietary and nutrient strategies have been studied as primary treatment in IBD. We review the nutritional consequences and therapy of IBD.

II. EPIDEMIOLOGY

A GENE–NUTRIENT INTERACTION

Incidence rates of IBD increased after 1940, but have remained stable over the past 30 years, with the prevalence of ulcerative colitis estimated at 214 cases per 100,000 and Crohn's disease at 174 per 100,000.[2] It is unclear if the increased incidence in IBD is due to improved diagnostic methods or as a response to changing environmental triggers. For example, the incidence of IBD has increased in Asian countries concurrent with increasing Westernized diets.[3] High-animal-fat, high-sugar, and low-fiber diets are proinflammatory and have been implicated in the development of IBD.[4–6] Though IBD has remained an idiopathic disease, it has been proposed that genetically susceptible individuals develop disease in response to an exaggerated immune response to an environmental trigger (i.e., infectious, dietary) in the gut microbiota. Since IBD is believed to be the result of a complex interaction between genetic, immune, microbial, and environmental factors as noted above, it is highly plausible that diet, as an environmental factor, may contribute to the pathogenesis of these diseases. For example, *Mycobacterium paratuberculosis* has reemerged as a possible infectious etiology for Crohn's disease. This infectious pathogen is found in unpasteurized cow's milk in Europe.[7] Furthermore, elemental diets will produce symptomatic relief and objective remission in up to 90% of patients, and may be considered as a first line in therapy for pediatric patients.[8] Elemental diets contain no intact protein, and dietary nitrogen is supplied as amino acids, while polymeric diets contain intact protein. In animal models of IBD, dietary protein increased intestinal

TABLE 14.1
Malnutrition in Inflammatory Bowel Disease

Deficiency	CD	UC	Treatment
Negative nitrogen balance	69%	Unknown	Adequate energy and protein
B12	48%	5%	1000 µg/day × 7 days, then monthly
Folate	67%	30–40%	1 mg/day
Vitamin A	11%	Unknown	5000–25,000 IU/day
Vitamin D	75%	35%	5000–25,000 IU/day
Calcium	13%	Unknown	1000–1200 mg/day
Potassium	5–20%	Unknown	Variable
Iron	39%	81%	Fe gluconate 300 mg TID
Zinc	50%	Unknown	Zn sulfate 220 mg qd or BID

permeability, which resolved with the institution of an elemental diet.[9] Since dietary constituents influence the composition and function of the intestinal microflora and the clinical course of IBD, nutrition appears to be an integral role in the pathogenesis and treatment.

III.   PATHOPHYSIOLOGY

OVERVIEW OF IBD PRESENTATION

Ulcerative colitis (UC) affects the colonic mucosa diffusely and is characterized by diarrhea, abdominal pain, and hematochezia. UC is categorized as *distal disease* (affecting rectum and/or sigmoid), *left-sided colitis* (up to splenic flexure), *extensive colitis* (up to hepatic flexure), or *pancolitis* (entire colon). Crohn's disease (CD) is characterized by transmural inflammation which is discontinuous and may affect any part of the gastrointestinal tract. The most common location of disease involvement is the small bowel, where most nutrients are assimilated and absorbed. Endoscopically, the mucosa is described as cobblestoned with evidence of apthous ulcerations. Radiographically, evidence of fistulae or stricturing disease may be present. CD is classified by location of disease and the pattern of disease (*inflammatory, fibrostenotic, or fistulizing*).[10] Patients with CD often have symptoms of abdominal pain, which limits nutrient intake, and diarrhea from severe mucosal injury causing malabsorption of fat and lipid-soluble vitamins, loss of fluids-electrolytes-minerals, and consequent weight loss. Despite aggressive evaluation with clinical, endoscopic, radiological, and pathological criteria, about 5% of patients with IBD affecting the colon are termed indeterminate colitis, whereby the disease is indistinguishable from either UC or CD.

CHRONIC INFLAMMATION

Chronic inflammation in IBD is characterized by infiltration of mononuclear cells and polymorphonuclear neutrophils into the wall of the intestine.[11] The inflammatory response is amplified as these cells are proinflammatory mediators that activate and recruit more inflammatory cells to the bowel. It is believed that mononuclear cells mediate this immune response via secretion of tumor necrosis factor (TNF), interferon-γ, interleukins, and eicosanoids (prostaglandin class 2, thromboxanes, leukotrienes class 4).[12] Activation of NFκB stimulates expression of these molecules, which are increased in active IBD, yet also stimulates expression of protective molecules that inhibit inflammatory responses.[13] This mechanism is not completely understood but is thought to play a key role in acute and chronic inflammation in IBD. Studies have shown that short chain fatty acids (SCFAs), such as butyrate, polyphenols, and omega-3 fatty acids can reduce NFκB activity and become possible nutraceutical therapeutic modalities for IBD.[14–16]

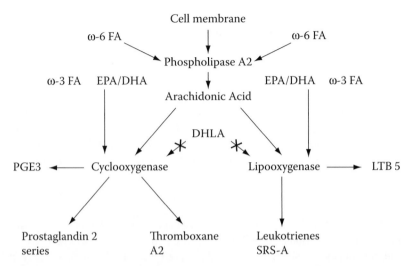

FIGURE 14.1 ω-3 Modulation of the arachidonic acid cascade. ω-6 Fatty acids appear to promote the production of phospholipase A2 (PLP A2), arachidonic acid (AA) and production of noxious proinflammatory eicosanoids such as prostaglandin-2 series (PGE2), leukotrienes (LTB) such as slow reactive releasing substance (SRS-A), and thromboxane A2 (TXA2). ω-3 Fatty acids, in contrast, down-regulate production of proinflammatory eicosanoids by competitive inhibition of the enzymes cyclooxygenase-2 (COX-2) and 5'-Lipoxygenase (5'LPO) for AA, thus leading to preferential production of the prostaglandin-3 series (PGE3) and leukotriene-5 series (LTB5). (From [15].)

Linoleic acid is an essential polyunsaturated fatty acid (PUFA) and is a substrate for eicosanoids. PUFAs are categorized into two main families: omega-6 and omega-3. Linoleic acid is the parent compound to the proinflammatory omega-6 fatty acids and is found in fairly high concentrations in corn, soybean, and safflower oils.[12] The other class of essential fatty acids are omega-3 PUFAs of which the parent compound is α-linoleic acid, which is synthesized into fatty acids important in immunomodulatory and anti-inflammatory effects via the production of prostaglandin class 3 and leukotriene B$_5$, and by inhibiting production of arachidonic acid[17] (see Figure 14.1). The omega-3 fatty acids are believed to compete with omega-6 fatty acids as precursors for eicosanoid synthesis.[18] Omega-3 fatty acids also reduce TNFα production by inhibiting protein kinase C activity.[19] Omega-3 PUFAs are found in flaxseed, canola, and walnuts, but oils from deep sea fish are a more advantageous source of omega-3 PUFAs since humans do not readily transform α-linoleic acid to eicosapentaenoic acid and docosahexaenoic acid, which are the main precursors for desirable eicosanoids.[12] Fish oil affects the gut immune system by suppressing T cell signaling, inhibiting proinflammatory cytokine synthesis, reducing inflammatory cell recruitment, and enhancing epithelial barrier function.[20,21]

Along with PUFAs, SCFAs are also thought to play a role in IBD pathogenesis. SCFAs are monocarboxylic hydrocarbons produced by the endogenous bacterial flora digestion of nonabsorbable carbohydrates reaching the colon, and include acetate, proprionate, and butyrate.[22] Nonabsorbable carbohydrates (e.g., dietary fibers) include, but are not limited to, nonstarch polysaccharides, resistant starch, cellulose, and pectins.[23] Butyrate is a major source of energy for colonocytes, and early studies demonstrated that rectal epithelial cells in patients with UC have impaired oxidation of butyrate, which may be caused by elevated levels of TNF.[24–26] Other studies have shown that SCFAs such as butyrate may have an anti-inflammatory effect by down-regulating cytokines.[27] Furthermore, SCFAs may promote colonic sodium absorption.[28] The therapeutic potential of SCFAs has been shown in both animal and human studies in IBD.[29]

IBD is thought to result from a complex interplay between genetic, immune, and environmental factors, including food and nutrients. While diets high in animal fats and sugar and low in fiber have been implicated in IBD, studies on the dietary role in IBD are challenging to interpret as other lifestyle or environmental factors may play a role.[1] Dietary microparticles have also been theorized to be involved in the etiology of IBD. Microparticles are bacterial-sized inorganic particles such as titanium, aluminum, and silicone, which are found in Western diets, often in food additives. They have been proposed to exacerbate inflammation via antigen-mediated immune responses and by increasing intestinal permeability, leading to increased immune exposure to antigens.[30,31] Specific foods can aggravate gastrointestinal symptoms in IBD, but do not indicate a causative role. Currently, there is no definitive evidence linking specific foods as a direct cause in IBD, therefore a diet rich in polyphenols, omega-3 fatty acids, along with prebiotic-rich foods coupled with a healthful lifestyle is recommended to patients with UC and CD to minimize the risk of malnutrition.

MALNUTRITION

Hospitalized patients with IBD have a higher prevalence of malnutrition than patients hospitalized with other benign conditions[32] (see Table 14.1). CD patients, in particular, are susceptible to protein-calorie malnutrition, which contributes to both increased length of stay and hospital costs.[33,34] Protein-calorie malnutrition in IBD is often manifested clinically by weight loss.[35] Up to 70% of adult patients with CD are underweight, while fewer patients with UC experience weight loss, and weight loss is more commonly seen in hospitalized UC patients.[36–38]

Not only do hospitalized CD patients experience weight loss, but it is common in outpatients as well, and up to 75% of patients with CD experience weight loss.[1,39–41] CD patients have significantly lower lean body mass.[42] Even when CD patients are in remission, 20% of patients were more than 10% below their ideal body weight.[43] Patients with IBD lose fat stores, and male patients with CD have been shown to have a significantly lower percentage of body fat and hamstring muscle strength compared to healthy controls.[38,44] The reasons for protein-calorie malnutrition in IBD stem from ongoing inflammation and catabolic cytokine production, hypothalamic pituitary adrenal (HPA) axis dysregulation, and malabsorption of nutrients, along with diminished intake from abdominal discomfort.

While malnutrition is common, obesity can be seen, which can lead to protein-calorie malnutrition. Often fat occurs in a distribution of mesenteric fat, though this is often independent of body mass index. "Creeping fat" is seen in CD and is described as fat hypertrophy and visceral fat wrapping around the small and large bowel.[1] It was originally thought that creeping fat simply results from transmural inflammation, but emerging data show that mesenteric fat itself is proinflammatory with increased synthesis of TNFα and proinflammatory adipocytokines.[45] Hyperinsulinism, cortisol, and catecholamine imbalance, along with enhanced proinflammatory cytokines, make obesity a special consideration in the setting of concurrent IBD. Prednisone therapy can contribute to weight gain by decreasing lipid oxidation and increasing protein oxidation while increasing fatty mass and depleting muscle protein.[46,47] Together, hypercortisolism, corticosteroids, and obesity are a dangerous combination for the IBD patient from both a nutritional and disease-outcome point of view.

MECHANISMS OF GROWTH RETARDATION AND MALNUTRITION

Growth impairment in IBD is multifactorial with poor nutrition, mediators of chronic inflammation, and complications of therapy all contributing.[48,49] Decreased oral intake is frequently seen in those with high disease activity, which may be due to anorexia or sitophobia.[50] Even while in remission, patients may have lower daily intake of nutrients such as fiber and phosphorus.[44] In addition to reduced dietary intake, maldigestion, malabsorption, enteric loss of nutrients, and rapid GI transit contribute to malnutrition, particularly in CD, as do increased basal caloric requirements from active inflammation with inherent catabolic proinflammatory cytokine production or sepsis. Disease activity and extent can markedly influence the prevalence and degree of malnutrition in CD.[40] Patients with diffuse small bowel involvement typically are at more risk for malnutrition due to impaired absorption of nutrients, which can be similarly seen in small bowel resection and small bowel bacterial overgrowth.[43,51-52] Genetic susceptibility may also play a role as children with NODII/ CARD15 variants in CD had lower height and weight percentiles.[53] The growth hormone, insulin-like growth factor (IGF)-1, has been found to be involved in metabolic derangements in both children and adults with IBD. Total and free IGF-1 levels are reduced in patients with both CD and UC when compared to healthy controls and may be partially, but not completely, reversed by steroid therapy and TNF inhibitors.[54-56] After inflammation and disease activity is controlled, patients' nutritional status usually improves. Biologic therapies improve weight and body mass index (BMI) in children with active CD who respond to treatment.[57] Four to 6 years after patients with UC undergo total proctocolectomy with ileal pouch-anal anastomosis, muscular strength is increased by 11%, total tissue mass by 4.5%, and bone mineral density by almost 2%, suggesting the role of inflammation in metabolic disturbance.[52]

IMPLICATIONS OF MALNUTRITION

Malnutrition has many detrimental effects. It is associated with deterioration in muscle, respiratory, and immune function, as well as delayed wound healing and recovery from illness.[58] In children, malnutrition leads to stunted growth, and in all ages leads to weight loss.[59,60] CD patients have a greater loss of muscle than fat, particularly in ileal and ileocolic disease.[40] Patients often develop hypoalbuminemia, which results from increased catabolism and decreased synthesis due to ongoing inflammation, intestinal protein loss, reduced hepatic protein synthesis, malabsorption, and anorexia.[61] In the hospitalized setting, hypoalbuminemia portends an adverse prognosis for the IBD patient. Villous atrophy may occur as a result of malnutrition leading to poor nutrient absorption.[62] Malnourished patients may experience a low quality of life, depression, and anxiety.[63,64] Malnutrition on admission to a hospital has been correlated with longer length of stay, higher costs, and increased mortality.[65-67] IBD patients admitted with hypoalbuminemia and evidence of malnutrition require a prompt nutritional evaluation and early intervention. Individuals who undergo an aggressive correction of their underlying malnutrition in the hospital setting have improved outcomes, lower morbidity, lower mortality rates, and shorter hospital stays.[68,69]

NUTRITION AND BONE HEALTH

Malnutrition and systemic inflammation contribute to the decreased bone mineral density that occurs in patients with IBD though other factors such as corticosteroid use likely contribute.[70-74] In IBD, the prevalence of osteopenia is 50% while the prevalence for osteoporosis is 15%.[75] Though both patients with CD and UC are at risk for decreased bone density, those with CD carry greater risk.[76] Studies have shown that osteopenia may be seen in newly diagnosed patients with IBD prior to any steroid therapy.[77] This is contrasted, however, with a study demonstrating that women who developed IBD prior to age 20 were likely to have normal bone mineral density as adults.[78] Though steroid use has often been blamed for reduced bone mineral density in IBD, it has been shown to be a weak predictor of osteopenia in CD patients. Age, BMI, serum magnesium, and history of bowel resections appear to be more important predictors for low bone mineral density.[79,80] Calcium and vitamin D supplementation has been shown to maintain and increase bone mineral density in patients with CD.[81,82] Vitamin D can help regulate cytokine responses and dampen inflammatory responses.[83] The ability of vitamin D to influence the immunopathogenesis of IBD is reviewed elsewhere and shown in Figure 14.2.[84,85] Biologic therapy with infliximab is associated with increased markers of bone formation without increasing bone resorption.[86] Weight-bearing exercise should be encouraged while smoking should be avoided. All women with IBD should be supplemented with calcium and vitamin D according to the Dietary Reference Intakes. However, most experts agree that given the prevalence of vitamin D insufficiency (25(OH)D levels < 32 ng/mL) in CD, supplementation should be individualized to meet individual needs.

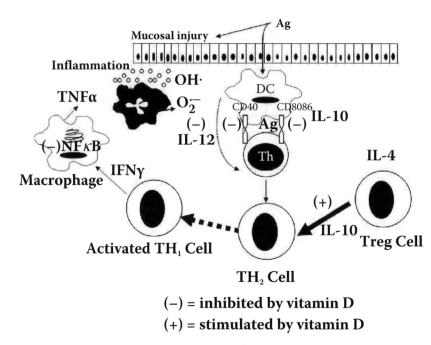

(−) = inhibited by vitamin D
(+) = stimulated by vitamin D

FIGURE 14.2 Potential role of vitamin D in CD: In CD, bacterial antigens drive antigen-presenting cells (DCs) to produce cytokines such as interleukin-12 (IL-12) to drive a T-helper (TH₁) proinflammatory response to induce macrophages, which produce TNFα and neutrophil chemoattractive agents that ultimately result in the production of noxious agents and tissue injury. The damaged intestinal tissue is more permeable to antigens, which drive the vicious cycle of antigen-presentation, local immune activation, and tissue injury. Anti-inflammatory cytokines such as interleukin-10 (IL-10), made by regulatory T cells (Tregs), antagonize TH₁ proinflammatory processes by stimulating T-helper 2 function. Vitamin D antagonizes TH₁ proinflammatory responses by interfering with antigen-presentation and TH₁ activation, up-regulating TH₂ cytokines, and down-regulating NFκB in macrophages. (From [85].)

NUTRIENT DEFICIENCIES

Vitamin and mineral deficiencies are commonly seen in IBD. Overall, low calcium and phosphorus levels occur in IBD as well as deficiencies in niacin, zinc, copper, and vitamins A and C.[87] In IBD, increased oxidative stress, oxidative damage to proteins and DNA, along with impaired antioxidant defenses in the form of mucosal zinc, copper, and superoxide dismutase has been shown in both serum and in the involved intestinal mucosa.[88] Every patient with IBD should be screened at least annually for vitamin and mineral deficiencies. The body systems most commonly impacted by nutrient inadequacies in IBD are summarized below.

Bone Health

The overall relative risk of fractures is 40% greater in IBD than in the general population—the prevalence of osteopenia and osteoporosis is 50% and 15%, respectively. The risk of fracture is similar for CD and UC and for both males and females with IBD. In relation to bone health, calcium, vitamin D, vitamin K, and magnesium deficiency occur. Vitamin D is not only important in bone health, but appears to have a role in immunomodulation as well. Vitamin D exerts its effects via vitamin D receptors on T-cells and antigen presenting cells. Vitamin D can antagonize T-helper 1 proinflammatory responses by interfering with antigen presentation and TH₁ activation, up-regulating TH₂ cytokines and down-regulation NFκB in macrophages.[85] (Figure 14.2.)

ANEMIA

In addition to vitamin D deficiency, anemia is frequently seen and may be related to iron, B12, and folic acid deficiency. Measurement of serum B12 should be performed annually in patients with ileal disease.[89] Methylmalonic acid (MMA) can be used as a more sensitive test for the diagnosis of cobalamin deficiency.[90] Hyperhomocysteinemia is seen in IBD and is associated with decreased levels of vitamin B12 and folate.[91]

IV. ROLE OF PARENTERAL NUTRITION

Previously, total parenteral nutrition (TPN) with bowel rest has been used as primary therapy for CD, though a key study in 1988 demonstrated that complete bowel rest was not a major factor in achieving clinical remission.[92] When feeding the gastrointestinal tract is not feasible, then TPN is used to provide nutritional support. TPN carries risks of sepsis and cholestatic liver disease (see Table 14.2). Complications are increased by overfeeding.[93] In animal models, long-term TPN use is associated with small intestine atrophy and increased intestinal permeability, while villous atrophy is not seen with enteral feeds, though this has not been uniformly seen in human studies.[94–97] A recent study of nationwide patterns of inpatient TPN utilization showed that usage was associated with higher in-hospital mortality, length of stay, and hospital costs ($51,729 vs. $19,563).[98] Total enteral nutrition can prevent malnutrition as well as TPN in patients with adequate bowel length, and thus should be favored over TPN due to preservation of mucosal integrity and favorable adverse effect profile relative to parenteral infusion.[99,100]

V. ROLE OF ENTERAL NUTRITION

The role of enteral nutrition as primary therapy is uncertain, particularly in adults. While enteral nutrition as primary therapy for active CD is less successful in inducing remission than steroid therapy, it has a better response than placebo.[101–103] Meta-analyses have shown that remission rates with enteral feeds in CD are approximately 60%.[102,104] Oral diet supplementation with low-residue nutrition has also been shown to improve nutritional status and decrease disease activity in CD.[105,106] One randomized control study showed that patients obtaining half of calories from an elemental diet and the remaining half from a polymeric diet was an effective strategy for reducing relapse compared to patients receiving all calories from a normal diet.[107] Often these studies are challenging to perform due to a large dropout rate from unpalatability or intolerance of the diet.[18] In terms of type of enteral feeds, elemental (amino acid-based) diets have not been shown to be more successful in inducing remission than nonelemental diets.[104,108] This is an important clinical pearl since elemental formulations are not palatable and noncompliance is an issue. In children, enteral nutritional support has a positive effect on growth and development and may help children avoid steroid use.[109,110]

TABLE 14.2
Complications of TPN

- Catheter-related infections
- Venous thrombosis
- Occlusion of catheter lumen
- Gallbladder stasis
- Hyperoxaluria
- Hepatic dysfunction

Source: [201].

MODE OF ACTION OF ENTERAL NUTRITION

It is unclear by what mechanism enteral nutrition acts to affect the inflammatory process in CD. Proposed mechanisms include provision of essential nutrients, reduction of antigenic load, alteration of bowel flora, and improved immune function.[111] The enteral diet may have an anti-inflammatory effect on the gastrointestinal mucosa, which may be related to the fatty acids in the feed or alteration of gut flora.[1,112–113] The feeds studied (AL110, Modulen IBD, and ACD004 [Nestle, Vevey, Switzerland]) all have casein as the protein source, are lactose free, and are rich in transforming growth factor beta (TGF-beta). They have all been shown to induce clinical remission associated with mucosal healing.[114] In the case of Modulen IBD, in addition to mucosal macroscopic and histological healing, there was a fall in mucosal proinflammatory cytokines: interleukin-1 mRNA in colon and ileum, interleukin-8 mRNA in colon and interferon gamma mRNA in ileum, but a rise in the regulatory cytokine TGF-beta mRNA in ileum. Taken together, these results indicate that these formulas are influencing the disease process itself, and thus suggest that the clinical remission achieved is a result of a reduction in inflammation, rather than a consequence of some other nutrition effect.

Clinical response to enteral nutrition is associated with mucosal healing and down-regulation of proinflammatory cytokines.[112] Modulen supplementation provided statistically significant protection against weight loss, hypoalbuminemia, acidosis, and GI damage in a rat model of IBD.[115] Though illustrative, future animal research of the mechanism of action of Modulen's protective effects is needed before further human trials are considered.

GLUTAMINE

The nonessential amino acid glutamine is a source of energy for intestinal epithelial cells, and it stimulates proliferation of intestinal epithelial cells.[116] In animal models of IBD, glutamine-enriched parenteral nutrition decreased bacterial translocation and stimulated IgA mucosal secretion.[117,118] New animal data have suggested that parenteral glutamine may have anti-inflammatory effects via the NFκB pathway with anti-TNFα properties.[119] These findings led to the hypothesis that glutamine-enriched parenteral nutrition may improve outcomes in patients with CD. Glutamine-enriched parenteral nutrition has failed to show a clinical benefit in patients with IBD compared to standard parenteral nutrition.[120] However, intestinal utilization of glutamine is impaired, thus mitigating attempts for restorative therapy.[121]

VI. OTHER DIETARY THERAPY IN IBD

As stated previously, though diet has been implicated in the pathogenesis of IBD, there is no definitive evidence linking a specific food or additive as a cause of IBD. Therefore, most patients are given a recommendation to follow a healthy, well-balanced diet. However, following are dietary strategies and management that have been studied further.

PUFAS

Dietary fat has been proposed to have a role in disease activity. One proposed mechanism for the efficacy of low-fat elemental diets is insufficient omega-6 fatty acids to synthesize proinflammatory eicosanoids.[122] The family of omega-3 fatty acids have the parent compound α-linoleic acid, which is synthesized into fatty acids important in immunomodulatory and anti-inflammatory effects via the production of prostaglandin class 3 and leukotriene B_5, and by inhibiting production of arachidonic acid and TNFα production.[17–19] These findings would suggest that a diet rich in omega-3 PUFAs may be protective against IBD while those rich in omega-6 PUFAs would promote inflammation. PUFAs may reduce the risk of recurrence in CD and may also have a role in UC.[123,124]

A controlled trial evaluated a polymeric enteral diet high in oleate acid (monounsaturated fat) versus an identical diet high in linoleate acid, and demonstrated that remission rates were better with the linoleate diet.[113] Elemental diets with increasing amounts of long-chain triglycerides (LCTs) had lower remission rates in active CD than the same diet with lower LCTs.[125] Soybean oil was used as the LCT with the principal fatty acids being oleic acid and linoleic acid. Based on the Cochrane Review, omega-3 fatty acids might be effective for maintenance therapy in CD, though this was not supported in UC (see Table 14.3).[126,127] Most recently, though, two randomized, placebo-controlled trials showed omega-3 fatty acids were not effective in the prevention of relapse in CD.[128]

SCFAs, LOW PARTICLE DIETS, AND POLYPHENOLS

In addition to PUFAs, other dietary strategies in IBD include SCFAs, low particle diets, and polyphenols.[15,27,123,124,129] The majority of studies on SCFAs have been performed in animals, but human studies have been performed. Though the studies were small, many prospective studies demonstrated clinical response or improvement with SCFA enemas (Table 14.4).[130–134] One small randomized controlled trial demonstrated a decrease in clinical index activity scores in patients with UC treated with 30 g of germinated barley, which increased luminal butyrate production.[29]

Microparticles have been proposed to exacerbate inflammation via antigen-mediated immune responses.[30] An initial pilot study of 20 patients showed that those on a diet low in microparticles had a significant improvement in CD activity index, though a follow-up multicenter randomized controlled trail showed no improvement in CD activity with reduced microparticle intake in the diet.[135,136]

Polyphenols are phytochemicals found in food substances produced from plants and have been found to be potentially immunomodulating.[137] Examples of polyphenols include resveratrol, epigallocatechin, and curcumin. Resveratrol is found most abundantly in the skin of red grapes.[138] Resveratrol appears to have anti-inflammatory and immunomodulatory effects, though the mechanism has not been clearly established.[15] In rodent models of inflammatory colitis, resveratrol has been shown to reverse weight loss, increase stool consistency, improve mucosal appearance, improve histology, decrease inflammatory infiltrate, and decrease mucosal levels of interleukin-1β, COX-2, and prostaglandin D_2.[139] To date, resveratrol has not been studied in human subjects with IBD.

TABLE 14.3

Omega-3 Fatty Acids for Maintenance of Remission in CD (from Cochrane Review)
Review: Omega-3 fatty acids (fish oil) for maintenance of remission in Crohn's disease
Comparison: Omega-3 versus placebo
Outcome: Relapse rate at 1 year (all studies)

Study	Treatment n/N	Control n/N	Relative Risk (Random) 95% CI	Weight (%)	Relative Risk (Random) 95% CI
Belluzzi 1996	11/39	27/39		26.3	0.41 [0.24, 0.70]
Belluzzi 1997	2/26	5/24		7.8	0.37 [0.08, 1.73]
Lorenz-Meyer 1996	40/70	36/65		34.3	1.03 [0.77, 1.39]
Romano 2005	11/18	19/20		31.6	0.64 [0.44, 0.94]
Total (95% CI)	153	148		100.0	0.64 [0.40, 1.04]

Total events: 64 (Treatment), 87 (Control)
Test for heterogeneity chi-square = w
  10.89 df = 3 p = 0.01 I^2 = 72.4%
Test for overall effect z = 1.80 p = 0.07

	0.1	0.2	0.5	1	2	5	10	
	Favors treatment				Favors control			

Source: [123, 126, 202, 203].

TABLE 14.4
Prospective Studies of Short Chain Fatty Acids for Left-Sided Ulcerative Colitis

Study	Design	No. Patients (Treatment)	Study Duration (wk)	Butyrate Dose	Results
Scheppach	Single-blind	10 (Butyrate enema)	2	100 mM	↓ Stool frequency, hematochezia, ↓ Endoscopic histologic score
Breuer	Crossover Open-label	10 (Placebo) 10 (SCFA enema)	6	100 mL bid 40 mM 100 mL bid	No change with placebo ↓ Disease activity index ↓ Mucosal histology score
Steinhart	Open-label	10 (Butyrate enema)	6	80 mM 60 mL qd	↓ Disease activity index 60% Response 40% Complete remission
Patz	Open-label	10 (SCFA enema)	6	40 mM 100 mL bid	5/10 Endoscopic and clinical improvement
Vernia	Open-label	10 (Butyrate + 5-ASA enema)	6	80 mM 100 mL bid	7/9 Endoscopic, clinical, and histologic improvement

Source: [130–134].

Catechins such as epigallocatechin gallate (EGCG) are abundant in green (nonfermented) tea.[140] Green tea has been linked to beneficial effects in prevention or treatment of cancers such as breast, lung, ovarian, prostate, and stomach, as well as in diseases such as hypertension and cardiovascular health.[15] EGCG can modulate and inhibit NFκB activity, which may affect inflammation.[141] Similar to resveratrol, green tea has been shown to improve disease activity in murine models of colitis.[142–144] An in vitro study involving human colonic tissues showed that EGCG administration resulted in decreased proinflammatory cytokine production, but to date, there are no in vivo human studies to evaluate the role of green tea extract in IBD.[145]

Another phytonutrient studied for its anti-inflammatory role is curcumin. Turmeric, from the herb *Curcuma longa*, is the major spice found in curry. Curcumin is the major chemical constituent of turmeric. Curcumin has been used as an oral and topical agent to treat a variety of ailments and has had an excellent safety profile.[146,147] Curcumin appears to have multiple mechanisms of action including NFκB inhibition, thereby likely down-regulating proinflammatory genes and cytokines.[148] Overall, in animal models of colitis, curcumin has demonstrated positive effects.[149–154] A randomized controlled trial of 89 patients with quiescent UC were administered 1 g of curcumin twice daily and had clinical improvement and a significant decrease in the rate of relapse.[155]

VII. SUPPORTING COLONIC MICROBES

PREBIOTICS AND PROBIOTICS

Disturbances in bacterial intestinal flora have been purported as a triggering factor for IBD.[156] Therapy with prebiotics and probiotics may present a treatment option with few side effects. Animal models suggest probiotics may be useful in the treatment of UC and CD.[157,158] Probiotics are living microbes that can benefit the host once introduced. Examples include lactobacilli, bifidobacteria, and yeast species such as *Saccharomyces boulardii*.[159] Based on animal models, probiotics can alter gastrointestinal flora and ameliorate disease.[160] Probiotics also produce SCFAs.[161] Pouchitis is a complication of surgery for UC and is typically treated effectively with antibiotics, suggesting a role of bacteria.[162] In patients with chronic pouchitis induced to remission with antibiotic therapy, VSL#3, a well-studied probiotic, was successful in maintaining remission.[163] VSL#3 may also have a role as primary prophylaxis of pouchitis in patients with ileal pouch-anal anastomosis.[164] There have been studies, however, that demonstrated no significant benefit of VSL#3 in maintaining remission induced by antibiotics.[165] Trials using a combination of probiotic species (such as VSL#3) have yielded more successful results than those using only a single species.[166] Prebiotics may also have a role in antibiotic-refractory or antibiotic-dependent pouchitis.

Probiotics have been shown to be efficacious in maintenance therapy in UC. Three randomized controlled trials showed that *Escherichia coli* Nissle 1917 equaled conventional 5-ASA treatment.[167–169] Studies using other probiotic species have yielded mixed results. Probiotics have also been studied in the treatment of active UC. VSL#3 used in combination with low-dose balsalazide had shorter time to remission than balsalazide alone.[170] Of note, the doses of balsalazide were lower than typically used in a clinical scenario. Probiotics have also been used as topical therapy with *E. coli* Nissle 1917 enemas and led to remission, with the time to remission being shortest with the highest dose of enema.[171]

Prebiotics are compounds that promote intestinal proliferation of probiotic bacteria (also metabolized into SCFAs). Most prebiotics are from the group of dietary fibers found in foods such as legumes, artichokes, onions, garlic, banana, soya and other beans.[172] Examples of prebiotics are inulin and oligofructose. When these prebiotics are given in sufficient amounts they selectively promote the growth of bifidobacteria.[173] Animal models of IBD have shown inulin to reduce inflammatory mediators and reduce histological damage scores.[174] Along with inulin, other prebiotics such as oligofructose and lactulose have shown anti-inflammatory effects in animal modes of IBD.[175,176] In clinical studies, inulin as compared to placebo was associated with improvement in inflammation in chronic pouchitis.[177] Combining probiotics and prebiotics as synbiotics may play a role in the treatment of IBD. In mild UC, a synbiotic preparation (oligofructose-enriched inulin and *Bifidobacterium longum*) compared to placebo showed a trend in reduction of mucosal expression of proinflammatory cytokines (TNFα), improvement in inflammation on a histological level and by clinical activity indices.[178]

Probiotics have been studied in CD as well. One studied showed patients using *S. boulardii* plus mesalazine had fewer relapses than those using mesalazine alone.[179] There have been other studies, however, that did not demonstrate probiotics to be effective in a maintenance strategy in CD.[180,181] Prebiotics and synbiotics have not been extensively studied in the maintenance of CD. In treating active CD, probiotics have not been shown to significantly have a role in treatment, though one study showed that prebiotics may reduce disease activity in active CD.[182] Research on probiotics and prebiotics in this area is limited for a number of reasons, including enrollment of small number of patients, variability in choice of probiotic or prebiotic used, and variability in patients' diets. Larger randomized controlled trials are needed to determine the role of probiotics and prebiotics in the treatment of IBD (see Tables 14.5 and 14.6).

VIII. FOOD INTOLERANCE AND IBD

Irritable bowel syndrome (IBS) occurs with increased frequency and severity given the underlying chronic inflammation in IBD, and physicians need to recognize this in order to avoid use of IBD therapy to treat symptoms resulting from IBS.[183] Patients may have intolerance to many foods, including but not limited to dairy products, caffeine, fried foods, and foods with high fiber content.[184] It is important to note that food intolerance is not a true allergic reaction; if foods cause a true allergic reaction they need to be completely avoided. Patients who have intolerance to certain foods should try to avoid specific triggers in order to minimize their symptoms.

GLUTEN

Celiac disease has been noted with increased frequency among patients with CD.[185] Rather than recommending a gluten-free diet for all, if patients continue to have ongoing symptoms despite

TABLE 14.5
Probiotics in Inflammatory Bowel Disease

Author	Year	Probiotic	Result
Kruis	1997	*E. coli* Nissle 1917	Equal to mesalamine
Rembacken	1999	*E. coli* Nissle 1917	Equal to mesalamine
Guslandi	2000	*S. boulardii*	Equal to mesalamine
Ishikawa	2003	*Bifidobacterium* milk	Superior to placebo
Borody	2003	Stool enema	Improved
Kruis	2004	*E. coli* Nissle	Superior to conventional
Kato	2004	*Bifidobacterium* milk	Superior to placebo
Furrie	2005	*Bifidobacterium* + fiber	Improved

Source: [167–169, 178–179, 204–206].

treatment for CD, testing for celiac disease should ensue. In general, only those with celiac disease should be given a gluten-free diet. Given that there is not enough data to support or refute a recommendation concerning gluten sensitivity testing for IBD, it is reasonable as experts for us to suggest that clinicians query patients as to their possible intolerance to gluten and if suspicious, IgG_1/IgG_4 antibody testing should be considered.

FIBER

IBD, particularly CD, can result in complications of intestinal strictures, fistulas, high-output ostomy, as well as short bowel syndrome. Though patients with nonstricturing CD do not benefit universally from a low residue diet, most experts in IBD would recommend a low residue diet in patients who have ongoing intestinal strictures.[186] As discussed previously, soluble fiber is fermented by enteric bacteria into short-chain fatty acids, which are crucial to the metabolism and healing of colonic enterocytes. Insoluble fiber products help serve as prebiotic products to facilitate population of beneficial enteric bacteria. Thus, continued intake of adequate fiber is helpful for patients with both forms of IBD; however, tolerance can limit intake based upon disease manifestations (i.e., stricturing). Patients with intestinal fistula, high-output ostomy, and short bowel syndrome

TABLE 14.6
Prebiotics in Ulcerative Colitis

Author	Year	Fiber	Study	Outcome
Fernandez-Banares	1999	Plantago ovata seed fiber 10 grams BID	Fiber +/− mesalamine in patients in remission	Equal to mesalamine in maintenance of remission
Kanauchi	2002 2003	Barley 20–30 grams	Mild to moderately active UC	Decreased disease activity
Hallert	2003	Oat bran 60 grams (fiber 20 grams)	Patients in remission	Decreased abdominal pain, increased fecal butyrate
Welters	2002	Inulin 24 grams	IPAA	Deceased pouch inflammation

Source: [29, 177, 207–209].
IPAA = ileal pouch–anal anastomosis

often are difficult to manage from a nutrition standpoint. Careful management of fluid and electrolyte disturbances is essential, and parenteral nutrition may be necessary in some cases.[187]

IX.   PATIENT EVALUATION

INFLAMMATION AND DISEASE ACTIVITY

In the evaluation of the patient with IBD, disease activity needs to be assessed. Inflammation plays a role in malnutrition as well as in potential complications of IBD such as osteoporosis and colorectal cancer. Medications need to be adjusted to maintain patients in remission. Often, if disease flare is suspected, markers of inflammation may be ordered, including erythrocyte sedimentation rate (ESR) and C-reactive protein (CRP).

MALNUTRITION

At each visit, the patient's weight and BMI should be recorded to assess for weight loss as a marker of protein-calorie malnutrition.

VOLUME DEPLETION/DEHYDRATION

Patients with intestinal fistula, high-output ostomy, and short bowel syndrome often are difficult to manage from a nutrition standpoint. Careful management of fluid and electrolyte disturbances is essential, and parenteral nutrition may be necessary in some cases.[187] If patients with CD have these complications, orthostatic vital signs should be performed to assess for adequate fluid hydration.

NUTRIENT DEFICIENCIES

Laboratory studies that should be followed periodically include vitamin B12 levels, particularly in patients with ileal CD. If there is evidence of anemia, iron studies and folic acid levels may need to be assessed. Since patients with IBD are at risk for osteoporosis, vitamin D levels should be ordered, and dual-energy x-ray absorptiometry (DEXA) should be assessed soon after diagnosis and repeated in about 1 year. Other fat-soluble vitamins may be deficient, such as vitamin A, E, and K. Minerals other than iron may be deficient in IBD; these include magnesium, selenium, zinc, and copper. Zinc is commonly deficient in CD, and copper status is unknown. In UC, these trace minerals are unlikely to be deficient unless patients have profuse diarrhea.[188] Selenium deficiency may be seen in patients on long-term parenteral nutrition or in patients who have undergone significant small bowel resections.[189] Serum levels should be checked as selenium is an essential cofactor for glutathione peroxidase, which helps detoxify hydroxyl free radicals, which are overabundant in inflamed tissues.

X.   TREATMENT APPROACHES

AVOID UNNECESSARY FOOD RESTRICTION

Most patients and some providers believe that diet influences their disease and this can lead to unnecessary food restriction.[190] It is important to establish food intolerance as a separate entity, not part of IBD itself. As such, one patient's food intolerance should not be generalized to a recommendation appropriate for IBD at large. For example, there is no evidence that a gluten-free diet is efficacious in CD if celiac disease is absent; however, if gluten sensitivity is suspected and confirmed via IgG testing or an elimination trial, removal is warranted.[191] Patients with IBD need to eat healthful diets with as few restrictions as possible. Unnecessary food restrictions can have harmful effects:

- *Removing spicy foods* from the diet would lessen the phytonutrient curcumin and other less studied nutrients known to temper inflammation.

- *Removing gluten-containing foods* as a general rule has been shown to result in unhealthful food selection that the patient may mistakenly consider healthful solely because it is gluten-free. Confirmation of gluten sensitivity, if suspected, should be done prior to removal from the diet.
- *Avoiding foods containing lactose* may not be necessary if the patient tolerates lactose. Following a lactose-free diet can reduce the intake of highly absorbable minerals, and fermented dairy products are a source of probiotics. Breath hydrogen testing should be performed if lactose intolerance is suspected.
- *Avoiding nuts and seeds* as a potential IBD trigger in patients who are not demonstrated to have allergies or sensitivities to these foods results in unnecessary restriction of monounsaturated fats, minerals, and protein. For example, walnuts are a rich source of omega-3 fatty acids, which are anti-inflammatory in nature and can benefit patients with IBD. Nuts and seeds are often substituted for processed snack foods known to be proinflammatory. Nuts and seeds may need to be avoided in patients with stricturing disease or ostomies.

Be Careful with Red Meat

Use caution with red meat, due to colorectal cancer risk. Topical nutrients are preferentially used by the gut mucosa to maintain structure and function. With the colon, topical nutrients are generated by the colonic microbiota to maintain mucosal health. As previously mentioned, SCFAs control proliferation and differentiation, thereby reducing colon cancer risk. Unfortunately, the microbiota may also elaborate toxic products from food residues such as genotoxic hydrogen sulfide by sulfur-reducing bacteria in response to a high-meat diet. Most nutritionists suggest abundant red meat in the diet of IBD patients due to microscopic blood loss from the chronic inflammation. Iron, although important to maintain sufficiency, can be a pro-oxidant by catalyzing superoxide anion formation. Thus, caution needs to be exercised with regard to iron intake in IBD patients.[88] Patients with both forms of IBD have an increased risk of acquiring colorectal cancer. Given the connection of red meat and processed meats to colorectal cancer, advising patients to consume an ad lib diet of red meat and or processed meats as is done in most hospital centers is concerning and should be scrutinized.[192-194]

Minimize Bone Loss

To minimize bone loss, calcium supplements should be given at doses of 1200 mg/day with vitamin D supplementation at 800 IU/day. If vitamin D deficiency is found, repletion and maintenance will be needed. Finally, patients may need bisphosphonates to treat osteoporosis.

Replenish Nutrient Deficiencies

1. Hypovitaminosis D: IBD, particularly small bowel CD, patients are susceptible to vitamin D deficiency. This often is manifested by low 25(OH)D levels. A target serum level of 32 ng/mL or greater is considered the optimal serum 25(OH)D level. For vitamin D deficiency (25(OH)D < 20 ng/mL), initial treatment should be 50,000 IU of vitamin D2 or D3 orally once per week for 6 to 8 weeks, then 800 to 1000 IU of vitamin D3 daily, thereafter.[195] For vitamin D insufficiency, 25(OH)D 20-30 ng/mL, 800 to 1000 IU of vitamin D3 should be given daily and this should bring levels within the target range in approximately 3 months. Vitamin D (25(OH)D) should be measured 3 months after beginning therapy. In patients with malabsorption, repletion will vary. These patients may need higher doses of vitamin D of 10,000 to 50,000 IU daily. Calcium supplementation of 1000 to 1200 mg should be given with vitamin D. Vitamin D toxicity can occur at levels of 88 ng/mL or greater, and the first signs of toxicity include hypercalciuria and hypercalcemia.[196,197]

2. Iron deficiency: Anemia is frequently seen in IBD, and iron status should be assessed. Iron deficiency in IBD is typically caused by chronic blood loss. Though oral iron supplementation has not been shown to worsen disease activity, patients may develop gastrointestinal side effects.[198] With oral supplementation, usually ferrous sulfate 325 mg three times daily is given, though if patients develop gastrointestinal upset, ferrous gluconate may be substituted. Other tips for patients suffering from side effects of iron therapy include gradually increasing the dose from one time per day to three times per day or taking it with food, though absorption will be decreased. Parenteral iron is usually given to patients who do not tolerate oral iron or where blood loss exceeds the ability of the GI tract to absorb iron.

3. Vitamin B12 deficiency: Patients with B12 deficiency do not always have evidence of anemia or it may be mild. Therefore, serum cobalamin should be assessed periodically, particularly in patients with ileal CD or following ileal resection. If the serum cobalamin level is greater than 300 pg/mL, this is normal and cobalamin deficiency is unlikely. Levels less than 200 pg/mL are consistent with cobalamin deficiency. If the level ranges between 200 to 300 pg/mL, cobalamin deficiency is possible and further testing may be needed with measurement of MMA and homocysteine levels. If both tests are normal with MMA levels of 70 to 270 nmol/L and homocysteine of 5 to 14 μmol/L, then cobalamin deficiency is unlikely. If MMA and homocysteine levels are increased, then cobalamin deficiency is likely, though folate deficiency may be present as well. If MMA is normal, but homocysteine is elevated, then folate deficiency is likely.[90] Patients with cobalamin deficiency are treated with a dose of cobalamin 1000 μg or 1 mg daily for 1 week followed by 1 mg/week for 4 weeks, then 1 mg/month. Serum cobalamin levels should be monitored after therapy.

4. Folate deficiency: Folate deficiency is frequently seen in both UC and CD and is multifactorial, with insufficiency dietary amounts of folic acid and side effects of medicine contributing. Serum folate levels reflect short-term folate balance, while red blood cell (RBC) folate is a more accurate measure of tissue folate.[199] However, if the serum folate is > 4 ng/mL, folate deficiency is unlikely. If serum folate is between 2 to 4 ng/mL, then RBC folate can be measured along with the metabolites described above (MMA and homocysteine). Serum folate < 2 ng/mL is essentially diagnostic of deficiency in the absence of recent fasting or anorexia, which may be frequent, particularly in hospitalized patients. Typically, folate is repleted with 1 mg of folic acid daily for 1 to 4 months or longer if needed. It is important to rule out cobalamin deficiency before treating a patient with folic acid. Recent literature suggests that repletion with folate in doses greater than 1 mg/day can actually be harmful.[200]

Receive Specialized Nutrition Support

In patients receiving TPN, serum electrolytes, glucose, calcium, magnesium, phosphate, aminotransferases, bilirubin, and triglycerides should be measured regularly. The catheter site needs to be monitored to assess for signs of infection. See Table 14.2 for complications related to TPN use. Avoid overfeeding to "catch up," as many patients with IBD are malnourished in the hospitalized setting. Overzealous feeding, termed "refeeding syndrome" is a particularly deadly complication of TPN that is under-recognized by physicians worldwide.

XI. SUMMARY

Given the challenges in research in the area of nutrition in IBD, there is no clear evidence that any specific diet either is a cause or a "cure" for IBD. Thus, in order to prevent food restriction, patients should be encouraged to follow a healthy diet as tolerated, but be mindful to follow an anti-inflammatory Mediterranean type diet whenever possible. When supplemental nutrition is necessary, enteral therapy should be used over parenteral therapy if the gut can be used. Medical therapy needs to be initiated to achieve remission to minimize inflammation, and this varies from 5-ASA medications to infliximab. Supplementation with polyphenols, probiotics, and fish oils should be considered as adjuncts to care. Patients should be counseled on the risk of osteopenia and osteoporosis and be encouraged to take calcium and vitamin D, if deficient. Other nutrients may be deficient as well, and should be evaluated and repleted when deficient.

REFERENCES

1. O'Sullivan M, O'Morain C. Nutrition in inflammatory bowel disease. *Best Practice & Research Clinical Gastroenterology*. 2006;20(3):561–573.
2. Loftus CG, Loftus EV, Jr, Harmsen WS, et al. Update on the incidence and prevalence of Crohn's disease and ulcerative colitis in Olmsted County, Minnesota, 1940–2000. *Inflamm Bowel Dis*. 2007;13(3):254–261.
3. Shoda R, Matsueda K, Yamato S, Umeda N. Epidemiologic analysis of Crohn disease in Japan: Increased dietary intake of n-6 polyunsaturated fatty acids and animal protein relates to the increased incidence of Crohn disease in Japan. *Am J Clin Nutr*. 1996;63(5):741–745.
4. Jarnerot G, Jarnmark I, Nilsson K. Consumption of refined sugar by patients with Crohn's disease, ulcerative colitis, or irritable bowel syndrome. *Scand J Gastroenterol*. 1983;18(8):999–1002.
5. Sakamoto N, Kono S, Wakai K, et al. Dietary risk factors for inflammatory bowel disease: A multicenter case-control study in Japan. *Inflamm Bowel Dis*. 2005;11(2):154–163.
6. Kelly DG, Fleming CR. Nutritional considerations in inflammatory bowel diseases. *Gastroenterol Clin North Am*. 1995;24(3):597–611.
7. Behr MA, Kapur V. The evidence for mycobacterium paratuberculosis in Crohn's disease. *Curr Opin Gastroenterol*. 2008;24(1):17–21.
8. Akobeng AK, Thomas AG. Enteral nutrition for maintenance of remission in Crohn's disease. *Cochrane Database Syst Rev*. 2007;(3):CD005984.
9. Suzuki H, Hanyou N, Sonaka I, Minami H. An elemental diet controls inflammation in indomethacin-induced small bowel disease in rats: The role of low dietary fat and the elimination of dietary proteins. *Dig Dis Sci*. 2005;50(10):1951–1958.
10. Chutkan RK. Inflammatory bowel disease. *Prim Care*. 2001;28(3):539–556, vi.
11. Podolsky DK. Inflammatory bowel disease. *N Engl J Med*. 2002;347(6):417–429.
12. Razack R, Seidner DL. Nutrition in inflammatory bowel disease. *Curr Opin Gastroenterol*. 2007;23(4):400–405.
13. Sartor RB. Mechanisms of disease: Pathogenesis of Crohn's disease and ulcerative colitis. *Nat Clin Pract Gastroenterol Hepatol*. 2006;3(7):390–407.
14. Hodin R. Maintaining gut homeostasis: The butyrate-NF-kappaB connection. *Gastroenterology*. 2000;118(4):798–801.
15. Clarke JO, Mullin GE. A review of complementary and alternative approaches to immunomodulation. *Nutr Clin Pract*. 2008;23(1):49–62.
16. Hudert CA, Weylandt KH, Lu Y, et al. Transgenic mice rich in endogenous omega-3 fatty acids are protected from colitis. *Proc Natl Acad Sci USA*. 2006;103(30):11276–11281.
17. Miura S, Tsuzuki Y, Hokari R, Ishii H. Modulation of intestinal immune system by dietary fat intake: Relevance to Crohn's disease. *J Gastroenterol Hepatol*. 1998;13(12):1183–1190.
18. Wild GE, Drozdowski L, Tartaglia C, Clandinin MT, Thomson AB. Nutritional modulation of the inflammatory response in inflammatory bowel disease—from the molecular to the integrative to the clinical. *World J Gastroenterol*. 2007;13(1):1–7.
19. Caughey GE, Mantzioris E, Gibson RA, Cleland LG, James MJ. The effect on human tumor necrosis factor alpha and interleukin 1 beta production of diets enriched in n-3 fatty acids from vegetable oil or fish oil. *Am J Clin Nutr*. 1996;63(1):116–122.
20. Zhang P, Kim W, Zhou L, et al. Dietary fish oil inhibits antigen-specific murine Th1 cell development by suppression of clonal expansion. *J Nutr*. 2006;136(9):2391–2398.
21. Whiting CV, Bland PW, Tarlton JF. Dietary n-3 polyunsaturated fatty acids reduce disease and colonic proinflammatory cytokines in a mouse model of colitis. *Inflamm Bowel Dis*. 2005;11(4):340–349.
22. Kles KA, Chang EB. Short-chain fatty acids impact on intestinal adaptation, inflammation, carcinoma, and failure. *Gastroenterology*. 2006;130(2 Suppl 1):S100–105.
23. James SL, Muir JG, Curtis SL, Gibson PR. Dietary fibre: A roughage guide. *Intern Med J*. 2003;33(7):291–296.

24. Dray X, Marteau P. The use of enteral nutrition in the management of Crohn's disease in adults. *JPEN J Parenter Enteral Nutr*. 2005;29(4 Suppl):S166–169; discussion S169–172, S184–188.

25. Roediger WE. The colonic epithelium in ulcerative colitis: An energy-deficiency disease? *Lancet*. 1980;2(8197):712–715.

26. Yamamoto T, Nakahigashi M, Umegae S, Kitagawa T, Matsumoto K. Impact of elemental diet on mucosal inflammation in patients with active Crohn's disease: Cytokine production and endoscopic and histological findings. *Inflamm Bowel Dis*. 2005;11(6):580–588.

27. Segain JP, Raingeard de la Bletiere D, Bourreille A, et al. Butyrate inhibits inflammatory responses through NFkappaB inhibition: Implications for Crohn's disease. *Gut*. 2000;47(3):397–403.

28. Binder HJ, Mehta P. Short-chain fatty acids stimulate active sodium and chloride absorption in vitro in the rat distal colon. *Gastroenterology*. 1989;96(4):989–996.

29. Kanauchi O, Suga T, Tochihara M, et al. Treatment of ulcerative colitis by feeding with germinated barley foodstuff: First report of a multicenter open control trial. *J Gastroenterol*. 2002;37 Suppl 14:67–72.

30. Lomer MC, Thompson RP, Powell JJ. Fine and ultrafine particles of the diet: Influence on the mucosal immune response and association with Crohn's disease. *Proc Nutr Soc*. 2002;61(1):123–130.

31. Korzenik JR. Past and current theories of etiology of IBD: Toothpaste, worms, and refrigerators. *J Clin Gastroenterol*. 2005;39(4 Suppl 2):S59–65.

32. Pirlich M, Schutz T, Kemps M, et al. Prevalence of malnutrition in hospitalized medical patients: Impact of underlying disease. *Dig Dis*. 2003;21(3):245–251.

33. O'Sullivan M, O'Morain C. Nutritional therapy in inflammatory bowel disease. *Curr Treat Options Gastroenterol*. 2004;7(3):191–198.

34. Harries AD, Jones L, Heatley RV, Rhodes J, Fitzsimons E. Mid-arm circumference as simple means of identifying malnutrition in Crohn's disease. *Br Med J (Clin Res Ed)*. 1982;285(6351):1317–1318.

35. Silk DB, Payne-James J. Inflammatory bowel disease: Nutritional implications and treatment. *Proc Nutr Soc*. 1989;48(3):355–361.

36. O'Keefe SJ. Nutrition and gastrointestinal disease. *Scand J Gastroenterol Suppl*. 1996;220:52–59.

37. Burke A, Lichtenstein G, Rombeau J. Nutrition and ulcerative colitis. *Bailliére's Clinical Gastroenterology*. 1997;11(1):153–174.

38. Powell-Tuck J. Protein metabolism in inflammatory bowel disease. *Gut*. 1986;27 Suppl 1:67–71.

39. Dyer NH, Dawson AM. Malnutrition and malabsorption in Crohn's disease with reference to the effect of surgery. *Br J Surg*. 1973;60(2):134–140.

40. Lanfranchi GA, Brignola C, Campieri M, et al. Assessment of nutritional status in Crohn's disease in remission or low activity. *Hepatogastroenterology*. 1984;31(3):129–132.

41. Heatley RV. Assessing nutritional state in inflammatory bowel disease. *Gut*. 1986;27 Suppl 1:61–66.

42. Jahnsen J, Falch JA, Mowinckel P, Aadland E. Body composition in patients with inflammatory bowel disease: A population-based study. *Am J Gastroenterol*. 2003;98(7):1556–1562.

43. Harries AD, Jones LA, Heatley RV, Rhodes J. Malnutrition in inflammatory bowel disease: An anthropometric study. *Hum Nutr Clin Nutr*. 1982;36(4):307–313.

44. Geerling BJ, Badart-Smook A, Stockbrugger RW, Brummer RJ. Comprehensive nutritional status in patients with long-standing Crohn disease currently in remission. *Am J Clin Nutr*. 1998;67(5):919–926.

45. Schaffler A, Scholmerich J, Buchler C. Mechanisms of disease: Adipocytokines and visceral adipose tissue—emerging role in intestinal and mesenteric diseases. *Nat Clin Pract Gastroenterol Hepatol*. 2005;2(2):103–111.

46. Al-Jaouni R, Schneider SM, Piche T, Rampal P, Hebuterne X. Effect of steroids on energy expenditure and substrate oxidation in women with Crohn's disease. *Am J Gastroenterol*. 2002;97(11):2843–2849.

47. Cabre E, Gassull MA. Nutritional and metabolic issues in inflammatory bowel disease. *Curr Opin Clin Nutr Metab Care*. 2003;6(5):569–576.

48. Baldassano RN, Piccoli DA. Inflammatory bowel disease in pediatric and adolescent patients. *Gastroenterol Clin North Am*. 1999;28(2):445–458.

49. Reilly J, Ryan J, Strole W, Fischer J. Hyperalimentation in inflammatory bowel disease. *The American Journal of Surgery*. 1976;131(2):192–200.

50. Rigaud D, Angel LA, Cerf M, et al. Mechanisms of decreased food intake during weight loss in adult Crohn's disease patients without obvious malabsorption. *Am J Clin Nutr*. 1994;60(5):775–781.

51. Sandstrom B, Davidsson L, Bosaeus I, Eriksson R, Alpsten M. Selenium status and absorption of zinc (65Zn), selenium (75Se) and manganese (54Mn) in patients with short bowel syndrome. *Eur J Clin Nutr*. 1990;44(10):697–703.

52. Jensen MB, Houborg KB, Vestergaard P, Kissmeyer-Nielsen P, Mosekilde L, Laurberg S. Improved physical performance and increased lean tissue and fat mass in patients with ulcerative colitis four to six years after ileoanal anastomosis with a J-pouch. *Dis Colon Rectum.* 2002;45(12):1601–1607.

53. Tomer G, Ceballos C, Concepcion E, Benkov KJ. NOD2/CARD15 variants are associated with lower weight at diagnosis in children with Crohn's disease. *Am J Gastroenterol.* 2003;98(11):2479–2484.

54. Grønbæk H, Thøgersen T, Frystyk J, Vilstrup H, Flyvbjerg A, Dahlerup JF. Low free and total insulinlike growth factor I (IGF-I) and IGF binding protein-3 levels in chronic inflammatory bowel disease: Partial normalization during prednisolone treatment. *The American Journal of Gastroenterology.* 2002;97(3):673–678.

55. Eivindson M, Grønbæk H, Flyvbjerg A, Frystyk J, Zimmermann-Nielsen E, Dahlerup JF. The insulin-like growth factor (IGF)-system in active ulcerative colitis and Crohn's disease: Relations to disease activity and corticosteroid treatment. *Growth Hormone & IGF Research,* 2007;17(1):33–40.

56. Eivindson M, Grønbæk H, Skogstrand K, et al. The insulin-like growth factor (IGF) system and its relation to infliximab treatment in adult patients with Crohn's disease. *Scand J Gastroenterol.* 2007;42(4):464–470.

57. Walters TD, Gilman AR, Griffiths AM. Linear growth improves during infliximab therapy in children with chronically active severe Crohn's disease. *Inflamm Bowel Dis.* 2007;13(4):424–430.

58. O'Sullivan MA, O'Morain CA. Nutritional therapy in Crohn's disease. *Inflamm Bowel Dis.* 1998;4(1):45–53.

59. Burbige EJ, Huang SH, Bayless TM. Clinical manifestations of Crohn's disease in children and adolescents. *Pediatrics.* 1975;55(6):866.

60. McCaffery TD, Nasr K, Lawrence AM, Kirsner JB. Severe growth retardation in children with inflammatory bowel disease. *Pediatrics.* 1970;45(3):386.

61. Stokes MA. Crohn's disease and nutrition. *Br J Surg.* 1992;79(5):391–394.

62. Winter TA, Lemmer ER, O'Keefe SJ, Ogden JM. The effect of severe undernutrition, and subsequent refeeding on digestive function in human patients. *Eur J Gastroenterol Hepatol.* 2000;12(2):191–196.

63. Norman K, Kirchner H, Lochs H, Pirlich M. Malnutrition affects quality of life in gastroenterology patients. *World J Gastroenterol.* 2006;12(21):3380–3385.

64. Addolorato G, Capristo E, Stefanini GF, Gasbarrini G. Inflammatory bowel disease: A study of the association between anxiety and depression, physical morbidity, and nutritional status. *Scand J Gastroenterol.* 1997;32(10):1013–1021.

65. Weinsier RL, Hunker EM, Krumdieck CL, Butterworth CE, Jr. Hospital malnutrition. A prospective evaluation of general medical patients during the course of hospitalization. *Am J Clin Nutr.* 1979; 32(2):418–426.

66. Chima C, Barco K, Dewitt MA, Maeda M, Teran JC, Mullen K. Relationship of nutritional status to length of stay, hospital costs, and discharge status of patients hospitalized in the medicine service. *Journal of the American Dietetic Association.* 1997;97(9):975–978.

67. Nguyen GC, Munsell M, Harris ML. Nationwide prevalence and prognostic significance of clinically diagnosable protein-calorie malnutrition in hospitalized inflammatory bowel disease patients. *Inflamm Bowel Dis.* 2008;14(8): 1105–1111.

68. Executive summary: Management of the critically ill patient with severe acute pancreatitis. *Proc Am Thorac Soc.* 2004;1(4):289–290.

69. Brugler L, DiPrinzio MJ, Bernstein L. The five-year evolution of a malnutrition treatment program in a community hospital. *Jt Comm J Qual Improv.* 1999;25(4):191–206.

70. Silvennoinen JA, Karttunen TJ, Niemela SE, Manelius JJ, Lehtola JK. A controlled study of bone mineral density in patients with inflammatory bowel disease. *Gut.* 1995;37(1):71–76.

71. Abitbol V, Roux C, Chaussade S, et al. Metabolic bone assessment in patients with inflammatory bowel disease. *Gastroenterology.* 1995;108(2):417–422.

72. Bjarnason I, Macpherson A, Mackintosh C, Buxton-Thomas M, Forgacs I, Moniz C. Reduced bone density in patients with inflammatory bowel disease. *Gut.* 1997;40(2):228–233.

73. Semeao EJ, Jawad AF, Stouffer NO, Zemel BS, Piccoli DA, Stallings VA. Risk factors for low bone mineral density in children and young adults with Crohn's disease. *J Pediatr.* 1999;135(5):593–600.

74. Ardizzone S, Bollani S, Bettica P, Bevilacqua M, Molteni P, Bianchi Porro G. Altered bone metabolism in inflammatory bowel disease: There is a difference between Crohn's disease and ulcerative colitis. *J Intern Med.* 2000;247(1):63–70.

75. Bernstein CN, Blanchard JF, Metge C, Yogendran M. The association between corticosteroid use and development of fractures among IBD patients in a population-based database. *Am J Gastroenterol.* 2003;98(8):1797–1801.

76. Jahnsen J, Falch JA, Aadland E, Mowinckel P. Bone mineral density is reduced in patients with Crohn's disease but not in patients with ulcerative colitis: A population based study. *Gut*. 1997;40(3):313–319.

77. Lamb EJ, Wong T, Smith DJ, et al. Metabolic bone disease is present at diagnosis in patients with inflammatory bowel disease. *Aliment Pharmacol Ther*. 2002;16(11):1895–1902.

78. Bernstein CN, Leslie WD, Taback SP. Bone density in a population-based cohort of premenopausal adult women with early onset inflammatory bowel disease. *Am J Gastroenterol*. 2003;98(5):1094–1100.

79. Habtezion A, Silverberg MS, Parkes R, Mikolainis S, Steinhart AH. Risk factors for low bone density in Crohn's disease. *Inflamm Bowel Dis*. 2002;8(2):87–92.

80. Jong DJ, Corstens FHM, Mannaerts L, Rossum LGM, Naber AHJ. Corticosteroid-induced osteoporosis: Does it occur in patients with Crohn's disease? *Am J Gastroenterol*. 2002;97(8):2011–2015.

81. Vogelsang H, Ferenci P, Resch H, Kiss A, Gangl A. Prevention of bone mineral loss in patients with Crohn's disease by long-term oral vitamin D supplementation. *Eur J Gastroenterol Hepatol*. 1995;7(7):609–614.

82. Siffledeen JS, Fedorak RN, Siminoski K, et al. Randomized trial of etidronate plus calcium and vitamin D for treatment of low bone mineral density in Crohn's disease. *Clin Gastroenterol Hepatol*. 2005;3(2):122–132.

83. Leal JY, Romero T, Ortega P, Amaya D. Serum values of interleukin-10, gamma-interferon and vitamin A in female adolescents. *Invest Clin*. 2007;48(3):317–326.

84. Ginanjar E, Sumariyono, Setiati S, Setiyohadi B. Vitamin D and autoimmune disease. *Acta Med Indones*. 2007;39(3):133–141.

85. Mullin GE, Dobs A. Vitamin D and its role in cancer and immunity: A prescription for sunlight. *Nutr Clin Pract*. 2007;22(3):305–322.

86. Abreu MT, Geller JL, Vasiliauskas EA, et al. Treatment with infliximab is associated with increased markers of bone formation in patients with Crohn's disease. *J Clin Gastroenterol*. 2006;40(1):55–63.

87. Dudrick SJ, Latifi R, Schrager R. Nutritional management of inflammatory bowel disease. *Surg Clin North Am*. 1991;71(3):609–623.

88. Lih-Brody L, Powell SR, Collier KP, et al. Increased oxidative stress and decreased antioxidant defenses in mucosa of inflammatory bowel disease. *Dig Dis Sci*. 1996;41(10):2078–2086.

89. Carter MJ, Lobo AJ, Travis SPL. Guidelines for the management of inflammatory bowel disease in adults. *Gut*. 2004;53(S5):v1–16.

90. Savage DG, Lindenbaum J, Stabler SP, Allen RH. Sensitivity of serum methylmalonic acid and total homocysteine determinations for diagnosing cobalamin and folate deficiencies. *Am J Med*. 1994;96(3):239–246.

91. Romagnuolo J, Fedorak RN, Dias VC, Bamforth F, Teltscher M. Hyperhomocysteinemia and inflammatory bowel disease: Prevalence and predictors in a cross-sectional study. *Am J Gastroenterol*. 2001;96(7):2143–2149.

92. Greenberg GR, Fleming CR, Jeejeebhoy KN, Rosenberg IH, Sales D, Tremaine WJ. Controlled trial of bowel rest and nutritional support in the management of Crohn's disease. *Gut*. 1988;29(10):1309–1315.

93. Jeejeebhoy KN. Enteral and parenteral nutrition: Evidence-based approach. *Proc Nutr Soc*. 2001;60(3):399–402.

94. Hughes CA, Bates T, Dowling RH. Cholecystokinin and secretin prevent the intestinal mucosal hypoplasia of total parenteral nutrition in the dog. *Gastroenterology*. 1978;75(1):34–41.

95. Guedon C, Schmitz J, Lerebours E, et al. Decreased brush border hydrolase activities without gross morphologic changes in human intestinal mucosa after prolonged total parenteral nutrition of adults. *Gastroenterology*. 1986;90(2):373–378.

96. Rossi TM, Lee PC, Young C, Tjota A. Small intestinal mucosa changes, including epithelial cell proliferative activity, of children receiving total parenteral nutrition (TPN). *Dig Dis Sci*. 1993;38(9):1608–1613.

97. Sedman PC, MacFie J, Palmer MD, Mitchell CJ, Sagar PM. Preoperative total parenteral nutrition is not associated with mucosal atrophy or bacterial translocation in humans. *Br J Surg*. 1995;82(12):1663–1667.

98. Nguyen GC, LaVeist TA, Brant SR. The utilization of parenteral nutrition during the in-patient management of inflammatory bowel disease in the United States: A national survey. *Aliment Pharmacol Ther*. 2007;26(11–12):1499–1507.

99. Dickinson RJ, Ashton MG, Axon AT, Smith RC, Yeung CK, Hill GL. Controlled trial of intravenous hyperalimentation and total bowel rest as an adjunct to the routine therapy of acute colitis. *Gastroenterology*. 1980;79(6):1199–1204.

100. Gonzalez-Huix F, Fernandez-Banares F, Esteve-Comas M, et al. Enteral versus parenteral nutrition as adjunct therapy in acute ulcerative colitis. *Am J Gastroenterol*. 1993;88(2):227–232.
101. King T. Meta-analysis of enteral nutrition as a primary treatment of active Crohn's disease. *Clinical Nutrition*. 1995;14(6):388–389.
102. Griffiths AM, Ohlsson A, Sherman PM, Sutherland LR. Meta-analysis of enteral nutrition as a primary treatment of active Crohn's disease. *Gastroenterology*. 1995;108(4):1056–1067.
103. Messori A, Trallori G, D'Albasio G, Milla M, Vannozzi G, Pacini F. Defined-formula diets versus steroids in the treatment of active Crohn's disease: A meta-analysis. *Scand J Gastroenterol*. 1996;31(3):267–272.
104. Fernandez-Banares F, Cabre E, Esteve-Comas M, Gassull M. How effective is enteral nutrition in inducing clinical remission in active Crohn's disease? A meta-analysis of the randomized clinical trials. *JPEN J Parenter Enteral Nutr*. 1995;19(5):356–364.
105. Harries AD, Danis V, Heatley RV, et al. Controlled trial of supplemented oral nutrition in Crohn's disease. *The Lancet*. 1983;321(8330):887–890.
106. Koga H, Iida M, Aoyagi K, Matsui T, Fujishima M. Long-term efficacy of low residue diet for the maintenance of remission in patients with Crohn's disease. *Nippon Shokakibyo Gakkai Zasshi*. 1993;90(11):2882–2888.
107. Takagi S, Utsunomiya K, Kuriyama S, et al. Effectiveness of an 'half elemental diet' as maintenance therapy for Crohn's disease: A randomized-controlled trial. *Aliment Pharmacol Ther*. 2006;24(9):1333–1340.
108. Verma S, Kirkwood B, Brown S, Giaffer MH. Oral nutritional supplementation is effective in the maintenance of remission in Crohn's disease. *Dig Liver Dis*. 2000;32(9):769–774.
109. Wilschanski M, Sherman P, Pencharz P, Davis L, Corey M, Griffiths A. Supplementary enteral nutrition maintains remission in paediatric Crohn's disease. *Gut*. 1996;38(4):543–548.
110. Newby EA, Sawczenko A, Thomas AG, Wilson D. Interventions for growth failure in childhood Crohn's disease. *Cochrane Database Syst Rev*. 2005;(3):CD003873.
111. Lewis JD, Fisher RL. Nutrition support in inflammatory bowel disease. *Med Clin North Am*. 1994;78(6):1443–1456.
112. Fell JM, Paintin M, Arnaud-Battandier F, et al. Mucosal healing and a fall in mucosal pro-inflammatory cytokine mRNA induced by a specific oral polymeric diet in paediatric Crohn's disease. *Aliment Pharmacol Ther*. 2000;14(3):281–289.
113. Gassull MA, Fernandez-Banares F, Cabre E, et al. Fat composition may be a clue to explain the primary therapeutic effect of enteral nutrition in Crohn's disease: Results of a double blind randomised multi-centre European trial. *Gut*. 2002;51(2):164–168.
114. Fell JM. Control of systemic and local inflammation with transforming growth factor beta containing formulas. *JPEN J Parenter Enteral Nutr*. 2005;29(4 Suppl):S126–128; discussion S129–133, S184–188.
115. Harsha WT, Kalandarova E, McNutt P, Irwin R, Noel J. Nutritional supplementation with transforming growth factor-beta, glutamine, and short chain fatty acids minimizes methotrexate-induced injury. *J Pediatr Gastroenterol Nutr*. 2006;42(1):53–58.
116. Bamba T, Kanauchi O, Andoh A, Fujiyama Y. A new prebiotic from germinated barley for nutraceutical treatment of ulcerative colitis. *J Gastroenterol Hepatol*. 2002;17(8):818–824.
117. Kudsk KA, Wu Y, Fukatsu K, et al. Glutamine-enriched total parenteral nutrition maintains intestinal interleukin-4 and mucosal immunoglobulin A levels. *JPEN J Parenter Enteral Nutr*. 2000;24(5):270–274.
118. Chen K, Okuma T, Okamura K, Torigoe Y, Miyauchi Y. Glutamine-supplemented parenteral nutrition improves gut mucosa integrity and function in endotoxemic rats. *JPEN J Parenter Enteral Nutr*. 1994;18(2):167–171.
119. Singleton KD, Beckey VE, Wischmeyer PE. Glutamine prevents activation of NF-kappaB and stress kinase pathways, attenuates inflammatory cytokine release, and prevents acute respiratory distress syndrome (ARDS) following sepsis. *Shock*. 2005;24(6):583–589.
120. Ockenga J, Borchert K, Stuber E, Lochs H, Manns MP, Bischoff SC. Glutamine-enriched total parenteral nutrition in patients with inflammatory bowel disease. *Eur J Clin Nutr*. 2005;59(11):1302–1309.
121. Sido B, Seel C, Hochlehnert A, Breitkreutz R, Droge W. Low intestinal glutamine level and low glutaminase activity in Crohn's disease: A rational for glutamine supplementation? *Dig Dis Sci*. 2006;51(12):2170–2179.
122. Fernandez-Banares F, Cabre E, Gonzalez-Huix F, Gassull MA. Enteral nutrition as primary therapy in Crohn's disease. *Gut*. 1994;35(1 Suppl):S55–59.
123. Belluzzi A, Brignola C, Campieri M, Pera A, Boschi S, Miglioli M. Effect of an enteric-coated fish-oil preparation on relapses in Crohn's disease. *N Engl J Med*. 1996;334(24):1557–1560.

124. Shimizu T, Fujii T, Suzuki R, et al. Effects of highly purified eicosapentaenoic acid on erythrocyte fatty acid composition and leukocyte and colonic mucosa leukotriene B4 production in children with ulcerative colitis. *J Pediatr Gastroenterol Nutr.* 2003;37(5):581–585.

125. Bamba T, Shimoyama T, Sasaki M, et al. Dietary fat attenuates the benefits of an elemental diet in active Crohn's disease: A randomized, controlled trial. *Eur J Gastroenterol Hepatol.* 2003;15(2):151–157.

126. Turner D, Zlotkin SH, Shah PS, Griffiths AM. Omega 3 fatty acids (fish oil) for maintenance of remission in Crohn's disease. *Cochrane Database Syst Rev.* 2007;(2):CD006320.

127. Turner D, Steinhart AH, Griffiths AM. Omega 3 fatty acids (fish oil) for maintenance of remission in ulcerative colitis. *Cochrane Database Syst Rev.* 2007;(3):CD006443.

128. Feagan BG, Sandborn WJ, Mittmann U, et al. Omega-3 free fatty acids for the maintenance of remission in Crohn disease: The EPIC randomized controlled trials. *JAMA.* 2008;299(14):1690–1697.

129. Lomer MC, Harvey RS, Evans SM, Thompson RP, Powell JJ. Efficacy and tolerability of a low microparticle diet in a double blind, randomized, pilot study in Crohn's disease. *Eur J Gastroenterol Hepatol.* 2001;13(2):101–106.

130. Scheppach W, Sommer H, Kirchner T, et al. Effect of butyrate enemas on the colonic mucosa in distal ulcerative colitis. *Gastroenterology.* 1992;103(1):51–56.

131. Breuer RI, Buto SK, Christ ML, et al. Rectal irrigation with short-chain fatty acids for distal ulcerative colitis: preliminary report. *Dig Dis Sci.* 1991;36(2):185–187.

132. Steinhart AH, Brzezinski A, Baker JP. Treatment of refractory ulcerative proctosigmoiditis with butyrate enemas. *Am J Gastroenterol.* 1994;89(2):179–183.

133. Patz J, Jacobsohn WZ, Gottschalk-Sabag S, Zeides S, Braverman DZ. Treatment of refractory distal ulcerative colitis with short chain fatty acid enemas. *Am J Gastroenterol.* 1996;91(4):731–734.

134. Vernia P, Cittadini M, Caprilli R, Torsoli A. Topical treatment of refractory distal ulcerative colitis with 5-ASA and sodium butyrate. *Dig Dis Sci.* 1995;40(2):305–307.

135. Lomer MC, Harvey RS, Evans SM, Thompson RP, Powell JJ. Efficacy and tolerability of a low microparticle diet in a double blind, randomized, pilot study in Crohn's disease. *Eur J Gastroenterol Hepatol.* 2001;13(2):101–106.

136. Lomer MC, Grainger SL, Ede R, et al. Lack of efficacy of a reduced microparticle diet in a multi-centred trial of patients with active Crohn's disease. *Eur J Gastroenterol Hepatol.* 2005;17(3):377–384.

137. Shapiro H, Singer P, Halpern Z, Bruck R. Polyphenols in the treatment of inflammatory bowel disease and acute pancreatitis. *Gut.* 2007;56(3):426–435.

138. Athar M, Back JH, Tang X, et al. Resveratrol: A review of preclinical studies for human cancer prevention. *Toxicol Appl Pharmacol.* 2007;224(3):274–283.

139. Martin AR, Villegas I, La Casa C, de la Lastra CA. Resveratrol, a polyphenol found in grapes, suppresses oxidative damage and stimulates apoptosis during early colonic inflammation in rats. *Biochem Pharmacol.* 2004;67(7):1399–1410.

140. Cabrera C, Artacho R, Gimenez R. Beneficial effects of green tea—a review. *J Am Coll Nutr.* 2006; 25(2):79–99.

141. Nomura M, Ma W, Chen N, Bode AM, Dong Z. Inhibition of 12-O-tetradecanoylphorbol-13-acetate-induced NF-kappaB activation by tea polyphenols -epigallocatechin gallate and theaflavins. *Carcinogenesis.* 2000;21(10):1885–1890.

142. Mazzon E, Muia C, Paola RD, et al. Green tea polyphenol extract attenuates colon injury induced by experimental colitis. *Free Radic Res.* 2005;39(9):1017–1025.

143. Oz HS, Chen TS, McClain CJ, de Villiers WJ. Antioxidants as novel therapy in a murine model of colitis. *J Nutr Biochem.* 2005;16(5):297–304.

144. Varilek GW, Yang F, Lee EY, et al. Green tea polyphenol extract attenuates inflammation in interleukin-2-deficient mice, a model of autoimmunity. *J Nutr.* 2001;131(7):2034–2039.

145. Porath D, Riegger C, Drewe J, Schwager J. Epigallocatechin-3-gallate impairs chemokine production in human colon epithelial cell lines. *J Pharmacol Exp Ther.* 2005;315(3):1172–1180.

146. Bengmark S. Curcumin, an atoxic antioxidant and natural NFkappaB, cyclooxygenase-2, lipooxygenase, and inducible nitric oxide synthase inhibitor: A shield against acute and chronic diseases. *JPEN J Parenter Enteral Nutr.* 2006;30(1):45–51.

147. Cheng AL, Hsu CH, Lin JK, et al. Phase I clinical trial of curcumin, a chemopreventive agent, in patients with high-risk or pre-malignant lesions. *Anticancer Res.* 2001;21(4):2895–2900.

148. Jobin C, Bradham CA, Russo MP, et al. Curcumin blocks cytokine-mediated NF-kappa B activation and proinflammatory gene expression by inhibiting inhibitory factor I-kappa B kinase activity. *J Immunol.* 1999;163(6):3474–3483.

149. Jian YT, Mai GF, Wang JD, Zhang YL, Luo RC, Fang YX. Preventive and therapeutic effects of NF-kappaB inhibitor curcumin in rats colitis induced by trinitrobenzene sulfonic acid. *World J Gastroenterol.* 2005;11(12):1747–1752.

150. Ukil A, Maity S, Karmakar S, Datta N, Vedasiromoni JR, Das PK. Curcumin, the major component of food flavour turmeric, reduces mucosal injury in trinitrobenzene sulphonic acid-induced colitis. *Br J Pharmacol.* 2003;139(2):209–218.

151. Sugimoto K, Hanai H, Tozawa K, et al. Curcumin prevents and ameliorates trinitrobenzene sulfonic acid-induced colitis in mice. *Gastroenterology.* 2002;123(6):1912–1922.

152. Zhang M, Deng C, Zheng J, Xia J, Sheng D. Curcumin inhibits trinitrobenzene sulphonic acid-induced colitis in rats by activation of peroxisome proliferator-activated receptor gamma. *Int Immunopharmacol.* 2006;6(8):1233–1242.

153. Salh B, Assi K, Templeman V, et al. Curcumin attenuates DNB-induced murine colitis. *Am J Physiol Gastrointest Liver Physiol.* 2003;285(1):G235–243.

154. Deguchi Y, Andoh A, Inatomi O, et al. Curcumin prevents the development of dextran sulfate sodium (DSS)-induced experimental colitis. *Dig Dis Sci.* 2007;52(11):2993–2998.

155. Hanai H, Iida T, Takeuchi K, et al. Curcumin maintenance therapy for ulcerative colitis: Randomized, multicenter, double-blind, placebo-controlled trial. *Clin Gastroenterol Hepatol.* 2006;4(12):1502–1506.

156. Campieri M, Gionchetti P. Probiotics in inflammatory bowel disease: New insight to pathogenesis or a possible therapeutic alternative? *Gastroenterology.* 1999;116(5):1246–1249.

157. Schultz M, Sartor RB. Probiotics and inflammatory bowel diseases. *The American Journal of Gastroenterology.* 2000;95(1):S19–S21.

158. Shanahan F. Probiotics in inflamatory bowel disease. *Gut.* 2001;48(5):609.

159. Fuller R. Probiotics in man and animals. *J Appl Bacteriol.* 1989;66(5):365–378.

160. Sartor RB. Therapeutic manipulation of the enteric microflora in inflammatory bowel diseases: Antibiotics, probiotics, and prebiotics. *Gastroenterology.* 2004;126(6):1620–1633.

161. Probert HM, Apajalahti JH, Rautonen N, Stowell J, Gibson GR. Polydextrose, lactitol, and fructo-oligosaccharide fermentation by colonic bacteria in a three-stage continuous culture system. *Appl Environ Microbiol.* 2004;70(8):4505–4511.

162. Sandborn W, Waters G, Gregory S, Pemberton J. Ileal pouch anal anastomosis and the problem of pouchitis. *Curr Opin Gastroenterol.* 1997;13(1):34–40.

163. Gionchetti P, Rizzello F, Venturi A, et al. Oral bacteriotherapy as maintenance treatment in patients with chronic pouchitis: A double-blind, placebo-controlled trial. *Gastroenterology.* 2000;119(2):305–309.

164. Gionchetti P, Rizzello F, Helwig U, et al. Prophylaxis of pouchitis onset with probiotic therapy: A double-blind, placebo-controlled trial. *Gastroenterology.* 2003;124(5):1202–1209.

165. Shen B, Brzezinski A, Fazio VW, et al. Maintenance therapy with a probiotic in antibiotic-dependent pouchitis: Experience in clinical practice. *Aliment Pharmacol Ther.* 2005;22(8):721–728.

166. Laake KO, Bjorneklett A, Aamodt G, et al. Outcome of four weeks' intervention with probiotics on symptoms and endoscopic appearance after surgical reconstruction with a J-configured ileal-pouch-anal-anastomosis in ulcerative colitis. *Scand J Gastroenterol.* 2005;40(1):43–51.

167. Kruis W, Schutz E, Fric P, Fixa B, Judmaier G, Stolte M. Double-blind comparison of an oral *Escherichia coli* preparation and mesalazine in maintaining remission of ulcerative colitis. *Aliment Pharmacol Ther.* 1997;11(5):853–858.

168. Kruis W, Fric P, Pokrotnieks J, et al. Maintaining remission of ulcerative colitis with the probiotic *Escherichia coli* Nissle 1917 is as effective as with standard mesalazine. *Gut.* 2004;53(11):1617–1623.

169. Rembacken BJ, Snelling AM, Hawkey PM, Chalmers DM, Axon AT. Non-pathogenic *Escherichia coli* versus mesalazine for the treatment of ulcerative colitis: A randomised trial. *Lancet.* 1999;354(9179):635–639.

170. Tursi A, Brandimarte G, Giorgetti GM, Forti G, Modeo ME, Gigliobianco A. Low-dose balsalazide plus a high-potency probiotic preparation is more effective than balsalazide alone or mesalazine in the treatment of acute mild-to-moderate ulcerative colitis. *Med Sci Monit.* 2004;10(11):PI126–131.

171. Matthes H, Krummenerl T, Giensch M, Wolff C, and Schulze J. Treatment of mild to moderate acute attacks of distal ulcerative colitis with rectally-administered *E. coli* Nissle 1917: Dose-dependent efficacy. *Gastroenterol.* 2006;130:A119.

172. Bengmark S. Pre-, pro- and synbiotics. *Curr Opin Clin Nutr Metab Care.* 2001;4(6):571–579.

173. Roberfroid MB. Introducing inulin-type fructans. *Br J Nutr.* 2005;93 (S1):S13–25.

174. Videla S, Vilaseca J, Antolin M, et al. Dietary inulin improves distal colitis induced by dextran sodium sulfate in the rat. *Am J Gastroenterol.* 2001;96(5):1486–1493.

175. Hoentjen F, Welling GW, Harmsen HJ, et al. Reduction of colitis by prebiotics in HLA-B27 transgenic rats is associated with microflora changes and immunomodulation. *Inflamm Bowel Dis*. 2005;11(11):977–985.

176. Madsen KL, Doyle JS, Jewell LD, Tavernini MM, Fedorak RN. Lactobacillus species prevents colitis in interleukin 10 gene-deficient mice. *Gastroenterology*. 1999;116(5):1107–1114.

177. Welters CF, Heineman E, Thunnissen FB, van den Bogaard AE, Soeters PB, Baeten CG. Effect of dietary inulin supplementation on inflammation of pouch mucosa in patients with an ileal pouch-anal anastomosis. *Dis Colon Rectum*. 2002;45(5):621–627.

178. Furrie E, Macfarlane S, Kennedy A, et al. Synbiotic therapy (bifidobacterium longum/Synergy 1) initiates resolution of inflammation in patients with active ulcerative colitis: A randomised controlled pilot trial. *Gut*. 2005;54(2):242–249.

179. Guslandi M, Mezzi G, Sorghi M, Testoni PA. Saccharomyces boulardii in maintenance treatment of Crohn's disease. *Dig Dis Sci*. 2000;45(7):1462–1464.

180. Prantera C, Scribano ML, Falasco G, Andreoli A, Luzi C. Ineffectiveness of probiotics in preventing recurrence after curative resection for Crohn's disease: A randomised controlled trial with lactobacillus GG. *Gut*. 2002;51(3):405–409.

181. Schultz M, Timmer A, Herfarth HH, Sartor RB, Vanderhoof JA, Rath HC. Lactobacillus GG in inducing and maintaining remission of Crohn's disease. *BMC Gastroenterol*. 2004;4:5.

182. Lindsay JO, Whelan K, Stagg AJ, et al. Clinical, microbiological, and immunological effects of fructo-oligosaccharide in patients with Crohn's disease. *Gut*. 2006;55(3):348–355.

183. Bayless TM, Harris ML. Inflammatory bowel disease and irritable bowel syndrome. *Med Clin North Am*. 1990;74(1):21–28.

184. MacDermott RP. Treatment of irritable bowel syndrome in outpatients with inflammatory bowel disease using a food and beverage intolerance, food and beverage avoidance diet. *Inflamm Bowel Dis*. 2007;13(1):91–96.

185. Tursi A, Giorgetti GM, Brandimarte G, Elisei W. High prevalence of celiac disease among patients affected by Crohn's disease. *Inflamm Bowel Dis*. 2005;11(7):662–666.

186. Levenstein S, Prantera C, Luzi C, D'Ubaldi A. Low residue or normal diet in Crohn's disease: A prospective controlled study in Italian patients. *Gut*. 1985;26(10):989–993.

187. Misiakos EP, Macheras A, Kapetanakis T, Liakakos T. Short bowel syndrome: Current medical and surgical trends. *J Clin Gastroenterol*. 2007;41(1):5–18.

188. Goldschmid S, Graham M. Trace element deficiencies in inflammatory bowel disease. *Gastroenterol Clin North Am*. 1989;18(3):579–587.

189. Rannem T, Ladefoged K, Hylander E, Hegnhoj J, Jarnum S. Selenium status in patients with Crohn's disease. *Am J Clin Nutr*. 1992;56(5):933–937.

190. Jowett SL, Seal CJ, Phillips E, Gregory W, Barton JR, Welfare MR. Dietary beliefs of people with ulcerative colitis and their effect on relapse and nutrient intake. *Clin Nutr*. 2004;23(2):161–170.

191. Schedel J, Rockmann F, Bongartz T, Woenckhaus M, Scholmerich J, Kullmann F. Association of Crohn's disease and latent celiac disease: A case report and review of the literature. *Int J Colorectal Dis*. 2005;20(4):376–380.

192. Kuhnle GG, Bingham SA. Dietary meat, endogenous nitrosation and colorectal cancer. *Biochem Soc Trans*. 2007;35(Pt 5):1355–1357.

193. Ryan-Harshman M, Aldoori W. Diet and colorectal cancer: Review of the evidence. *Can Fam Physician*. 2007;53(11):1913–1920.

194. Santarelli RL, Pierre F, Corpet DE. Processed meat and colorectal cancer: A review of epidemiologic and experimental evidence. *Nutr Cancer*. 2008;60(2):131–144.

195. Dawson-Hughes B, Heaney RP, Holick MF, Lips P, Meunier PJ, Vieth R. Estimates of optimal vitamin D status. *Osteoporos Int*. 2005;16(7):713–716.

196. Gertner JM, Domenech M. 25-hydroxyvitamin D levels in patients treated with high-dosage ergo- and cholecalciferol. *J Clin Pathol*. 1977;30(2):144–150.

197. Vieth R. Vitamin D supplementation, 25-hydroxyvitamin D concentrations, and safety. *Am J Clin Nutr*. 1999;69(5):842–856.

198. de Silva AD, Mylonaki M, Rampton DS. Oral iron therapy in inflammatory bowel disease: Usage, tolerance, and efficacy. *Inflamm Bowel Dis*. 2003;9(5):316–320.

199. Galloway M, Rushworth L. Red cell or serum folate? Results from the national pathology alliance benchmarking review. *J Clin Pathol*. 2003;56(12):924–926.

200. Kim YI. Does a high folate intake increase the risk of breast cancer? *Nutr Rev*. 2006;64(10 Pt 1):468–475.

201. Montalvo-Jave EE, Zarraga JL, Sarr MG. Specific topics and complications of parenteral nutrition. *Langenbecks Arch Surg.* 2007;392(2):119–126.
202. Lorenz-Meyer H, Bauer P, Nicolay C, et al. Omega-3 fatty acids and low carbohydrate diet for mainte-nance of remission in Crohn's disease. A randomized controlled multicenter trial. study group members (German Crohn's disease study group). *Scand J Gastroenterol.* 1996;31(8):778–785.
203. Romano C, Cucchiara S, Barawbino A, Annese V, Sferlazzas C. Usefulness of omega-3 fatty acid supple-mentation in addition to mesalazine in maintaining remission in pediatric Crohn's disease: A double-blind, randomized, placebo-controlled study. *World J Gastroenterol.* 2005;11(45):7118–7121.
204. Ishikawa H, Akedo I, Umesaki Y, Tanaka R, Imaoka A, Otani T. Randomized controlled trial of the effect of bifidobacteria-fermented milk on ulcerative colitis. *J Am Coll Nutr.* 2003;22(1):56–63.
205. Borody TJ, Warren EF, Leis S, Surace R, Ashman O. Treatment of ulcerative colitis using fecal bacterio-therapy. *J Clin Gastroenterol.* 2003;37(1):42–47.
206. Kato K, Mizuno S, Umesaki Y, et al. Randomized placebo-controlled trial assessing the effect of bifidobacteria-fermented milk on active ulcerative colitis. *Aliment Pharmacol Ther.* 2004;20(10):1133–1141.
207. Fernandez-Banares F, Hinojosa J, Sanchez-Lombrana JL, et al. Randomized clinical trial of plantago ovata seeds (dietary fiber) as compared with mesalamine in maintaining remission in ulcerative colitis. Spanish group for the study of Crohn's disease and ulcerative colitis (GETECCU). *Am J Gastroenterol.* 1999;94(2):427–433.
208. Kanauchi O, Mitsuyama K, Homma T, et al. Treatment of ulcerative colitis patients by long-term admin-istration of germinated barley foodstuff: Multi-center open trial. *Int J Mol Med.* 2003;12(5):701–704.
209. Hallert C, Bjorck I, Nyman M, Pousette A, Granno C, Svensson H. Increasing fecal butyrate in ulcerative colitis patients by diet: Controlled pilot study. *Inflamm Bowel Dis.* 2003;9(2):116–121.

15 Food Reactivities

Diagnosing and Treating Food Allergies, Intolerances, and Celiac Disease

Russell Jaffe, M.D., Ph.D.

I. INTRODUCTION

Food reactivities include the sum of diet-related acute allergy, hypersensitivity (delayed allergy), and intolerance.[1-3] Celiac disease incorporates all aspects of food reactivity into a perfect storm of suffering too often overlooked in practice. Careful history and recently available predictive diagnostic tests are recommended to properly include or exclude food reactivities.[1-4] This chapter reviews the link between the varieties of food reactions and their clinical relevance to inflammatory, autoimmune, and degenerative conditions.[1]

II. EPIDEMIOLOGY

"... food intolerances affect nearly everyone at some point."

NIAID/NIH/HHS, 2/16/08, National Institute of Allergy and Infectious Diseases (NIAID), U.S. Department of Health & Human Services (HHS)

The incidence and prevalence of food reactivities are increasing. Current understanding of the pathophysiology of food reactivities provides a robust basis to explain the increase in disease. Ecologic data presented in Table 15.1 also provide perspective.

Developed countries have a greater prevalence of types I and III allergies due in part to the dietary changes concurrent with industrialization, age of onset, and time from onset to diagnosis point, and to processes that take time to acquire and reach clinical significance. Gender differences may be due in part to hormone variances that are evident as early as perinatally.

Celiac disease epidemiologic surveys suggest celiac disease to have a prevalence of 1/250 Caucasians. Celiac disease is exceedingly rare in patients of pure Japanese, Chinese, or Afro-Caribbean descent. Prevalence of celiac disease has substantially increased at the same time that human diets have become more highly refined and processed.[2] Celiac disease is rare in people who are adequately breastfed and allowed to wean to traditional foods for infants, including fruits, vegetables, pulses, herbs, and fermented foods.[3] Most studies are based on screening for anti-gliadin, a protein component of gluten, and/or anti-endomysial antibodies.[4]

TABLE 15.1
Ecologic Data and Characteristics of Food Reactivities

	Type I	Type II	Type III	Type IV	Intolerance
Demographics	Developed countries	Global	Developed countries	Global	Global
Age of onset	Any	Adult	Any	Any	Any
Gender	F > M	F > M	F > M	F > M	M > F
Time to diagnosis	<1 yr	2–5 yrs	4–8 yrs	3–6 yrs	2–4 yrs

III. PATHOPHYSIOLOGY

Recent advances in basic and molecular sciences have substantially changed our understanding of both the causes and the management of food reactivities.[5] While often overlooked or misunderstood for lack of awareness of recent scientific evidence, food reactivities are more than acute histaminic reactions.[6,7] Food reactivities are antecedents to most inflammatory syndromes,[8] which include digestive, degenerative, and autoimmune chronic conditions.[9]

Food reactivities are absent from fully healthy people who maintain immune tolerance and homeostasis and occur only in people who have lost healthy tolerance and self-rebalancing homeostasis due to acquisition of dysbiosis, xenotoxins, or maldigestion.[10]

Dysbiosis refers to unhealthful microbes in the intestinal tract.[11] Clinically, a stool digestive analysis will reveal culturable organisms. The proportion, species, and antimicrobial sensitivity of culturable microbes can be assessed clinically with a stool digestive analysis.

Xenotoxin burdens can disrupt digestion.[12] Detergent and solvent residues disperse and disrupt digestive systems. Biocides and hormone disrupters inhibit receptors and enzyme systems. Toxic minerals are easily taken up in too many people, mostly those who are magnesium deficient, mildly and significantly metabolically acidotic, and deficient in metallothionein. Together they make up the xenotoxins that are often involved in food reactivities yet are undetected until included in clinical evaluations.[13]

Maldigestion is the failure to sufficiently process food before it reaches the intestinal lumen. Digestion relies heavily on adequate mucins and secretory IgA to avoid absorbing immunoreactive material across the permeable gut membrane and overloading the intestinal immune system.[14] Maldigestion promotes formation and absorption of the following promoters of ill health:

- Digestive remnants: immune reactive material introduced to the intestinal mucosal system
- Lectins: food glycosides specifically activate lymphocytes or macrophages
- Neuroimmunotoxic residue: pesticides, fumigants, or growth regulators
- Oxidants such as sulfites used in food storage or processing
- Intrinsic toxicants such as alkaloids, oxidized essential oils, or mutagens
- Endotoxins such as immune response amplifiers and pyrogens
- Pathogen and parasite products such as cyclosporin-type immune response inhibitors produced by yeast and fungi that are induced by digestive remnants entering the colon

The importance of processing foreign antigens is reflected in the largest part of the immune system in the submucosa of the digestive tract.[15] While thought vestigial until recently, we now recognize that the Peyer's patches are critical to maintaining homeostasis and tolerance.[16] This mucosally associated lymphoid tissue and gut-associated lymphoid tissue are part of our primary defense against foreign invaders, including food digestive remnants.[17] Since the immune system is highly amplified, once the intestinal tract is sensitized with an initial large dose, subsequent tiny amounts of a compound can incite a large and clinically significant response.[18]

Maldigestion results in inflammation that can be understood as cumulative repair deficits. These repair deficits accrue when we take in too little of any of the essential nutrients needed for healthy immune function. Immune system responsibilities include defense and repair. Human immune systems are particularly vulnerable to lack of protective antioxidants, buffering minerals, essential amino acids, essential fats, cofactors, or any needed factor that must be taken in through diet because internal manufacture does not occur or is not occurring.

When lack of essential nutrients or excess of toxins occurs, immune cells shift from protective to survival mode.

Repair deficits launch a vicious cycle of catabolic illness, metabolic acidosis, and loss of homeostasis. The body cannibalizes itself due to impaired essential nutrients needed for healthy metabolism, usually due to metabolic stress or surgical causes. Metabolic acidosis ensues due to acid-forming diet choices or metabolic defects. Loss of homeostasis and neurohormonal rhythms ensues and leads to cortisol and DHEA imbalances. This can lead to attendant endogenous suppression of immune defense and repair responses.

Diet and nutrient deficits along with nutrient depleting, free-radical oxidizing, and xenotoxin bioaccumulation result in maldigestion that predisposes one to food reactivities.[19] Allergies, hypersensitivities, and intolerances taken together are linked through complex, subtle, yet manageable mechanisms presented in Table 15.2 and below.

Type I: Acute Allergy

Histaminic reactivities are seen with type I reactions. A food allergy occurs when the immune system responds defensively to a partially digested food antigen.[20] Dendritic, first-line responder cells are designed to ingest and recycle any foreign antigen that transgresses a mucosal barrier.[21] Once developed, the IgE antibodies are poised to react, releasing large amounts of histamine in an effort to expel the "foreign invader" from the body.[22] Histamine is a powerful chemical that can affect the respiratory system, gastrointestinal tract, skin, or cardiovascular system.[23] People with adaptive immune systems increase IgG4 antibodies to counterbalance IgE antibodies.[24] People who are atopic do not increase IgG4 antibodies in response to IgE induction.[25]

Type II: Delayed Hypersensitivity Antibodies

Type II reactivities are characterized by complement fixation. Lectins bind to various cells including erythrocytes and cells comprising the intestinal wall symptom, provoking antibody reactivities seen with type II reactions. In the absence of maldigestion, lectins were considered unlikely mediators of food allergies because they are broken down by food preparation and digestion. Food reactivites associated with anemia can be partially mediated by lectins that bind to erythrocytes, making them targets for IgG, killer cells, and subsequent destruction.

Type III: Immune Complexes

In type III reactivities, immune complexes, that is, IgM-anti-IgG-antigen complexes, provoke reactions. In contrast to type I allergies where IgE binds to mast cells, in type III reactions IgM binds directly to food antigens and IgG against that antigen. These form immune complexes that circulate and can deposit in various tissues.

Type IV: Direct T-Cell Responses

Type IV reactivities are T-cell mediated, delayed responses. In food reactivities macrophages engulf food allergens that they then process and present to T-cells. T-cells which have had prior contact with a sensitizing antigen and macrophages release cell-signaling interleukins, which induce the immune cascade leading to inflammation and repair deficits and to comorbid conditions.

TABLE 15.2
Classification of Food Reactivities

	Common Term	Antibody Associated	Assay	Synonyms
Type I	Hives Anaphylaxis	IgE	RadioAllergoSorbed Technique; IntraDermal Skin Tests	Reagin; Ishizaka Antigen
Type II	Delayed allergy	IgM, IgA, IgG	IgG ELISA/EIA; Lymphocyte Response Assay by ELISA/ACT	Late phase Delayed allergies
Type III	Serum sickness	IgM anti-IgG Antigen complex	Raji cell Lymphocyte Response Assay	Immune complex diseases; Arteritis
Type IV	Thymus-derived helper 1 / Thymus-derived helper 2 lymphocyte balance	T cell (IgD)	Lymphocyte Response Assay; Memory Lymphocyte Immunostimulation Assay (MELISA®)	Schwartzman reaction Arthus reaction
Intolerance	Maldigestion Stress- or toxin-associated loss of protective molecules	Multiple mechanisms	Various digestive function tests; therapeutic dietary trials	Dysbiosis Enteropathy Host hospitality

Source: Modified from [6].

FOOD INTOLERANCES: FUNCTIONAL CHANGES IN DIGESTIVE MECHANISMS

Food intolerances include dysbiosis due to unhealthful microflora in the gut, lactose intolerance due to lactase deficiency, celiac disease, IgA deficiency, sIgA deficiency, and maldigestion leading to immunoreactive remnants. Also, oxidants link sulfite, which increases antioxidant requirements.[26] Several protective molecules are lost due to stress, toxins, and failed nutrient-dependent epigenetic processes:

- Lactase deficiency is responsible for lactose intolerance and other elective, inducible digestive enzymes.[27]
- Mucins trap toxins to prevent their reabsorption from the gut.[28]
- sIgA is a mucosal antibody designed to trap reactive food remnants to prevent them from being absorbed and then burden immune defense and repair systems.[29]
- Trophic opsonins such as mucin and nutrient production by probiotic flora reflect the symbiotic relationship between the gut and host mucosal immune defense and repair systems.[30]
- Metallothioneins are a magnesium- and zinc-rich Gly-Cys polypeptides that trap toxic minerals in plasma, CSF, stool, and urine. Produced only in healthy, energetic cells, they are down-regulated or turned off during persisting stress, toxin overload, and essential nutrient deficit.[31]

Food and nutrients have newly emerging roles in causation and perpetuation of food reactivities. The following are examples:

- Intake of foods and nutrients in excess or deficit relative to individual essential requirements[32]

- Epigenetic phenotypic modulation, especially during the pre-, neo-, and post-natal period[33]
- Impaired uptake, usually acquired due to enteropathy[34]
- Medications that reduce healthy probiotic microflora[35]
- Diets deficient in fiber content[36]
- Occupational or environmental exposure to toxins that interrupt digestion[37]
- Circadian disruption that leads to loss of restorative sleep[38]

Knowledge of the pathophysiology can help better direct disease management toward the underlying causes of food reactivities in clinical practice.

IV. CELIAC DISEASE, SPECIAL CONSIDERATIONS

The following is a hypothetical case presentation of a patient with celiac disease and is intended as a teaching tool:

> A 50-year-old Caucasian engineer father of two presented with complaints of "My get up and go got up and went; I just don't have the energy to do what I want to do." He experienced no prior problem with his energy, sleep, or mood level until about a year ago. His weight has been stable despite the 2500–3500 calories he says he eats daily. He reported no other complaints. His past medical and social history is noncontributory; he does not provide any pertinent family history of illness, particularly denying any family history of cancer. Physical examination reveals a well-developed individual with nothing out of the normal range except some slight conjunctival pallor. Laboratory examination reveals a significant microcytic anemia and mild transaminitis. Three stool samples sent to assess for occult blood were negative. Despite this, he underwent a colonoscopic exam, which revealed a 3 mm sigmoid polyp, and an esophagogastroduodenoscopy, which appeared normal, except for mild gastric erythema. Biopsies were taken from his gastric antrum and the mid-body, greater curve of his stomach, as well as from the normal-appearing duodenal mucosa. The histologic appearance of the gastric biopsies was normal, but the duodenal biopsies revealed severe blunting of the villi, crypt hypertrophy, with lymphocytic infiltration of the mucosa. The pathologist suggested that the findings were consistent with celiac disease, a diagnosis that was confirmed by a positive IgA tissue transglutaminase antibody. The patient continued to experience no gastrointestinal symptoms.

The variability and nonspecific nature of symptoms experienced by patients with celiac disease frequently lead to delayed and missed diagnoses of this increasingly common condition. As many as 85% of cases go undiagnosed and thus many patients are subject to comorbidity and mortality due to untreated disease. The biggest obstacle to diagnosing celiac disease is lack of clinical awareness.

Described first in 1888, celiac disease, also known as nontropical sprue or gluten-sensitive enteropathy, is an autoimmune inflammatory condition mostly triggered by gliadin, a hard-to-digest component of gluten found in several different grains (wheat, barley, and rye). While most common among northern Europeans, it is found around the world and has a strong genetic predisposition. HLA types DQ2 and DQ8 are more at risk to develop the condition. In classic celiac disease, continued ingestion of gluten-containing products leads to mucosal inflammation that often results in a syndrome of malabsorption with slowly progressive vitamin and mineral deficiencies, weight loss, and diarrhea. Though malabsorption and diarrhea are classical features of celiac disease, this case illustrates that many patients report neither diarrhea nor constipation.

A multitude of diverse extra-intestinal symptoms may dominate or complicate the clinical picture of celiac disease. Among these are neuropsychiatric disorders, iron-deficiency anemia, arthritis, osteoporosis, abnormal liver function tests, and infertility. Other autoimmune conditions are often concurrent. Type 1 diabetes mellitus, thyroid and liver disease, connective tissue diseases, and dermatitis herpetiformis are more common in celiac disease. The associated autoantibodies, particularly anti-endomysial antibodies and anti-tissue transglutaminase antibodies, have been well studied and are increasingly reliable aids in screening for the condition. The gold standard remains small bowel biopsy where villous atrophy associated with intra-epithelial lymphocytes and crypt hyperplasia are prototypic. With the increased incidence of selective IgA deficiency among patients with celiac disease, screening for IgA and salivary sIgA before serological testing for IgA anti-endomysial and IgA anti-tissue transglutaminase antibodies is recommended. The majority of patients improve symptomatically with meticulous removal of gluten from the diet. Avoiding even small amounts of antigen is important because the immune responses are highly amplified.

In a study by Hin and colleagues, 2000 patients were prospectively studied upon referral for an endoscopic biopsy for suspicion of celiac disease.[39] All patients had serology performed for anti-tissue transglutaminase (tTG antibodies) and underwent small bowel biopsy. Patients were classified as high or low risk for celiac disease based on the presence or absence of any one of the following:

1. Weight loss
2. Diarrhea or stool changes
3. Anemia of unexplained etiology

In total 77 (~4% of 2000) cases of celiac disease were diagnosed.[43] The sensitivity and negative predictive value of antibody testing alone was 90.9% and 99.6% respectively. The sensitivity and negative predictive value of the clinical decision tool was 100% and 100% respectively. The results of this study suggest that small bowel biopsy of patients with a positive serology or high-risk features will capture all cases of celiac disease, and biopsy can be safely deferred among those with negative serologies and the absence of high-risk features.

V. PHARMACOLOGY

Medications can predispose to food reactivities by mechanisms beyond nutrient deficiencies. Examples include

1. Cyclooxygenase inhibitors are painkillers that contribute to maldigestion by preventing repair that depends upon cyclooxigenase enzymes.
2. Antibiotics kill gut flora as collateral damage. When the gut's health-promoting denizens are not replenished, the antibiotic assault leaves hospitality to pathogens or parasites.[40] Prebiotic and probiotic interventions can compensate for ensuing dysbiosis.
3. Histamine antagonists (H_2 blockers) and proton pump inhibitors reduce stomach acid, with the untoward effects of impairing B12 absorption and digestive efficiency.[41] Betaine and l-histidine are digestive aides that promote healthy stomach acid balance to create the low pH where pepsin functions optimally and healthier protein digestion occurs.

VI. COMORBID CONDITIONS

"With more than two in three of the general population suffering from chronic ill-health conditions that have not fully responded to conventional therapies, there is a likelihood that [hidden] food allergy plays an etiologic role."

Public Perception of Food Allergy, ACAAI working group, 1996.

Food reactivities are associated with a diverse group of comorbid conditions. These are presented in Table 15.3. Once the food reactivity is diagnosed and treated, the associated comorbidities generally improve. Food reactivities underlie and complicate the management of most inflammatory and autoimmune chronic illness.[42]

VII.   PATIENT EVALUATION

PATIENT HISTORY

Use of the medications and presence of the comorbidities described earlier in this chapter should direct attention to the presence of food reactivities, which are greatly underdiagnosed. The following additional findings also increase the probability of food reactivities.

Hypertension

Tyramines in cheeses are linked to hypertension, particularly in those patients on anti-hypertensive medications.[43] This includes carefully modifying diet when medication complications are commonly induced by dietary substrates.

Lactose Intolerance

Lactose in dairy products is due to lactase enzyme electively produced in healthy digestive tracts. Enzyme production is down-regulated under oxidative stress or with nutritional compromise, suggestive of an underlying repair deficit.[44]

TABLE 15.3
Comorbid Conditions Associated with Food Reactivities

Type I	Type II	Type III	Type IV	Intolerances
Rhinitis	Asthma	Asthma	Addison's	Dysbiosis
Sinusitis	Celiac disease	Bronchitis (allergic)	hypoadrenalism	Lactose
Asthma	Glomerulonephritis	Celiac disease	Biliary cirrhosis	Celiac disease
Anaphylaxis	Hyperthyroidism	Fibromyalgia	Celiac disease	Gluten/gliadin
Mastocytosis	Irritable bowel	FICA	Chronic fatigue	IgA deficiency
Anyphylactoid	syndrome	Glomerulonephritis	Connective tissue	sIgA deficiency
histaminic	Myasthenia gravis	Hemolytic anemia	diseases	Maldigestion
reactions	Neutropenia	Hepatitis	Enteropathy	Oxidants
Celiac disease	Pemphigus vulgaris	Allergic infertility	Fibromyalgia	(e.g., sulfite)
	Pernicious anemia	Lupus (SLE)	Hepatitis	
	Rhinitis	Multiple sclerosis	Hyperthyroidism	
	Sinusitis	Pemphigus vulgaris	Irritable bowel	
	Sjogen's syndrome	Pneumonitis	syndrome	
	Thyroiditis	Psoriasis	Lupus	
	Type 1 diabetes	Rheumatoid Arthritis	Pemphigus vulgaris	
	Type 2 diabetes	Sjogren's rhinitis sica	Pernicious anemia	
		syndrome	Psoriasis	
		Thrombocytopenia	Rhinitis	
		ITP	Sinusitis	
		Type 2 diabetes	Sjogren's syndrome	
			Thyroiditis,	
			Hashimoto's	
			Type 1 diabetes	
			Type 2 diabetes	
			Vitiligo	

Source: [1–4, 9–14].

Low Stomach-Acid Production Secondary to Atrophy, Pharmacologic Interventions, or Other Causes

Hypochlorhydria interferes with protein digestion and reduces the stimulation of bicarbonate and digestive enzymes from the pancreas after the chyme passes from the stomach to the duodenum.[45] It leads to increased digestive remnants.

Cholecystectomy or Gallbladder Symptoms

Lipotropics as bile acids, released from the gall bladder and produced in the liver, are necessary for the uptake of lipids and fat-soluble vitamins by the body. Impaired gallbladder function can result in reduced and insufficient uptake of fat-soluble nutrients including vitamins A, D, and E.[46]

Type I Immediate Food Allergies

Type I immediate food allergies are diagnosed in childhood. Symptoms can include a tingling sensation of the mouth, swelling of the tongue and throat, hives, skin rashes, vomiting, abdominal cramps, difficulty breathing, diarrhea, a drop in blood pressure, or even a loss of consciousness. Some individuals can develop a rash in areas that come in contact with foods. There are people who are so sensitive to food allergens that the odor of that particular food can cause a reaction.[47] Primarily eight foods cause over 90% of acute food allergies: milk, eggs, peanuts, wheat, soy, fish, shellfish, and tree nuts such as walnuts, cashews, and almonds.[48]

DIET MODIFICATION AS A DIAGNOSTIC TOOL

A food diary may help determine the foods that could trigger allergies. Eliminate all reactive foods and then add them back to your diet one at a time to see if they prompt any reaction after digestive competence has been restored.[49] See discussion of avoidance-provocation testing below. An accurate diet diary can be useful to identify nutrient density and diet idiosyncrasies. Accurate diet records are difficult to obtain in primary practice. People tend to record what they think is better more than accurately what they have eaten. A dietician can be effective in assisting patients with diet diaries.[50]

Elimination diets remove common reactors and slow-to-digest foods with antigens. The eliminated foods tend to contain hard-to-digest antigens or endorphin-like molecules that influence gut and central nervous system functions. Typical foods to exclude on elimination diets are grains, cow dairy, chicken eggs, soy, chocolate, nightshade foods, and corn. By contrast, easy-to-digest foods are recommended. These include uncontaminated fruits and vegetables, pulses and herbs, sprouts and nut butters, along with several quarts daily of mineral-rich water.

Limitations of the elimination diet are that avoiding certain foods leads to a broader change in diet with fewer food additives and artificial sweeteners, and more whole foods. The ancillary changes may be the basis for improvement rather than the foods eliminated. Elimination diets can narrow food selection to the point that they can exacerbate underlying nutrient deficiencies. Often several foods cause delayed reactivities, leading to a challenging interpretation of results.

For some individuals, careful avoidance of sulfite, monosodium glutamate, and other food additives or preservatives in prepared foods is helpful.[51] Therefore reading labels carefully and enlisting the assistance of a knowledgeable nutritionist can help to discover hidden sources of food allergens in the diet.[52]

LABORATORY TESTING (TABLE 15.4)

Type I Allergy Testing

In regard to client evaluation for acute (type I) allergies, there are two different approaches to testing: blood and skin tests.[53] RAST (radioallergosorbent test) is the blood test that compares with properly performed intradermal skin tests (IDT).[57] In the United States, 20% of acute allergy is tested by RAST while 80% of tests are performed using IDT. Outside the United States this proportion reverses, with 80% of tests by RAST and the remaining 20% by IDT.[54]

Lymphocyte Response Assays

Lymphocyte response assays (LRA) can be done ex vivo as the enzyme-linked immuno-sensitive antibody test (ELISA/ACT) or in vitro as the memory lymphocyte immunostimulation assay (MELISA®). These assays expose purified antigens from the food or item being tested to cell-rich plasma containing functional lymphocytes. After a suitable incubation period the reactions are read. Nonreactive substances show no reaction. Reactive items induce mitogenic transformations that are measured to determine the result.[55] Individualized tests for food sensitivies are available using lymphocyte response assays. Avoidance of one or more of these is often helpful in clinical management of food reactivities.[56]

Biopsy

Biopsy in someone with food reactivities, including special studies, usually finds[57]

1. Gross morphology is rarely revealing of the problem; hyperemia is commonly observed but not diagnostic.

TABLE 15.4
Laboratory Tests for Food Reactivities

Assessment/Diagnostic Test	Specimen	Reference Labs	Comment/Note
Digestive stool analysis	Stool	Specialty stool & parasitology lab; ARUP Laboratories	3 + purged specimen for parasite detection
Conjugated toxins: Mercapturates, glucuronidies, hippurates, & sulfites/sulfates	Urine	Doctors Data, Inc. Mayo Clinic	24° specimen best
Lymphocyte response assays	Whole blood	ELISA/ACT Biotechnologies Lab; MELISA® Laboratories	
Metabolic acidosis: 1st AM urine assessment	Urine	Self-test; 1st AM urine	
Stress hormones: Free cortisol & DHEA at 4 times during day	Saliva *or* plasma	Neurosciences Lab; Mayo Clinic	Free hormones are more predictive of outcome
Ascorbate antioxidant need: Ascorbate calibration protocol	Stool	Self-test (stool); Quest Diagnostics (Nichols Institute) (plasma ascorbate levels)	
sIgA: mucosal immune defense	Saliva *or* Stool	Neurosciences lab; ARUP Laboratories	See Mucosal Immunity by Strober *et al.* for details
Transglutaminase	Serum	Great Plains Laboratory; Quest Diagnostics (Nichols Institute)	Factor XIII; transligase
Small bowel biopsy for celiac enteropathy	Tissue	Pathology lab	Light & electron microscopy suggested

Source: [1–5, 9–18, 68–73].

2. Microscopic views often show mononuclear cellular infiltrates, which suggests lymphocytes and dendritic cells are migrating to stimulate repair by recycling the tissue that needs to be repaired.

3. Ultrastructure is often revealing of abnormalities although rarely is the specific cause identified.

Predictive Tests

CT and MRI scans of the gut show increased water retention as shown in thickened intestinal walls. With treatment, diagnostic imaging tests improve, making them a useful monitoring tool. When comparing one person's tests over time, more precise outcomes can be discerned.[58]

Transglutaminase and a Diagnostic Approach to Celiac Disease

Advances in immunology and screening have made celiac diagnosis more reliable.[59] Since disease onset can be insidious and often presents with only subtle multisystem dysfunctions,[60] developing a diagnostic approach such as that presented in Figure 15.1 can be helpful.[61] Clinicians should consider celiac disease in patients who present with confounding symptoms or paradoxic responses. In people with IgA or sIgA deficiency, the risk of acquiring celiac enteropathy is substantially increased.[62]

Celiac disease onset in children manifests as failure to thrive with abdominal distention and steatorrhea with onset shortly after grain is introduced into the diet. Such textbook cases are rare today.[63] Nausea and vomiting are more common in children. Subtle symptoms and signs can include unexplained edema, anemia, growth retardation, and/or defective tooth enamel. In older children, recurrent abdominal pain, fall in growth percentile, or iron deficiency should suggest the possibility of celiac disease.[64]

Adults are more likely to have milder symptoms or evanescent symptoms. Comparing IBS symptoms and celiac disease, recent reports show 20% of celiac patients fulfilled the Rome criteria for

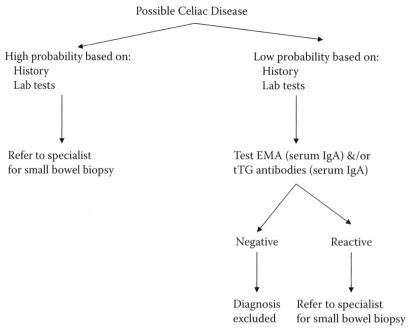

Legend:
EMA, endomysial antibodies; tTG, tissue transglutaminase antibodies

FIGURE 15.1 Celiac disease diagnosis: A flow chart. (Modified from [63].)

IBS, with small bowel biopsy recommended to confirm and differentiate the diagnoses.[65] While more study of this link is needed, it underscores the importance of considering celiac disease in patients with nonspecific gastrointestinal complaints.

VIII. TREATMENT

DIET

Several diets and food patterns have been developed to treat food allergies. The diets presented here may be most suited to different individuals, based on factors such as food reactivity types, food preferences, and meal preparation. What the different diets have in common is that they reduce aberrant immune system reactivity.

The diet used primarily for type I, IgE-mediated food allergies acquired in childhood is avoiding any exposure to the food allergen. Often the avoidance needs to extend beyond food consumption and may involve not using the same cookware for preparing foods containing the food allergen.

The elimination diet previously described for its diagnostic usefulness can be used as a treatment approach. Gradually the foods that are eliminated are returned to the diet one at a time, while the patient logs symptoms in a food diary. A concern about chronic use of elimination diets is that it narrows food selection and can lead to further deficits in nutrient needs.

Rotation diets strive to reduce symptoms to a useful endpoint in managing food reactivities.[66] Rotation diets are used in conjunction with nutritional strategies to treat the patient's repair deficit. Rotation diets may be helpful in patients who experience mild food reactivities with many different foods. Using diet diaries or careful histories, meals are selected so that foods are eaten no more often than every 3 to 7 days. Some rotation diets avoid the food group or food family so that cross-reactive antigens within food families can be avoided.[67]

Substitution diets replace reactive foods as determined by LRA tests, food provocation, or diet history. The goal is to substitute comprehensively for items found reactive, so as to prevent dietary imbalances or nutrient deficiencies. The desired clinical endpoint is to restore digestive competence so that oral tolerance in the immune system is also restored. A typical program to achieve digestive restoration takes 6 to 12 months. Retesting every 6 months until delayed allergen reactions are no longer detected is part of the long-term treatment plan.[68] This indicates that food is being digested to small enough units that what is taken up through the mucosa are not laden with immunoreactive digestive remnants. Following a period of recovery and resetting of hypersensitivity responses, homeostasis and immune tolerance can be restored.[69]

The alkaline diet presented in Chapter 31, "Osteoporosis" is an evidence-based, sustainable diet designed to enhance or restore digestive competence. The alkaline diet is used as part of a comprehensive, integrative health promotion plan that meets all nutrient, fiber, and dietary balance goals. The alkaline diet has a favorable glycemic index and encourages different cuisine choices based on preference while adhering to the principles of a more digestible diet.

NUTRIENT-SPECIFIC RECOMMENDATIONS TO COMPLEMENT DIET

For most people supplements are needed because of low essential nutrient density of most available diet choices, however calorie-rich they may be.[70] Specific nutrients have demonstrated roles in modulating inflammation and improving maldigestion, two mechanisms which in a vicious-cycle fashion contributed to nutrient deficits in the first place.

1. Omega-3/omega-6 essential fats become the communication prostaglandins and thromboxanes. They are both needed. We recommend supplementation primarily with omega-3 fats such as EPA and DHA at 1 to 4 grams daily or with balanced combinations of EFAs for health maintenance and to improve treatment outcomes of all inflammatory conditions.[71]

2. Enzyme-activating minerals also buffer metabolic acids, particularly magnesium. Blocks to magnesium uptake are common and can be overcome by concurrent intake of choline citrate, 1300 mg in water or juice to accompany 220 mg elemental magnesium as glycinate, ascorbate, and aspartate.[72]

3. Antioxidants meet oxidative stress needs.[73] Comprehensive, 40-component essential nutrient supplements are available to form a platform of nutrient adequacy.[74] Ascorbate is a substrate for many reactions, helps protect from oxidative stress, and sets cell oxidation-reduction potential. Half-life and consumption rate for ascorbate are higher than for any other cell component. All metabolically active cells of the body concentrate ascorbate 30-fold over plasma levels.[75] Clinically, ascorbate needs can be determined by the ascorbate calibration protocol (Table 15.4) since ascorbate consumption rates vary widely across individuals.[76]

4. Prebiotic fibers can be supplemented as 80% soluble and 20% insoluble as found in unprocessed whole grain complex carbohydrates. Healthful intake is 40 to 100 grams daily. Typically Americans consume 5 to 10 grams daily on a standard American diet.[77]

5. Probiotic organisms replenish digestive organisms. Probiotics can be dosed at 5 to 40 billion colony-forming units daily of multiple strains showing high activity in humans. Multiple strains of acidophilus, bifidus, and thermophilus with high viability organisms are recommended. Active probiotics are usually kept cold during storage to prolong shelf life.[78]

6. Detoxification factors, from oxidative phosphorylation to conjugation, can be measured in the urine. Impaired detoxification is a common comorbid condition for all food reactivities.[79]

7. Coenzyme Q10, 60 to 600 mg/day in micellized rice bran oil for high uptake, facilitates energy production in the mitochondria.[80] Enterocytes have a high turnover rate and their function and repair can be supported with coenzyme Q10.

8. Structural joint repair components such as soluble glucosamines, chondroitins, and hyaluronates can be supplemented at 1500 mg one to four times daily.[81] See Chapter 33, "Osteoarthritis."

9. Essential or conditionally essential aminoacids such as recycled l-glutamine plus Pyridoxyl-Alpha-Ketoglutarate at 1.5 to 6 grams daily.[82] This is clinically equivalent to 15 to 60 grams daily of free l-glutamine. Glutamine is a principal energy source for intestinal and other cells with particularly high metabolism.[83]

TREATMENT CONSIDERATION WITH CELIAC DISEASE

The foundation of celiac treatment is avoidance of reactive antigens such as gluten and gliadin from all sources. Until recently, avoidance of gluten and symptomatic treatment provided the best available care. Recently, availability of comprehensive lymphocyte response assays that can determine the full range of delayed reactions have come into clinical practice. These are acquired due to digestive remnants transgressing the intestinal mucosa and, when host defense are depleted, entering the systemic circulation. Proactive treatments that include comprehensive substitution for all reactive items along with a repair-inducing alkaline diet (Chapter 31, "Osteoporosis"), targeted supplementation, and behavioral actions aimed at evoking the human healing responses are now available in practice. This opens a new age in proactive treatment. The goal is to repair intestinal digestive competences, improve host immune defense and repair systems, and restore tolerance.[1–5,60–72]

IX. SUMMARY

This chapter reviews the multiple aspects and opportunities to more clearly understand food reactivities based on recent breakthroughs in understanding and practice. Food allergies, hypersensitivities, and intolerances are common, contingent aspects of chronic diseases. Effective management of food reactivities results in better outcomes at lower cost due to addressing the causes rather than treating based on suppressing symptomatic consequences. However, food reactivities remain vastly under-diagnosed and the underlying causes under-recognized and therefore under-treated. Advances in assessment and treatment of food reactivities allow us to achieve better outcomes and better quality of life at sustainable costs for our patients.

REFERENCES

1. Cohen, IR, The self, the world, and autoimmunity, *Sci Am.* 1988; 258: 52–60.
2. Al-toma A, Verbeek W, Mulder C. The management of complicated celiac disease. *Dig Dis.* 2007; 25:230–236.
3. Lewis Mehl-Madrona, MD, PhD, personal communication, 5/5/1998.
4. Ozgenc F, Aksu G, Akman S, Genel F, Kutukculer N, Alkanat MB, Vural Yagci R. Association between anti-endomysial antibody and total intestinal villous atrophy in children with celiac disease. *J Postgrad Med.* 2003; 49:21–24.
5. Ronchetti R, Kaczmarski MG, Haluszka J, Jesenak M, Villa MP. Food allergies, cross-reactions and agroalimentary biotechnologies. *Adv Med Sci.* 2007; 52:98–103.
6. *Clinical Aspects of Immunology*, by PG Gel, RR Coombs, PJ Lachman. Blackwell, 1975.
7. Sampson HA, Metcalfe DD. Food allergies. *JAMA.* 1992; 268:2840–2844.
8. Cardoso CR, Teixeira G, Provinciatto PR, Godoi DF, Ferreira BR, Milanezi CM, Ferraz DB, Rossi MA, Cunha FQ, Silva JS. Modulation of mucosal immunity in a murine model of food-induced intestinal inflammation. *Clin Exp Allergy.* 2008 Feb; 38(2):229–232.
9. Fasano A, Shea-Donohue T. Mechanisms of disease: the role of intestinal barrier function in the pathogenesis of gastrointestinal autoimmune diseases. *Nat Clin Pract Gastroenterol Hepatol.* 2005; 2(9):416–422.
10. *Robbins and Cotran's Pathologic Basis of Disease,* 7th ed., by V Kumar, N Fausto, A Abbas. Saunders, 2004.
11. Ebert E C. Maldigestion and malabsorption. *Dis Mon.* 2001; 47(2):49–68.
12. *Drug-Induced Liver Disease,* 2nd ed., edited by N Kaplowitz, LD DeLeve. Informa Science, 2007.
13. *A Textbook of Modern Toxicology,* by E Hodgson. Wiley-Interscience, 2004.
14. Owens S R, Greenson J K. The Pathology of Malabsorption: Current Concepts. *Histopathology.* 2007; 50(1):64–82.
15. Rautava S, Walker WA. Commensal bacteria and epithelial cross talk in the developing intestine. *Curr Gastroenterol Rep.* 2007; 9(5):385–392.
16. Izcue A, Powrie F. Special regulatory T-cell review: Regulatory T cells and the intestinal tract—patrolling the frontier. *Immunology.* 2008; 123(1):6–10.
17. Ang W, Kudsk KA. Is there evidence that the gut contributes to mucosal immunity in humans? *J Parenter Enteral Nutr.* 2007; 31(3):246–258.
18. *Information Handbook for Use with Your Immune Enhancement Program,* 11th ed. Health Studies Collegium, 1990.
19. Deitch EA, Xu D, Qi L, Berg RD. Bacterial translocation from the gut impairs systemic immunity. *Surgery,* 1991; 109:269–276.
20. *The New Dictionary of Cultural Literacy,* 3rd ed., by ED Hirsch, Jr., JF Kett, J Trefil. Houghton Mifflin Co, 2002.
21. Swanson, J. Immunology: The pick of the nibbled bits. *Nature.* 2006; 440:750–751.
22. S. MacDonald, T Rafnar, J Langdon, Lichtenstein L. Molecular identification of an IgE-dependent histamine-releasing factor. *Science.* 1995; 269(5224): 688–690.
23. Maintz L, Novak N. Histamine and histamine intolerance. *Am J Clin Nutr.* 2007; 85(5):1185–1196.
24. Turnera JD, Faulknera H, Kamgnob J, Kennedyc M W, Behnkea J, Boussinesqb M, Bradley J E. Allergen-specific IgE and IgG4 are markers of resistance and susceptibility in a human intestinal nematode infection. *Microbes and Infection.* 2005; 7:990–996.
25. Moneret-Vautrin DA, Kanny G, Frémont S. Laboratory tests for diagnosis of food allergy: advantages, disadvantages and future perspectives. *Eur Ann Allergy Clin Immunol.* 2003; 35(4):113–119.
26. Assa'ad AH. Gastrointestinal food allergy and intolerance. *Pediatr Ann.* 2006; 35(10):718–726.
27. Bahna SL. Cow's milk allergy versus cow milk intolerance. *Ann Allergy Asthma Immunol.* 2002; 89(6 Suppl 1):56–60.

28. *Mucosal Immunity*, by J Mestecky, J Bienenstock, ME Lamm, W Strober, J McGhee, L Mayer. Academic Press, 2005.

29. Brandtzaeg P. Do salivary antibodies reliably reflect both mucosal and systemic immunity? *Ann N Y Acad Sci.* 2007; 1098:288–311.

30. Guarner F, Malagelada JR. Gut flora in health and disease. *Lancet.* 2003; 361(9356):512–519.

31. Formigari A, Irato P, Santon A. Zinc, Antioxidant Systems and Metallothionein in Metal Mediated-Apoptosis: Biochemical and Cytochemical Aspects. *Comp Biochem Physiol C Toxicol Pharmacol.* 2007; 146(4):443–459.

32. *Biochemical Individuality,* by RJ Williams. Keats Publishing, 1956.

33. Snykers S, Vinken M, Rogiers V, Vanhaecke T. Differential role of epigenetic modulators in malignant and normal stem cells: a novel tool in preclinical in vitro toxicology and clinical therapy. *Arch Toxicol.* 2007; 81(8):533–544.

34. NIH Consensus Development Conference on Celiac Disease. *NIH Consens State Sci Statements.* 2004, Jun 28-30; 21(1):1–23.

35. Snydman DR. The safety of probiotics. *Clin Infect Dis.* 2008; 46 Suppl 2:S104–11; discussion S144–151.

36. Wolever TM, Jenkins DJ. What is a high fiber diet? *Adv Exp Med Biol.* 1997; 427:35–42.

37. *Hormone Deception: How Everyday Foods and Products Are Disrupting Your Hormones—and How to Protect Yourself and Your Family*, by D Lindsey Berkson. McGraw Hill, 2001.

38. Zisapel N. Sleep and sleep disturbances: biological basis and clinical implications. *Cell Mol Life Sci.* 2007; 64(10):1174–1186.

39. Hin H, Bird G, Fisher P, Mahy N, Jewell D. Coeliac disease in primary care: case finding study. *Brit Med J.* 1999; 318:164–167.

40. *When Antibiotics Fail: Restoring the Ecology of the Body,* by M Lappé. North Atlantic Books, 1986.

41. Streeter AM, Goulston KJ, Bathur FA, Hilmer RS, Crane GG, Pheils MT. Cimetidine and malabsorption of cobalamin. *Dig Dis Sci.* 1982; 27(1):13–16.

42. Gruenewald TL, Seeman TE, Ryff CD, Karlamangla AS, Singer BH. Combinations of biomarkers predictive of later life mortality. *Proc Natl Acad Sci USA.* 2006; 103(38):14158–14163.

43. Da Prada M, Zurcher G, Wuthrich I, Haefely WE. Tyramine, Food, beverages and the reversible MAO inhibitor moclobemide. *J Neural Transm.* 1988; 26 (Suppl):31–56.

44. Bayless TM, Christopher NL. Disaccharidase deficiency. *Am J Clin Nutr.* 1969; 22(2):181–190.

45. Schubert ML. Gastric Secretion. *Curr Opin Gastroenterol.* 2003; 19(6):519–525.

46. Cornatzer, WE. Lipotropic agents and lipid transport. *Am J Clin Nut.* 1960; 8:306–309.

47. Amaro C, Goossens A. Immunological occupational contact urticaria and contact dermatitis from proteins: a review. *Contact Dermatitis.* 2008; 58:67–75.

48. http://www.fda.gov/FDAC/features/2001/401_food.html

49. Krall EA, Dwyer JT. Validity of a food frequency questionnaire and a food diary in a short-term recall situation. *J Am Diet Assoc.* 1987; 87(10):1374–1377.

50. Friedenreich C M, Slimani N, Riboli E. Measurement of past diet: review of previous and proposed methods. *Epidem Rev.* 1992; 14:177–191.

51. Lau K, McLean W G, Williams D P, Howard C V. Synergistic interactions between commonly used food additives in a developmental neurotoxicity test. *Toxocological Sciences.* 2006; 90(1):178–187.

52. Halpern GM, Scott JR. Non-IgE antibody mediated mechanisms in food allergy. *Ann Allergy.* 1987; 58(1):14–27.

53. Meriney DK. Comparison of the radioallergosorbent test (RAST) with other diagnostic techniques in clinical allergy. *Cutis.* 1976; 17(6):1045–1048.

54. Chinoy B, Yee E, Bahna S L. Skin testing versus radioallergosorbent testing for indoor allergens. *Clin Mol Allergy.* 2005; 3:4–11.

55. Simms PE, Ellis TM. Utility of flow cytometric detection of CD69 expression as a rapid method for determining poly-and oligoclonal lymphocyte activation. *Clin Diagn Lab Immunol.* 1996; 3:301–304.

56. Ferguson LR, Shelling AN, Browning BL, Huebner C, Petermann I. Genes, diet and inflammatory bowel disease. *Mutat Res.* 2007; 622(1–2):70–83.

57. Rosekrans PC, Meijer CJ, Cornelisse CJ, van der Wal AM, Lindeman J. Use of morphometry and immunohistochemistry of small intestinal biopsy specimens in the diagnosis of food allergy. *J Clin Path.* 1980; 33:125–130.

58. Eliakim R, Fischer D, Suissa A, Yassin, K, Katz, D, Guttman, N, Migdal, M. Wireless capsule video endoscopy is a superior diagnostic tool in comparison to barium follow-through and computerized tomography in patients with suspected Crohn's disease. *Eur J of Gastroenterol & Hepatol.* 15(4):363–367.

59. Barton SH, Kelly DG, Murray JA. Nutritional deficiencies in celiac disease. *Gastroenterol Clin North Am.* 2007; 36(1):93–108.

60. See J, Murray JA. Gluten-free diet: the medical and nutrition management of celiac disease. *Nutr Clin Pract.* 2006; 21(1):1–15.

61. Devlin SM, Andrews CN, Beck PL. Celiac disease: CME update for family physicians. *Can Fam Physician.* 2004; 50:719–725.

62. Esposito C, Caputo I, Troncone R. New therapeutic strategies for celiac disease: tissue transglutaminase as a target. *Curr Med Chem.* 2007; 14(24):2572–2580.

63. Presutti RJ, Cangemi JR, Cassidy HD, Hill DA. Celiac disease. *Am Fam Physician.* 2007; 76(12):1795–1802.

64. Hopper AD, Hadjivassiliou M, Butt S, Sanders DS. Adult coeliac disease. *BMJ.* 2007; 335:558–562.

65. Frissora CL, Koch KL. Symptom overlap and comorbidity of irritable bowel syndrome with other conditions. *Curr Gastroenterol Rep.* 2005; 7(4):264–271.

66. Taylor J P, Krondl M M, Spidel M, Csima A C. Dietary adequacy of the rotary diversified diet: As a treatment for environmental illness. *Canadian J Dietetic Pract Res.* 2002; 63, 198–201.

67. http://www.drsallyrockwell.com/

68. Deuster PA, Jaffe R. A Novel Treatment for Fibromyalgia Improves Clinical Outcomes in a Community-Based Study. *J Musculo Pain.* 1998; 6:133–149.

69. Jaffe R. Clinical importance of delayed immune reactions to antigens and haptens detected by functional Lymphocyte Response Assays in primary management of chronic disease—part II—LRA by ELISA ACT tests. *Townsend Letter for Doctors and Patients.* 2004; 246:68–73.

70. http://www.cdc.gov/nchs/products/elec_prods/subject/nhanes3.htm

71. *Know Your Fats: The Complete Primer for Understanding the Nutrition of Fats, Oils and Cholesterol,* 1st ed., by M Enig. Bethesda Press, 2001.

72. Jaffe R, Enhancement of Magnesium Uptake in Mammals, USPTO, PCT/US2004/026007.

73. Aviram M. Review of human studies on oxidative damage and antioxidant protection related to cardiovascular diseases. *Free Radic Res.* 2000; 33 Suppl:S85–97.

74. Singh A, Moses FM, Deuster PA. Vitamin and mineral status in physically active men: effects of a high-potency supplement. *Am J Clin Nutr.* 1992; 55(1):1–7.

75. Linster CL, Van Schaftingen E. Vitamin C. Biosynthesis, recycling and degradation in mammals. *FEBS J.* 2007; 274(1):1–22.

76. Englard S, Seifter S. The biochemical functions of ascorbic acid. *Annu Rev Nutr.* 1986; 6:365–406.

77. Abrams SA, Griffin IJ, Hawthorne KM, Ellis KJ. Effect of prebiotic supplementation and calcium intake on body mass index. *J Pediatr.* 2007; 151(3):293–298.

78. Tappenden KA, Deutsch AS. The physiological relevance of the intestinal microbiota—contributions to human health. *J Am Coll Nutr.* 2007; 26(6):679S–683S.

79. Lampe JW. Diet, genetic polymorphisms, detoxification, and health risks. *Altern Ther Health Med.* 2007; 13(2):S108–111.

80. Bhagavan HN, Chopra RK. Plasma coenzyme Q10 response to oral ingestion of coenzyme Q10 formulations. *Mitochondrion.* 2007; 7 Suppl:S78–88.

81. McAlindon TE, LaValley MP, Gulin JP, Felson DT. Glucosamine and chondroitin for treatment of osteoarthritis: a systematic quality assessment and meta-analysis. *JAMA.* 2000 Mar 15; 283(11):1469–75.

82. http://www.freepatentsonline.com/6545044.html

83. Buchman AL. Glutamine for the Gut: mystical properties or an ordinary amino acid? *Curr Gastroenterol Rpts.* 1999; 1:417–423.

Section IV

Endocrine and Dermatologic Disorders

16 Hypothyroidism

Optimizing Function with Nutrition

Sherri J. Tenpenny, D.O.

I. INTRODUCTION

The key nutritional needs of patients with hypothyroidism are iodine and selenium. The sufficient daily intake of iodine ranges from 50 µg/day to more than 200 mg/day. Physicians may not be aware of recent changes in diet, lifestyle, the environment, and related medical conditions that predispose patients to suboptimal levels of iodine.

Population studies suggest that the prevalence of iodine deficiency warrants increased clinical vigilance. The First National Health and Nutrition Examination Survey (NHANES I) performed between 1971 and 1974 found 2.6% of U.S. citizens were iodine deficient (32 µg/L). NHANES III, conducted between 1988 and 1994, found 11.7% of those in the United States to be iodine deficient (14.5 µg/L) and that women of childbearing age are disproportionately affected.[1] The results from NHANES 2000 indicated the median urinary iodine level of the population 6 to 74 years of age was 16.1 µg/L.[2]

Currently an estimated 27 million Americans have known thyroid disease and many millions more are under-diagnosed and under-treated. The presence of goiter can represent a profoundly late stage of iodine deficiency. Methods of early stages of detection are presented in this chapter, including dietary and nutritional treatment strategies. Optimizing iodine status has health implications beyond thyroid function.

II. REVIEW OF THYROID PHYSIOLOGY

Thyroid hormones T4 and T3 demonstrate the essential role of dietary nutrients, particularly the halogen iodine. T3 is composed of the amino acid tyrosine and three molecules of iodine. T4 has an additional fourth iodine molecule.

Hormone synthesis begins with up-regulation of the sodium/I-symporter, located on the basal membrane of thyroid cells. Active transport is necessary because iodine must enter thyroglobulin against a concentration gradient. Once inside the thyroglobulin, inorganic iodide (I^-) is oxidized by hydrogen peroxide into reactive iodine (I_2). Each molecule of iodine is subsequently coupled to tyrosine though a multistep process catalyzed by thyroid peroxidase (TPO). The pre-hormones monoiodo-tyrosine (MIT) and diiodo-tyrosine (DIT) are stored in the follicular space of the thyroid gland until TPO combines MIT and DIT to form T3, and DIT and DIT to form T4. Lysosomes digest the thyroglobulin, releasing both hormones into circulation.

More than 99% of T4 and T3 travel through the body bound to serum proteins: thyroid binding globulin (TBG, 70%), albumin (15%), and transthyretin (10% to 15%). Homeostatic mechanisms

TABLE 16.1
Foods for Hypothyroidism

	Meat/Dairy Source	Vegetable/Fruit Source
Omega-3 fatty acids	Coldwater fish (salmon, cod, herring, mackerel, anchovies, sardines), grass-fed beef, fish oils, eggs	Flax seed (aka linseed), flax oil, krill oil, walnuts, canola, whole grains, legumes, green leafy vegetables, Acai palm fruit, kiwi fruit, black raspberries, wakame (sea vegetable)
Tyrosine	Red meat, most fish and dairy products	Almonds, avocado, banana, lima beans, pumpkin seeds, sesame seeds, wheat, oats
Vitamin A	Organ meats, herring	Carrots, carrot juice, pumpkin, spinach, chard, collards, kale, turnip greens, winter squash, dandelion greens, mustard greens, red sweet pepper, Chinese cabbage, broccoli, broccoli rabe, bok choy, sweet potato, peas, parsley, acorn squash, yellow corn, brussels sprouts, apricots, cantaloupe, mango, watermelon, peaches, papaya
Vitamin D	Cod liver oil, salmon, mackerel, sardines, fortified milk (100 IU), liver, eggs	Green leafy vegetables, fortified cereals
Vitamin E	Sardines, Atlantic herring, blue crab	Almonds, sunflower seeds, safflower oil, hazelnuts, turnip greens, pine nuts, peanuts, peanut butter, tomato, wheat germ, avocado, carrot juice, olive oil, corn oil, peanut oil, spinach, dandelion greens, Brazil nuts
Zinc	Grass-fed beef, crabmeat, oysters, lamb, pork, turkey, salmon, chicken, clams, lobster	Brown rice, spinach, beans, rye bread, whole wheat bread, lentils, lima beans, oatmeal, peas, baked potato
Selenium	Dairy products, liver, coldwater fish, shellfish	Asparagus, broccoli, garlic, onions, mushrooms, grains, sea vegetables, Brazil nuts
Biologically available iodine	Fish (amounts variable between species), yogurt, cow's milk, eggs, mozzarella cheese	Strawberries, dried fruit, molasses, sea vegetables (alaria, dulse, kelp, laver, sea lettuce, and bladderwrack)

are designed to maintain normal serum-free hormone concentrations. Protein-bound hormones contribute to this balance.

The iodinated tyrosines are responsible for the basal metabolic rate of most tissues in the body. Insufficient iodine and tyrosine from low intake of the foods listed in Table 16.1 can impair normal thyroid function. Tyrosine is manufactured in the liver from phenylalanine. The mental retardation that occurs with phenylketonuria may result in tyrosine deficiency and defective thyroid hormone production. Iodine deficiency is a known cause of goiter and congenital hypothyroidism with mental retardation.

III. DIAGNOSING HYPOTHYROIDISM

LABORATORY TESTING

In the 1970s, the TSH blood test became the gold standard for diagnosing thyroid problems and the normal range for the test has long been 0.5 to 5.5 mIU/L. Subclinical hypothyroidism is defined as a TSH $\geq$ 4.0 mIU/L and a normal free T4 level.

There are several problems with using only the TSH to screen for hypothyroidism:

- TSH has a diurnal variation and a pulsatile secretion; random samples can show a wide variation.[3]

- Individual variability and hormonal requirements are not considered.
- TSH does not measure sensitivity of the TSH receptor.
- TSH does not assess the functionality of the Na^+/I^- symporter and TPO.
- TSH is associated with central control of thyroid hormones but T3 conversion in local can only be indirectly assessed.
- TSH does not factor in tyrosine and iodine levels.

These are among the concerns that prompted the 2002 American Association of Clinical Endocrinologists (AACE) decision to revise the normal range for TSH to 0.3 to 3.0 mIU/L.[4] The lower TSH is intended to identify thyroid hypofunction before it contributes to more serious conditions as in the following evidence.[5]

- A study of more than 1100 postmenopausal women found that the 0.8% with subclinical hypothyroidism had a greater age-adjusted prevalence of aortic atherosclerosis and myocardial infarction.[6]
- In a study of 9403 women with singleton pregnancies, the 209 (2.2%) with TSH measurements of 6 mIU/L or greater in the second trimester had a significantly higher incidence of fetal death.[7]
- Up to 10% of the 98 million Americans diagnosed with elevated cholesterol levels have undiagnosed thyroid conditions.[8] Normalization of thyroid function lowered total and LDL cholesterol concentrations; no impact on HDL or triglyceride concentrations was observed.[9]
- Mild thyroid dysfunction worsens the symptoms and course of inflammatory bowel disease.[10]

Subclinical hypothyroidism can be the direct result of insufficient total body iodine. A TSH ≥ 2.0 mIU/L is an independent risk factor for developing overt hypothyroid disease at some point in the next 20 years.[11] The risk factor can be reduced when iodine is replenished. Iodine deficiency can be overlooked since L-thyroxine alone improves symptoms in 25% to 50% of patients with iodine-deficient hypothyroidism.[12]

The over-reliance and misinterpretation of TSH leads to medical treatment of subclinical hypothyroidism instead of recognizing that the pattern may represent suboptimal iodine and selenium in the diet.[13]

Physical Examination

Physical findings should prompt diagnostic testing. Additionally, a TSH ≥ 2 suggests looking closely for any of the following findings:

- Hair to be dry, brittle, and thinning.
- Outer third of the eyebrow missing.
- Swelling or puffiness under the eyes.
- Thick and swollen tongue.
- Rough, dry, and flaky skin.
- Nails that tend to be brittle and break easily.
- Palpably enlarged thyroid gland.
- Hands and feet that are cold to the touch.
- Persistent constipation.
- Slow pulse rate even though the patient is not a well-trained athlete.
- Slow or absent recovery phase of Achilles reflexes. This clinical sign was used for years as the diagnostic sign of hypothyroidism.

BASAL BODY TEMPERATURE MEASUREMENT

Instructions for taking basal body temperatures are relatively easy. Menstruating women should take the basal temperature test for thyroid function on the first through fourth day of menses, preferably beginning on the second day. Males, pre-pubertal girls, and postmenopausal or nonmenstruating women may take basal temperatures any day of the month. Women taking progesterone should not take the medication on the day before, and the day of, temperature taking.

- Use an oral glass thermometer.
- Shake the thermometer down before going to bed, and leave it on the bedside table within easy reach.
- Immediately upon awakening, and with as little movement as possible, place the thermometer firmly in the armpit next to the skin.
- Take temperature for 10 minutes with eyes open and lights on in the room. The presence of bright, ambient light is important to suppress nocturnal melatonin.
- Record the readings for three consecutive days.

If the average axillary temperature is below 97.8°F, the diagnosis of a low-functioning thyroid system is likely. An average temperature between 97.8°F and 98.2°F is considered normal.

IV. GOITROGENIC FOODS TO AVOID IN HYPOTHYROIDISM

Goitrogens are naturally occurring substances that can interfere with thyroid function by blocking the activity of TPO. Isoflavones in legumes and soybeans are considered to be potent phytoestrogens and hormone disruptors and have goitrogenic effects. Soy isoflavones have a structural similarity to 17β-estradiol. Actions that have been identified include:

- Activation of estrogen receptors
- Stimulation of sex hormone-binding globulin
- Reduction of bioavailable sex steroids
- Irreversible inactivation of TPO, contributing to goiter, hypothyroidism, and autoimmune thyroiditis[14]

In 1991, Japanese researchers reported that consumption of as little as 30 g (two tablespoons) of soybeans per day for 1 month resulted in a significant increase in TSH. Diffuse goiter and hypothyroidism appeared in some subjects and many complained of constipation, fatigue, and lethargy.[15]

In 2002, two researchers from the FDA's National Center for Toxicological Research, Daniel Sheehan, Ph.D., and Daniel Doerge, Ph.D., published warnings on the goitrogenic and estrogenic properties of soy isoflavones.[16] These officials opposed soy health claims over concerns that isoflavones demonstrated toxicity to the thyroid."[17] Doerge warned that TPO could be irreversibly damaged from soy supplements and soy foods.[18]

Evaluating medical literature about soy is complex. Soy foods are divided into three categories: genetically modified, fermented, and nonfermented. Most research does not identify which soy was used during the trial. Up to 89% of soybeans grown in the United States are *genetically modified* (GM) and approximately 60% of processed foods contain GM soy as filler or oil. Much has been written by concerned scientists on the health problems associated with GM soy. *Nonfermented soy foods* include green and dry soybeans, soy nuts, soy sprouts, soymilk, and soymilk products tofu, okara, and yuba. Nonfermented soy contains trypsin inhibitors, which can affect protein digestibility, and phytates. Phytates can inhibit the absorption of calcium, magnesium copper, iron, and most importantly, zinc. Cooking reduces, but does not eliminate, these compounds. *Fermented soy foods* include tempeh, miso, soy sauces (shoyu), natto, and fermented tofu and some soymilk products. The fermentation process, which can take up to 2 years, mitigates the effects of proteases and phytates.

Iodine deficiency increases the antithyroid effects of soy. Incubation of isoflavones with TPO in the presence of H_2O_2 causes irreversible inactivation of the enzyme; the presence of iodide blocks the inactivation.[19] While occasional consumption of tofu and other soy products is not problematic, the overall effect of soy on the thyroid function is dependent upon iodine status. For example, Asians may be protected from the adverse effects of soy by the cultural consumption of large quantities of iodine-containing sea vegetables and fish.

In the mid-1960s, iodine-supplemented infant soy formulas were introduced by commercial manufacturers. Children have demonstrated plasma phytoestrogen concentrations up to 7000 nm/L compared to an average of 744 nm/L in adult Japanese women.[20] Infant plasma concentrations of isoflavones in soy formulas were 13,000 to 22,000 times higher than endogenous estrogen concentrations.[21] While small studies report no statistically significant differences between soy-fed versus cow's-milk-fed infants,[22] large-scale, longitudinal studies have not been done. Additional cautions with soy formulas are advised in children with congenital hypothyroidism.[23]

Cruciferous vegetables are potentially goitrogenic foods. Crucifers classified as thioglucosides belong to the *Brassica* family and include broccoli, cauliflower, brussels sprouts, cabbage, mustard, rutabagas, kohlrabi, and turnips. Cyanoglucosides are also goitrogens and include cassava (manioc), maize, bamboo shoots, sweet potatoes, and lima beans. After ingestion, both groups release cyanide, which converts to thiocyanate, a powerful goitrogenic substance with the same molecular size as iodine. Thiocyanate inhibits TPO, which blocks accumulation of iodide and prevents iodination of tyrosine. The determining factor involved in the goitrogenic action of these foods is the presence of adequate dietary iodine.[24]

Cooking inactivates most goitrogenic compounds found in cruciferous vegetables. Two to three servings of cruciferous vegetables per week are well tolerated by individuals with hypothyroidism. Adding sea vegetables to the diet may also counteract goiterogens from crucifers and soy.

V. FOODS THAT SUPPORT THYROID FUNCTION

When subclinical hypothyroidism is identified in asymptomatic patients, first remove goitrogenic foods and increase thyroid-supportive foods, particularly those high in iodine and selenium.

Mild thyroid enlargement occurs due to the need for iodine trapping. There is less iodine in goiterous tissue than normal tissue. Therefore hypothyroidism and the development of goiter correlate with low iodine states. The effective treatment of patients with endemic goiter with iodine alone is convincing. According to the AACE, several vitamins and nutrients have been shown to be beneficial for improving thyroid function (see Table 16.1).

IODINE

Iodine was first discovered in the 1800s as a residue from burning seaweed. In 1920, the administration of a small amount of iodinated salt prevented the development of goiters in schoolchildren in Akron, Ohio. Iodinated salt has been used throughout the United States since 1924.

Iodine deficiency is a global problem including in the United States where body iodine stores in the population appear to be trending downward. Potential factors are presented in Table 16.2.

Approximately 150 µg of iodine per day is sufficient to prevent goiter. Unfortunately, the total body RDA for iodine remains unknown, even though substantial amounts of iodine are necessary for the health of other organs. Peroxidase and symporter activity incorporates iodide into salivary glands, gastric mucosa, ovaries, thymus, joints, the choroid plexus, and the ciliary body of the eye. Both lactating and nonlactating[25] mammary tissue accumulates iodine. The amount of iodine necessary to protect the breasts from fibrocystic disease and cancer is 20 to 40 times more than is needed to prevent goiter, or as much as 6000 µg/day.[26]

TABLE 16.2
Factors That Reduce Body Iodine Stores

Cause for Iodine Deficiency	Reason
Decreased salt consumption	Concerns over hypertension
Decreased egg consumption	Concerns over cholesterol
Decreased fish consumption	Dislike of food; concerns over mercury
Decreased iodine in milk	Changes in dairy industry
Removal of iodine from bread products	Commercial bread production replacement of iodine with potassium bromate
Minimal access to sea vegetables	Unaware or no access to the food; dislike of food
Soil iodine depletion	Accelerated deforestation and soil erosion
Heavy daily sweating through athletic training[38]	May be part of a physician-prescribed fitness program
Frequent use of saunas and steam rooms[39]	Sweat loss can range from 11.6 to 99.8 μg for 1 hour of heavy sweating during activity
Chronic inflammatory bowel disease[40]	Decreased absorption; see Chapter 14, "Inflammatory Bowel Disease"

A false sense of security exists over iodized salt as an adequate iodine source because:

- The amount of iodine added during the iodization process is variable.
- Large amounts of iodine are lost by incomplete binding due to salt impurities.
- Displacement and loose chemical binding are due to another halogen, chloride.
- There is uneven distribution within salt batches and between individual packages.
- Containers left open can lose 10% to 100% of iodine, especially in humid environments.[27]

In 1948, Wolff and Chaikoff published a landmark paper[28] on the thyroid effect of increasing amounts of potassium iodide injected intraperitoneally in rats. The authors stated, "Organic binding of iodine within the thyroid gland can be almost completely blocked by raising the level of plasma inorganic iodine above a certain critical level, which for the rat amounts to about 20 to 35 percent." This became known as the Wolff-Chaikoff (W-C) effect. When extrapolated to humans, excess iodine became defined as more than 200 μg/day, or slightly above the amount necessary to prevent the development of a goiter. The W-C effect is the most cited for limiting or avoiding iodine intake.

However, the following year, Wolff and Chaikoff reported that the maximum duration of the inhibitory effect of iodine was about 50 hours. Within 2 days, even in the presence of continued high plasma iodide, an "escape," or adaptation, occurs and normal hormone biosynthesis resumes.[29] This finding was reconfirmed by Braverman in 1963.[30]

Maternal Low Iodine

In the NHANES III, 14.9% of women of childbearing age had low urinary iodine concentration compared to 11.7% of the general population.[31] If pregnancy reduces maternal iodine stores, the depletion confers iodine deficiency to the fetus and more than thyroid function is compromised. A sufficient supply of iodine is essential for normal fetal brain development, and deficiency may result in mental retardation. In adults, iodine deficiency can be associated with apathy, depression, and reduced mental function due to cerebral hypothyroidism. The brain makes its own T3 as peripheral T3 does not cross the blood-brain barrier.[32]

Iodine Deficiency and Hyperthyroidism

One consequence of longstanding iodine deficiency can be the development of hyperthyroidism, especially in multinodular goiters with autonomous nodules. Longstanding iodine deficiency leads to thyroid hyperplasia and an altered pattern of thyroid hormone production. Preferential production is shunted toward the release of T3 over T4. Synthesis of T3 requires 25% less iodine even though the hormone possesses about four times the metabolic potency of T4. The shift toward T3 is an adaptation and survival response.

An inverse relationship exists between iodine supply and thyroidal uptake of iodide. The more iodine deficient a person is, the faster the gland uptakes iodine. This offers an explanation why sudden increases in iodine, such as radioisotope infusions during medical testing, have been reported to cause hyperthyroid crisis. According to Delange, iodine-induced hyperthyroidism is an iodine deficiency disease.[33]

Can iodine tablets recommended for travel medicine induce hyperthyroidism? Iodine is frequently recommended as a simple, cost-efficient means to disinfect water during travel or work in areas where municipal water is not reliable. The generally recommended 2 mg/day dose for a maximum of 3 weeks maximum does not have a firm basis. An occasional unmasking of underlying thyroid disease can occur; however, most people can use iodine for water treatment in excess of recommended daily dietary consumption over a prolonged period without concern.[34] Iodine-treated water has a foul taste. It has been reported that adding one teaspoon of activated charcoal per liter of water will remove most of the taste.

Radiation and Iodine

Epidemiological studies obtained after the Chernobyl reactor accident in 1986 provide the best-documented example of massive radiation exposure in a large number of people. Approximately 4 years after the accident, a sharp increase in the number of thyroid cancers emerged. In countries where adults received immediate doses of potassium iodide (KI) at 70 mg/kg, the incidence of cancer was substantially less. Transient thyroid symptoms, including hypo- and hyperthyroidism, were managed medically. The protective effect of KI lasts approximately 24 hours and optimal prophylaxis should be continued daily, throughout the period of exposure risk.[35]

Testing for Iodine Deficiency

The kidneys excrete approximately 90% of unused iodine. Therefore, the best diagnostic test is a 24-hour urine iodine collection. If 24-hour urine collection is not practical or feasible, a random urine iodine-to-creatinine ratio can be used and interpreted as in Table 16.3. This test is generally used in population-based studies and should be considered an estimate of deficiency. No test can reliably diagnose iodine deficiency in individual patients.

High Iodine Foods

The Institute of Medicine (IOM) recommended dietary allowance (RDA) is 150 μg/day of iodine for adults and adolescents, 220 μg/day for pregnant women, 290 μg/day for lactating women, and 90 to 120 μg/day for children ages 1 to 11 years. Two grams of iodized salt (about ½ teaspoon) provides approximately 150 μg of iodine.

The best source of iodine is whole foods. Forms of edible kelp, also known as sea vegetables, contain the highest concentrations of iodine of all foods. Sea vegetables can be obtained in health food stores, Asian groceries, and through the Internet from high-quality manufacturers who assure the plants are harvested from clean waters (see Table 16.4). Multivitamins may contain iodine, usually in the amount of less than 150 μg. Drinking water is generally not a significant source of ionized iodine.

TABLE 16.3
Iodine Testing

Iodine Deficiency	None	Mild	Moderate	Severe
Spot urine iodine, μg/L	>100	50–99	20–49	<20

TABLE 16.4

Sea Vegetables and Iodine Content

Sea Vegetable	How Provided	How Used	Amount of Iodine in a Serving	Amount Needed to Provide 150 µg/day
Sea Salt	Formed from evaporation of ocean water. Contains trace minerals. Unlike salt mined from land sources, sea salt does not contain added sugar.	Beyond food, sea salt is also used in cosmetics, deodorants, antiperspirants and other skin care products.	0.065 mg per 1 gram	About ½ teaspoon
Dulce	Can be powdered in a condiment, used in chunks for cooking.	Plain food source. Used in soups and stews. Chewy texture when cooked. Often included in packaged foods as a thickener or stretcher.	0.135 mg per 1 g	About ⅓ teaspoon
Whole leaf kelp	There are many different types of kelp, constituting around 30 genera.	Used as a flavoring, a garnish, a vegetable, or a snack food. Dried sheets used to wrap sushi and other foods such as broth.	0.450 mg per 1 g	About ¹⁄₁₀ teaspoon
Nori	Type of edible red algae. Dried into thin sheets.	Wrap for sushi, edible garnish, flavoring in noodles and soups.	40 µg per sheet	4 sheets
Kombu	Edible kelp from China, Korea, and Japan. Comes as green, thick strips.	Soup stock, eaten fresh as sashimi	1450 µg per 1-inch piece	¹⁄₁₀ inch
Wakame	Edible kelp from China, Korea, and Japan. Green leaves, sweet flavor, slippery texture.	Miso soup, salads, served alone like a cucumber. High in calcium, thiamine, niacin, vitamin B12, and omega-3 essential fatty acids	82 µg/tablespoon	2 tablespoons
Arame	Edible kelp from China, Korea, and Japan. Brown strands, mild flavor, firm texture.	Soups, muffins, rice dishes. High in iron and calcium.	732 µg/tablespoon	½ teaspoon

SELENIUM

Selenium deficiency may have profound effects on thyroid hormone metabolism and possibly on the thyroid gland itself. Type I deiodinase, a selenium-dependent enzyme, plays a major role in T4 deiodination in peripheral tissues. When iodine and selenium are both deficient and only selenium is supplemented, as in multivitamins or excess selenium-containing foods, serum T4 decreases. Therefore, adding selenium in the presence of iodine deficiency can lead to clinical hypothyroidism with lowered T4 and increased TSH.

Selenium deficiency reduces the function of the selenium-dependent enzyme glutathione peroxidase. Glutathione peroxidase detoxifies H_2O_2, the oxidant used by TPO to produce MIT and DIT. In the absence of selenium, H_2O_2 accumulates within the thyroglobin and can lead to thyroid cell death. The accumulation may contribute to Hashimoto's thyroiditis and may explain why selenium has been reported to significantly improve this condition.[36,37]

Nutrient Repletion Plan

The significance and duration of iodine deficiency in each person are unknown. Reintroduction of high-iodine foods needs to begin slowly. Add one or two teaspoons of sea vegetables per week. Always couple high-iodine foods with high-selenium foods listed in Table 16.1. Monitor patient's TSH every 8 weeks. Thyroid medication dosages may need to be adjusted up or down, based on laboratory assessment and clinical assessment. Dietary interventions can sometimes be sufficient to restore normal thyroid function.

VI. SUMMARY

- TSH and free T4 should not be the only parameters for assessing hypothyroidism.
- A biochemical picture of a mildly elevated serum TSH, normal serum T4 and T3 is called subclinical hypothyroidism and deserves assessment for low iodine.
- Patients who complain of hypothyroid symptoms may benefit from dietary recommendations that increase iodine, selenium, and other nutrients prior to treating with medication.
- Asymptomatic patients with new onset TSH elevation should have soy removed from their diet first before additional tests are recommended.
- Iodine deficiency can lead to development of goiter, hypo-, and/or hyperthyroidism.
- Hypothyroidism can worsen in the presence of selenium deficiency.

REFERENCES

1. Hollowell JG, et al., Iodine excretion data from NHANES I and NHANES III. *J Clin Endocrinol and Metab.* 1998; 88:3401–3410.
2. National Center for Health Statistics, "Iodine level, United States." 2000. http://www.cdc.gov/nchs/products/pubs/pubd/hestats/iodine.htm.
3. Weeke J, Gundersen HJ, Circadian and 30 minute variations in serum TSH and thyroid hormones in normal subjects. *Acta Endocrinol.* 1978; 89:659–672.
4. Baskin HJ, et al., American Association of Clinical Endocrinologists Medical Guidelines for Clinical Practice for the Evaluation and Treatment of Hyperthyroidism and Hypothyroidism. *Endocrine Practice.* 2002; 8(6):457–469.
5. Crapo LM, Subclinical hypothyroidism and cardiovascular disease. *Arch Intern Med.* 2005 Nov 28; 165(21):2451–2452.
6. Hak AE, et al., Subclinical hypothyroidism is an independent risk factor for atherosclerosis and myocardial infarction in elderly women: the Rotterdam Study. *Ann Intern Med.* 2000 Feb 15; 132(4):270–278.
7. Allan WC, et al., Maternal thyroid deficiency and pregnancy complications: implications for population screening. *J Med Screen.* 2000; 7(3):127–130.
8. Michalopoulou G, Alevizaki M, Piperingos G, et al., High serum cholesterol levels in persons with 'high normal' TSH levels: should one extend the definition of subclinical hypothyroidism. *Eur J Endocrinol.* 1998; 138:141–145.
9. Danese MD, et al., Clinical review 115: effect of thyroxine therapy on serum lipoproteins in patients with mild thyroid failure: a quantitative review of the literature. *J Clin Endocrinol Metab.* 2000 Sep; 85(9):2993–3001.
10. Shah SA et al., Autoimmune (Hashimoto's) thyroiditis associated with Crohn's disease. *J Clin Gastro.* March 1998; 26(2):117–120.
11. Vanderpump MP, Tunbridge WM, French JM, Appleton D, Bates D, Clark F, Grimley Evans J, Hasan DM, Rodgers H, Tunbridge F, et al., The incidence of thyroid disorders in the community: a twenty-year follow-up of the Whickham Survey. *Clin Endocrinol (Oxf).* 1995 Jul; 43(1):55–68.
12. Cooper DS, et al., L-Thyroxine therapy in subclinical hypothyroidism. A double-blind, placebo-controlled trial. *Ann Intern Med.* 1984 Jul; 101(1):18–24.
13. Mastorakos G, Nezi M, Papadopoulos C, *The Iodine Deficiency Disorders,* Chapter 20, pages 23–24.
14. Divi RL, Chang HC, Doerge DR. Anti-thyroid isoflavones from soybean: isolation, characterization, and mechanisms of action. *Biochem Pharmacol.* 1997 Nov 15; 54(10):1087–1096.
15. Ishizuki Y, Hirooka Y, Murata Y, Togashi K, The effects on the thyroid gland of soybeans administered experimentally in healthy subjects. *Nippon Naibunpi Gakkai Zasshi.* 1991 May 20; 67(5):622–629.

16. Doerge DR, Inactivation of thryoid peroxidase by genistein and daidzein in vitro and in vivo; mechanism for anti-thyroid activity of soy, presented at the November 1999 Soy Symposium in Washington, DC. National Center for Toxicological Research, Jefferson, AR, 72029

17. Sheehan D, Doerge D, "Scientists protest soy approval." Posted on ABC.com website. http://www.wellnesswithin.com/articles/ScientistsProtestSoy.pdf.

18. Doerge DR, Sheehan DM, Goitrogenic and estrogenic activity of soy isoflavones. *Environ Health Perspect.* 2002 Jun; 110 Suppl 3:349–353.

19. Divi RL, Chang HC, Doerge DR, Anti-thyroid isoflavones from soybean: isolation, characterization, and mechanisms of action. *Biochem Pharmacol.* 1997 Nov 15; 54(10):1087–1096.

20. Badger TM, et al., The health consequences of early soy consumption. *J. Nutr.* 132: 559S–565S.

21. Setchell KD, et al., Exposure of infants to phyto-oestrogens from soy-based infant formula. *Lancet.* 350:23–27.

22. Strom BL, et al., Exposure to soy-based formula in infancy and endocrinological and reproductive outcomes in young adulthood. *JAMA.* 286:807–814.

23. Conrad SC, Chiu H, Silverman BL, Soy formula complicates management of congenital hypothyroidism. *Arch Dis Child.* 2004 Jan; 89(1):37–40.

24. Wollman SH, Inhibition by thiocyanate of accumulation of radioiodine by thyroid gland. *Am J of Physiol.* 203, 517–524.

25. Strum JM, Phelps PC, McAtee MM, Resting human female breast tissue produces iodinated proteins. *J Ultrastruc Res.* 84:130–139.

26. Ghent W, Iodine replacement in fibrocystic disease of the breast. *Can J Surg.* 36:453–460.

27. Iodine Deficiency Diseases WHO Manual. http://www.sph.emory.edu/PAMM/IDD/whomanual/factors.pdf.

28. Wolff J, Chaikoff IL, Plasma inorganic iodide as a homeostatic regulator of thyroid function. *J Biol Chem.* 174:555–564.

29. Wolff J, Chaikoff IL, Goldberg RC, Meier JC, The temporary nature of the inhibitory action of excess iodide on organic iodide synthesis in the normal thyroid. *Endocrinology.* 45:504.

30. Braverman LE, Ingbar SH, Changes in thyroidal function during adaptation to large doses of iodine. *J Clin Invest.* 1963 August; 42(8):1216–1231.

31. Hollowell JG, et al., Iodine excretion data from NHANES I and NHANES III. *J Clin Endocrinol and Metab.* 1998; 88:3401–3410.

32. Leonard JL, Koehrle J. 2000. Intracellular pathways of iodothyronine metabolism. In *The thryoid: A fundamental and clinical text, 8th ed.*, 147. Philadelphia: Lippincott Williams & Wilkins.

33. Delange FM. 2000. Iodine deficiency. In *The thyroid: A fundamental and clinical text, 8th ed.*, 312. Philadelphia: Lippincott Williams & Wilkins.

34. Backer H, Hollowell J, Use of iodine for water disinfection: iodine toxicity and maximum recommended dose. *Environ Health Perspect.* 2000 August; 108(8):679–684.

35. Department of Health and Human Services, FDA CDER, "Guidance potassium iodide as a thyroid blocking agent in radiation emergencies. http://www.dfa.gov/cder/guidance/index.htm.

36. Duntas LH, Mantzou E, Koutras DA, Effects of a six month treatment with selenomethionine in patients with autoimmune thyroiditis. *Eur J Endocrinol.* 2003 Apr; 148(4):389–393.

37. Mazokopakis EE, et al., Effects of 12 months treatment with L-selenomethionine on serum anti-TPO levels in patients with Hashimoto's thyroiditis. *Thyroid.* 2007 Jul; 17(7):609–612.

38. Smyth PP, Duntas LH, Iodine uptake and loss—Can frequent strenuous exercise induce iodine deficiency? *Horm Metab Res.* 2005 Sep; 37(9):555–558.

39. Mao IF, Chen ML, Ko YC, Electrolyte loss in sweat and iodine deficiency in a hot environment. *Arch Environ Health.* 2001 May–Jun; 56(3):271–277.

40. Järnerot G, The thyroid in ulcerative colitis and Crohn's disease. I. Thyroid radioiodide uptake and urinary iodine excretion. *Acta Med Scand.* 1975 Jan–Feb; 197(1–2):77–81.

17 Hyperparathyroidisms

Michael F. Holick, M.D., Ph.D.

I. INTRODUCTION

Parathyroid hormone (PTH) is essential for maintaining calcium homeostasis.[1-8] It accomplishes this by regulating calcium mobilization from the skeleton, controlling calcium excretion in the kidneys, and stimulating the kidneys to activate vitamin D. Hyperparathyroidism is a consequence of the excess production of PTH by the parathyroid glands. This can be caused by a benign or malignant tumor in the parathyroid gland(s), or stimulation of the parathyroid glands by vitamin D deficiency, hypocalcemia, or hyperphosphatemia. The consequences of hyperparathyroidism include hypercalciuria, hypercalcemia, hypophosphatemia, osteopenia/osteoporosis, osteomalacia, and kidney stones.[1-7] The major causes of hyperparathyroidism are a benign adenoma in a parathyroid gland causing primary hyperparathyroidism, and vitamin D deficiency and chronic kidney disease (CKD) causing secondary hyperparathyroidism.[1-5]

II. PARATHYROID PHYSIOLOGY

The Chief cells in the parathyroid glands produce PTH. The calcium sensor (calcium receptor, CaR) in the plasma membrane of the Chief cells is constantly monitoring blood ionized calcium levels.[4-6] In response to a decrease in serum ionized calcium, there is an immediate increase in the receptor activity leading to signal transduction resulting in the stimulation of nuclear expression of the PTH mRNA, which increases the transcription and translation for PTH.[2,6] PTH is transcribed into a 115 amino acid peptide often called the prepro form.[2,6] It undergoes posttranslational modification to the 84 amino acid PTH and is then incorporated into secretionary granules that release PTH into the circulation. The first 34 amino acids in the N-terminal region of PTH are responsible for most if not all of the calcium regulating properties of PTH.[2,6] PTH interacts with its receptor PTH receptor 1 (PTHR-1) in the kidneys, which stimulates proximal and distal tubular reabsorption of calcium from the ultrafiltrate and decreases tubular reabsorption of phosphorus (Figure 17.1). PTH interacts with its receptor on the osteoblasts to increase the expression of RANKL (receptor activator of NFκB ligand).[8] RANKL, which is on the plasma membrane of the osteoblast, interacts with its receptor RANK present on the monocytic precursor of the osteoclast and stimulates it to become a mature osteoclast to mobilize calcium from the skeleton (Figure 17.2).

PTH enhances the renal adenylate cyclase to increase cAMP for inducing signal transduction in the renal tubular cell. This results in an increase in urinary levels of cAMP. PTH also stimulates the kidneys to convert 25-hydroxyvitamin D [25(OH)D] to its active form 1,25-dihydroxyvitamin D [1,25(OH)$_2$D].[3,10] 1,25(OH)$_2$D interacts with its nuclear receptor (VDR) in the small intestine to increase the efficiency of intestinal calcium absorption. Thus, PTH indirectly is responsible for enhancing intestinal calcium absorption to help maintain serum calcium levels within the normal physiologic range of 8.6 to 10.2 mg%.[3,10]

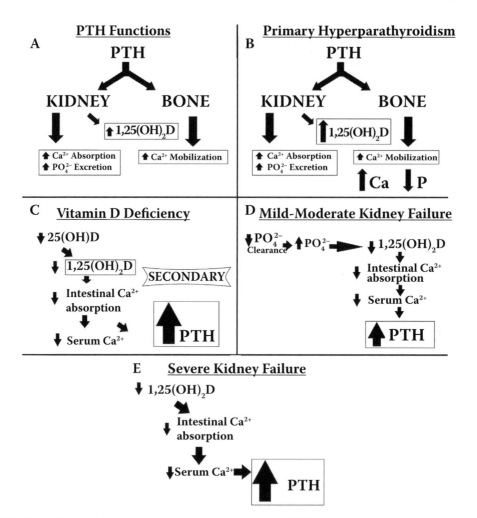

FIGURE 17.1 The physiologic functions of parathyroid hormone (PTH) on calcium phosphorus and vitamin D metabolism. The consequences of vitamin D deficiency and chronic kidney disease (CKD) on PTH level and its effects on calcium and phosphorus metabolism are schematically presented. (From [11]. With permission.)

The CaR that is present in the parathyroid glands is a seven transmembrane receptor.[4, 6] Unlike most receptors, where binding its ligand stimulates receptor activity and signal transduction, the CaR works in an opposite manner: The less calcium binding to the CaR the more active the CaR is in enhancing signal transduction for stimulating the parathyroid cell to produce PTH (Figure 17.3).

Magnesium and Parathyroid Function and Activity

Magnesium plays a major role in parathyroid function.[12] The CaR recognizes magnesium. If the magnesium is elevated, it will shut down the production of PTH similar to high serum calcium (Figure 17.3). However, more important is that hypomagnesemia leads to a marked decrease in the production and secretion of PTH and also prevents PTH from acting on the skeleton[13] (Figure 17.3). As a result, hypomagnesemia causes functional hypoparathyroidism, that is, the parathyroid glands cannot increase the production of PTH and the PTH that is made is unable to carry out its physiologic functions on both the skeleton and in the kidneys.[12] Alcohol causes magnesium loss into the

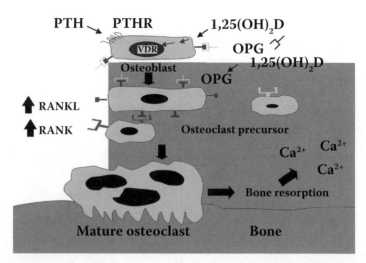

FIGURE 17.2 Both parathyroid hormone (PTH) and 1,25-dihydroxyvitamin D [1,25(OH)₂D] interact with their respective receptors in osteoblasts resulting in the expression of RANKL. The receptor RANK on the preosteoclast interacts with RANKL inducing the cell to become a mature osteoclast. The mature osteoclasts release collagenases and hydrochloric acid to destroy the matrix and release calcium into the extra cellular space. Osteoprotegerin (OPG) is a decoy RANKL that can bind to the RANK of the preosteoclast, preventing it from becoming a mature osteoclast. (From [11]. With permission.)

urine. Alcoholics who present to an emergency room with seizure, carpal pedal spasms, and severe hypocalcemia are also severely magnesium deficient. Thus, repleting the calcium as well as the magnesium deficits are important in restoring calcium metabolism. Most magnesium is intracellular, and, thus, a serum magnesium level does not provide any insight into the magnesium status of an individual. The only method to determine whether patients are magnesium deficient or sufficient is to give them a loading dose of 1 gram of magnesium oxide and then to collect the 24 hour urine magnesium. If magnesium is spilled into the urine, then the magnesium tank is likely to be full and the magnesium status normal. However, if there is very little magnesium excreted into the urine, then there is a magnesium deficit even if the serum magnesium is normal. This is the reason why it is often advertised that it is necessary to take magnesium with calcium in order to maximize calcium absorption. Magnesium has no direct influence on calcium absorption. It indirectly influences intestinal calcium absorption by maintaining the production of PTH, which stimulates the kidneys to produce 1,25(OH)₂D, which stimulates intestinal calcium absorption. Magnesium also is important for PTH and 1,25(OH)₂D to stimulate bone calcium mobilization when dietary sources of calcium are inadequate to satisfy the body's calcium needs.[13]

PRIMARY HYPERPARATHYROIDISM AND ITS HEALTH CONSEQUENCES

Approximately one in 1000 adults will develop a benign tumor in one or more of their parathyroid glands resulting in the autonomous production of PTH.[1,14] The chronic elevation in PTH results in an increase in osteoclastic activity that causes loss of matrix and mineral from the skeleton. Cortical bone is more sensitive to PTH than trabecular bone and, thus, cortical bone wasting is greater than trabecular bone wasting. The consequence for patients with primary hyperparathyroidism is that they are at higher risk of fracturing their wrist or hip than their spine.[1,7,14] (See Figure 17.4.) Thus, primary hyperparathyroidism will precipitate and exacerbate osteopenia and osteoporosis. The elevated serum calcium and increased calcium in the urine can increase risk of nephrocalcinosis and kidney stones.[14]

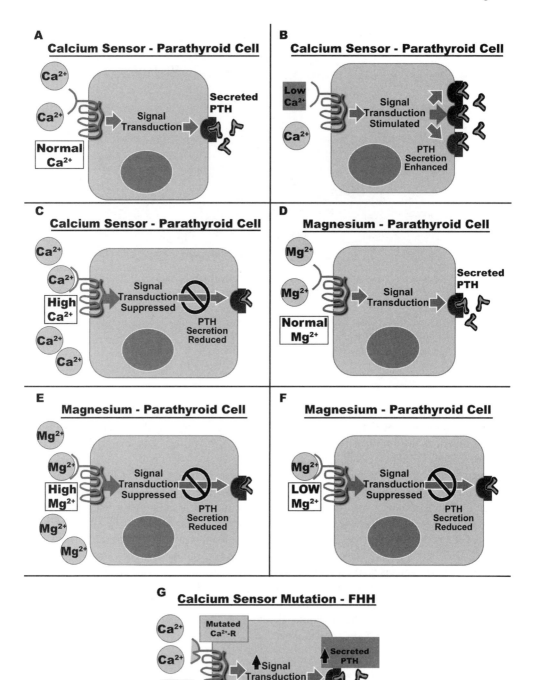

FIGURE 17.3 These schematics portray how calcium and magnesium interact with the calcium sensor (calcium receptor; CaR) on the parathyroid cell resulting in either an increase, decrease, or normal expression and secretion of PTH. (From [11]. With permission.)

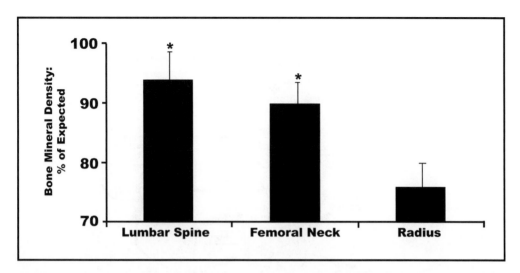

FIGURE 17.4 Bone mineral density in postmenopausal women with primary hyperparathyroidism. (Adapted from [7]. With permission.)

Patients with hyperparathyroidism have elevated PTH, which is associated with fasting hypercalcemia, hypophosphatemia, and high normal or elevated levels of $1,25(OH)_2D$. Since the PTH increases the metabolism of $25(OH)D$ to $1,25(OH)_2D$, often the patients with hyperparathyroidism have vitamin D deficiency, low serum levels of $25(OH)D$.[3,10] (See Figures 17.2 and 17.5.)

Approximately 85% of patients with primary hyperparathyroidism have a benign tumor, that is, a single adenoma. Ten percent of these patients can have a second adenoma in a different parathyroid gland. Most people have four parathyroid glands; however, as many as six can be present. Often the parathyroid adenoma can be visualized by using a sestamibi scan, which helps the surgeon locate and easily remove the adenoma.[1,14] Once the adenoma is removed, these patients often have remarkable improvement in their bone mineral density and restoration of the calcium metabolism to normal.

INHERITED CAUSES OF HYPERPARATHYROIDISM

Approximately 15% of patients who present with hyperparathyroidism have hyperplasia of all four parathyroid glands. The two major inherited causes for parathyroid gland hyperplasia are the multiple endocrine neoplasia (MEN) syndromes type 1 and type 2[15] and familial hypocalciuric hypercalcemia (FHH).[4,16] The MEN syndromes are due to a mutation in the genes that regulate the proliferation and differentiation not only of parathyroid cells but other cells of endocrine origin.[15]

When evaluating patients with mild to moderate elevation in serum calcium with elevated PTH, it is important to rule out FHH. Although this disease is relatively rare, it should not be missed. The cause is due to a point mutation of the CaR in the parathyroid glands making the parathyroid glands less responsive to serum calcium levels. As a result, the serum calcium levels are chronically mildly elevated and there is an elevation in serum PTH levels. Since the calcium sensor in the kidney is also defective, this results in a marked increase in tubular resorption of calcium in the kidney. Thus, distinguishing primary hyperparathyroidism from FHH can be accomplished by obtaining a 24-hour urine for calcium and creatinine and a blood for calcium and creatinine at the same time. A calcium clearance should be determined. A calcium clearance of < 1% is considered consistent with FHH and not primary hyperparathyroidism because patients with FHH have hyperplasia of all their hyperparathyroid glands. If the surgeon removes 3¾ glands, remnant parathyroid tissue will once again become hyperplastic and cause the same problem. Most patients with FHH do not have

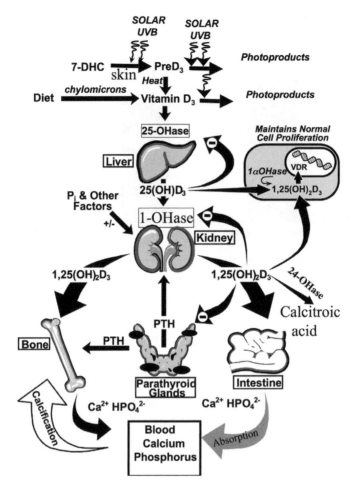

FIGURE 17.5 Schematic diagram of cutaneous production of vitamin D and its metabolism and regulation for calcium homeostasis and cellular growth. During exposure to sunlight, 7-dehydrocholesterol (7-DHC) in the skin absorbs solar UVB radiation and is converted to previtamin D_3 (preD_3). Once formed, previtamin D_3 undergoes thermally induced transformation to vitamin D_3. Additional exposure to sunlight converts previtamin D_3 and vitamin D_3 to biologically inert photoproducts. Vitamin D originating from the diet or from the skin enters the circulation and is metabolized to 25(OH)D_3 in the liver by vitamin D 25-hydroxylase (25-OHase). 25(OH)D_3 reenters the circulation and is converted to 1,25(OH)$_2$D$_3$ in the kidney by 25(OH)D$_3$ 1α-hydroxylase (1-OHase). A variety of factors, including serum phosphorus (P$_i$) and PTH, regulate the renal production of 1,25(OH)$_2$D and calcium metabolism through interactions with its major target tissues, that is, bone and intestine. 1,25(OH)$_2$D$_3$ also induces its own destruction by enhancing the expression of 25(OH)D 24-hydroxylase (24-OHase). 25(OH)D is metabolized in other tissues for regulation of cellular growth. (From [10]. With permission.)

any deleterious effects on either their skeleton or calcium metabolism, and, thus, do not need any intervention. The only intervention is to make the diagnosis and prevent the patient from seeing a surgeon to have a parathyroidectomy.

SECONDARY HYPERPARATHYROIDISM ASSOCIATED WITH VITAMIN D DEFICIENCY AND ITS HEALTH CONSEQUENCES

The major cause of hyperparathyroidism is due to vitamin D deficiency. Vitamin D deficiency is defined as a low circulating level of 25(OH)D of < 20 ng/mL.[3,17] This results in a decrease of efficiency of intestinal calcium absorption leading to a decrease of ionized calcium, which is recognized by the CaR in the parathyroid glands resulting in an increase in the synthesis and secretion of PTH (Figure 17.1).

Like primary hyperparathyroidism, the elevated PTH levels result in increased osteoclastic activity. This causes osteopenia and osteoporosis and increases risk of fracture. The secondary hyperparathyroidism also causes a loss of phosphorus into the urine, resulting in low normal or low serum phosphorus. The consequence is an inadequate calcium-phosphate product in the circulation preventing the normal mineralization of the collagen matrix laid down by osteoblasts. The defect is known as osteomalacia.[3,10] Patients with osteomalacia often present with isolated or generalized aches and pains in their bones and muscles. These patients have a normal sedimentation rate, and, thus, no rheumatologic disorder and often are misdiagnosed as having fibromyalgia, chronic fatigue syndrome, or depressive symptoms.[18-20] The unmineralized collagen matrix is hydrated, thus pushing upward on the periosteal covering of the bones, which is heavily innervated with sensory fibers. These patients complain of throbbing, aching bone pain, and when their periosteum is depressed, they complain of bone pain. This can happen when patients are sitting or lying in bed and complain of painful bones. The diagnosis can be made by pressing with a thumb or forefinger with moderate pressure on the sternum or anterior tibia. If the patient winces with pain, it's likely that their periosteal bone discomfort is caused by osteomalacia.[3,20]

To make the diagnosis of secondary hyperparathyroidism associated with vitamin D deficiency, a fasting blood chemistry reveals a normal serum calcium, low normal or low serum phosphorus, elevated PTH, and a low 25(OH)D of < 20 ng/mL (Figure 17.1). The $1,25(OH)_2D$ levels are often normal or elevated for several reasons.[3] $1,25(OH)_2D$ levels are 1000 times less in concentration compared to 25(OH)D. The elevated PTH levels stimulate the kidneys to produce $1,25(OH)_2D$. The reason that patients are vitamin D deficient is that there is an inadequate amount of $1,25(OH)_2D$ that is being made to satisfy the small intestine's requirement. Thus, even though the blood level of $1,25(OH)_2D$ can be normal or elevated, it is not a reflection of the intestinal levels of $1,25(OH)_2D$. This is the reason why measurement of $1,25(OH)_2D$ should never be used in evaluating patients for vitamin D deficiency.[3]

SECONDARY HYPERPARATHYROIDISM ASSOCIATED WITH CKD

It is outside the scope of this chapter to review in any detail the causes and treatment for secondary hyperparathyroidism associated with CKD. See Kidney Disease Outcomes Quality Intiative (K/DOQI) Guidelines and recent reviews for more details.[3,21-24] It was obvious after it was realized that the kidneys were responsible for producing $1,25(OH)_2D$ why patients with severe CKD had severe abnormalities in their calcium metabolism and had associated metabolic bone disease.[3,22,23] However, patients with mild to moderate CKD also have abnormalities in their calcium and bone metabolism and often suffer from secondary hyperparathyroidism. There are several reasons for this. In mild to moderate CKD, the patients are unable to efficiently excrete phosphorus (Figure 17.1). The increase in serum phosphorus levels results in a marked inhibition in renal production of $1,25(OH)_2D$.[3,22,23] This is thought to be due to an increase in fiberblast growth factor 23 that is produced by the osteoblasts and causes a suppression of the production of $1,25(OH)_2D$ in the kidneys. In addition, the high serum phosphorus suppresses the expression of the CaR in the parathyroid cell and enhances TGFα/EGFR activation to enhance proliferation and stimulate the parathyroid glands to produce PTH.[22] Thus, most patients with mild to moderate CKD use a phosphate binder such as calcium carbonate or a resin to prevent excess dietary phosphorus from being absorbed and to help keep the serum phosphorus level within the normal range.[3,22,23]

In CKD disease where more than ~ 60% of the kidney function is lost, the kidneys no longer have the capacity to produce an adequate amount of $1,25(OH)_2D$ to satisfy the body's requirement. As a result, intestinal calcium absorption is decreased, resulting in a decrease in ionized calcium stimulating the parathyroid glands to produce PTH. These patients benefit by receiving either $1,25(OH)_2D_3$ or one of its active analogues.[3,21-25] (See Figure 17.1.)

Patients with CKD disease benefit from maintaining a serum 25(OH)D of > 30 ng/mL, which is what is recommended by the K/DOQI guidelines.[3,21–25] There are at least two reasons for this. The first is that the parathyroid glands have the enzymatic machinery, 25-hydroxyvitamin D-1-hydroxylase (1-OHase), to produce 1,25(OH)$_2$D in the parathyroid cells, which locally suppress PTH expression and production.[3,22,26] (See Figure 17.5.) Increasing serum 25(OH)D > 30 ng/mL suppresses PTH synthesis.[22–27] In addition 25(OH)D may be converted to 1,25(OH)$_2$D in many other tissues in the body including colon, breast, and prostate for the purpose of regulating cell growth and a wide variety of other cellular functions.[3,10,24,25] Thus, maintaining serum 25(OH)D > 30 ng/mL helps reduce risk of cancers, infectious diseases, heart disease, and autoimmune diseases.[3,10,24,25]

Tertiary Hyperparathyroidism and Health Consequences

Chronic secondary hyperparathyroidism leads to marked hyperplasia, increased cellular growth of the parathyroid glands that can markedly increase their size. Often these glands become hypercellular and develop islands of nodules.[22] The cells within these nodules have less CaR expression and also lack a vitamin D receptor (VDR), making the cells less responsive to the regulatory activities that calcium and 1,25(OH)$_2$D have on suppressing PTH production.[3,10,22,24,25,27] Thus, patients with chronic severe secondary hyperparathyroidism due to vitamin D deficiency or CKD can have autonomous activity within the parathyroid glands. As a result, the serum calcium becomes elevated, and with an elevated PTH level, this is now no longer considered to be secondary hyperparathyroidism, but tertiary hyperparathyroidism.[3,10,22,27,28] By definition, tertiary hyperparathyroidism is associated with an elevated serum calcium, elevated PTH, low normal or low phosphorus with a low or normal serum 25(OH)D level. For patients with CKD, their serum calcium can be controlled by dialysis three times a week with a low calcium dialysis bath. When these patients receive a renal transplant, their transplanted kidney makes 1,25(OH)$_2$D. Some of these patients who have marked parathyroid gland hyperplasia will have autonomous parathyroid cell activity resulting in hypercalcemia, and, thus, tertiary hyperparathyroidism.[3,28]

III. TREATMENT STRATEGIES

Most patients with primary hyperparathyroidism who have a single adenoma often go to surgery to have the adenoma removed with good outcomes.[1,2,14] However, if the patient has hyperplasia, 3¾ glands are removed. This usually preserves parathyroid function, but markedly diminishes the parathyroid tissue burden resulting in reduced or normal levels of PTH with normal calcium homeostasis.[14] Less than 1% of patients with primary hyperparathyroidism have a malignant carcinoma that needs to be aggressively treated.[14] Sometimes these patients with metastatic disease and who have elevated PTH levels benefit by using a CaR mimetic cinacalcet.[14]

There is no need to treat FHH unless the hypercalcemia causes nonspecific constitutional symptoms including fatigue, depression, constipation, and so on. From my clinical experience, a trial of cinacalcet may be helpful. Patients with MEN 1 and 2 require parathyroid surgery and need to be evaluated for other endocrine tumors.[14]

Patients with mild to moderate CKD should control their serum phosphorus levels with a calcium binder.[3,21–27] In addition, they need to be vitamin D sufficient with 25(OH)D of > 30 ng/mL. Patients with more severe kidney disease and who are unable to produce adequate 1,25(OH)$_2$D need to be treated with either 1,25(OH)$_2$D$_3$ therapy or one of its active analogues including paricalcitol and doxercalciferol.[3,21–27]

The most common cause of hyperparathyroidism is vitamin D deficiency. Vitamin D deficiency is defined as a 25(OH)D of < 20 ng/mL. However, many studies have reported that PTH levels will continue to decrease until 25(OH)D levels are > 30 ng/mL.[29–31] Thus, vitamin D sufficiency is now considered to be a 25(OH)D of > 30 ng/mL and is the level believed to maximize child and adult bone health and prevent secondary hyperparathyroidism.[3,32,33] To achieve this level, at least 1000 IU of vitamin D a day is needed when inadequate sun exposure cannot provide the body with its vitamin D requirement.[3,10] The rule of thumb is that for every 100 IU of vitamin D ingested, there is an increase in 25(OH)D of 1 ng/mL.[3,11,34] Although it has been reported that vitamin D_2 is less effective than vitamin D_3 in maintaining serum 25(OH)D levels[35] and that vitamin D_2 enhanced the destruction of vitamin D_3,[36] a recent report suggests that 1000 IU of vitamin D_2 is equally effective as 1000 IU of vitamin D_3 in maintaining serum 25(OH)D levels.[11]

Patients who are vitamin D deficient need to be aggressively repleted. This can be accomplished by giving 50,000 IU of vitamin D_2 once a week for 8 weeks to fill the empty vitamin D tank.[3,16] If the blood level of 25(OH)D does not reach above 30 ng/mL, the tank may be so empty that it requires an additional 8 week course of 50,000 IU of vitamin D_2. Since treatment for vitamin D deficiency does not correct the cause of the vitamin D deficiency, once I have corrected their vitamin D deficiency and raised their blood level of 25(OH)D > 30 ng/mL, I give all of my patients 50,000 IU of vitamin D_2 once every two weeks forever. A recent analysis of more than 100 of my patients who received this therapy for up to 6 years showed that they maintained blood levels of 25(OH)D of between 30 to 60 ng/mL with no untoward consequences. An alternative is to give 2000 to 3000 units of vitamin D_2 or vitamin D_3 a day for at least 2 to 3 months followed by at least 1000 IU of vitamin D_2 or vitamin D_3 daily thereafter. It has also been reported that taking 100,000 IU of vitamin D_3 every 3 months can help reduce risk of fracture and maintain 25(OH)D above 20 ng/mL.[37]

Patients with CKD with a renal transplant who develop tertiary hyperparathyroidism and patients with chronic vitamin D deficiency and tertiary hyperparathyroidism often benefit by treating their vitamin D deficiency and raising blood levels of 25(OH)D > 30 ng/mL.[3] There has been concern that patients with primary or tertiary hyperparathyroidism who have elevated levels of serum calcium would increase their serum calcium to a greater extent if vitamin D were given to them. Patients with primary hyperparathyroidism who received vitamin D to treat their vitamin D deficiency did not experience an increase in the serum calcium levels.[3,38] From my own experience, patients with both primary and tertiary hyperparathyroidism often benefit by correcting their vitamin D deficiency. Correcting vitamin D deficiency can significantly reduce PTH levels, especially in patients with tertiary hyperparathyroidism, and can sometimes prevent the need for surgical debulking of the parathyroid glands.

IV. CONCLUSIONS

Patients are routinely screened with their blood chemistries for a serum calcium level. Most patients with a primary hyperparathyroidism are picked up by the primary care physician who finds an elevated serum calcium. If further workup reveals an elevated PTH level, this is diagnostic of primary hyperparathyroidism. The only time this is not true is when a patient has tertiary hyperparathyroidism or FHH.

The major cause of secondary hyperparathyroidism is vitamin D deficiency. Besides causing osteopenia and osteoporosis with increased risk of fracture, most patients with vitamin D deficiency and secondary hyperparathyroidism have nonspecific aches and pains in their bones and muscles due to osteomalacia.[3] These patients often have dramatic improvement of their nonspecific complaints by correction of their vitamin D deficiency. Since the serum calcium is normal in patients with secondary hyperparathyroidism, primary care physicians will not easily pick up this diagnosis unless they routinely screen for 25(OH)D levels. From a cost-benefit perspective, it would be much better to obtain a 25(OH)D on patients suspected of vitamin D deficiency and to forego the PTH analysis unless there is an extenuating circumstance that requires it. Only when the calcium is elevated should a PTH level be determined to rule out primary or tertiary hyperparathyroidism.

ACKNOWLEDGMENT

This work was supported in part by NIH grant M01RR00533.

REFERENCES

1. Silverberg, S.H., Bilezikian, J.P. 1997. Primary hyperparathyroidism: still evolving? *J Bone Miner Res* 12(5):856–862.
2. Kronenberg, H.M., Bringhurst, F.R., Segre, G.V., Potts, Jr., J.T. 1994. Parathyroid hormone biosynthesis and metabolism. In *The parathyroids: basic and clinical concepts*, eds. J.P. Bilezikian, R. Marcus, M.A. Levine, 125–137. New York: Raven Press.
3. Holick, M.F. 2007. Vitamin D deficiency. *N Eng J Med* 357:266–281.
4. Tfelt-Hansen, J., Yano, S., Brown, E.M., Chattapadyay, N. 2002. The role of the calcium-sensing receptor in human pathophysiology. *Current Medicinal Chemistry—Immunology, Endocrine & Metabolic Agents* 2(3):175–193.
5. Slatopolsky, E., Brown, A., Dusso, A. 2001. Role of phosphorus in the pathogenesis of secondary hyper-parathyroidism. *Am J Kidney Dis* 37(1 suppl 2):S54–57.
6. Brown, E.M, Juppner, H. 2006. Parathyroid hormone: synthesis, secretion, and action. In *Primer on the metabolic bone diseases and disorders of mineral metabolism*, ed. M.J. Favus, MD, 6th edition, 90–99. Washington, DC: American Society for Bone and Mineral Research.
7. Silverberg, S.J., Shane, E., de la Cruz, L., et al. 1989. Skeletal disease in primary hyperparathyroidism. *J Bone Miner Res* 4(3):283–291.
8. Bell, N.H. 2003. RANK ligand and the regulation of skeletal remodeling. *J Clin Invest* 111(3): 1120–1122.
9. Holick, M.F. 2004. Sunlight and vitamin D for bone health and prevention of autoimmune diseases, cancers, and cardiovascular disease. *Am J Clin Nutr* 80:1678S–1688S.
10. Holick, M.F., Garabedian, M. 2006. Vitamin D: photobiology, metabolism, mechanism of action, and clinical applications. In *Primer on the metabolic bone diseases and disorders of mineral metabolism*, ed. M.J. Favus, MD, 6th edition, 129–137. Washington, DC: American Society for Bone and Mineral Research.
11. Holick, M.F., Biancuzzo, R.M., Chen, T.C., et al. 2008. Vitamin D_2 is as effective as vitamin D_3 in maintaining circulating concentrations of 25-hydroxyvitamin D. *J Clin Endocrinol Metab* 93(3):677–681.
12. Rude, R.K. 2006. Magnesium depletion and hypermagnesemia. In *Primer on the metabolic bone diseases and disorders of mineral metabolism*, ed. M.J. Favus, MD, 6th edition, 230–233. Washington, DC: American Society for Bone and Mineral Research.
13. Holick, M.F. 1996. Evaluation and treatment of disorders in calcium, phosphorus, and magnesium metabolism. In *Primary Care and General Medicine*, ed. J. Noble, 2nd edition, Chapter 37, 545–557. St. Louis: Mosby.
14. Bilezikins, J.P., Silverberg, S.J. 2006. Primary hyperparathyroidism. In *Primer on the metabolic bone diseases and disorders of mineral metabolism*, ed. M.J. Favus, MD, 6th edition, 181–185. Washington, DC: American Society for Bone and Mineral Research.
15. Arnold, A. 2006. Familial hyperparathyroid syndromes. In *Primer on the metabolic bone diseases and disorders of mineral metabolism*, ed. M.J. Favus, MD, 6th edition, 185–188. Washington, DC: American Society for Bone and Mineral Research.
16. Marx, S. 2006. Familial hypocalciuric hypercalcemia. In *Primer on the metabolic bone diseases and disorders of mineral metabolism*, ed. M.J. Favus, MD, 6th edition, 188–190. Washington, DC: American Society for Bone and Mineral Research.
17. Malabanan, A., Veronikis, I.E., Holick, M.F. 1998. Redefining vitamin D insufficiency. *Lancet* 351: 805–806.
18. Glerup, H., Middelsen, K., Poulsen, L., et al. 2000. Hypovitaminosis D myopathy without biochemical signs of osteomalacia bone involvement. *Calcif Tissue Int* 66:419–424.
19. Plotnikoff, G.A, Quigley, J.M. 2003. Prevalence of severe hypovitaminosis D in patients with persistent, nonspecific musculoskeletal pain. *Mayo Clin Proc* 78:1463–1470.
20. Holick, M.F. 2003. Vitamin D deficiency: What a pain it is. *Mayo Clin Proc* 78(12):1457–1459.
21. K/DOQI. 2003. Clinical practice guidelines for bone metabolism and disease in chronic kidney disease. *Am J Kidney Dis* 42(suppl 3):S1–S201.

22. Dusso, A.S., Sato, T., Arcidiacono, M.V., et al. 2006. Pathogenic mechanisms for parathyroid hyperplasia. *Kidney Int Suppl* 70:S8–S11.

23. Martin, K.J. Al-Aly, Z., Gonzalez, E. 2006. Renal osteodystrophy. In *Primer on the metabolic bone diseases and disorders of mineral metabolism*, ed. M.J. Favus, MD, 6th edition, 359–368. Washington, DC: American Society for Bone and Mineral Research.

24. Dusso, A.S., Brown, A.J., Slatopolsky, E. 2005. Vitamin D. *Am J Physiol Renal Physiol* 289(1): F8–F28.

25. Jones, G. 2007. Expanding role for Vitamin D in chronic kidney disease: Importance of blood 25-OH-D levels and extra-renal 1α-hydroxylase in the classical and nonclassical actions of 1α,25-dihydroxyvitamin D$_3$. *Seminars in Dialysis* 20(4):316–324.

26. Correa, P., Segersten, U., Hellman, P., Akerstrom, G., Westin, G. 2002. Increased 25-hydroxyvitamin D$_3$, 1α-hydroxylase and reduced 25-hydroxyvitamin D$_3$, 24-hydroxylase expression in parathyroid tumors—new prospects for treatment of hyperparathyroidism with vitamin D. *J Clin Endorcrinol Metab* 87:5826–5829.

27. Holick, MF. 2005. Vitamin D for health and in chronic kidney disease. *Seminars in Dialysis* 18: 266–275.

28. Prince, R.L. 2006. Secondary and tertiary hyperparathyroidism. In *Primer on the metabolic bone diseases and disorders of mineral metabolism*, ed. M.J. Favus, MD, 6th edition, 190–195. Washington, DC: American Society for Bone and Mineral Research.

29. Chapuy, M.C., Preziosi, P., Maaner, M., et al. 1997. Prevalence of vitamin D insufficiency in an adult normal population. *Osteopor Int* 7:439–443.

30. Thomas, K.K., Lloyd-Jones, D.M., Thadhani, R.I., et al. 1998. Hypovitaminosis D in medicine in patients. *N Engl J Med* 338:777–783.

31. Holick, M.F., Siris, E.S., Binkley, N., Beard, M.K., Khan, A., Katzer, J.T., et al. 2005. Prevalence of vitamin D inadequacy among postmenopausal North American women receiving osteoporosis therapy. *J Clin Endocrinol Metab* 90:3215–3224.

32. Vieth, R., Bischoff-Ferrari, H., Boucher, B.J., et al. 2007. The urgent need to recommend an intake of vitamin D that is effective. *Am J Clin Nutr* 85(3):649–650.

33. Bischoff-Ferrari, H.A., Giovannucci, E., Willett, W.C., Dietrich, T., and Dawson-Hughes, B. 2006. Estimation of optimal serum concentrations of 25-hydroxyvitamin D for multiple health outcomes. *Am J Clin Nutr* 84:18–28.

34. Heaney, R.P., Davies, K.M., Chen, T.C., Holick, M.F., Barger-Lux, M.J. 2003. Human serum 25-hydroxycholecalciferol response to extended oral dosing with cholecalciferol. *Am J Clin Nutr* 77: 204–210.

35. Tang, H.M., Cole, D.E.C., Rubin, L.A., Pierratos, A., Siu, S., Vieth, R. 1998. Evidence that vitamin D$_3$ increases serum 25-hydroxyvitamin D more efficiently than does vitamin D$_2$. *Am J Clin Nutr* 68: 854–858.

36. Armas, L.A.G., Hollis, B., Heaney, R.P. 2004. Vitamin D$_2$ is much less effective than vitamin D$_3$ in humans. *J Clin Endocrino Metab* 89:5387–5391.

37. Trivedi, D.P., Doll, R., Khaw, K.T. 2003. Effect of four monthly oral vitamin D$_3$ (cholecalciferol) supplementation on fractures and mortality in men and women living in the community: Randomized double blind controlled trial. *BMJ* 326:469–475.

38. Grey, A.G., Lucas, J., Horne, A., Gamble, G., Davidson, J.S., Reid, I.R. 2005. Vitamin D repletion in patients with primary hyperparathyroidism and coexistent vitamin D insufficiency. *J Clin Endocrinol Metab* 90:2122–2126.

18 Diabetes

Food and Nutrients in Primary Practice

Russell Jaffe, M.D., Ph.D., and Jayashree Mani, M.S.

I. INTRODUCTION

This chapter provides a contemporary overview of diabetes. Dietary patterns and nutrients that can improve glucose-insulin-energy function are emphasized. Strategic food choices and adequate essential nutrients improve outcomes in people with the continuum from metabolic syndrome to diabetes. Cellular metabolic homeostasis is disrupted long before diabetes becomes clinically apparent by elevated blood glucose or insulin. A direct consequence of these metabolic disturbances is free radical oxidative damage secondary to nutrient deficits detailed in this chapter.

II. EPIDEMIOLOGY AND DISEASE DEFINITIONS

One in every three children born today is likely to develop diabetes based on current trends [1]. Diabetes afflicts over a quarter of a billion people worldwide, 10% of them within the United States. It is the leading source for all-cause mortality in many industrialized countries. The epidemiology points to different types of diabetes intersecting and causing more aggressive disease in those who are overfed yet undernourished:

1. Type 1 diabetes (5% to 10% of cases) is deficiency of insulin production usually following an autoimmune destruction of pancreatic islets (insulitis). Genetic and immunologic markers are being developed.
2. Type 2 diabetes (90% to 95% of cases) is usually due to insulin resistance and inadequate compensatory insulin secretion from the pancreas [2].
3. Gestational diabetes is a variant of type 2 diabetes, occuring in about 4% of all pregnancies. Gestational diabetes increases offspring risk of developing diabetes [3]. Tight glycemic control before and during pregnancy can decrease the risk of adverse outcomes. Low birthweight has been linked to an increased risk for type 2 diabetes in later life.
4. Latent autoimmune diabetes of the adult (LADA) occurs in nonobese, anti-insulin antibody positive patients, and can be diagnosed decades before they become frankly diabetic [4, 5]. Metabolic syndrome and insulin resistance are prevalent in people with LADA.
5. Type 1.5 diabetes is a new syndrome that includes anti-insulin antibody-positive patients with phenotypic type 2 diabetes. These patients are usually obese and insulin resistant [5].

6. Type 3 diabetes is the emerging link between insulin resistance and neurodegeneration. The brain makes insulin. Insulin resistance in the brain results in accelerated nerve cell oxidative stress, cell damage, poor function, and early death [6]. The hippocampus, frontal cortex, hypothalamus, and other regions of the brain responsible for memory have measurably lower levels of insulin and insulin-like growth factor in patients with Alzheimer's-type dementia. Several lines of research now indicate that Alzheimer's-type dementia is diabetes on the other side of the blood-brain barrier.

III. PATHOPHYSIOLOGY

In utero nutrition may be as powerful as genetics in determining future diabetes risk.

The rate of increase in diabetes is too rapid to be explained by genetics. Emerging epigenetic studies suggest that risk acquired *in utero* is primarily mediated nutritionally [7, 8]. A mother with diabetes therefore confers not only heritable susceptibility but a nutritionally induced epigenetic susceptibility, where the fetus misgauges the energy availability in the outside world. Gestational diabetes, short of optimal treatment, creates an unfavorable *in utero* environment, which confers risk of diabetes later in life to the fetus, superimposed on any genetic risk.

Therefore, prevention of type 2 diabetes would ideally begin *in utero* and continue for life [2–4, 9, 10]. Diabetes management of women of childbearing age is both disease treatment of a future mother and disease prevention for the next generation. To primary care physicians, the emerging science of epigenetics poses what may be the greatest challenge and opportunity in diabetes management, for which nutrition has a powerful and underutilized role.

Diabetes Is an Energy Crisis

Feast in the midst of famine is a common metaphor for diabetes [2]. However "feast" is not necessarily synonomous with overeating. Feast means too much sugar in the bloodstream; cell famine means too little sugar converted to energy to keep up with cell needs. In molecular terms, diabetes is sugar-hormone-electron transport dysregulation.

Blood sugar levels are regulated by hormones such as insulin and insulin-like growth factors counterbalanced by glucagon, growth hormones, adrenaline, and autocoids [2, 4]. A relative or absolute deficit of insulin tips metabolic balance from protective to defensive. Plasma glucose reflects cell energy turnover. Cells generally extract energy from foods in the following order:

1. Glucose
2. Fructose, which is isomerized to glucose
3. Amino acids are cannibilized from protein and turned into keto acids
4. Fat is beta oxidized from two carbon units

Generally fat is metabolized where sugar and amino acids leave off so that cell energy production can be sustained. Hyperlipidemia is a consequence of impaired cell energy production [3]. Heart muscle, in contrast to other tissues, derives most of its energy from beta oxidation of fats. Intestinal lining cells use butyrate and 1-glutamine as primary energy sources.

The hormone insulin is largely responsible for regulating sugar uptake by cells. Insulin resistance is a decrease in sensitivity or response to the metabolic actions of insulin [2, 11]. Hyperinsulinism is the adaptive response. If maintained over a prolonged period, refractive hyperinsulinism leads to pancreatic beta cell exhaustion and insulin deficits. Insulin resistance plays a central role in the pathogenesis of diabetes, obesity, hypertension, dyslipidemia, and atherosclerotic cardiovascular diseases, commonly referred to as metabolic syndrome, syndrome X, and insulin resistance syndrome [11]. Appreciable pancreatic beta cell destruction has already occurred by the time glucose intolerance is present [4].

DIABETES IS CHARACTERIZED BY IMMUNE SYSTEM DYSREGULATION AND OXIDATIVE STRESS

The immune system is responsible for both repair and defense. Autoimmune pancreatic insulitis leads to type 1 diabetes [2]. Autoimmunity is also important in the pathogenesis of LADA [5]. Circulating antibodies to pancreatic antigens are typified by anti-glutamic acid decarboxylase antibodies. Loss of immune tolerance in the gut potentiates diabetes [12]. Improvement in gut tolerance improves glucose tolerance [13]. At the same time, diabetes includes immune system dysregulation with loss of protective immunity, activation of cytokine cascades, increased free radical mediated injury, and impaired healing and repair [14]. Further, protein glycation depresses the activities of antioxidant scavengers and enzymes. This altered redox equilibrium accentuates inflammatory injury, in which antioxidants may therefore have a therapeutic role.

The clinical consequences of these deficits are inflammation, as measured by elevated C-reactive protein (CRP), tumor necrosis factor, fibrinogen, ferritin, and inflammatory cytokines.

Oxidative stress plays a major role in the pathogenesis of diabetic macro- and microvascular complications [15]. Ascorbate is of particular importance as it protects serum lipids from oxidation as reflected in plasma oxidized cholesterol. It is associated with both blood lipid and HbA_1C reduction, perhaps reflecting its pro-repair and antioxidant functions. Improving glycemic control enhances the action of ascorbate since high glucose concentrations can reduce ascorbic acid uptake by as much as 40% [16–21].

DIABETES BEGINS AT THE MOLECULAR LEVEL BUT QUICKLY IMPOSES MULTI-ORGAN COMPROMISE

Atherosclerosis accelerates in poorly controlled diabetes and manifests as endothelial or dendritic cell injury, hyperlipidemia, and hypertension, as well as increased myocardial infarction, strokes, aortic aneurysms, and peripheral vascular disease. Organ-specific microvascular complications include macular degeneration, optic neuritis, nephropathy, peripheral neuropathy, and autonomic neuropathy including gastrointestinal, genitourinary, and cardiovascular symptoms, and sexual dysfunction. Macrovascular and microvascular pathologies are prominent in diabetes.

Diabetes involves simultaneous muscle compromise and fat accumulation. Obesity, particularly abdominal fat, suggests the presence of insulin resistance with release of nonesterified fatty acids, glycerol, hormones, fibrinogen, pro-inflammatory cytokines, and C-reactive protein [22]. The inflammatory state perpetuated by fat also reflects an ongoing deterioration in lean tissue. As protein is directed to cellular energy production, less is available for repair functions. In a healthy state muscle turnover is approximately 2% a day but decreases during metabolic compromise. At the same time inflammation causes more muscle damage and need to repair. The ongoing repair deficit and diversion of dietary protein to energy production eventually results in physical changes of muscle atrophy and obesity.

Diabetes and obesity are important determinants of fatty liver disease and steatohepatitis [23]. Of note, the hepatitis C virus (HCV) also induces insulin resistance due to the enhanced production of tumor necrosis factor by the HCV core antigen. Routine glucose tolerance testing has been suggested in patients with chronic hepatitis C [24].

Diabetes frequently involves renal compromise. Since the kidneys help regulate blood pH, when people with nephropathy eat a diet high in acidifying foods such as sugar, starch, and meat, the kidneys may be slow to adapt to it. Avoiding excess dietary protein is one way of slowing the progression of diabetic renal disease [25]. Reduction in protein intake improves insulin sensitivity and has beneficial influences on different steps of carbohydrate metabolism. Low glycemic index (GI) and low phosphate diets are also recommended in these patients [25–27].

People with diabetes also develop a more recently appreciated neurodegeneration of the central nervous system. Vascular consequences related to carotid and cerebrovascular disease, hypertension, and changes in the blood-brain barrier are common. Metabolic consequences that arise are related to repeated hypoglycemic episodes, hyperglycemia, hyperosmolarity, acidosis, ketosis, uremia, neuroendocrine, or neurochemical changes [6, 28]. The newly emerging link between neurodegeneration and diabetes may focus future nutritional interventions on reducing inflammation and preventing cognitive decline. Diets high in fat, especially *trans* and saturated fats, and high copper, abundant in processed foods and high GI foods, adversely affect cognition [29, 30], while those high in fruits, vegetables, cereals, and fish are associated with better cognitive function and lower risk of dementia [31–35].

Gastrointestinal symptoms as a consequence of autonomic neuropathy also result. Delayed gastric emptying is observed in 40% of patients with longstanding type 1 and type 2 diabetes. Accelerated gastric emptying, on the other hand, is manifested in about 20% of recently diagnosed patients [36]. This usually results from loss of glycemic control. Gastroesophageal reflux, dyspepsia, dysbiosis, maldigestion, impaired uptake of nutrients from the GI tract, and unhealthfully long transit times also exist [36–38]. The recently developed ^{13}C-octanoic acid breath test (OBT) can be useful in detecting and studying gastric emptying [39]. Major symptoms of gastroparesis include nausea, vomiting, postprandial fullness, early satiety, bloating, belching, and vague abdominal discomfort. Restoring hydration, glycemic, and electrolyte status are the main goals of therapy. Hyperglycemia slows gastric emptying whereas hypoglycemia may accelerate it and optimizing glycemic control is the key [40].

Polycystic ovary syndrome (PCOS) is a complex disorder affecting up to 10% of all American women. It is the leading cause of female infertility and comprises both hormonal and metabolic abnormalities that include impaired glucose tolerance, type 2 diabetes, vascular disease, dyslipidemia, and obstructive sleep apnea. A post-receptor-binding defect in insulin action leads to insulin resistance, which is the central pathogenic issue. This leads to an imbalance of the hypothalamic-pituitary-adrenal axis to which there is usually increased compensatory cortisol production. The high stress and high cortisol cycle is linked to increased refined carbohydrate and sweet foods cravings and this underlies glucose dysregulation [41–43].

SLEEP IMPROVES GLYCEMIC CONTROL

Getting sufficient sleep has been shown to improve insulin sensitivity. Glucose metabolism and insulin sensitivity are implicated in sleep disorders such as restless leg syndrome and sleep apnea [44, 45]. People with diabetes are therefore in a conundrum, with a condition that is treated by adequate sleep and side effects that undermine quality sleep. Screening and diagnosis create the opportunity for treating sleep disorders. Sleep disturbance is often responsive to supplementation with select amino acids and the cofactors needed to synthesize neurotransmitters [46–48].

IV. EVALUATION

The ADA guideline for plasma glucose is 70 to 100 mg/dL fasting, and not more than 140 mg/dL 2 hours after a meal [3]. Table 18.1 details the interpretation of blood glucose levels and conveys the often gradual onset of diabetes.

Laboratory tests such as plasma glucose are the basis of diagnosing diabetes, maintaining glycemic control, as well as identifying risks [3, 49, 50]. Glucose to insulin ratio, fasting insulin levels, and homeostatic model assessment are common indices of insulin sensitivity in clinical practice [11, 51]. Insulin-like growth factor binding protein-1 (IGF1) is emerging as a useful marker of insulin resistance [51].

Progressive dysfunction of the hypothalamic-pituitary-adrenal axis, with elevated levels of circulating cortisol, is implicated in visceral and abdominal obesity risk [52]. Measurement of salivary cortisol and dehydroepiandrosterone can identify underlying adrenal stress and help in diabetes management [53]. Saliva is an ultrafiltrate and therefore may more closely reflect tissue levels, although certain conditions common among those with diabetes may limit its accuracy in some circumstances.

Recent research findings on sleep and insulin resistance suggest that administering a brief sleep survey to patients with diabetes would be a useful diagnostic screening tool.

TABLE 18.1
Diabetes Diagnostic Criteria

Category	Fasting Plasma Glucose	2-hr Plasma Glucose
Usual	<100 mg/dL (<5.6 mmol/L)	<140 mg/dL (<7.8 mmol/L)
Healthy	<85 mg/dL (<5 mmol/L)	<115 mg/dL (<6.3 mmol/L)
Impaired fasting glucose (prediabetes, metabolic syndrome)	100–125 mg/dL (5.6–6.9 mmol/L)	—
Impaired glucose tolerance (prediabetes, syndrome X)	—	140–199 mg/dL (7.8–11.0 mmol/L)
Diabetes*	≥126 mg/dL (≥7.0 mmol/L)	≥200 mg/dL (≥11.1 mmol/L)

Source: From the Expert Committee on Diagnosis & Classification of Diabetes Mellitus, including suggested healthy range values [3].

* A diagnosis of diabetes needs to be confirmed on at least two occasions to avoid transient, stress-related hyperglycemia being misunderstood as diagnostic of diabetes.

Information available on neurodegeneration and diabetes might suggest more frequent use of a cognitive screening tool.

The role of oral tolerance and the immunotoxic effects of xenobiotics and anthropogenics in potentiating and maintaining the diabetic state have only recently been recognized. Immune reactivities to food and environmental antigens in diabetics are clinically important and patient specific. Food reactivities to dairy are common and may partly explain why diabetes is less common in nonmilk drinkers and insulin resistance is more common in milk drinkers [13, 54, 55]. Diagnostic tests are available to evaluate for food reactivities and to guide treatment (Chapter 15, "Food Reactivities").

Evaluation of B12, folate, and other B vitamins (including metabolites such as homocysteine) could be valuable in patient workup due to the risk of dementia and peripheral neuropathy. This may be especially important in hypochlorhydria and in patients on metformin, which interacts with these nutrients.

CRP, fibrinogen, and ferritin assessed for separate clinical indications can gauge systemic inflammation. Since inflammation is mediated in part by the balance of omega-3 and omega-6 fats, red cell fatty acid analysis can help guide supplemental fatty acids.

A self-assessment monitoring tool that some patients find useful is the first morning urine pH. A urine pH of 6.5 to 7.5 suggests that the body's buffering systems are adequate and there is not a net acid excess, and it may correlate with glycemic control in some patients. A target pH can reinforce the recommended daily dietary intake of 13 servings of fruits and vegetables [56] or the equivalent.

V. TREATMENT

DIET PATTERNS

Diet management of diabetes is shifting from a focus on calorie quantity and caloric excess to a focus on lifelong diet quality and essential nutrient sufficiency to avoid or correct deficit.

Diets should include 13 servings daily of fresh fruits and vegetables or the equivalent in antioxidant protection. Diets with optimal antioxidants are also high in fiber and alkalinizing.

We review alkalinizing diets. The internal acid-base balance of the body is tightly controlled in health and is maintained in a slightly alkaline state (pH 7.4). Acids produced as a result of metabolism are buffered by bicarbonate, intracellular magnesium, potassium, calcium, and sodium. Diets prominent in refined sugars, fat, and protein result in increased cell acid production. This saturates the cell's buffering capacity. Over time, if these mineral buffers are not replenished, net acid excess (NAE) can lead to depletion of mineral stores from tissues to bone and result in chronic metabolic acidosis. Repair mechanisms and resilience are reduced and the organism is more susceptible to fatigue, illness, disease, and pain when cells are acidotic. Oats, quinoa, lentils and other pulses, vegetables with the exception of peas and carrots, herbs, and nonsodium spices are alkalinizing and low glycemic [57].

The preferred distribution for a diabetic patient's diet would be comprised of 45% to 65% of energy intake from carbohydrates, 10% to 35% from protein, and 20% to 35% from fat [58]. Emphasis is placed on the type and quality of each macronutrient, which is emerging as more important than the precise distribution of each.

CARBOHYDRATES

Although many current popular weight-loss diets advocate low carbohydrate diets [59], the Food and Nutrition Board suggests a minimum recommended dietary allowance (RDA) of 130 g carbohydrates, in part due to brain dependence on glucose to meet energy needs [60].

Carbohydrates are broadly divided into simple sugars, complex carbohydrates known as starches, and fiber. Each has a different effect on blood glucose. It is this response of food on blood glucose levels that is known as the Glycemic Index (GI) [61, 62]. (See Table 18.2.) A GI of above 75 is considered high and foods below 50 have a favorably low GI [61–64]. GI is most applicable to whole foods. It becomes less helpful and even confusing when applied to food components. For example, fructose in the diet should be minimized, but it has a low GI because it converts to glucose once inside the cell. In contrast, D-ribose is a 5 carbon sugar rather than a 6 carbon sugar like fructose and glucose, which gives it a negligible effect on glycemic level. It is a sugar energy source that can regenerate low ATP levels in both the skeletal and cardiac muscle [65]. GI is also unhelpful when portion size is disregarded. Large portions of a low GI food can represent a large glycemic load (GL), which undesirably increases the need for insulin. Food preparation also alters GI. In general the more breakdown there is in the food structure, the higher the GI. For example wild, minimally cooked, long-grain rice has approximately half the GI of rice crackers. This brings us to the very important and frequently overlooked role of fiber.

Preferred fibers are unprocessed and provide 80% soluble or fermentable and 20% insoluble or viscous fiber content. Foods with low GI and a high fiber content such as dried peas, beans, and lentils lower postprandial glucose and insulin response, reduce insulin resistance, reduce weight, improve blood lipid levels, and reduce markers of inflammation such as C-reactive protein thus decreasing the risk of developing diabetes and cardiovascular disease [63, 66].

High fiber foods have a low GI. People who eat 3+ servings per day of whole grain foods have a 20% to 30% reduced risk of developing type 2 diabetes [63, 66]. The ADA recommends a daily intake of at least 14 g fiber/1000 kcal and foods with whole grains to prevent diabetes [67]. The extent to which the structure of grains and legumes is kept intact, method of cooking, type of starch, satiety, and nutrient retention also play a role [68]. Foods high in fiber also tend to provide more magnesium and antioxidants. We suggest 40+ grams of total dietary fiber to improve digestive transit and to improve glycemic response. Oat bran flour and barley are good examples of fibers high in beta-glucan and can decrease postprandial glycemic response in diabetes [69–71]. It is essential that the fibers are minimally processed to maintain fiber integrity [72].

Many patients in our clinical practice need to transition into a high fiber diet due to barriers in food preparation, taste acquisition, and gastrointestinal tolerance. In such settings supplemental fiber can be used to achieve target levels and can confer similar benefits.

PROTEINS

Protein restriction is not generally recommended in diabetes unless there is nephropathy; even so it is wise to limit proteins to < 20% of the total energy intake, within the usual Western diet range of 15% to 20% of energy intake [67]. Protein has increasing metabolic cost when taken above 50 to

TABLE 18.2
Glycemic Index of Certain Traditional and Contemporary Foods

Food	GI with Glucose as 100	GI with White Bread as 100	Serving Size (g)	Amount of Carbohydrate g/serving	GL per Serving
Grains/cereals					
Cornflakes (Kellogg's)	92	130	30	26	24
Doughnut	76	108	47	23	17
Bagel, white	72	103	70	35	25
White flour	70	100	—	—	—
Angel food cake	67	95	50	29	19
Coca Cola, soft drink	63	90	250 mL	26	16
White rice	56	80	150	41	23
Brown rice	55	79	150	33	18
Muesli bread, made from packet mix	54	77	30	12	7
Bulgur wheat	48	68	150	26	12
Oat bran bread	47	68	30	18	9
Barley kernel bread	43	62	30	20	9
Whole wheat	41	59	50 (dry)	34	14
All-Bran (Kellogg's)	38	54	45	30	23
High amylase rice	38	54	150	39	15
Rye kernels	34	48	50 (dry)	38	13
Dairy					
Milk, skim	32	46	250	13	4
Milk, full fat	27	38	250	12	3
Fruits					
Banana	52	74	120	24	12
Apple raw	38	52	120	15	6
Apricot (dried)	31	44	60	28	9
Grapefruit, raw	25	36	120	11	3
Pulses/Peas/Beans					
Chickpeas	28	39	150	30	8
Kidney beans	28	39	150	25	7
Red lentils	26	36	150	18	5
Soya beans	18	25	150	6	1
Sweeteners					
Sucrose (table sugar)	68	97	10	10	7
Honey	55	78	25	18	10
Fructose	19	27	10	10	2
Organic agave cactus nectar	10	14	10	8	1
Xylitol	8	11	10	10	1
Lactitol	2	3	10	10	0
Vegetables					
Russet potato	85	121	150	30	26
Instant mashed potato	85	122	150	20	17
Peas	48	68	80	7	3
Carrots	47	68	80	6	3

Source: [61, 62].

Note: Glycemic index is based on whole foods. Food components should be evaluated in the context of the foods in which they are eaten. Variations in food preparations also alter glycemic index.

60 g/day, typically about 15% of caloric intake. Protein-containing foods tend to increase net acid load. People with diabetes also commonly have trouble digesting and absorbing protein due to hypochlorhydria and maldigestion. The body is also likely to use additional, metabolically expensive protein in place of carbohydrates for energy. Requirement for taurine, carnitine, and tryptophan go up in response to increased protein intake. Diabetes is associated with impaired protein synthesis, wound healing, and all needed repair functions. Higher protein intake can improve glycemic control. In sum, protein is necessary but metabolically costly.

Strategies to optimize protein intake in patients with diabetes include the following:

- Digestive enzymes are reported as helpful in increasing absorption of dietary protein, particularly in those who have functional hypochlorhydria.
- Most protein should be derived from plant sources.
- Animal protein should be lean, not charbroiled, and preferably from grass-fed animals.
- Protein should be consumed with ample alkalinizing minerals, adequate ascorbate, and with other antioxidants.
- Supplementation can be used to bring select amino acids into healthful range.

FATS

Fat intake and the body's ability to process these dietary fats into the necessary energy and structural components are critical. Diet and strategic supplementation can help compensate for deficits in fat metabolism associated with diabetes:

- *Trans* fats from processed food need to be avoided at any dose.
- Saturated animal fats should be used but in moderation [73].
- Omega-6 fats should be reduced and omega-3 fats increased to move the omega-6 to omega 3 ratio from a proinflammatory state of 20–30:1 to 4:1 [73, 74].
- Elevated blood glucose impairs the delta-6-desaturase enzyme that converts omega-3 and omega-6 essential fatty acids into eicosapentaenoic acid (EPA) and subsequently docosahexaenoic acid (DHA), which are omega-3 fats, and gamma linolenic acid (GLA), which is an omega-6 fat. Patients with diabetes have a demonstrated benefit from supplementation with all three of these fats even though GLA is an omega-6 fat. Evening primrose and borage oils are supplemental sources of GLA. Fish oil, which is a source of EPA and DHA, helps normalize glucose metabolism and modify the fatty acid composition of membrane phospholipids. In isolated beta cells, lipid contents and glucose oxidation return to normal. All these effects contribute to the normalization of glucose-stimulated insulin secretion and muscle insulin sensitivity in diabetes and metabolic syndrome [75, 76].
- Fat-soluble phytonutrients such as lycopene, lutein, quercetin, zeaxanthines, and all eight forms of vitamin E are partly or even completely removed during extensive food processing. This is a disadvantage of partially hydrogenated, hydrogenated, and inter-esterified fats even if the label reads "contains zero grams *trans* fats."
- Conjugated linoleic acid (CLA) contains a *trans* isomer of oleic acid that is produced by microorganisms in ruminant animals. Conjugated linoleic acid enters the human diet when the meat and dairy products of ruminant animals are consumed. Unlike the synthetic *trans* fats CLA may provide biochemical advantage in reducing insulin resistance and is available as a supplement taken 1 to 6 g/day. The salient point may be that CLA is produced in higher concentrations in ruminant animals fed grass than in those fed grain, so that by altering agricultural practices we are altering the nutrient content of our own food.
- In addition, incorporation of foods rich in oleic acid (omega-9), as found in extra virgin olive oil, helps produce a more fluid lipid cell membrane with less prothrombotic risk of blood clotting [77, 78].

- Carnitine's metabolic role is to bring fatty acids to the mitochondria for ATP synthesis. Supplemental carnitine may facilitate fat metabolism in patients with diabetes. Carnitine reduces total fat mass with an increase in lean mass.
- Medium chain triglycerides are derived from plant sources of fatty acids and may be absorbed directly from the intestine. Their use is limited by gastrointestinal intolerance, but can be effectively used in small, frequent doses.

MINERALS AND VITAMINS

Magnesium

Magnesium is the second most abundant intracellular cation and appears to modulate hormonal and biochemical aspects of cellular glucose utilization and carbohydrate metabolism. Magnesium is critical in regulating insulin sensitivity, vascular tone, and blood pressure homeostasis. Magnesium deficiency is a common feature of diabetic, cardiovascular, and other metabolic processes such as aging. Serum magnesium levels have a bearing on morbidity in patients with diabetes [79]. Magnesium, which is ionized with citrate, malate, succinate, fumarate, glycinate, or ascorbate, is more bioavailable than magnesium oxide or magnesium chelated with soy peptides [80–82]. Magnesium absorption can be further enhanced with choline citrate. Neutral micellar droplets form in the gut and facilitate magnesium uptake through neutral pores even when the usual calcium–magnesium ATPase enzymes are inhibited by toxic minerals or hormone disrupters [80–82].

Chromium

Extensive studies have been conducted on the effect of chromium on glycemic control, because chromium increases lean body mass, reduces weight, decreases visceral fat, and improves free fatty acid levels and insulin sensitivity, when used in addition to oral anti-hyperglycemic agents [83], and low chromium concentrations can precipitate diabetes. Urinary losses of chromium occur during pregnancy, strenuous exercise, infection, physical trauma, steroid medication, and high cortisol states in general. Iron given in supplemental doses reduces chromium absorption by competitive inhibition. Because chromium is a trace mineral in concentrations two orders of magnitidue less than iron, direct measurements are not clinically available. Chromium supplementation in doses of 800 to 1000 µg/day has been shown to improve glucose and insulin metabolism in patients with insulin resistance [84].

Iodine

Fortifying table salt with iodine might not be providing many Americans with optimal body iodine stores. People with diabetes have a higher prevalence of thyroid disorders [85] and may be disproportionately affected, because they may be low in several other trace minerals and often try to adhere to the recommended treatment of low salt intake and fresh foods whenever possible. Patients with a TSH greater than 2.5 should be given a trial of iodine supplementation, avoid goiterogenic soy foods, and consume sea vegetables as described in Chapter 16, "Hypothyroidism."

Vanadium

Ever since vanadium salts were discovered to stimulate glucose uptake in rats without raising insulin levels [86], vanadium has been shown to mimic the metabolic effects of insulin, thereby influencing glucose metabolism in diabetes. In addition, vanadium improves myocardial function by regulating metabolic processes. Side effects of vanadium supplementation include diarrhea, nausea, and flatulence in a few cases. Products with high bioavailability have minimal side effects [87]. Other trace minerals with potential roles in diabetes management include zinc, molybdenum, manganese, and selenium.

Taurine

Taurine is a semi-essential beta amino acid with antihyperglycemic, antihyperlipidemic, and hyperinsulinemic effects. In diabetes, increased intracellular accumulation of sorbitol can deplete taurine. Altered taurine metabolism is linked to the development of cellular dysfunction in diabetes complications including retinopathy, neuropathy, nephropathy, cardiomyopathy, platelet aggregation, endothelial dysfunction, and atherosclerosis [88]. Combinations of taurine and vanadium have synergistic effects [89].

Biotin

Biotin is thought to improve abnormal glucose metabolism by stimulating glucose-induced insulin secretion by pancreatic beta cells and by accelerating glycolysis in the liver and pancreas. Biotin also enhances muscle insulin sensitivity by increasing guanylate cyclase activity. Combining chromium and biotin can have added effect in maintaining optimal glycemic control and in improving cardiometabolic risk factors [90].

Alpha Lipoic Acid

Alpha lipoic acid is a fat-soluble and water-soluble antioxidant that may be directly insulin sensitizing. It may also improve diabetes outcomes by acting on hepatocytes to help repair the sugar-hormone-electron transport dysregulation. Alpha lipoic acid has been shown to reduce diabetes-related peripheral neuropathy [91].

Quercetin

Quercetin is a bioflavonoid found in several fruits, most notably apples. Quercetin dihydrate administration (10 mg/kg) improves vascular function in diabetes, reduces blood glucose levels, and shows antiatherogenic effects [92].

BOTANICALS

Overview

Coupled with vitamins and minerals and other nutrients, certain botanicals are emerging as valuable adjuncts to diabetes risk reduction and clinical management (see Table 18.3). They add to our arsenal of novel glucose-regulating agents. Phytonutrients with better evidence of efficacy are outlined later.

Fenugreek

Perhaps the most studied herb in the management of diabetes, fenugreek has been found to lower both blood glucose and lipids [94]. Fenugreek decreases insulin resistance and triglyceride levels. Fenugreek can safely be used as an adjunct and in combination with sulfonylureas in the treatment of type 2 diabetes [95].

Bitter Melon

Bitter melon contains various hypoglycemic extracts that work on increasing glucose utilization by the liver, decreasing gluconeogenesis and enhancing the cellular uptake of glucose. It also promotes insulin release, potentiates its effect, and increases the number of insulin-producing beta cells in diabetic animals. Dietary use of bitter melon and its juice decreases blood glucose levels, increases HDL-cholesterol, and decreases triglyceride levels, thus exhibiting antiatherogenic qualities [96].

Banaba

Corosolic acid (CRA), an active component of Banaba leaves (*Lagerstroemia speciosa L.*), has been shown to decrease blood glucose levels in diabetic animals and humans. Banaba is a medicinal plant

TABLE 18.3
Foods, Botanicals, and Supplemental Nutrients in Diabetes

Nutrients	Role in Diabetes
Vinegar (acetic acid)	Acetate alters glycolysis/gluconeogenic cycle in liver, reduces fasting hyperglycemia.
Ginger	Source of active thiols to increase detoxification substrates and enzyme activators; similar to onions, garlic, brassica sprouts & eggs; one or more as staple in the diet recommended.
Red wine (also dealcoholized)	High resveratrol content.
Apples	High quercetin flavanoids, with vascular benefits.

Fiber

Oat bran, beta glucan rich gum acacia, insoluble fiber glucomannan, freeze dried dextrans, low molecular weight prebiotics	Low glycemic, sterol binding, transit time shortening, and probiotic promoting 40+ g/day total fiber intake recommended; 80% soluble & 20% insoluble. Supplementation can help achieve intake goals.
Nuts and seeds	Fiber and mineral rich; low glycemic.
Berries	Rich in anthocyanidins and other polyphenolic flavanoids, especially if vine-ripened.
Cinnamon	Polyphenolics in cinnamon have demonstrated improvements in fasting glucose, glucose tolerance & insulin sensitivity.
Rosemary, green tea, cranberries, blueberries, lemon balm	These foods contain polyphenolic compounds, which are natural alpha amylase inhibitors. They can lower postprandial blood glucose level and have been recommended in the supplementary glycemic treatment management of diabetes.

Foods to avoid

Fructose-rich foods	Bypasses glucose/insulin control yet converts back to glucose inside the cell.
Trans fat–containing foods	Impair cell membrane actions.
Empty calorie, nutrient poor foods	Increase cortisol, contribute to nutrient deficiencies.

Botanicals

Trigonella foenum–graecum (fenugreek)	Decreases insulin resistance and triglyceride levels.
Momordica charantia (marah, bitter melon)	Increases glucose utilization by liver; decreases blood glucose levels and increases HDL cholesterol.
Lagerstromia speciosa (corosolic acid)	48 mg/day in a 1% standardized extract: effective blood glucose reduction.
Galega officinalis (French lilac)	The active ingredient galegine reduces insulin resistance. Metformin is a galegine derivative.
Vaccinium myrtillis (bilberry)	Leaf extract shown to lower blood sugar.
Gymnema sylvestre	The active group polyphenolics of gymnemicates has antihyperglycemic hypoglycemic properties.
Zizyphus spina-christi	Insulinotropic and hypoglycemic effects of the Egyptian *Zizyphus spina-christi* leaves are attributed to a possible sulfonylurea-like activity.
Catharanthus roseus	Hypoglycemic action of the leaves has been attributed to increased glucose metabolism & reduces oxidative stress.

Nutrients

Betaine (trimethylglycine), and l-histidine	Protein digestion enhancers; 50–100 mg betaine with each meal and 500 mg l-histidine 30 min before each meal can improve stomach protein digestion by helping maintain or restore adequate stomach digestive acid; Heidelberg test recommended to confirm stomach acid status; unwell people likely to be functionally hypochlorhydric.

continued

TABLE 18.3 *(continued)*

Nutrients	Role in Diabetes
Magnesium	400–1000 mg daily as glycinate, citrate, ascorbate, or other fully ionized forms. Uptake is enhanced with concurrent choline citrate to form neutral charge droplet easily taken up by small intestine.
Chromium: can be enhanced with biotin, taurine, vanadium	800–1000 µg/day as picolinate or citrate. Improves lean body mass and insulin sensitivity.
Iodine	Thyroid disorders more likely with diabetes; need for iodine levels.
Zinc	With other antioxidants useful for diabetic retinopathy.
Ascorbate	Adequate to quench free radicals and keep C-reactive protein < 0.5.
Vitamin E	400–3200 IU/day only as mixed natural tocopherols. D-alpha tocopherol acetate or succinate not recommended.
Alpha lipoic acid	600 mg alpha lipoic acid twice daily can be neuroprotective in diabetes.
Acetyl carnitine	500–1000 mg/day can improve nerve conduction and pain reduction.

Source: [86–107].

that grows in India, Southeast Asia, and the Philippines. The antidiabetic properties of CRA include inhibition of gluconeogenesis and promotion of glycolysis. Forty-eight mg of CRA daily as a 1% standardized extract has shown to be effective in blood glucose reduction [97].

PHARMACOLOGY

The average glucose-lowering effect of the major classes of oral antidiabetic agents is broadly similar, averaging a 1% to 2% reduction in HbA1c with alpha-glucosidase inhibitors being rather less effective. Of note, neither sulphonylureas nor biguanides appreciably alter the rate of progression of complications in patients with type 2 diabetes [108]. Drug interactions have been extensively reviewed elsewhere [109].

Drug-Nutrient Interactions

Oral antidiabetic agents and nutrient interactions are reviewed in Table 18.4.

Metformin use increases homocysteine and decreases folate and vitamin B12 concentrations [110]. Older diabetics are more prone to this complication, since vitamin B12 deficiency affects at least a fifth of the elderly and may present as accelerated cognitive decline and neuropathy [110, 111]. Diabetics often have slow intestinal transit causing bacterial overgrowth and vitamin B12 malabsorption. Vitamin B12-intrinsic factor complex uptake by ileal cell membrane receptors is calcium dependent, and metformin affects calcium-dependent membrane action. Management options include calcium, folate, and hydroxocobalamin supplementation since hydroxocobalamin does not require intrinsic factor for absorption or withdrawal of metformin.

Fixed-dose pioglitazone-metformin combination tablets are best taken with food to reduce gastrointestinal side effects [112]. Rosiglitazone given alone can be administered without regard to meals unlike glipizide (glucotrol) [113]. Grapefruit juice is rich in polyphenolics that induce cytochromes and thereby alter kinetics of statins, dihydropyridines, and repaglinide in particular, increasing hypoglycemia risk [114].

TABLE 18.4
Diabetes Pharmacology and Nutrients

Pharmacological Agent	Mechanism of Action	Clinical Considerations	Nutrient Considerations	Food Interactions
Sulfonylureas: first generation (chlorpropamide, tolbutamide) and second generations (glyburide, glipizide & glimepiride)	Stimulate insulin secretion by binding to receptors on the pancreatic beta cell. Metabolized in the liver via the cytochrome P450 system.	Secondary benefit: decrease LDL, increase HDL to normal levels. Risks: weight gain, hypoglycemic episodes.	Minor	To be avoided with alcohol. For glipizide: 30 minutes before a meal recommended for optimum results.
Meglitinides: repaglinide and nateglinide (glinides)	Similar to sulfonylureas. Metabolized in the liver via the cytochrome P450 system.	More favorable safety profile than sulfonylureas, especially in patients with renal failure. Specific caution with the following medications: Rifampicin, Ciclosporin, gemfibrozil, and repaglinide. Also, statins such as simvastatin and lovastatin.	Minor	They have a rapid elimination rate, so recommended to be taken at the beginning of a meal Not to be taken with grapefruit juice as it can enhance its effect precipitating hypoglycemia.
Biguanides (metformin)	Reduce hepatic glucose production	Metformin: Reduction in TG, LDL, total cholesterol, HbA1C and insulin, reducing oxidative stress. GI discomfort, rare lactic acidosis.	Folate and vitamin B12. Intrinsic factor is calcium dependent so supplementation of calcium may be indicated too. Increase in homocysteine levels. Due to risk of bone loss, bone nutrient supplementation is recommended	To minimize GI disturbances, recommended to be taken with food.

continued

TABLE 18.4 (*continued*)

Pharmacological Agent	Mechanism of Action	Clinical Considerations	Nutrient Considerations	Food Interactions
Thiazolidinediones (rosglitazone, pioglitazone)	Improve insulin action. Metabolized in the liver via the cytochrome P450 system.	Decrease in homocysteine. Rosglitazone: reduction in TG, LDL, total cholesterol, HbA1C and insulin, reducing oxidative stress; increased risk of myocardial infarction and heart failure; fracture risk in women, and, for rosiglitazone, more rapid bone loss. To be used with caution in people with hepatic dysfunction. Specific caution when combined with statins.		No effect of food on action
Incretin analogues: exenatide and rimonabant (injectable)	Stimulate insulin secretion from pancreatic beta cell; slower absorption of carbohydrate from the gut.	Accelerated weight loss. Nausea, diarrhea, vomiting.	No specific interactions yet identified.	Not to be taken after meals.

Source: [110–116].

Pancreatic/Islet Transplantation and Stem Cell Research

A successful whole pancreas or islet transplant offers the advantages of attaining normal or near normal blood glucose control and normal HbA$_1$C levels without causing severe hypoglycemia that is associated with intensive insulin therapy. Pancreatic transplantation, however, carries with it a significant risk of surgical and postoperative complications. Although islet transplantation is less invasive it may not always achieve the sustained level of tight glucose control [117]. Due to the limited number of donor islet cells available, stem cell research is being actively investigated [118,119]. There is potential for synergistic treatment between nutrient interventions and stem cell research.

VI. CONCLUSIONS

Prevention is important with any disease, but none more poignant than diabetes. With an epidemic that causes disease earlier in life, women of childbearing age are increasingly affected by diabetes. Newly emerging research on epigenetics suggests that the *in utero* nutritional environment is a significant risk factor in the development of diabetes, and the clinical implications are profound.

Diabetes can be predicted by laboratory testing years before clinical manifestations occur and nutritional therapies have been demonstrated to be effective throughout the disease course. Dietary patterns, foods, phytonutrients, minerals, and vitamins can improve glycemic control. Diets with high antioxidant capacity, rich in fiber, and alkalinizing are recommended. The quality of the macronutrients in the diet may be more important than the precise ratio of fats, carbohydrates, and protein.

Physicians should be aware of food and nutrient-drug interactions with antihyperglycemic agents (Table 18.4). Both the disease process and the medications used to treat it place patients with diabetes at added risk of nutrient deficiencies. Adjuncts to medical treatment are listed in Table 18.3 [86–107]. Both diagnostic tests and the presence of specific organ damage can guide nutrient recommendations for a specific patient. Nutritional medicine should be patient centered and comprehensive.

ACKNOWLEDGMENT

The authors thank Dow Chemical for their professional development support.

REFERENCES

1. American Diabetes Association economic costs of diabetes in the U.S. in 2007: ADA statement. *Diabetes Care.* 2008;31:1–20.
2. Nelson DL, Cox MM, *Lehninger Principles of Biochemistry,* 4th Ed, 2005. WH Freeman and Company: 909.
3. Diagnosis and classification of diabetes mellitus: American Diabetes Association. *Diabetes Care.* 2007 Jan;30 Suppl 1:S42–47.
4. Fowler MJ, Diabetes: Magnitude and mechanisms. *Clinical Diabetes.* 2007;25:25–28.
5. Palmer JP, Hirsch IB, What's in a name? Latent autoimmune diabetes of adults, type 1.5, adult-onset, and type 1 diabetes. *Diabetes Care.* 2003;26:536–553.
6. de la Monte SM, Tong M, Lester-Coll N, Plater M Jr, Wands JR. Therapeutic rescue of neurodegeneration in experimental type 3 diabetes: relevance to Alzheimer's disease. *J Alzheimers Dis.* 2006 Sep;10(1):89–109.
7. Gluckman P, Hamson M, *Fetal Matrix: Evolution Development and Disease,* 2000, Cambridge University Press.
8. See WC, Gilberto P, *Early Environments: Fetal and Infant Nutrition,* in Scientific Evidence for Musculoskeletal, Bariatric, and Sports Nutrition, Ed. Kohlstadt I, 2005 Taylor & Francis, 2005:43.
9. Arch JR, Cawthorne MA, Stocker CJ. Fetal origins of insulin resistance and obesity. *Proc Nutr Soc.* 2005 May;64(2):143–151.
10. Woolley SL, Saranga S. Neonatal diabetes mellitus: A rare but important diagnosis in the critically ill infant. *Eur J Emerg Med.* 2006 Dec;13(6):349–351.

11. Ye J, Kraegen T. Insulin resistance: central and peripheral mechanisms. The 2007 Stock Conference Report Obesity Reviews. 2008;9(1):30–34.

12. Solly NR, Honeyman MC, Harrison LC. The mucosal interface between 'self' and 'non-self' determines the impact of environment on autoimmune diabetes. *Curr Dir Autoimmun.* 2001;4:68–90.

13. Jaffe R, Mani J, DeVane J, Mani H. Tolerance loss in diabetics: association with foreign antigen exposure. *Diabet Med.* 2006 Aug;23(8):924–925.

14. Jaffe R, Mani J, Trocki T, Mehl-Madrona L. First line comprehensive care. The diabetes continuum of insulin, glucose, energy dysregulation: better clinical management of causes improves outcomes, reduces risks and vascular complications. *Original Internist.* 2004;11(3):11–27.

15. Peerapatdit T, Patchanans N, Likidlilid A, Poldee S, Sriratanasathavorn C. Plasma lipid peroxidation and antioxidiant nutrients in type 2 diabetic patients. *J Med Assoc Thai.* 2006 Nov;89 Suppl 5:S147–155.

16. Jariyapongskul A, Rungjaroen T, Kasetsuwan N, Patumraj S, Seki J, Niimi H. Long-term effects of oral vitamin C supplementation on the endothelial dysfunction in the iris microvessels of diabetic rats. *Microvasc Res.* 2007 Jul;74(1):32–38.

17. Connor KM, SanGiovanni JP, Lofqvist C, Aderman CM, Chen J, Higuchi A, Hong S, Pravda EA, Majchrzak S, Carper D, Hellstrom A, Kang JX, Chew EY, Salem N Jr, Serhan CN, Smith LE. Increased dietary intake of omega-3-polyunsaturated fatty acids reduces pathological retinal angiogenesis. *Nat Med.* 2007 Jul;13(7):868–873.

18. Age-Related Eye Disease Study Research Group, SanGiovanni JP, Chew EY, Clemons TE, Ferris FL 3rd, Gensler G, Lindblad AS, Milton RC, Seddon JM, Sperduto RD. The relationship of dietary carotenoid and vitamin A, E, and C intake with age-related macular degeneration in a case-control study: AREDS Report No. 22. *Arch Ophthalmol.* 2007 Sep;125(9):1225–1232.

19. Cangemi FE. TOZAL Study: an open case control study of an oral antioxidant and omega-3 supplement for dry AMD. *BMC Ophthalmol.* 2007 Feb 26;7:3.

20. Moustafa SA. Zinc might protect oxidative changes in the retina and pancreas at the early stage of diabetic rats. *Toxicology and Applied Pharmacology.* 1 December 2004;201(2):149–155.

21. Siepmann M, Spank S, Kluge A, Schappach A, Kirch W. The pharmacokinetics of zinc from zinc gluconate: a comparison with zinc oxide in healthy men. *Int J Clin Pharmacol Ther.* 2005 Dec;43(12):562–565.

22. Haffner SM. Abdominal adiposity and cardiometabolic risk: do we have all the answers? *Am J Med.* 2007 Sep;120(9 Suppl 1):S10–16; discussion S16–17.

23. Yeh MM, Brunt EM. Pathology of nonalcoholic fatty liver disease. *Am J Clin Pathol.* 2007 Nov; 128(5):837–847.

24. Lonardo A, Carulli N, Loria P. HCV and diabetes. A two-question-based reappraisal. *Dig Liver Dis.* 2007 Aug;39(8):753–761.

25. Robertson L, Waugh N, Robertson A. Protein restriction for diabetic renal disease. *Cochrane Database Syst Rev.* 2007 Oct 17;(4):CD002181.

26. Taketani Y, Shuto E, Arai H, Nishida Y, Tanaka R, Uebanso T, Yamamoto H, Yamanaka-Okumura H, Takeda E. Advantage of a low glycemic index and low phosphate diet on diabetic nephropathy and aging-related diseases. *J Med Invest.* 2007 Aug;54(3–4):359–365.

27. Lee EY, Lee MY, Hong SW, Chung CH, Hong SY. Blockade of oxidative stress by vitamin C ameliorates albuminuria and renal sclerosis in experimental diabetic rats. *Yonsei Med J.* 2007 Oct 31;48(5): 847–855.

28. Mooradian AD. Pathophysiology of central nervous system complications in diabetes mellitus. *Clin Neurosci.* 1997;4(6):322–326.

29. Morris MC, Evans DA, Tangney CC, Bienias JL, Schneider JA, Wilson RS, Scherr PA. Dietary copper and high saturated and *trans* fat intakes associated with cognitive decline. *Arch Neurol.* 2006 Aug;63(8):1085–1088.

30. Greenwood CE, Kaplan RJ, Hebblethwaite S, Jenkins DJ. Carbohydrate-induced memory impairment in adults with type 2 diabetes. *Diabetes Care.* 2003 Jul;26(7):1961–1966.

31. Parrott MD, Greenwood CE, Dietary influences on cognitive function with aging: from high-fat diets to healthful eating. *Ann N Y Acad Sci.* 2007 Oct;1114:389–397.

32. Sun Y, Lai MS, Lu CJ. Effectiveness of vitamin B12 on diabetic neuropathy: systematic review of clinical controlled trials. *Acta Neurol Taiwan.* 2005 Jun;14(2):48–54.

33. Vanotti A, Osio M, Mailland E, Nascimbene C, Capiluppi E, Mariani C. Overview on pathophysiology and newer approaches to treatment of peripheral neuropathies. *CNS Drugs.* 2007;21 Suppl 1:3–12; discussion 45–46.

34. Várkonyi T, Kempler P. Diabetic neuropathy: new strategies for treatment. *Diabetes Obes Metab.* 2008 Feb;10(2):99–108.

35. Head KA. Peripheral neuropathy: pathogenic mechanisms and alternative therapies. *Altern Med Rev.* 2006 Dec;11(4):294–329.

36. Tomi S, Płazińska M, Zagórowicz E, Ziółkowski B, Muszynski J . Gastric emptying disorders in diabetes mellitus. *Pol Arch Med Wewn.* 2002 Sep;108(3):879–886.

37. Kuo P, Rayner CK, Jones KL, Horowitz M. Pathophysiology and management of diabetic gastropathy: a guide for endocrinologists. *Drugs.* 2007;67(12):1671–1687.

38. Wang X, Pitchumoni CS, Chandrarana K, Shah N. Increased prevalence of symptoms of gastroesophageal reflux diseases in type 2 diabetics with neuropathy. *World J Gastroenterol.* 2008 Feb 7;14(5):709–712.

39. Nohara S, Iwase M, Imoto H, Sasaki N, Nakamura U, Uchizono Y, Abe S, Doi Y, Iida M. Gastric emptying in patients with Type 2 diabetes mellitus and diabetes associated with mitochondrial DNA 3243 mutation using 13C-octanoic acid breath test. *J Diabetes Complications.* 2006 Sep–Oct;20(5):295–301.

40. Gentilcore D, O'Donovan D, Jones KL, Horowitz M. Nutrition therapy for diabetic gastroparesis. *Curr Diab Rep.* 2003 Oct;3(5):418–426.

41. Hoffman LK, Ehrmann DA. Cardiometabolic features of polycystic ovary syndrome. *Nat Clin Pract Endocrinol Metab.* 2008 Apr;4(4):215–222.

42. Miller JE, Bray MA, Faiman C, Reyes FI, Characterization of 24-h cortisol release in obese and non-obese hyperandrogenic women. *Gynecol Endocrinol.* 1994 Dec;8(4):247–254.

43. Epel E, et al. Stress may add bite to appetite in women: a laboratory study of stress-induced cortisol and eating behavior. *Psychoneuroendocrinology.* 2001 Jan;26(1):37–49.

44. Tasali E, Leproult R, Ehrmann DA, Van Cauter E, Slow-wave sleep and the risk of type 2 diabetes in humans. *Proc Natl Acad Sci USA.* 2008 Jan 2 [Epub ahead of print].

45. Chasens ER. Obstructive sleep apnea, daytime sleepiness, and type 2 diabetes. *Diabetes Educ.* 2007 May–Jun;33(3):475–482.

46. Paredes SD, Terrón MP, Cubero J, Valero V, Barriga C, Reiter RJ, Rodríguez AB. Tryptophan increases nocturnal rest and affects melatonin and serotonin serum levels in old ringdove. *Physiol Behav.* 2007 Mar 16;90(4):576–582.

47. Hvas AM, Juul S, Bech P, Nexø E, Vitamin B6 level is associated with symptoms of depression. *Psychother Psychosom.* 2004 Nov–Dec;73(6):340–343.

48. Chollet D, Franken P, Raffin Y, Henrotte JG, Widmer J, Malafosse A, Tafti M. Magnesium involvement in sleep: genetic and nutritional models. *Behav Genet.* 2001 Sep;31(5):413–425.

49. Ferrannini E. Insulin resistance is central to the burden of diabetes. *Diabetes Metab Rev.* 1997; 13:81–86.

50. Huerta MG. Adiponectin and leptin: potential tools in the differential diagnosis of pediatric diabetes? *Rev Endocr Metab Disord.* 2006 Sep;7(3):187–196.

51. Borai A, Livingstone C, Ferns GA. The biochemical assessment of insulin resistance. *Ann Clin Biochem.* 2007 Jul;44(Pt 4):324–342.

52. Rosmond R. Stress induced disturbances of the HPA axis: a pathway to Type 2 diabetes? *Med Sci Monit.* 2003 Feb;9(2):RA35–39.

53. Gallagher P, Leitch MM, Massey AE, Hamish McAllister-Williams R, Young AH. Assessing cortisol and dehydroepiandrosterone (DHEA) in saliva: effects of collection method. *J Psychopharm.* 2000;20(5): 643–649.

54. Lawlor DA, Ebrahim S, Timpson N, Davey Smith G. Avoiding milk is associated with a reduced risk of insulin resistance and the metabolic syndrome: findings from the British Women's Heart and Health Study. *Diabet Med.* 2005 Jun;22(6):808–811.

55. Brostoff J, Challacombe SJ. Diagnosis of food allergy and intolerance in food allergy and intolerance, *Balliere Tindall.* 1987:795–968.

56. U.S. Department of Health and Human Services and U.S. Department of Agriculture. *Dietary Guidelines for Americans, 2005,* 6th Edition, 2005 Washington, DC: U.S. Government Printing Office.

57. Brown S. *Better Bones, Better Body* 2000 Keats Publishing:294–303.

58. Food and Nutrition Board, Institute of Medicine, *Dietary Reference Intakes for Energy, Carbohydrate, Fiber, Fat, Fatty Acids, Cholesterol, Protein, and Amino Acids (Macronutrients),* 2005, Washington, DC: National Academy Press.

59. Dyson PA, Beatty S, Matthews DR. A low-carbohydrate diet is more effective in reducing body weight than healthy eating in both diabetic and non-diabetic subjects. *Diabet Med.* 2007 Dec;24(12):1430–1435.

60. Nutrition Recommendations and Interventions for Diabetes. A position statement of the American Diabetes Association. *Diabetes Care.* 2007;30:S48–S65.

61. Jenkins DJ, Kendall C, Marchie A, Augustin L. Too much sugar, too much carbohydrate, or just too much? *Am J Clin Nutr.* May 2004;79(5):711–712.

62. Foster-Powell K, Holt SHA, Brand-Miller JC. International table of glycemic index and glycemic load values. *Am J Clin Nutr.* 2002;76(1):5–56.

63. Riccardi G, Rivellese AA, Giacco R. Role of glycemic index and glycemic load in the healthy state, in prediabetes, and in diabetes. *Am J Clin Nutr.* 2008 Jan;87(1):269S–274S.

64. Meyer KA, Kushi LH, Jacobs DR, Jr, Slavin J, Sellers TA, Folsom AR. Carbohydrates, dietary fiber, and incident type 2 diabetes in older women. *Am J Clin Nutr.* 2000 Apr;71(4):921–930.

65. Fenstad ER, Gazal O, Shecterle LM, St. Cyr JA, Seifert JG. Dose effects of D-ribose on glucose and purine metabolites. *Internet J Nutr Wellness.* 2008;5(1).

66. Krishnan S, Rosenberg L, Singer M, Hu FB, Djoussé L, Cupples LA, Palmer JR. Glycemic index, glycemic load, and cereal fiber intake and risk of type 2 diabetes in US Black women. *Arch Intern Med.* 2007 Nov 26;167(21):2304–2309.

67. Bantle W-RJJP, Albright AL, Aprovian CM, Clark NG, Franz MJ, Hoogwerf BJ, Lichtenstein AH, Mayer-Davis E, Mooradian AD, Wheeler ML. Nutrition recommendations and interventions for Diabetes-2006: a position statement of the American Diabetes Association. *Diabetes Care.* 2006;29(9):2140–2157.

68. Salmerón J, Ascherio A, Rimm EB, Colditz GA, Spiegelman D, Jenkins DJ, Stampfer MJ, Wing AL, Willett WC. Dietary fiber, glycemic load, and risk of NIDDM in men. *Diabetes Care.* 1997 Apr;20(4):545–550.

69. Queenan KM, Stewart ML, Smith KN, Thomas W, Fulcher RG, Slavin JL. Concentrated oat β-glucan, a fermentable fiber, lowers serum cholesterol in hypercholesterolemic adults in a randomized controlled trial. *Nutr J.* 2007 Mar 26;6:6.

70. Maki KC, Carson ML, Miller MP, Turowski M, Bell M, Wilder DM, Reeves MS. High-viscosity hydroxypropylmethylcellulose blunts postprandial glucose and insulin responses. *Diabetes Care.* 2007 May;30(5):1039–1043.

71. Mäkeläinen H, Anttila H, Sihvonen J, Hietanen RM, Tahvonen R, Salminen E, Mikola M, Sontag-Strohm T. The effect of beta-glucan on the glycemic and insulin index. *Eur J Clin Nutr.* 2007 Jun;61(6):779–785.

72. Hlebowicz J, Wickenberg J, Fahlström R, Björgell O, Almér LO, Darwiche G. Effect of commercial breakfast fibre cereals compared with corn flakes on postprandial blood glucose, gastric emptying and satiety in healthy subjects: a randomized blinded crossover trial. *Nutr J.* 2007 Sep 17;6:22.

73. American Diabetes Association. Nutrition Principles and Recommendations in Diabetes. *Diabetes Care.* 2004;27:S36.

74. Sanders TA, Lewis F, Slaughter S, Griffin BA, Griffin M, Davies I, Millward DJ, Cooper JA, Miller GJ. Effect of varying the ratio of n-6 to n-3 fatty acids by increasing the dietary intake of alpha-linolenic acid, eicosapentaenoic and docosahexaenoic acid, or both on fibrinogen and clotting factors VII and XII in persons aged 45-70 y: the OPTILIP study. *Am J Clin Nutr.* 2006 Sep;84(3):513–522.

75. Lombardo YB, Hein G, Chicco A. Metabolic syndrome: effects of n-3 PUFAs on a model of dyslipidemia, insulin resistance and adiposity. *Lipids.* 2007 May;42(5):427–437.

76. Harris GD, White RD. Diabetes management and exercise in pregnant patients with diabetes. *Clinical Diabetes.* 2005;23:165–168.

77. Lopez-Miranda J, Delgado-Lista J, Perez-Martinez P, Jimenez-Gómez Y, Fuentes F, Ruano J, Marin C. Olive oil and the haemostatic system. *Mol Nutr Food Res.* 2007 Oct;51(10):1249–1259.

78. Carpentier YA, Portois L, Malaisse WJ. n-3 fatty acids and the metabolic syndrome. *Am J Clin Nutr.* 2006 Jun;83(6 Suppl):1499S–1504S.

79. Sales CH, Pedrosa Lde F. Magnesium and diabetes mellitus: their relation. *Clin Nutr.* 2006 Aug;25(4):554–562.

80. Walker AF, Marakis G, Christie S, Byng M. Mg citrate found more bioavailable than other Mg preparations in a randomised, double-blind study. *Magnes Res.* 2003 Sep;16(3):183–191.

81. Schuette SA, Lashner BA, Janghorbani M. Bioavailability of magnesium diglycinate vs magnesium oxide in patients with ileal resection. *JPEN J Parenter Enteral Nutr.* 1994 Sep–Oct;18(5):430–435.

82. Coudray C, Rambeau M, Feillet-Coudray C, Gueux E, Tressol JC, Mazur A, Rayssiguier Y. Study of magnesium bioavailability from ten organic and inorganic Mg salts in Mg-depleted rats using a stable isotope approach. *Magnes Res.* 2005 Dec;18(4):215–223.

83. Cefalu WT, Hu FB. Role of chromium in human health and in diabetes. *Diabetes Care.* 2004. 27:2741–2751.

84. Balk EM, Tatsioni A, Lichtenstein AH, Lau J, Pittas AG. Effect of chromium supplementation on glucose metabolism and lipids: a systematic review of randomized controlled trials. *Diabetes Care.* 2007 Aug;30(8):2154–2163.

85. Johnson JL. Diabetes control in thyroid disease. *Diabetes Spectrum.* 2006;19:148–153.

86. Kent H. Vanadium for diabetes. *CMAJ.* 1999 January 12;160(1):17.

87. García-Vicente S, Yraola F, Marti L, González-Muñoz E, García-Barrado MJ, Cantó C, Abella A, Bour S, Artuch R, Sierra C, Brandi N, Carpéné C, Moratinos J, Camps M, Palacín M, Testar X, Gumà A, Albericio F, Royo M, Mian A, Zorzano A. Oral insulin-mimetic compounds that act independently of insulin. *Diabetes.* 2007 Feb;56(2):486–493.

88. Hansen SH. The role of taurine in diabetes and the development of diabetic complications. *Diabetes Metab Res Rev.* 2001 Sep–Oct;17(5):330–346.

89. Tas S, Sarandol E, Ayvalik SZ, Serdar Z, Dirican M. Vanadyl sulfate, taurine, and combined vanadyl sulfate and taurine treatments in diabetic rats: effects on the oxidative and antioxidative systems. *Arch Med Res.* 2007 Apr;38(3):276–283.

90. Albarracin CA, Fuqua BC, Evans JL, Goldfine ID. Chromium picolinate and biotin combination improves glucose metabolism in treated, uncontrolled overweight to obese patients with type 2 diabetes. *Diabetes Metab Res Rev.* 2008 Jan;24(1):41–51.

91. Head KA. Peripheral neuropathy: pathogenic mechanisms and alternative therapies. *Altern Med Rev.* 2006 Dec;11(4):294–329.

92. Machha A, Achike FI, Mustafa AM, Mustafa MR. Quercetin, a flavonoid antioxidant, modulates endothelium-derived nitric oxide bioavailability in diabetic rat aortas. *Nitric Oxide.* 2007 Jun;16(4):442–447.

93. Sima AA, Calvani M, Mehra M, Amato A. Acetyl-L-Carnitine Study Group. Acetyl-L-carnitine improves pain, nerve regeneration, and vibratory perception in patients with chronic diabetic neuropathy: an analysis of two randomized placebo-controlled trials. *Diabetes Care.* 2005 Jan;28(1):89–94.

94. Gupta A, Gupta R, Lal B. Effect of Trigonella foenum-graecum (fenugreek) seeds on glycaemic control and insulin resistance in type 2 diabetes mellitus: a double blind placebo controlled study. *J Assoc Physicians India.* 2001 Nov;49:1057–1061.

95. Lu FR, Shen L, Qin Y, Gao L, Li H, Dai Y. Clinical observation on trigonella foenum-graecum L. total saponins in combination with sulfonylureas in the treatment of type 2 diabetes mellitus. *Chin J Integr Med.* 2008 Jan 25 (Epub ahead of print).

96. [No authors listed] Momordica charantia (bitter melon). Monograph. *Altern Med Rev.* 2007 Dec;12(4):360–363.

97. Fukushima M, Matsuyama F, Ueda N, Egawa K, Takemoto J, Kajimoto Y, Yonaha N, Miura T, Kaneko T, Nishi Y, Mitsui R, Fujita Y. Yamada Y, Seino Y. Effect of corosolic acid on postchallenge plasma glucose levels. *Diabetes Res Clin Pract.* 2006 Aug;73(2):174–177.

98. Witters LA. The blooming of the French lilac. *J Clin Invest.* 2001;108:1105–1107.

99. Savickiene N, Dagilyte A, Lukosius A, Zitkevicius V. Importance of biologically active components and plants in the prevention of complications of diabetes mellitus. *Medicina (Kaunas).* 2002;38(10):970–975.

100. Kanetkar P, Singhal R, Kamat M. Gymnema sylvestre: A memoir. *J Clin Biochem Nutr.* 2007 Sep;41(2):77–81.

101. Abdel-Zaher AO, Salim SY, Assaf MH, Abdel-Hady RH. Antidiabetic activity and toxicity of Zizyphus spina-christi leaves. *J Ethnopharmacol.* 2005 Oct 3;101(1–3):129–138.

102. Anderson RA. Chromium and polyphenols from cinnamon improve insulin sensitivity. *Proc Nutr Soc.* 2008 Feb;67(1):48–53.

103. White AM, Johnston CS. Vinegar ingestion at bedtime moderates waking glucose concentrations in adults with well-controlled type 2 diabetes. *Diabetes Care.* 2007 Nov;30(11):2814–2815. [Epub 2007 Aug 21].

104. Singh SN, Vats P, Suri S, Shyam R, Kumria MM, Ranganathan S, Sridharan K. Effect of an antidiabetic extract of Catharanthus roseus on enzymic activities in streptozotocin induced diabetic rats. *J Ethnopharmacol.* 2001 Aug;76(3):269–277.

105. Al-Amin ZM, Thomson M, Al-Qattan KK, Peltonen-Shalaby R, Ali M. Anti-diabetic and hypolipidaemic properties of ginger (Zingiber officinale) in streptozotocin-induced diabetic rats. *Br J Nutr.* 2006 Oct;96(4):660–666.

106. Su HC, Hung LM, Chen JK. Resveratrol, a red wine antioxidant, possesses an insulin-like effect in streptozotocin-induced diabetic rats. *Am J Physiol Endocrinol Metab.* 2006;290(6):E1339–1346.

107. Boyer J, Liu RH. Apple phytochemicals and their health benefits. *Nutr J.* 2004 May 12;3:5.

108. Krentz AJ. Bailey CJ. Oral antidiabetic agents: current role in type 2 diabetes mellitus. *Drugs.* 2005;65(3):385–411.

109. Scheen AJ. Drug interactions of clinical importance with antihyperglycaemic agents: an update. *Drug Saf.* 2005;28(7):601–631.

110. Sahin M, Tutuncu NB, Ertugrul D, Tanaci N, Guvener ND. Effects of metformin or rosiglitazone on serum concentrations of homocysteine, folate, and vitamin B12 in patients with type 2 diabetes mellitus. *J Diabetes Complications.* 2007 Mar–Apr;21(2):118–123.

111. Pongchaidecha M, Srikusalanukul V, Chattananon A, Tanjariyaporn S. Effect of metformin on plasma homocysteine, vitamin B12 and folic acid: a cross-sectional study in patients with type 2 diabetes mellitus. *J Med Assoc Thai.* 2004 Jul;87(7):780–787.

112. Karim A, Slater M, Bradford D, Schwartz L, Laurent A. Oral antidiabetic drugs: effect of food on absorption of pioglitazone and metformin from a fixed-dose combination tablet. *J Clin Pharmacol.* 2007 Jan;47(1):48–55.

113. Wåhlin-Boll E, Melander A, Sartor G, Scherstén B. Influence of food intake on the absorption and effect of glipizide in diabetics and in healthy subjects. *Eur J Clin Pharmacol.* 1980 Oct;18(3):279–283.

114. Bailey DG, Dresser GK. Interactions between grapefruit juice and cardiovascular drugs. *Am J Cardiovasc Drugs.* 2004;4(5):281–297.

115. Schwartz AV, Sellmeyer DE. Effect of thiazolidinediones on skeletal health in women with Type 2 diabetes. *Expert Opin Drug Saf.* 2008 Jan;7(1):69–78.

116. Green JB, Feinglos MN. Exenatide and rimonabant: new treatments that may be useful in the management of diabetes and obesity. *Curr Diab Rep.* 2007 Oct;7(5):369–375.

117. Meloche RM. Transplantation for the treatment of type 1 diabetes. *World J Gastroenterol.* 2007 Dec 21;13(47):6347–6355.

118. Iskovich S, Kaminitz A, Yafe MP, Mizrahi K, Stein J, Yaniv I, Askenasy N. Participation of adult bone marrow-derived stem cells in pancreatic regeneration: neogenesis versus endogenesis. *Curr Stem Cell Res Ther.* 2007 Dec;2(4):272–279.

119. Abraham NG, Li M, Vanella L, Peterson SJ, Ikehara S, Asprinio D. Bone marrow stem cell transplant into intra-bone cavity prevents type 2 diabetes: Role of heme oxygenase-adiponectin. *J Autoimmun.* 2008 Feb 1;30(3):128–135.

19 Obesity

Primary Care Approaches to Weight Reduction

Ingrid Kohlstadt, M.D., M.P.H.

I. INTRODUCTION

A 10% reduction in weight improves overall health among obese and overweight individuals. This vital public health message raises an important question. What is the physician's role in helping patients lose weight?

Since advice from health care professionals can significantly increase patient motivation and a medical doctor is perceived as the best source of health information [1], it is sometimes recommended that physicians add dietary counseling to already full office visits. The U.S. Preventive Services Task Force found fair to good evidence for intensive behavioral dietary counseling where obesity increases disease risk [2]. However, nutritionists, dieticians, and specifically trained nurses also provide dietary counseling, often more cost-effectively than physicians [2].

This chapter refocuses the physician's role in weight management on diagnosing and treating underlying metabolic disturbances. The emerging epidemiology and pathophysiology build a basis for the recommended food and nutrient therapies.

II. EPIDEMIOLOGY

Epidemiologic trends can help physicians assess risk of obesity and its complications:

- Obesity consistently affects women at higher rates than men.
- All racial and ethnic groups appear vulnerable despite unique dietary and genetic factors.
- The rapid rise in obesity exceeds what can be explained by genetic factors alone. The *in utero* environment and neonatal nutrition exert influences on genetic expression, not previously known to be possible.
- Not only is obesity affecting more people than ever before, its onset is also occurring at younger ages, giving rise to subepidemics of previously rare medical conditions such as slipped capital femoral epiphysis, polycystic ovary syndrome, precocious puberty, and childhood onset of type 2 diabetes.

There is growing evidence for a causal role between obesity and the risk factors in Table 19.1.

TABLE 19.1
Modifiable Risk Factors for Obesity, Suggested by Epidemiologic Data

- Increased caloric intake from beverages
- Heightened adrenocortical response (stress) in daily living
- Shift in dietary fat quality toward saturated and processed fats
- Decreased intake of dietary fiber
- Forfeiting lactation's protection against obesity for both mother and infant
- Stressors in the fetal environment that increase nongenetic heritable risk factors for obesity
- Exposure to chemicals that act as endocrine disruptors
- Iatrogenic factors such as drug-nutrient interactions
- Indoor living, which is generally accompanied by declining physical activity, altered circadian pattern, insidious dehydration from drier air, and less sun exposure

III. PATHOPHYSIOLOGY

Obesity is not a caloric accounting error. It cannot be fully explained by overeating and underexercising. Pathophysiology points to complex, redundant, multifactorial disturbances.

MALNUTRITION

Overconsumption of calories does not imply adequate nutrition. Data from a representative sample of the U.S. population demonstrates the opposite: Obesity increases the pretest probability of several correctable micronutrient deficiencies [3]. Poor nutrient intake can partially explain micronutrient

TABLE 19.2
Common Medications Known to Alter Nutrients Central to Metabolism

Medication	Nutrient	Mechanism
Coumadin	Vitamin K	Blocks enzyme that synthesizes vitamin K. Avoidance
	Lutein	of dark green leafy vegetables.
Iron	Chromium	Competitive absorption.
Antibiotics	Vitamins K and B	Destroy intestinal flora that synthesize these vitamins.
Corticosteroids	Calcium; Vitamin D;	Reduce active D; decrease calcium absorption; increase
	Chromium	chromium losses.
Bile acid sequestrants; Orlistat	Fat-soluble vitamins	Decrease absorption and low-fat diet.
Diuretics	Magnesium, Zinc	Increase urinary losses.
Digoxin	Calcium; Magnesium	Increases urinary losses.
Beta Blockers	Coenzyme Q10	Antagonize enzyme needed for synthesis.
HMG-CoA reductase inhibitors	Coenzyme Q10	Block enzyme needed for synthesis.
Sulfonylureas	Coenzyme Q10	Inhibit NADH-oxidase enzyme.
Biguanides	Vitamin B12	Competitive absorption.
NSAIDs	Folate	Competes with enzymatic synthesis.
H₂ blockers and proton pump inhibitors	B12, Calcium, Protein	Decrease absorption by increasing gastric pH.
Theophylline	Vitamin B6	Inhibits enzyme.
Anticonvulsants (most) and lithium	Vitamin D; Folate; L-carnitine	Interfere with metabolism; low serum levels.

Source: Adapted from [53]. With permission.

inadequacies. Obesity is associated with consuming highly processed fats and refined carbohydrates sometimes called "empty calories." Childhood diets high in sucrose are low in nutrients [4]. Additionally, obesity requires higher amounts of several nutrients because of inflammation, oxidative stress, mitochondrial dysfunction, malabsorption, and biophysical factors. Frequently overlooked in clinical practice are iatrogenic causes of micronutrient deficiencies, such as medication side effects (Table 19.2).

INFLAMMATION AND INSULIN RESISTANCE

Many of obesity's comorbidities (Table 19.3) are diseases of inflammation and impaired insulin signaling. Abdominal obesity is associated with unfavorable elevations in laboratory markers such as C-reactive protein, oxidized LDL [5], liver function tests, glycosylated hemoglobin, triglycerides,

---

TABLE 19.3
Medical Complications of Obesity and Obesity-Exacerbating Conditions

Medical Complications of Obesity	Obesity-Exacerbating Conditions Responsive to Food and Nutrients
Idiopathic intracranial hypertension	Chemosensory disorders
Stroke	Asthma
Alzheimer's disease	Hypochlorhydria
Parkinson's disease	Nonalcoholic fatty liver disease:
Cataracts	Elevated triglycerides
Coronary heart disease:	Steatosis
Hypertension	Steatohepatitis
Diabetes	Depression
Dyslipidemia	Sleep disturbance:
Obstructive sleep apnea	Obstructive sleep apnea
Hypoventilation syndrome	Restless leg syndrome
Asthma	Dyssynchronosis
Gastroesophageal reflux disease	Subclinical hypothyroidism
Nonalcoholic fatty liver disease	Type 2 diabetes
Pancreatitis	Polycystic ovary syndrome
Cholecystitis	Osteomalacia
Nephrolithiasis	Muscle atrophy
Chronic kidney disease	Peripheral edema
Reproductive health:	
Male infertility	
Female infertility in general	
Polycystic ovary syndrome (PCOS)	
Complications of pregnancy	
Difficulty in lactation	
Compromised *in utero* environment	
Precocious puberty	
Cancers	
Delayed wound healing and skin infections	
Phlebitis	
Gout	
Orthopedic conditions:	
Osteoarthritis, especially of the knee	
Slipped capital femoral epiphysis	
Nerve entrapment syndromes	

and glucose. Laboratory markers are intermediate outcome measures that can guide the management of obesity as well as its comorbidities.

DISPROPORTIONATE (ALLOMETRIC) GROWTH OF ADIPOSE

Obesity poses biophysical challenges. When adipose tissue exceeds lean tissue there are several downstream consequences for the metabolism:

1. Paucity of body water
Fat is relatively anhydrous. While a healthy weight adult has 60% to 65% body water, someone who is extremely obese may have a total body water of 30%. Disproportionate (allometric) growth of adipose may increase vulnerability to dehydration [6].

2. Suppressed metabolic rate
Body water is involved in removing heat and chemical by-products from metabolic reactions. In order to satisfy the physiologic priorities of temperature and pH, exothermic, acid-producing, metabolic reactions such as fat oxidation may be suppressed, which could help explain why proportional metabolic rate decreases with extreme obesity [7].

3. Transport of fat-soluble nutrients and toxins
Vitamin D travels from the epidermis where it is synthesized to the liver where it becomes partially activated. Obesity is associated with low levels of vitamin D in the serum and adequate levels in adipose tissue. Other fat-soluble vitamins such as lutein, xeoxanthin, and lycopene may be similarly stored in adipose, rendering the nutrients unavailable elsewhere. Also inadequately studied are the adverse effects of fat-soluble toxins released into circulation during weight reduction.

ATROPHY

Muscle loss can cause and often heralds obesity. Skeletal muscle has approximately three times the metabolic rate of adipose tissue, so muscle loss without reduced calorie intake is likely to lead to weight gain.

- Obesity is associated with inflammation, nutrient deficiencies, inefficient use of dietary protein, and impaired IGF-1, all of which damage muscle tissue.
- Obesity may limit the physical activity needed for maintenance of lean tissue.
- Losing weight and regaining it (yo-yo dieting) nets muscle loss because adipose is regained more quickly than muscle.
- Obesity can mask muscle atrophy and delay diagnosis of sarcopenic obesity.
- Obesity may have resulted from medications that simultaneously increase adipose and decrease lean tissue.
- Obesity alters protein usage, leaving inadequate protein for anabolic functions.
- In striking contrast to dieting humans, hibernating mammals and aestivating frogs preserve skeletal muscle, suggesting there is more to learn about the molecular controls of muscle and fat accumulation [8].

HOMEOSTASIS

The most successful diets are those to which patients can adhere. Adhering to a diet generally takes more than willpower [9]. Willpower is swimming in a riptide of homeostatic mechanisms involving the gut-brain axis, interrelated hypothalamic centers, and other regions of the brain that evolutionarily predate the neocortex.

While the body strives for a state of biochemical balance known as metabolic homeostasis, obesity is homeostasis at the wrong benchmark. Successful weight reduction must overcome the body's internal workings and create "unhomeostasis" until a new benchmark can be obtained and

TABLE 19.4
Neuroendocrine Messengers of Appetite Regulation

	Increase Appetite Promote Weight Gain	Decrease Appetite Promote Weight Loss
Neuropeptides	• Neuropeptide Y • Galanin	• Bombesin • Enterostatin (central action) • Corticotrophin releasing hormone • Melanocyte stimulating hormone • Peptide analogues and antagonists (under development)
Neurotransmitters	• Serotonin antagonists • Dopamine antagonists • Mu and Kappa opioids • Gamma amino butyric acid • Histamine H1 antagonists • Norepinephrine α receptor agonists	• Serotonin agonists and reuptake inhibitors • Dopamine agonists and reuptake inhibitors • Mu and Kappa opioid antagonists (under development) • Histamine H1 receptor agonists • Norepinephrine β receptor agonists
Central Action of Peripheral Hormones	• Insulin • Ghrelin (potentiating role) • Glucocorticoids • Adipocytokines (other than adiponectin) • Androgens • Progestins	• Glucagon-like peptide-1 • Leptin • Cholecystokinin • Adiponection • Estrogen • Gut hormone peptide YY [55]

Source: Adapted from [54]. With permission.

maintained. Subtle cues of circadian patterns, neurotransmitter sufficiency, meal timing, rate of eating, smell and taste as appetite stimulants, the glycemic index of foods, the extent to which food extends the stomach, and the availability of digestive enzymes can become important factors in diet adherence during "unhomeostasis." During "unhomeostasis" patients can be more vulnerable to medications that influence appetite and satiety (Table 19.4).

EARLY ENVIRONMENTAL FACTORS

Adulthood risk for obesity is greatly influenced *in utero*. Heritable factors are often mistaken to be synonymous with genetic factors and the powerful influence of the *in utero* nutritional environment is therefore overlooked. The *in utero* environment could be more hazardous now. Because obesity is occurring at younger ages, women of childbearing age may be passing obesity on to their children, not primarily because of genetics, but epigenetics, the nutritional milieu in which the genes are "read." Several lines of evidence have recently converged to conclude that healthful choices prior to and during pregnancy confer on the fetus lifelong protection against obesity.

- Animal research models: When mice inherit a gene known to cause obesity, they vary in the degree this gene is expressed based on their *in utero* environment. For example, bisphenol-A is a toxin from plastics detected in most Americans. Bisphenol-A can cause the obesity gene to be expressed, while genisten found in soy and folate found in vegetables can counteract the toxin and switch the obesity gene off [10, 11].
- Studies of twins that have traditionally been used to distinguish nature from nurture are limited in separating genetic influences from the *in utero* environment, because two-thirds of monozygotic twins have a shared placenta. The monozygotic twins with a shared placenta have not only common DNA but also a common nutrient supply line. Twins with a

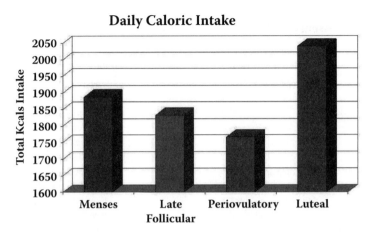

FIGURE 19.1 Calorie intake fluctuates with the phases of the menstrual cycle. (Adapted from [42]. With permission.)

shared placenta may be more likely to have similar adult weight than either dizygotic twins or monozygotic twins with separate placentas.
- Maternal starvation during the first half of pregnancy confers a greater risk of obesity and diabetes on the adult children [12].
- Women of childbearing age with type 2 diabetes have offspring who are at greater risk of childhood obesity and insulin resistance [13].
- Lactation, often considered an extension of the *in utero* environment, is protective against obesity in adulthood.

SEX HORMONE IMBALANCES

Testosterone, estrogen, and progesterone greatly influence muscle accretion and fat oxidation. Surgery, diseases, medications, and toxin exposures can contribute to obesity by disrupting sex hormones from age- and gender-appropriate levels. Obesity in turn can exacerbate the hormone imbalance. Adipose tissue is an endocrine organ that converts androgens to estrogen. Steatohepatitis compromises the liver's ability to neutralize foreign estrogens and interconvert endogenous hormones. Medical efforts directed at restoring age- and gender-appropriate hormone levels can help patients adhere to their diets.

Influence of sex hormones on appetite is subtle but measurable. Women's monthly hormone fluctuations influence calorie intake (Figure 19.1). During obesity and weight reduction the propensity to overeat during the luteal (premenstrual) phase can be exaggerated. Familiarity with this biologic tendency can help women avoid overeating.

IV. PATIENT EVALUATION

PATIENT HISTORY

Concise and clinically useful questions include the following:

1. What do you eat for breakfast?
Eating breakfast improves metabolic rate. Patients who skip breakfast miss out on boosting their metabolic rate and may have underlying insulin resistance and elevated triglycerides. Food selection at breakfast can prevent or promote food cravings throughout the day.

2. How is your digestion?

Irregular bowel patterns, heartburn, and constipation influence food selection. Impaired digestion can point to gallbladder disease, use of artificial sweeteners, food reactivities, and an opportunity to increase fiber, magnesium, vitamin C and hydration.

3. What has helped you lose weight in the past?

Diet patterns, nutritional programs, supplements, prescription medications, surgeries, and fitness programs that have been helpful in the past are likely to be helpful again as the patient's metabolism is optimized. Nonmedically advised weight loss, eating disorders, depressed mood, and risks for muscle atrophy might also be identified.

PHYSICAL EXAM

The following components of a comprehensive physical exam tend to be underutilized in weight management.

1. Monitoring fat reduction instead of weight reduction

Body mass index (BMI) is a well-established screening tool for adult obesity, but an insufficient monitoring tool since it does not distinguish between adipose and lean tissue. As a patient's weight changes or is anticipated to change, an assessment of body composition is a meaningful benchmark. Reduction in adipose tissue can be estimated by monitoring waist circumference, waist to hip ratio, bioimpedence [14], and resting metabolic rate. Clinical assessment can be supported by imaging studies. Dual energy x-ray absorptiometry (DEXA) can technically assess bone densitometry and body composition in the same scan, although not all facilities utilize both features.

2. Examining the oral cavity

Dental pain and poor dentition greatly influence food selection and a patient's ability to carry out dietary recommendations. Saliva that promotes poor dentition is likely to lack the salivary enzymes that digest food. Deficiencies in nutrients intrinsic to metabolism can sometimes be detected or suspected by visualizing the oral cavity. Periodontal disease indicates systemic inflammation and measurably increases risk of cardiovascular disease and cancer [15].

3. Assessing hydration status

Dry mucus membranes, pedal edema, poor skin turgor, and a dry mouth generally indicate intracellular dehydration. A lack of improvement in bioimpedence monitoring can also suggest inadequate hydration. Since muscle is more hydrous than fat it conducts a current more quickly. Similarly, being well hydrated improves bioimpedence results.

4. Screening for chemosensory disorders

Hyposmia alters taste and food selection. Impaired function of cranial nerve I can be diagnosed using the Alcohol Sniff Test (Chapter 3, "Chemosensory Disorders").

MEDICATION REVIEW

Medications alter appetite (Table 19.4) and reduce nutrient availability (Table 19.2).

LABORATORY EVALUATION

Laboratory tests can guide patient-centered weight management (Table 19.5).

OBESITY-EXACERBATING CONDITION EVALUATION

Obesity-exacerbating conditions (OECs) (Table 19.3) cause obesity by unfavorably altering metabolism or interfering with diet and exercise programs. OECs are often underdiagnosed and untreated despite effective medical and nutritional therapies.

1. Sleep apnea

Obesity has long been known to cause sleep apnea. Recent research has demonstrated that sleep apnea contributes to insulin resistance and even in patients with a healthful weight, sleep apnea is obesigenic [16]. The adverse metabolic effects of apnea predispose children ages 2 to 4 years to adult obesity [17]. Treatment with positive airway pressure should not be delayed due to intended weight reduction, but used in conjunction [18].

2. Chemosensory disorders

Diminished or altered taste and smell can be acquired during disease states, from medications, and following cancer treatment. Patients are often unaware that they are salting and sweetening their food in excess. Sometimes the diagnosis alone can provide sufficient impetus for a patient to reestablish healthful eating habits. Use of tastants and spices, and restoring healthful levels of phosphotidyl choline, zinc, and B vitamins, can also improve symptoms [19, 20].

3. Polycystic ovary syndrome (PCOS)

PCOS is associated with dietary obstacles such as sweet cravings, obesigenic fertility medications, bulimia nervosa, central adiposity, low cholecystokinin (a satiety peptide), and insulin resistance [21, 22]. Nutritional strategies that improve insulin sensitivity can be effectively applied to patients with PCOS.

4. Gastroesophageal reflux disease (GERD)

Obesity exacerbates GERD and medications that treat reflux can reduce vitamin B12 [23]. There are several methods to assay vitamin B12 status (Table 19.5). Restoring vitamin B12 also improves occult peripheral nerve damage, which can limit exercise, predispose to injury, and make physical activities painful.

5. Osteomalacia

Low-fat diets, increased body fat, and fat-malabsorbing obesity treatments lower serum vitamin D levels and may contribute to the high pretest probability of low vitamin D among overweight women [3]. Low vitamin D in turn can forestall weight loss by perpetuating insulin resistance, lowering mood, making physical activity more difficult, and causing musculoskeletal pain known as osteomalacia [3, 24, 25]. Even though it is a relatively late manifestation of vitamin D deficiency, osteomalacia is frequently misdiagnosed.

6. Subclinical hypothyroidism

The NHANES III data suggest that 1 in 10 Americans are deficient in iodine [26]. Iodine deficiency as a contributing cause of subclinical hypothyroidism is frequently overlooked and undertreated. Weight reduction diets are frequently low in iodine-fortified salt and high in goiterogenic soy products, which therefore potentially worsen iodine deficiency. Ethnic diets high in soy are also high in iodine-rich seaweed. Seaweed and selenium-rich foods can effectively provide thyroid support (Chapter 16, "Hypothyroidism").

7. Nonalcoholic fatty liver disease

Even in its earliest stages, fatty liver interferes with weight loss. As triglycerides accumulate in the bloodstream in excess of 100 mg/dL, the attached fatty acids become less available for energy production. Avoidance of *trans* fats and refined carbohydrates can improve metabolism. Eventually steatosis impairs the liver's metabolism of sex hormones and detoxification of fat-soluble toxic chemicals.

8. Muscle atrophy

Obesity and muscle atrophy can coexist in a condition known as sarcopenic obesity, which suggests obesity more advanced than indicated by BMI alone. Obese people with greater lean tissue and fitness had measurably lower mortality than people with an equally high BMI who were less fit [27]. Nutritional interventions can reduce sarcopenia in a high-risk population [28].

TABLE 19.5
Nutritional Diagnostic Tests to Guide Weight Reduction

Test	Interpretation	Mechanism	Treatment	Why Optimize
Resting metabolic rate (RMR)	RMR lower than predicted may suggest thyroid dysfunction or loss of lean tissue.	Protein malabsorption; iodine insufficiency.	Establish plan for preventing further muscle atrophy with exercise and adequate protein. Evaluate for iodine deficiency–related hypothyroidism.	Maintain lean body mass; restore thyroid function.
Thyroid-stimulating hormone	Above 2.5 mIU/L consider iodine deficiency and further evaluation.	Iodine deficiency from impaired absorption and decreased intake.	Eat seaweed, not soy; iodine and selenium supplementation.	Maintain optimal metabolic rate.
Vitamin B12	Serum concentration under 540 pg/mL and elevated urine methylmalonate excretion suggest deficiency.	Impaired absorption often due to a nutrient-drug interaction.	Oral or IM B12 supplementation.	Energy metabolism.
Homocysteine	Elevation signifies deficiency in B12, folate, or B6.	Impaired absorption and inadequate intake.	Supplementation and dietary intake.	Energy metabolism.
C-reactive protein	High sensitivity CRP below 10 mg/L, ideally below 5 mg/L; further evaluation for food reactivities may be indicated.	Inflammation.	Supplemental fiber; alkaline diet; avoidance of reactive foods; supplemental curcumin 2–4 g/day.	Monitor improvement in inflammatory component of obesity.
Vitamin D	25(OH)D in the range of 30–40 ng/mL; interpret keeping seasonal variation in mind.	Malabsorption, decreased activation.	50,000 IU of vitamin D_2 weekly for eight weeks to achieve 30 ng/mL 25(OH)D; sunlight and dietary sources; fish, dairy, and mushrooms.	Maintain insulin sensitivity and avoid seasonal low mood often associated with overeating.
Triglycerides	Fasting values above 100 mg/dL suggest impaired fat metabolism.	Steatosis, increased oxidative stress, impaired fat metabolism.	Diet low in refined carbohydrates and no *trans* or highly processed fats; liver support; supplemental l-carnitine 2 g/day.	Improve fat oxidation and spare lean tissue; preserve detoxification.
DEXA	Body composition and bone mineral density.	Sarcopenia and osteopenia from various causes.	Dietary protein; supplemental amino acids; digestive enzymes; alkaline diet; supplemental bone nutrients in a personalized plan; combine diet strategies with physical activity.	Screen and monitor musculoskeletal integrity.

Tests Recommended in Patients With Underlying Medical Conditions

Test	Interpretation	Mechanism	Treatment	Why Optimize
Fatty acids	Erythrocyte fatty acid profile can identify isolated fatty acid deficiencies and impaired enzyme function.	Skewed dietary intake, variable absorption, impairment of delta-6-desaturase due to zinc deficiency.	Balance dietary intake of mono- and polyunsaturated fatty acids; supplemental polyunsaturates.	Maintain intracellular hydration, improve oxidative phosphorylation, reduce comorbidities.

continued

TABLE 19.5 *(continued)*

Test	Interpretation	Mechanism	Treatment	Why Optimize
Magnesium	Erythrocyte (RBC) magnesium.	Impaired absorption, inadequate dietary intake, competitive absorption with calcium which is supplemented postbariatric surgery.	Increase fruit and vegetable intake; supplement calcium and magnesium in a ratio of 2:1.	Hydration; fat metabolism.
Coenzyme Q10	Low serum CoQ10 signifies depletion of tissue CoQ10; high levels of pyruvate, succinate, fumarate and malate in the urine suggests insufficient CoQ10 to meet energy pathway demands.	Fat metabolism increases demand for this conditionally essential vitamin; drug–nutrient interactions.	Supplemental CoQ10 up to 300 mg.	Fat metabolism; electron transport and membrane antioxidant.
Carnitine	Deficiency if low plasma carnitine or elevated urinary excretion of adipic, suberic, and ethylmalonic acids.	Impaired absorption; Decreased synthesis; high demand during fat metabolism.	Supplemental l-carnitine.	Fat metabolism.
Serum albumin	Low suggests protein malnutrition.	Inadequate intake, malabsorption.	Dietary protein; supplemental amino acids; digestive enzymes.	Maintain lean body mass.
Iron studies	Low ferritin and % saturation ≤15 suggest iron-deficient erythropoesis even when HCT is normal; elevation can suggest hemochromatosis.	Impaired absorption or inadequate intake; primary hemochromatosis is a nutrient-gene interaction.	Supplemental minerals, not only supplemental iron; hemochromatosis is managed medically and by minimizing dietary iron intake.	Often coexists with other mineral deficiencies such as chromium, vanadium, and iodine; hemochromatosis contributes to the inflammatory component of obesity.
Mineral/toxic elements	Second day 24 hr urine after d-penicillamine provocation; compare results to reference ranges.	Impaired absorption of minerals; impaired excretion of toxicants and greater uptake during mineral deficiency state.	Supplemental intake of minerals; further assessment of metal toxicant exposure.	Weight reduction may release toxicants into circulation; minerals influence food selection.
Fractionated serum or plasma carotenes	α-Carotene: 9–101 µg/L. β-Carotene: 42–373 µg/L. Lutein: 50–250 µg/L. Zeaxanthin: 8–80 µg/L.	Impaired absorption; increased oxidative stress.	Green leafy vegetables for prevention of age-related macular degeneration, cataracts, and cancer.	Systemic benefit from optimal protection against oxidation.

9. Peripheral edema

Edema is worsened by excessive dietary intake of sodium, which is primarily an extracellular electrolyte. Inadequate dietary intake of the primarily intracellular electrolytes magnesium and potassium also exacerbates edema. Supplemental magnesium and potassium can reduce edema, improve hydration, and relieve symptoms that hinder lifestyle management of obesity and require obesigenic medications [6].

10. Depression and emotional eating

Depression and emotional eating are both associated with insufficiency of the neurotransmitters serotonin, dopamine, and possibly gamma-aminobutyric acid (GABA). Newer antidepressants and anticonvulsants [29] that potentiate the same neurotransmitters are being used, sometimes off-label, for weight management. A similar role for the amino acid precursors of neurotransmitters is posited here. Treating depression (Chapter 29, "Depression") with amino acids can improve patient adherence. Sometimes patients initiate amino acids, which are available as supplements. Medical supervision is urged.

11. Asthma

Asthma interferes with aerobic exercise. Clinical management often requires obesigenic medications. Nutritional strategies (Chapter 8, "Asthma") can reduce the dosage and number of medications required.

SPECIAL CIRCUMSTANCES

1. Lactation

Breastfeeding helps mothers shed the weight gained during pregnancy. At the same time breastfeeding protects the infant from obesity later in life. However, mothers with a BMI over 30 are less likely to initiate lactation. They have delayed onset of lactation, experience less prolactin response to suckling, and are prone to early cessation of breastfeeding. Anticipation of and adequate preparation for these barriers can help overcome them. Interventions include optimizing prenatal weight gain, limiting maternal-newborn separation, and massage or pumping of the breasts [30].

2. Childhood obesity

Childhood onset of obesity adds urgency to weight reduction. Eighty percent of obese children become obese adults, comorbidities appear earlier in adults who were obese as children, and obesity in childhood reduces overall life expectancy [13]. While special attention is important to the social and behavioral components of eating, food and nutrient interventions should be early and intensive. When small children are unable to innately regulate calorie intake, it usually signals a metabolic disturbance. Often overlooked are the opportunity to correct metabolic disturbances secondary to OECs, especially musculoskeletal disorders, delayed healing time from injuries [31], depression, asthma, sleep disorders, and vitamin D deficiency.

3. Prior bariatric surgery

Surgical treatment of obesity extends life [32, 33]. A 10-year follow-up study identified surgical weight reduction as 10-fold more effective than lifestyle intervention and medication [34]. Bariatric surgery is no longer limited to permanent procedures. Reversible banding has achieved successful results as part of a comprehensive treatment of lifestyle modification, nutritional medicine, and surgery. Addressing nutrient deficiencies (Table 19.5) following bariatric surgery can help prevent weight recidivism [35, 36]. Bariatric surgery does not exclude nutritional interventions. On the contrary, surgical outcomes are enhanced by nutrient optimization and presurgical weight loss [36].

V. TREATMENT RECOMMENDATIONS

Consider starting by diagnosing and treating obesity-exacerbating conditions. A nutritional deficiency, medical disorder, or necessary medication can interfere with weight reduction. Diagnosing and treating the underlying metabolic problem can help a patient succeed. Success improves diet adherence.

Communicate the "big picture" of needed dietary change and decide which diet to use. The Alkaline Diet (Chapter 31, "Osteoporosis") is low in sugar, high in fiber, low glycemic index, and appropriate in amount and sources of dietary fat. The Alkaline Diet in contrast to many popular diets offers latitude in dietary selection. The Mediterranean Diet is a popular Alkaline Diet and can be recommended to patients who enjoy and have access to Mediterranean foods. However, alkaline diets can be assembled from most ethnic foods. People are more likely to adhere to diets they enjoy and those that honor their ethnic traditions.

Diet

Substitutions

An effective method for shifting a patient's dietary pattern is by implementing a series of substitutions. Substitutions can break down a complex shift in diet into small manageable steps and are one of the least difficult forms of change. Ideally these changes will be implemented by all those who share meals with the patient.

- Replace *trans* and other processed fats with unrefined oils.
- Replace starches with whole grains, vegetables, berry fruits, and other fiber sources [37].
- Replace sugar with flavor.
- Replace calories with volume [38, 39].
- Replace caloric beverages with water, herbal tea, and highly diluted juices [40].
- Replace routine with variety by rotating diets, meal plans, and dining venues to help eating remain an enjoyable, portion-appropriate, and multi-sensory experience.

One commonly used substitution that is unlikely to be beneficial long term is replacing sugar with a low calorie, high intensity (artificial) sweetener. Several medically related problems can arise:

- The first ingredient in the sweetener packets is usually dextrose. Consuming several packets a day can impede glucose control in patients with diabetes.
- Artificial sweeteners are orders of magnitude sweeter than sugar. They tend to accustom the palette to a very sweet taste and may thereby increase total calorie intake long-term.
- People may not be aware that certain diet foods contain artificial sweeteners, making the source of potential side effects such as flatus and diarrhea difficult to diagnose.
- Non-absorbed chemicals in the intestinal lumen create an osmotic effect, which commonly contributes to dehydration. Sweeteners do not facilitate water uptake by enterocytes the way glucose does.
- Weight control during pregnancy is important, but the safety and potential side effects of sweeteners on fetal development are poorly established.
- Artificial sweeteners and other poorly understood additives may underlie or trigger migraine headaches, attention deficit hyperactivity disorder, food reactivities, and irritable bowel syndrome.

Xylitol and ribose (Chapter 34, "Fibromyalgia and Chronic Fatigue Syndrome") are sugars with unique health benefits and can be used instead of sucrose and artificial sweeteners. Spices such as vanilla and cinnamon can also infuse sweet flavors, requiring less sugar. Diagnosing and treating chemosensory disorders (Chapter 3, "Chemosensory Disorders") can also reduce excess sugar intake.

Calorie Restriction

Food quality should take precedence over calorie counting and macronutrient ratios. However, attention to the following can help patients more easily achieve the necessary calorie restriction.

1. Eating breakfast reduces total calorie intake and late night eating increases it. Meal timing may extend beyond calorie intake, with breakfast favoring fat metabolism and late night eating reducing fat metabolism [41].
2. Eating mindfully reduces total calorie intake, mostly by giving the body sufficient time to experience satiety before overeating.
3. Increasing dietary fiber to 40 g/day increases the volume of food, which increases satiety and reduces overall food intake.
4. Eating calories rather than drinking calories also reduces total calorie intake.
5. Women of childbearing age can monitor calorie intake more closely as their menstrual cycle approaches (Figure 19.1) [42].

NUTRIENTS AND SUPPLEMENTS

Dietary supplements are not evaluated for safety and efficacy by the Food and Drug Administration (FDA) before marketing. Neither are dietary supplements safer than over-the-counter (OTC) or prescription medications. Judicious selection of therapeutic foods and supplemental nutrients often falls to patients. Physicians can correct patient misperceptions about dietary supplements [43] and recommend patients discontinue any dietary supplements that increase metabolic rate at the expense of lean tissue, may be of compromised quality, or are taken at inappropriately high doses.

Supplemental nutrients used appropriately can help patients achieve weight maintenance. Supplemental nutrients are usually not called diet supplements because they don't "rev up" metabolism. Instead they are used by skilled clinicians to restore optimal metabolic functioning. Supplemental nutrients can be used short term and transition patients to nutrient-rich foods.

Fiber

Low-fiber intake is a key mediator of the obesity epidemic. In the United States the population averages 10 to 15 g of fiber a day, less than half of the recommended 25 g for women and 38 g for men. Reversing the low-fiber trend can be an effective component of weight loss [44]:

- Low glycemic index foods are generally high in fiber [45].
- Fiber adds volume to food, and mechanically stretching the stomach releases gut-synthesized satiety peptides [38, 39].
- Fiber improves lipid profiles and insulin sensitivity, which enables patients to improve comorbidities and avoid obesigenic nutrient-drug interactions [46].
- Fiber reduces inflammation [47, 48].
- There are other hypothesized benefits that are not easy to quantify. Fiber may reduce intake of endocrine-disrupting fat-soluble toxicants by the same mechanism by which fiber reduces colon cancer risk. Fiber may improve nutrient-synthesizing, pathogen-fighting gastrointestinal microflora, which may additionally exert satiety signals.

Gastrointestinal symptoms frequently limit fiber's therapeutic use. Like a fitness program, one can work up to higher fiber intake, often called improving bowel tolerance. Supplementing dietary fiber in gradually increasing doses can improve bowel tolerance and make use of fiber's dietary benefits. Hydroxypropylmethylcellulose (HPMC) can be supplemented as 2.5 g added to an 8 oz beverage twice daily. While HPMC can be taken with or between meals [49], just before meals or during meals is likely to maximize the satiety effect of fiber. Fiber powders that also contain digestive enzymes and vitamins can serve as snacks or meal substitutes (Chapter 12, "Viral Hepatitis, Nonalcoholic Steatohepatitis, and Postcholecystectomy Syndrome").

Polyunsaturated Fatty Acids

Supplemental polyunsaturated fats effectively prevent and treat many of obesity's comorbidities, increase the fluidity of mitochondrial membranes thereby facilitating fat oxidation, preserve lean tissue during calorie restriction, compensate for impaired delta-6-desaturase enzyme activity, and balance the oxidation of highly saturated adipose tissue.

Supplements can be initiated as follows:

1. Emphasize complete avoidance of *trans* and other highly processed fats.
2. Initiate a starting dose, often eicosapentaenoic acid (EPA) 240 mg, docosahexaenoic acid (DHA) 160 mg, and gamma-linolenic acid (GLA) 160 mg. Fish oil and evening primrose oil can be used.
3. Recommend fish and evening primrose oils over flax oil, which contains alpha-linolenic acid and linoleic acid. Conversion to EPA and GLA depends on delta-6-desaturase, an enzyme often impaired by obesity.
4. Include GLA even though it is an omega-6 fat. Suboptimal levels can be further impaired by supplemental EPA and DHA.
5. Hold off on conjugated linoleic acid (CLA), which is sometimes promoted for weight reduction. It is presently unclear who benefits from this microbially derived *trans* fat. A dietary shift away from dairy products and changes in agricultural practice may cause low dietary intake of CLA, but other changes in dietary fat are more compelling and warrant prioritization.
6. Several disease states and malabsorption may prompt a red blood cell fatty acid analysis (Chapter 24, "Seizures") to more precisely guide dietary intake and supplement dosage.
7. The supplemental dosing can serve as a transition to a diet rich in fish, nuts, seeds, and varied high-quality cooking oils.

Chromium

Body stores of chromium are two orders of magnitude less than iron and too small to measure clinically. Chromium is found in diverse foods, and low chromium is generally not due to inadequate intake so a diet history is unhelpful in establishing a chromium deficiency state. Chromium uptake is competitively inhibited by iron, posing hypotheses that supplemental iron and hemochromatosis may lower body stores of chromium. Stress and steroid medications appear to increase urinary loss of chromium, another mechanism by which a deficiency state may occur.

Chromium facilitates glucose uptake by the muscles. Deficiency is more likely in diabetes where urinary losses of chromium may be significant. A randomized clinical trial found that chromium reduces body fat in those with diabetes when added to conventional oral antihyperglycemic agents [50]. There was no demonstrated benefit in women with a healthy weight on a balanced diet [51]. The average chromium dose in clinical trials is 400 µg/day and duration of treatment 79 days [52]. Patients with insulin resistance and polycystic ovary syndrome may find chromium helpful in managing food cravings. Rather than on a scheduled dosing, 200 µg can be taken twice daily as needed for food cravings.

Protein

Obesity makes getting adequate dietary protein more difficult: Greater total protein requirements are due to larger size, calorie restriction for weight loss, decreased absorption from impaired digestive enzyme function, increased demand due to inflammation and exercise, and reallocation for energy production rather than anabolic functions. However, protein is metabolically expensive. Protein sources are usually acidifying, high in saturated fat, and energy dense. Clinical interventions can therefore be directed at improving protein absorption.

Some amino acid combinations are utilized more readily for anabolic function than other amino acid combinations. Eggs (white and yolk together) are the single best protein source for promoting anabolic function. Eggs have a net nitrogen utilization approximately 60% greater than lean meats and approximately 150% that of whey and soy protein powders. Patients using soy in high doses during dieting may experience goiterogenic effects.

Supplemental essential amino acids are well-absorbed, low-calorie, and more readily utilized for anabolic functions. Five grams can be taken twice daily on an empty stomach. Amino acids are neurotransmitter precursors. Insufficient amino acid precursors for dopamine, serotonin, and possibly GABA may be a significant component of food cravings. Medications that potentiate the action of neurotransmitters are sometimes used in weight reduction [29]. The amino acids L-tyrosine and 5-hydroxytryptophan can be supplemented per Chapter 29, "Depression." Some patients will experience reduction in food cravings.

Carnitine

L-carnitine is an organic acid that transports fatty acids to the inner mitochondria for fat oxidation. The body's ability to synthesize adequate l-carnitine may not be sufficient during the phase of active weight reduction. While found primarily in meats, it can also be supplemented during weight reduction where it has been shown to be beneficial [36]. L-carnitine can be dosed at 1 g twice daily (Chapter 6, "Congestive Heart Failure and Cardiomyopathy"). Two grams twice daily can lead to gastrointestinal symptoms. Purified l-carnitine should be chosen, not a racemic mixture. L-carnitine should be combined with avoidance of *trans* fats and refined carbohydrates.

L-carnitine is most likely to benefit patients with impaired fat oxidation, identified early as triglycerides in excess of 100 mg/dL. Vegetarians may benefit from l-carnitine due to low dietary intake. A clinical assay for l-carnitine is available (Table 19.5).

Vitamin D

Outdoor exercise throughout the year, fat oxidation, and fish consumption can be recommended alongside supplemental vitamin D administered to maintain 25(OH)D above 30 ng/mL.

Magnesium

Magnesium plays a critical role in fat oxidation. Suboptimal dietary intake, competitive absorption with supplemental calcium, and impaired absorption with various gastrointestinal conditions make magnesium deficiency common. Pedal edema and constipation are often responsive to supplemental magnesium [31]. Magnesium supplementation can be initiated at 250 mg/day, generally as chelated minerals, especially magnesium citrate, which is highly alkalinizing.

Phosphatidyl Choline

Phosphatidyl choline reduces cholesterol, improves membrane pliability, and enhances the uptake of magnesium. Obese patients are likely to have suboptimal levels of phosphatidyl choline from low dietary intake of nuts, seeds, and egg yolk. Prior cholecystectomy and low-functioning digestive enzymes can reduce absorption. Supplementation at 4 g/day may be beneficial alongside higher dietary intake (Chapter 24, "Seizures").

Iodine

Patients should optimize thyroid function by eating sea vegetables. Iodine and selenium supplementation is sometimes indicated (Chapter 16, "Hypothyroidism").

HYDRATION

Physicians can help patients overcome medically related barriers to hydration. Barriers include edema, prolonged urination with prostate hypertrophy, bladder incontinence, and urinary frequency from diuretics.

The health importance of avoiding dry indoor air, drinking more water when at higher elevation or low air cabin pressure, and avoiding beverages with calories can also be underscored. For example, while a 2% glucose solution promotes the uptake of water by enterocytes, beverages sweeter than this offer no added advantage. Sports drinks generally contain 6% glucose.

Sweating can be considered a form of regional hydration, since one of the biophysical challenges of obesity is delivery of nutrients through and to adipose tissue. Sweating may be an overlooked advantage of exercise. For patients unable to work up a sweat, steam rooms and saunas may have some, albeit sparsely studied, benefit to hydrating tissue and facilitating removal of toxicants.

WEIGHT LOSS MEDICATIONS

Patients with excess adipose accumulation may wish to choose pharmacotherapy as part of their weight management program. This may be appropriate since the risk profiles of rimonabant, sibutramine, and orlistat are very low. There is no evidence from clinical practice that phentermine and diethylpropion have addiction potential while there is some evidence of addiction potential with phendimetrazine. Unfortunately, clinical results show but modest benefit [34].

The opportunity costs of medication use may be high and are sometimes overlooked. Expense may preclude some patients from using both nutrients and medications. Medications can unfavorably alter food selection such as avoiding healthful dietary fats and increasing intake of refined carbohydrates. Medication may prevent adequate fiber intake since both can cause gastrointestinal discomfort. Medications can increase demand and impair absorption of nutrients that may already be at suboptimal levels.

VI. SUMMARY

Epidemiology, pathophysiology, and limited clinical data shape a unique role for medical doctors in managing obesity. Clinical practice can incorporate the following:

- Distinguish between muscle and fat, rather than focusing on weight alone.
- Screen for obesity-exacerbating conditions such as vitamin D deficiency, vitamin B12 deficiency, sleep apnea, chemosensory disorders, depression, and iodine deficiency, which are treatable and under-diagnosed dieting saboteurs.
- Implement an alkalinizing diet by using a stepwise series of substitutions.
- Consider potential medical side effects of artificial sweeteners, frequently used to help restrict calorie intake (Chapter 13, "Irritable Bowel Syndrome"; Chapter 15, "Food Reactivities"; Chapter 25, "Attention Deficit Hyperactivity Disorder"; Chapter 26, "Migraine Headaches").
- Help patients optimize thyroid function with a dietary intervention. Eat seaweed and avoid soy when subclincial hypothyroidism is suspected.
- Reduce refined carbohydrates, eliminate *trans* fats, and consider supplemental dosing of l-carnitine when triglycerides are elevated.
- Be aware that chromium deficiency may exist, albeit difficult to assess. Supplemental chromium can be used on an as-needed basis to help manage food cravings.
- Use supplemental fiber to transition patients to eating optimal dietary fiber.
- Consider supplemental amino acids. Essential amino acids may help maintain lean tissue. The amino acids 5-hydroxytryptophan and tyrosine (Chapter 29, "Depression") may help relieve food cravings by enhancing the neurotransmitters for which they are precursors.
- Emphasize quality of dietary fat. Supplemental polyunsaturated fats EPA, DHA, and GLA can help transition patients to a dietary oil change.

REFERENCES

1. Hiddink, G.J., et al. *Consumers' expectations about nutrition guidance: the importance of primary care physicians.* Am J Clin Nutr, 1997. 65(6 Suppl): p. 1974S–1979S.
2. *Screening for obesity in adults: recommendations and rationale.* Ann Intern Med, 2003. 139(11): p. 930–32.
3. Kimmons, J.E., et al. *Associations between body mass index and the prevalence of low micronutrient levels among US adults.* Med Gen Med, 2006. 8(4): p. 59.
4. Ruottinen, S., et al. *High sucrose intake is associated with poor quality of diet and growth between 13 months and 9 years of age: the special Turku Coronary Risk Factor Intervention Project.* Pediatrics, 2008. 121(6): p. 1676–85.
5. Holvoet, P., et al. *Association between circulating oxidized low-density lipoprotein and incidence of the metabolic syndrome.* Jama, 2008. 299(19): p. 2287–93.
6. Batmanghelidj, F., and I. Kohlstadt. *Water: a driving force in the musculoskeletal system.* In *Scientific Evidence for Musculoskeletal, Bariatric, and Sports Nutrition*, I. Kohlstadt, Editor. 2006, CRC Press, Taylor & Francis Group: Boca Raton, FL. p. 127–36.
7. Livingston, E.H., and I. Kohlstadt. *Simplified resting metabolic rate-predicting formulas for normal-sized and obese individuals.* Obes Res, 2005. 13(7): p. 1255–62.
8. Shavlakadze, T., and M. Grounds. *Of bears, frogs, meat, mice and men: complexity of factors affecting skeletal muscle mass and fat.* Bioessays, 2006. 28(10): p. 994–1009.
9. Badman, M.K., and J.S. Flier. *The gut and energy balance: visceral allies in the obesity wars.* Science, 2005. 307(5717): p. 1909–14.
10. Dolinoy, D.C., and R.L. Jirtle. *Environmental epigenomics in human health and disease.* Environ Mol Mutagen, 2008. 49(1): p. 4–8
11. Dolinoy, D.C., et al. *Maternal genistein alters coat color and protects Avy mouse offspring from obesity by modifying the fetal epigenome.* Environ Health Perspect, 2006. 114(4): p. 567–72.
12. Gluckman, P.D., and M.A. Hanson. *The fetal matrix: evolution, development, and disease.* 2005, Cambridge, UK; New York: Cambridge University Press. xiv, 257 p.
13. Salbe, A., M.B. Schwartz, and I. Kohlstadt. *Childhood obesity.* In *Scientific evidence for musculoskeletal, bariatric, and sports nutrition*, I. Kohlstadt, Editor. 2006, CRC Press, Taylor & Francis Group: Boca Raton, FL. p. 253–69.
14. Heber, D., et al. *Clinical detection of sarcopenic obesity by bioelectrical impedance analysis.* Am J Clin Nutr, 1996. 64(3 Suppl): p. 472S–477S.
15. Michaud, D.S., et al. *Periodontal disease, tooth loss, and cancer risk in male health professionals: a prospective cohort study.* Lancet Oncol, 2008. 9(6): p. 550–58.
16. Punjabi, N.M., and V.Y. Polotsky. *Disorders of glucose metabolism in sleep apnea.* J Appl Physiol, 2005. 99(5): p. 1998–2007.
17. Al Mamun, A., D.A. Lawlor, S. Cramb, et al. *Do childhood sleeping problems predict obesity in young adulthood? Evidence from a prospective birth cohort study.* Am J Epidemiol, 2007. 12(166): p. 1368–73.
18. Trenell, M.I., et al. *Influence of constant positive airway pressure therapy on lipid storage, muscle metabolism and insulin action in obese patients with severe obstructive sleep apnoea syndrome.* Diabetes Obes Metab, 2007. 9(5): p. 679–87.
19. Wrobel, B.B., and D.A. Leopold. *Clinical assessment of patients with smell and taste disorders.* Otolaryngol Clin North Am, 2004. 37(6): p. 1127–42.
20. Hirsch, A.R. *Weight reduction through inhalation of odorants.* J Neurol Orthop Med Surg, 1995. 16: p. 28–31.
21. Hirschberg, A.L., et al. *Impaired cholecystokinin secretion and disturbed appetite regulation in women with polycystic ovary syndrome.* Gynecol Endocrinol, 2004. 19(2): p. 79–87.
22. Hirschberg, A.L. *Hormonal regulation of appetite and food intake.* Ann Med, 1998. 30(1): p. 7–20.
23. Valuck, R.J., and J.M. Ruscin. *A case-control study on adverse effects: H2 blocker or proton pump inhibitor use and risk of vitamin B12 deficiency in older adults.* J Clin Epidemiol, 2004. 57(4): p. 422–28.
24. Holick, M. *Vitamin D: Importance for musculoskeletal function and health.* In *Scientific Evidence for Musculoskeletal, Bariatric and Sports Nutrition*, I. Kohlstadt, Editor. 2006, CRC Press, Taylor & Francis Group: Boca Raton, FL. p. 153–174.
25. Wicherts, I.S., et al. *Vitamin D status predicts physical performance and its decline in older persons.* J Clin Endocrinol Metab, 2007. 92(6): p. 2058–65.
26. Hollowell, J.G., et al. *Iodine nutrition in the United States. Trends and public health implications: iodine excretion data from National Health and Nutrition Examination Surveys I and III (1971–1974 and 1988–1994).* J Clin Endocrinol Metab, 1998. 83(10): p. 3401–8.

27. Sui, X., et al. *Cardiorespiratory fitness and adiposity as mortality predictors in older adults.* Jama, 2007. 298(21): p. 2507–16.

28. Demark-Wahnefried, W., et al. *Preventing sarcopenic obesity among breast cancer patients who receive adjuvant chemotherapy: results of a feasibility study.* Clin Exerc Physiol, 2002. 4(1): p. 44–49.

29. Miller, S. *Pharmacotherapy for weight loss.* US Pharmacist, 2006. 12: p. 75–85.

30. Jevitt, C., I. Hernandez, and M. Groer. *Lactation complicated by overweight and obesity: supporting the mother and newborn.* J Midwifery Womens Health, 2007. 52(6): p. 606–13.

31. Kohlstadt, I. *Scientific evidence for musculoskeletal, bariatric, and sports nutrition.* 2006, Boca Raton: CRC Taylor & Francis. xx, 621 p.

32. Sjostrom, L., et al. *Effects of bariatric surgery on mortality in Swedish obese subjects.* N Engl J Med, 2007. 357(8): p. 741–52.

33. Adams, T.D., et al. *Long-term mortality after gastric bypass surgery.* N Engl J Med, 2007. 357(8): p. 753–61.

34. Sjostrom, L., et al. *Lifestyle, diabetes, and cardiovascular risk factors 10 years after bariatric surgery.* N Engl J Med, 2004. 351(26): p. 2683–93.

35. Bralley, J.A. *Laboratory evaluations in molecular medicine.* 2001: Institute for Advances in Molecular Medicine.

36. Kohlstadt, I. *Bariatric surgery: More effective with nutrition.* In *Scientific Evidence for Musculoskeletal, Bariatric, and Sports Nutrition*, I. Kohlstadt, Editor. 2006, CRC Press, Taylor & Francis Group: Boca Raton, FL. p. 271–82.

37. Ledikwe, J.H., et al. *Dietary energy density is associated with energy intake and weight status in US adults.* Am J Clin Nutr, 2006. 83(6): p. 1362–68.

38. Rolls, B.J., E.A. Bell, and M.L. Thorwart. *Water incorporated into a food but not served with a food decreases energy intake in lean women.* Am J Clin Nutr, 1999. 70(4): p. 448–55.

39. Rolls, B.J., L.S. Roe, and J.S. Meengs. *Reductions in portion size and energy density of foods are additive and lead to sustained decreases in energy intake.* Am J Clin Nutr, 2006. 83(1): p. 11–17.

40. Rolls, B.J., and L.S. Roe. *Effect of the volume of liquid food infused intragastrically on satiety in women.* Physiol Behav, 2002. 76(4–5): p. 623–31.

41. de Castro, J.M. *The time of day of food intake influences overall intake in humans.* J Nutr, 2004. 134(1): p. 104–11.

42. Gong, E.J., D. Garrel, and D.H. Calloway, *Menstrual cycle and voluntary food intake.* Am J Clin Nutr, 1989. 49(2): p. 252–58.

43. Pillitteri, J.L., et al. *Use of dietary supplements for weight loss in the United States: results of a national survey.* Obesity (Silver Spring), 2008. 16(4): p. 790–96.

44. Rigaud, D., et al. *Effect of psyllium on gastric emptying, hunger feeling and food intake in normal volunteers: a double blind study.* Eur J Clin Nutr, 1998. 52(4): p. 239–45.

45. Thomas, D.E., E.J. Elliott, and L. Baur. *Low glycaemic index or low glycaemic load diets for overweight and obesity.* Cochrane Database Syst Rev, 2007(3): p. CD005105.

46. Jenkins, D.J., et al. *Dietary fibres, fibre analogues, and glucose tolerance: importance of viscosity.* Br Med J, 1978. 1(6124): p. 1392–94.

47. King, D.E., et al. *Effect of psyllium fiber supplementation on C-reactive protein: the trial to reduce inflammatory markers (TRIM).* Ann Fam Med, 2008. 6(2): p. 100–106.

48. King, D.E., et al. *Effect of a high-fiber diet vs a fiber-supplemented diet on C-reactive protein level.* Arch Intern Med, 2007. 167(5): p. 502–6.

49. Maki, K.C., et al. *High-molecular-weight hydroxypropylmethylcellulose taken with or between meals is hypocholesterolemic in adult men.* J Nutr, 2000. 130(7): p. 1705–10.

50. Martin, J., et al. *Chromium picolinate supplementation attenuates body weight gain and increases insulin sensitivity in subjects with type 2 diabetes.* Diabetes Care, 2006. 29(8): p. 1826–32.

51. Lukaski, H.C., W.A. Siders, and J.G. Penland. *Chromium picolinate supplementation in women: effects on body weight, composition, and iron status.* Nutrition, 2007. 23(3): p. 187–95.

52. Pittler, M.H., C. Stevinson, and E. Ernst. *Chromium picolinate for reducing body weight: meta-analysis of randomized trials.* Int J Obes Relat Metab Disord, 2003. 27(4): p. 522–29.

53. Joseph, V.A., and I. Kohlstadt. *Preparing for orthopedic surgery.* In *Scientific Evidence for Musculoskeletal, Bariatric, and Sports Nutrition*, I. Kohlstadt, Editor. 2006, CRC Press, Taylor & Francis Group: Boca Raton, FL. p. 507–20.

54. Contoreggi, C., and I. Kohlstadt. *Neuroendocrine regulation of appetite.* In *Scientific Evidence for Musculoskeletal, Bariatric, and Sports Nutrition*, I. Kohlstadt, Editor. 2006, CRC Press, Taylor & Francis Group: Boca Raton, FL. p. 211–29.

55. le Roux, C.W., et al. *Attenuated peptide YY release in obese subjects is associated with reduced satiety.* Endocrinology, 2006. 147(1): p. 3–8.

20 Acne

The Underlying Influences of Nutrition

Valori Treloar, M.D.

I. INTRODUCTION

In the early 20th century, dermatologists believed that diet could have a profound influence on acne [1]. However, in 1969 and 1971, two studies authored by prominent dermatologists proclaimed the opposite [2, 3] and since that time the major textbooks of dermatology [4, 5] have denied that diet affects acne by citing those two papers. "Acne is caused by diet" is still second on the list of "Acne Myths" posted on the Web site of the American Academy of Dermatology [6]. The pendulum has remained suspended in that position, defying the gravity of scrutiny for nearly 40 years. However, over the past few years, studies have started trickling in that challenge the present acne-diet dogma.

Over the same time period, the science of nutrition has evolved into a much more sophisticated field, unfortunately still rarely accessed by practicing physicians. This chapter reviews the scientific evidence for the acne-diet link and concludes with a dietary treatment program for acne patients.

II. EPIDEMIOLOGY

Observational and epidemiologic studies support a diet-acne connection. Schaeffer, who worked among the Inuit for 30 years, observed that acne, absent in that population, became prevalent as the people acculturated from a fish-based diet to one rich in bread, sweets, pastries, and soft drinks. [7] The low rate of acne among Japanese teens, half that of American teens in 1964 [8], could be attributed to genetics except that a recent study shows that with the displacement of part of the traditional Japanese diet by Western fast foods, the rates are now equal [9]. Acne is nearly unknown in the Kitavan and Ache tribes still living in their hunter-gatherer tradition with a diet rich in wild game, fish, and plants, while those sharing the same ethnic background but living in cities suffer acne at rates seen in the West [10].

In Western cultures, acne appears to be increasing in incidence and occurring in older people and/or persisting longer. Goulden and others noted that the mean age of acne patients referred to their department increased from 20.5 to 26.5 from 1989 to 1999 [11]. A study of male students at the University of Glasgow found an increase in the incidence of acne over the period 1948 to 1968 [12]. The authors state: "We suggest that environmental exposure may underlie this, as changes in the prevalence of germ-line genetic variants are very unlikely to occur in such a short time period."

If our genes have not changed, some change in our environment must account for the striking increase in acne. The uniform worldwide response does not correlate with any known industrial pollutant. On the other hand, diet, one of the most powerful nongenetic influences on physiology, has changed dramatically over the past few decades around the world. This "nutrition transition," characterized by "the introduction of fast-food chains and Westernized dietary habits . . . seems to be a marker of the increasing prevalence of obesity" and its related complications [13]. To understand the influence of dietary change on acne, we must first review the pathophysiology of the disease.

III. OVERVIEW OF ACNE PATHOPHYSIOLOGY[1]

Acne = plugs + oil + bugs + red swelling

The pathophysiology of acne encompasses four problems:

1. Abnormal hyperkeratinization in the hair follicle (plugs);
2. Increased sebum production by the sebaceous glands (oil);
3. Overgrowth of *Propionibacterium acnes (P. acnes)* in the follicle (bugs); and
4. Inflammation (red swelling) [14].

The conventional approach is to find pharmaceutical agents that quell the symptoms. For example, retinoids slow hyperkeratosis and decrease sebum production while the tetracycline antibiotics suppress both *P. acnes* and inflammation (see Figure 20.1).

The more salient question is, Why do hyperkeratinization, excessive sebum, bacterial overgrowth, and inflammation occur in the first place? Understanding the antecedents and triggers of the disease process may give us insight into the mechanisms of the dietary effects on acne.

Abnormal follicular keratinization plugs the follicle by increased proliferation of the basal keratinocytes and decreased apoptosis and separation of the corneocytes. Rather than being shed, the cells remain in place and thicken the lining of the follicle. This crowding of the follicular lumen

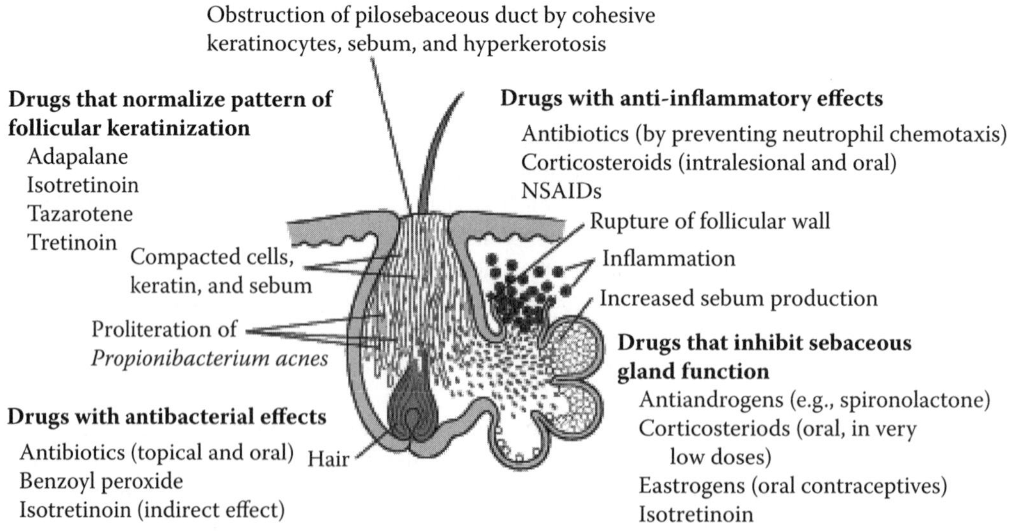

Obstruction of pilosebaceous duct by cohesive keratinocytes, sebum, and hyperkerotosis

Drugs that normalize pattern of follicular keratinization
Adapalane
Isotretinoin
Tazarotene
Tretinoin
    Compacted cells,
    keratin, and sebum

Proliteration of
Propionibacterium acnes

Drugs with antibacterial effects
Antibiotics (topical and oral)   Hair
Benzoyl peroxide
Isotretinoin (indirect effect)

Drugs with anti-inflammatory effects
Antibiotics (by preventing neutrophil chemotaxis)
Corticosteroids (intralesional and oral)
NSAIDs
    Rupture of follicular wall
    Inflammation
    Increased sebum production

Drugs that inhibit sebaceous gland function
Antiandrogens (e.g., spironolactone)
Corticosteriods (oral, in very
    low doses)
Eastrogens (oral contraceptives)
Isotretinoin

FIGURE 20.1 The four elements of acne pathophysiology. Hyperkeratosis, increased sebum production, proliferation of *P. acnes* and inflammation are targets for pharmacologic and nutrient-based treatment. (From www.merck.com, accessed March 31, 2008. With permission.)

---

[1] Refer to F. William Danby's Web site, www.acnemilk.com/acne_animation, for an excellent animation of the process.

may contribute to tearing and rupture of the wall with attendant inflammation. Plugging also seals the lumen contributing to the anaerobic environment ideal for *P. acnes*. The plugging has been attributed to:

- Localized insufficient action of vitamin A [15]
- Localized deficiency of linoleic acid (LA) [16]
- Increased inflammation [17, 18]
- Increased insulin-like growth factor (IGF-1) [19]
- Decreased peroxisome-proliferator activated receptor-gamma (PPAR-γ) [20]
- Disturbance of desmosomes and tonofilaments [21]
- Increased dihydroepiandrostendione sulfate (DHEA-S) [22]

Increased sebaceous gland activity leads to not only an increase in the amount of sebum, but also alters the composition of the secretion. The amount of LA decreases as the quantity of oil increases. As a nutrient source for the bacteria, sebum feeds an increasing population of the organisms. Breakdown of the oils by the bacteria produces inflammatory free fatty acids. The increased sebum that produces the oiliness of the skin so characteristic of acne has been ascribed to:

- Increased testosterone, dihydrotestosterone (DHT) [23]
- Increased insulin [24]
- Increased IGF-1 [25]
- Increased PPAR-α [26]
- Decreased PPAR-γ [26]
- Increased corticotropin releasing hormone (CRH) [27]
- Increased Substance P [21]
- Localized insufficient action of vitamin A [15]

P. acnes, the "bug" thought to contribute to acne, is a normal inhabitant of our skin and its role in acne is not well understood. However, the numbers of this organism increase in acne and tend to decrease as treatment produces clinical improvement. Recent research shows that *P. acnes* activates toll-like receptor 2 (TLR2) in the innate immune system, triggering an inflammatory cascade [28]. Overgrowth of *P. acnes* appears to be triggered by:

- Decreased LA
- Increased sebum (nutrient supply)
- Abnormally desquamated follicular keratinocytes (increasing anaerobic conditions) [29]

Inflammation accounts for the characteristic redness, swelling, and pustule and nodule formation in acne. The following factors may account for the inflammation (red swelling) seen in acne:

- TLR-2 activation by *P. acnes* [28]
- Omega-6 fatty acids and eicosanoids [30]
- Oxidative stress [31, 32]
- Insulin [33]
- Adiposity [34]
- Testosterone [35]
- PPAR-γ [36]

Note that these lists tend to overlap, that is, the same proximate causes contribute to more than one of the four pathophysiologic factors of acne. Not only do the same elements repeat among our lists, the causes and factors perform an intricate interactive dance. Inflammation increases the hyperproliferation of keratinocytes; the excess cellular debris makes a more anaerobic environment optimal for *P. acnes*; *P. acnes* binds TLR-2 triggering further inflammation. We like to think of pathophysiology as a list of linear processes, but we are instead faced with a messy soup of inter-twining, tangled, chaotic actions. Four recurring themes that deserve particular attention include disturbances of:

- Fatty acids and fatty acid signaling via PPARs
- Testosterone and its analogs
- Insulin and IGF-1
- Adrenal stress and oxidative stress

IV. PATHOPHYSIOLOGY TRIGGERS AND DIET

Fatty Acids and Fatty Acid Signaling via PPARs

Fatty acids serve as precursors for inflammatory mediators, the prostaglandins (PG) and leukot-rienes (LT). Classically, the omega-6 fatty acid arachidonic acid (AA) is the most prevalent fatty acid in cellular membranes and is most likely to be plucked out by phospholipase A and shunted down the mediator cascade. The end products include the highly inflammatory PGE2 and LTB4, both of which have been shown to participate in acne [32, 37]. Our membranes also contain the omega-3 fatty acids that travel through the same path and produce mediators in the odd-numbered series that have far less inflammatory action [38]. (See Figure 20.2.) If we produce more of the even-numbered mediators relative to the odd-numbered ones, our internal milieu will be more inflamed.

Long chain unsaturated fatty acids also act on our genes by binding the PPARs, members of the family of nuclear receptors that act on the genes for inflammatory cytokines. PPARs inhibit the nuclear transcription factor, NFκB, thereby down-regulating the production of inflammatory cytokines IL-1, IL-6, TNF-alpha [39]. Again some fatty acids ramp the process up, while others keep things calmer. The PPAR ligands have also been shown to affect lipogenesis by sebocytes in culture [40].

Dietary fatty acids play a few more astonishingly relevant roles. Omega-3 fatty acids actually block TLR-2, the innate immunity trigger specifically activated by *P. acnes* [41]. (Zinc may also act at this site [42].) Omega-3 fatty acids also appear to attenuate the proinflammatory response to psy-chogenic stress [43]. Gamma linolenic acid (GLA) inhibits 5-alpha reductase (5AR), the enzyme that converts testosterone to its more acneigenic form [44]. *Trans* fats exacerbate essential fatty acid defi-ciency symptoms, increasing hyperkeratosis in a rat model [45] and contributing to inflammation.

The role played by LA is complex and incompletely understood. LA suppresses *P. acnes* growth. *P. acnes* protects itself by biohydrogenating LA rendering it incapable of its suppressive action [46]. LA also controls keratinocyte proliferation and in its absence, hyperkeratosis occurs. The propor-tion of LA decreases as sebum production increases. The follicular plugging of acne has been attributed to "localized LA deficiency" [47]. On the other hand, LA increases sebum production in cell culture [48].

Fatty acids and fatty acid signaling via PPARs play important roles in all four of the compo-nents of acne pathogenesis: hyperkeratinization, sebum overproduction, *P. acnes* overgrowth, and inflammation.

Does Diet Affect the Fatty Acids in the Skin and Follicle?

The lipid bilayer cell membranes can be envisioned as sacks made from fatty acid fabric composed of the fats in the diet. Arachidonic acid, dominant in the American diet, is the dominant fatty acid in the bodies of most Americans. LA from vegetable oils converts readily to AA. Enriching the diet with foods containing omega-3 fatty acids will incorporate more eicosapentaenoic acid (EPA) and docosahexaenoic acid (DHA) in cell membranes while decreasing AA [49]. A diet rich in hydrogenated vegetable oils will weave a stiff fabric containing straight *trans* fatty acids.

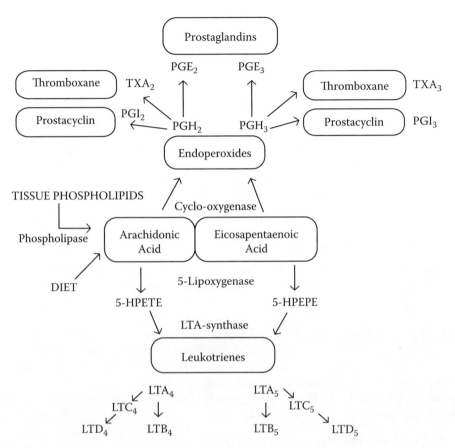

FIGURE 20.2 Arachidonic acid and eicosapentaenoic acid follow parallel pathways in the production of inflammatory mediators, but mediators derived from AA have far greater inflammatory activity. (From [53]. With permission.)

In contrast to carbohydrates and proteins, which humans digest into their saccharide and amino acid components, when it comes to fats, "you are what you eat."

Since cell membranes serve as the reservoir for the building blocks of inflammatory mediators, a stockpile of AA will produce a wealth of inflammatory odd-numbered eicosanoids. Omega-3 fatty acids compete for the same enzyme pathways and produce eicosanoids with lower activity. The PPAR and TLR-2 actions of fatty acids may also help explain why higher serum levels of omega-3 fatty acids correlate with lower serum levels of proinflammatory markers and higher levels of anti-inflammatory markers [38, 50]. Eating fish and seaweed and taking omega-3 supplements will create a less inflammatory internal milieu.

Man-made hydrogenated vegetable oils brought *trans* fatty acids into our food supply in the early 20th century and have achieved a dominant position over the past few decades. Intake of hydrogenated vegetable oil, the major source of dietary *trans* fats, has increased from 10 g/day in 1960 to 30 g/day in 1993 [51]. In women, *trans* fatty acid intake correlates directly with serum levels of inflammatory markers [52]. The same eicosanoid and PPAR mechanisms previously discussed probably explain why eating less hydrogenated vegetable oil will help decrease inflammation.

Concurrent with increased intake of *trans* fat, the dietary ratio of omega-6 to omega-3 fatty acids changed. When human metabolism evolved, diets were rich in hunted wild animal and bird meat, fish, and gathered root vegetables, greens, fruits, nuts, seeds, and eggs. The whole vegetable, nut, or seed accompanied by fiber and antioxidant vitamins and plant polyphenols served as the dietary source of omega-6 fats. The ratio of omega-6 to omega-3 was about 1:1.

Today much of the fat in the American diet comes from sophisticated, powerful presses squeezing omega-6-rich oils from plant seeds: canola, safflower, sunflower, peanut, soy, and cottonseed. LA, one of the dominant plant seed fatty acids, is an omega-6 fatty acid that is readily converted to AA in our bodies. The heat from the pressing produces oxidized moieties, many not found in nature. Further processing includes degumming, refining, bleaching, deodorizing, additives, and winterization in order to produce the clear oil with a prolonged shelf life that we find in the grocery stores. It is devoid of the polyphenolic compounds that provide color, flavor, and antioxidant protection. The modern omega-6 to omega-3 ratio is about 16:1 [53]. Given that we experience about a 1% change in our genome every 10,000 years or so, we have not had time to adapt to this dietary change. Given the acneigenic effects of an increased omega-6 to omega-3 ratio and increased dietary *trans* fats, knowledgeable observers might have predicted the "acne epidemic" [54] that has accompanied this change in the Western diet over the past several decades.

TESTOSTERONE AND ITS ANALOGS

Androgens are the long-recognized "bad boys" of acne. Acne begins as testosterone levels rise (notably, eunuchs do not develop acne) [55]. DHEAS, an adrenal precursor to testosterone, is elevated in many women with acne [56]. The sebaceous glands contain all the enzymatic machinery required to generate and interconvert the "male hormones." Testosterone is converted to the more active DHT via 5-alpha-reductase (5AR) and activity of this enzyme plays an important role in acne [57]. Androgens stimulate proliferation and differentiation of the sebocytes as well as up-regulating lipid production [58]. Androgens also appear to increase inflammation in wound healing, which suggests that they may contribute to the inflammation of acne [35].

The androgens impact two of the four components of acne pathophysiology: sebum overproduction and inflammation.

Does Diet Influence Androgen Levels or Activity?

In the sebaceous gland, the enzyme 5AR ramps up testosterone's action by converting it to the more active dihydrotestosterone (DHT) and some pharmaceutical agents (e.g., spironolactone) are aimed at this target. Dietary input also affects the activity of 5AR. Decreased activation can be seen with green tea catechins in a rat model [59], with zinc and vitamin B6 in an in vitro human skin model [60], and as noted above by GLA in cell culture. While none of these interventions were tested via human ingestion, the biochemistry is convincing and the risk of prudent supplementation is negligible.

Testosterone travels in the blood in both an active, free form and in an inactive form, bound to sex hormone binding globulin (SHBG). Higher levels of SHBG decrease the pool of active hormone, resulting in less testosterone activity. Hepatic production of SHBG is influenced by diet. Both human and animal studies show a rise in SHBG with a low-protein diet [61]. A high-fiber diet is associated with higher levels of SHBG. A diet with decreased fat and refined carbohydrates, an increased ratio of omega-3 to omega-6 plus saturated fatty acids, and an increase in foods rich in "phytoestrogens" and fiber raised SHBG, lowered serum testosterone and insulin levels, and reduced waist circumference [62]. While many sources attribute this effect to insulin, it appears that dietary monosaccharides, especially fructose, may also have a large impact on slowing SHBG production [63].

INSULIN/IGF-1

A little-recognized, but well-documented phenomenon of adolescence is the rise and fall of insulin resistance that mirrors acne activity. Insulin resistance peaks at about Tanner stage 3 and returns to normal at the end of the teen years [64]. Insulin is one of our major anabolic hormones and tends to rise with elevation of growth hormone (GH); an increase in insulin levels during a period of rapid growth and development should come as no surprise. Insulin, GH, and IGF-1 interweave in their physiologic activity. Insulin and IGF-1 can bind each other's receptors and may stimulate similar processes, albeit in different concentrations [24].

IGF-1 levels reflect GH levels and are used as the surrogate marker for the elusive GH. Elevation during adolescence is normal and expected. Less expected is the elevation of IGF-1 in adult women with acne that was noted by Cappel and colleagues [56]. While men's IGF-1 levels do not correlate with acne severity, they do match DHEAS and androstendione levels. The authors suggest that the effects of androgens were "dependent on the influence of IGF-1." Patients with longstanding acne have increases in IGF-1 and decreased levels of the protein that binds IGF-1 and takes it out of the action, IGF binding protein-3 (IGFBP-3) [65].

What Roles Do These Factors Play in Acne?

Insulin appears to decrease hepatic production of SHBG, which leads to higher circulating levels of unbound, active androgen, triggering all the androgen effects listed above. Although the correlation has not been shown in acne, insulin can increase systemic inflammatory markers [33]. Insulin and IGF-1 directly increase sebum production; insulin largely through differentiation, and IGF-1 through proliferation of the sebocytes [24]. Free IGF-1 directly stimulates basal keratinocyte proliferation, thereby contributing to the follicular hyperkeratosis, whereas IGFBP-3 inhibits it [19, 66]. Also, IGFBP-3 and tretinoin, a mainstay of acne therapy, bind the same retinoid X nuclear receptor (RXR alpha) [67].

Insulin/IGF-1 affect three of the four pathophysiologic steps in acne: hyperkeratinization, inflammation, and sebum overproduction.

Does Diet Have an Effect on Insulin and IGF-1?

Insulin levels are driven by diet. Sugars digested and absorbed into the bloodstream must be directed into cells to be used as energy or stored. The health ravages of diabetes show why our bodies strive to keep blood glucose levels within a tight range and this is insulin's primary job. Insulin levels chase blood sugar levels, rising fast and high in response to rapidly absorbed refined carbohydrate and more slowly and lower when foods contain more fiber, fat, and protein, all of which slow the absorption of sugar into the blood.

The glycemic index (GI) is an attempt to measure how fast and high blood sugar is pushed by different foods. The glycemic load (GL) takes the usual size of a portion into consideration. The insulinemic response tends to track the glycemic response, so low GI foods eaten at regular intervals will help keep insulin levels even throughout the day. A typical American diet tends to result in spiking insulin levels and the area under the curve tends to be high [68].

In a recent Australian study, young men with acne were randomized to either a low GI diet or a standard Western diet. Statistically significant clinical improvement in acne paralleled improved insulin sensitivity, body mass index (BMI), decreased free androgen index, and increased IGFBP-1 [69, 70].

Dairy products are a special case; the insulinemic response is higher than predicted from the GI [71]. This may be part of the explanation for the association between dairy intake and acne found in a series of studies from the Harvard School of Public Health [72–74].

Diet affects IGF-1 and IGFBP-3. Insulin raises IGF-1 levels. IGFBP-3, on the other hand, falls after ingestion of high GI foods and rises after eating low GI foods [75]. Lower levels of IGF-1 and higher levels of IGFBP-3 are associated with greater intake of omega-3 fatty acids, tomatoes, vegetables, and dietary fiber. In contrast, higher levels of IGF-1 are associated with dietary saturated fat, vegetable oils, milk, and dairy products [76, 77].

ADRENAL STRESS AND OXIDATIVE STRESS

Using McEwen's concept of allostatic load, stress becomes problematic when the forces impinging on an individual overwhelm the capacity to compensate for the disturbance or when the compensatory mechanisms begin to cause problems themselves [78]. For example, in the former case, UV light causes oxidative damage to cell membranes in the dermis. Vitamin E can reduce the oxidized fatty acid in the membrane, but unless the vitamin E is replaced or reduced back to its normal state by vitamin C, the capacity to contain the oxidative damage becomes overwhelmed and injury ensues. An example of the latter is cortisol levels that rise in response to sleep deprivation. In the short term, this keeps the metabolism running fairly smoothly, but over time, excessive cortisol causes central obesity, periphery muscle wasting, and hyperglycemia (see Chapter 30, "Sleep Disturbance").

Several lines of evidence suggest that adrenal stress plays a role in acne. Examination stress appears to increase acne severity [79, 80]. Stress has been shown to elicit the release of the neuropeptide Substance P, which appears to increase lipogenesis in sebocytes and also inflammation via mast cells [81]. CRH generated in the sebaceous gland increases sebocyte lipogenesis. This is thought to be a localized stress response analogous to that of the central hypothalamic-pituitary-adrenal axis [27]. CRH released centrally may have a similar effect.

More than 20 years ago, Swedish researchers noted that in men with severe acne, red blood cells carried far less of one of our most powerful antioxidants, glutathione [82]. Recently, measurement of markers of oxidative injury and activity of antioxidant enzymes showed significant oxidative damage in acne patients compared to controls [31, 83]. Reactive oxygen species (ROS) generated by neutrophils contribute to follicular wall injury and inflammation. ROS can serve as regulators of NFκB, a transcription factor that up-regulates expression of genes for inflammatory cytokines including TNF-alpha, IL-1, IL-8, and IL-6. AP-1 is another redox-sensitive transcription factor that generates inflammatory cytokines [84]. Among the genes reported to be up-regulated in acne, the most strongly induced included IL-1, IL-8, and MMP1—all known to be generated through ROS-activated pathways. IL-1 may actually "trigger the keratinocyte activation cycle" perhaps serving as one of the very first steps in the formation of an acne lesion [54]. Matrix metalloproteinases (MMPs) degrade IGFBP-3, interfering with its protective effect against hyperkeratinization and its action at the retinoid X receptor [85].

Stress impacts three of four components of acne pathophysiology: hyperkeratinization, sebum overproduction, and inflammation.

Does Diet Affect Oxidative or Adrenal Stress?

Psychological stress induces the production of proinflammatory cytokines, IFN-gamma, TNF-alpha, and IL-6. University students with lower serum omega-3 levels or with a higher omega-6/omega-3 ratio had significantly greater examination-induced TNF-alpha and IFN-gamma responses [43]. Given that the gene for TNF-alpha is one of those found to be activated in acne, we are not surprised to find that examination stress increases acne. On the other hand, the fact that dietary intake of different fatty acids can alter the immunologic response to stress is an unexpected and welcome surprise.

Oxidative stress is a condition of life in our earthly atmosphere. To contend with the ROS generated by our normal metabolism we provide our bodies with antioxidants by eating them. The richest dietary sources of antioxidants are vegetables and fruits. Not only do they contain high levels of antioxidant vitamins, but all the polyphenolic compounds that give produce its colors, fragrances, and tastes appear to have even more powerful antioxidant activity than vitamins do [86].

While some foods offer antioxidant benefit, other foods are prooxidants, compounding the problem. Dietary *trans* fats increase markers of oxidative damage [87]. High fructose intake enhances ROS generation and the protein and lipid damage it causes [88]. In fact, a high fructose diet is used in experimental models to create insulin resistance in rats. Zinc alone and in combination with selenium and vitamin E decreased both the degree of insulin resistance and the oxidative damage sustained [89]. To round out the discussion, oxidative stress appears to be instrumental in triggering insulin resistance, the biochemical finding in teens that most closely parallels acne [90]. Following the syllogism, high fructose intake (e.g., sports drinks sweetened with high fructose corn syrup) increases ROS generation and exacerbates the normal insulin resistance of adolescence, perhaps contributing to acne.

Based on their findings of increased oxidation markers and decreased antioxidant enzyme activity in acne patients, the researchers stated: "Drugs with antioxidative effects might be valuable in treatment" [91]. More prudent perhaps would be the suggestion to increase intake of foods rich in antioxidants and decrease intake of prooxidant foods.

V. CONCLUSION

Diet can influence the antecedents and triggers of acne—the proximate causes behind the four pathophysiologic elements of acne. Why did two widely accepted clinical trials conclude otherwise? We return to these two landmark studies that turned the tide away from the acne-diet connection. Through the lens of modern nutritional science, the two studies that form the foundation of the current diet-acne dogma demonstrate significant weaknesses, the most glaring being that neither took the underlying diet into consideration. Anderson's open study included only 27 subjects and no controls; it would not be accepted for publication under today's more stringent peer review [3]. Fulton and colleagues [2] concluded that chocolate had no influence on acne by comparing a chocolate bar to a pseudochocolate bar composed of 28% hydrogenated vegetable oil, a food known to increase inflammatory markers, and 14% nonfat milk solids, the acneigenic potential of which is demonstrated by three studies from the Harvard School of Public Health. The sugar content of the bars was 44.3% and 53% respectively, both likely to induce a rapid and high insulin response. The evidence for a dietary effect on acne is a young and growing body of knowledge, but it is far more robust than the evidence against such an effect.

In spite of the dearth of the controlled, blinded, human trials that clinicians rely on most heavily, the risk-benefit ratio of dietary strategies for acne remains far more favorable than any pharmaceutical agent. The implementation of a dietary treatment for acne does not preclude conventional treatment and is likely to complement it. Even when advised that these suggestions are based on biochemistry and physiology, cell culture, and animal studies, but very few human clinical trials, many of our patients will jump at the opportunity to try this approach. Especially for patients whose response to conventional dermatology has been disappointing, we can open a whole new tool box. Proactive patients who opt for healthy lifestyle choices seek doctors with this knowledge and expertise.

VI. CLINICAL RECOMMENDATIONS

DIET

- Try a dairy-free diet for 3 to 6 months. No milk, cream, yogurt, ice cream, cheese of any kind, including cream and cottage. Decrease your use of butter or switch to ghee (clarified butter).
- Eat three nutrient-dense meals and two "mini-meal" snacks daily.
- Eat 5 to 8 servings of vegetables and 2 servings of fruit per day.
- Eat 2.5 to 3 palm-sized servings of protein-rich foods (meat, poultry, eggs, fish) daily; include fish twice weekly.
- Minimize refined carbohydrates, such as candy, sweets, baked goods, crackers, white bread, white rice, white potatoes, pasta, unless you are performing very high intensity exercise more than an hour a day on a regular basis.
- Eat vegetable carbohydrates, such as squash, sweet potatoes, beans, and, if you tolerate them, legumes and grains.
- Eliminate hydrogenated vegetable oil; decrease liquid oil rich in omega-6 fatty acids (safflower, sunflower, peanut, soy, cottonseed).
- Eliminate high fructose corn syrup.
- Do not drink liquid calories, such as soda, sports drinks, undiluted juice, chocolate.

- Drink filtered water, green tea, diluted juice, herbal teas, juiced vegetables.
- Limit alcohol intake. If you are under legal drinking age, do not drink.

SUPPLEMENTS

Consider nutritional supplements on a patient-by-patient basis. These are administered under medical supervision and may be contraindicated in some patients.

- High-quality fish oil capsules, with a maximum of 4g/day
- Zinc gluconate (or other readily absorbed form), 15 to 20 mg daily
- Vitamin E with natural mixed tocopherols, 100 to 200 IU daily
- Black currant seed oil, 500 mg (90 mg GLA), one capsule daily
- Pyridoxal-5-phosphate (B6), 25 to 50 mg daily
- Vitamin C, 500 mg daily
- Selenium, 100 micrograms daily
- Vitamin, A 5000 IU daily

LIFESTYLE

Complement nutritional intervention with a lifestyle that helps reduce adrenal stress.

- Aim to sleep 7 to 8 uninterrupted hours nightly.
- Practice an exercise that induces the relaxation response every day, such as meditation, yoga, tai chi, self-hypnosis, or progressive muscle relaxation.
- Participate in strength, aerobic, and flexibility exercise at least three times weekly. Aim to do at least one of the three every day.

For greater detail in clinical recommendations and specific guidelines written in a style targeting patients, refer to *The Clear Skin Diet* [92].

REFERENCES

1. Stokes, J.H. *Fundamentals of Medical Dermatology*. Seventh Revision ed. 1942, Philadelphia: University of Pennsylvania Department of Dermatology Book Fund.
2. Fulton, J.E., Jr., G. Plewig, and A.M. Kligman. *Effect of chocolate on acne vulgaris.* JAMA, 1969. 210(11): p. 2071–74.
3. Anderson, P.C. *Foods as the cause of acne.* Am Fam Physician, 1971. 3(3): p. 102–3.
4. Freedberg, I. *Fitzpatrick's Dermatology in General Medicine*. 6th ed. 2003: McGraw-Hill.
5. Burns, T., S. Breathnach, N. Cox, and C. Griffiths. *Rook's Textbook of Dermatology,* 7th edition. 2004: John Wiley and Sons, Inc.
6. *Acne Myths* [Web site]. Available from: http://www.skincarephysicians.com/acnenet/myths.html.
7. Schaefer, O. *When the Eskimo comes to town.* Nutr Today, 1971. 6: p. 8–16.
8. Hamilton, J.B., H. Terada, and S.E. Mestler. *Greater tending to acne in white Americans than in Japanese populations.* J Clin Endocrinol Metab, 1964. 24: p. 267–72.
9. Hayashi, N., M. Kawashima, S. Watanabe, and T. Nakata. *An epidemiological study of Acne vulgaris in Japan by questionnaire.* Jpn J Dermatol, 2001. 111: p. 1347–55.
10. Cordain, L., et al. *Acne vulgaris: a disease of Western civilization.* Arch Dermatol, 2002. 138(12): p. 1584–90.
11. Goulden, V., G.I. Stables, and W.J. Cunliffe. *Prevalence of facial acne in adults.* J Am Acad Dermatol, 1999. 41(4): p. 577–80.

12. Galobardes, B., et al. *Has acne increased? Prevalence of acne history among university students between 1948 and 1968. The Glasgow Alumni Cohort Study.* Br J Dermatol, 2005. 152(4): p. 824–25.

13. Astrup, A., et al. *Nutrition transition and its relationship to the development of obesity and related chronic diseases.* Obes Rev, 2008. 9 Suppl 1: p. 48–52.

14. Webster, G. *Mechanism-based treatment of acne vulgaris: the value of combination therapy.* J Drugs Dermatol, 2005. 4(3): p. 281–88.

15. Orfanos, C.E., et al. *Current use and future potential role of retinoids in dermatology.* Drugs, 1997. 53(3): p. 358–88.

16. Cunliffe, W.J., et al. *Comedogenesis: some aetiological, clinical and therapeutic strategies.* Dermatology, 2003. 206(1): p. 11–16.

17. Plewig, G. *Follicular keratinization.* J Invest Dermatol, 1974. 62(3): p. 308–20.

18. Jeremy, A.H., et al. *Inflammatory events are involved in acne lesion initiation.* J Invest Dermatol, 2003. 121(1): p. 20–27.

19. Bol, D.K., et al. *Overexpression of insulin-like growth factor-1 induces hyperplasia, dermal abnormalities, and spontaneous tumor formation in transgenic mice.* Oncogene, 1997. 14(14): p. 1725–34.

20. Demerjian, M., et al. *Topical treatment with thiazolidinediones, activators of peroxisome proliferator-activated receptor-gamma, normalizes epidermal homeostasis in a murine hyperproliferative disease model.* Exp Dermatol, 2006. 15(3): p. 154–60.

21. Toyoda, M., and M. Morohashi. *Pathogenesis of acne.* Med Electron Microsc, 2001. 34(1): p. 29–40.

22. Harper, J.C., and D.M. Thiboutot. *Pathogenesis of acne: recent research advances.* Adv Dermatol, 2003. 19: p. 1–10.

23. Deplewski, D., and R.L. Rosenfield. *Role of hormones in pilosebaceous unit development.* Endocr Rev, 2000. 21(4): p. 363–92.

24. Deplewski, D., and R.L. Rosenfield. *Growth hormone and insulin-like growth factors have different effects on sebaceous cell growth and differentiation.* Endocrinology, 1999. 140(9): p. 4089–94.

25. Smith, T.M., et al. *Insulin-like growth factor-1 induces lipid production in human SEB-1 sebocytes via sterol response element-binding protein-1.* J Invest Dermatol, 2006. 126(6): p. 1226–32.

26. Trivedi, N.R., et al. *Peroxisome proliferator-activated receptors increase human sebum production.* J Invest Dermatol, 2006. 126(9): p. 2002–9.

27. Zouboulis, C.C., et al. *Corticotropin-releasing hormone: an autocrine hormone that promotes lipogenesis in human sebocytes.* Proc Natl Acad Sci U S A, 2002. 99(10): p. 7148–53.

28. Jugeau, S., et al. *Induction of toll-like receptors by Propionibacterium acnes.* Br J Dermatol, 2005. 153(6): p. 1105–13.

29. Leyden, J.J., K.J. McGinley, and B. Vowels. *Propionibacterium acnes colonization in acne and nonacne.* Dermatology, 1998. 196(1): p. 55–58.

30. Alestas, T., et al. *Enzymes involved in the biosynthesis of leukotriene B4 and prostaglandin E2 are active in sebaceous glands.* J Mol Med, 2006. 84(1): p. 75–87.

31. Arican, O., E.B. Kurutas, and S. Sasmaz. *Oxidative stress in patients with acne vulgaris.* Mediators Inflamm, 2005. 2005(6): p. 380–84.

32. Ottaviani, M., et al. *Peroxidated squalene induces the production of inflammatory mediators in HaCaT keratinocytes: a possible role in acne vulgaris.* J Invest Dermatol, 2006. 126(11): p. 2430–37.

33. Fishel, M.A., et al. *Hyperinsulinemia provokes synchronous increases in central inflammation and beta-amyloid in normal adults.* Arch Neurol, 2005. 62(10): p. 1539–44.

34. Pou, K.M., et al. *Visceral and subcutaneous adipose tissue volumes are cross-sectionally related to markers of inflammation and oxidative stress: the Framingham Heart Study.* Circulation, 2007. 116(11): p. 1234–41.

35. Gilliver, S.C., et al. *Androgens modulate the inflammatory response during acute wound healing.* J Cell Sci, 2006. 119(Pt 4): p. 722–32.

36. Zhang, Q., et al. *Involvement of PPAR gamma in oxidative stress-mediated prostaglandin E(2) production in SZ95 human sebaceous gland cells.* J Invest Dermatol, 2006. 126(1): p. 42–48.

37. Tehrani, R., and M. Dharmalingam, *Management of premenstrual acne with Cox-2 inhibitors: a placebo controlled study.* Indian J Dermatol Venereol Leprol, 2004. 70(6): p. 345–48.

38. Bagga, D., et al. *Differential effects of prostaglandin derived from omega-6 and omega-3 polyunsaturated fatty acids on COX-2 expression and IL-6 secretion.* Proc Natl Acad Sci U S A, 2003. 100(4): p. 1751–56.

39. Jump, D.B. *The biochemistry of n-3 polyunsaturated fatty acids.* J Biol Chem, 2002. 277(11): p. 8755–58.

40. Downie, M.M., et al. *Peroxisome proliferator-activated receptor and farnesoid X receptor ligands differentially regulate sebaceous differentiation in human sebaceous gland organ cultures in vitro.* Br J Dermatol, 2004. 151(4): p. 766–75.

41. Lee, J.Y., et al. *Differential modulation of Toll-like receptors by fatty acids: preferential inhibition by n-3 polyunsaturated fatty acids.* J Lipid Res, 2003. 44(3): p. 479–86.

42. Jarrousse, V., et al. *Zinc salts inhibit in vitro Toll-like receptor 2 surface expression by keratinocytes.* Eur J Dermatol, 2007. 17(6): p. 492–96.

43. Maes, M., et al. *In humans, serum polyunsaturated fatty acid levels predict the response of proinflammatory cytokines to psychologic stress.* Biol Psychiatry, 2000. 47(10): p. 910–20.

44. Liang, T., and S. Liao. *Inhibition of steroid 5 alpha-reductase by specific aliphatic unsaturated fatty acids.* Biochem J, 1992. 285 (Pt 2): p. 557–62.

45. Hill, E.G., S.B. Johnson, and R.T. Holman. *Intensification of essential fatty acid deficiency in the rat by dietary trans fatty acids.* J Nutr, 1979. 109(10): p. 1759–65.

46. Verhulst, A., G. Janessen, G. Parmentier, and H. Eyssen. *Isomerization of polyunsaturated long chain fatty acids by propionobacteria.* System Appl Microbiol, 1987. 9: p. 12–15.

47. Downing, D.T., et al. *Essential fatty acids and acne.* J Am Acad Dermatol, 1986. 14(2 Pt 1): p. 221–25.

48. Makrantonaki, E., and C.C. Zouboulis. *Testosterone metabolism to 5alpha-dihydrotestosterone and synthesis of sebaceous lipids is regulated by the peroxisome proliferator-activated receptor ligand linoleic acid in human sebocytes.* Br J Dermatol, 2007. 156(3): p. 428–32.

49. Calder, P.C. *Dietary modification of inflammation with lipids.* Proc Nutr Soc, 2002. 61(3): p. 345–58.

50. Ferrucci, L., et al. *Relationship of plasma polyunsaturated fatty acids to circulating inflammatory markers.* J Clin Endocrinol Metab, 2006. 91(2): p. 439–46.

51. Enig, M. *Trans Fatty Acids in the Food Supply: A Comprehensive Report Covering 60 Years of Research.* 2nd ed. 1995, Silver Spring, MD: Enig Associates, Inc.

52. Mozaffarian, D., et al. *Dietary intake of trans fatty acids and systemic inflammation in women.* Am J Clin Nutr, 2004. 79(4): p. 606–12.

53. Simopoulos, A.P. *Essential fatty acids in health and chronic disease.* Am J Clin Nutr, 1999. 70(3 Suppl): p. 560S–569S.

54. Silverberg, N.B., and J.M. Weinberg. *Rosacea and adult acne: a worldwide epidemic.* Cutis, 2001. 68(2): p. 85.

55. Thiboutot, D. *Regulation of human sebaceous glands.* J Invest Dermatol, 2004. 123(1): p. 1–12.

56. Cappel, M., D. Mauger, and D. Thiboutot. *Correlation between serum levels of insulin-like growth factor 1, dehydroepiandrosterone sulfate, and dihydrotestosterone and acne lesion counts in adult women.* Arch Dermatol, 2005. 141(3): p. 333–38.

57. Darley, C.R. *Recent advances in hormonal aspects of acne vulgaris.* Int J Dermatol, 1984. 23(8): p. 539–41.

58. Rosignoli, C., et al. *Involvement of the SREBP pathway in the mode of action of androgens in sebaceous glands in vivo.* Exp Dermatol, 2003. 12(4): p. 480–89.

59. Liao, S., and R.A. Hiipakka. *Selective inhibition of steroid 5 alpha-reductase isozymes by tea epicatechin-3-gallate and epigallocatechin-3-gallate.* Biochem Biophys Res Commun, 1995. 214(3): p. 833–38.

60. Stamatiadis, D., M.C. Bulteau-Portois, and I. Mowszowicz. *Inhibition of 5 alpha-reductase activity in human skin by zinc and azelaic acid.* Br J Dermatol, 1988. 119(5): p. 627–32.

61. Longcope, C., et al. *Diet and sex hormone-binding globulin.* J Clin Endocrinol Metab, 2000. 85(1): p. 293–96.

62. Kaaks, R., et al. *Effects of dietary intervention on IGF-I and IGF-binding proteins, and related alterations in sex steroid metabolism: the Diet and Androgens (DIANA) Randomised Trial.* Eur J Clin Nutr, 2003. 57(9): p. 1079–88.

63. Selva, D.M., et al. *Monosaccharide-induced lipogenesis regulates the human hepatic sex hormone-binding globulin gene.* J Clin Invest, 2007. 117(12): p. 3979–87.

64. Moran, A., et al. *Insulin resistance during puberty: results from clamp studies in 357 children.* Diabetes, 1999. 48(10): p. 2039–44.

65. Kaymak, Y., et al. *Dietary glycemic index and glucose, insulin, insulin-like growth factor-I, insulin-like growth factor binding protein 3, and leptin levels in patients with acne.* J Am Acad Dermatol, 2007. 57(5): p. 819–23.

66. Edmondson, S.R., et al. *Epidermal homeostasis: the role of the growth hormone and insulin-like growth factor systems.* Endocr Rev, 2003. 24(6): p. 737–64.

67. Cordain, L. *Implications for the role of diet in acne.* Semin Cutan Med Surg, 2005. 24(2): p. 84–91.
68. Brand-Miller, J.C., et al. *Physiological validation of the concept of glycemic load in lean young adults.* J Nutr, 2003. 133(9): p. 2728–32.
69. Smith, R.N., et al. *The effect of a high-protein, low glycemic-load diet versus a conventional, high glycemic-load diet on biochemical parameters associated with acne vulgaris: a randomized, investigator-masked, controlled trial.* J Am Acad Dermatol, 2007. 57(2): p. 247–56.
70. Smith, R.N., et al. *A low-glycemic-load diet improves symptoms in acne vulgaris patients: a randomized controlled trial.* Am J Clin Nutr, 2007. 86(1): p. 107–15.
71. Hoyt, G., M.S. Hickey, and L. Cordain. *Dissociation of the glycaemic and insulinaemic responses to whole and skimmed milk.* Br J Nutr, 2005. 93(2): p. 175–77.
72. Adebamowo, C.A., et al. *Milk consumption and acne in teenaged boys.* J Am Acad Dermatol, 2008. 58(5): p. 787–793.
73. Adebamowo, C.A., et al. *Milk consumption and acne in adolescent girls.* Dermatol Online J, 2006. 12(4): p. 1.
74. Adebamowo, C.A., et al. *High school dietary dairy intake and teenage acne.* J Am Acad Dermatol, 2005. 52(2): p. 207–14.
75. Brand-Miller, J.C., et al. *The glycemic index of foods influences postprandial insulin-like growth factor-binding protein responses in lean young subjects.* Am J Clin Nutr, 2005. 82(2): p. 350–54.
76. Gunnell, D., et al. *Are diet-prostate cancer associations mediated by the IGF axis? A cross-sectional analysis of diet, IGF-I and IGFBP-3 in healthy middle-aged men.* Br J Cancer, 2003. 88(11): p. 1682–86.
77. Probst-Hensch, N.M., et al. *Determinants of circulating insulin-like growth factor I and insulin-like growth factor binding protein 3 concentrations in a cohort of Singapore men and women.* Cancer Epidemiol Biomarkers Prev, 2003. 12(8): p. 739–46.
78. McEwen, B. *Protective and damaging effects of stress mediators.* New England J Med, 1998. 338: p. 171–79.
79. Chiu, A., S.Y. Chon, and A.B. Kimball. *The response of skin disease to stress: changes in the severity of acne vulgaris as affected by examination stress.* Arch Dermatol, 2003. 139(7): p. 897–900.
80. Yosipovitch, G., et al. *Study of psychological stress, sebum production and acne vulgaris in adolescents.* Acta Derm Venereol, 2007. 87: p. 135–39.
81. Toyoda, M., and M. Morohashi. *New aspects in acne inflammation.* Dermatology, 2003. 206(1): p. 17–23.
82. Michaelsson, G., and L.E. Edqvist. *Erythrocyte glutathione peroxidase activity in acne vulgaris and the effect of selenium and vitamin E treatment.* Acta Derm Venereol, 1984. 64(1): p. 9–14.
83. Kurutas, E.B., O. Arican, and S. Sasmaz. *Superoxide dismutase and myeloperoxidase activities in polymorphonuclear leukocytes in acne vulgaris.* Acta Dermatovenerol Alp Panonica Adriat, 2005. 14(2): p. 39–42.
84. Briganti, S., and M. Picardo. *Antioxidant activity, lipid peroxidation and skin diseases. What's new.* JEADV, 2003. 17: p. 663–69.
85. Fowlkes, J.L., et al. *Matrix metalloproteinases degrade insulin-like growth factor-binding protein-3 in dermal fibroblast cultures.* J Biol Chem, 1994. 269(41): p. 25742–46.
86. Arts, I.C., and P.C. Hollman. *Polyphenols and disease risk in epidemiologic studies.* Am J Clin Nutr, 2005. 81(1 Suppl): p. 317S–325S.
87. Tomey, K.M., et al. *Dietary fat subgroups, zinc, and vegetable components are related to urine F2a-isoprostane concentration, a measure of oxidative stress, in midlife women.* J Nutr, 2007. 137(11): p. 2412–19.
88. Sakai, M., M. Oimomi, and M. Kasuga. *Experimental studies on the role of fructose in the development of diabetic complications.* Kobe J Med Sci, 2002. 48(5–6): p. 125–36.
89. Faure, P., et al. *Comparison of the effects of zinc alone and zinc associated with selenium and vitamin E on insulin sensitivity and oxidative stress in high-fructose-fed rats.* J Trace Elem Med Biol, 2007. 21(2): p. 113–19.
90. Evans, J.L., et al. *Are oxidative stress-activated signaling pathways mediators of insulin resistance and beta-cell dysfunction?* Diabetes, 2003. 52(1): p. 1–8.
91. Basak, P.Y., F. Gultekin, and I. Kilinc. *The role of the antioxidative defense system in papulopustular acne.* J Dermatol, 2001. 28(3): p. 123–27.
92. Logan, A.C., and V. Treloar. *The Clear Skin Diet: A Nutritional Plan for Getting Rid of and Avoiding Acne.* 2007, Nashville, TN: Cumberland House Publishing Company.

Section V

Renal Diseases

21 Renal Calculi

Nutrient Strategies for Preventing Recurrence

Laura Flagg, C.N.P., and Rebecca Roedersheimer, M.D.

I. INTRODUCTION

Nephrolithiasis affects approximately 10% of the American population, with men affected about twice as often as women. Fifty percent of patients who have one incident of symptomatic stones will have another within 5 to 7 years. It appears that the incidence is increasing, but it is unclear whether or not this is due to changes in the American diet [1]. Stone formation can be life-alteringly chronic. In patients such as athletes, soldiers, and astronauts, even the risk of one recurrence may be unacceptably large.

There exist many different physiologic mechanisms that promote stone formation. Over the last decade, refinements to prior understanding of dietary management have led to improved dietary recommendations for fluids and nutrients. Dietary recommendations can be refined based on family history, stone type, and urine testing. This chapter equips providers to analyze stone type and prescribe diets shown to reduce stone formation.

II. EPIDEMIOLOGY

DIET-GENE INTERACTIONS

Epidemiology has been helpful to establish recurrent stone formation as a diet-gene interaction. Men form symptomatic stones approximately twice as often as do women. Stones are associated with periods of dehydration and lower fluid intake, as well as higher intake of meat, sodium, and ascorbic acid. Yet clearly not all men who follow these dietary patterns form symptomatic stones. Stone formation is recognized in some patients as a result of multiple inherited metabolic disorders. Hypercalciuria, the most commonly identified anomaly found in kidney stone formation, results from multiple factors, including genetics. The genetics of hypercalciuria are complex and defy simple description by Mendelian genetics. In addition, many inheritable conditions can coexist within one individual, leading to stone production as a result of more than one disorder. Examples include congenital lactase deficiency, an autosomal recessive disorder, multiple endocrine neoplasia syndrome type 1 with hyperparathyroidism, hypophosphatemia, and absorptive hypercalciuria [2]. Hyperoxaluria, defined as urinary excretion of more than 45 mg of oxalate per day, also has genetic underpinnings. Primary hyperoxaluria results from a deficiency in peroxisomal alanine:glyoxalate aminotransferase (AGT), and there have been 50 mutations identified in the gene responsible for AGT production [3]. Individualized recommendations are based on 24-hour urine and serum biochemistry rather than genetic markers for the foreseeable future, until the field of genetics allows for more practical clinical application. In summary, the field of genetics uncoupled with diet has not led to satisfactory understanding of stone formation.

INCIDENCE

One in 10 adults in the United States develops a renal stone. Two-thirds of the patients are men. Calcium oxalate (CaOx) stones are the most common stone type. CaOx stones account for 60% of all symptomatic stones in American adults. Uric acids stones represented 7% to 10% of all stone occurrences in the United States in the 1980s [4, 5]. This demographic may be increasing with the increasing prevalence of obesity. See Figure 21.1 for the percentage rates of the different stone types.

III. PATHOPHYSIOLOGY

CaOx stone formation is recognized as not a single disease entity, but rather one finding associated with a whole host of metabolic disturbances. *Hypercalciuria,* defined as urinary calcium that exceeds 200 mg in 24 hrs, can result from one or more of three basic types of disorders of calcium metabolism: from a disorder of calcium *absorption* from the gut; from *renal hypercalciuria,* which results from impaired renal tubular absorption of calcium, leading to increased excretion in the urine; and from *resorptive* hypercalciuria, which can be a secondary result of primary hyperparathyroidism [6].

Understanding the physiology of uric acid stone formation provides insights into prevention as well as the reasoning behind specific dietary recommendations. The formation of any type of stone depends on the solubility of the particular substance in urine. Two main factors influence the solubility of uric acid in urine: uric acid concentration and solution pH [7]. Either high uric acid concentration or low urine pH can lead to uric acid crystallization. The pKa of uric acid is 5.5, and uric acid becomes highly soluble in pH ranges greater than this value [8]. As pH values rise above 5.5, increasing amounts of uric acid are converted to urate—the ionized form of uric acid, which is 20 times more soluble than uric acid itself [9]. Therefore, alkalinizing urine can prevent uric acid crystallization and has even been shown to dissolve preformed uric acid stones 70% to 80% of the time [10–11].

Uric acid concentration in the urine depends on the total body uric acid pool. This pool is made up of endogenous production and exogenous sources. Since uric acid is the end product of purine

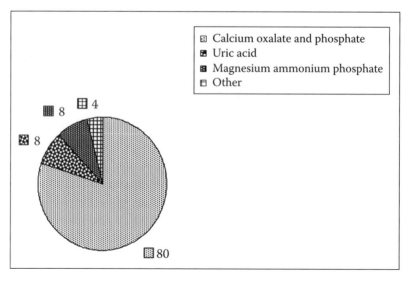

FIGURE 21.1   Classification of stones by chemical composition. (From [5].)

metabolism in humans [7], it has been hypothesized that eating food rich in purines will increase the uric acid pool. Foods rich in purines such as meat, seafood, yeast products, tea, coffee, and cola lower the exogenous purine synthesis, and will increase the total pool of uric acid and subsequently the risk of stone formation [12]. Clinical studies of dietary interventions to reduce exogenous purine sources have been marginally effective. Limiting dietary intake of purine has also been but marginally effective in gout, another condition associated with hyperuricemia.

A newly emerging hypothesis is that over time, diet influences endogenous production of uric acid from de novo purine synthesis and tissue catabolism. The baseline production of uric acid is usually 300 to 400 mg/day [7]. The rapid cell turnover seen in myeloproliferative disorders and Lesch-Nyhan syndrome increase de novo purine synthesis [13]. Extreme weight loss can increase breakdown of lean tissue thereby increasing uric acid. By mechanisms that are less well understood, obesity, diabetes, and insulin resistance appear to cause hyperuricemia, which predisposes patients to gout as well as uric acid stones [14]. Diets that treat the metabolic disturbances of diabetes and insulin resistance appear to reduce hyperuricemia.

IV. DIAGNOSTIC TESTING AND CLINICAL EVALUATION

To allow for individualized dietary recommendations, 24 hour urine studies are at the heart of diagnostic testing. Laboratory studies including urine volume, calcium, oxalate, uric acid, citrate, magnesium, phosphate, sodium, and pH can be obtained with a second stone occurrence. These urine studies should be done with concurrent serum calcium, uric acid, phosphate, potassium, chloride, bicarbonate, albumin, and creatinine. These test results, plus biochemical analysis of the stone, allow the clinician to identify metabolic aberrations commonly occurring with the particular stone type. It is virtually impossible to counsel a patient in diet management of stones when the type of stone is not known, nor the urinary properties in which the stone was formed. For example, recognizing the urinary specific gravity of 1.030 or greater, and a 24-hour urinary volume of 900 mL, easily suggests low fluid intake, and is significant for any stone type. But recognizing urinary properties such as hyperoxaluria or low pH allows for more specific recommendations. Recommendations for fluid intake, hyperoxaluria, acidic urine, and other recommendations for application of diet and laboratory testing are offered below.

V. DIET

FLUID INTAKE

Low fluid intake is recognized as the single most important dietary factor in stone formation. Supersaturation of common components of urine causes crystal formation, and crystal nucleation and growth are positively associated with low fluid intake. High fluid intake promotes higher urinary volumes, which wash out small, formed crystals before larger, symptomatic stones can form. Pak and colleagues in 1980 [15] were perhaps the first to scientifically show that increasing fluid intake to 2.5 L/day would reduce the risk of stone formation. A large, prospective, epidemiologic study of 45,000 male physicians and other health professionals reinforced this finding in 1993 [16]. Three years later, Borghi et al. [17] performed a large 5-year randomized, prospective study of 199 stone formers showing convincingly that higher fluid intake does indeed promote a continued stone-free state. Another prospective self-reporting epidemiologic study of 91,000 female registered nurses found that a fluid intake of 2.5 liters daily reduced a woman's relative risk of symptomatic stone formation compared with women whose fluid intake was less [18].

Increasing fluid intake can lower uric acid concentration in urine, possibly by lowering endogenous production of uric acid as well as by dilution of the urine. The decreased formation of stones with increased fluid intake has been proven in both scientific and large-scale prospective studies that have been previously discussed [15, 19–20]. The composition of the incident stones in these studies was not recorded, however, so direct conclusions on uric acid nephrolithiasis cannot be made. Uric acid stone incidence has been found to increase in times of dehydration, such as in warmer climates and hot working conditions [21–22]. The effect of fluid intake on the incidence of uric acid stone formation, specifically, has not been studied, but one can conclude from the above-mentioned studies that increased fluid intake is likely beneficial in the prevention of uric acid nephrolithiasis.

CALCIUM INTAKE

Contrary to previously held beliefs, studies in the last 10 or more years have shown that lower calcium intake actually raises a patient's risk of CaOx stone formation. This finding is counterintuitive, and has effectively reversed previous recommendations for calcium reduction to reduce stone risk. Stone formation relies on factors other than simple ingestion of nutrients. Calcium and oxalate are known to filter into the urine with variations based more on metabolic disturbances than dietary intake of these elements alone. Curhan and colleagues [16] studied the effects of calcium intake via questionnaires on the incidence of symptomatic stone formation over the course of 4 years. The men with the highest calcium intake (1050 mg daily or more) had the lowest rate of symptomatic stone formation, with a relative risk (RR)=0.66, 95% CI, compared to those with the lowest calcium intake of 605 mg daily or less. A similar study of women in 1997 also confirmed this pattern [18]. Similarly, Borghi and colleagues [23] studied 60 stone-forming men who followed a low-calcium diet and 60 men who followed a low-protein and low-sodium diet in this randomized study in 2002, and found that the men who limited calcium had twice the rate of symptomatic stones as the men who followed a low-protein and low-sodium diet. Given the additional risk of osteopenia and osteoporosis with low-calcium diets, these studies represent more cautionary warnings against calcium restriction among those at risk for stones by personal or family history.

The data would suggest that all forms of calcium intake are not equivalent regarding the risk of stone formation, particularly in women. Women who took calcium supplementation in a modest dose (500 mg daily) had a greater rate of symptomatic stones than women who obtained their daily calcium via diet only, 1.20 times the rate of the women without supplementation [18]. Yet this finding of greater risk with supplementation did not also hold true in men in a similar epidemiologic study [16] of 45,000 men. Calcium supplementation was thought to be actually protective in an experimental study [24] of men with known low-oxalate intake. Thirty-two men who were given calcium supplementation responded with urinary qualities thought to promote a lower stone risk (increased urinary citrate, decreased urinary oxalate, increased urinary calcium). In discussion of the finding of higher stone risk with calcium supplementation among women, researchers noted that potentially some other factor besides calcium, such as the natural phosphorous present in dietary sources of calcium, may have actually been responsible for the protective effect of the dietary calcium as opposed to supplemental calcium. They also theorized that the time of ingestion of supplement may be responsible for the added risk of stones with supplemental calcium, and recommended that the supplement be taken with a meal in which oxalate ingestion would naturally be higher [18]. It is noted that there was no attempt to identify the type of calcium supplementation used (calcium carbonate vs. calcium citrate). Perhaps calcium citrate would be better since it is alkalinizing. Calcium supplements that contain vitamin D and magnesium may also diminish any impact of calcium on stone formation [25].

OXALATE INTAKE

Dietary oxalate intake has been studied to a lesser degree than calcium intake. Variations in urinary oxalate levels are derived from three known mechanisms: exogenous or dietary intake, which is at least theoretically modifiable; the rate of intestinal absorption, which is in some cases related to gastrointestinal disease; and the rate of endogenous oxalate production during metabolism of nutrients via the Krebs cycle. The quantities of oxalate in the urine are much smaller than quantities of urinary calcium; therefore, alterations in the quantity of oxalate have a much greater effect on stone risk than the quantity of calcium. Alterations in urinary oxalate are less dependent on oxalate intake; rather, variations are often based in errors in nutrient metabolism [26].

Hyperoxaluria is defined as urinary excretion of oxalate greater than 45 mg/day. Metabolic disorders known to predispose to hyperoxaluria include renal tubular acidosis, hyperparathyroidism, sarcoidosis, inflammatory bowel disease, and Crohn's disease, and are thought to increase a person's stone risk [6]. A study of 93 stone-forming patients with idiopathic hyperoxaluria and 93 stone formers with normooxaluria underwent dietary modifications to determine the changes made in urinary characteristics thought to affect stone formation. Researchers found that there were no significant differences in dietary oxalate between those with hyperoxaluria and those with normooxaluria [27]. However, in another experimental study with strict dietary modifications, 12 normal (no history of renal stones) men and women ingested three different controlled diets that were altered based on oxalate content, showing that oxalate intake did significantly alter urinary oxalate, and theoretically, the risk of stone formation [28]. A large cohort study of male health professionals found no significant difference in risk of stone formation based on self-reported oxalate intake [16]. Oxalate is present in most foods to some degree and most highly concentrated in tea, chocolate, spinach, nuts, and rhubarb. In summary, recommending reduction in oxalate intake may be both difficult and unnecessary. Given oxalate's ubiquitous presence in the human diet and its concentration in otherwise health-promoting foods, instead of avoiding intake, a clinically more successful approach may be to drink a glass of water when eating a spinach salad.

Vitamin C Intake

Vitamin C is broken down during carbohydrate digestion into oxalate, and is possibly one dietary source responsible for higher risk of some renal stone formation. Review of data from the Health Professionals Follow-Up Study of over 50,000 men found that ascorbic acid intake in either dietary or supplement form increased the risk of symptomatic stones in men. In this study, the highest level of intake was associated with the highest risk (RR 1.41, P = 0.01, 95% CI) for intake of greater than 1000 mg daily compared with the lowest intake of 99 mg daily or less [19]. In another study of 186 stone formers, there was a significant positive association between high levels of dietary ascorbic acid in the form of fruits and vegetables and excretion of oxalate among those patients with known hyperoxaluria compared to those with normooxaluria. Vitamin C intake through fruits and vegetables among the hyperoxaluric group was 80% higher than recommended. Researchers concluded that in the hyperoxaluric group, high levels were associated with high absorption levels of oxalate from the intestines, probably from metabolism of higher dietary intake of ascorbic acid [27]. Baxmann and colleagues [29] altered the diets of 47 stone formers and 20 controls by administration of 1 g and 2 g of vitamin C supplements, measuring urinary properties afterwards. The urine of stone formers and controls showed increases in urinary oxalate and other risk factors measured by the Tiselius Index. Another experimental crossover study of 29 stone formers and 19 non-stone formers identified increases in urinary oxalate levels after supplementation with ascorbic acid: Significant increases in urinary oxalate were found among the stone formers and non-stone formers alike [30].

Specific Beverage Intake

Various Fruit Juices

Research of the association between vitamin C and renal stones underscores the importance of studying specific foods and not only the nutrients in isolation. In a study of specific beverages, grapefruit juice has been shown to significantly increase stone risk (RR 1.44, P=0.008, 95% CI). No such increase in risk was seen in other juices containing ascorbic acid, including apple, orange, tomato, and other fruit juices relative to water despite their ascorbic acid content [20]. The peculiarities of grapefruit juice have been well studied with respect to its effect upon drug absorption and metabolism. However, to date, the particular elements responsible for juice-drug interactions that affect drug availability and metabolism are not completely understood [31]. It may be that these not yet understood elements implicated in pharmaceutical alterations are also responsible for changes in absorption and metabolism of dietary nutrients, including those involved in stone formation.

In contrast to grapefruit juice, cranberry juice may lower stone risk despite its vitamin C and oxalate content. Cranberry juice decreased urinary oxalate and phosphate, while increasing urinary citrate, which is also thought to decrease stone risk [32]. Cranberry juice is a widely recognized homeopathic treatment for urinary tract infections [33], and the authors have noted for patients to ask about this specific treatment. It is important to urge moderation in intake of a calorie-laden simple carbohydrate such as fruit juice of any kind. Clinicians should remind patients that a serving of cranberry juice is a mere 6 ounces, and that most fluid intake should be water.

Alcohol and Caffeine Intake

Some of the same epidemiologic studies discussed earlier investigating the link between dietary patterns and stone formation also studied the risk of stones with caffeine and alcohol intake. Curhan and colleagues found that among women, increased coffee, tea, wine, and beer reduced the risk of stone formation over the course of 8 years [20]. The most marked reduction in risk was found with wine, showing a 45% reduction in risk for women who drank one or more glasses of wine daily compared with those who drank less than one glass per month (RR = 0.41, 95% CI). Less impressive but still significant reductions were also noted with coffee, tea, and surprisingly, decaffeinated coffee. Researchers theorized that despite significant oxalate content in tea and coffee, the unexpected inverse relationship between these beverages and stone formation was likely due to the diuretic effect of caffeine and alcohol through anti-diuretic hormone (ADH) inhibition, which theoretically offset the increased oxalate content. They could not adequately identify a mechanism by which the decaffeinated coffee also improved stone risk, simply calling for further study [20]. More recent works suggest that polyphenolic compounds present in coffee, tea, and decaffeinated coffee improve carbohydrate metabolism. Pereira found lower risk of diabetes among postmenopausal women who drank both regular and decaffeinated coffees [34]. Since diabetics are recognized as more frequent stone formers, improved carbohydrate metabolism may result in lower risk of stone formation.

Similar to the women's findings, coffee, tea, beer, and wine were also associated with decreased risk of stone formation over the course of 6 years among men [35]. As an epidemiologic study, there was no attempt to further identify the physiology behind these findings, or to positively identify the stone types involved.

With regard to alcohol intake and the risk of uric acid stones, beer, specifically, should be mentioned. Beer contains purines that are metabolized to uric acid [36]. An epidemiological study looking at uric acid stones, specifically, showed increased alcohol consumption in patients with uric acid stones as opposed to other stone types [37]. Furthermore, increased plasma and urine uric acid levels have been seen after several nights of increased beer ingestion [38–39]. With this in mind, moderation of beer consumption is recommended in patients who suffer from recurrent uric acid stones, again in contrast to the recommendations for those with known calcium oxalate stones.

SODIUM INTAKE

Sodium intake is thought to have a negative impact on urinary properties for the stone former. Sodium is reabsorbed in the kidney's proximal tubule with water and provides for calcium to reabsorb with sodium and water into the bloodstream during filtration by the kidney. An overabundance of sodium in the diet provides for less sodium reabsorption in the proximal tubule, and with it, less calcium reabsorption. This is thought to be the mechanism by which high sodium intake is responsible for hypercalciuria, and therefore the increased risk of stones. A study of 91,000 female nurses indeed showed that those with a dietary sodium intake of more than 4081 mg sodium/

day had an RR of 1.30 (P < 0.001, 95% CI) for stone formation over those with a sodium intake of less than 1965 mg/day [18]. However, a similar large epidemiologic study of men did not show significant risk of symptomatic stone formation based on dietary sodium intake [19]. In support of a low-sodium diet recommendation, Borghi and colleagues manipulated the diets of 120 men with history of stones and known hypercalciuria. They did find that a normal calcium, low sodium, and low animal protein diet protected 60 men from recurrent stone formation more effectively than the lower calcium diet without modifications for protein and sodium prescribed for 60 other stone-forming men [23].

MAGNESIUM INTAKE

Magnesium is recognized as another important element in reduction of CaOx kidney stone risk. Hypomagnesuria (excretion of less than 50 mg magnesium/24 hours) is a finding in 24-hour testing that increases the risk of CaOx stones. Magnesium intake is thought to improve stone risk by reducing dietary oxalate absorption and increasing the solubility of calcium oxalate in the urine, preventing stone formation [40–41].

Hypomagnesuria is thought to be primarily rooted in dietary deficiency. To that end, a study of 24 healthy (non-stone-forming) adults underwent separate dietary loads of oxalate with either calcium carbonate, magnesium oxide, or no dietary supplement intake to determine the response on urinary oxalate. The subjects who took magnesium supplementation as well as calcium supplementation both demonstrated improvements in their urinary properties. Magnesium supplementation was nearly as effective as calcium carbonate in reduction of urinary oxalate [40].

A 3-year double-blind study of 64 patients with known CaOx stone disease reduced their recurrent stone risk by ingestion of potassium-magnesium citrate. Compared with controls who received placebo, those who took the supplementation reduced their risk of recurrent symptomatic stone incidence by 84% (95% CI) [42].

PROTEIN INTAKE

Protein intake is thought to be positively associated with calcium and uric acid stone risk. Stones are relatively rare among vegetarians, and more common among more affluent societies and populations with animal-based rather than plant-based diets. Protein intake is thought to increase calcium oxalate stone risk through increases in urinary calcium levels. Epidemiologic studies of men's and women's protein intake and the risk of symptomatic stones showed that for men, a protein intake of greater than 77 g daily was associated with an RR of 1.33 compared to men with a protein intake of less than 50 g daily [16]. For women in a similar study, there was no such association. Researchers were unable to explain this finding, but theorized that perhaps problems with the questionnaire's design gave inaccurate results [18]. In a study of 18 stone-forming men and women with idiopathic hypercalciuria, subjects underwent protein intake restriction to determine the diet's effect on urinary qualities thought to affect stone risk. After subjects were given a diet modestly restricted in protein (0.8 g protein/kg body weight) for 15 days, urine showed significant reductions in calcium, phosphate, uric acid, and oxalate, and significant improvement in citrate levels, all thought to improve the risk of stones in patients with hypercalciuria [43].

Uric acid is the end product of protein metabolism. Increased protein consumption has been shown to increase endogenous acid load with a subsequent increase in the net renal acid excretion [44]. Due to decreased urine pH and increased urine levels of uric acid, high purine intake, especially from animal protein, has been considered to increase the risk of stone formation. Despite this common recommendation, solid evidence regarding the risk of uric acid stones is lacking. Two large epidemiological studies regarding dietary habits and stone incidence were contradictory in regard to protein. One showed decreased stone incidence in men with protein intake less than 50 g/day after 4 years, but when it was carried out for 14 years, this was only significant for men with BMI less than 25 kg/m² [16, 19]. The other study did not show any association between protein intake and stone incidence in women [45].

Several small studies have clarified the effect of protein intake on urine parameters, which increases the risk for stone formation. In a comparison of 12 days of a diet high in vegetable protein versus a diet high in animal protein in 15 healthy subjects, Breslau found among the animal protein group an increased excretion of undissociated uric acid and an increased risk of uric acid stone formation on in vitro crystallization studies [46]. This finding was confirmed in 2002 with a comparison of urine parameters after 5 days of a vegetarian versus a Western diet and an omnivorous diet. Uric acid excretion was significantly lower after the vegetarian diet with a 93% reduction in the risk of uric acid crystallization as compared to the Western diet [47]. In yet another comparison of diets with varying amounts of protein, patients with protein intake greater than 2 g/kg/day had significantly higher levels of urinary uric acid [48].

From these studies we can conclude that high animal protein diets may increase a patient's risk for uric acid stone formation as it has been proven that such diets certainly alter urine parameters. An actual increased incidence of uric acid stones in patients with high protein intake has not been proven in a large, prospective study. Therefore protein intake in moderation is recommended, but restriction of protein to less than the current RDA cannot be recommended currently.

Fruit and Vegetable Intake

Increasing fruit and vegetable intake has been suggested to reduce the risk of nephrolithiasis. In contrast to meat intake, which has an acidifying effect, the intake of fruits and vegetables provides an alkaline load that theoretically protects against uric acid stone formation. Both the biologic basis and the clinical applications of the alkaline diet are discussed in Chapter 31, "Osteoporosis." Vegetarian diets, those generally thought to be high in fruit and vegetable intake, have been found to change urine parameters in the direction of decreased risk for uric acid crystallization [46–49]. Increased fruit and vegetable consumption was found to have a protective effect on kidney stone formation in a retrospective review of self-reported stone incidence and dietary habits [50].

Fruit juices, specifically citrus juices, have often been touted to prevent kidney stone formation and several authors have investigated this claim. Orange juice may be beneficial in the prevention of uric acid stones. Two studies showed an increase in urine pH and a decrease in undissociated uric acid levels in urine compared to baseline after several days of orange juice ingestion (1.2 L/day) [51–52]. Another study showed a significant increase in urine pH after 0.5 L/day of orange juice ingestion, but no change in uric acid excretion [53]. Urinary uric acid and pH were not affected by lemonade intake in two separate studies [54–55]. Earlier, we discussed the positive effect of cranberry juice on urinary qualities thought to inhibit calcium oxalate stones. Inversely, however, cranberry juice has been found to decrease urine pH and increase the concentration of undissociated uric acid, thus likely increasing the risk of uric acid stones [56]. Thus increased consumption of fruits and vegetables is likely protective in uric acid nephrolithiasis and given the myriad additional health benefits of fruit and vegetable intake, this should be recommended to patients wishing to prevent further episodes of uric acid stones. These recommendations highlight the importance of biochemical analysis of stone type before giving specific recommendations for some dietary changes. Although orange juice consumption may be protective, the large amounts of calorie-filled juice necessary to initiate a small effect on urinary parameters constrain the recommendation for orange juice to one glass a day.

VI. COMORBID CONDITIONS

Obesity

Recommendations for weight loss to reduce stone risk are largely based on epidemiologic findings of cohort studies of men and women in the Health Professionals Follow-up Study, the Nurses' Health Study, and the Nurses' Health Study II, which incorporate findings of 45,000 men and

194,000 women; this information, like many of the findings discussed previously, is offered without the benefit of knowledge of the type of stone that subjects formed in these three studies. In men, the risk of symptomatic stones was significantly larger for men weighing 220 lbs than for men weighing less than 150 lbs (RR 1.44, P = 0.002, 95% CI). Other measurements related to obesity, specifically degrees of weight gain and higher body mass index (BMI), were significantly and positively related to stone risk [57].

The same trends found in men also held true in women. In younger women, the relative kidney stone risk rose to 1.92 (P < 0.001, 95% CI) for those with a body weight of over 220 lbs relative to women with a body weight of less than 150 lbs. Similar risk was found for older women. For younger women who gained 35 lbs or more after age 21, the relative risk was 1.82 (P < 0.001, 95% CI) of those whose weight remained unchanged. Older women's risk of stones with the same weight gain was 1.7 times the risk of women who did not gain weight (P < 0.001, 95% CI). BMI and waist circumference showed similar significant associations with stone risk among women [57].

A study that reviewed 24-hour urine studies of 4883 stone patients found a strong inverse association between obesity and urinary pH, and proposed that insulin resistance is at the heart of the metabolic findings [58]. Increasing urinary acidity is found to be associated with formation of uric acid stones, and will be discussed in the following. This may represent the physiologic basis for the findings in the three cohort studies above, though without information specific to the type of stone, it is not possible to determine whether there is another association between obesity and calcium oxalate stones.

DIABETES MELLITUS

Increased incidence of uric acid nephrolithiasis has been seen in both diabetic and obese patients [59]. Insulin resistance results in lower urine pH through impaired ammoniagenesis, so it has been hypothesized that type 2 diabetes favors the formation of uric acid stones. This was confirmed in two large studies that showed an increased proportion of uric acid stones among diabetics as compared to nondiabetic stone formers [60–61]. Obesity increases urine acidity due to insulin resistance. Indeed urine pH has been found to be inversely associated with body weight [62, 58]. Because urine is more acidic in obese patients, one would presume these patients have an increased risk of uric acid stones specifically. This was confirmed in a study that showed that the proportion of uric acid stones increases with BMI in both males and females. Obesity and diabetes appear to be risk factors for uric acid nephrolithiasis, thus patients with recurrent uric acid stones should be counseled to control weight and consider screening for diabetes.

URINARY TRACT INFECTION

Another comorbid condition frequently associated with kidney stones is urinary tract infection (UTI). Certain stones form specifically in urine infected with urea-splitting organisms such as proteus or klebsiella. These stones, composed of magnesium ammonium phosphate, then become the source of recurrent urinary tract infections because they harbor bacteria that are not susceptible to antibiotic therapy. These stones should be treated surgically to decrease the risk of recurrent infections and life-threatening urosepsis. Once the stones have been cleared, dietary prevention of urinary tract infection can be recommended. Cranberry juice and cranberry products are perhaps the most common recommendation. Cranberries have been shown to prevent bacteria (particularly *E. coli*) from attaching to the bladder epithelium, thus theoretically preventing infection [63–64]. A recent review from the Cochrane Database regarding evidence for the use of cranberry products to prevent UTIs concludes that there is some evidence to recommend cranberries in the prevention of UTIs, particularly in women with recurrent infections [65]. The authors note, however, that the dose and duration of treatment have not been established and that a significant number of subjects dropped out of the reviewed studies, indicating that the treatment may not be acceptable to all patients. Again, patients should be cautioned regarding the caloric content of juice and should recognize that the acidifying effect of the juice may increase uric acid stone risk, although this has not been specifically studied.

In addition to cranberry juice, the role of probiotics in the prevention of UTI has been gaining interest in recent years. Theoretically, probiotics help to maintain a normal, healthy vaginal flora and thus prevent overgrowth and urogenital ascension of pathogenic organisms. Probiotic vaginal suppositories have been shown to reduce the rate of recurrent UTIs in two studies [66–67]. Studies on orally administered probiotics and the prevention of UTIs have been conflicting [68]. Currently, there are no commercially available probiotics in the United States that have been proven to reduce urinary tract infection. One comparative study did show that women with more frequent consumption of fresh berry juices and fermented milk products containing probiotic bacteria, such as yogurt, sour milk, and cheese, had a lower incidence of UTIs [69].

Hyperparathyroidism

Approximately 2% to 3% of patients with recurrent stone disease have hyperparathyroidism. While this percentage is small, it should cause suspicion when a patient with recurrent CaOx stones has exaggerated urinary and blood measurements suggestive of oversecretion of parathyroid hormone (PTH). Such findings include normocalcemia or hypercalcemia with hypercalciuria, hypophosphatemia, elevated PTH, bone demineralization evidenced by DEXA scan, and/or concurrent irritable bowel syndrome, depression, or other central nervous disorders [70]. Such patients may be diagnosed with the more common secondary hyperparathyroidism, resulting from chronic overstimulation of the parathyroid glands due to, for example, use of calcium-wasting diuretics such as furosemide, as well as chronic renal failure, malabsorption syndrome, and inadequate vitamin D. In such patients, an elevated ratio of chloride to phosphate (33:1 or greater) is also indicative of hyperphosphatemia [72]. The less common primary hyperparathyroidism can be caused by a benign adenoma of one or more parathyroid glands, however, and is cured by parathyroidectomy. As a matter of practice, referring patients with known elevated PTH to endocrinologists can more easily diagnose and treat the underlying defect. Patients with recurrent CaOx stones can benefit from serum PTH measurement to detect one more underlying mechanism that, when properly treated, can make a significant improvement in the risk for recurrence of CaOx stones, as well as fractures associated with the disease [70, 72].

VII.   SPECIAL CONSIDERATIONS

Several medications can contribute to kidney stone formation. Some medications themselves crystallize in urine and others contribute to stone formation due to their effects on urine pH and composition. Indinivir, trimaterene, and over-the-counter combinations of guaifenesin and ephedrine can all crystallize in urine leading to stone formation [73–76]. Crystallization of ciprofloxacin and sulfa medications has also been reported [77–78]. Patients who need these medications for other medical problems should be advised to maximize fluid intake in order to prevent stone formation. Loop diuretics lead to a hypercalciuric state by inhibiting the resorption of both calcium and sodium in the thick ascending limb of the loop of Henle. Carbonic anhydrase inhibitors, such as acetazolamide, may contribute to calcium phosphate stone formation by causing a chronic acidosis with resultant high urine pH, hypercalciuria, and low urinary citrate levels [76]. Topiramate has a similar effect on urine composition with a reported incidence of stones in patients taking this medication ranging from 1.5% to 5% [79–80]. Laxative abuse has also been associated with kidney stone formation [81]. If possible, these medications should be discontinued. Otherwise, general dietary recommendations of increased fluid intake and moderation of sodium and protein are recommended in these specific situations.

VIII. CONCLUSION

In conclusion, this chapter offers guidance for dietary recommendations in the treatment of the most common types of recurrent kidney stones, namely, calcium oxalate and uric acid stones. Because these are, by far, the most common stone types, most of the available literature focuses on calcium oxalate and uric acid stones. The reader should note that many other less common types of stones exist including calcium phosphate stones, cystine stones, and struvite (magnesium ammonium phosphate) stones. General recommendations, such as increased fluid intake, can be given for all stone formers. More specific recommendations, however, depend on the chemical composition of the stones that are formed by a particular patient. Further individualized recommendations regarding dietary management may be made confidently only after stone type is known. Twenty-four hour urine testing can further delineate metabolic irregularities that can be at least partially modified by diet. Examples of how this may be approached are found in Table 21.1.

TABLE 21.1
Diet Recommendations for Stone Type and Urinary Properties

Stone Type	Urinary Property	Recommendation
All stone types		Increase fluid intake to 2500 mL/24 hours; mostly water intake.
		Promote optimal weight through diet, exercise.
		Monitor for insulin resistance.
		Monitor for signs of hyperparathyroidism.
CaOx		Maintain protein intake of 30% of total caloric intake. No need for further restriction, however.
		Maintain adequate calcium intake for age, gender.
		If supplement used, take with meals. Calcium citrate may be preferable to calcium carbonate.
		Monitor serum vitamin D levels. High levels may increase stone formation; low levels decrease calcium absorption, increasing risk.
		Evaluate drug interactions promoting stone formation.
	Hyperoxaluria	Moderate fruits and vegetables. Do not restrict calcium. Consider magnesium oxide or magnesium citrate supplementation. No real need for oxalate restriction.
		Encourage moderate vitamin C intake by dietary sources. Caution with use of supplemental vitamin C; take with meals.
	Hypomagnesuria	Increase dietary sources of magnesium. Consider supplementation with magnesium oxide or magnesium citrate.
	Hypocitraturia	Consider calcium citrate or magnesium citrate supplementation. Lemon water (lemon or lime wedge in water) encouraged.
	Hypercalciuria	Sodium restriction to 2 g/24 hours or less. Do not restrict calcium intake below recommendations for age and gender.
Uric Acid		Increase fruits and vegetables.
		Decrease excessive protein intake to no more than 30% of total caloric intake.
		Limit intake of cranberry juice. Promote moderate use of orange juice.
		No concerns for intake of coffee, tea, decaffeinated coffee; may improve carbohydrate metabolism, reduce stones in diabetics.
		Beer intake reduced or eliminated.

REFERENCES

1. Stamatelou KK, Francis FE, Jones CA, Nyberg LM, Curhan GC: Time trends in reported prevalence of kidney stones in the United States: 1976–1994. *Kidney Int* 63:1817–1823, 2003.
2. Moe OW, Bonny O: Genetic hypercalciuria. *J Amer Soc Neph* 16:729–745, 2005.
3. Coulter-Mackie MB: Preliminary evidence for ethnic differences in primary hyperoxaluria type 1 genotype (abstract). *Am J Neph* 25:264–268, 2005.
4. Mandel NS, Mandel GS: Urinary tract stone disease in the United States veteran population. I. Geographical frequency of occurrence. *J Urol* 142:1513–1515, 1989.
5. Gault MH, Chafe L: Relationship of frequency, age, sex, stone weight and composition in 15,624 stones: Comparison of Results for 1980 to 1983 and 1995 to 1998. *J Urol* 164:302–307, 2000.
6. Parmar M: Kidney stones. *Brit Med J* 328:1420–1424, 2004.
7. Shekarriz B, Stoller ML: Uric acid nephrolithiasis: Current concepts and controversies. *J Urol* 168:1307–1314, 2002.
8. Finlayson B, Smith A: Stability of the first dissociable proton of uric acid. *J Chem Engl Data* 19:94–97, 1974.
9. Menon M, Resnick MI: *Urinary lithiasis: Etiology, diagnosis, and medical management*. In *Campbell's Urology*. P. Walsh, et al. Eds. 8th ed. Philadelphia, PA: Saunders, 2002. 3257–8.
10. Kursh ED, Resnick MI: Dissolution of uric acid calculi with systemic alkalization. *J Urol* 132:286–287, 1984.
11. Moran ME, Abrahams HM, Burday DE, Greene TD: Utility of oral dissolution therapy in the management of referred patients with secondarily treated uric acid stones. *Urology* 59:206–210, 2002.
12. Schlesinger N: Dietary factors and hyperuricaemia. *Curr Pharm Des* 11:4133–4138, 2005.
13. Ngo TC, Assimis DG: Uric acid nephrolithiasis: recent progress and future directions. *Rev Urol* 9:17–27, 2007.
14. Helman A: *Gout*. In *Scientific Evidence for musculoskeletal, bariatric, and sports nutrition,* I. Kohlsteadt, Ed. 2006, CRC Press, Taylor & Francis Group, Boca Raton, FL: 425–430.
15. Pak CYC, Sakhaee K, Crowther C, Brinkley L: Evidence justifying a high fluid intake in treatment of nephrolithiasis. *Ann Int Med* 93:36–39, 1980.
16. Curhan GC, Willett WC, Rimm EB, Stampfer MJ: A prospective study of dietary calcium and other nutrients and the risk of symptomatic kidney stones. *N Engl J Med* 328:833–838, 1993.
17. Borghi L, Meschi T, Amato F, Briganti A, Novarini A, Giannini A: Urinary volume, water and recurrences in idiopathic calcium nephrolithiasis: A 5 year prospective study. *J Urol* 155:839–843, 1996.
18. Curhan GC, Willett WC, Speizer FE, Spiegelman D, Stampfer MJ: Comparison of dietary calcium with supplemental calcium and other nutrients as factors affecting the risk for kidney stones in women. *Ann Int Med* 126:497–504, 1997.
19. Taylor EN, Stampfer MJ, Curhan GC: Dietary factors and the risk of incident kidney stones in men: New insights after 14 years of follow-up. *J Am Soc Nephrol* 15:3225–3232, 2004.
20. Curhan GC, Willett WC, Speizer FE, Stampfer MJ: Beverage use and risk for kidney stones in women. *Ann Int Med* 128:534–540, 1998.
21. Borghi L, Meschi T, Amato F, Novarini A, Romanelli A, Cigala F: Hot occupation and nephrolithiasis. *J Urol* 150:1757–1760, 1993.
22. Atan L, Andreoni C, Oriz V, Silva EK, Pitta R, Atan F, Srougi M: High kidney stone risk in men working in steel industry at hot temperatures. *Urology* 65:858–861, 2005.
23. Borghi L, Schanchi T, Meschi T, Guerra A, Allegra F, Maggiore U, et al.: Comparison of diets for the prevention of recurrent stones in idiopathic hypercalciuria. *N Engl J Med* 346:77–83, 2002.
24. Stitchantrakul W, Sopassathit W, Prapaipanich S, Domrongkitchaiporn S: Effects of calcium supplements on the risk of renal stone formation in a population with low oxalate intake (abstract). *Southeast Asian J Trop Med Public Health* 35:1028–33, 2004.
25. Brown S: *Bone Nutrition*. In *Scientific Evidence for musculoskeletal, bariatric and sports nutrition,* I. Kohlsteadt, Ed. 2006, CRC Press, Taylor & Francis Group, Boca Raton, FL: 443–472.
26. Morton AR, Iliescu EA, Wilson JWL: Nephrology: 1. Investigation and treatment of recurrent kidney stones. *Can Med Assoc J* 166:213–218, 2002.
27. Siener R, Ebert D, Nicolay C, Hesse A: Dietary risk factors for hyperoxaluria in calcium oxalate stone formers. *Kidney Int* 63:1037–1043, 2003.
28. Holmes RP, Goodman HO, Assimos DG: Contribution of dietary oxalate to urinary oxalate excretion. *Kidney Int* 59:270–276, 2005.

29. Baxmann AC, De OG, Mendonça C, Heilberg IP: Effect of vitamin C supplements on urinary oxalate and pH in calcium stone-forming patients. *Kidney Int* 63:1066–1071, 2003.

30. Massey LK, Liebman M, Kynast-Gales SA: Ascorbate increases human oxaluria and kidney stone risk. *J Nut* 135:1673–1677, 2005.

31. Kiani J, Imam S: Medicinal importance of grapefruit juice and its interaction with various drugs. *Nut J* 6:33, 2007.

32. McHarg T, Rodgers A, Charlton K: Influence of cranberry juice on the urinary risk factors for calcium oxalate kidney stone formation. *BJU Int* 92:765–768, 2003.

33. Jepson RG, Craig JC: A systematic review of the evidence for cranberries and blueberries in UTI prevention. *Molecular Nutr & Food Res* 51(6):738–745, 2007.

34. Pereira MA: Coffee intake linked to lower diabetes risk. *Ann Int Med* 166:1311–1316, 2006.

35. Curhan GC, Willett WC, Speizer FE, Speigelman D, Stampfer MJ: Prospective study of beverage use and the risk of kidney stones. *Amer J Epidemiol* 143:240–247, 1996.

36. Gibson T, Rodgers AV, Simmonds HA, Toseland P: Beer drinking and its effect on uric acid. *Br J Rheumatol* 23:203–209, 1984.

37. Zechner O, Pfluger H, Scheiber V: Idiopathic uric acid lithiasis: epidemiologic and metabolic aspects. *J Urol* 128:1219–1223, 1982.

38. Ka T, Moriwaki Y, Takahashi S, Yamamoto A, Tsutsumi Z, Inokuchi T, Yamamoto T: Effects of long term beer ingestion on plasma concentrations and urinary excretion of purine bases. *Horm Metab Res* 37:641–645, 2005.

39. Moriwaki Y, Ka T, Takahashi S, Tsutsumi Z, Yamamoto T: Effect of beer ingestion on the plasma concentrations and urinary excretion of purine bases: one-month study. *Nucleosides Nucleotides Nucleic Acids* 25:1083–1085, 2006.

40. Liebman M, Costa G: Effects of calcium and magnesium on urinary oxalate excretion after oxalate loads. *J Urol* 163:1565–1569, 2000.

41. Colella J, Kochis E, Galli B, Munver R: Urolithiasis/nephrolithiasis: What's It All About? *Urol Nurs* 25:427–448, 2005.

42. Ettinger B, Pak CYC, Citron JT, Thomas C, Adams-Huet B, Vangessel A: Potassium-magnesium citrate is an effective prophylaxis against recurrent calcium oxalate nephrolithiasis. *J Urol* 158:2069–2073, 1997.

43. Giannini S, Nobile M, Sartori L, Carbonare LD, et al.: Acute effects of moderate dietary protein restriction in patients with idiopathic hypercalciuria and calcium nephrolithiasis. *Am J Clin Nut* 69:267–271, 1999.

44. Remer T, Manz F: Estimation of the renal net acid excretion by adults consuming diets containing variable amounts of protein. *Am J Clin Nutr* 59:1356–1361, 1994.

45. Curhan GC, Willett AC, Knight EL, Stampfer, MJ: Dietary factors and the risk of incident kidney stones in younger women. *Arch Intern Med* 164:885–891, 2004.

46. Breslau NA, Brinkley L, Hill KD, Pak CY: Relationship of animal protein-rich diet to kidney stone formation and calcium metabolism. *J Clin Endocrinol Metab* 66:140–146, 1988.

47. Siener R, Hesse A: The effect of a vegetarian and different omnivorous diets on urinary risk factors for uric acid stone formation. *Eur J Nutr* 42:332–337, 2003.

48. Kok DJ, Iestra JA, Doorenbos CJ, Papapoulos SE: The effects of dietary excesses in animal protein and in sodium on the composition and the crystallization kinetics of calcium oxalate monohydrate in urines of healthy men. *J Clin Endocrinol Metab* 71:861–867, 1990.

49. Liatsikos EN, Barbalias GA: The influence of a low protein diet in idiopathic hypercalciuria. *Int Urol Nephrol* 31:271–276, 1999.

50. Goldfarb DS, Fischer ME, Keich Y, Goldberg J: A twin study of genetic and dietary influences on nephrolithiasis: A report from the Vietnam Era Twin Registry. *Kidney Int* 67:1053–1061, 2005.

51. Wabner CL, Pak CY: Effect of orange juice consumption on urinary stone risk factors. *J Urol* 149:1405–1408, 1993.

52. Odvina CV: Comparative value of orange juice versus lemonade in reducing stone forming risk. *Clin J Am Soc Nephrol* 1:1269–1274, 2006.

53. Honow R, Laube N, Schneider A, Kessler T, Hesse A: Influence of grapefruit-, orange- and apple-juice consumption on urinary variables and risk of crystallization. *Br J Nutr* 90:295–300, 2003.

54. Seltzer MA, Low RK, McDonald M, Shami GS, Stoller ML: Dietary manipulation with lemonade to treat hypocitraturic calcium nephrolithiasis. *J Urol* 156:907–909, 1996.

55. Koff SG, Paquette EL, Cullen J, Gancarczyk KK, Tucciarone PR, Schenkman NS: Comparison between lemonade and potassium citrate and impact on urine pH and 24 hour urine parameters in patients with kidney stone formation. *Urology* 69:1013–1016, 2007.

56. Gettman MT, Ogan K, Brinkley LJ, Adams-Huet B, Pak CY, Pearle MS: Effect of cranberry juice consumption on urinary stone risk factors. *J Urol* 174:590–594, 2005.

57. Taylor EN, Stampfer MJ, Curhan GC: Obesity, weight gain, and the risk of kidney stones. *JAMA* 293 (4): 455–462, 2005.

58. Maalouf NM, Sakhaee K, Parks JH, Coe FL, Adams-Huet B, Pak CY: Association of urinary pH with body weight in nephrolithiasis. *Kidney Int* 65:1422–1425, 2004.

59. Lieske JC, de la Vega LS, Gettman MT, Slezak JM, Bergstralh EJ, Melton LJ 3rd, Liebson CL: Diabetes mellitus and the risk of urinary tract stones: a population-based case control study. *Am J Kidney Dis* 48:897–904, 2006.

60. Daudon M, Traxer O, Conort P, Lacour B, Jungers P: Type 2 diabetes increases the risk for uric acid stones. *J Am Soc Nephrol* 17:2026–2033, 2006.

61. Pak CY, Sakhaee K, Moe O, Preminger GM, Poindexter JR, Peterson RD, Pietrow P, Ekeruo W: Biochemical profile of stone forming patients with diabetes mellitus. *Urology* 61:523–527, 2003.

62. Cameron MA, Maalouf NM, Adams-Huet B, Moe OW, Sakhaee K: Urine composition in type 2 diabetes: predisposition to uric acid nephrolithiasis. *J Am Soc Nephrol* 17:1422–1428, 2006.

63. Zafriri D, Ofek I, Adar R, Pocino M, Sharon N: Inhibitory activity of cranberry juice on adherence of type 1 and type P fimbriated Escherichia coli to eukaryotic cells. *Antimicrob Agents Chemother* 33:92–98, 1989.

64. Gupta K, Chou MY, Howell A, Wobbe C, Grady R, Satpleton AE: Cranberry products inhibit adherence of P-fimbriated Escherichia coli to primary cultured bladder and vaginal epithelial cells. *J Urol* 177:2357–2360, 2007.

65. Jepson RG, Craig JC: Cranberries for preventing urinary tract infections. *Cochrane Database Syst Rev* 23:CD001321, 2008.

66. Reid G, Bruce AW, Taylor M: Influence of three day antimicrobial therapy and Lactobacillus suppositories on recurrence of urinary tract infection. *Clin Ther* 14:11–16, 1992.

67. Reid G, Bruce AW, Taylor M: Instillation of Lactobacillus and stimulation of indigenous organisms to prevent recurrence of urinary tract infections. *Microecol Ther* 23:32–45, 1995.

68. Reid G, Bruce AW: Probiotics to prevent urinary tract infections: the rationale and evidence. *World J Urol* 24:28–32, 2006.

69. Kontiokari T, Laitinen J, Jarvi L, Pokka T, Sundqvist K, Uhari M: Dietary factors protecting women from urinary tract infection. *Am J Clin Nutr* 77:600–604, 2003.

70. Favus MJ: Chapter 14: Nephrolithiasis. Diseases of bone and metabolism. Retrieved on February 19, 2008 from www.endotext.org/parathyroid/parathyroid14/parathyroidframe14.htm.

71. Holick M. *Vitamin D: Importance for Musculoskeletal Function and Health.* In *Scientific Evidence for musculoskeletal, bariatric, and sports nutrition,* I. Kohlsteadt, Ed. 2006, CRC Press, Taylor & Francis Group, Boca Raton, FL:153–174.

72. Allerheiligen DA, Schoeber J, Houston RE, Mohl VK, Wildman KM: Hyperparathyroidism. *Amer Fam Phys* 57, April 1998.

73. Satel E, Angel JB, Futter NG, Walsh WG, O'Rourke K, Mahoney JE: Increased prevalance and analysis of risk factors for indinavir nephrolithiasis. *J Urol* 164:1895–1897, 2000.

74. Kohan AD, Armenakas NA, Fracchia JA: Indinavir urolithiasis: an emerging cause of renal colic in patients with human immunodeficiency virus. *J Urol* 161:1765–1768, 1999.

75. Sorgel F, Ettinger B, Benet LZ: The true composition of kidney stones passed during triamterene therapy. *J Urol* 134:871–873, 1985.

76. Matlage BR, Shah OD, Assimos DG: Drug induced urinary calculi. *Rev Urol* 5: 227–231, 2003.

77. Chopra N, Fine PL, Price B, Atlas I: Bilateral hydronephrosis from ciprofloxacin induced crystalluria and stone formation. *J Urol* 164:438, 2000.

78. Siegel WH: Unusual complication of therapy with sulfamethoxazole-trimethoprim. *J Urol* 117:397, 1977.

79. Reid G, Bruce AW: Probiotics to prevent urinary tract infections: the rationale and evidence. *World J Urol* 24:28–32, 2006.

80. Kontiokari T, Laitinen J, Jarvi L, Pokka T, Sundqvist K, Uhari M: Dietary factors protecting women from urinary tract infection. *Am J Clin Nutr* 77:600–604, 2003.

81. Dick WH, Lingeman JE, Preminger GM, Smith LH, Wilson DM, Shirrell WL: Laxative abuse as a cause for ammonium urate renal calculi. *J Urol* 143:244–247, 1990.

22 Chronic Kidney Disease

Overview and Nutritional Interventions

Allan E. Sosin, M.D.

I. INTRODUCTION

Chronic kidney disease is underdiagnosed and underappreciated as a cause of illness and mortality. Fundamental changes in lifestyle predispose people in Western societies to compromised renal integrity and progressive deterioration of renal function. It is important to include the proper evaluation of renal status in overall health assessment. Prompt diagnosis provides an opportunity to implement the strategies presented in this chapter and improve the current statistics.

II. EPIDEMIOLOGY

At present 350,000 are people on dialysis therapy in the United States, and that number is increasing at the rate of 7% yearly.[1] Hemodialysis, peritoneal dialysis, and renal transplantation are the methods of treatment for chronic renal failure. Although they permit survival in an otherwise uniformly fatal condition, they are difficult and costly procedures, and impact quality of life.

The major causes of end-stage renal disease (ESRD) are diabetes mellitus, accounting for 45% of cases, and hypertension, accounting for 27%.[2] Since the majority of cases of diabetes and hypertension are preventable, and nearly all can be mitigated, optimal clinical management would greatly reduce the prevalence of end-stage renal disease.

There are five stages of kidney disease, comprising a total of nearly 20 million affected individuals:

Stage 1: Chronic kidney disease with normal or increased glomerular filtration rate (GFR >90)
Stage 2: Mild loss of kidney function (GFR 60–89)
Stage 3: Moderate loss of kidney function (GFR 30–59)
Stage 4: Severe loss of kidney function (GFR 15–29)
Stage 5: Kidney failure (GFR <15 or on dialysis)

One-third of patients with stage 4 disease will develop ESRD within 3 years. The median age of patients beginning dialysis in the United States is 65 years. The mortality rate of dialysis is high, 24% per year, primarily due to heart disease and stroke, approaching that of lung cancer.

III. PATIENT EVALUATION

Two measurements of kidney function should be made: glomerular filtration rate (GFR) and the degree of albuminuria. A routine chemistry panel provides the level of creatinine, a protein metabolite. Utilizing this number along with age, weight, and sex in the Cockroft-Gault equation, GFR can be calculated.

GFR (cc/min) = (140–age) × (weight in kg) × (0.85 for women or 1.0 for men) / 72 × creatinine

Serum creatinine alone is not sufficient to estimate GFR. Creatinine production reflects muscle mass, which is less in older people, thinner people, those who are inactive, and women. Thus, a creatinine of 1.0 indicates normal kidney function in a 300-pound football lineman, but signifies substantial renal compromise in an 85-pound, 80-year-old woman. This distinction becomes especially important when administering drugs to older people, whose serum creatinine level does not reflect the degree of renal disease, and whose prescription selections and dosages should be modified.

Albuminuria, or protein loss through the kidneys, is a marker for the degree of renal damage. Protein loss, especially in diabetics, occurs prior to the rise of serum creatinine. This is most easily assessed by measuring the ratio of albumin to creatinine, preferably in the first morning urine. Monitoring albuminuria offers information on the rate of loss of renal function, since the rate of loss of GFR increases with the rate of protein loss. Additionally, the degree of albuminuria correlates with the risk of cardiovascular complications, including myocardial infarction, stroke, and congestive heart failure. Albuminuria can be reduced, and this reduction is accompanied by a lessening of cardiovascular events. In diabetics, suppression of albuminuria helps to preserve kidney function. As we will discuss, this can be achieved with medication, dietary protein restriction, and specific nutrient supplementation.

Urinary albumin losses greater than 3 g/day are accompanied by edema and hyperlipidemia, defining the nephrotic syndrome. Albumin itself may be toxic to renal tissue, and accelerate renal disease. Other compounds may be lost, including 1,25-dihydroxyvitamin D, and clotting factors IX, XI, and XII, leading to coagulation defects. Loss of antithrombin III may cause increased thrombosis. A quarter of patients with nephrotic syndrome will have clotting disorders.

IV. PATHOPHYSIOLOGY

REVIEW OF RENAL PHYSIOLOGY

The kidneys have multiple functions, the loss of which impacts other system operations:

1. Waste product excretion—renal impairment leads to metabolic acidosis, anorexia, nausea, loss of muscle protein and general depletion, neurologic dysfunction due to accumulated toxins, and soft tissue deposition of oxalates and phosphates.
2. Exquisite regulation of electrolyte concentrations and fluid volumes—impairment leads to hyponatremia, hyperkalemia, hypocalcemia, hyperphosphatemia, hypermagnesemia, and intolerance to electrolyte or mineral loading.
3. Blood pressure regulation—impairment leads to hypertension and cardiovascular disease, and accelerates the progression of renal disease.
4. Endocrine mediators:
   a. Erythropoietin—deficiency leads to anemia.
   b. Renin system activation—leads to hypertension and damage to arterial walls.
   c. 1,25-dihydroxyvitamin D production—decline leads to osteoporosis and immune dysfunction.
   d. Secondary hyperparathyroidism due to hyperphosphatemia and hypocalcemia, leading to metabolic bone disease and disseminated soft tissue calcification.

e. Prolonged half-lives of peptide hormones due to reduced degradation, including insulin, glucagon, growth hormone, parathyroid hormone, prolactin, gastrin, and follicle-stimulating hormone.

Pathophysiologic Mechanisms

Symptoms and signs of renal impairment often do not occur until disease is advanced. It is therefore important to detect abnormalities prior to the onset of clinical manifestations. The progression of renal disease can be modified, but in most cases it is not possible to restore renal function once lost. Exceptions include auto-immune disease such as lupus erythematosus or idiopathic nephrotic syndrome, and acute renal failure.

The following factors contribute to the progression and initiation of renal disease:

1. Uncontrolled diabetes mellitus
2. Hypertension
3. Nephrotoxic medicines
4. High protein diet
5. High phosphorus diet
6. Proteinuria
7. Acidemia
8. Inflammatory renal response, with release of cytokines
9. Calcium oxalate or calcium phosphate deposition in the kidney
10. Lead and cadmium toxicity
11. Hyperuricemia
12. Platelet aggregation in the kidney

V. PHARMACOLOGIC CONSIDERATIONS IN NEPHROTOXICITY

Prescription and nonprescription drugs frequently damage renal function. Acute interstitial nephritis is largely a consequence of pharmaceuticals, including antibiotics (penicillins, rifampin, sulfa drugs, vancomycin, ciprofloxacin, cephalosporins, erythromycin, acyclovir), diuretics (furosemide, thiazides, triamterene), and nonsteroidal anti-inflammatory drugs (NSAIDs). NSAIDs cause both acute and chronic interstitial nephritis, and should be avoided, along with acetaminophen and aspirin, in patients with renal impairment. Despite having reduced kidney function, it is common for patients to employ NSAIDs or acetaminophen, without receiving cautionary advice from their physicians.

Osteoarthritis is ubiquitous in older people, and NSAIDs, acetaminophen, and aspirin are often prescribed or purchased over the counter. It is crucial that individuals with impaired renal function be told the risk of taking these drugs, kept on minimal required doses for the briefest period, and monitored for a rise in serum creatinine. Combinations of nephrotoxic drugs should be avoided. Other drugs known to provoke toxic kidney effects include the anti-seizure drugs phenytoin, phenobarbital, sodium valproate, and carbamazepine. Lithium, allopurinol, ranitidine, omeprazole, interferon, cyclosporin, methotrexate, and cisplatin are other medications frequently causing kidney damage.

It was recently discovered that the magnetic resonance imaging contrast injectable gadolinium may cause a severe systemic reaction in people with preexisting renal disease. Called nephrogenic systemic fibrosis, the disease involves induration and hyperpigmentation of the skin, with fibrosis of skeletal muscles, heart, lungs, liver, and central nervous system.[3] The condition is progressive and usually irreversible, and no treatment is effective. It is crucial to measure serum creatinine prior to injecting gadolinium in any patient. Gadolinium should be withheld from any patient with GFR less than 30, if possible.

Aristolochia, a Chinese herb used primarily for weight loss, may cause chronic interstitial nephritis. It also causes urologic malignancies, and was responsible for the deaths of over 60 people in China, and several cases of renal failure in Belgium, England, and other European countries.[4]

The use of statin drugs (HMG-CoA reductase inhibitors) is controversial in kidney disease. Statins may cause rhabdomyolysis with heme pigment tubular toxicity.[5] Nevertheless, because renal disease is a cardiac equivalent, statins are often prescribed to those with renal failure. Recent studies, however, reveal no significant reduction of cardiovascular events in dialysis patients receiving statins, despite the lowering of cholesterol.[6]

Radiologic contrast dyes are a frequent cause of renal toxicity. Contrast-induced nephropathy, defined as an increase of creatinine greater than 0.5 mg/dL within 3 days of contrast administration without alternative cause, is the third most common cause of acute renal failure in hospitalized patients. Nephropathy occurs in up to 10% of patients with normal renal function, but in up to 25% of those with preexisting kidney disease or other risk factors such as diabetes, congestive heart failure, older age, and concomitant use of nephrotoxic drugs. Although the kidneys may eventually recover, permanent damage requiring chronic dialysis therapy may occur.

Prevention of contrast-induced nephropathy includes adequate hydration with intravenous saline before and after the procedure, a dose of 100 cc/hour for a total of 6 to 12 hours. N-acetylcysteine is also provided, 600 to 1200 mg orally, the day before and the day after the procedure.[7] N-acetylcysteine is an inexpensive nutritional supplement with virtually no side effects, and should likely be provided to all patients receiving intravenous contrast dyes.

The profusion of pharmaceutical agents, along with rampant prescribing of multiple drugs by some physicians, sets the stage for undesirable drug interactions and adverse patient reactions. Doctors should assess their patients' vulnerabilities prior to offering drug therapy, caution patients about risks, monitor the metabolic effects of these agents, and rapidly terminate drug use when organ deterioration appears. Renal effects may be progressive and irreversible, and when the patient enters stage 4 or 5 kidney disease, dialysis may be inevitable. Safe nutritional alternatives to drugs exist for the treatment of diabetes and hypertension, the two major causes of renal failure, and these should be employed in combination with, or in preference to, drugs whenever possible.

VI. COMORBIDITIES

Hypertension

Hypertension is not only a major cause of kidney disease, but also determines the rate of progression and the risk of kidney failure.[8] Blood pressure of less than 130/80 is the recommended target blood pressure for individuals with chronic kidney disease.[9]

Patients with greater proteinuria derived more benefit from tighter blood pressure control in the National Institutes of Health–funded study, Modification of Diet in Renal Disease.[10,11] Nutritional and lifestyle modifications included restrictions in dietary sodium and alcohol intake, along with exercise and weight loss. In 840 adults with chronic kidney disease of various origins, the usual blood pressure goal was a mean arterial pressure of <107 mm Hg, while the low blood pressure goal was a mean arterial pressure of <92 mm Hg. After 10 years, the incidence of kidney failure in the low blood pressure group was only 0.68 the incidence in the usual blood pressure group. The low blood pressure group also had a reduced risk of all-cause mortality. The type of medication used to lower blood pressure did not influence the results. In general, angiotensin-converting enzyme (ACE) inhibitors and angiotensin receptor blockers (ARBs) are used preferentially for blood pressure control in patients with renal impairment because of their superior effects on proteinuria. Patients taking these medications must be monitored for hyperkalemia.

Protein intake also influences blood pressure. The International Study of Macronutrients and Blood Pressure confirmed that more vegetable protein, but not animal protein, was associated with lower blood pressure.[12]

The Dietary Approaches to Stop Hypertension (DASH) Study revealed that salt restriction and an increase in protein intake from 14% to 18% of calories reduced systolic and diastolic blood pressure in both hypertensive and nonhypertensive patients.[13] In another study, Chinese adults with prehypertension or mild hypertension were given a diet high in soy protein.[14] Both systolic and diastolic blood pressures fell significantly. Soy protein may reduce blood pressure by increasing insulin sensitivity, or by increasing nitric oxide production from arginine.

High blood pressure affects one-third of adults in industrialized societies. Excess sodium intake is a notorious contributor to hypertension. Primary and age-related hypertension are almost unknown in populations with sodium chloride intake of less than 50 mmol (about 3g) per day. The median urinary sodium excretion in a study involving 32 countries and 10,000 participants was 170 mmol/day, representing a salt intake of 10g.[15]

Processed foods are high in sodium and low in potassium. A cup of canned chicken noodle soup contains 48 mmol of sodium and 1.4 mmol of potassium, while an orange contains no sodium and 6.0 mmol of potassium. Primitive populations eating unprocessed foods have an intake of potassium greater than 150 mmol/day, a sodium intake of 20 to 40 mmol/day, and a ratio of dietary potassium to sodium of 3–10/1. By contrast, people in industrialized societies ingest foods with a potassium to sodium ratio less than 0.4.[16]

Low potassium aggravates the hypertensive effect of high sodium. Increasing potassium intake in rats has lowered blood pressure and reduced stroke and renal damage. Potassium supplementation reduces the requirement for antihypertensive medication. In one study, increasing potassium intake reduced the dose of antihypertensive medication by over half in 81% of patients, and allowed for termination of medication in 38%.[17]

The kidneys eliminate 90% of potassium, the rest exiting by the fecal route. The kidneys are not well adapted to handle a high-sodium diet. A low-potassium diet results in greater sodium retention. High sodium intake increases renal losses of potassium. The long-term effect of potassium depletion is to further promote sodium retention. Thus, our aberrated modern diet of high sodium and low potassium promotes a vicious cycle of physiologic impairment leading to hypertension, arterial wall thickening and rigidity, and arterial thrombosis and atherosclerosis.

Potassium intake should be at least 5 g/day, twice our current intake. The forms of potassium not containing chloride, such as those found in fruits and vegetables, allow more effective cellular exchange of sodium for potassium, and a better antihypertensive effect.[18]

In our practice, nutrients used for blood pressure control include:

1. Fish oils, 1500 to 3000 mg/day of combined EPA/DHA.
2. Magnesium chelate or citrate containing 400 to 800 mg of elemental magnesium (monitor blood levels in renal disease).
3. Potassium citrate containing 400 to 800 mg/day of elemental potassium (monitor blood levels in renal disease).
4. Calcium chelate, malate, or aspartate, containing 400 to 1000 mg/day of elemental calcium.
5. L-arginine, 2000 to 4000 mg/day. L-arginine promotes formation of nitric oxide, a vasodilator.

Metabolic Syndrome

The metabolic syndrome is defined as three or more of the following factors:

1. Elevated blood sugar
2. Low HDL cholesterol
3. High triglycerides
4. Elevated blood pressure
5. Abdominal obesity

The metabolic syndrome has long been recognized to be a significant risk factor for heart disease, stroke, and diabetes. A recent study has identified metabolic syndrome as a risk factor for the development of chronic renal disease as well.[19] In Chen et al. the odds ratio of chronic kidney disease (GFR less than 60) was 2.6 in persons with metabolic syndrome compared to normals. The odds ratio of kidney disease for individuals with four components of the metabolic syndrome was 4.2, and for those with five components it was 5.8. The risk for microalbuminuria (urinary albumin-creatinine ratio of 30 to 300 mg/gm) increased in a similar fashion.

Individually and collectively, low HDL and high triglycerides, obesity, high blood pressure, and elevated blood sugar in the prediabetic range, correlate strongly with the development of renal disease. In fact, it is uncommon to find renal disease in people without any element of the metabolic syndrome.

Thus, lifestyle measures employed for the management of obesity, hypertension, diabetes, and cardiovascular disease will be effective for the prevention and slowing of renal disease. In our practice we recommend a Mediterranean-style diet, low in salt, high in fiber, with protein predominantly vegetable in origin. Compared with a low-fat diet, the Mediterranean diet has superior effects on systolic blood pressure, glucose levels, and cholesterol/HDL ratio.[20] A Mediterranean diet also tends to be an alkalinizing diet as described in Chapter 31, "Osteoporosis."

There is controversy regarding the implementation of soy products in nutritional programs, related to the fact that most soy products in the United States are derived from genetically modified seeds, and possible connections between soy and thyroid disease and bladder cancer.[21] Soy protein, however, has demonstrated benefits in rat studies of aging nephropathy and polycystic kidney disease. Soy modified all components of renal remodeling, proliferation, inflammation, and fibrosis. These favorable changes may result from reduced arachidonic acid synthesis in favor of the anti-inflammatory prostaglandins.[22]

Nutrients used for blood sugar control in our practice include:

1. Chromium—up to 1000 µg/day. Facilitates glucose uptake into cells.[23]
2. Vanadium—50 mg/day. Enhances insulin action. No evidence of toxicity at this dose.[24]
3. Alpha lipoic acid—300 to 1800 mg/day. Improves insulin sensitivity, also effective in treating diabetic neuropathy. It is a strong anti-oxidant and detoxifier, regenerates vitamins C and E, and glutathione.[25]
4. Biotin—3000 µg/day. Improves both insulin sensitivity and diabetic neuropathy.[26]
5. *Gymnema sylvestre*—400 mg/day, which may act to increase insulin release.[27] *Gymnema sylvestre* is an herbal product. There have been numerous reports of problems found in various herbal preparations, including contamination with heavy metals and pesticides, lower dosage than stated, or even the wrong ingredient. It is best to obtain these products from a reputable source, and to verify the absence of contaminants and correct identification of the product.
6. Cinnamon as a spice and in supplemental doses of cinnaminic acid supplements, Cinnulin™, 150 mg/day.

The medical literature indicates that over 50% of diabetes type 2 is preventable using lifestyle changes in individuals with impaired glucose tolerance.[28]

VII.   TREATMENT INTERVENTIONS

CHELATION AND RENAL DISEASE

Chelation therapy with EDTA has been offered as a treatment for cardiovascular disease with the proviso that chelation therapy should not be employed in the presence of elevated creatinine. Recent evidence indicates that chelation therapy may actually delay the progression of renal disease.

Investigators in Taiwan studied patients with chronic renal insufficiency (creatinine 1.5 to 3.9 mg/dL).[29] One gram of calcium disodium ethylenediaminetetraacetic acid (EDTA) was infused over 2 hours, and urine lead was measured in a 72-hour collection. Patients with urinary lead excretion over 80 μg were assigned to either weekly chelation therapy or placebo. Chelation therapy was provided weekly for 24 months.

GFR increased by 11.9% in the chelation therapy group, while it declined in the control group. The body lead burden prior to therapy was similar to that in the general population. Results suggested that chronic low-level environmental lead exposure may aggravate the progression of chronic renal disease, and that chelation therapy may delay progression in patients with chronic renal disease.

Fish Oil for Glomerular Disease

IgA nephropathy is the most common type of glomerulonephritis, and leads to kidney failure in about 25% of patients. Disease recurs in transplanted kidneys, and causes graft failure in half of them. Fish oil therapy reduces proteinuria and protects kidney function. In one case, proteinuria recurred 5 years after renal transplantation. In that patient, proteinuria was quantified at 3299 mg/day prior to therapy. Six capsules of fish oil were given twice daily, for a total dose of 4320 mg eicosapentaenoic acid (EPA) and 2880 mg docosahexaenoic acid (DHA). Proteinuria declined to 458 mg/day, and did not worsen over the next 5 years.[30]

The action of fish oil is thought to be a reduction of vasoconstrictive and proinflammatory eicosanoids, and a decrease in cytokine release.

In another study, fish oils were given to 10 patients with focal sclerosis or membranous glomerulonephritis.[31] The dosage was 10 g/day of combined EPA and DHA, as ethyl esters. Platelet thromboxane declined 25%, triglycerides fell 30%, and bleeding time increased by 2 minutes. Proteinuria declined from 3.7 g/day to 2.6 g/day at week 6, when treatment was stopped. The decline in proteinuria persisted for another 12 weeks, and then returned to prior levels.

Chronic Renal Failure

Dietary protein restriction is the mainstay of therapy in chronic renal failure. When animals with renal injury were fed a high-protein diet, renal failure ensued, while a low-protein diet slowed the progression. High-protein diets may aggravate renal disease by:

1. Stimulating nephron cell hypertrophy and proliferation, and glomerular scarring
2. Increasing reactive oxygen species
3. Creating an acid load, causing ammonium production and complement formation
4. Increasing urea formation, causing hypertrophy of renal tubules
5. Generating aldosterone and angiotensin II

Low-protein diets result in less uremic toxicity, so patients fed these diets may be able to avoid dialysis therapy at lower levels of renal function than patients on high-protein regimens.[32] Soy protein, compared with casein, an animal protein, more effectively slowed progression of renal disease.[33]

When glomerular filtration rate falls to between 25 and 70 mL/1.73m^2/minute, recommended protein intake is 0.6 g/kg/day. With GFR below 25 mL/1.73m^2/minute, it becomes increasingly important to pursue protein restriction. The low-protein diet generates fewer toxic nitrogenous byproducts, and has the additional benefit of lower potassium and phosphorus content. At this stage, renal excretion of potassium, magnesium, and phosphorus is usually impaired, and blood levels may rise excessively. When GFR falls below 5 mL/1.73m^2/minute, the risk of malnutrition and uremic toxicity is high, and renal replacement therapy through transplantation or dialysis should be pursued. Hemodialysis patients should receive 1.1 to 1.2 g of protein/kg/day. Peritoneal dialysis patients lose about 9 g of protein daily into the dialysate, as well as 2.5 to 4.0 g of amino acids. They should receive 1.2 to 1.3 g protein/kg/day.

In nephrotic syndrome, seen in glomerular diseases and common in diabetic renal disease, the heavy urinary protein loss is accompanied by the loss of protein-bound nutrients, including iron, copper, and vitamin D. Heavy proteinuria potentiates renal failure, perhaps through the irritative effect of proteins on glomerular tissue.

Renal failure causes weakness, nausea, and vomiting, weight loss, anemia, itching, muscle cramps, tremors, neuropathy, irritability, and cognitive dysfunction, eventuating in coma. Potassium, magnesium, and phosphorus levels rise, calcium declines due to hyperphosphatemia, and bicarbonate falls due to retained acids. Aluminum, mercury, and other toxic metals may accumulate due to the loss of usual renal excretion. Deficiencies of vitamin B6, vitamin C, and folic acid occur. 1,25-dihydroxyvitamin D production by the kidneys is greatly impaired.

Amino acid metabolism changes. Taurine levels are low, and l-carnitine levels are depressed in dialysis patients, impairing the metabolism of long-chain fatty acids in mitochondria and perhaps affecting energy production. L-carnitine supplementation is often provided either intravenously or orally, mainly to patients with muscle weakness, cramps, cardiomyopathy, anemia, and hypotension. The oral dose is 0.5 g/day.

Uremia is invariably fatal without intervention in the form of renal transplantation or dialysis, either hemo- or peritoneal dialysis. The success rate of transplantation has greatly improved, now 90% at 1 year, but there is a shortage of donor kidneys. The majority of patients are treated with dialysis, but long-term survival is limited, and dialysis itself is sometimes poorly tolerated. Daily dialysis therapy offers an improved quality of life.

Cardiovascular mortality in dialysis patients is extremely high, 25% per year, somewhat related to preexisting disease. Homocysteine levels are markedly elevated. Treatment with high doses of folic acid, vitamin B12, and vitamin B6, while reducing homocysteine levels, has not affected cardiovascular complications significantly.[34] Cholesterol levels are also often elevated in dialysis patients, but treatment with statin drugs has not improved survival.[35] The results suggest a different pathophysiology of cardiovascular disease in dialysis patients, perhaps related to the dialysis process itself.

Phosphorus levels rise in chronic renal failure, lowering serum calcium and leading to hyperparathyroidism. This causes increased morbidity and mortality. Reduced phosphorus intake, a concomitant of the low-protein diet, slows the advance of chronic renal failure. Phosphorus levels should be kept between 2.7 to 4.6 mg/dL. Aluminum-containing phosphate binders, once commonly employed, should be avoided, because aluminum may induce a syndrome of osteomalacia, anemia, weakness, and dementia. Instead, calcium carbonate, citrate, or acetate can effectively lower phosphorus levels.

Calcium requirements increase in renal failure because of impaired renal production of 1,25-dihydroxyvitamin D and resistance to vitamin D actions. Further, the low-protein and low-phosphorus diet is also low in calcium. Most renal failure patients on low-protein diets require supplemental calcium of 1000 to 1400 mg/day. If the 25-hydroxyvitamin D level is less than 30 ng/mL, replacement should be provided with vitamin D2 (ergocalciferol). In addition, for patients with high parathyroid hormone levels (over 300 pg/mL of the intact hormone), the hyperparathyroidism can be suppressed using 1,25-dihydroxyvitamin D (calcitriol) or a related compound such as alpha-calcidol or paricalcitol.

Table 22.1 recommends nutrient intakes in chronic renal failure and dialysis patients. Patients with advanced renal disease or on dialysis may be depleted of water-soluble vitamins and certain minerals. Anorexia, poor food intake, and the protein-limited diet cause these deficiencies, along with altered metabolism, prescribed medications, and the dialysis process itself. Vitamin B6, vitamin C, and folic acid are most often deficient. Vitamin B12 is stored in the body, is protein-bound and not lost in dialysis, so that deficiency is uncommon. Vitamin C should not be given in doses higher than 60 mg/day. Ascorbic acid may be converted to oxalate, which is highly insoluble and may be deposited in tissues, thus aggravating renal insufficiency. A 31-year-old renal failure patient had been taking 2 g of vitamin C daily for 3 years while on dialysis. Her kidney transplant initially functioned well but later failed, and she had widespread deposition of calcium oxalate crystals in the transplanted kidney.[36]

TABLE 22.1

Recommended Nutrient Intake for Nondialyzed Patients With Chronic Renal Failure and Patients Undergoing Maintenance Hemodialysis or Chronic Peritoneal Dialysis[37]

Nutrients	Chronic Renal Failure	Maintenance Dialysis	Comments
Protein	0. 60–0.75 g/kg/d	Hemodialysis 1.1–1.2 g/kg/d Chronic peritoneal dialysis 1.2–1.3g/kg/d, up to 1.5 g/kg/d if indicated	Over half should be high biologic value protein.
Energy	35 kcal/kg/d	35 kcal/kg/d	Reduce if the patient's relative body weight is >120% or the patient gains unwanted weight.
Fat (as percent of total energy intake)	30–40	30–40	If triglyceride levels are markedly elevated, percentage of fat in the diet may be increased to 40%. Otherwise, 30% is preferable.
Carbohydrate	Remainder of nonprotein calories	Remainder of nonprotein calories	Should be primarily complex carbohydrates.
Fiber	20–25 g/d	20–25 g/d	Total intake.

Minerals (Diets to be supplemented with these quantities)

Sodium	1000–3000 mg/d	750–1000 mg/d	
Potassium	40–70 meq/d	40–70 meq/d	
Phosphorus	5–10 mg/kg/d	8–17 mg/kg/d	
Calcium	1400–1600 mg/d	1400–1600 mg/kg/d	
Magnesium	200–300 mg/d	200–300 mg/d	
Iron	10–18 mg/d	variable	
Zinc	15 mg/d	15 mg/d	
Water	~1500 mL/d, as tolerated	usually 750–1500 mL/d	

Vitamins (Diets to be supplemented with these quantities)

Thiamin	1.5 mg/d	1.5 mg/d	
Riboflavin	1.8 mg/d	1.8 mg/d	
Pantothenic acid	5 mg/d	5 mg/d	
Niacin	20 mg/d	20 mg/d	
Pyridoxine HCl	15 mg/d	5–10 mg/d	
Vitamin B12	3 µg/d	3 µg/d	
Vitamin C	60 mg/d	60 mg/d	
Folic acid	1–10 mg/d	1–10 mg/d	Determine dose by serum homocysteine level.
Vitamin A	No addition	No addition	
Vitamin D	Variable	Variable	Dose depends on phosphorus and calcium levels. Provided as 1,25-dihydroxyvitamin D3 or synthetic.
Vitamin E	15 IU/d	15 IU/d	
Vitamin K	None	None	May be necessary if malnutrition present or patient is on antibiotics.

Source: [37].

Vitamin A levels are elevated in uremia, and vitamin A should not be supplemented. Doses above 7500 IU/day may cause bone toxicity.

Nutritional modifications in renal failure are so substantial and difficult to implement that patients should not be confronted with all requirements at once. Of primary importance is restriction of dietary protein, phosphorus, potassium, and magnesium, and supplementation of calcium. Fluid and sodium control, increased dietary fiber, and reduced saturated fat and refined carbohydrate intake are of secondary importance.

VIII. SUMMARY

Kidney disease is largely a consequence of hypertension, obesity, diabetes, metabolic syndrome, and drug and environmental toxicities. The same factors are underlying causes of many chronic degenerative diseases. Correction and prevention of these conditions will yield a reduced incidence of renal failure.

Medical professionals should pay greater attention to the signs of altered renal function. These are:

- Increasing serum creatinine, even within the normal range.
- Proteinuria—measure urine microalbumin in all patients with hypertension, diabetes, and prediabetes. Repeat this test at regular intervals. The level of proteinuria correlates with the presence and the advance of kidney disease.
- Increasing hypertension.
- Possible drug toxicities—patients taking one or more drugs known to cause kidney damage, especially NSAIDS and antibiotics.

Kidney disease is often not discovered until it is advanced, and the opportunity to reverse the damage has become remote. If renal impairment is detected early, and corrective measures are implemented, it need not progress.

Proteinuria can be reversed, with concomitant preservation of renal function, by using fish oils in high dosage, and preferentially using ACE inhibitors and ARBs for the management of hypertension and proteinuria.

A low-protein diet, consisting mainly of vegetable protein, slows the progression of kidney disease. The diet should also be alkalinizing.

The additive effect of reno-toxic medications, given in consort, should be considered when prescribing medications. Doses should be lower when there is evidence of renal compromise. Renal status should be monitored during the course of therapy, and drugs should be stopped if renal impairment intervenes.

Reno-protective measures should be followed under all circumstances, and not reserved only for those with known kidney impairment. Adequate hydration and N-acetylcysteine prevent contrast-induced nephropathy, have no risks, and should be routinely provided.

Perhaps the most effective means of protecting renal integrity is yet the most difficult to implement—lowering blood pressure by reversing the sodium/potassium ratio in the Western diet. Potassium content is high in plant-based, whole-foods diets, while sodium content is low. Refined foods and packaged products contain sodium in excess. Doctors should instruct their patients on ways to establish potassium dominance in meal planning.

REFERENCES

1. Goldman L, et al. *Cecil Medicine 23rd edition.* Philadelphia: Saunders Elsevier. 2008 p. 936.
2. Goldman L, et al. *Cecil Medicine 23rd edition.* Philadelphia: Saunders Elsevier. 2008 p. 922.
3. Kay J, Bazari H, Avery L, et al. Case 6-2008—A 46-Year-Old Woman with Renal Failure and Stiffness of the Joints and Skin. *NEJM.* 2008; 358:827–839.

4. Nortier J, Muniz-Martinez M, Schmeiser H, et al. Urothelial Carcinoma Associated with the Use of a Chinese Herb (Aristolochia fangchi). *NEJM*. 2000; 342:1682–1692.
5. Goldman L, et al. *Cecil Medicine 23rd edition,* Saunders Elsevier. 2008 p. 863.
6. Wanner C, Krane V, März W, et al. Atorvastatin in Patients with Type 2 Diabetes Mellitus Undergoing Hemodialysis. *NEJM*. 2005; 353:238–248.
7. Kelly A, Dwamena B, Cronin P, et al. Meta-analysis: Effectiveness of Drugs for Preventing, Contrast-Induced Nephropathy. *Ann Intern Med*. 2008; 148:284–294.
8. Sarnak M, Greene T, Wang X, et al. The Effect of a Lower Target Blood Pressure on the Progression of Kidney Disease: Long-Term Follow-up of the Modification of Diet in Renal Disease Study. *Ann Intern Med*. 2005; 142:342–351.
9. Initiative KDOQ: K/DOQI Clinical Practice Guidelines on Hypertension and Antihypertensive Agents in Chronic Kidney Disease. *Am J Kidney Dis*. 2004; 43:S1–S290.
10. Klahr S, Levey A, Beck G, et al. The Effects of Dietary Protein Restriction and Blood-Pressure Control on the Progression of Chronic Renal Disease. *NEJM*. 1994; 330:877–884.
11. Levey A, Caggiula A, et al. Effects of Dietary Protein Restriction on the Progression of Advanced Renal Disease in the Modification of Diet in Renal Disease Study. *Am J Kidney Dis*. 1996; 27:652–663.
12. Elliot P, Stamler J, Dyer A, et al. Association Between Protein Intake and Blood Pressure: The INTERMAP Study. *Arch Intern Med*. 2006; 166:79–87.
13. Sacks F, Svetkey L, Vollmer W, et al. Effects on Blood Pressure of Reduced Dietary Sodium and the Dietary Approaches to Stop Hypertension (DASH) Diet. *NEJM*. 2001; 344:3–10.
14. He J, Gu D, Wu X, et al. Effect of Soybean Protein on Blood Pressure: A Randomized, Controlled Trial. *Ann Intern Med*. 2005; 143:1–9.
15. Intersalt Cooperative Research Group. Intersalt: An International Study of Electrolyte Excretion and Blood Pressure. Result for 24 Hour Urinary Sodium and Potassium Excretion. *BMJ*. 1988; 297:319–328.
16. Standing Committee on the Scientific Evaluation of Dietary Reference Intakes. *Dietary Reference Intakes for Water, Potassium, Sodium, Chloride, and Sulfate*. National Academies Press, 2005.
17. Sinai A, Strazzullo P, Giacco A, et al. Increasing the Dietary Potassium Intake Reduces the Need for Antihypertensive Medication. *Ann Intern Med*. 1991; 115:753–759.
18. Adrogué H, Madias N. Sodium and Potassiumin the Pathogenesis of Hypertension. *NEJM*. 2007; 356:1966–1978.
19. Chen J, Munter P, Hamm L, et al. The Metabolic Syndrome and Chronic Kidney Disease in U.S. Adults. *Ann Intern Med*. 2004; 140:167–174.
20. Estruch R, Martínez-Gonzalez MA, Corella D, et al. Effects of a Mediterranean-Style Diet on Cardiovascular Risk Factors: A Randomized Trial. *Ann Intern Med*. 2006; 145:1–11.
21. Sun C, Yuan J, Arakawa K, et al. Dietary Soy and Increased Risk of Bladder Cancer: the Singapore Chinese Health Study. *Cancer Epidemiol Biomarkers Prev*. 2002; 11:1674–1677.
22. Ogborn M, Nitschmann E, Weiler H, et al. Modification of Polycystic Kidney Disease and Fatty Acid Status by Soy Protein Diet. *Kidney International*. 2000; 57:159–166.
23. Anderson RA, Cheng N, Bryden NA, et al. Elevated Intakes of Supplemental Chromium Improve Glucose and Insulin Variables in Individuals with Type 2 Diabetes. *Diabetes*. 1997; 46:1786–1791.
24. Boden G, Chen X, Ruiz, et al. Effects of Vanadyl Sulfate on Carbohydrate and Lipid Metabolism in Patients with Non-Insulin-Dependent Diabetes Mellitus. *Metabolism*. 1996; 45:1130–1135.
25. Jacob S, Russ P, Hermann R, et al. Oral Administration of RAC-alpha-lipoic Acid Modulates Insulin Sensitivity in Patients with Type-2 Diabetes Mellitus: A Placebo Controlled Pilot Trial. *Free Radic Biol Med*. 1999; 27:309–314.
26. Koutsikos D, Agroyannis B, Tazanatos-Exarchou H. Biotin for Diabetic Peripheral Neuropathy. *Biomed Pharmacother*. 1990; 44:511–514.
27. Baskaran K, Ahmath BK, Shanmugasundaram KR, et al. Antidiabetic Effect of a Leaf Extract From Gymnema Sylvestre in Non-Insulin-Dependent Diabetes Mellitus Patients. *J Ethnopharmacol*. 1990; 30:295–305.
28. Tuomilehto J, Lindstrom J, Eriksson J, et al. Prevention of Type 2 Diabetes Mellitus by Changes in Lifestyle among Subjects with Impaired Glucose Tolerance. *NEJM*. 2001; 344:1343–1350.
29. Lin J, Lin-Tan D, Hsu K, et al. Environmental Lead Exposure and Progression of Chronic Renal Disease in Patients without Diabetes. *NEJM*. 2003; 348:277–286.
30. Ng R. Fish Oil Therapy in Recurrent IgA Nephropathy. *Ann Intern Med*. 2003; 138:1011.
31. De Caterina R, Caprioli R, Giannessi D, et al. n-3 Fatty Acids Reduce Proteinuria in Patients with Chronic Glomerular Disease. *Kidney International*. 1993; 44:843–850.

32. Shils M, et al. *Modern Nutrition in Health and Disease, 10th Edition.* Baltimore, MD: Lippincott Williams and Wilkins. 2006; pp. 1475–1501.

33. Damico G, Gentile MG, Manna G, et al. Effect of Vegetarian Soy Diet on Hyperlipidaemia in Nephrotic Syndrome. *Lancet.* 1992; 339:1131–1134.

34. Jamison R, Hartigan P, Kaufman J, et al. Effect of Homocysteine Lowering on Mortality and Vascular Disease in Advanced Chronic Kidney Disease and End-stage Renal Disease. *JAMA.* 2007; 298:1163–1170.

35. Wanner C, Krane V, März W, et al. Atorvastatin in Patients with Type 2 Diabetes Mellitus Undergoing Hemodialysis. *NEJM.* 2005; 353:238–248.

36. Nankivell BJ, Murali KM. Renal Failure from Vitamin C after Transplantation. *NEJM.* 2008; 358:e4.

37. Shils M, et al. *Modern Nutrition in Health and Disease, 10th Edition.* Baltimore, MD: Lippincott Williams and Wilkins. 2006; 1487.

Section VI

Neurologic and Psychiatric Disorders

23 Autistic Spectrum Disorder

Dynamic Intervention for Neuronal Membrane Stabilization

Patricia C. Kane, Ph.D., Annette L. Cartaxo, M.D., and Richard C. Deth, Ph.D.

I. INTRODUCTION

Autistic spectrum disorder (ASD) is a neurodevelopmental disorder characterized by impairments in social interaction, communication, behavioral stereotypes, and a range of cognitive deficits. Clinical signs of autism are frequently present at 3 years of age, but many toddlers demonstrate abnormalities in social, communication, and play behavior as early as 14 months. These impairments are considered to arise as a consequence of a disturbed neural network during pre- or postnatal development.

Children within the realm of ASD exhibit a systemic presentation that has forced us to look deeper, to embrace the whole person—the brain, the nervous system, the gastrointestinal system, the immune system, the endocrine system, the hepatic system. Children with autism will teach us as no patient ever has before.

A new autism model is emerging[1] with a major shift in emphasis from genetic causality to environmental factors that act upon individual genetic vulnerability, to systemic insult, to cellular function. This chapter approaches autism by discarding the old model of autism as a static or "fixed" condition, and embracing autism as a dynamic condition with changeable features, where significant improvements and recoveries are reachable. By carefully examining the state of the cell membrane, the relevant neurochemistry, and the essential fatty acid status, we have a metabolic window into attaining an individualized biomedical approach toward food and nutrient-based interventions.

II. EPIDEMIOLOGY

Autism was initially described in the U.S. and European medical literature in the 1940s, and was deemed to be rare until the 1980s, when the prevalence was determined to be no more than 5 per 10,000 persons. Today the prevalence of ASDs is understood to be many times greater, second only to mental retardation among the most common serious developmental disabilities in the United States,[2] occurring in 1 in 150 children.

In 2007, in the most recent government survey on the rate of autism, the Centers for Disease Control and Prevention (CDC) found that the rate is higher than the rates found from studies conducted in the United States during the 1980s and early 1990s. The debate continues about whether or not this represents a true increase in the prevalence of autism or a change in criteria used to diagnose it. Increased recognition of the disorder by health care professionals and the general public may be a contributing factor to the increasing rates.

Nonetheless, the CDC report confirms other recent epidemiologic studies documenting that more children are being diagnosed today than ever before.

Epidemiological surveys of ASD have now been carried out in several countries yielding some common characteristics, including an association with cognitive deficits in ~60% of the cases of idiopathic autism, and ~30% with autism spectrum taken as a whole. The three diagnoses of ASD include Autistic disorder, Asperger's disorder, and Pervasive Developmental Disorder Not Otherwise Specified (PDD-NOS).

The male-to-female ratio of children with autism is 4.3:1 among those with comorbid mental retardation. While approximately 70% of individuals with ASD have IQs measured below 70, it is considered "functional retardation"; some individuals with ASD have very high IQ readings in specific subtests or overall. ASD is a condition separate from mental retardation and there exists a clear distinction between the two disorders. Estimates of the occurrence of epilepsy associated with autism vary, but the latest consensus is 30%.[3] There is a 5% to 10% association with rare and genetic medical conditions, but no correlation with social class, race, and ethnicity.[4]

III. PATHOPHYSIOLOGY

The new biological model for autism contends that there are many "autisms" and that the etiology of the disorder is based on biology, not behavior. Autism has been modeled as a brain-based, strongly genetic disorder, but emerging findings and hypotheses support a broader model of this condition as being genetically influenced and systemic. The rising incidence of autism warrants a closer look at both preventable causes and potential solutions related to genetic, environmental, and nutritional factors. The new autism paradigm (Table 23.1) proposed by Martha Herbert[1,9] attempts to reconcile the controversy.

Herbert views multiple levels of understanding of autism that point us toward an integration of basic and practical research:

- Chronicity—Autism now appears to be not simply a result of something abnormal before a child is born, but instead a result of processes that are ongoing and active.
- Plasticity—We have a greater appreciation of dynamic, changeable features of autism and the possibility of sustained improvement.
- Complexity—New knowledge is illuminating the many levels of autism within each individual as neurological, medical, metabolic, molecular, and genetic, existing alongside communication and behavior.

Reports of rate increases and improvement or recovery support a role for modulation of the condition by controlling environmental factors, according to Herbert and other prominent investigators. Altered neurodevelopment is widely recognized as the underlying neuropathological cause of

TABLE 23.1
Changing Models of Autism

Old Model	New Model
Genetically determined	Environmentally triggered; genetically influenced
Brain based	Both brain and body are involved
Hard wired	Metabolic abnormalities play a big role
Treatable but not curable	Treatable and recovery possible

ASD. There is evidence of postnatal evolution and chronic persistence of brain, behavior, and tissue changes, along with physical illness and symptomatology such as gastrointestinal, immune, and hepatic involvement. Autistic features may overlap with other disorders:

Fragile X syndrome, tuberous sclerosis, Landau-Kleffner syndrome, Angelman's syndrome, Lesch-Nyhan syndrome, adrenoleukodystrophy, ornithine transcarbamylase deficiency, Huntington's chorea, glutaric aciduria, phenylketonuria, hyperasparaginemia, propionic acidemia, systemic carnitine deficiency, purine disorders, cobalamin metabolism defects, sulfite oxidase deficiency, cytomegalovirus, West Nile virus, herpes encephalitis, Rett's syndrome, congenital rubella, phenosulphotransferase-P deficiency, porphyria, and Smith-Lemli-Optiz syndrome.

Investigations into the etiology of autism include genetic and epigenetic factors, environmental toxicity, errors in metabolism, acquired errors in metabolism resulting in metabolic disturbance, hepatic dysfunction, endocrine imbalance, disturbed membrane stability, and neuroinflammation as focal points. The cause of autism is very likely a common pathophysiologic sequence that is triggered in various ways by epigenetic and/or environmental factors. The biomedical approach in the treatment of ASD considers that the brain and body can be injured together, that behavioral problems stem from altered tissue properties, that biomedical treatments focused toward stabilizing cellular function can help heal tissue, and that healthier tissue generates healthier behaviors.

NEUROINFLAMMATION

Zimmerman and colleagues, at Johns Hopkins,[10–12] identified neuroinflammation in autism in 2005. In essence, they hypothesize that environmental factors such as neurotoxins, infections, and maternal infections; genetic susceptibility; and the immunogenetic background of the child affect the development of aberrations in cortical organization and neuronal circuitry. Consequently, neuroinflammatory changes occur, resulting in the eruption of autistic symptoms. Their research has demonstrated neuroglial and innate neuroimmune system activation, as evidenced by neuroinflammation in the brains studied, with marked activation of microglia and astroglia.

Neuroinflammatory processes were isolated in the cerebral cortex, white matter, and notably, in the cerebellum. The neuroinflammation appears to reflect innate CNS response, but not to involve the adaptive immune system with lymphocytes. Classical descriptions of inflammatory processes involve a vascular component. Autism lacks both a vascular component and a classical inflammatory response. The immune system appears activated exclusively within the brain and in aspects only of its innate components, astrocytes and microglial cells, and the influx of macrophages. Cytokine profiling revealed elevations in a number of proinflammatory cytokines in brain tissue, particularly macrophage chemoattractant protein (MCP-1) and tumor growth factor-beta 1, derived from neuroglia. The cerebellum was isolated as the focus of an active and chronic neuroinflammatory process. Cerebral spinal fluid (CSF) showed a unique proinflammatory profile of cytokines, including a marked increase in MCP-1, as noted in the Vargas et al. studies, while recently Chez and colleagues[13] identified elevation of tumor necrosis-α (TNFα) in CSF.

Cytokines and chemokines play important roles as mediators of inflammatory reactions in the CNS and in the neuronal-neuroglial interactions.[14] The immune and nervous systems are complex, highly evolved networks that transmit signals through the release of chemical mediators such as cytokines and neuropeptides. The neuronal synapse and the contact interface between T cells and antigen-presenting cells share a similar architecture. There is continual communication between the immune and nervous systems, with many peptides playing a role in both. It has been proposed that abnormalities in the levels and actions of neurotransmitters or neuroactive compounds during early critical windows of neurodevelopment may lead to the onset of autism. Neurotransmitters and neuropeptides not only have crucial roles in the development and organization of neural tissue, but also have a systemic impact on almost all body functions, including immunity. Numerous transmitter systems, including acetylcholine, dopamine, glutamate, serotonin (5-HT), epinephrine, norepinephrine, oxytocin, vasopressin, and γ-aminobutyric acid (GABA), have been studied in autism,[15] revealing a 48% to 61% decrease in glutamic acid decarboxylase, an enzyme that converts glutamate into GABA, in the parietal and cerebellar regions of the brain, compared with controls.[16] In autism, this may suppress the GABA-ergic system, resulting in seizures due to the heightened stimulation of the glutamate system. In addition, excitotoxic damage of neurons may result in abnormal structural development of the brain due to glutamate hyperactivity.[17]

Two early biomarkers of neuronal toxicity are mitochondrial dysfunction (depolarization, decreased ATP synthesis, structural collapse, and potential opening of the permeability transition pore) and the formation of focal swellings (termed dendritic beads) along the length of dendrites. The appearance of dendritic beads is indicative of dysfunctional (depolarized and morphologically collapsed) mitochondria due to toxic exposure.[18]

Mitochondrial dysfunction and dendritic beading are both initiated by glutamate excitotoxicity. However, these events can also be induced by a combination of mitochondrial depolarization (or the subsequent failure of ATP synthesis) and ion (sodium and/or calcium) influx involving an increase in intracellular NaCl (osmotically driven H_2O) following the rapid failure of active Na^+ efflux or Ca^{2+}-dependent excitotoxicity. Kane and Cartaxo have observed frequent elevation of serum calcium in 90% of children with ASD in ~10,000 analyses of blood chemistries over the past 25 years.

Mitochondria are highly dynamic organelles with their trafficking and elongated morphology being regulated by neuronal and mitochondrial activity. Mitochondrial transport, morphology, and function are affected by physiological activity such as synaptic transmission and pathological processes, as manifested in excitotoxicity.

Dendrites are especially vulnerable to neuronal injury under pathological conditions. Given that excitatory synaptic contacts are made predominantly on dendritic arbors, the dendrites have been demonstrated to be the initial site of glutamate-mediated excitotoxic injury.[19]

Mitochondria exhibit changes in both mobility and morphology during excitotoxicity. Under normal physiological conditions, mitochondria within neuronal dendrites appear elongated and undergo extensive directional and lateral movement. However, following exposure of neurons to glutamate[20] or synaptic activity,[21] an inhibition of mitochondrial movement is observed. This is accompanied by a change in mitochondrial shape from an elongated to a rounded/swollen morphology.[20–24]

Although mitochondrial induction of delayed calcium deregulation (DCD) involves the generation of cell-damaging reactive oxygen species (ROS) by calcium-loaded mitochondria, which some might suggest to be "oxidative stress," it has been demonstrated that levels of ROS only increase significantly following the induction of DCD, implying that the release of ROS is a *consequence rather than a cause* of calcium deregulation[25] Recently, it has been reported that the critical factor responsible for the induction of DCD appears to be bioenergetic insufficiency and downstream failure of plasma membrane ion pumps.[26] This mechanism is supported by observations that mitochondrial ATP production is impaired during excitotoxic insults and neuronal ATP levels are diminished rapidly.[27,28] There is also indication that dendritic beading results from disruption of the cytoskeleton, which has been viewed during ultrastructural studies of human cortical biopsies, which revealed disrupted microtubules in dendritic beads.[29]

To attempt to stabilize mitochondrial function and production of ATP it would be necessary to optimize mitochondrial membrane morphology, which is dependent upon cardiolipin. Cardiolipin (CL) is an acidic phospholipid present almost exclusively in membranes of mitochondria, which generate an electrochemical potential gradient for ATP synthesis, providing stability to respiratory chain supercomplexes. Cardiolipin structurally appears as the joining of two phospholipids at their respective head groups. Appearing as a "Siamese twins" structure, cardiolipin has two lipid tails on each phospholipid, but with the connection, has four lipid tails. Cardiolipin's four acyl chains are composed of ~80% linoleic acid (18:2ω6), a polyunsaturated fatty acid of the ω6 series.

Cardiolipin is found only in the inner matrix of the mitochondria, and has one specific function, that of slowing down the high activity level that is characteristic of all active membrane lipids. It is especially useful in its particular location on the inner leaflet of the mitochondria, considering the critical demands of the electron chain transfer of the Krebs cycle. Cardiolipin biosynthesis is regulated by the mitochondrial transmembrane pH gradient. The disruption of the pH gradient, but not membrane potential or ATP synthesis, results in decreased cardiolipin synthesis.[30] Therefore, the pathway for cardiolipin biosynthesis is regulated by the transmembrane pH component of the proton-motive force generated by the mitochondrial respiratory chain, thus the alteration of subcellular pH as a mechanism of regulation of phospholipid biosynthesis.

Recent attention has focused on mitochondrial involvement in ASD by Zimmerman and colleagues[31] after identifying that a 19-month-old girl developed ASD associated with mitochondrial dysfunction following nine vaccinations at one time at 18 months of age. Muscle biopsy revealed an increased lipid content and reduced cytochrome c oxidase activity, along with marked reductions in enzymatic activities for complex I and III. To determine the frequency of routine laboratory abnormalities in similar patients, tests were performed on 159 patients with autism. Aspartate aminotransferase was elevated in 38% of patients with autism compared with 15% of controls ($P < .0001$). The serum creatine kinase level also was abnormally elevated in 22 (47%) of 47 patients studied with autism. Elevation of creatine kinase is directly linked to suppression of phosphatidylcholine in the cell membrane.

In 2002, Fillano and colleagues[32] found that children with a clinical constellation of symptoms, including hypotonia, epileptic seizures, autism, and developmental delay, had mitochondrial dysfunction, including extensive abnormalities in specific enzyme activities, mitochondrial structure, and mitochondrial DNA integrity, and termed the condition HEADD syndrome.

Kane and Cartaxo view ASD as a disturbance in cellular function due to toxic insult. It is apparent that there is marked impairment in peroxisomal function due to the characteristic buildup of very long chain fatty acids.[33–46] Ceramides, or lipid rafts, can accumulate[47] after toxic insult, impairing cell structure and function. Phospholipid architecture and cell membrane integrity can be distorted if there is an overexpression of ceramides, so that peptides, receptors, and ion channels are compromised. Mitochondrial function may also be involved due to global cellular derangement and inefficient metabolism. Yechiel and Barenholtz[48] describe the phenomenon of an overall swollen morphology of the cell if it is deprived of phosphatidylcholine, or is subject to toxic insult. In addition, these researchers found that the higher the level of creatine kinase, the lower the phosphatidylcholine (PC) level in the cell. Control of mitochondrial respiration must be achieved through cardiolipin homeostasis. Phosphatidylcholine supports the stabilization of the mitochondrial (cardiolipin) and cell (phospholipid) membranes with oral and intravenous use, and may be the mechanism by which ASD patients have positive responses to the Membrane Stabilizing Protocol.[42] Dendritic beading does not always result in cell death, *and* some cells recover from the original toxic insult.[28] Perhaps this is the pivotal point whereby ASD is not a static condition, but rather a dynamic one where a child's neurological status can improve. By approaching ASD from a cell membrane perspective we have a treatment regime that targets the core of this disorder.

NEUROTOXICITY, ALTERED NEUROTRANSMISSION, AND FALSE NEUROTRANSMITTERS

Consideration must be given to the possibility that various classes of environmental factors contribute to the etiology of neuroinflammation in autism, since low-dose persistent toxic exposures may prove relevant, especially where genetics plays a role in modulating the threshold for vulnerability.[49]

An intriguing hypothesis is that brain-specific autoantibodies[50,51] found in serum may be increased through pathways that induce neuronal degeneration and dysfunction in the absence of any immune-mediated mechanism. Among these pathways are chronic, subclinical infection or the sequelae of past infection;[52–55] the consequence of maternal infection, such as influenza[16,56–59] or exposure to a naturally occurring feline-borne or equine-borne pathogen, such as Borna disease virus.[60–63]

These autoantibodies may eventually serve as diagnostic markers for autism. Neonatal Borna disease virus (BDV) appears to be linked to neuronal loss in the hippocampus, neocortex, and cerebellum, with hallmark Purkinje cell degeneration and predominant dendritic abnormalities.[3] Similarly, Margaret Bauman found the same areas of the brain affected in ASD as in Borna virus-associated abnormalities, along with "stunting of dendritic arbors" after detailed examination of ASD brains.[64,65] In both BDV and ASD, behavioral anomalies include deficient social behaviors, cognitive deficits, hyperactivity, and stereotypy. The similarities of BDV and ASD are reviewed in Bauman's book, *The Neurobiology of Autism*,[64] stating that there are a striking number of parallel symptoms and features, including brain pathology, neurochemical alterations, and behavioral deficits that closely link autism and Borna disease virus.[66]

Fatemi and colleagues[16] have identified a sharp elevation of 5-HIAA (hydroxyindoleacetic acid) and serotonin via neurochemical analysis of the brains of mice whose mothers were injected with human influenza virus. Thus, increased 5-HIAA may have a strong link to the genesis of ASD.

Kane[33] proposed in 1996 that ASD may be the aftermath of a toxic insult (viral infection, acetaminophen overdose, heavy metal toxicity) evoking hepatic encephalopathy, resulting in hyperammonemia and suppression of several key enzymes, such as carbamylphosphate synthetase, glutamine synthetase, and ornithine transcarbamylase. In addition, alteration in serotonin and dopamine metabolism could occur with characteristic elevation of metabolites 5-HIAA (5-hydroxyindoleacetic acid), DOPAC (3,4-dihydroxyphenylacetic acid), and IAA (indole-3-acetic acid). Kane[33] found that children with ASD consistently have elevated serum blood urea nitrogen (BUN) levels that normalize as their symptoms of autism resolve with oral and IV phospholipid therapy.

Both Page and Coleman found organic acidemia in artifacts such as elevated uric acid and orotic acid in urine depicting purine autism[67–69] and poor nitrogen clearance involving hyperammonemic states. Folate deficiency causes massive incorporation of uracil into DNA and subsequently chromosome breaks due to disturbed methylation. Both high DNA uracil levels and elevated micronucleus frequency (a measure of chromosome breaks) are reversed by folate (folinic acid or tetrahydrobiopterin, not folic acid) administration.[70]

Orotic acid found in urine may indicate an ornithine transcarbamylase deficiency with an accompanying state of hyperammonemia and susceptibility to seizures. Impairment or damage of the orthithine transcarbamylase hepatic enzyme may be exacerbated by exposure to heavy metals such as mercury, or by toxic doses of acetaminophen.

It is conceivable that, rather than the full expression of hepatic encephalopathy, a milder form, termed metabolic or subclinical encephalopathy, may result in autistic features. Brain abnormalities in hepatic encephalopathy include astrocytic rather than neuronal changes,[71] whereby astrocytes take on a characteristic swollen shape distinctive in Alzheimer's disease.[9,18,72,73] This phenomenon is described in autism, and appears quite similar to the neuroinflammation in Alzheimer's disease.

The metabolites of altered serotonin metabolism and ammonia are a result of postviral insult. The hallmark of hepatic encephalopathy, hyperammonemia, produces an increase in brain glutamine, which results in an increase in brain water and a deterioration in neuropsychological function.[74]

In the brain, the astrocyte is the main arena for ammonia detoxification, during the conversion of glutamate to glutamine. Astrocytes maintain and regulate the extracellular environment, and influence neuronal excitability and neurotransmission.[75] The swelling of astrocytes activates extracellular regulated protein kinases, elevates intracellular calcium concentration, up-regulates the expression of peripheral benzodiazepine receptors, affects multiple ion channels and amino acid transport, affects receptor densities and neurotransmitter processing, and increases the synthesis of neurosteroids, which are potent modulators of neuronal GABA receptor activity. These mechanisms induce changes in multiple neurotransmitter systems, which produce the neuropsychiatric disturbances.

Astrocytes belong to the macrophage lineage, thus they have the potential repertoire of cytokine responses. They contain most cytokines and have the ability to synthesize interleukin-1beta (IL-1β) in response to peripheral inflammation,[76] which may induce mediators such as nitric oxide, superoxide, and prostaglandins, thereby making the brain more vulnerable to the effects of hyperammonemia.

Ammonia causes neurotransmitter abnormalities, and induces injury to astrocytes that are partially mediated by oxidative stress. Viral infections can stimulate nitric oxide synthase, which synthesizes NO, leading to increases in free radical production and to oxidative stress. Recently, there has been a reemergence of discussion of oxidative stress involvement with the etiology of autism; however, any toxic exposure (infection, heavy metals) evokes a similar response and the consequent free radical production. Thus oxidative stress would be present as the aftermath of a toxic event, not the cause of autism. An analogy would be that, if a house burned to the ground, and the following day water was poured on the remains of the house, it would not "re-build" the house. Loading a patient with antioxidants is a futile gesture, as the damage has already occurred. Treatment should be centered on rebuilding membrane structure and thereby stabilizing membrane function. Membranes can be repaired by supplying balanced essential fatty acids, phosphatidylcholine, and phenylbutyrate orally and intravenously.[42]

Hepatic encephalopathy is a disease process that is accompanied by a constellation of CNS derangements, and can evoke altered dopamine and serotonin metabolism, modifications of neurotransmission, and activation of the brain opioid system.[77,78] In 1971, Fischer and Baldessarini found that abnormalities of the metabolism of amines and amino acids may explain behavioral and neurologic changes in hepatic dysfunction. Accumulations of false or substitute neurotransmitters may mediate neuropsychiatric phenomena in states of inborn or acquired metabolic error.[79,80]

Research has indicated that disturbed brain metabolism and altered functions of the neurotransmitters dopamine, noradrenaline, serotonin, and GABA, and the false neurotransmitters phenylethanolamine, octopamine, and synephrine, may be of high importance in the pathomechanism of hepatic encephalopathy.[81] Octopamine was found to be the primary false neurotransmitter formed in the CNS, and it competes with dopamine for uptake and release in central nerve endings, hence leading to encephalopathy.[82] Recently, Deshpande and colleagues[78] found increased extracellular concentration of DOPAC in an animal model of liver ischemia with no change in dopamine itself. They administered branched chain amino acids (BCAA) to suppress DOPAC successfully; however, neither serotonin nor its metabolite 5-HIAA were affected by treatment with BCAAs.

High concentrations of free tryptophan and indolyl acrylic acid correlate with subclinical encephalopathy and the development of disordered neurotransmission and mental disturbance.[77,83] In 1961, Schain and Freedman first reported elevation of platelet serotonin in children with autism. Researchers have continued until the present to query hyperserotoninemia as a causal or noncontributory entity in autism.

In 1998, both Shattock[84] and Marklova[85] published papers on increased levels of indole excretion in urine as indolyl-3-acryloylglycine (IAcrGly) and indoleacrylic acid (IAcrA). Bergeron also noted in 1998 that 5-HIAA, the major metabolite of serotonin (5-hydroxytryptamine, 5-HT), is increased in the prefrontal cortex and in the caudate nucleus of brain tissue[86] in hepatic encephalopathy.

Indole-3-acetic acid (IAA) was found to inhibit tryptophan binding to human serum albumin. Elevation of free tryptophan and IAA correlate with hepatic encephalopathy and deranged neurotransmission, and may be directly linked to autistic features.[77,83] Research failed to elucidate altered tryptophan and serotonin metabolism for many years due to false negative test results occurring if the patient had exposure to sunlight. IAcrGly undergoes isomerization with in vivo sunlight exposure and will not appear in the urine or blood during the summer months. See Table 23.2 for the abnormal lab results suggestive of metabolic encephalopathy and the corresponding treatment regimes.

The neurological and immune systems are inextricably intertwined from the beginning of life. Pre- or perinatal immune dysregularities are capable of altering levels of cytokines, chemokines, neurotransmitters, and neuropeptides, as well as hormones. Each of these biomarkers may influence the course of development in the nervous and/or immune systems.[14] A developmental perturbation may be the beginning of a continual cycle of damage to or disruption of both systems. Numerous pathways may lead to the development of autism, including, but not limited to, genetic susceptibility, toxicity, aberrant lipid metabolism, infection, or immune abnormalities playing primary roles. Research in understanding the reciprocal actions of the nervous, immune, hepatic, and endocrine systems is beginning to unravel the mystery of autism.

TABLE 23.2

Abnormal Lab Results Depicting Involvement of Metabolic Encephalopathy

- Elevation of 5-hydroxyindoleacetic acid (5-HIAA)
- Elevation of 3,4-dihydroxyphenylacetic acid (DOPAC)
- Elevation of indole-3-acetic acid (IAA)
- Elevation of urinary false neurotransmitters: phenylethanolamine, octopamine, synephrine
- Elevation of serum calcium
- Elevation of BUN and ammonia

Treatment Regimes Suggested for Metabolic Encephalopathy to Clear Ammonia

- Butyrate, phenylbutyrate (oral or IV), phenylacetate
- Phosphatidylcholine (oral or IV)
- L-carnitine
- Sodium benzoate
- L-ornithine-L-aspartate (oral or IV)
- Lactulose
- Branched chain amino acids (to reduce DOPAC only)
- Sunlight

BIG BRAINS, INCREASED WHITE MATTER VOLUME, AND DISTURBED CONNECTIVITY

Autism has been found to be associated with an overall enlargement of brain volume, while being further associated with increased subcortical white matter in the frontal lobe, with abnormal patterns of growth in the cerebral cortex, amygdala, and hippocampal formations.[73] The clinical onset of autism appears to be preceded by two phases of brain growth abnormalities: a reduced head size at birth, followed by a sudden and excessive increase between 1 to 2 months and 6 to 14 months of age.[87] Neuroimaging studies have shown that an abnormal pattern of brain overgrowth also occurs in areas of the frontal lobe,[90,91] cerebellum, and limbic structures between 2 and 4 years of age, a pattern that is followed by retardation of brain growth.[87–89] Other studies of cortical and cerebral white matter volumes are indicative of interregional disconnectivity,[90,91] potentially resulting in poor integration within and across neurobehavioral developmental domains.[88,92] All of these brain regions are intimately involved in the development of social, communication, and motor abilities, which are impaired in ASD.

White matter enlargement is initially greater, and persists longer, than cerebral or cerebellar cortical involvement, suggesting that the white matter enlargement is less likely a function of an increase in neuronal number and more likely to be a consequence of changes intrinsic to white matter, such as through increased myelination.[73] Bauman hypothesizes[65] that the most likely explanation for the increase in brain size is the presence of improperly formed or chemically abnormal myelin, or atypical up-regulation in the normal early production of myelin during the first few years of life, resulting in a disturbance of myelin that could lead to dysfunctional processing of information throughout the brain. This phenomenon was described further by Kohl as a "possible quantitative difference" in myelin phospholipids, proteolipid protein, and glycolipids that could be aberrant in autism.[93,94] The finding of membrane-enclosed brain glycolipids in adult presentations described by Simon[95] may support Kohl's hypothesis, especially since the siblings Simon describes present with symptoms that parallel autism.

Simon[95] and colleagues describe a unique familial leukodystrophy with adult-onset dementia in a brother and sister whose manifestation of symptoms occurred after the age of 30. The patients presented with progressive cognitive decline, paucity of speech, limited thought content, blunted affect, motor restlessness, poor judgment, liability, and with progression of the nonverbal presentation.

Extensive laboratory investigation was unrevealing; however, a right frontal brain biopsy showed "scattered cortical neurons containing coarse, irregular, densely osmophilic material and round lipid droplets (lipofuscin) described as a leukodystrophy with membrane enclosed glycolipoid inclusions."

Kane reported overmyelination in autism and hyperactivity in 1996 based on red cell fatty acid analyses that depicted sharp elevation of the myelin markers, dimethyl acetyls (DMA) from plasmalogens as 16:0 DMA, 18:1 DMA, and 18:0 DMA. High-dose intravenous phosphatidylcholine, used as part of a broader treatment called the Membrane Stabilizing Protocol,[42] has normalized DMAs in red cell pediatric patients with ASD in 6 to 9 months. Adult patients with amyotrophic lateral sclerosis (ALS) often have gross elevations of DMAs, which have been shown to normalize with treatment generally in 1 year.[39,42,96]

The observed association between increased white matter volume and functional impairment may be representative of global patterns of brain abnormality, reflecting deficits in socialization and communication that define the disorder. Investigators have proposed that the pattern on impairments associated with autism, as well as some relative strengths in perceptual processing is secondary to abnormalities in structural and functional connectivity.[91,97,98]

Overgrowth of localized cortical connections and undergrowth of more distant connections between the cerebral cortical regions and within subcortical structures[91,98] have been hypothesized to cause impaired complex information processing[99] and "weak central coherence."[100] Increased volume of localized cortical connections contributes to functional impairment in children with autism.

Casanova's[101] studies of individuals with autism suggest abnormalities in cortical minicolumns, vertical clusters of large neurons delimited by cell-sparse areas on either side, reflected as a bias toward shorter connecting fibers, which are localized to radiate white matter, at the expense of longer fibers connecting distant cortical and cortical-subcortical regions. Nitric oxide insufficiency has been proposed as one potential causal mechanism for autism that could cause narrow minicolumns postnatally.[102]

White matter growth is not synonymous with the connectivity at all histological levels. Although autism is a developmental disorder characterized by white matter overgrowth, it is very different from a disorder associated with damage to white matter, such as cerebral palsy. The increase in white matter volume and poor clinical and brain function highlights the dissociation between white matter tract overgrowth and dendritic and synaptic underdevelopment. White matter fiber pathways may be larger without actual dendritic or synaptic connections having been established. Thus, the appropriate interpretation may be that the white matter pathways are enlarged, not that connectivity is increased.[3]

In a series of proton (1H) MR spectroscopy (MRS) studies, Minshew identified the cerebral cortex as the site of origin of neurological abnormalities.[3] These imaging studies have revealed a lack of increased white matter in the corpus callosum, suggesting that the primary pathophysiology is intrahemispheric and not specific to white matter. Minshew further delineates decreased gray matter concentrations of choline-containing compounds, and of myoinositol in the Friedman imaging studies,[103] are indicative of decreased cellularity and synaptosome density. Sokol[104] found an increase in the choline/creatinine ratio associated with membrane degeneration. Minshew hypothesizes[3] that the primary event might have been neuronal, occurring in the cerebral cortex, and that the white matter changes are expressions or consequences of that event.

Imaging of patients with ASD has unveiled the neural systems related to social interaction, gaze and motion processing, face identity and emotion, visual perception, higher-order perceptual processing, and the difference between automatic processing and deliberate conscious or cognitive processing.[3] Due to the constellation of symptoms of ASD, various genetic and epigenetic mechanisms are beginning to be identified that account not only for multi-organ involvement, but also for the diversity of findings within the central nervous system in ASD.

Cellular Lipid Aberrations, Low Cholesterol, EFA Insufficiency, and VLCFAs

In 1993, Minshew[3] found evidence of enhanced membrane degradation and decreased levels of high-energy phosphate compounds in early ^{31}P MRS spectroscopy studies of the prefrontal cortex of high-functioning ASD males from ages 11 to 36. These early findings revealed disturbed membrane phospholipid metabolism, which Kane had observed in lab results of patients with ASD, after interpretation of their red cell fatty acid analysis. In 1996, Ann Moser, of the Peroxisomal Diseases Laboratory at Kennedy Krieger Institute, was able to precisely analyze red cell specimens of patients with autism, so that it was possible to accurately assess aberrations in membrane structure and function.

Kane observed a sharp elevation of very long chain fatty acids (VLCFAs) in patients with autism and neurological difficulties,[33] which may reflect disordered lipid membrane metabolism in myelin as well as in neuronal structures. Bauman and Kemper consistently found enlarged neurons (described as "big fat neurons") in the brains (specifically in the deep cerebellar nuclei, inferior olive, and nucleus of the diagonal bond of Broca in the septum) of children aged 5 to 13 years, while, in contrast, older brains had neurons that were markedly reduced in size.[64] Bauman hypothesizes that there may be various causative factors, such as "neuronal swelling which may be followed by atrophy due to transaction of an axon." However, in 1994, Kane discussed with Bauman the sharp elevation of VLCFAs in autism, which would engorge peroxisomes paralleling the "big fat" neurons with "big fat" peroxisomes, and that this phenomenon could be a possible etiology of ASD. Interestingly, in peroxisomal disorders the phenomenon of engorgement of very long chain fatty acids in the peroxisome occurs in the initial phase, but eventually is atrophied as the individual neurologically deteriorates or survives the metabolic disorder into adulthood.[105,106]

Peroxisomal disorders are characterized by an accumulation in tissue and body fluids of renegade fatty acids: saturated and mono-unsaturated VLCFAs, odd chain fatty acids, and branched chain fatty acids, pristanic and phytanic, which are normally degraded within the peroxisome, but instead can accumulate and form lipid rafts, or ceramides, which derange cell membrane structures. The accumulation of renegade or VLCFAs reflects blocked detoxification and methylation pathways, and may be characteristic in autism, PDD, seizure disorders, stroke, neurological disease, and states of neurotoxicity.[35,45,46,96]

Research on inherited peroxisomal disorders, such as neuroinflammatory X-linked adrenoleukodystrophy (X-ALD), has been inspired by the work of Hugo and Ann Moser.[107] X-ALD has a typical clinical onset of 2.75 to 10 years of age, presenting with strikingly similar symptoms to ASD, including behavioral changes, intellectual deterioration, poor school performance, verbal apraxia, attention deficit, hyperactivity, impaired auditory discrimination, fatigue, anorexia, alternating diarrhea and constipation, abdominal pain, vomiting, and visual impairment (visual field cuts).

The hallmark of X-ALD is an accumulation of C24:0 and C26:0 fatty acids in plasma and tissues. Degradation of VLCFAs occurs in peroxisomes via beta oxidation. Since the accumulation of VLCFAs[108] can form ceramides and has been clearly established to be deleterious to the brain and CNS,[109] it is possible that autism may mimic pseudo-neonatal adrenoleukodystrophy[105,106,110] as a peroxisomal disorder with enlarged peroxisomes, suppressed peroxisomal ß-oxidation, and a compromised neurological system.

Aberrations in the red cell fatty acid analysis of patients with autism include:

- Buildup of renegade fatty acids, including VLCFAs, branched chain fatty acids, and odd chain fatty acids, leading to compromised membrane integrity, as these rigid VLCFAs form ceramides, which can traverse the cell and deform the membrane phospholipid structure, thereby altering the position of receptors, peptides, and ion channels.
- Enzymes involved in peroxisomal oxidation are suppressed by the elevation of VLCFAs and subsequently, inflammatory cytokines.[111] Riboflavin (vitamin B2) is pivotal in lipid metabolism,[110] especially during cytokine expression and exposure to endotoxins[112] and may be used intravenously and/or orally to address inflammation and detoxification, and to stimulate peroxisomal function.

- Low total lipid content due to poor nutrition, digestive difficulties, or deviant fatty acid metabolism.
- Grossly imbalanced ω-6 and ω-3 essential fatty acids due to overzealous supplementation of fish oil. Overdosing with ω-3 suppresses ω-6 by competitive inhibition.
- Deficiency of EFAs due to failure to obtain EFAs from a poor quality diet, or a digestive problem involving the gall bladder's release of bile and/or the release of lipase from the pancreas.
- Sharp elevation of DHA, indicative of the formation of aberrant inflammatory lipid metabolites, which occurs after a toxic exposure to pesticides, microbes, heavy metals, or chemicals.

Kane[33] reported in 1996 that children with ASD had elevation of DHA in their RBCs without fish oil supplementation. UMDNJ researchers discovered the same abnormality, and researcher Bernd Spur linked elevation of DHA to toxic exposure. He notes that subsequent aberrant lipid metabolism leads to inflammatory pathways, which may be identified by a buildup of VLCFAs. The use of IV phenylbutyrate can attenuate this inflammatory process; however, intravenous phosphatidylcholine must also be administered to stabilize membrane function and to prevent the reformation of VLCFAs and aberrant inflammatory responses, which in ASD involve neuroinflammation. DHA supplements should not be administered to children and adults with autism.

In states of toxicity via biotoxins, chemicals, or heavy metals, there is a sharp increase in phospholipase A2 (PLA2) activity.[113] A spike in PLA2 profoundly disrupts the lipid bilayer of the membrane because fatty acids are uncoupled from the phospholipids. Membrane integrity is sacrificed and control of prostaglandins, involving vital management of bodily processes, is in disarray.[114,115] Accelerated loss of EFA results in an inflammatory immune response due to the release of arachidonic acid in the presence of an overexpression of PLA2. A prolonged increase in PLA2 results in altered membrane permeability and ion homeostasis, loss of ATP, degeneration of essential membrane phospholipids, and release of free fatty acids, which may result in inflammation, including neuroinflammation. Severe neurodegeneration may occur in the brain[115] if PLA2 activity is not controlled. Carbohydrate consumption, as one of the strongest stimulators of PLA2, must be restricted to control the insulin response and the subsequent loss of EFAs.

Zimmerman and colleagues[116] recently verified improvement in aberrant behavior including irritability, hyperactivity, stereotypy, and inappropriate speech in children with autism during febrile episodes. However, they were not able to elucidate the underlying biological mechanism.

Fever is initiated by circulating PGE2 synthesized by macrophages of the LPS-processing organs (lungs and liver) via phosphorylation of cPLA2 and transcriptional up-regulation of COX-2.[117] Prostaglandin (PG) E2 is a principal downstream mediator of fever. By increasing the blood-brain gradient of PGE2, this mechanism likely facilitates penetration of PGE2 into the brain.[22]

Eicosanoid biosynthesis is initiated by the activation of phospholipase A2 and the release of arachidonic acid (AA) from membrane phospholipids.[118] Thus, fever affects lipid metabolism by the release of EFAs, which are the substrates to prostaglandins and modulators of behavior, immunologic and neurobiological pathways, intracellular signaling, and synaptic plasticity.

Bukelis and colleagues[119] published a paper describing patients with an inborn error of cholesterol synthesis, Smith-Lemli-Opitz syndrome, as having abnormalities strikingly characteristic of ASD. Phospholipids, sphingomyelin, cholesterol, cerebrosides, gangliosides, and sulfatides are the most predominant lipids in the brain residing within the architectural bilayers.[48,120] Cholesterol is a major membrane component, and along with the wax-like saturated palmitic and stearic acids, is responsible for the rigidity and strength of the membrane.

EFAs, including both polyunsaturated fatty acids (PUFAs) and highly unsaturated fatty acids (HUFAs), are liquid, which increases the fluidity index of the cell membrane. Phospholipids and their essential fatty acid components provide second messengers and signal mediators. The proper balance of EFAs, phospholipids, cholesterol, and saturated fatty acids is paramount to establish an optimal index of membrane fluidity.

In essence, phospholipids and their EFA components play a vital role in cell signaling systems in the neuron. The functional behavior of neuronal membranes largely depends upon the ways in which individual phospholipids are aligned, interspersed with cholesterol, and associated with proteins. All neurotransmitters are stored in phospholipid vesicles, and the release and uptake of the neurotransmitters depend upon the realignment of the phospholipid molecules. The nature of the phospholipid is a factor in determining how much neurotransmitter or metal ion will pass out of a vesicle or be taken back in. Phospholipid remodeling may be accomplished by supplying generous amounts of balanced lipids and catalysts via nutritional intervention and the use of intravenous phospholipids as oral and intravenous phosphatidylcholine.

Having tested thousands of patients with ASD over the past 25 years, Kane and Cartaxo[36] (unpublished data) note that about one-third have low cholesterol. Low cholesterol is indicative of poor cell membrane integrity, but supplementation of cholesterol can be easily accomplished by the use of organic egg yolk, which contains 250 mg of cholesterol per yolk.

Candidate Susceptibility Genes for Autism

A polygenetic theory of ASD is emerging, while the possibility of a single-gene disorder is fading and is being replaced with the concept of an expression of multiple abnormal genes acting in concert with a currently unspecified environmental factor.

The identification of chromosomal abnormalities in autism[2,121,122] has helped reinforce the view that genetic influences are important in the development of this disorder. There are numerous reports in the literature documenting chromosomal abnormalities, but there is a lack of consistent findings. Regions of interest identified on chromosomes include 1p, 2q, 5q, 7a, 7q, 15q, 16p, and Xq. One promising region is on chromosome 7q, which has been substantiated by the identification of chromosomal anomalies in this area in individual autism cases. Other candidate genes for autism risk have been identified in the same location. Additional candidate genes that have received much attention are the serotonin transporter gene on chromosome 17q, the HOX genes on chromosome 2, the reelin gene and engrailed gene on 7q, and neuroligin genes on Xp and Xq.

Autism has been linked with autoimmunity, and an association has been established with immune-based genes including human leukocyte antigen HLA-DR B1 phenotype[123] and complement C4 alleles. There is potential that aberrant immune activity during vulnerable and critical periods of neurodevelopment could participate in the generation of neurological dysfunction characteristic of ASD. Specific alleles of the human leukocyte antigen (HLA) system, such as the DR4 allele, occur more often in ASD children, and frequently in their mothers. A fetus possessing a DR4 allele may have increased immune reactivity due to the mother's exposure to toxins, which could create an increased susceptibility to forming autoantibody or cytokines that cross-react with antigens in the fetal brain.

The numerous and complex modes of gene-environment and system impacts are aligned with systemwide findings (e.g., gastrointestinal, hepatic, immune) in ASD.[121] Kane and Cartaxo[36] have had several patients with exposure to arsenic (city water supply in Australia) and methylmercury (daily consumption of white albacore tuna or swordfish) during fetal development who had gross developmental abnormalities with acquired, not inherited, chromosome abnormalities. Liberal administration of EFAs, phosphatidylcholine, phenylbutyrate, and support with methylation catalysts (folinic, methylcobalamin, tetrahydrobiopterin, riboflavin, pyridoxine) and nutrient-dense diet have yielded positive outcomes for these patients with the development of speech and normal cognitive processes.

Epigenetic Aspects

Epigenetics is the study of heritable changes in gene expression that are not mediated at the DNA sequence level. Molecular mechanisms that mediate epigenetic regulation include DNA methylation and chromatin/histone modifications. The science of epigenetics is the study of all those mechanisms that control the unfolding of the genetic program for development, and that determine the phenotypes of differentiated cells. The best-known and most thoroughly studied epigenetic mechanism is DNA methylation,[124] which provides a basis both for the switching of gene activities, and for maintaining the stability of differentiated cells. Developmental insults or epigenetic interactions can unmask underlying genetic vulnerabilities, and probably are at the core of the development of ASD.

DISTURBED METHYLATION, DOPAMINE RECEPTOR–MEDIATED PHOSPHOLIPID METHYLATION

From the earliest origins of life, the unique chemical reactivity of sulfur compounds has given them a central role in maintaining homeostasis and adapting to environmental threats. Important examples include the antioxidant activity of glutathione, detoxification of heavy metals and xenobiotics, redox-dependent modifications of cysteine residues in proteins, and more than 150 methylation reactions, each depending upon the sulfur amino acid methionine, as a source of methyl groups. Since available sulfur resources are limited, these activities functionally compete with each other, requiring dynamic adaptive responses within pathways of sulfur metabolism.

Four major components of sulfur metabolism can be recognized:

- Glutathione synthesis
- Sulfation
- Transsulfuration
- Methylation

Dopamine-stimulated phospholipid methylation represents a unique example of methylation that appears to be involved in synchronization of neuronal networks, particularly during attention. Among these four activities, synthesis of the cysteine-containing tripeptide glutathione is arguably the most fundamental, since it controls the cellular potential for oxidation or reduction,[125–127] affecting essentially every biochemical reaction and supporting the very survival of cells.

All cells contain the same chromosomes, and the same potential for gene expression. Differentiation of distinct cell types during development reflects a time-dependent progression of variable gene expression. This progression is orchestrated by shifts in the methylation pattern of both DNA and histone proteins, which tightly bind DNA and sequester genes so they cannot be transcribed into mRNA or protein products. Thus, methylation must function normally during development to maintain normal epigenetic control over gene expression. Toxic exposure during gestation or infancy can impair methylation, and is, therefore, a threat to normal development, and may lie at the root of autism, as well as of other developmental disorders that lie within this interface between metabolism and gene function.

If ASD patients have polymorphisms in 5,10-methylenetetrahydrofolate reductase (MTHFR), modeling predicts that there will be a decrease in MTHFR activity reducing concentrations of S-adenosylmethionine and 5-methyltetrahydrofolate, as well as DNA methylation, while modestly increasing S-adenosylhomocysteine and homocysteine concentrations and thymidine or purine synthesis.[128] Decreased folate, together with a simulated methyl-B12 deficiency, result in decreases in DNA methylation and purine and thymidine synthesis. Decreased MTHFR activity superimposed on the methyl-B12 deficiency appears to reverse declines in purine and thymidine synthesis.[128]

When dysfunctional methylation is caused by genetic abnormalities, it influences early fetal development, often with devastating consequences. One example is Down's syndrome, caused by chromosome 21 trisomy with excess transsulfuration. The coincident appearance of an extra copy of the cystathionine-beta-synthase (CBS) gene[129] causes neural tube defects, at least partly due to inadequate levels of active folate (methylfolate),[130] which is a source of methyl groups for methionine synthase. Angelman/Prader-Willi, Rett, and fragile-X syndromes are also linked to methylation-related genetic origins.[131,132] Thus impaired methylation is a common coincident of neurodevelopmental disorders.

Dysfunctional methylation from environmental (i.e., nongenetic) causes can arise either from exposures during gestation or during postnatal development or both.

Examples of gestational exposure include:

- Alcohol exposure resulting in fetal alcohol syndrome, where consumption lowers glutathione levels leading to impaired methylation.[133]
- Methylmercury exposure from frequent consumption of white albacore tuna.[134]
- Terbutaline administration to delay preterm labor crosses the placenta and can disrupt the replication and differentiation of developing neurons.[135,136]
- Corn contaminated with a mycotoxin, fumonisin, can cause neural tube defects by interfering with methylation.[137] Fumonisins have been shown to inhibit the biosynthesis of sphingolipids,[138] which interferes with the uptake of 5-methyltetrahydrofolate and decreases total folate binding.[139]

Postnatal xenotoxin exposure may play an important role in the current "autism epidemic," although the offending agent(s) remains to be identified. This is particularly true in cases of regressive autism, where a shift in cellular metabolism can result in a loss of previously acquired abilities. Of further concern is the fact that epigenetic effects (i.e., changes in methylation patterns) can be passed across generations, allowing environmental exposures to exert cumulative ramifications.[140]

Concern has been raised over childhood vaccinations being a cause of autism. The connection of autism to vaccination remains to be elucidated, but a review of the vaccine schedule often reveals that vaccinations are often given too soon and/or too many vaccinations are given at one time. Most frequently the MMR vaccination is given at 1 year of age, rather than the suggested 15 to 18 months, and it is often combined with up to six other vaccines on the same day.

Vaccinations should never be given at the time of illness, which is often the case when the chart notes from the pediatrician's office are matched to the vaccination schedule. Previously, acetaminophen was often suggested to be given to children before and/or after vaccination at a time when vaccine contained thimerosal, a mercury preservative. Acetaminophen can lower glutathione levels in the blood; thus the exposure to mercury in combination with reduction in the amount of available glutathione may have made the child more susceptible to mercury toxicity, since glutathione can chelate mercury safely from the body.

To address the aftermath of heavy metal toxicity, glutathione cannot be used orally (or topically) as it breaks down into individual amino acids, one of which is excitatory glutamate. Glutathione can be infused into the bloodstream but it will not pass through the cell membrane or blood-brain barrier unless it is given with phosphatidylcholine, in the form of Lipostabil.

During cognitive activity, networks of neurons fire synchronously in specific frequency ranges (e.g., theta, alpha, beta, and gamma), and neurotransmitters such as dopamine are responsible for modulating shifts in frequency during attention and awareness. In autism, the ability to synchronize brain activity is impaired, in association with deficits in attention and awareness. Among dopamine receptors, as well as among all receptors, only the D4 receptor subtype is capable of carrying out methylation of membrane phospholipids in response to dopamine, and D4 receptors are involved in synchronization of neuronal activity in the gamma frequency range (30 to 80 Hz).[141] Since gamma activity is reduced in autism, this has led to the proposal that dopamine-stimulated phospholipid methylation (PLM) may be impaired in autism.[142,143]

Dopamine stimulation of D4 receptors activates a cycle of methylation that is supported by methylfolate, as provided by the vitamin B12–dependent enzyme methionine synthase. Vitamin B12 (cobalamin) receives the folate-derived methyl group and transfers it to a homocysteine in the receptor, in a manner parallel to folate-dependent methylation of free homocysteine. While it awaits the next methyl group, cobalamin is vulnerable to oxidation, depending upon cellular redox status, which temporarily halts activity until the cobalamin is either reduced or replaced with methylcobalamin.

Methylcobalamin synthesis requires glutathione, so methionine synthase activity functions as a sensor of cellular redox status and cellular glutathione status. Methionine synthase in neuronal cells is completely dependent upon methylcobalamin for reactivation, which may underlie the therapeutic benefit of methylcobalamin treatment in autism.

Supporting disturbed methylation pathways with targeted nutrient support is paramount to improving the condition of the child with autism. To verify that there may be a disturbance in methylation, national laboratories now offer testing of methylene tetrahydrofolate reductase (MTHFR) for polymorphism on A1298C and C677T. If there is an abnormality, then supportive supplementation would include riboflavin (vitamin B2), folinic acid (or Leucovorin), tetrahydrobiopterin,[144] pyridoxine (vitamin B6), and methylcobalamin (administered by subcutaneous injection).

The pathophysiology of autism is intimately related to a metabolic disturbance, probably induced by exposure to one or more xenotoxins. The resulting shifts in sulfur metabolism decrease the capacity for methylation, with adverse consequences for gene expression during development, and for dopamine-dependent neuronal synchronization during attention.

IV. PATIENT EVALUATION

Physical examination of a patient with ASD can be quite a challenge for the practitioner since children often have acute tactile defensiveness and sensory processing and integration problems, along with hyper- and/or hypoactivity. To a child with autism, a firm grasp or a gentle touch could be perceived as painful; therefore, ask the parents if the child likes rough play and deep pressure or prefers a gentle touch. Further, sensitivities to loud noises, smells, and lighting may also be a challenge for ASD patients. Review of the history in advance of the patient visit may be particularly helpful as can inviting families to bring a patient's favorite toy or activity to reduce anxiety.

PATIENT HISTORY FOR ASD

A complete medical history along with a comprehensive physical examination is critical to address the vast differences, and hence the variable needs of patients diagnosed with ASD. There is no lab test or x-ray to confirm the diagnosis of ASD. The diagnosis is based on clinical judgment regarding observations of the individual's behavior, as well as information from family members and other observers. The primary care physician may, however, order tests to rule out other conditions that might be confused with ASD, such as mental retardation, deafness, metabolic, or genetic diseases. A comprehensive evaluation of a child with ASD might include a complete medical and family history, physical exam, formal audiology evaluation, vision exam, and diagnostic tests. Complete medical records should be obtained on the patient along with a detailed history of development, and detailed toxic, nutritional, and medical history. The health professional should ask about the mother's pregnancy, the child's development, aspects of eating, vaccine reactions, and recurrent illness. Referral may be necessary for adequate evaluation of the child's social communication, communication skills, motor skills, play skills, interests and behaviors, past and present therapies, and family history.

PHYSICAL EXAMINATION FOR ASD

Table 23.3 presents the signs and symptoms commonly seen in ASD, which have possible underlying biochemical and nutritional deficiencies.

Since the pathophysiology suggests that exposure to toxins can precipitate ASD in vulnerable individuals, screening for potential toxin exposures is important especially if the exposure is ongoing or its sequaele are treatable. See Table 23.4 for a screening questionnaire that can guide further evaluation and diagnostic testing.

TABLE 23.3
Physical Exam Manifestations of Metabolic Imbalance

Physical Exam Finding	Potential Cause
Failure to thrive, low percentile measurements in weight and height	Methylation defect, poor diet, poor absorption, infectious etiologies, inflammatory bowel disorders, autoimmune disorders, metabolic diseases, and genetic disorders.
Tender scalp—pulling of the child's hair elicits screams of pain	May need vitamin D.
Flaky dandruff; dry straw-like hair	May be due to too much refined sugar, essential fatty acid deficiency; also is best treated with a balance of essential fats and may be related to dehydration (most children do not drink enough water).
Cracked skin behind the ears	Usually more zinc is needed, along with essential fatty acids.
Dilated pupils	Salicylate sensitivity (not only aspirin but artificial colors and flavorings), mercury toxicity or neurotransmitter imbalance.
Dark circles under the eyes/horizontal creases in the lower eyelids ("allergic shiners"/ "Dennies lines")	Allergies, poor circulation.
Macrocephaly or microcephaly—some children with ASD develop macrocephaly	Some children with ASD develop macrocephaly by the age of 2. At later stages of development the rate of brain growth in the ASD child may be less than that of typically developing children.
Hard or excessive ear wax	May indicate the need of essential fatty acids.
Poor eye contact	Many children with autism have poor eye contact, which is related to poor membrane integrity and disturbed methylation.
Hyperkeratosis pilaris ("white bumps") on the backs of the upper arms and front of the thighs	Vitamin A deficiency or hypothyroidism (which leads to inability to convert beta-carotene to vitamin A).
Yellow cast to the skin on the palms of hands, soles of feet, around the mouth and nose or the entire face	May be from consuming too many orange vegetables (carrots), impaired hepatic function, or low functioning thyroid. Hypothyroid is also seen with dry skin, dry hair, brittle nails, low body temperature.
White spots, ridged, brittle nails	Minerals are low, especially zinc.
Eczema, dry skin	Essential fatty acid deficiency (usually ω-6 in evening primrose oil), atopic allergies, digestive impairment involving the gall bladder, or hepatic dysfunction. Balanced essential fatty acids, digestive support, and zinc are supportive.
Aphthous ulcer "canker sore"	Food allergies, deficiency of niacin (B3).
Cracked corners of the mouth	Riboflavin (B2) deficiency.
Geographic tongue	Folinic acid, methylcobalamin, and zinc.
Red cheeks and ears	Allergies, magnesium deficiency, sulfation defect.
Tan stool	Gall bladder problem (not releasing bile).
Constipation, diarrhea, poorly formed stools, pellet-type stools, foul odor to the stool, bulky stools, grainy stools	All relate to dysbiosis, poor digestion, food intolerance, allergies, and poor diet and respond to an organic, pure diet with the removal of common food allergens (wheat, milk), increased fiber (ground flaxseed, raw crunchy vegetables), probiotics, magnesium carbonate, enzymes (protease, lipase, amylase), bile salts.
Red ring around the anus	Infection, dysbiosis.
Excessive thirst	Essential fatty acid deficiency.
Light sensitivity	Magnesium deficiency.
Sleep disturbances	Deficiencies in folinic acid, magnesium, potassium, riboflavin (B2), niacinamide (B3).
Irritability	Deficiencies of essential fatty acids, folinic acid, magnesium, methylcobalamin B12, magnesium, manganese, electrolyte imbalance, and elevated phosphorus levels.
Abdominal distention	Digestive impairment, food allergies (usually gluten).

TABLE 23.4
Screening Questionnaire for Toxic Exposure

- History of travel outside the country.
- Vaccine reactions, list of dates vaccines were given, any vaccines for travel.
- Toxic mold exposure, age of home, leaks or floods causing mold.
- Corn consumption (possible fumonisin exposure, which is a toxic mold that can impair methylation).
- Tylenol exposure.
- Aspartame intake, diet soda.
- Surgeries requiring anesthesia.
- Hospitalizations.
- History of all infections, including ear infections.
- List of all past and present medications.
- Head trauma from falls or car accidents.
- Pesticide exposure: Are pesticides sprayed in the home or yard, does patient live near a golf course or farmland or vineyards where there is aerial spraying?
- Fish intake such as tuna, especially large predator fish like swordfish or shark.
- Chemical or solvent exposure from parents' work on autos, artwork, or photo processing.
- Home renovation in an old or moldy home.
- Heavy metal exposure from lead and mercury in old homes.
- Well water exposure may be a source of heavy metals including copper.
- Tick bite history, bull's eye rash, joint pain, light sensitivity, mosquito, spider, or other insect bites that became infected.
- Pets with illnesses such as parvo, lyme, and parasites.
- Electrical low frequency exposure from high tension wires near home or school.
- Wild game consumption such as venison and wild boar.
- Chewing on toys with lead paint or inappropriate objects such as batteries, pencils.
- Firearms used on a shooting range are an antimony exposure.
- Sleeping garments with flame retardant used can be an antimony exposure.
- Sensitivity to perfume or chemicals suggests a sulfation deficit.

TESTING

In addition to nitrogen markers, electrolyte panel, liver enzymes, total creatine kinase, and a complete blood count (Table 23.5), specialty diagnostic tests can guide individualized dietary intervention (Table 23.6).

V. TREATMENT

Intervention with children and adults with ASD is quite complicated since these patients are acutely sensitive to medication, nutrients, and even foods that are introduced. Authors Kane and Cartaxo have each seen patients clinically with ASD for more than 25 years and have learned that slow introduction of simple changes yields the best outcome in regard to compliance and positive patient outcomes. Treatment should be oriented to an evidence-based approach with targeted nutritional intervention that meets the needs of the individual patient.

MEDICATION

No drug is specific in treating the core symptoms of ASD, but medication may serve as an adjunctive therapy for aberrant symptoms, such as self-destructive behavior. Generally, medications

TABLE 23.5
Chemistry Panel and Blood Count Findings Can Help Direct Treatment

Lab Result	Clinical Significance	Potential Treatment
Acidosis	Elevated CO_2	Support with magnesium carbonate.
Hyperammonemia	Elevated BUN	Clear with butyrate and PC.
Immune incompetence	High or low globulin, WBC, neutrophils, lymphocytes	Support with balanced EFAs trace minerals, especially zinc.
Hepatic toxicity	High bilirubin, high BUN, high liver enzymes	Clear with butyrate and PC.
Electrolyte imbalance	High or low Na, K, Cl, P, CO_2, Ca	Add oral balanced electrolyte solution.
Renal insufficiency	Elevation of creatinine, BUN, potassium	Clear with butyrate and PC.
Low protein intake	Low albumin	Increase protein intake.
Dehydration	High sodium, high albumin	Encourage more fluids.
Anemia	Low hemoglobin, high RDW	Support with folinic acid, methylcobalamin.
GI inflammation	High monocytes	Support with probiotics, organic food; remove possible food allergens such as wheat or milk.
Poor membrane integrity	Low cholesterol, high potassium	Support with EFAs, egg yolk, phosphatidylcholine-PC, balanced electrolyte solution.
Blood sugar problems	High or low glucose, high triglycerides	If the triglycerides are high it is a clear depiction of a diet that is too high in carbohydrate; carbohydrates must be reduced and balanced in the diet with more protein and EFAs. Many children have low blood glucose, which is an indication that they are deficient in trace minerals and that they need to eat frequently.

TABLE 23.6
Additional Diagnostic Tests To Guide Treatment in Patients With ASD

Red Cell Fatty Acids*
Analysis of red cell fatty acids depicts 4 to 6 months of cellular metabolism, myelination status (DMAs as dimethyl acetyls), cellular stability, hepatic and brain function (if compromised there will be an elevation of VLCFAs). An individualized clinical treatment intervention of balanced fatty acids and coenzymes is included with the analysis according to the evidence-based medical literature.

Urinary Organic and Amino Acids**
5-Hydroxyindoleacetic acid (5-HIAA), uracil, orotic acid, oxalic acid
Investigation into inborn errors in metabolism with detailed analysis of organic and amino acids may give insight into the etiology of the patient's ASD. If abnormalities are identified, coenzymes as vitamins and minerals may be given to stimulate suppression of particular enzymes.

Urinary Neurotransmitters***
Glutamate, aspartic acid, serotonin, epinephrine, norepinephrine, dopamine, 5-HIAA (5-hydroxyindoleacetic acid), DOPAC (3, 4 dihydroxyphenylacetic acid), and future testing for phenylethanolamine octopamine, synephrine.
    Obtaining urinary neurotransmitters may reflect the balance of neurotransmitters and be indicative of states of excitation and impaired methylation if norepinephrine is elevated and epinephrine is decreased. The administration of IV and oral lipid therapy often balances urinary neurotransmitters, but in some cases oral amino acids or natural foods may be utilized if there is severe depletion of an individual neurotransmitter. If serotonin was grossly depleted, for example, the patient may be given 5-hydroxytryptophan or encouraged to consume turkey frequently. Elevations of false neurotransmitters such as DOPAC (from dopamine) and 5-HIAA (from serotonin) are depiction of posthepatic encephalopathy, involving viral infection.

TABLE 23.6 *(continued)*

Serum Hormones****

DHEA, IGF-1 (growth hormone marker), pregnenolone, ACTH, cortisol, alpha melanocyte stimulating hormone, thyroid panel- T3, T4, TSH, testosterone or estrogen panel (E1, E2, E3)

Energy metabolism, neurohormone levels (pregnenolone), hormone balance, and the ability to beta oxidize VLCFAs may be indicated by expanded hormonal testing. Low levels of IGF-1 may serve as a marker for suppression of methionine synthase. Many patients with neurotoxicity present with suppression of serum hormones. As the patient receives oral and IV phosphatidylcholine and balanced EFAs, hormonal balance is often naturally reestablished.

Toxic Screen****

Urinary porphyrins, beta-2-microglobulin, cholinesterase panel (plasma, RBC, serum), viral antibodies (Parvo 19, West Nile, HHV6, CMV, EBV, herpes simplex, hepatitis panel), CD26 or also termed Dipeptidyl Peptidase IV (DPP-IV), Anti-DNase B Strep antibodies, Anti-streptolysin, Lyme Western Blot IgG and IgM, Bartonella henselae PCR, Apolipoprotien A-1, B, and E.

Patients with ASD often present with chronic microbial infections. If the history indicates exposure to pesticides and other fat-soluble chemical toxins, a cholinesterase panel may reflect this exposure by a decrease in the enzyme level while exposure to heavy metals may be reflected in urinary porphyrins and beta-2-microglobulin, suppression of CD26 is linked to hepatic toxicity while an increase in CD26 may be indicative of exposure to pesticides or diabetes, elevations on Strep biomarkers may reveal Pediatric Autoimmune Neuropsychiatric Disorders Associated with Streptococcal infections (PANDAS), a low level of Apolipoprotein B which is the main protein component of LDL and has been connected to ASD by the MIND Institute, Apolipoprotein A-1 which is the main protein component of HDL, and Apolipoprotein E genotype, which is a marker for mercury toxicity.

Immune and Inflammatory Markers****

Lipoprotein(a), C-Reactive Protein, IgM, IgA, IgE, IgG + subclasses, T-cells and T-cell subsets, Erythropoietin, Lipoprotein-associated Phospholipase A2, C3a, C2, C3, C4, Auto-antibodies for Myelin Basic protein, Neuronal Filament protein, Brain-Derived Neurotrophic Factor & Thyroid, Blood type, Gliadin and Casein antibodies IgG & IgA, urinary 8-hydroxy-2-deoxyguanosine, LDL, Beta-casomorphin, gliadinomorphin.

Evaluation of immune function by checking Lipoprotein (a) and C-Reactive protein for inflammation, immune status by testing Total IgM, IgA, IgE, IgG + subclasses, T-cells and T-cell subsets, C3a, C2, C3, C4, autoantibodies for myelin basic protein, neuronal filament protein, brain-derived neurotrophic factor and thyroid, check free radical status by checking LDL but for an additional test if needed urinary 8-Hydroxy-2-deoxyguanosine, blood type as most ASD individuals are A+ as it was the last blood type to evolve and individuals with this type have the most sensitive immune systems, gluten and casein sensitivity with Gliadin and Casein antibodies IgG & IgA, Beta-casomorphin, gliadinomorphin and membrane stability status with lipoprotein-associated PLA2 whereby an increase of PLA2 acts as a lipid scissors and aggressively deteriorates the membrane; elevation of PLA2 occurs with exposure to neurotoxins. Erythropoietin reflects rejuvenation capacity.

Gene Nutrient Interactions-MTHFR (A1298C, C677T) and HLA-DR B1****

Screening for the two currently known genetic polymorphisms of methylene tetrahydrofolate reductase (A1298C and C677T) can reveal a potential gene-nutrient interaction. Presence of either or both of these polymorphisms suggests an inherited impairment of detoxification, neurotransmitters, growth, cognitive and cellular function. Polymorphisms may be addressed with oral nutrients as methylcobalamin, folinic acid or Leucovorin Rx, tetrahydrobiopterin, and riboflavin. Testing specific alleles of the human leukocyte antigen (HLA) system, the DR4 allele, which is linked to autoimmune disorders, occurs most often in ASD children and their mothers. The fetus with DR4 allele may have increased immune reactivity due to the mother's exposure to toxins, which could create an increased susceptibility to forming autoantibody or cytokines that crossreact with antigens in the fetal brain. If the DR4 is positive, support can be given with balanced essential fatty acids, phenylbutyrate and phosphatidylcholine for detoxification and stabilization of immune function.

* Lab kits may be obtained from Body Bio for the Kennedy Krieger Institute Peroxisomal Diseases Laboratory and biomedical interpretation for individualized metabolic modeling.
** Saint Louis University Metabolic Screening Laboratory under the direction of Dr. James Shoemaker in St. Louis, MO.
*** Neuroscience Laboratory in Osceola, WI, offers a wide array of urinary neurotransmitters.
**** National laboratories such as Quest and LabCorp now have availability of the above suggested lab tests.

administered in ASD are aimed at treating comorbid behaviors and problematic symptoms such as anxiety, insomnia, seizures, obsessive compulsive behaviors, short attention span, hyperactivity, repetitive or perseverative behaviors, psychoses, rage, and self-injurious behaviors. Commonly prescribed in patients with ASD are antipsychotic drugs, antidepressants, stimulants, and anticonvulsants. Therefore, medications that are used are individualized and directed to specific symptoms superimposed upon, or comorbid with, autism, and are not directed at the autistic process per se.

Few of these drugs have been tested in scientific studies in individuals with ASD and many of these medications have significant side effects. These medications should only be prescribed by a medical professional experienced in treating patients with ASD who have severely aggressive behavior toward themselves and/or others. Close monitoring, attention to interactions with other medications, nutrients, and foods, short- and long-term effects, and especially the use of pediatric dosages, are only some of the issues to be concerned about.

Current treatment approaches to modify neuroimmune response are nonspecific and may evoke more potential problems than benefits. The use of steroids, intravenous immunoglobulin,[145] and cytotoxic drugs may complicate and possibly exacerbate neuroinflammtory response as these medications act mostly in cellular and humoral responses that are part of the adaptive or innate immune responses, which are not targeted to modify neuroglial activation and neuroinflammation in ASD.

APPROACHES TO AVOID

First and foremost, do no harm. Approaches to avoid include:

- Detoxification with intravenous use of EDTA is well documented in its use for adults with cardiovascular disease in a 3 hour drip; while in children with autism someone changed the EDTA drip to 30 minutes. The use of intravenous EDTA in this fast drip technique can cause kidney damage and in one documented case led to cardiac arrest (after administration of Na EDTA).
- Detoxification of heavy metals with DMPS, EDTA, or DMSA (oral) such as lead from paint on toys made in China or frequent consumption of white albacore tuna cannot remove heavy metals from inside the cell or the brain since they are bound to the peptide metallothionien in the cell membrane.
- The use of excessive amounts of fish oil can cause gross imbalance of the EFAs; some children have been prescribed 6 tablespoons of cod liver oil, which contains a gross overdose of vitamin A. Overdosing vitamin A, a fat-soluble vitamin, can cause increased intracranial pressure, among other side effects.
- Restrictive diets can lead to severe malnutrition.
- The use of hyperbaric oxygen (HBO) beta oxidizes or burns off VLCFAs, yet initial exposure for about 1 month can be positive in some instances. Unfortunately, all the fatty acids, including the EFAs, are burned off at the same time and there can be destabilization of the cell membranes, which has led to stroke and seizure activity with the use of HBO unless treatment is under the direction of a qualified physician, preferably a neurologist.
- The prolonged use of high-dose, potent antibiotic therapy such as IV or IM Rocephin and other antibiotics has been used for "Lyme" disease without acquiring abnormal, acute (IgM+), or other lab results. This places the patient at risk for suppressed immunocompetence and further complications of ASD.

NUTRIENT INTERVENTION

Research and clinical application have shown promise that specific nutrients, especially fatty acids, targeted to the individual disturbances in biochemistry, may play a key role in the treatment and management of ASD. A general approach to nutrient supplementation in ASD is presented in Table 23.7.

TABLE 23.7
Nutrients Recommended for Treatment of ASD

Nutrients	Dosage	Administration
Balanced 4:1 ω-6 to ω-3 oil	1 to 2 tablespoons bid	Add to food
Evening primrose oil	1 to 2 tablespoons bid	Add to food
Phosphatidylcholine	1 to 2 tablespoons bid	Dilute with water and flavoring
Liquid trace minerals with ascorbic acid	¼ ounce liquid mineral solution, add ⅛ teaspoon of ascorbic acid	Mix in diluted fresh juice
Electrolyte formula	1 tablespoon tid	Mix in foods normally salted
Magnesium carbonate or citrate	200 mg qd	Add to food
Folinic acid or Rx Leucovorin	5 mg qd	Add to food, no taste
Phenylbutyrate Rx	1 teaspoon to 1 tablespoon bid	Can be obtained as a liquid with flavoring added

The introduction of supplementation should begin with nutrients that are easy for the patient to take; therefore, they must not have much taste, and must be mixable into foods that are enjoyed.

After the basic nutrients have been introduced for a few weeks, nutrients can be added that have been targeted to abnormal test results. For example, if the MTHFR comes back positive for polymorphisms then IM injections of methylcobalamin and oral pyridoxine and riboflavin could be administered. Children with ASD cannot handle B complex supplements due to the choline, cyanocobalamin, and folic acid that interrupt methylation. Phosphatidylcholine will replace choline, folinic acid can replace folic acid, and methylcobalamin injections will replace cyanocobalamin. B complex formulas that many children with ASD do tolerate are available without choline, folic acid, and cyanocobalamin. If a child cannot swallow capsules, parents can mix a tiny amount of the B vitamins into a small amount of juice and administer in an oral syringe. Other nutritional supplements are added upon completion of test results. Tables 23.5 and 23.6 review diagnostic tests and results that could guide nutrient therapy for individual patients. Additionally if the screen for toxic exposure identifies a likely exposure, nutrient interventions specific to that exposure would be important to address.

Dietary Modification

The child's diet needs to consist of simple foods made from scratch, organic whenever possible. Not every parent is ready to make the change to a natural food type diet and in this case it will be necessary to take small steps. The general concept for the change in diet is that it should be shifted to a high fat and oil and high protein diet. If oils and fats are increased in the diet, the child has satiety and stops craving sweet, empty "filler foods."

The Membrane Stabilizing Protocol Diet[42] was created by Kane for stabilization of cellular function by balancing EFAs with targeted oral lipids after red cell analysis along with a restriction of carbohydrates. See Chapter 24, "Seizures," Table 24.1.

Most children dislike green vegetables. It is not a good idea ever to force a child to eat anything, but to introduce new foods slowly and to "run out" of particularly detrimental foods, such as those that are processed and highly sugared. The parents can remove all *trans* fats from the cupboards and refrigerator as soon as they arrive home from their visit to your clinic. Protein foods can be encouraged and balanced oil, evening primrose oil, and butter can be mixed into foods. Power drinks can be made with nut milk, eggs or egg protein powder, electrolyte, balanced 4:1 oil, and unsweetened cocoa powder, using stevia or glycerin to sweeten. The most difficult foods to remove are bread and pasta. Rice bread and rice pasta can be the first step away from gluten-based food.

Encourage the parents to make slow but deliberate changes. Laugh with them about how hard it is to avoid donuts and candy even in their own diet. Help them find acceptable substitutes for favorite foods.[42]

GASTROINTESTINAL SUPPORT

Patients with ASD often have impaired gastrointestinal health. Gershon[146] describes the GI system, including the liver, pancreas, and gall bladder, as the "Second Brain," with more serotonin produced in the GI tract then in the mainframe brain. Care should be taken to optimize the function of the GI system as it is responsible for the digestion of foods, absorption of nutrients, and prevention of toxic agents from reaching the circulation. GI health is often severely impaired with disturbed gut pathology in patients with ASD. The most important objective is to heal the GI tract and restore the integrity of the gut wall. A large part of the body's immune system develops and resides in the gastrointestinal tract and it functions as the first line of defense in neutralizing infectious microbes and toxic agents, thereby providing a natural resistance to these harmful agents.

The first step is to eliminate foods that are highly allergic for that individual, and to avoid foods containing simple sugars, artificial sweeteners, and additives.

Start simply by replacing these harmful foods with organic foods, wholesome proteins, healthy fats, and increased fiber. Many positive anecdotal reports are from parents who implemented a gluten-free and casein-free diet in their children with autism. More recently, there have been favorable reports on various other diets, such as the Specific Carbohydrate Diet, a diet that eliminates all starch, processed sugars, and complex carbohydrates. The Membrane Stabilizing Protocol Diet[42] is the easiest to follow and the most nourishing as it includes a wide array of recipes for cakes, pies, cookies, and muffins that are made from egg protein powder, glycerin or stevia, and ground nuts and seeds, instead of regular flour and sugar.

Probiotics, digestive enzymes, bile salts, magnesium carbonate, and ground flaxseed are supportive interventions for individuals with ASD who need digestive support.

INTRAVENOUS THERAPY FOR NEUROLOGICAL MEMBRANE STABILIZATION AND DETOXIFICATION

The Membrane Stabilizing IV Protocol[42] may be administered with weekly and biweekly infusions as detailed in Chapter 24, "Seizures."

VI. SUMMARY

Although ASD presents us with an extremely complicated medical condition due to its systemic nature, it also offers us a unique opportunity to approach illness from a membrane perspective.

- ASD prevalence is increasing, yet traditional approaches have failed to uncover effective solutions.
- ASD is now being approached from the new model of a systemic disorder that can be treated with individualized nutritional intervention.
- There exists the possibility of recovery from ASD with evidence-based, nutritional intervention.
- Supplementation with balanced EFAs as Yehuda's 4:1 ratio of ω-6 to ω-3 oil and phosphatidylcholine is supportive to cell membrane integrity.
- Catalysts supportive to methylation and cellular metabolism are crucial adjuncts to addressing disturbed neurochemistry in ASD presentations and include folinic acid, methylcobalamin, tetrahydrobiopterin, riboflavin, pyridoxine, and trace minerals.

- Appropriate testing can identify the impaired metabolic, immune, hepatic, toxic, and gastrointestinal difficulties that are present and that require nutritional support. Some individuals with ASD have impaired detoxification pathways and need intravenous support for alteration of sulfation and methylation pathways using infusions of phosphatidylcholine, folinic acid, glutathione, and phenylbutyrate.
- Caution should be used to apply clinical therapies that are safe and effective using natural interventions due to the acute sensitivities in individuals with ASD.
- The diet should be changed to a nutrient-dense, organic, high-protein, high-EFA diet called the Membrane Stabilizing Diet.

ACKNOWLEDGMENTS

We gratefully acknowledge assistance in preparation of this manuscript from Thomas Wnorowski, Ph.D., and Edward Kane.

REFERENCES

1. Herbert MR, Anderson MP. An expanding spectrum of autism models: from fixed developmental defects to reversible functional impairments. In Zimmerman, A (Ed.), *Autism: Current Theories and Evidence.* Totowa, NJ: Humana Press, 2008.
2. Newschaffer CJ, Croen LA, Daniels J, Giarelli E, Grether JK, Levy SE, Mandell DS, Miller LA, Pinto-Martin J, Reaven J, Reynolds AM, Rice CE, Schendel D, Windham C. The epidemiology of autism spectrum disorders. *Annu Rev Public Health.* 28:235–258; 2007.
3. Williams DL, Minshew NJ. Understanding autism and related disorders: what has imaging taught us? *Neuroimaging Clin N Am.* 17:4:495–509, ix; Nov 2007.
4. Fombonne E. Epidemiological studies of pervasive developmental disorders. In Volkmar F, Paul R, Klin A, Cohen D (Eds.), *Handbook of Autism and Pervasive Developmental Disorders*, pp. 42–69. Hoboken, NJ: Wiley, 2005.
5. Gupta AR, State MW. Recent advances in the genetics of autism. *Biol Psychiatry.* 61(4):429–437; Feb 2007.
6. Bailey A, Le Couteur A, Gottesman I, Bolton P, Simonoff E, Yuzda E, Rutter M. Autism as a strongly genetic disorder: evidence from a British twin study. *Psychol Med.* 25:1:63–77; Jan 1995.
7. Le Couteur A, Bailey A, Goode S, Pickles A, Robertson S, Gottesman I, Rutter M. A broader phenotype of autism: the clinical spectrum in twins. *J Child Psychol Psychiatry.* 37:7:785–801; Oct 1996.
8. Piven J, Palmer P, Jacobi D, Childress D, Arndt S. Broader autism phenotype: evidence from a family history study of multiple-incidence autism families. *Am J Psychiatry.* 154:2:185–190; Feb 1997.
9. Anderson M, Hooker B, Herbert MR. Bridging from cells to cognition in autism pathophysiology: biological pathways to defective brain function and plasticity. *Am J Biochem and Biotech.* 4:2: 167–176; 2008.
10. Pardo CA, Vargas DL, Zimmerman AW. Immunity, neuroglia and neuroinflammation in autism. *Int Rev Psychiatry.* 17:6:485–495; Dec 2005.
11. Zimmerman AW, Jyonouchi H, Comi AM, Connors SL, Milstien S, Varsou A, Heyes MP. Cerebrospinal fluid and serum markers of inflammation in autism. *Pediatr Neurol.* 33(3):195–201; Sep 2005.
12. Vargas DL, Nascimbene C, Krishnan C, Zimmerman AW, Pardo CA. Neuroglial activation and neuroinflammation in the brain of patients with autism. *Ann Neurol.* 57(1):67–81; Jan 2005.
13. Chez MG, Dowling T, Patel PB, Khanna P, Kominsky M. Elevation of tumor necrosis factor-alpha in cerebrospinal fluid of autistic children. *Pediatr Neurol.* 36(6):361–365; Jun 2007.
14. Ashwood P, Wills S, Van de Water J. The immune response in autism: a new frontier for autism research. *J Leukoc Biol.* 80(1):1–15; Jul 2006. Epub 2006 May 12.
15. Lam KS, Aman MG, Arnold LE. Neurochemical correlates of autistic disorder: a review of the literature. *Res Dev Disabil.* 27(3):254–289; May–Jun 2006. Epub 2005 Jul 5.
16. Fatemi SH, Reutiman TJ, Folsom TD, Huang H, Oishi K, Mori S, Smee DF, Pearce DA, Winter C, Sohr R, Juckel G. Maternal infection leads to abnormal gene regulation and brain atrophy in mouse offspring: implications for genesis of neurodevelopmental disorders. *Schizophr Res.* 99:1–3:56–70. Feb 2008. Epub Jan 2008.

17. Bittigau P, Ikonomidou C. Glutamate in neurologic diseases. *J Child Neurol.* 12(8):471–485; Nov 1997.
18. Greenwood SM, Connolly CN. Dendritic and mitochondrial changes during glutamate excitotoxicity. *Neuropharmacology.* 53(8):891–898. Dec 2007. Epub 2007 Oct 14.
19. Bindokas VP, Miller RJ. Excitotoxic degeneration is initiated at non-random sites in cultured rat cerebellar neurons. *J Neurosci.* 15(11):6999–7011. Nov 1995.
20. Rintoul GL, Filiano AJ, Brocard JB, Kress GJ, Reynolds IJ. Glutamate decreases mitochondrial size and movement in primary forebrain neurons. *J Neurosci.* 23(21):7881–7888; Aug 2003.
21. Li Z, Okamoto K, Hayashi Y, Sheng M. The importance of dendritic mitochondria in the morphogenesis and plasticity of spines and synapses. *Cell.* 119(6):873–87; Dec 2004.
22. Isaev NK, Zorov DB, Stelmashook EV, Uzbekov RE, Kozhemyakin MB, Victorov IV. Neurotoxic glutamate treatment of cultured cerebellar granule cells induces $Ca2^+$-dependent collapse of mitochondrial membrane potential and ultrastructural alterations of mitochondria. *FEBS Lett.* 392:2:143–147; Aug 1996.
23. Pivovarova NB, Nguyen HV, Winters CA, Brantner CA, Smith CL, Andrews SB. Excitotoxic calcium overload in a subpopulation of mitochondria triggers delayed death in hippocampal neurons. *J Neurosci.* 24:24:5611–5622; Jun 2004.
24. Shalbuyeva N, Brustovetsky T, Bolshakov A, Brustovetsky N. Calcium-dependent spontaneously reversible remodeling of brain mitochondria. *J Biol Chem.* 281(49):37547–37558. Dec 2006. Epub Oct 2006.
25. Vesce S, Kirk L, Nicholls DG. Relationships between superoxide levels and delayed calcium deregulation in cultured cerebellar granule cells exposed continuously to glutamate. *J Neurochem.* 90:3:683–693; Aug 2004.
26. Nicholls DG, Budd SL. Mitochondria and neuronal survival. *Physiol Rev.* 80:1:315–360; Jan 2000.
27. Kushnareva YE, Wiley SE, Ward MW, Andreyev AY, Murphy AN. Excitotoxic injury to mitochondria isolated from cultured neurons. *J Biol Chem.* 280:32:28894–28902. Aug 12 2005. Epub Jun 2005.
28. Greenwood SM, Mizielinska SM, Frenguelli BG, Harvey J, Connolly CN. Mitochondrial dysfunction and dendritic beading during neuronal toxicity. *J Biol Chem.* 282:36:26235–26244. Sep 7 2007. Epub Jul 2007.
29. Purpura DP, Bodick N, Suzuki K, Rapin I, Wurzelmann S. Microtubule disarray in cortical dendrites and neurobehavioral failure. I. Golgi and electron microscopic studies. *Brain Res.* 281:3:287–297; Nov 1982.
30. Gohil VM, Hayes P, Matsuyama S, Schägger H, Schlame M, Greenberg ML. Cardiolipin biosynthesis and mitochondrial respiratory chain function are interdependent. *J Biol Chem.* 279(41):42612–42618. Oct 8 2004. Epub Jul 2004.
31. Poling JS, Frye RE, Shoffner J, Zimmerman AW. Developmental regression and mitochondrial dysfunction in a child with autism. *J Child Neurol.* 2:2:170–172; Feb 2006.
32. Fillano JJ, Goldenthal MJ, Rhodes CH, Marín-García J. Mitochondrial dysfunction in patients with hypotonia, epilepsy, autism, and developmental delay: HEADD syndrome. *J Child Neurol.* 17(6):435–439; Jun 2002.
33. Kane PC. *The Neurochemistry and Neurophysics of ASD.* Millville, NJ: BodyBio, 1996, updated 2001.
34. Kane PC. Peroxisomal disturbances in children with epilepsy, hypoxia and autism. *Prostaglandins, Leukotrienes and Essential Fatty Acids.* 57:2:265; Aug 1997.
35. Kane PC, Kane E. Peroxisomal disturbances in ASD. *J Ortho Med.* 12:4:207–218, 1997.
36. Kane PC, Cartaxo AL. Clinical data, 1998 to present.
37. Kane PC. The neurobiology of lipids in ASD. *J Ortho Med.* 14:2:103–109, 1999.
38. Kane PC. Suppression of peroxisomal respiration in children with ASD: pattern recognition and neurobiological role of treatment protocol. *Johns Hopkins Int Conference Brain Uptake and Utilization of Fatty Acids.* Presented March 2–3, 2000.
39. Kane PC, Foster JS. Clinical data. *Wellspring Clinic,* 2000–2002.
40. Kane PC, Foster JS, Cartaxo AL. Clinical detoxification of neurotoxins and heavy metals in ASD. *Autism, Genes and the Environment UMDNJ,* October 2002.
41. Kane PC, Foster JS, Cartaxo AL. Lipid treatment for brain fatty acid abnormalities in ASD. *IMFAR, International Meeting for Autism Research.* Orlando, FL, November 1–2, 2002.
42. Kane PC, Foster JS, Braccia D, Kane E. *The Detoxx Book: Detoxification of Biotoxins in Chronic Neurotoxic Syndromes, The Detoxx Book for Patients and The PK Protocol.* Millville, NJ: BodyBio, 2002, updated 2007.
43. Kane PC, Cartaxo AL, Braccia D, Kane E. Disturbed Peroxisomal Function in ASD, *22nd Int Neurotoxicology Conference,* Research Triangle Park, NC, September 11–14, 2005.
44. Kane PC, Cartaxo AL, Braccia D, Kane E. Neurotoxicity and Disturbed Membrane in Autism, *24th Int Neurotoxicology Conference,* San Antonio, TX, November 11–14, 2007.

45. Kane PC. Essential fatty acids and membrane stability in neurological disease. *Royal College of Physicians,* Nov 2007.

46. Kane PC, Foster JS, Cartaxo, AL, Speight N. Clinical data, The PK Protocol. 2000–2008.

47. Haughey NJ. Department of Neurology, The Johns Hopkins University School of Medicine, personal communication, March 2005.

48. Yechiel E, Barenholz Y. Relationships between membrane lipid composition and biological properties of rat myocytes. Effects of aging and manipulation of lipid composition. *J Biol Chem.* 260:16:9123–9131; Aug 1985.

49. Pletnikov MV, Moran TH, Carbone KM. Borna disease virus infection of the neonatal rat: developmental brain injury model of autism spectrum disorders. *Front Biosci.* 7:d593–607; Mar 2002.

50. Cabanlit M, Wills S, Goines P, Ashwood P, Van de Water J. Brain-specific autoantibodies in the plasma of subjects with ASD. *Ann N Y Acad Sci.* 1107:92–103; Jun 2007.

51. Wills S, Cabanlit M, Bennett J, Ashwood P, Amaral D, Van de Water J. Autoantibodies in autism spectrum disorders (ASD). *Ann N Y Acad Sci.* 1107:79–91; Jun 2007.

52. Patterson PH. Maternal infection: window on neuroimmune interactions in fetal brain development and mental illness. *Curr Opin Neurobiol.* 12:1:115–118; Feb 2002.

53. Fatemi SH, Halt AR, Stary JM, Kanodia R, Schulz SC, Realmuto GR. Glutamic acid decarboxylase 65 and 67 kDa proteins are reduced in autistic parietal and cerebellar cortices. *Biol Psychiatry.* 52:8: 805–810; Oct 2002.

54. Dalton P, Deacon R, Blamire A, Pike M, McKinlay I, Stein J, Styles P, Vincent A. Maternal neuronal antibodies associated with autism and a language disorder. *Ann Neurol.* 53:4:533–537; Apr 2003.

55. Shi L, Fatemi SH, Sidwell RW, Patterson PH. Maternal influenza infection causes marked behavioral and pharmacological changes in the offspring. *J Neurosci.* 23:1:297–302; Jan 2003.

56. Watanabe M, Lee BJ, Yamashita M, Kamitani W, Kobayashi T, Tomonaga K, Ikuta K. Borna disease virus induces acute fatal neurological disorders in neonatal gerbils without virus- and immune-mediated cell destructions. *Virology.* 310(2):245–253; Jun 2003.

57. Singer HS, Morris CM, Gause CD, Gillin PK, Crawford S, Zimmerman AW. Antibodies against fetal brain in sera of mothers with autistic children. *J Neuroimmunol.* 194(1–2):165–172. Feb 2008. Epub 2008 Feb 21.

58. Martin LA, Ashwood P, Braunschweig D, Cabanlit M, Van de Water J, Amaral DG. Stereotypies and hyperactivity in rhesus monkeys exposed to IgG from mothers of children with autism. *Brain Behav Immun.* 2008 Feb 7 [Epub ahead of print].

59. Braunschweig D, Ashwood P, Krakowiak P, Hertz-Picciotto I, Hansen R, Croen LA, Pessah IN, Van de Water J. Autism: maternally derived antibodies specific for fetal brain proteins. *Neurotoxicology.* 29(2):226–231. Mar 2008. Epub Nov 2007.

60. Carbone KM, Rubin SA, Pletnikov M. *Borna disease virus (BDV)-induced model of autism: application to vaccine safety test design.* Mol Psychiatry. 7 Suppl 2:S36–37; 2002.

61. Lancaster K, Dietz DM, Moran TH, Pletnikov MV. Abnormal social behaviors in young and adult rats neonatally infected with Borna disease virus. *Behav Brain Res.* 176(1):141–148. Jan 2007. Epub Jul 2006.

62. Nishino Y, Kobasa D, Rubin SA, Pletnikov MV, Carbone KM. Enhanced neurovirulence of borna disease virus variants associated with nucleotide changes in the glycoprotein and L polymerase genes. *J Virol.* 76:17:8650–8658; Sep 2002.

63. Williams BL, Yaddanapudi K, Hornig M, Lipkin WI. Spatiotemporal analysis of purkinje cell degeneration relative to parasagittal expression domains in a model of neonatal viral infection *J Virol.* 81(6):2675–2687. Mar 2007. Epub Dec 2006.

64. Bauman ML, Kemper TL. Structural brain anatomy in autism: what is the evidence? In *The Neurobiology of Autism*, 2nd edition, pp. 121–135. Baltimore, MD: The Johns Hopkins University Press, 2005.

65. Bauman ML, Kemper TL. Neuroanatomic observations of the brain in autism: a review and future directions. *Int J Dev Neurosci.* 23(2–3):183–187. Apr–May 2005.

66. Pletnikov MV, Carbone KM. An animal model of virus-induced autism: borna disease virus infection of the neonatal rat. In *The Neurobiology of Autism*, 2nd edition. Bauman ML, Kemper TL (Eds.), pp. 190–201. Baltimore, MD: The Johns Hopkins University Press, 2005.

67. Page T, Coleman M. De novo purine synthesis is increased in the fibroblasts of purine autism patients. *Adv Exp Med Biol.* 431:793–796; 1998.

68. Page T, Coleman M. Purine metabolism abnormalities in a hyperuricosuric subclass of autism. *Biochim Biophys Acta.* 1500:3:291–296; Mar 2000.

69. Page T, Moseley C. Metabolic treatment of hyperuricosuric autism. *Prog Neuropsychopharmacol Biol Psychiatry.* 26:2:397–400; Feb 2002.

70. Blount BC, Mack MM, Wehr CM, MacGregor JT, Hiatt RA, Wang G, Wickramasinghe SN, Everson RB, Ames BN. Folate deficiency causes uracil misincorporation into human DNA and chromosome breakage: implications for cancer and neuronal damage. *Proc Natl Acad Sci USA.* 94:7:3290–295; Apr 1997.

71. Hazell AS, Butterworth RF. Hepatic encephalopathy: an update of pathophysiologic mechanisms. *Proc Soc Exp Biol Med.* 222:2:99–112; Nov 1999.

72. Herbert MR. Large brains in autism: the challenge of pervasive abnormality. *Neuroscientist.* 11:5:417–424; Oct 2005.

73. Herbert MR, Kenet T. Brain abnormalities in language disorders and in autism. *Pediatr Clin North Am.* 54:3:563–583, vii; Jun 2007.

74. Jalan R, Shawcross D, Davies N. The molecular pathogenesis of hepatic encephalopathy. *Int J Biochem Cell Biol.* 35:8:1175–1181; Aug 2003.

75. Norenberg MD. A light and electron microscopic study of experimental portal-systemic (ammonia) encephalopathy. Progression and reversal of the disorder. *Lab Invest.* 36:6:618–627; Jun 1977.

76. Licinio J, Wong ML. Pathways and mechanisms for cytokine signaling of the central nervous system. *J Clin Invest.* 100:12:2941–2947; Dec 1997.

77. Greco AV, Mingrone G, Favuzzi A, Bertuzzi A, Gandolfi A, DeSmet R, Vanholder R, Gasbarrini G. Subclinical hepatic encephalopathy: role of tryptophan binding to albumin and the competition with indole-3-acetic acid. *J Investig Med.* 48:4:274–280; Jul 2000.

78. Deshpande G, Adachi N, Liu K, Motoki A, Mitsuyo T, Nagaro T, Arai T. Recovery of brain dopamine metabolism by branched-chain amino acids in rats with acute hepatic failure. *J Neurosurg Anesthesiol.* 19:4:243–248; Oct 2007.

79. Fischer JE, Baldessarini RJ. False neurotransmitters and hepatic failure. *Lancet.* 2:7715:75–80; Jul 1971.

80. Baldessarini RJ, Fischer JE. Substitute and alternative neurotransmitters in neuropsychiatric illness. *Arch Gen Psychiatry.* 34:8:958–964; Aug 1997.

81. Fogel WA, Andrzejewski W, Máslínski C. Neurotransmitters in hepatic encephalopathy. *Acta Neurobiol Exp (Wars).* 50:4–5:281–293; 1990.

82. Lam KC, Tall AR, Goldstein GB, Mistilis SP. Role of a false neurotransmitter, octopamine, in the pathogenesis of hepatic and renal encephalopathy. *Scand J Gastroenterol.* 8:6:465–472; 1973.

83. al Mardini H, Harrison EJ, Ince PG, Bartlett K, Record CO. Brain indoles in human hepatic encephalopathy. *Hepatology.* 17:6:1033–1040; Jun 1993.

84. Mills MJ, Savery D, Shattock PE. Rapid analysis of low levels of indolyl-3-acryloylglycine in human urine by high-performance liquid chromatography. *J Chromatogr B Biomed Sci Appl.* 712:1–2:51–58; Aug 1998.

85. Marklová E. Where does indolylacrylic acid come from? *Amino Acids.* 17:4:401–413; 1999.

86. Bergeron M, Reader TA, Layrargues GP, Butterworth RF. Monoamines and metabolites in autopsied brain tissue from cirrhotic patients with hepatic encephalopathy. *Neurochem Res.* 14:9:853–859; Sep 1989.

87. Courchesne E, Redcay E, Kennedy DP. The autistic brain: birth through adulthood. *Curr Opin Neurol.* 17:4:489–496; Aug 2004.

88. Courchesne E, Pierce K. Why the frontal cortex in autism might be talking only to itself: local over-connectivity but long-distance disconnection. *Curr Opin Neurobiol.* 15:2:225–230; Apr 2005.

89. Schumann CM, Hamstra J, Goodlin-Jones BL, Lotspeich LJ, Kwon H, Buonocore MH, Lammers CR, Reiss AL, Amaral DG. The amygdala is enlarged in children but not adolescents with autism; the hippocampus is enlarged at all ages. *J Neurosci.* 24:28:6392–6401; Jul 2004.

90. Herbert MR, Ziegler DA, Deutsch CK, O'Brien LM, Lange N, Bakardjiev A, Hodgson J, Adrien KT, Steele S, Makris N, Kennedy D, Harris GJ, Caviness VS, Jr. Dissociations of cerebral cortex, subcortical and cerebral white matter volumes in autistic boys. *Brain.* 126(Pt 5):1182–1192; May 2003.

91. Herbert MR, Ziegler DA, Makris N, Filipek PA, Kemper TL, Normandin JJ, Sanders HA, Kennedy DN, Caviness VS, Jr. Localization of white matter volume increase in autism and developmental language disorder. *Ann Neurol.* 55:4:530–540; Apr 2004.

92. Korvatska E, Van de Water J, Anders TF, Gershwin ME. Genetic and immunologic considerations in autism. *Neurobiol Dis.* 9:2:107–125; Mar 2002.

93. Koul O. Myelin and autism. Paper presented at the International Meeting for Autism Research in November 2001.

94. Greenfield EA, Reddy J, Lees A, Dyer CA, Koul O, Nguyen K, Bell S, Kassam N, Hinojoza J, Eaton MJ, Lees MB, Kuchroo VK, Sobel RA. Monoclonal antibodies to distinct regions of human myelin proteolipid

protein simultaneously recognize central nervous system myelin and neurons of many vertebrate species. *J Neurosci Res.* 83(3):415–431; Feb 15 2006.

95. Simon DK, Rodriguez ML, Frosch MP, Quackenbush EJ, Feske SK, Natowicz MR. A unique familial leukodystrophy with adult onset dementia and abnormal glycolipid storage: a new lysosomal disease? *J Neurol Neurosurg Psychiatry.* 65:2:251–254; Aug 1998.

96. Kane PC, Braccia D, Kane E. *Phospholipid therapy in ALS, The PK Protocol.* Johns Hopkins Int Conference on Brain Uptake and Utilization of Fatty Acids. Presented Oct 2004.

97. Minshew NJ, Goldstein G, Dombrowski SM, Panchalingam K, Pettegrew JW. A preliminary 31P MRS study of autism: evidence for undersynthesis and increased degradation of brain membranes. *Biol Psychiatry.* 33(11–12):762–773. Jun 1–15 1993.

98. Happé F, Frith U. The weak coherence account: detail-focused cognitive style in autism spectrum disorders. *J Autism Dev Disord.* 36(1):5–25; Jan 2006.

99. Minshew NJ, Goldstein G, Siegel DJ. Neuropsychologic functioning in autism: profile of a complex information processing disorder. *J Int Neuropsychol Soc.* 3:303–316; 1997.

100. Shah A, Frith U. Why do autistic individuals show superior performance on the block design task? *J Child Psychol Psychiatry.* 34:8:1351–1364; Nov 1993.

101. Casanova MF, van Kooten IA, Switala AE, van Engeland H, Heinsen H, Steinbusch HW, Hof PR, Trippe J, Stone J, Schmitz C. Minicolumnar abnormalities in autism. *Acta Neuropathol.* 112(3):287–303. Sep 2006. Epub Jul 2006.

102. Gustafsson L. Comment on "Disruption in the inhibitory architecture of the cell minicolumn: implications for autism." *Neuroscientist.* 10:3:189–191; Jun 2004.

103. Friedman SD, Shaw DW, Artru AA, Dawson G, Petropoulos H, Dager SR. Gray and white matter brain chemistry in young children with autism. *Arch Gen Psychiatry.* 63:7:786–794; Jul 2006.

104. Sokol DK, Kunn DW, Edwards-Brown M, Feinberg J. Hydrogen proton magnetic resonance spectroscopy in autism: preliminary evidence of elevated choline/creatinine ratio. *J Child Neurol.* 17:245–249; 2002.

105. Poll-The BT, Roels F, Ogier H, Scotto J, Vamecq J, Schutgens RB, Wanders RJ, van Roermund CW, van Wijland MJ, Schram AW, et al. A new peroxisomal disorder with enlarged peroxisomes and a specific deficiency of acyl-CoA oxidase (pseudo-neonatal adrenoleukodystrophy). *Am J Hum Genet.* 42:3:422–434; Mar 1988.

106. Kyllerman M, Blomstrand S, Mansson JE, Conradi NG, Hindmarsh T. Central nervous system malformations and white matter changes in pseudo-neonatal adrenoleukodystrophy. *Neuropediatrics.* 21:4:199–201; Nov 1990.

107. Moser AB, Rasmussen M, Naidu S, Watkins PA, McGuinness M, Hajra AK, Chen G, Raymond G, Liu A, Gordon D, et al. Phenotype of patients with peroxisomal disorders subdivided into sixteen complementation groups. *J of Pediatr* 127:1:13–22; July 1995.

108. Wanders RJ. Peroxisomes, lipid metabolism, and peroxisomal disorders. *Mol Genet Metab.* 83:1–2:16–27; Sep–Oct 2004.

109. Moser HW, Moser AB. Peroxisomal disorders: overview. *Ann N Y Acad Sci.* 804:427–441. Review; Dec 1996.

110. Araki E, Kobayashi T, Kohtake N, Goto I, Hashimoto. A riboflavin-responsive lipid storage myopathy due to multiple acylCoA cehydrogenase deficiency: an adult case. *J of the Neurological Sciences* 126:202–205; 1994.

111. Beier K, Volkl A, Fahimi HD. Suppression of peroxisomal lipid ß-oxidation enzymes by TNF-alpha. *FEBS Lett.* 310:273–278; 1992.

112. Kodama K, Suzuki M, Toyosawa T, Araki S. Inhibitory mechanisms of highly purified vitamin B2 on the productions of proinflammatory cytokine and NO in endotoxin-induced shock in mice. *Life Sci.* 78:2:134–139. Nov 26 2005. Epub Aug 2005.

113. Verity MA, Sarafian T, Pacifici EH, Sevanian A. Phospholipase A2 stimulation by methyl mercury in neuron culture. *J Neurochem.* 62(2):705–714; Feb 1994.

114. Shanker G, Syversen T, Aschner M. Astrocyte-mediated methylmercury neurotoxicity. *Biol Trace Elem Res.* 95:1:1–10; Oct 2003.

115. Farooqui AA, Ong WY, Horrocks LA. Biochemical aspects of neurodegeneration in human brain: involvement of neural membrane phospholipids and phospholipases A2. *Neurochem Res.* 29:11:1961–1977; Nov 2004.

116. Curran LK, Newschaffer CJ, Lee LC, Crawford SO, Johnston MV, Zimmerman AW. Behaviors associated with fever in children with autism spectrum disorders. *Pediatrics.* 120(6):e1386–1392; Dec 2007.

117. Steiner AA, Ivanov AI, Serrats J, Hosokawa H, Phayre AN, Robbins JR, Roberts JL, Kobayashi S, Matsumura K, Sawchenko PE, Romanovsky AA. Cellular and molecular basis of the initiation of fever. *PLoS Biol.* 4:9:e284; Sept 2006.

118. Khanapure SP, Garvey DS, Janero DR, Letts LG. Eicosanoids in inflammation: biosynthesis, pharmacology, and therapeutic frontiers. *Curr Top Med Chem.* 7:3:311–340; 2007.

119. Bukelis I, Porter FD, Zimmerman AW, Tierney E. Smith-Lemli-Opitz syndrome and autism spectrum disorder. *Am J Psychiatry.* 164:11:1655–1661; Nov 2007.

120. Bazan NG, Murphy MG, Toffano G. Neurobiology of essential fatty acids. In *Advances in Experimental Medicine and Biology.* Vol 318 from the proceedings July 10–12, 1991, Australia. NY: Plenum Publishing, 1992.

121. Herbert MR, Russo JP, Yang S, Roohi J, Blaxill M, Kahler SG, Cremer L, Hatchwell E. Autism and environmental genomics. *Neurotoxicology.* 27(5):671–684. Sep 2006. Epub Mar 2006.

122. Persico AM, Bourgeron T. Searching for ways out of the autism maze: genetic, epigenetic and environmental clues. *Trends Neurosci.* 29(7):349–358. Jul 2006. Epub Jun 2006.

123. Lee LC, Zachary AA, Leffell MS, Newschaffer CJ, Matteson KJ, Tyler JD, Zimmerman AW. HLA-DR4 in families with autism. *Pediatr Neurol.* 35(5):303–307; Nov 2006.

124. Santos KF, Mazzola TN, Carvalho HF. The prima donna of epigenetics: the regulation of gene expression by DNA methylation. *Braz J Med Biol Res.* 38(10):1531–1541. Oct 2005. Epub Sep 2005.

125. James SJ, Cutler P, Melnyk S et al. Metabolic biomarkers of increased oxidative stress and impaired methylation capacity in children with autism. *Am J Clin Nutr.* 80(6):1611–1617; Dec 2004.

126. Kern JK, Jones AM. Evidence of toxicity, oxidative stress, and neuronal insult in autism. *J Toxicol Environ Health B Crit Rev.* 9:485–499; 2006.

127. James SJ, Melnyk S, Fuchs G, Reid T, Jernigan S, Pavliv O, Hubanks A, Chambers N, Simshauser D, Gaylor DW. Efficacy of methylcobalamin and folinic acid treatment on glutathione redox status and core behaviors in children with autism. *Ped. Res.* (In Press.)

128. Reed MC, Nijhout HF, Neuhouser ML, Gregory JF 3rd, Shane B, James SJ, Boynton A, Ulrich CM. A mathematical model gives insights into nutritional and genetic aspects of folate-mediated one-carbon metabolism. *J Nutr.* 136(10):2653–2661; Oct 2006.

129. Chadefaux B, Rethoré MO, Raoul O, Ceballos I, Poissonnier M, Gilgenkranz S, Allard D. Cystathionine beta synthase: gene dosage effect in trisomy 21. *Biochem Biophys Res Commun.* 128(1):40–44; Apr 16 1985.

130. Scott JM, Weir DG, Molloy A, McPartlin J, Daly L, Kirke P. Folic acid metabolism and mechanisms of neural tube defects. *Ciba Found Symp.* 181:180–187; discussion 187–191; 1994.

131. Robertson KD, Wolffe AP. DNA methylation in health and disease. *Nat Rev Genet.* 1:1:11–19; Oct 2000.

132. Jiang YH, Bressler J, Beaudet AL. Epigenetics and human disease. *Annu Rev Genomics Hum Genet.* 5:479–510; 2004.

133. Henderson GI, Devi BG, Perez A, Schenker S. In utero ethanol exposure elicits oxidative stress in the rat fetus. *Alcohol Clin Exp Res.* 19(3):714–720; Jun 1995.

134. Murata K, Grandjean P, Dakeishi M. Neurophysiological evidence of methylmercury neurotoxicity. *Am J Ind Med.* 50(10):765–771; Oct 2007.

135. Slotkin TA, Tate CA, Cousins MM, Seidler FJ. Imbalances emerge in cardiac autonomic cell signaling after neonatal exposure to terbutaline or chlorpyrifos, alone or in combination. *Brain Res.* 160(2):219–230. Dec 7 2005. Epub Oct 2005.

136. Zerrate MC, Pletnikov M, Connors SL, Vargas DL, Seidler FJ, Zimmerman AW, Slotkin TA, Pardo CA. Neuroinflammation and behavioral abnormalities after neonatal terbutaline treatment in rats: implications for autism. *J Pharmacol Exp Ther.* 322(1):16–22. Jul 2007. Epub Mar 2007.

137. Missmer SA, Suarez L, Felkner M, Wang E, Merrill AH, Jr, Rothman KJ, Hendricks KA. Exposure to fumonisins and the occurrence of neural tube defects along the Texas-Mexico border. *Environ Health Perspect.* 114(2):237–241; Feb 2006.

138. Wang E, Norred WP, Bacon CW, Riley RT, Merrill AH, Jr. Inhibition of sphingolipid biosynthesis by fumonisins. Implications for diseases associated with Fusarium moniliforme. *J Biol Chem.* 266:22:14486–14490; Aug 1991.

139. Stevens VL, Tang J. Fumonisin B1-induced sphingolipid depletion inhibits vitamin uptake via the glycosylphosphatidylinositol-anchored folate receptor. *J Biol Chem.* 272:29:18020–18025; Jul 1997.

140. Anway MD, Cupp AS, Uzumcu M, Skinner MK. Epigenetic transgenerational actions of endocrine disruptors and male fertility. *Science.* 308(5727):1466–1469; Jun 2005.

141. Demiralp T, Herrmann CS, Erdal ME, Ergenoglu T, Keskin YH, Ergen M, Beydagi H. DRD4 and DAT1 polymorphisms modulate human gamma band responses. *Cereb Cortex.* 17(5):1007–1019. May 2007. Epub June 2 2006.

142. Kuznetsova AY, Deth RC. A model for modulation of neuronal synchronization by D4 dopamine receptor-mediated phospholipid methylation. *J Comput Neurosci*. Oct 11 2007. [Epub ahead of print].

143. Deth R, Muratore C, Benzecry J, Power-Charnitsky VA, Waly M. How environmental and genetic factors combine to cause autism: a redox/methylation hypothesis. *Neurotoxicology*. 29(1):190–201, 2008v. Jan 2008. Epub Oct 2007.

144. Danfors T, von Knorring AL, Hartvig P, Langstrom B, Moulder R, Stromberg B, Torstenson R, Wester U, Watanabe Y, Eeg-Olofsson O. Tetrahydrobiopterin in the treatment of children with autistic disorder: a double-blind placebo-controlled crossover study. *J Clin Psychopharmacol*. 25:5:485–489; Oct 2005.

145. Gupta S. Treatment of children with autism with intravenous immunoglobulin. *J Child Neurol*. 14(3): 203–205; Mar 1999.

146. Gershon MD. *The Second Brain: The Scientific Basis of Gut Instinct and a Groundbreaking New Understanding of Nervous Disorders of the Stomach and Intestines*. NY: Harper Collins, 1998.

24 Seizures

Balancing Fatty Acids in the Diet to Stabilize Brain Activity

Patricia C. Kane, Ph.D., and Annette L. Cartaxo, M.D.

I. INTRODUCTION

Seizure activity involves deranged lipids, primarily disturbed phospholipid structures within the cell membrane. Stabilizing membrane function is paramount to seizure disorder management. A targeted nutritional clinical treatment plan can address the cellular disturbance, aberrant lipid accumulation, and imbalance of essential fatty acids (EFAs) that are linked to seizure activity. This chapter probes the biological basis of seizure presentations, and offers measurable analyses and therapies that may be applied in a clinical setting.

II. EPIDEMIOLOGY

Worldwide incidence of acute symptomatic seizures is 29–39 per 100,000 per year with predominance in males <12 months of age and >65 years.[1] Seizures are a symptom of an underlying disorder that may be due to genetic, traumatic, metabolic, infectious, toxic, malignant, or pharmacologic factors. The most common causes of seizure onset are traumatic brain injury, cerebrovascular disease, drug withdrawal, infarction, and metabolic insult. Due to multiple underlying causes, any changes in disease prevalence from changes in food and diet patterns would be difficult to identify.

III. PATHOPHYSIOLOGY

DEFINITION

Seizures result from an abnormal and excessive discharge of a set of neurons in the brain impacting neuronal activity. Sudden and transitory abnormal phenomena may include alterations of consciousness, or motor, sensory, autonomic, or psychic events. Sensory manifestations may include somatosensory, auditory, visual, olfactory, gustatory, and vestibular senses, perceptual distortions, or psychic manifestations. Seizure presentation depends on the location of onset in the brain, patterns of propagation, maturity of the brain, environmental exposures, disease processes, sleep-wake cycle, medication, nutritional content of the diet, balance of EFAs, and cellular function. The impact of seizures may involve sensory, motor, and autonomic function; consciousness; emotional state; memory; cognition; and behavior.

FOOD AND NUTRIENT-RELATED ETIOLOGIES

Food has diverse roles in seizure pathology and management. Thus investigation as to the cause of a seizure presentation requires consideration of environmental exposures such as those with a foodborne origin:

- Food contamination can cause seizures, as is the case with neurocysticercosis. Cysticercosis arises when humans instead of pigs become the aberrant host for the larval stage of the pork tapeworm. Cysticercosis is acquired from ingesting the eggs of the pork tapeworm, from fecal oral contamination. Cysticercosis is not acquired from eating pork, which can be an important distinction for religious and diagnostic criteria.
- Dietary patterns emphasizing certain categories of food and nutrients can precipitate seizures in those with genetic vulnerability. Adrenoleukodystrophy is an inherited metabolic aberration where high consumption of foods containing very long chain fatty acids such as peanut butter, canola oil, and mustard exacerbate the expression of the disorder.
- Food can create a toxic insult in susceptible individuals, with excessive consumption of aspartame in foods and liquids provoking excitation in the brain.
- Frequent consumption of large body predator fish such as shark and swordfish or white albacore tuna can lead to methylmercury exposure. Methylmercury can suppress enzymes such as ornithine transcarbamylase and methionine synthase, which leads to liver impairment, hyperammonemia, and poor methylation, all of which increase the risk of seizures.

Food and isolated nutrients can compensate for genetic susceptibility such as vulnerability toward seizures observed in methylene tetrahydrofolate reductase deficiency (MTHFR), the most common inborn error of folate metabolism, presenting with neurological signs as developmental delay and seizures.[2] Clinical testing is now widely available to isolate MTHFR polymorphisms. With MTHFR identified, appropriate nutritional intervention may be applied to stabilize methylation, which is supported with the administration of methylcobalamin, folinic acid, tetrahydrobiopterin, and riboflavin.

MEMBRANE PATHOPHYSIOLOGY

Bruce Lipton writes in his book *The Biology of Belief*[3] that the cell membrane, comprising 50% phospholipid content, is paramount to the examination of healthy cellular function. Stabilization of cellular function is dependent not on the deoxyribonucleic acid but rather on the nourishment that the cell receives, and the avoidance of toxic insult such as chemicals, microbes, and heavy metals.

Disturbances in lipid metabolism play a pivotal role in seizure presentations. The membrane and organelles within the cell are the primary focus of electrical discharge within the central nervous system. The mitochondria have been a focal point for many researchers in brain function.

Another organelle, the peroxisome, plays a critical role in cellular lipid metabolism in the biosynthesis of fatty acids via ß-oxidation and ultimately, stabilization of seizure activity. The peroxisome is a primary site of detoxification within the cell. Peroxisomes are present in almost all cells, and they are most concentrated in liver and kidney cells. Clearance of neurotoxins may be compromised in states of suppressed peroxisomal ß-oxidation due to the interrelationship between the peroxisome and the cytochrome P450s. With exposure to a toxin the P450s are crucial for clearance of exogenous compounds,[4] and for the biotransformation of endogenous compounds including fatty acids, steroids, prostaglandins, and leukotrienes.

PEROXISOMAL β-OXIDATION AND FATTY ACIDS

Peroxisomal disorders are characterized by an accumulation in tissue and body fluids of renegade fatty acids: saturated and mono-unsaturated very long chain fatty acids (VLCFAs), odd chain fatty acids, and branched-chain (pristanic, phytanic) fatty acids. Renegade fatty acids are normally degraded within the peroxisome through a process known as ß-oxidation, but when peroxisomal function is impaired they accumulate in membrane structures throughout the body and can be measured most simply by analyzing the membranes of red blood cells. VLCFAs constitute a minor part of overall fatty acid content in red cells, yet their accumulation is deleterious to the brain and CNS, as is demonstrated in peroxisomal disorders.[5,6] Renegade fatty acids block detoxification and methylation pathways and may be characteristic of seizure disorders, autism, pervasive developmental delay, stroke, metabolic disorders involving the CNS, MS, ALS, Alzheimer's, Parkinson's disease, and states of neurotoxicity. Derangement of red cell lipids pertaining to suppression of peroxisomal ß-oxidation in children with autistic spectrum disorder and seizure disorders was discovered and presented at medical conferences in 1995,[7] but the hypothesis was not published until 1997.[8]

Inherited peroxisomal disorders, such as X-linked adrenoleukodystrophy (X-ALD), have been hallmarked by the research of Hugo and Ann Moser.[9] X-ALD has a typical clinical onset of 2.75 to 10 years of age, presenting with behavioral disturbances, poor school performance, difficulty understanding speech, attention deficit, hyperactivity, deterioration of vision (visual field cuts), impaired auditory discrimination, fatigue, anorexia, alternating diarrhea and constipation, abdominal pain, and vomiting. X-ALD is a neuroinflammatory, demyelinating disease. The course of some forms of X-ALD is relentlessly progressive. The biomarkers for ALD are most notably an accumulation of C24:0 (Carbon 24:0) and C26:0 (Carbon 26:0) in plasma and tissues. The ultimate result of disorders of peroxisomal ß-oxidation is most notably the accumulation of VLCFAs.[10] Suppressed ß-oxidation, revealed by a buildup of renegade VLCFAs in red cells, may be indicative of toxic exposure. These renegade VLCFAs serve as a substrate in the formation of ceramides, and have been established to be deleterious to the brain and CNS. It is possible that seizure disorders, autism, pervasive developmental delay, and adult neurological syndromes may mimic pseudo-neonatal adrenoleukodystrophy,[11] atypical ALD, asymptomatic ALD, and other variations of ALD, as peroxisomal disorders with enlarged peroxisomes, suppressed peroxisomal ß-oxidation, and a compromised neurological system.

CLINICAL APPLICATIONS THAT ALTER PEROXISOMAL ACTIVITY

The liberal use of potent antioxidants is contraindicated in the presence of elevated VLCFAs, odd chain fatty acids, and branched chain fatty acids in red cells.[12] Antioxidants are essential nutrients, but they slow cellular metabolism and must remain in the proper balance with all the essential nutrients and substrates (EFAs) to maintain metabolic equilibrium. Inappropriate use (megadosing) of antioxidants, such as vitamin E, will inhibit ß-oxidation[13] impacting the production of prostaglandins (the synthesis of a prostaglandin is an oxidative event) and cellular metabolism.[14]

Steroids are suggested as an intervention for infants with infantile spasms, which may link to disturbances in ß-oxidation of VLCFAs, as ALD disorders frequently have involvement with overt or subclinical adrenocortical insufficiency (Addison's disease) along with seizure activity.[15] Typically, low DHEA levels have been identified in patients expressing clinical ALD symptoms,[16] which parallels an increase in serum VLCFAs. Oral administration of hormones such as pregnenolone, DHEA, or thyroid[17] all stimulate peroxisomal proliferation via the ß-oxidation of renegade fatty acids as do nutrients (riboflavin, manganese), oxidative therapies, starvation states, and diets that suppress phospholipase A2 as the Membrane Stabilizing Diet Protocol[18] or the ketogenic diet.

Oral administration of hormones such as pregnenolone, DHEA, or thyroid[17] all stimulate peroxisomal proliferation via the ß-oxidation of renegade fats, as do the B vitamin riboflavin, the trace mineral manganese, and oxidative therapies. Diet and food also influence this process. For example, starvation states, the ketogenic diet, and the Membrane Stabilizing Diet Protocol (Table 24.1)[18] suppress phospholipase A2 thereby stimulating peroxisomal proliferation.

The limitation of aggressive stimulation of ß-oxidation, however, is that not only are VLCFAs ß-oxidized, but EFAs also are oxidized in the process and must be repleted and balanced. The introduction of oral and/or IV phenylbutyrate, along with phosphatidylcholine and the Membrane

TABLE 24.1

The Membrane Stabilizing Diet

Foods permitted on the diet

- Protein at each meal—organic meat, poultry, eggs, fish (wild salmon, sardines)
- Organic raw seeds and nuts (may use in place of flour)
- Organic 4:1 omega 6/omega 3 rich oils/4–6 tablespoons daily
- Free range, organic eggs
- Organic butter, ghee, cream, sour cream, full fat organic yogurt or homemade kefir
- Organic 4:1 omega-6/omega-3 oil, grape seed oil mayonnaise, coconut butter (to fry foods), homemade salad dressing, cold pressed/organic oils and dressing (no canola or peanut oil)
- Soft organic cheeses—cottage, ricotta, sheep milk feta, mozzarella
- Green/low carbohydrate vegetables—organic cucumber, chives, chard, cauliflower, cabbage, sprouts, celery, onion, leeks, zucchini, broccoli, asparagus, snow peas, bok choy, eggplant, green beans, kale, collard greens, Chinese cabbage, brussels sprouts
- Green leafy vegetables—one or more servings daily (no spinach—contains high oxalates)
- Salads daily—organic greens, sprouts, cucumber, celery, mache, cilantro/other fresh herbs, peppers, tomato, avocado, homemade dressing of pure oils, vinegar (Eden Plum), lemon juice
- Fresh herbs/spices, natural flavoring to flavor foods
- Lemonade or limeade made with fresh lemon/lime with water + dry stevia to sweeten drinks
- Organic unsweetened berries/fresh whipped cream or organic yogurt with stevia to sweeten
- Soy chips (taste like tortilla chips)
- Tofu spaghetti or fettuccine (drain, rinse, boil on high 30 minutes)
- Ice cream and low-carbohydrate desserts permitted from Patient Detoxx Book recipes[18]

Allowed but limited to one small serving of ONE of the following daily:

- Starchy vegetables—*potatoes*
- Low-carbohydrate fruit—*berries, kiwi*
- Beans, legumes as *refried beans, bean soup, bean dip*

Must completely remove from the diet:

- Grains—wheat, rice, oat, barley, millet, rye, corn—*no pasta, bread, crackers, flour, cereal*
- Starchy vegetables—*no carrots, sweet potatoes, parsnips, beets*
- High-carbohydrate fruits—*no bananas, grapes, raisins*
- Fruit juice as *bottled or canned fruit or fruit juice*
- No foods sweetened with glucose, dextrose, sucrose, corn syrup, honey, sugar
- No processed (white flour, white sugar) fast foods, no soft drinks
- No diet drinks, aspartame, sorbitol, mannitol, Maltitol
- No hydrogenated vegetable oil, margarine, processed oils
- No canola oil (often in processed foods/dressing)
- No peanut butter, peanuts, peanut oil
- No mustard
- No spinach (contain oxalates)—okay to eat chard, kale, collard, and mustard greens
- No MSG (contained in commercial soups, dressing, bouillon)
- No commercial mayonnaise or salad dressing
- No corn chips, popcorn, or corn flour

Stabilizing Protocol[18] for our patients with seizure disorders, serves to stabilize metabolic function without disruption of cellular phospholipid structure.[19]

SODIUM PHENYLBUTYRATE (PBA)

Sodium phenylbutyrate (PBA), a short 4-carbon chain fatty acid, has a long history of treatment for hyperammonemia and urea cycle disorders (ornithine transcarbamylase deficiency) without adverse effects. The hallmark of many seizure presentations is that of hyperammonemia, thus the introduction of oral or IV sodium phenylbutyrate will clear ammonia and may stabilize seizure activity. When ß-oxidation of renegade fatty acids is impaired, as is the case in neurological disorders, phenylbutyrate has been utilized[19,20] in breaking apart VLCFAs and degrading lipid rafts or ceramides. In ALS models, phenylbutyrate addresses the formation of lipid rafts,[21,22] suppresses neuroinflammation, has neuroprotective effects as a histone deacetylase inhibitor, prolongs survival, and regulates expression of anti-apoptotic genes. The use of sodium phenylbutyrate or calcium/magnesium butyrate is of striking benefit[23] in lowering glutamate[24] and aspartate,[25] decreasing neuronal excitability,[26] sequestering ammonia,[27,28] suppressing seizure activity,[29] clearing biotoxins,[18] preventing cerebral ischemic injury,[30] and has a neuroprotective effect.[31]

Phenylbutyrate and butyrate may play a pivotal role in the efficacy of the ketogenic diet, which may be considered as a treatment for seizure disorders. Gilbert[32] reported in 2000 that "seizure control correlates better with serum beta-hydroxybutyrate than with urine ketones." Characteristic findings in ornithine transcarbamylase deficiency of increased blood ammonia levels leading to seizure activity and stroke is responsive to phenylbutyrate therapy. The etiology of the ketogenic diet may be that it offers increased availability of butyrate, which is anti-inflammatory, stimulates peroxisomal function and the beta-oxidation of VLCFAs, and detoxifies ammonia, which is directly linked to seizure activity. The Membrane Stabilizing Protocol,[18] however, offers a sharper increase in availability of metabolic support by the oral and/or IV use of phenylbutyrate or butyrate than the ketogenic, low carbohydrate, or modified Atkins diets.

CERAMIDES AND PHOSPHATIDYLCHOLINE (PC)

Cellular membranes are comprised of bilipid layers of opposing phospholipids that line up soldier fashion and organize themselves spherically to provide the protective outer layer of every cell and the organelles within the cell.[13] In the mammalian plasma membrane the two choline-containing phospholipids, phosphatidylcholine (PC) and sphingomyelin, constitute more than 50% of the total phospholipid content of the membrane.[33]

VLCFAs can group together to form lipid rafts or ceramides in states of disease or following toxic exposure. The smaller head group of the ceramide, as well as the predominantly saturated fatty acids, encourages a tighter packing of the fatty acid chains in the membrane, creating the formation of solid micro-domains or ceramides.[34] The geometry of the membrane is highly sensitive to the size of the lipid chains. The width of the fatty acid portion of the membrane is ~3 nm and ~4.5 nm including the head group,[33] which must be maintained for stability. Saturated or monounsaturated fatty acids with a length of 16 or 18 carbons, and polyunsaturated fatty acids of 18 to 22 carbons, are preferred to permit the structure to maintain optimal horizontal fluidity. VLCFAs, comprising lipid rafts or ceramides ranging from 20 to 30 or more carbons, force the parallel dimensions vertically or invade the opposing leaflet, thereby destabilizing the membrane. Ceramides can sensitize neurons to excitotoxic damage and thereby promote apoptosis.[35] Accumulation of ceramides is associated with the death of motor neurons in amyotrophic lateral sclerosis,[36] neurons in Alzheimer's disease,[37] stroke, seizures, and autism.[38,39]

An increase in ceramide generation results in the subsequent loss of phosphatidylcholine (PC). Cui and Houweling, in their 2002 review on PC and cell death,[40] discuss a variety of cellular disease states that perturb PC and lead to cell death. Toxicity and infections alter PC homeostasis in mammalian cells, which can progress to cell death. Cui and Houweling further state that in a majority of studies of PC perturbation, exogenous PC rescues cells from apoptosis.

PHOSPHOLIPASE A2 (PLA2)

In states of brain injury, hypoxia, and toxicity via biotoxins, chemicals, or heavy metals, there is a sharp elevation in phospholipase A2 (PLA2) activity.[41] Increases in PLA2 activity result in premature

TABLE 24.2

Factors That Influence Phospholipase A2 Activity

PLA2 Stimulators	PLA2 Inhibitors
Insulin	Reduction in carbohydrate intake
Pancreatic juice	Phosphatidylcholine/PC
Mercury and heavy metal exposure	IV Fast Push Glutathione
High carbohydrate intake	Hyaluronic acid
Aspartic acid	Lithium
Glutamic acid	Glucocorticoids (and inhibits PG synthesis)
Biotoxins—bacteria, virus, dinoflageliates,	Bilobalide/Ginkgo (stimulates glutamate)
fungi, parasites	Niacin, nicotinic acid
Aspartame/Equal	
Hypoxia/brain injury	
Inflammatory fluids—platelets, mast cells	
Bee, cobra or snake venom	
Heparin	

uncoupling of the EFAs from phospholipids in the cell membrane.[42–44] At low concentrations PLA2s act on membrane phospholipids and are involved with intracellular membrane trafficking, proliferation, differentiation, and apoptotic processes. At high concentrations, however, PLA2s are cytotoxic.[45] Severe neurodegeneration can occur in the brain[44,46] if PLA2 activity is not controlled. Factors that influence PLA2 activity are listed in Table 24.2.

Mercury is one of the most potent stimulators of PLA2.[41,47,48] Elevation of TNFα is also a major contributor to the release of PLA2 and destabilization of the membrane lipids.[49,50] Glucose-induced insulin secretion via high consumption of refined carbohydrates[51,52] is a strong stimulator of PLA2 and must be restricted to control the wasting of EFAs released from the phospholipids. Of further concern is that excessive carbohydrate consumption, as is the case in the dietary intake for a majority of children, may lead to periods of hyperinsulinism, which may inhibit hepatic peroxisomal beta-oxidation.[53]

Potent inhibitors of PLA2,[43] in states of overexpression, include intravenous glutathione,[54] phosphatidylcholine,[55] and limited carbohydrate consumption,[51–53] thus the Membrane Stabilizing Protocol,[18] or other restricted carbohydrate diet such as the ketogenic diet, is pivotal to controlling PLA2.

IV. PATIENT EVALUATION

Collection of pertinent blood specimens is necessary for analysis of blood chemistry, hematology, red cell membrane fatty acids, polymorphism of MTHFR, hormonal balance, creatine kinase, urinary organic acids, amino acids, and neurotransmitters. Complete medical records should be obtained on the patient along with a detailed history of development, and detailed toxic, nutritional, and medical history:

- Screening questionnaires for toxic exposures, present diet, and detailed history
- Physical exam with neurological emphasis
- Comprehensive chemistry panel with complete blood count
- Electrolyte panel
- Nitrogen markers: blood urea nitrogen, creatinine, uric acid, albumin, ammonia
- Hepatic assessment: liver enzymes including alkaline phosphatase, GGT, SGOT, SGPT, and LDH
- Total creatine kinase: elevation may suggest low phosphatidylcholine content in cell membranes

The following specialty diagnostic tests can guide individualized dietary intervention for patients:[a]

RED CELL FATTY ACIDS

Analysis of red cell fatty acids depict 4 to 6 months of cellular metabolism, myelination status, cellular stability, hepatic and brain function. If compromised there will be an elevation of VLCFAs. An individualized clinical treatment intervention of balanced fatty acids and coenzymes is included with the analysis according to the evidence-based medical literature (see Figure. 24.1).

URINARY ORGANIC AND AMINO ACIDS[b]

Investigation into inborn errors in metabolism with detailed analysis of organic and amino acids may give insight into the etiology of the patient's seizure disorder. If abnormalities are identified, coenzymes as vitamins and minerals may be given to stimulate suppression of particular enzymes.

SERUM HORMONES[c] AS DHEA, IGF-1 (GROWTH HORMONE MARKER), PREGNENOLONE, ACTH, ALPHA MELANOCYTE STIMULATING HORMONE, THYROID PANEL- T3, T4, TSH, TESTOSTERONE OR ESTROGEN PANEL (E1, E2, E3)

Energy metabolism, neurohormone levels (pregnenolone), hormone balance, and the ability to beta-oxidize VLCFAs may be indicated by expanded hormonal testing. Low levels of IGF-1 may serve as a marker for suppression of methionine synthase. Many patients with neurotoxicity present with suppression of serum hormones. As the patient receives oral and IV phosphatidylcholine and balanced EFAs, hormonal balance is often naturally reestablished.

TOXIC SCREEN AS URINARY PORPHYRINS, BETA-2-MICROGLOBULIN, CHOLINESTERASE PANEL (PLASMA, RBC, SERUM), VIRAL ANTIBODIES (PARVO 19, WEST NILE, HHV6, CMV, EBV, HERPES SIMPLEX, HEPATITIS PANEL)

Patients with seizure disorders often present with chronic microbial infections, primarily viral in nature. If the history indicates exposure to pesticides and other fat-soluble chemical toxins, a cholinesterase panel may reflect this exposure by a decrease in the enzyme level while exposure to heavy metals may be reflected in urinary porphyrins and beta-2-microglobulin.

GENE NUTRIENT INTERACTIONS-MTHFR (A1298C, C677T)

Screening for the two currently known genetic polymorphisms of the methylene tetrahydrofolate reductase A1298C and C677T can reveal a potential gene-nutrient interaction. Presence of either or both of these polymorphisms suggests an inherited impairment of detoxification, neurotransmitters, growth, cognitive, and cellular function. Polymorphisms may be addressed with oral nutrients as methylcobalamin, folinic acid or Leucovorin Rx, tetrahydrobiopterin, riboflavin.

V. TREATMENT

MEDICATIONS

Anti-convulsant medication, the mainstay of treatment for seizure disorders, can have unpredictable therapeutic and toxic effects due to the pharmacodynamics of drug intervention. Response to

---

[a] Lab kits may be obtained from Body Bio for the Kennedy Krieger Institute Peroxisomal Diseases Laboratory and biomedical interpretation for individualized metabolic modeling.

[b] Saint Louis University Metabolic Screening Laboratory under the direction of Dr. James Shoemaker in St. Louis, MO.

[c] National laboratories such as Quest and LabCorp now have availability of the above suggested lab tests.

Red Cell Lipid Biomarkers

UNCONTROLLED EPILEPSY: Male Child

The % Status is the weighted deviation of the lab result and will show no graph when the research does not support negative values.

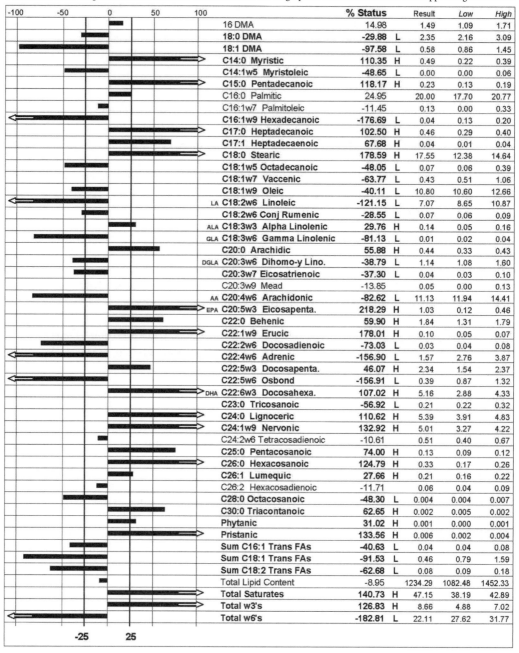

	% Status		Result	Low	High
16 DMA	14.98		1.49	1.09	1.71
18:0 DMA	-29.88	L	2.35	2.16	3.09
18:1 DMA	-97.58	L	0.58	0.86	1.45
C14:0 Myristic	110.35	H	0.49	0.22	0.39
C14:1w5 Myristoleic	-48.65	L	0.00	0.00	0.06
C15:0 Pentadecanoic	118.17	H	0.23	0.13	0.19
C16:0 Palmitic	24.95		20.00	17.70	20.77
C16:1w7 Palmitoleic	-11.45		0.13	0.00	0.33
C16:1w9 Hexadecanoic	-176.69	L	0.04	0.13	0.20
C17:0 Heptadecanoic	102.50	H	0.46	0.29	0.40
C17:1 Heptadecaenoic	67.68	H	0.04	0.01	0.04
C18:0 Stearic	178.59	H	17.55	12.38	14.64
C18:1w5 Octadecanoic	-48.05	L	0.07	0.06	0.39
C18:1w7 Vaccenic	-63.77	L	0.43	0.51	1.06
C18:1w9 Oleic	-40.11	L	10.80	10.60	12.66
LA C18:2w6 Linoleic	-121.15	L	7.07	8.65	10.87
C18:2w6 Conj Rumenic	-28.55	L	0.07	0.06	0.09
ALA C18:3w3 Alpha Linolenic	29.76	H	0.14	0.05	0.16
GLA C18:3w6 Gamma Linolenic	-81.13	L	0.01	0.02	0.04
C20:0 Arachidic	55.88	H	0.44	0.33	0.43
DGLA C20:3w6 Dihomo-y Lino.	-38.79	L	1.14	1.08	1.60
C20:3w7 Eicosatrienoic	-37.30	L	0.04	0.03	0.10
C20:3w9 Mead	-13.85		0.05	0.00	0.13
AA C20:4w6 Arachidonic	-82.62	L	11.13	11.94	14.41
EPA C20:5w3 Eicosapenta.	218.29	H	1.03	0.12	0.46
C22:0 Behenic	59.90	H	1.84	1.31	1.79
C22:1w9 Erucic	178.01	H	0.10	0.05	0.07
C22:2w6 Docosadienoic	-73.03	L	0.03	0.04	0.08
C22:4w6 Adrenic	-156.90	L	1.57	2.76	3.87
C22:5w3 Docosapenta.	46.07	H	2.34	1.54	2.37
C22:5w6 Osbond	-156.91	L	0.39	0.87	1.32
DHA C22:6w3 Docosahexa.	107.02	H	5.16	2.88	4.33
C23:0 Tricosanoic	-56.92	L	0.21	0.22	0.32
C24:0 Lignoceric	110.62	H	5.39	3.91	4.83
C24:1w9 Nervonic	132.92	H	5.01	3.27	4.22
C24:2w6 Tetracosadienoic	-10.61		0.51	0.40	0.67
C25:0 Pentacosanoic	74.00	H	0.13	0.09	0.12
C26:0 Hexacosanoic	124.79	H	0.33	0.17	0.26
C26:1 Lumequic	27.66	H	0.21	0.16	0.22
C26:2 Hexacosadienoic	-11.71		0.06	0.04	0.09
C28:0 Octacosanoic	-48.30	L	0.004	0.004	0.007
C30:0 Triacontanoic	62.65	H	0.002	0.005	0.002
Phytanic	31.02	H	0.001	0.000	0.001
Pristanic	133.56	H	0.006	0.002	0.004
Sum C16:1 Trans FAs	-40.63	L	0.04	0.04	0.08
Sum C18:1 Trans FAs	-91.53	L	0.46	0.79	1.59
Sum C18:2 Trans FAs	-62.68	L	0.08	0.09	0.18
Total Lipid Content	-8.95		1234.29	1082.48	1452.33
Total Saturates	140.73	H	47.15	38.19	42.89
Total w3's	126.83	H	8.66	4.88	7.02
Total w6's	-182.81	L	22.11	27.62	31.77

FIGURE 24.1   Red cell fatty acid laboratory results from a 12-year-old male with uncontrolled seizures. From © 1994-2008 BodyBio Inc. Patented, US Patents 5,746,204, 6,063,026, 6,277,070, 6,273,854. Other US & Foreign Patents Pending. All Rights Reserved.

medication varies widely with seizure type and syndrome. Polytherapy (combination, adjunctive, or add-on therapy) is often required in 30% to 50% of patients who fail to respond to single drug therapy. For many patients with breakthrough seizures, pharmacologic therapy currently does not offer sufficient control. Dietary intervention may be a viable consideration for those patients who fail to have stabilization with medication.

KETOGENIC DIET

The ketogenic diet, with or without adjunctive medication, is noted by Freeman[56] to be "perhaps more effective than most of the newer medications" in addressing seizure disorders. The primary negative reason for not using the ketogenic diet is the complex initiation (hospitalization) and highly restrictive dietary requirements; however, modification of the diet can eliminate these limitations.

Since the time of Hippocrates, fasting was considered an effective short-term treatment for seizures. Starvation generates ketone bodies, which can be used as metabolic fuel instead of glucose. The ketogenic diet is a high-fat, low-carbohydrate, and low-protein diet that mimics starvation by generating ketone bodies. Used since the 1920s to treat patients with intractable epilepsy, the diet has proven efficacy in controlling seizure activity. There are several types of ketogenic diets. The most frequently utilized is the Johns Hopkins traditional diet described by Wilder[57] in 1921, which is based on long chain saturated fats (butter, cream, meat fat, bacon) and utilizes a low percentage of protein and carbohydrate. The ketogenic ratio is 4:1 with four parts fat to one part of a combination of protein and carbohydrate. The ketogenic diet protocol requires an inpatient hospital setting whereby the patient is placed in a state of ketonuria by fasting for 24 hours. It has been noted that some patients have immediate improvement in seizure frequency and severity after the initial fasting period, while others experience improvement many weeks after the onset of the diet.[58] Overall, estimates indicate that complete cessation of all seizures occurs in about 16% of patients, with a greater than 90% reduction in seizures occurring in 32%, and a greater than 50% reduction in seizures occurring in 56%.[56]

The concept of the ketogenic diet is that it provides sufficient protein for growth but insufficient amount of carbohydrates for all the metabolic needs of the body. Energy is derived largely from fatty acid oxidation rather than from carbohydrates. During high rates of fatty acid oxidation, large amounts of acetyl-CoA are generated, leading to the synthesis, primarily in the liver, of the three ketone bodies (1) beta-hydroxybutyrate, (2) acetoacetate, and (3) acetone. The metabolic efficiency of the Krebs cycle is reduced, and excess acetyl-CoA is shunted to the production of ketone bodies. Ketone bodies spill into the circulation, causing serum levels to rise several-fold, and are then utilized as an energy (ATP) source in extrahepatic tissues, including the brain. Glucose is ordinarily the sole fuel for the human brain, but it is hypothesized that ketone bodies enter the brain in proportion to the degree of ketosis. Utilization of ketones by the brain is usually minimal but with the ketogenic diet, ketone bodies partly replace glucose as fuel for the brain.

Side effects of the ketogenic diet may include persistent metabolic acidosis, hypoglycemia, hyperlipidemia, hypertriglyceridemia, dehydration, nausea/vomiting, diarrhea, constipation, gastritis, fat intolerance, increased bruising, transient hyperuricemia, hypoproteinemia, hypomagnesemia, repetitive hyponatremia, low HDL, iron-deficiency anemia, and reduction in quality of life—unable to participate fully in celebrations and gatherings. Late-onset complications may include delayed growth, osteopenia, renal calculi, renal stones, cardiomyopathy, secondary hypocarnitinemia, lipoid pneumonia due to aspiration, hepatitis, ulcerative colitis, and acute pancreatitis.

Most early- and late-onset complications are described by Freeman and colleagues[59] as "transient and successfully managed by careful follow-up and conservative strategies"; however, this may not be the case in extended use of the diet, which may produce health risks. In addition, there are patients who simply cannot tolerate the ketogenic diet due to aberrant fatty acid oxidation involving both the mitochondrial and peroxisomal function. Detailed testing of red cell and plasma fatty acids can prevent health challenges and target the proper diet and balance of fatty acids for the individual patient.

Modified Ketogenic Diets

In the last several years papers have emerged stating that it is not necessary to comply to the rigid confines of the ketogenic diet and that it may be liberalized into a low-glycemic-index (LGIT) diet[60,61] or a modified Atkins diet[62] instead. Hospitalization is required to attain ketosis and maintenance of a low-carbohydrate, high-fat diet with unlimited protein and fats, green vegetables, salad, ~15 g of carbohydrate daily as vegetables or fruit such as berries is far easier for the patient to follow and results in similar clinical outcomes in regard to reduction in seizure activity achieved by the ketogenic diet. The LGIT and modified Atkins diets, however, do not address fatty acid imbalances or altered lipid metabolism that are at the core of a seizure presentation.

The Membrane Stabilizing Protocol

The Membrane Stabilizing Protocol[18] includes a Membrane Stabilizing Diet that was created for stabilization of cellular function by balancing EFAs with targeted oral lipids after red cell analysis along with a restriction of carbohydrates. The Membrane Stabilizing Diet Protocol is organic and nutrient dense, consisting of protein (meat, poultry, fish), green vegetables, seeds, nuts, cold pressed oil, and dairy products, with limited use of berries, potato, and legumes. Processed food, sugar, juice, grains, high-carbohydrate fruits, and starchy vegetables are not allowed (see Table 24.1).

Evaluating Red Cell Lipids to Establish a Membrane Stabilizing Protocol

The mechanism by which the ketogenic diet protects against seizures is described as "remaining elusive"; however, research on the etiology of the diet has never been integrated with current fatty acid literature. As the focus of a study is usually on one or limited variables, there is restriction into the scientific exploration of the complex nature of cellular and membrane function involving the brain.

It is paramount that the content of fatty acids be examined in red cells so that stabilization of brain function via lipids in regard to seizure activity may be realized. Red cell lipid analysis offers a reflection of neuronal fatty acid content that is noninvasive. The results of detailed fatty acid analysis have not been applied in individualized protocols in hospital-based ketogenic diet regimes. In clinical work, however, the results of red cell fatty acid analysis have been successfully applied to pediatric and adult populations with seizure disorders for more than a decade.[8,19,63]

Detailed examination of red cell fatty acids from the Peroxisomal Diseases Laboratory at Kennedy Krieger Institute over the past 12 years has demonstrated that our patient population[19,64] with seizure disorders has characteristic moderate to severe elevation of red cell very long chain fatty acids (VLCFAs) above C20 (carbon 20) indicating deranged peroxisomal involvement.[7,8,18,39,65–72] Altered peroxisomal function represents cellular membrane disturbance, neurological dysfunction, hepatic derangement in regard to detoxification, the potential for an increase in ceramide production, and impaired synthesis of prostaglandins, which may be a complication, or possible etiology of, seizure presentations. See the red cell lipid biomarkers presented in Figure 24.1.

Membrane phospholipid abnormalities with elevation of VLCFAs are indicative of altered cellular function resulting in suppressed peroxisomal ß-oxidation of VLCFAs. Numerous neurological disorders have also been identified with the buildup of VLCFAs including adrenoleukodystrophy, autism, ALS, Parkinson's disease, multiple sclerosis, pervasive developmental delay, brain injury, stroke, and Alzheimer's disease.[18,72–75] The origin of this cellular derangement may involve exposure to neurotoxins. The use of oral and IV lipids facilitates stabilization of phospholipids in cellular membranes thereby addressing hepatic and CNS clearance of microbes, chemicals, and heavy metals, ultimately resulting in optimal cellular and nervous system function.

Balancing EFAs and the Specific Ratio 3 (SR3)

Renowned lipid researcher Michael Crawford defines the dry weight of the human brain as 60% lipid,[76] with dendrites and synapses up to 80% lipid content. Phospholipids, cholesterol, cerebrosides, gangliosides, and sulfatides are the lipids most predominant in the brain, residing within the bilayers.[77] The phospholipids and their EFA components provide second messengers and signal mediators[78] and play a vital role in the cell signaling systems in the neuron.[79] The functional behavior of neuronal membranes largely depends upon the ways in which individual phospholipids are aligned, interspersed with cholesterol, and associated with proteins. Neurotransmitters are wrapped up in phospholipid vesicles. The release and uptake of the neurotransmitters are dependent upon the realignment of the phospholipid molecules. The nature of the phospholipid is a factor in determining how much of a neurotransmitter or metal ion will pass out of a vesicle or be taken back in. Phospholipid remodeling may be stimulated by supplying oral or IV phospholipids, principally PC, as well as balanced EFAs and catalysts via nutritional intervention.

The optimal function of the membrane, and consequently the organism, is intimately dependent upon lipid substrates. The EFAs *must* be ingested, and in a preferred proportion to one another, which involves the two basic EFA families, ω6 and ω3.

In 1993 Yehuda and a colleague[80] published their findings on an optimal EFA ratio of 4 parts ω6 linoleic acid to 1 part ω3 alpha linolenic acid, termed the SR-3 ratio, with reported benefits as improved learning and elevation of pain threshold. Continuation of Yehuda's research has elucidated that the SR-3 improves seizure control and anti-convulsant efficiency,[81-85] cognitive function,[86-89] sleep,[90] and stabilization of brain structure and function.[91,92]

Yehuda's SR-3 provides the EFAs linoleic acid (LA) and alpha linolenic acid (ALA) which, in themselves, are critical components to stable neurochemistry even though they are lower order fatty acid metabolites.[85] Clinical application of Yehuda's SR-3 oil has proven efficacy in seizure disorders in our patient population.[19] EFAs consist of two levels and are categorized as:

1.   Lower order fatty acids, or polyunsaturated fatty acids (PUFAs), linoleic acid (found in sunflower and safflower oil), and alpha linolenic acid (found in flax and soy oil).
2.   Higher order EFAs, or highly unsaturated fatty acids (HUFAs), gamma linolenic acid (GLA) found in evening primrose oil, dihomogamma linolenic acid (DGLA), arachidonic acid (AA) found in meat fat, butter, egg yolk, eicosapentaenoic acid (EPA) found in coldwater fish and fish oil, and docosahexaenoic acid (DHA) found in coldwater fish and fish oil.

All the EFAs must be a part of a balanced lipid regime for individuals with seizure presentations. Although an optimum balance of HUFAs or eicosanoids has not yet been elucidated in the literature, our access to a database of 15,000 red cell fatty acid analyses, extensive clinical experience with detailed history of patients' oral intake, and subsequent testing after aggressive supplementation of EFAs has led us to the creation of a targeted EFA-balance based on individual red cell fatty acid analysis. Liberal access to dietary and balanced oral supplementation of HUFAs must be supplied as meat fat, evening primrose oil, cream, butter, egg yolk, and coldwater, wild fish. PUFAs, however, should also be utilized as organic, cold-pressed sunflower oil and flax oil as in the SR-3 linoleic to alpha linolenic (4:1) ratio.

Indiscriminate use of marine oil, as is the case in a surprising number of patients presenting at our clinic, has resulted in gross distortion of the red cell fatty acid analysis. Over the past 12 years we have frequently observed the phenomenon of an "omega-3 overdose syndrome" after overzealous use of fish oil. Common symptoms in children are hypotonia and lethargy if a fish oil supplement with high EPA is overused without omega-6 supplementation. Eczema, mental confusion, learning difficulties, delusional behavior, irritability, inflammation, and exacerbation of autistic features and seizures may develop if a fish oil supplement with high DHA or cod liver oil is overused without omega-6 supplementation.

Patients with seizure disorders appear to have significant restabilization of their EFA balance upon retesting their red cell fatty acids when aggressive oral-balanced HUFA lipid therapy with egg yolk, meat fat, butter, and evening primrose oil is applied over ~6 months when marine oil has been overdosed.[19,63] The addition of IV phosphatidylcholine therapy appears to expedite stabilization of balanced phospholipids in the membrane in both our adult and pediatric populations along with oral-balanced EFAs.

CLEARING NEUROINFLAMMATION AND NEUROTOXINS

We have observed that patients with seizure disorders, autism, and pervasive developmental delay often have both a heavy metal burden coexisting with the additional complication of the presence of other toxins. Heavy metals may coexist within the cell membrane and fatty tissues requiring consideration of a variety of toxins: pesticides, petrochemicals, neurotoxic mold, bacteria, viruses, parasites, and chemicals such as acetaminophen. Thus intervention must address all aspects of possible toxic exposures involved in the presentation.

Introduction of a phospholipid emulsion, phosphatidylcholine (PC), as Lipostabil Rx may clear lipid-soluble microbes and toxins from the body as noted by Goldfarb and others.[93–95] Initially, research was conducted on animals whereby meningitis and systemic sepsis were cleared by the use of intravenous bolus PC. Human trials were later conducted on the use of PC in bolus IV drips to establish the safety of multi-gram doses in which no side effects were observed. Gordon and colleagues reported[95] on the first human study whereby bolus PC was administered intravenously followed by *Escherichia coli* endotoxin (2 ng/kg) intravenously, revealing that the subjects who received the bolus PC did clear the endotoxin while the subjects who received the placebo of medium chain triglycerides did not and had an immune response to the endotoxin. Presently, over 200 studies are being conducted on the use of bolus PC in regard to its medical efficacy in addressing toxic exposure.[95]

We have embarked on a clinical treatment plan for the past 6 years of therapy including both oral and intravenous lipid therapy to attenuate the accumulation of ceramides and renegade fatty acids that can compromise hepatic and CNS function. Identifying and treating methylation[97,98] and sulfation[99] deficits facilitate stabilization of phospholipids in cellular membranes, detoxification, gene expression, and stabilization of the dopamine response. Oral and IV phospholipids and phenylbutyrate therapy may modify the neuronal and hepatic membrane distortion by displacing the subsequent early expression of sphingomyelin, which follows the rise of ceramide synthesis.[40]

The Membrane Stabilizing[18] IV Protocol is initiated with a phospholipid exchange or bolus phospholipid drip followed by IV folinic acid to support methylation. In the last step of the protocol reduced glutathione (diluted with sterile H_2O, not saline) is infused. In administering glutathione with PC we are attempting to achieve a lipid-soluble glutathione to chelate heavy metals bound to metallothionein,[100–104] support immune function, and suppress PLA2,[43,54] thereby stabilizing the phospholipids in the membrane. Glutathione can form metal complexes via nonenzymatic reactions and is a versatile and pervasive metal-binding ligand. The sulfhydryl group of the cysteine moiety of glutathione has a strong affinity for mercury, silver, cadmium, arsenic, lead, gold, zinc, and copper.

The cellular impact of toxins and heavy metal burdens can result in disturbed prostaglandin synthesis, poor cellular integrity, increased cytokine release,[105] decreased glutathione levels,[106] suppression of ω6 arachidonic acid,[107,108] and marked elevation of renegade fats. Our clinical recourse is to address cellular derangement with PC, both orally and by infusion, to potentially offset the accumulation of ceramides, influence membrane fluidity, clear neurotoxins, and stabilize the integrity of the lipid membrane leaflets.

ORAL AND IV THERAPY OF THE MEMBRANE STABILIZING PROTOCOL

The Membrane Stabilizing Protocol,[18] involving diet, supplementation and IV therapy, is initiated after analysis of the patient's red cell fatty acids is completed, so that a targeted individualized approach toward stabilizing cell membrane function can be established. The core of therapy is controlling the lipid enzyme PLA2 (phospholipase A2) with the Membrane Stabilizing Diet Protocol, which is a nutrient-dense, balanced-EFA, low-carbohydrate diet to address the phospholipid architecture in the membrane. Additional benefit is derived from oral and intravenous administration of PC, balanced EFA therapy, and individualized oral regimen of EFAs specific to the aberrations in the patient's red cell fatty acid test. Additionally, membrane traffic is addressed by balancing electrolyte disturbances with an oral Ringers-type electrolyte solution; hepatic and neuroinflammatory function is augmented with butyrate (oral), phenylbutyrate (intravenous and oral), and glutathione (intravenous only); myelination is supported with fatty alcohols, which can pass the blood brain barrier (oral), supportive catalysts as coenzymes are utilized as trace minerals, macrominerals, vitamins, coenzyme Q10, carnitine, and carnosine; and methylation support is addressed with IV and oral folinic acid, riboflavin, tetrahydrobiopterin, and injectable or sublingual methylcobalamin.

The majority of sources of renegade fatty acids are removed in the Membrane Stabilizing Diet Protocol, which is accomplished by the avoidance of foods and oils that contain VLCFAs such as mustard, canola oil, peanuts, and peanut oil that can challenge patients with liver and CNS toxicity. Dr. Hugo Moser's original diet for adrenoleukodystrophy (ALD) consisted of removing oral intake of VLCFA[9] in food. The Membrane Stabilizing Diet Protocol is an expansion of Dr. Moser's diet to suppress PLA2 (phospholipase A2) but it is not as restrictive as the diet for patients with ALD or the ketogenic diet. The Membrane Stabilizing Protocol[18] establishes a PLA2 suppressive diet with the focus on nutrient density (reduced carbohydrate, high fats/oils/protein) and is also utilized to help stabilize membrane phospholipid integrity and peroxisomal function.

Many of our pediatric patients with seizure disorders have presented with complex symptomatology, including failure to thrive. Nourishing the body with EFAs, phospholipids, and a nutrient-dense diet usually results in weight stabilization and increased growth.

Weekly and biweekly infusions of phosphatidylcholine as lipostabil (natterman) may be administered by phospholipid exchange followed by folinic acid (leucovorin) and reduced glutathione (rGSH) diluted with sterile water by fast push. Only sterile water or dextrose in water can be used as a diluent for lipids as electrolytes, such as saline, will form a soap and are contraindicated. Intravenous dosing is adjusted to the age and weight of pediatric patients.

Bolus dosing of phosphatidylcholine is adjusted to the patient's test results and presentation. A detailed description of the Membrane Stabilizing Protocol including both IV and oral lipid therapy may be found in the medical book *The Detoxx Book—Detoxification of Biotoxins in Chronic Neurotoxic Syndromes*.[18]

Application of phospholipid exchange and/or bolus phosphatidylcholine as Lipostabil followed by folinic acid and glutathione by fast push has been successfully utilized in our clinical setting[109] with marked improvement in seizure control, cognition, IQ scores, focus, attention, mood, coordination, and speech as noted in our medical chart notes.[109]

VI. SUMMARY

Detailed examination of red cell fatty acids of patients with seizure presentations has revealed a characteristic elevation of VLCFAs within red cells, which may result from altered cellular function with suppressed peroxisomal ß-oxidation due to toxic insult or genetic vulnerability. Stabilizing membrane function is paramount to approaching seizure disorders and a targeted clinical treatment plan can address the cellular disturbance of the accumulation of aberrant lipids. Supplementation with balanced EFAs as Yehuda's 4:1 ratio omega-6 to omega-3 oil and phosphatidylcholine is supportive to cell membrane integrity. Catalysts supportive to methylation and cellular metabolism are crucial adjuncts to addressing disturbed neurochemistry in seizure presentations as is a low-carbohydrate, high-balanced fatty acid and high-protein diet.

To navigate the care of patients with seizure disorders it is crucial to:

- Obtain pertinent laboratory studies initially.
- Instruct patients and/or their parents in dietary changes that are reasonable for their lifestyle. Diet may need to be changed slowly to organic, fresh food.
- Begin with removal of refined sugar/flour and a sharp increase in oils containing balanced EFAs and protein foods. Carbohydrate foods may need to be slowly reduced and replaced with appropriate nutrient dense substitutes.

- Begin supplementation of nutrients slowly with phosphatidylcholine (9 capsules or 1 table-spoon daily), butyrate (may be obtained by Rx in a liquid form for pediatric patients), evening primrose oil, SR-3 balanced 4:1 omega-6 to omega-3 oil (3 to 6 tablespoons daily), folinic acid, thiamin, riboflavin, sublingual methylcobalamin, biotin, pyridoxine, niacin-amide, inositol, PABA, tetrahydrobiopterin, balanced electrolytes, magnesium, trace minerals (zinc, chromium, selenium, manganese, iodine).
- Application of phospholipid exchange and/or bolus phosphatidylcholine as Lipostabil fol-lowed by folinic acid and glutathione by fast push has been successfully utilized in our clinical setting[109] with marked improvement in seizure control, cognition, IQ scores, focus, attention, mood, coordination, and speech. Subcutaneous injection of methylcobalamin once weekly may also be indicated.

Diet has been demonstrated to be an effective treatment in the management of seizure disorders. We have investigated the biological validity of various low-carbohydrate, high-fat diets and suggest a modification of the ketogenic diet as the nutrient-dense Membrane Stabilizing Diet Protocol (see Table 24.1) so that compliance is not challenged and rather, food may be enjoyed.

ACKNOWLEDGMENTS

Thomas Wnorowski, Ph.D., and Edward Kane were supportive in the preparation of this manuscript.

REFERENCES

1. Hauser WA, Beghi E. First seizure definitions and worldwide incidence and mortality. *Epilepsia* 49, S1:8–12, 2008.
2. Fattal-Valevski A, Bassan H, Korman SH, Lerman-Sagie T, Gutman A, Harel S. Methylenetetrahydrofolate reductase deficiency: importance of early diagnosis. *J Child Neurol* 15:8:539–543, Aug 2000.
3. Lipton B. *The Biology of Belief.* Santa Rosa, CA: Mountain of Love/Elite Books, 2005.
4. Guengerich FP. Reactions and significance of cytochrome P-450 enzymes. *J Biol Chem* 266:16:10019–10022. Review. Jun 5, 1991.
5. Moser HW, Moser AB. Peroxisomal disorders: overview. *Ann N Y Acad Sci* 804:427–441. Review. Dec 27, 1996.
6. Moser AB, Kreiter N, Bezman L, Lu S, Raymond GV, Naidu S, Moser HW. Plasma very long chain fatty acids in 3,000 peroxisome disease patients and 29,000 controls. *Ann Neurol* 45:1:100–110, Jan 1999.
7. Kane PC. Unpublished data, 1995.
8. Kane PC. Peroxisomal disturbances in children with epilepsy, hypoxia and autism. *Prostaglandins, Leukotrienes and EFAs* 57:2:265, Aug 1997.
9. Moser HW, Raymond GV, Dubey P. Adrenoleukodystrophy: new approaches to a neurodegenerative disease. *JAMA* 294:24:3131–3134, Dec 28, 2005.
10. Wanders RJ. Peroxisomes, lipid metabolism, and peroxisomal disorders. *Mol Genet Metab* 83:1–2:16–27, Sep–Oct 2004.
11. Poll-The BT, Roels F, Ogier H, Scotto J, Vamecq J, Schutgens RB, Wanders RJ, van Roermund CW, van Wijland MJ, Schram AW, et al. A new peroxisomal disorder with enlarged peroxisomes and a specific deficiency of acyl-CoA oxidase (pseudo-neonatal adrenoleukodystrophy). *Am J Hum Genet* 42:3: 422–434, Mar 1988.
12. Akasaka K, Shichijyukari S, Matsuoka S, Murata M, Meguro H, Ohrui H. Absolute configuration of a ceramine with a novel branched-chain fatty acid isolated from the Epiphytic Dinoflagellate, Coolia monotis. *Biosci Biotechnol Biochem* 64:9:842–846, Sep 2000.
13. Rudin DO. Unpublished manuscript: *The Omega Factor: Our Nutritional Missing Link*, 1985, Chapter 7, p.18.
14. Gurr ML, Harwood JL, Frayn KN. *Lipid Biochemistry: An Introduction.* 5th Edition, Malden, MA: Blackwell Science, Inc, 2002.
15. Chang YC, Huang CC, Huang SC, Hung FC. Neonatal adrenoleukodystrophy presenting with seizure at birth: a case report and review of the literature. *Pediatr Neurol* 38:2:137–139, Feb 2008.

16. Assies J, Haverkort EB, Lieverse R, Vreken P. Effect of dehydroepiandrosterone supplementation on fatty acid and hormone levels in patients with X-linked adrenoleukodystrophy. *Clin Endocrinol (Oxf)* 59:4:459–466, Oct 2003.

17. Di Santo E, Foddi MC, Ricciardi-Castagnoli P, Mennini T, Ghezzi P. DHEAS inhibits TNF production in monocytes, astrocytes and microglial cells. *Neuroimmunomodulation* 3:5:285–288, Sept–Oct 1996.

18. Kane PC, Foster JS, Braccia D, Kane E. *The Detoxx Book: Detoxification of Biotoxins in Chronic Neurotoxic Syndromes, The Detoxx Book for Patients and The PK Protocol.* Millville, NJ: BodyBio, 2002.

19. Kemp S, Wei HM, Lu JF, Braiterman LT, McGuinness MC, Moser AB, Watkins PA, Smith KD. Gene redundancy and pharmacological gene therapy: implications for X-linked adrenoleukodystrophy. *Nat Med* 4:11:1261–1268, Nov 1998.

20. Gondcaille C, Depreter M, Fourcade S, Lecca MR, Leclercq S, Martin PG, Pineau T, Cadepond F, ElEtr M, Bertrand N, Beley A, Duclos S, De Craemer D, Roels F, Savary S, Bugaut M. Phenylbutyrate up-regulates the adrenoleukodystrophy-related gene as a nonclassical peroxisome proliferator. *J Cell Biol* 169:1:93–104, Apr 11, 2005.

21. Ryu H, Smith K, Camelo SI, Carreras I, Lee J, Iglesias AH, Dangond F, Cormier KA, Cudkowicz ME, Brown RH, Jr, Ferrante RJ. Sodium phenylbutyrate prolongs survival and regulates expression of anti-apoptotic genes in transgenic amyotrophic lateral sclerosis mice. *J Neurochem* 93:5:1087–1098, Jun 2005.

22. Petri S, Kiaei M, Kipiani K, Chen J, Calingasan NY, Crow JP, Beal MF. Additive neuroprotective effects of a histone deacetylase inhibitor and a catalytic antioxidant in a transgenic mouse model of amyotrophic lateral sclerosis. *Neurobiol Dis* 22:1:40–49, Apr 2006.

23. Yin L, Laevsky G, Giardina C. Butyrate suppression of colonocyte NF-kappa B activation and cellular proteasome activity. *J Biol Chem* 276:48:44641–44646, Nov 2001.

24. Daikhin Y, Yudkoff M. Ketone bodies and brain glutamate and GABA metabolism. *Dev Neurosci* 20: 358–364, 1998.

25. Yudkoff M, Daikhin Y, Nissim I, Lazarow A, Nissim I. Brain amino acid metabolism and ketosis. *J Neurosci Res* 66:2:272–281, Oct 15, 2001.

26. Leite M, Frizzo JK, Nardin P, de Almeida LM, Tramontina F, Gottfried C, Goncalves CA. Beta-hydroxy-butyrate alters the extracellular content of S100B in astrocyte cultures. *Brain Res Bull* 64:2:139–143, Aug 30, 2004.

27. Maestri NE, Brusilow SW, Clissold DB, Bassett SS. Long-term treatment of girls with ornithine transcar-bamylase deficiency. *N Engl J Med* 335:12:855–859, Sep 19, 1996.

28. Burlina AB, Ogier H, Korall H, Trefz FK. Long-term treatment with sodium phenylbutyrate in ornithine transcarbamylase-deficient patients. *Eur J Paediatr Neurol* 7:3:115–121, 2003.

29. Bogdanovic MD, Kidd D, Briddon A, Duncan JS, Land JM. Late onset heterozygous ornithine tran-scarbamylase deficiency mimicking complex partial status epilepticus. *J Neurol Neurosurg Psychiatry* 69:6:813–815, Dec 2000.

30. Qi X, Hosoi T, Okuma Y, Kaneko M, Nomura Y. Sodium 4-phenylbutyrate protects against cerebral isch-emic injury. *Mol Pharmacol* 66:4:899–908, Oct 2004.

31. Gardian G, Yang L, Cleren C, Calingasan NY, Klivenyi P, Beal MF. Neuroprotective effects of phenylbu-tyrate against MPTP neurotoxicity. *Neuromolecular Med* 5:3:235–241, 2004.

32. Gilbert DL, Pyzik PL, Freeman JM. The ketogenic diet: seizure control correlates better with serum beta-hydroxybutyrate than with urine ketones. *J Child Neurol* 15:12:787–790, Dec 2000.

33. Boal D. *Mechanics of a Cell*. Boston: Cambridge University Press, 2002, pp. 10.

34. Mouritsen OG. *Life—As a Matter of Fat, the Emerging Science of Lipidomics*. Berlin Heidelberg, Germany: Springer-Verlag, 2005.

35. Hofmann K, Tomiuk S, Wolff G, Stoffel W. Cloning and characterization of the mammalian brain-spe-cific Mg2+-dependant neutral sphingomyelinase. *Proc Natl Acad Sci USA* 97:5895–5900, 2000.

36. Cutler RG, Pedersen WA, Camandola S, Rothstein JD, Mattson MP. Evidence that accumulation of cer-amides and cholesterol esters mediates oxidative stress-induced death of motor neurons in amyotrophic lateral sclerosis. *Ann Neurol* 52:4:448–457, Oct 2002.

37. Cutler RG, Kelly J, Storie K, Pedersen WA, Tammara A, Hatanpaa K, Troncoso JC, Mattson MP. Involvement of oxidative stress-induced abnormalities in ceramide and cholesterol metabolism in brain aging and Alzheimer's disease. *Proc Natl Acad Sci* 101:7:2070–2075, Feb 17, 2004.

38. Haughey N, personal communication, March 2005.

39. Kane PC. *The Neurochemistry and Neurophysics of Autistic Spectrum Disorder*. Millville, NJ: BodyBio, 1996.

40. Cui A, Houweling M. Phosphatidylcholine and cell death. *Biochim Biophys Acta* 1585:2–3:87–96, Dec 30, 2002.

41. Verity MA, Sarafian T, Pacifici EHK, Seranian A. Phospholipase A2 stimulation by methyl mercury in neuron culture. *J of Neurochem* 62:705–714, 1994.

42. Shanker G, Hampson RE, Aschner M. Methylmercury stimulates arachidonic acid release and cytosolic phospholipase A2 expression in primary neuronal cultures. *Neurotoxicology.* 25:3:399–406, Mar 2004.

43. Farooqui AA, Litsky ML, Farooqui T, Horrocks LA. Inhibitors of intracellular phospholipase A2 activity: their neurochemical effects and therapeutic importance of neurological disorders *Brain Res Bull* 49:3:139–153, Jun 1999.

44. Farooqui AA, Ong WY, Horrocks LA. Biochemical aspects of neurodegeneration in human brain: involvement of neural membrane phospholipids and phospholipases A2. *Neurochem Res* 29:11:1961–1977, Nov 2004.

45. Farooqui AA, Horrocks LA. Excitatory amino acid receptors, neural membrane phospholipid metabolism and neurological disorders. *Brain Res Brain Res Rev* 16:2:171–191, May–Aug 1991.

46. Farooqui AA, Ong WY, Horrocks LA. Inhibitors of brain phospholipase A2 activity: their neuropharmacological effects and therapeutic importance for the treatment of neurologic disorders. *Pharmacol Rev* 58:3:591–620, Sep 2006.

47. Aschner M. Astrocytic swelling, phospholipase A2, glutathione and glutamate: interactions in methylmercury-induced neurotoxicity. *Cell Mol Biol (Noisy-le-grand)* 46:4:843–854, Jan 2000.

48. Marchi B, Burlando B, Moore MN, Viarengo A. Mercury- and copper-induced lysosomal membrane destabilisation depends on [Ca2+]i dependent phospholipase A2 activation. *Aquat Toxicol* 66:2:197–204, Feb 10, 2004.

49. Vivekananda J, Smith D, King RJ. Sphingomyelin metabolytes inhibit sphingomyelin synthase and CTP: phosphocholine cytidyltransferase. *Am J Physiol Lung Cell Mol Physiol* 281:L98–L107, 2001.

50. Awasthi S, Vivekananda J, Awasthi V, Smith D, King RJ. CTP: phosphocholine cytidylyltransferase inhibition by ceramide via PKC-alpha, p38 MAPK, cPLA2, and 5-lipoxygenase. *Am J Physiol Lung Cell Mol Physiol* 281:1:L108–118, Jul 2001.

51. Metz SA. Is phospholipase A2 a "glucose sensor" responsible for the phasic pattern of insulin release? *Prostaglandins* 1:147–58, Jan 1984.

52. Dunlop M, Clark S. Glucose-induced phosphorylation and activation of a high molecular weight cytosolic phospholipase A2 in neonatal rat pancreatic islets. *Int J Biochem Cell Biol* 27:11:1191–1199, Nov 1995.

53. Xu L, Ash M, Abdel-aleem S, Lowe JE, Badr M. Hyperinsulinemia inhibits hepatic peroxisomal beta-oxidation in rats. *Horm Metab Res* 27:2:76–78, Feb 1995.

54. Kramer BC, Yabut JA, Cheong J, Jnobaptiste R, Robakis T, Olanow CW, Mytilineou C. Toxicity of glutathione depletion in mesencephalic cultures: a role for arachidonic acid and its lipoxygenase metabolites. *Eur J Neurosci* 19:2:280–286, Jan 2004.

55. Arrigoni E, Averet N, Cohadon F. Effects of CDP-choline on phospholipase A2 and cholinephosphotransferase activities following a cryogenic brain injury in the rabbit. *Biochem Pharmacol* 36:21:3697–3700, Nov 1, 1987.

56. Freeman JM, Kossoff EH, Hartman AL. The ketogenic diet: one decade later. *Pediatrics* 119:535–543, 2007.

57. Wilder RM. The effect of ketonemia on the course of epilepsy. *Mayo Clin Bull* 2:307, 1921.

58. Vining EP. Clinical efficacy of the ketogenic diet. *Epilepsy Res* 37:181–190, 1999.

59. Hemingway C, Freeman JM, Pillas DJ, Pyzik PL. The ketogenic diet: A 3- to 6-year follow-up of 150 children enrolled prospectively. *Pediatrics* Oct 2001:108:4:898–905.

60. Pfeifer HH, Thiele EA. Low-glycemic-index treatment: a liberalized ketogenic diet for treatment of intractable epilepsy. *Neurology* 65:1810–1812, 2005.

61. Kang HC, Lee HS, You SJ, Kang DC, Ko TS, Kim HD. Use a modified Atkins diet in intractable childhood epilepsy. *Epilepsia* 48:182–186, 2007.

62. Kossoff EH, McGrogan JR, Bluml RM, Pillas DJ, Rubenstein JE, Vining EP. A modified Atkins diet is effective for the treatment of intractable pediatric epilepsy. *Epilepsia* 47:2:421–424, 2006.

63. Kane PC, Foster JS. Clinical data, Wellspring Clinic, 2000–2002.

64. Kane PC, Cartaxo AL. Clinical data, 1998.

65. Kane PC, Kane E. Peroxisomal disturbances in autistic spectrum disorder. *J Ortho Med* 12:4:207–218, 1997.

66. Kane PC. The neurobiology of lipids in autistic spectrum disorder. *J Ortho Med* 14:2:103–109, 1999.
67. Kane PC. Suppression of Peroxisomal Respiration in Children with Autistic Spectrum Disorder: Pattern Recognition and Neurobiological Role of Treatment Protocol. *Johns Hopkins Int Conference Brain Uptake and Utilization of Fatty Acids.* Presented March 2–3, 2000.
68. Kane PC, Foster JS, Cartaxo AL. Clinical detoxification of neurotoxins and heavy metals in autistic spectrum disorder. *Autism, Genes and the Environment UMDNJ*, October 2002.
69. Kane PC, Foster JS, Cartaxo AL. Lipid treatment for brain fatty acid abnormalities in ASD. *IMFAR, International Meeting for Autism Research.* Orlando, Florida, November 1–2, 2002.
70. Kane PC. EFAs and membrane stability in neurological disease. *Royal College of Physicians,* Nov 2007.
71. Kane PC. *It's all in the fat: the role of EFAs in health.* University of North Carolina at Chapel Hill, Conference, March 3, 2003.
72. Kane PC, Braccia D, Kane E. Phospholipid therapy as a treatment protocol in ALS. Poster Presentation in the 15th Annual Int ALS/MND Conference, Oct 2004.
73. Kane PC, Braccia D, Kane E. *Phospholipid therapy in ALS, The PK Protocol.* Johns Hopkins Int Conference on Brain Uptake and Utilization of Fatty Acids. Presented Oct 2004.
74. Kane PC, Speight N, Drisko J. *Phospholipids and ALS: The PK Protocol.* Compendium for the University of Kansas, October 2004.
75. Kane PC, Braccia D, Kane E. *Phospholipid therapy as a treatment protocol in ALS.* Poster in the 15th Annual Int ALS/MND Conference, Dec 2–3, 2004.
76. Crawford MA, Costeloe K, Ghebremeskel K, Phylactos A, Skirvin L, Stacey F. Are deficits of arachidonic and docosahexaenoic acids responsible for the neural and vascular complications of preterm babies? *Am J Clin Nutr* 66:4 Suppl:1032S–1041S, Oct 1997.
77. Bazan NG, Murphy MG, Toffano G. Neurobiology of EFAs. In: *Advances in Experimental Medicine and Biology* Vol. 318 from the proceedings July 10–12, 1991 Australia. New York: Plenum Publishing, 1992.
78. Schachter D, Abbott RE, Cogan U, Flamm M. Lipid fluidity of the individual hemileaflets of human erythrocyte membranes. *Ann N Y Acad Sci* 414:19–28, 1983.
79. Rapoport SI. In vivo fatty acid incorporation into brain phospholipids in relation to signal transduction and membrane remodeling. *Neurochem Res* 24:11:1403–1415, Nov 1999.
80. Yehuda S, Carasso RL. Modulation of learning pain thresholds, and thermoregulation in the rat by preparations of free-purified alpha linolenic and linoleic acids: determination of the optimal w3-to-w6 ratio. *Proc Natl Acad Sci USA* 90:10345–10349, 1993.
81. Yehuda S, Carasso RL, Mostofsky DI. EFA preparation (SR-3) raises the seizure threshold in rats. *Eur J Pharmacol* 254:1–2:193–198, Mar 11, 1994.
82. Yehuda S, Rabinovitz S, Carasso RL, Mostofsky DI. Fatty acids and brain peptides. *Peptide* 19:2:407–419, 1998.
83. Yehuda S, Rabinovitz S, Mostofsky DI. Treatment with a polyunsaturated fatty acid prevents deleterious effects of Ro4-1284. *Eur J Pharmacol* 365:1:27–34, Jan 1999.
84. Yehuda S, Rabinovitz S, Mostofsky DI. EFAs and the brain. From infancy to aging. *Neurobiol Aging* 26S:S98–S102, 2005.
85. Yehuda S, Mostofsky DI. *Nutrients, Stress and Medical Disorders.* Totawa, NJ: Humana Press, Inc. 2006.
86. Yehuda S, Carraso RL, Mostofsky DI. EFA preparation (SR-3) rehabilitates learning deficits induced by AF64A and 5,7-DHT. *Neuroreport* 6:3:511–515, Feb 1995.
87. Yehuda S, Rabinovitz S, Mostofsky DI, Huberman M, Sredni B. EFA preparation improves biochemical and cognitive functions in experimental allergic encephalomyelitis rats. *Eur J Pharmacol* 328:1:23–29, Jun 1997.
88. Yehuda S, Rabinovitz S, Mostofsky DI. Effects of EFA preparation (SR-3) on brain lipids, biochemistry and behavioral and cognitive functions. In: Yehuda A, Mostofsky DI, Eds. *Handbook of EFA biology, biochemistry physiology, and behavioral neurobiology.* New York: Humana Press, 1997, pp. 427–452.
89. Yehuda S, Rabinovitz S, Mostofsky DI. Modulation of learning and neuronal membrane composition in the rat by EFA preparation: timecourse analysis. *Neurochem Res* 2:5:627–634, May 1998.
90. Yehuda S, Rabinovitz S, Mostofsky DI. EFAs and sleep: minireview and hypothesis. *Med Hypoth* 50:2:139–145, Feb 1998.
91. Yehuda S, Rabinovitz S, Mostofsky DI. EFAs are mediators of brain biochemistry and cognitive functions. *J Neurosci Res* 56:6:565–570, Jun 1999.
92. Mostofsky DI, Yehuda S, Rabinovitz S, Carasso RL. The control of blepharospasm by EFAs. *Neuropsychobiology* 41:3:154–157, 2000.

93. Goldfarb RD, Parker TS, Levine DM, Glock D, Akhter I, Alkhudari A, McCarthy RJ, David EM, Gordon BR, Saal SD, Rubin AL, Trenholme GM, Parrillo JE. Protein-free phospholipid emulsion treatment improved cardiopulmonary function and survival in porcine sepsis. *Am J Physiol Regul Integr Comp Physiol* 28:2:R550–557, Feb 2003. Epub Oct 24, 2002.

94. Gordon BR, Parker TS, Levine DM, Saal SD, Hudgins LC, Sloan BJ, Chu C, Stenzel KH, Rubin AL. Safety and pharmacokinetics of an endotoxin-binding phospholipid emulsion. *Ann Pharmacother* 37: 7–8:943–950, Jul–Aug 2003.

95. Gordon BR, Parker TS, Levine DM, Feuerbach F, Saal SD, Sloan BJ, Chu C, Stenzel KH, Parrillo JE, Rubin AL. Neutralization of endotoxin by a phospholipid emulsion in healthy volunteers. *J Infect Dis* 191:9:1515–522, May 1, 2005. Epub 2005 Mar 24.

96. Gordon BR, personal communication, June 2005.

97. Deth RC. *Molecular Origins of Human Attention: The Dopamine-Folate Connection.* Norwell, MA: Kluwer Academic Publishers, 2003.

98. James SJ, Cutler P, Melnyk S, Jernigan S, Janak L, Gaylor DW, Neubrander JA. Metabolic biomarkers of increased oxidative stress and impaired methylation capacity in children with autism. *Am J Clin Nutr* 80:6:1611–1617, Dec 2004.

99. Dentico P, Volpe A, Buongiorno R, Grattagliano I, Altomare E, Tantimonaco G, Scotto G, Sacco R, Schiraldi O. Glutathione in the treatment of chronic fatty liver diseases. *Recenti Prog Med* 86:7–8: 290–293, Jul–Aug 1995.

100. Nordberg M, Nordberg GF. Toxicological aspects of metallothionein. *Cell Mol Biol (Noisy-le-grand).* 46:2:451–463, Mar 2000. Review.

101. Ebadi M, Iversen PL, Hao R, Cerutis DR, Rojas P, Happe HK, Murrin LC, Pfeiffer RF. Expression and regulation of brain metallothionein. *Neurochem Int* 27:1:1–22, Jul 1995.

102. Sato M, Sasaki M, Oguro T, Kuroiwa Y, Yoshida T. Induction of metallothionein synthesis by glutathione depletion after *trans-* and *cis-*stilbene oxide administration in rats. *Chemico-Biological Interactions* 98:15–25, 1995.

103. Aschner M, West AK. The role of MT in neurological disorders. *J Alzheimers Dis* 8:2:139–145; discussion 209–215, Nov 2005.

104. Watanabe H, Shimojo N, Sano K, Yamaguchi S. The distribution of total mercury in the brain after the lateral ventricular singe injection of methylmercury and glutathione. *Res Commun Chem Pathol Pharmacol* 60:1:57–69, Apr 1988.

105. Davidson J, Abul HT, Milton AS, Rotondo D. Cytokines and cytokine stimulate prostaglandin E2 entry into the brain. *Pfugers Arch* 442:4:526–533, Jul 2001.

106. Miles AT, Hawksworth GM, Beattie JH, Rodilla V. Induction, regulation, degradation, and biological significance of mammalian metallothioneins. *Crit Rev Biochem Mol Biol* 35:1:35–70, 2000.

107. Yiin SJ, Lin TH. Effects of metallic antioxidants on cadmium-catalyzed peroxidation of arachidonic acid. *Ann Clin Lab Sci.* 28:1:43–50, Jan–Feb 1998.

108. Grandjean P, Weihe P. Arachidonic acid status during pregnancy is associated with polychlorinated biphenyl exposure. *Am J Clin Nutr* 77:3:715–719, Mar 2003.

109. Kane PC, Braccia D, Foster JS, Speight N. Clinical data, The PK Protocol. Haverford Wellness Center, 2000–2008.

25 Attention Deficit Hyperactivity Disorder

Valencia Booth Porter, M.D., M.P.H.

I. INTRODUCTION

Attention Deficit Hyperactivity Disorder (ADHD) is the most common behavioral disorder in children, affecting approximately 2 to 3 million children in the United States.[1] Behavioral measures and pharmacotherapy are the cornerstones of medical management of ADHD, with stimulant drugs the mainstay of treatment for more than 60 years. Newer nonstimulant medications have also shown benefit in ameliorating symptoms of ADHD and comorbid disorders. However, with approximately 65% to 70% of patients reporting medication side effects[2,3] and up to 30% of children who may not respond to medication,[4] many families and physicians alike look to diet and nutrient interventions as an adjunct in long-term management of the disorder.[5]

A number of studies have shown the importance of omega-3 fatty acids in brain development and function. Carbohydrates are essential for brain fuel. Proteins are needed for amino acids and neurotransmitters. Vitamins and minerals serve as cofactors to create these building blocks. Certain food components can negatively impact behavior in certain children who appear vulnerable and have reactivities to these foods. Food colorings, flavorings, preservatives, and refined sugars have been linked to ADHD, with parents and other observers frequently reporting dramatic improvements in hyperactive children on a variety of defined diets.[6–8]

II. BACKGROUND

In the United States, the prevalence of ADHD in school-age children is estimated between 3% and 10%.[1] Onset is typically between age 4 and 7 years, with boys affected six times more than girls. ADHD may persist into adulthood in 40% to 60%. Although clinically heterogeneous, those suffering from ADHD have core features including developmentally inappropriate inattention, impulsivity, and hyperactivity. Currently recognized subtypes include predominantly inattentive, predominantly hyperactive and impulsive, or combined-type.[1] Comorbid conditions include oppositional defiant disorder, conduct disorder, both unipolar and bipolar mood disorders, anxiety disorders, and learning disorders.[9,10] Traditional treatment includes behavior modification, educational techniques, psychotherapy, and pharmacotherapy, most commonly with stimulant medications. In the United States and United Kingdom, use of stimulant medication for this condition has dramatically increased since the 1990s.

While the precise cause of ADHD remains unknown, it appears to have a multifactorial etiology including genetic, biologic, and environmental contributors. Family, twin, and adoption studies provide evidence that genes and *in utero* environmental factors (epigenetics) play a strong role in susceptibility to ADHD, with evidence pointing toward dopaminergic and adrenergic systems as well as fatty acid metabolism.[11]

Evidence from pharmacological effects and brain imaging studies highlight frontal lobe and subcortical regions of the brain as being affected in ADHD. The dopaminergic anterior system is thought to be related to behavioral inhibition and executive functions, whereas the noradrenergic posterior system may play a role in selective attention.[10,12] Stimulant drugs that modulate dopaminergic and noradrenergic systems, such as methylphenidate, have been successful at reducing core ADHD symptoms.[10,13] In addition, the nonstimulant drug atomoxetine works by inhibiting noradrenaline transport.[14] By contrast, serotonergic drugs have demonstrated little effect in treatment of ADHD despite interaction between serotonin and dopamine systems.[15]

Environmental exposures may also play a role in the development of ADHD, with associations found between exposure to lead and prenatal exposure to maternal cigarette smoking and alcohol use.[16,17] Although lead toxicity does not account for the majority of cases of ADHD and not all children with high lead exposure develop ADHD symptoms, lead has been shown in some children to cause distractibility, hyperactivity, restlessness, and lower intellectual functioning.[17] Environmental exposures to neurodevelopmental toxins such as heavy metals and organohalide pollutants have also risen with increased industrial pollutants.[17,18]

Thyroid problems such as hyperthyroidism are often included in the differential diagnosis, but studies have not shown a clear association between thyroid function and ADHD. Abnormal thyroid function has been found to occur more often in children with ADHD than in the general population.[19,20] A large proportion of children with generalized resistance to thyroid hormone (GRTH), where target tissues are less responsive to thyroid hormone, have also been found to have ADHD.[21,22] It is also possible that environmental thyrotoxicants such as PCBs may play a role in the etiology of ADHD.[23] *In utero*, maternal hypothyroxinemia has known neurodevelopmental consequences and recently Roman hypothesized that maternal exposure to environmental antithyroid and goitrogenic agents and insufficient dietary iodine intake can result in fetal brain changes.[24]

Food and nutrients from early childhood and on also play a role in the pathophysiology of this condition. In early life, children given soy-based formula due to food reactivities may be at added risk due to the goitrogenic properties of soy isoflavones as well as high levels of manganese.[25,26] Iodine deficiency is found in approximately 12% of the U.S. population and up to 15% of women of child-bearing age.[27] The recommended daily intake is 100 to 150 µg and one teaspoon of iodized table salt contains 400 µg. Patients choosing to reduce processed foods may unknowingly be reducing their iodine intake; however, this is preventable by supplementation or by eating other foods high in iodine such as fish, seaweed, kelp, and chicken eggs. The iodine content of vegetables and grains is dependent upon the content of the soil it is grown in. Sea salt is a poor source of iodine with less than 2 µg/g. It should be noted also that excessive iodine intake can also lead to thyroid dysfunction and the upper limit for safe intake is 1100 µg/day for adults and even less for children.[28] In addition to nutrients affecting thyroid function, over the last century, dietary changes have included dramatic changes in the ratio of essential fatty acids and a shift toward low-protein/high-carbohydrate diets.[29-31] Food additives with the potential for reactivities in the diet have also drastically increased, with over 2300 now approved for use.

III. FOOD ADDITIVES

In the diet, exposure to food additives and other substances has been commented on extensively in the literature. Differences and inadequacies in controlled trials make analysis difficult, but studies do indicate a limited positive association between defined diets and decrease in hyperactivity. A 1983 NIH Consensus Panel on defined diets and childhood hyperactivity stated that "defined diets should not be universally used in the treatment of childhood hyperactivity at this time. However, the Panel recognizes that initiation of a trial of dietary treatment or continuation of a diet may be warranted in patients whose family and physicians perceive benefits."[32]

With domestic production of food dyes increasing four-fold between 1955 and 1998, more than 2000 food additives are approved by the Food and Drug Administration (FDA).[33] While preservatives such as benzoates serve to increase shelf-life of food, artificial food colorings have no nutritional value or other benefits to consumers and are mainly used for cosmetic purposes, often to make non-nutritious foods more appealing to children. An unpublished study by the FDA in 1976 noted that the average American child consumed 27 mg of artificial food colors daily.[34] These substances are generally regarded as safe, but hypersensitivity responses or idiosyncratic reactions could have effects on central nervous system functioning.

A recent study has re-ignited interest in the influence of food additives on children's behavior. Replicating an earlier study showing that ingestion of usual amounts of food colorings and additives may significantly increase hyperactivity in some 3-year-old children, McCann and colleagues showed similar effects in 8- to 9-year-old children.[8] In the first study, 3-year-old children from the general population given a diet free of artificial dyes and benzoate preservatives had reduction in hyperactive behavior. When challenged with a mix containing commonly used additives sodium benzoate and Sunset Yellow, carmoisine, tartrazine, and Ponceau 4R, hyperactivity increased.[35]

The new study evaluated 153 3-year-olds and 144 8- to 9-year-olds from the general population initially placed on an elimination diet free of challenge elements for 6 weeks.[8] Elements tested included those in the original study (mix A) and mix B containing: sodium benzoate plus the dyes Sunset Yellow, carmoisine, Quinolone Yellow, and Allura Red AC. These elements were typical of the artificial food colors and additives currently found in some children's foods and were given in amounts representative of average daily intake of these additives by young children in the United Kingdom. In both age groups, small but significant increases in hyperactivity as assessed by parents, teachers, and trained observers were seen with mix A. Mix B was also associated with a small significant increase in hyperactivity in the older children, but not in the 3-year-olds, who exhibited a wider range of responses. This corresponds to the clinical observation that some hyperactive children are highly sensitive to food colorings and additives, while other children are not. On the basis of this study, the British Food Standards Agency advised parents of hyperactive children to consider eliminating the additives used in the study from their diets. Further study is needed to determine what may account for individual differences in response as well as to determine the specific compounds or combination of compounds responsible for these effects.

These findings are consistent with a recent meta-analysis of 15 double-blind placebo-controlled trials of artificial food colorings that showed increase in hyperactivity as measured by behavioral rating scales in hyperactive children.[36] A prior review that was not supportive included trials of hyperactive and nonhyperactive children and various methodologies.[37]

As one hypothesis for these reactions is a potential hypersensitivity to these compounds, additional studies have looked at children with ADHD who were also atopic. In one study using an elimination diet, 73% of 26 children with ADHD had behavioral improvement and atopic children responded more than those who were not atopic.[38] In addition, a dose-response effect of the food coloring tartrazine was observed in some hyperactive children and all of those who reacted were also found to have atopy.[39]

FEINGOLD DIET

In the 1970s Dr. Benjamin Feingold, a pediatrician and allergist, popularized the idea of diet affecting children's hyperactive behavior. He originally hypothesized that hyperactivity was a symptom of salicylate intolerance in genetically predisposed individuals and because many of these people also had hypersensitivity to tartrazine (Yellow Dye No. 5) he suggested that this additive as well as several artificial flavors similar in structure to salicylates were involved.

The original Feingold Diet, also known as Kaiser-Permanente or K-P diet, eliminates all foods containing artificial (synthetic) colors and/or flavors and all foods high in naturally occurring salicylates, a category that includes some fruits and vegetables (almonds, cucumbers, tomatoes, berries, apples, oranges, and several other fruits). The role of salicylates was later diminished and preservatives sodium benzoate, butylated hydroxyanisole (BHA), and butylated hydroxytoluene (BHT) were added to the exclusion list.[40–42] After several weeks on the elimination diet, salicylate-containing foods are gradually reintroduced, looking for adverse reactions.[38] Feingold reported anecdotally that 40% to 70% of children who strictly adhere to the diet have a marked reduction in hyperactive behavior and suggested that younger children tended to respond more rapidly and more completely.[42]

For the most part, other researchers evaluating the Feingold hypothesis yielded inconclusive results and suffer from small sample sizes and methodological deficiencies.[34] However, a subgroup of hyperactive children may show improvement on the diet, although it is uncertain what component of the dietary change is responsible, be it lack of additives, salicylate avoidance, placebo effect, change in nutrient status, or other variables including family dynamics.[34,43] It is possible that salicylates accounted for more cases in the 1970s than in current times in which the intake of sugar and other additives is much higher and ADHD has reached epidemic levels. While the potential for food reactivities is great with thousands of artificial compounds in use, the amount of testing needed to assess the role in ADHD would likely take decades. On the other hand, motivated parents may find that their child benefits from this approach and the Feingold Association* provides ample resources to support them in this endeavor.[43]

OLIGOANTIGENIC/FEW FOODS DIET

In addition to food additives, common foods including sugar, milk, corn, wheat, chocolate, eggs, and oranges have also been implicated as factors responsible for behavioral problems in ADHD. Dr. William Crook, an allergist and pediatrician, reported parent-noted food triggers in 70% of 182 hyperactive patients and with dietary elimination of these substances, an excellent or good response was reported by nearly 80%.[44]

Similar to the Feingold Diet, the rationale behind the very restrictive oligoantigenic or few foods diet is to eliminate foods and ingredients that may provoke adverse behavioral reactions, including additives and artificial colorings as well as other substances assumed to be antigenic such as cereal proteins and citrus fruits. As first described by Egger, this diet consists of two types of meats (lamb, turkey/chicken), two carbohydrate sources (rice, potatoes), two types of vegetables (*Brassica*, carrots), and two fruits (apple, banana). For preparing the meals, oil, margarine, salt, and water are allowed. Beverages include apple juice and mineral water and calcium and multivitamins are given as supplements.[45]

In the original study of 76 children, 62 improved, with the behavior of 21 normalizing. Other symptoms such as headaches and abdominal pain often improved as well. When re-exposed in a double-blind, crossover, placebo-controlled trial, symptoms returned or were exacerbated within 2 to 3 days. Artificial colorings (tartrazine) and preservatives (benzoates) were the most common provoking substances, but all children had multiple sensitivities.[45] Other studies of children with ADHD or hyperactivity have shown that at least in some children, hyperactivity may be a manifestation of food intolerance and behavior may improve with an oligoantigenic or few foods diet.[46-48]

SUGAR

It is commonly believed that foods high in refined sugar exacerbate behavioral problems in children.[49] Anecdotal and observational studies have supported this belief, showing deteriorations in attention or behavior after sucrose challenge versus placebo in children with and without ADHD.[50-54]

Interestingly, it may not only be the sugar, but the relationship to other food components. Changes in behavior have been correlated with the amount of sugar ingested, with the ratio of sugar products to other foods, and with the ratio of carbohydrate to protein in the diet.[51] In a challenge study, behavioral deteriorations in normal and hyperactive children were seen when sucrose was given after a breakfast consisting of mostly carbohydrates, but not after fasting or a high-protein breakfast.[55] Another study showed that declines in attention and memory seen in children in a fasting condition or given a glucose drink were not seen when a breakfast of complex carbohydrates was given.[56] Indeed, a higher ratio of sugar to total energy has been found to be associated with increases

---

* www.feingold.org.

in activity, off-task behaviors, and attention problems.[57] As drops in blood sugar can trigger sympathetic nervous system response, it is hypothesized that altering the carbohydrate:protein ratio might influence neurotransmitters, leading to these behavioral symptoms.[58,59] Serum levels of precursor amino acids (tyrosine, phenylalanine, and tryptophan) for neurotransmitters affected in hyperactivity are increased by dietary consumption and lowered by carbohydrate load.[58]

A number of controlled studies in the literature do not support the notion that sugar intake leads to increase in activity.[49,60–63] Some even reported a decrease in activity levels after sucrose or glucose ingestion.[63,64] One should note, however, that many of these negative studies use another sweetener such as aspartame or saccharin as the placebo challenge, with unknown behavioral effects in general and some associations emerging that food reactivities and these synthetic compounds may be linked.[66–69]

Specific Nutrients

Essential Fatty Acids

Fatty acids have fundamental structural and functional roles in the central nervous system, comprising key components of neuronal membranes, neurotransmitter receptor sites, as well as second messenger systems.[70,71] Essential fatty acids (EFAs) cannot be synthesized by the body and therefore must be provided in the diet. Sometimes dietary intake is inadequate; however, other times further metabolic processing of EFAs is impaired. The conversion is dependent on precursor levels and can also be influenced by environmental factors.[72,73] The omega-6 linoleic acid (LA) and omega-3 alpha-linolenic acid (ALA) undergo desaturation and elongation to become the omega-6s arachidonic acid (AA) and dihomo-gamma-linolenic acid (DGLA), a metabolite of gamma-linolenic acid (GLA), and omega-3s eicosapentaenoic acid (EPA) and docosahexaenoic acid (DHA).[74] AA and DHA are key components of neuronal membranes, accounting for up to 15% to 20% of the brain's dry mass. AA additionally plays a role in cellular processes underlying learning and memory. DGLA, AA, and EPA are also important eicosanoid precursors thus affecting many other biochemical processes.[74]

While both the omega-3s and omega-6s are crucial to brain development and function, the omega-3s in particular are often lacking in diets of developed countries where dramatic increases in consumption of processed foods have led to relative deficiencies in certain EFAs and a change in the omega-6:omega-3 ratio from approximately 3:1 to more than 20:1 in some cases.[70,75] These dietary changes may have contributed to the increased incidence of many diseases including neurodevelopmental disorders.[70] Dietary omega-3 sources include fish and shellfish, as well as plant sources such as flax oil, hemp oil, soy oil, canola oil, pumpkin seeds, sunflower seeds, leafy vegetables, and walnuts, which do not contain EPA or DHA.

Various behavioral and developmental problems including ADHD have been linked to deficiencies or imbalances of fatty acids.[76] Hyperactive and ADHD children have been noted to have symptoms of EFA deficiency such as dry hair and skin, excessive thirst and urination, and other findings including follicular keratoses, brittle nails, and symptoms of eczema, asthma, and other atopic conditions.[76,77] In addition to physical signs of fatty acid deficiency, plasma and erythrocyte fatty acid levels, particularly omega-3s, have been found to be decreased in subjects with ADHD.[78–81] Recent studies have shown that genes involved in fatty acid metabolism can influence tissue concentrations and these may have a potential role in ADHD.[82] A deficiency in omega-3s can further disrupt the dopaminergic mesocorticolimbic pathway by reducing dopamine vesicle density.[72]

EFA Supplementation

Supplementation with omega-3s changes blood levels and can lead to changes in mood and behavior. A 4:1 ratio of omega-6:omega-3 has been found to be optimal for neuronal membrane functioning although this has not yet been applied specifically to ADHD.[83] Early intervention studies of supplementation with evening primrose oil (primarily GLA) in children with ADHD had mixed, but unsatisfactory outcomes.[84,85] Further studies of DHA supplementation alone also failed to demonstrate improvement in ADHD symptoms.[86,87] As neither serum nor erythrocyte DHA was found to be related to ADHD symptom severity in adults, this may be an inadequate intervention.[80]

Children with ADHD given a 15 week intervention of polyunsaturated fatty acids (PUFAs) alone or PUFAs with micronutrients showed significant medium to strong positive effects over placebo on parent-rated but not teacher-rated inattention and hyperactivity/impulsivity.[88] The PUFA capsules contained 400 mg fish oil and 100 mg evening primrose oil with 93 mg EPA, 29 mg DHA, 10 mg GLA and 1.8 mg vitamin E. No additional effects of the micronutrients were seen. Results were replicated in the placebo group after all groups crossed over for another 15 weeks on PUFAs, with treatment groups continuing to show significant improvements on core ADHD symptoms. Another study showed that supplementation with flax oil (200 mg ALA) with 25 mg vitamin C twice a day for 3 months increased erythrocyte EPA and DHA levels and improved parent-rated impulsivity, restlessness, inattention, and self-control over controls.[89] Psychosomatic, social, and learning problems also improved. Pre-supplementation levels of fatty acids measured in red blood cell membranes were significantly lower in ADHD patients as compared to normal controls. Post-supplementation levels of EPA and DHA significantly increased and AA decreased.

A further study of 50 children with ADHD as well as symptoms suggestive of fatty acid deficiency (thirst and skin problems) were randomized to receive 4 months of either olive oil or a mixture of 480 mg DHA, 80 mg EPA, 40 mg AA, 96 mg GLA, and 24 mg alpha-tocopherol acetate.[90] Changes in plasma and erythrocyte FA composition as well as improvements in ADHD behaviors were consistently observed for the treatment group more than the control group, with significant changes on parent-rated conduct problems and teacher-rated attention symptoms. Also, more children had improvement in oppositional defiant behaviors with the PUFA mixture compared with olive oil. For both groups, biochemical changes were related to improvements in behavior. Significant correlations were found for increasing erythrocyte EPA levels and decreasing parent-rated disruptive behavior, and for erythrocyte EPA and DHA levels and teacher-rated attention. Interestingly, significant correlations were also observed between a decrease in scores for all four teacher subscales (hyperactivity, attention, conduct, and oppositional/defiant disorder) and increase in erythrocyte alpha-tocopherol concentrations, suggesting an additional role for vitamin E.

L-Carnitine

Both l-carnitine and its esterified form, acetyl-l-carnitine, have potential neuroprotective, neuro-modulatory, and neurotrophic properties and have demonstrated improvements in cognitive processes such as memory and learning.[90] Frank carnitine deficiency is known to have major deleterious effects on the central nervous system as well as other organ systems. L-carnitine has an important role in fatty acid metabolism and regulation.[91,92] Acetyl-l-carnitine is more efficiently incorporated into PUFA and is an important constituent of brain phospholipids.

Looking at this potential, l-carnitine was given to 26 boys with ADHD in an 8-week double-blind, placebo-controlled, double-crossover study.[92] Doses of 100 mg/kg daily were given twice after meals with a maximum of 4 grams daily. Improvements of 30% or more on two objective measures were seen in approximately half of the children. Of note, plasma-free carnitine and acetyl-l-carnitine levels were significantly different between responders and nonresponders after treatment ($p < 0.03$ and $p < 0.05$).

Most people obtain enough carnitine from their diet, but some may have dietary deficiencies or cannot properly absorb it from food. Common food sources include red meat (particularly lamb) and dairy products. Carnitine is also found in fish, poultry, tempeh (fermented soybeans), wheat, asparagus, avocados, and peanut butter. Certain medications and low dietary levels of the amino acids lysine and methionine may cause deficiencies. Dietary supplementation of l-carnitine does not appear to cause significant side effects. Nausea, vomiting, diarrhea, and body odor have been reported in higher doses above 3 g/day.

Iron

Iron plays a role in regulation of dopaminergic activity and may therefore contribute to the physiopathology of ADHD.[93] Children with ADHD have been shown to have lower mean serum ferritin levels than age and sex-matched controls.[94] In addition, low serum ferritin levels corresponded to more severe behavioral symptoms.[95,96] Even in the absence of anemia, iron supplementation may have an impact on ADHD symptoms. A pilot study of 14 boys with ADHD showed that administration of an iron preparation (Ferrocal) 5 mg/kg/day for 30 days had significant increase in serum ferritin levels and significant decreases on parent but not teacher rating scores.[97] A recent 12-week placebo-controlled study of oral ferrous sulfate 80 mg/day for 23 non-anemic children with low serum ferritin levels (<30 ng/mL) showed improvement on parent- but not teacher-rated ADHD behavior on iron versus placebo.[98]

Restless legs syndrome (RLS) frequently occurs with iron deficiency anemia and improves with iron supplementation.[99] Pharmacologic and PET studies show that RLS is related to impaired dopaminergic transmission, in which iron plays a role. Given that RLS and ADHD may share common pathophysiological mechanisms it is not surprising that up to 26% of subjects with RLS have been found to have ADHD or ADHD symptoms and up to 44% of subjects with ADHD have been found to have RLS or RLS symptoms.[100] In a small study of seven children with both ADHD and RLS, four of whom failed prior stimulant therapy, treatment with dopaminergic monotherapy improved both RLS symptoms as well as behavior and neuropsychological assessments.[101]

Manganese

Manganese (Mn) is an essential trace mineral that is obtained through the diet and excreted in bile. Some reports have shown high levels of Mn in hair of children with ADHD and studies have shown that Mn toxicity compromises dopamine metabolism.[26,102] With soy-based infant formula having concentrations of Mn more than 2 to 50 times (depending on brand) the level of human milk and a high absorption in the neonate,[103] the potential for neurotoxic consequences needs to be further evaluated.

Zinc

Zinc (Zn) is an important cofactor for metabolism related to neurotransmitters such as dopamine, fatty acids, prostaglandins, and melatonin.[104,105] With a role in synthesis of complex omega-3 and omega-6 FAs, zinc deficiency may further exacerbate problems related to these EFAs in children with ADHD.

In a population study, nearly one-third of children with ADHD had significantly lower serum zinc levels than age- and sex-matched controls.[106] This could not be explained by obvious factors concerning diet, health, or medication status. Another study also found significantly lower mean serum FA and mean serum zinc levels in 48 children with ADHD versus 45 children without ADHD.[107]

Other evidence suggests that zinc deficiencies may also reduce the treatment response to stimulants such as methylphenidate.[105] A small study looking at 18 ADHD subjects by zinc status, showed a linear relationship with response to d-amphetamine whereas response to evening primrose oil yielded benefit only in those with borderline zinc status.[105] With mild zinc deficiency, effect size for both treatments was diminished. Zinc sulfate may be useful as an adjunct to treatment with methylphenidate as shown in a double-blind placebo-controlled trial with significant differences in both parent- and teacher-rated behaviors.[108]

Dietary zinc can be found in high-protein foods such as organ meats, seafood, especially shellfish, whole grains, and legumes.

Magnesium

In Poland, children with ADHD were commonly found to have deficiency of magnesium in the hair, erythrocytes, and less often in plasma.[109] Magnesium deficiency also occurred more often among hyperactive children than among healthy children.[110] When children with hyperactivity who were found to have magnesium deficiency were given magnesium supplementation 200 mg/day for 6 months, a decrease in hyperactivity was seen in those supplemented versus those who did not receive supplementation.[111] In another study, 40 children with ADHD showed significantly lower erythrocyte Mg levels than controls.[112] When given 6 mg/kg/d Mg with 0.6 mg/kg/d vitamin B6 (pyridoxine) for 8 weeks, hyperactivity and aggressiveness were significantly reduced and school attention increased along with an increase in erythrocyte Mg levels. Within a few weeks of stopping treatment, symptoms returned and Mg levels again decreased.

Amino Acids

Amino acids are the building blocks for neurotransmitters; therefore, low levels can lead to neurotransmitter deficiency. Pharmacological doses of dietary amino acids can increase brain levels of specific neurotransmitters,[113] thus they can be used as a stand-alone treatment or to maintain effectiveness of medication.

Prior published trials using L-dopa alone, dl-phenylalanine alone, and l-tyrosine alone did not result in lasting therapeutic effect.[114–116] In an unpublished abstract, Dr. Robert Neff reports retrospectively on 85 children using amino acid therapy with 70% reporting some relief from ADHD symptoms over 8 weeks. Thirty percent reported complete relief by week 5 and 33% by week 8. Although some of these children were taking stimulant medications as well, 35% not taking medication also reported full symptom relief by week 8.[117]

Increased production of dopamine is the main goal of amino acid therapy; however, preliminary studies suggest that amino acids need to be balanced in order to avoid depletion of other key neurotransmitters. For example, the enzyme amino acid decarboxylase works to convert both L-dopa to dopamine and 5-HTP to serotonin. In addition, monoamine oxidase and catecholamine-O-methyl transferase enzymes metabolize both serotonin and dopamine. Therefore, administration of unopposed L-dopa will deplete serotonin as a result of increased metabolism without increased production. L-dopa can be administered exogenously, but it is also synthesized from tyrosine which can keep dopamine levels stable. Tyrosine is also an important precursor, with reduced stimulant effects of amphetamines observed in individuals who had been made tyrosine deficient.[118]Further evaluation of amino acid therapy is needed. A double-blind placebo-controlled trial using balanced amino acids (tyrosine/5-HTP with cofactors including cysteine and selenium to prevent sulfur amino acid depletion) is underway in a large school district in Texas.

Measurement of urinary neurotransmitters reflects those synthesized by the kidneys and excreted into the urine. Urinary neurotransmitters do not necessarily correlate with CNS levels; however, they can show response to administration of amino acids precursors. Optimal time for collection of urinary NT samples is 4 to 6 hours prior to bedtime due to diurnal variation with a low point at this time. As more is learned about testing for neurotransmitters and their amino acid precursors, better defined therapies may arise, but one must always treat the patient and not the lab value.

Other

Initial studies of other dietary supplements and nutritional products such as phosphatidylserine, pyridoxine, and thiamin have shown some promise, but should be studied more rigorously before recommending their use routinely.[24,25,119-122]

IV. PHARMACOLOGY

Numerous studies of stimulant medication for ADHD have demonstrated increased attention span, improved concentration, decreased excessive motor behavior, and improved social behavior when used alone or in conjunction with behavioral and cognitive interventions. Despite these robust benefits, however, long-term academic performance does not appear to be improved.[123] Approximately 70% of patients will respond to the first stimulant taken, with at least 80% responding if medications are tried systematically. Other medications used in treatment include amoxetine, tricyclic antidepressants (TCA), non-TCA antidepressants, clonidine, and buproprion.[124]

Up to 30% may not respond to stimulants. Side effects are common, including appetite suppression, headache, sleep disturbance, mood difficulties, or exacerbation of tic disorders.[125] In a study examining attitudes of 40 students on medication ages 11 to 18 years regarding ADHD medications, 64% reported some side effects.[2] Reports of sudden death with stimulant use generated understandable concern, but the majority of reported cases occurred in children with preexisting structural cardiac abnormalities.

As some of the drugs used to treat ADHD are dopamine and norepinephrine reuptake inhibitors, chronic use of these medications may lead to increase in dopamine and norepinephrine metabolism. Therefore, amino acid precursors prevent further depletion by these drugs.[*]

Dextroamphetamine can increase blood levels of magnesium, which causes lowering of calcium to magnesium ratio in blood; therefore, one should also pay attention to micronutrients.

V. PATIENT EVALUATION

Initial evaluation of the patient should include interview, physical exam, and basic laboratory tests to assure the diagnosis and look for comorbid conditions. Initial tests may include evaluation for lead, iron status, and thyroid function. One may also consider additional laboratory tests to evaluate for potential nutrient deficiencies such as zinc, magnesium, and carnitine. Measures of phospholipid metabolism looking for fatty acids in red blood cells and in plasma are offered through several commercial labs (Chapter 24, "Seizures"). Questionnaires highlighting symptoms of EFA deficiency may be useful clinically.[77] A few laboratories offer IgA, IgG, and IgM food sensitivity testing and non-IgE mediated food sensitivity may also be assessed with an elimination diet followed by controlled provocation.

Screening questionnaires focusing on the symptoms of inattention, hyperactivity, and impulsivity are useful in the initial evaluation as well as in following treatment effects. A large number of rating scales are available for assessment of ADHD, with each having unique characteristics.[126]

VI. TREATMENT RECOMMENDATIONS

Aside from standard pharmacologic and behavioral treatments, dietary recommendations should be addressed in the primary treatment plan. Additionally some alternative treatments of ADHD are effective or probably effective, but mainly for certain patients.

Many parents are ready to adopt diet as a treatment for their child's behavior although adherence to a strict and demanding diet is a burden to the family. To prevent the child from feeling different, to reduce temptation, and to provide motivation, the whole family should be encouraged to participate. Initial dietary recommendations include eating a well-balanced, whole-foods diet, with minimal processed and artificial foods. A consultation with a nutritionist may be helpful in reinforcing nutrient needs: complex carbohydrates as brain fuel, proteins for amino acids and neurotransmitters, vitamins and minerals as cofactors, healthful (non-*trans*), balanced (omega-3:6) fats, and water.

Encouraging families to pay attention to foods rich in the EFAs has the potential for a multitude of health benefits. The omega-3 fats should be emphasized and they are found in coldwater fish such as salmon. It is important, however, to avoid contamination of fish and fish oil products by methylmercury, polychlorinated biphenyls, and dioxin. ALA is found in green vegetables and some nuts and seeds including flax, but conversion to EPA and DHA is limited in some individuals. Omega-6 fats are generally abundant in the standard American diet with most vegetable oils rich in LA and dairy and meat products providing AA.

If food reactivities are suspected, an elimination or few foods diet may be employed as both a diagnostic and therapeutic tool. Such an approach takes dedication from the parent and child, and eating out such as in a school cafeteria or restaurant is practically impossible. The Feingold Association provides a helpful website that provides practical information on navigating eating both at home and out of the home using the Feingold Diet.

---

[*] http://www.neuroassist.com/DiseaseHomePage1.htm.

VII. SUMMARY

- Initial workup should address potential underlying medical conditions, considering the potential for lead toxicity and thyroid disorders as well as evaluation of iron status.
- When making dietary changes, do not single out the child unless there are specific allergies. Instead, encourage the whole family to eat healthier.
- Reinforce eating a well-balanced whole-foods-based diet, with minimal processed and artificial foods.
- Reduce sugary foods and beverages. Breakfast with complex carbohydrates and protein can help maintain steady blood sugar levels.
- If potential food reactivities are suspected, consider an elimination diet that is both diagnostic and therapeutic. Other approaches are discussed in detail in Chapter 15, "Food Reactivities."
- Consider supplementation with omega-3 fatty acids with EPA and DHA 1 to 2 g/day and/ or encourage eating fatty fish three times a week. Chapter 24, "Seizures," details a comprehensive diet and nutrient approach to balance fatty acids in cell membranes.
- A trial of acetyl-l-carnitine 100 mg/kg daily with a maximum of 4 g daily may be helpful, particularly if plasma carnitine is low.
- Zinc and erythrocyte magnesium levels can be checked or add a high-quality multivitamin with trace minerals especially if diet is poor.
- Consider supplementation with B complex as essential cofactors for neurotransmitter production, which are especially depleted in stress.
- Evaluate sleep quality and quantity. Behavioral therapy and mind-body approaches can be employed. Nutrients for sleep including an emerging role for amino acid interventions are detailed in Chapter 29, "Depression," and Chapter 30, "Sleep Disturbance."

All of the above may be used in combination with pharmacologic management. Physicians may also wish to utilize online patient resources and laboratory testing information.[*]

REFERENCES

1. Root RW, Resnick RJ. An update on the diagnosis and treatment of attention-deficit/hyperactivity disorder in children. *Prof Psychol Res Pr,* 2003; 34:34–41.
2. Moline S, Frankenberger W. Use of stimulant medication for treatment of attention-deficit/hyperactivity disorder: a survey of middle and high school students' attitudes. *Psychol Sch,* 2001; 38:569–584.
3. Kemper KJ. Dietary supplements for attention-deficit/hyperactivity disorder—a fishy business? *J Pediatr,* 2001; 139:173–174.
4. Garber SW, Garber MD, Spizman RF. *Beyond Ritalin.* 1997. New York: Harper Collins.
5. Sinha D, Efron D. Complementary and alternative medicine use in children with attention deficit hyperactivity disorder. *J Paediatr Child Health,* 2005; 41:23–26.
6. Schnoll R, Burshteyn D, Cea-Aravena J. Nutrition in the treatment of attention-deficit hyperactivity disorder: a neglected but important aspect. *Appl Psychophysiol Biofeedback,* 2003; 28:63–75.
7. Stevenson J. Dietary influences on cognitive development and behaviour in children. *Proc Nutr Soc,* 2006; 65:361–365.
8. McCann A, Barrett A, Cooper A, Crumpler D, Dalen L, Grimshaw K, Kitchin E, Lok K, Porteous L, Prince E, Sonuga-Barke E, Warner JO, Stevenson J. Food additives and hyperactive behaviour in 3-year-old and 8/9-year-old children in the community: a randomised, double-blinded, placebo-controlled trial. *Lancet,* 2007; 370:1560–1567.
9. Spencer T, Biederman J, Wilens T. Attention-deficit/hyperactivity disorder and comorbidity. *Pediatr Clin North Am,* 1999; 46:915–927.

---

[*] www.neuroassist.com; www.feingold.org; www.metamatrix.com—amino acid profiles, fatty acid profiles, IgG and IgE food allergy; www.neurorelief.com—urinary neurotransmitter testing, food sensitivity testing IgA, IgG, IgM; www.labDBS.com—neurotransmitter testing.

10. Pliszka SR, McCRacken JT, Maas JW. Catecholamines in attention-deficit/hyperactivity disorder: current perspectives. *J Am Acad Child Adolesc Psychiatry,* 1996; 35:264–272.

11. Comings DE. Clinical and molecular genetics of ADHD and Tourette syndrome. Two related polygenic disorders. *Ann N Y Acad Sci,* 2001; 931:50–83.

12. Barkley RA. Behavioral inhibition, sustained attention, and executive functions: constructing a unifying theory of ADHD. *Psychol Bull,* 1997; 121:65–94.

13. Zametkin AJ, Liotta W. The neurobiology of attention-deficit/hyperactivity disorder. *J Clin Psychiatry,* 1998; 59(suppl 7)1986:17–23.

14. Michelson D, Adler L, Spencer T, Reimherr FW, West SA, Allen AJ, Kelsey D, Wernicke J, Dietrich A, Milton D. Atomoxetine in adults with ADHD: two randomized, placebo-controlled studies. *Biol Psychiatry,* 2003; 53:112–120.

15. Zametkin AJ, Rapoport JL. Noradrenergic hypothesis of attention deficit disorder with hyperactivity: a critical review. In: *Psychopharmacology: The Third Generation of Progress.* 1987. Meltzer HY, ed. New York: Raven, 837–842.

16. Biederman J. Attention-deficit/hyperactivity disorder: a selective overview. *Biol Psychiatry,* 2005; 57:1215–1220.

17. Rowland AS, Lesesne CA, Abramowitz AJ. The epidemiology of attention-deficit/hyperactivity disorder (ADHD): a public health view. *Ment Retard Dev Disabil Res Rev,* 2002; 8:162–170.

18. Weiss RE, Stin MA, Trommer B, Refetoff S. Attention-deficit hyperacitivity disorder and thyroid function. *J Pediatr,* 1993; 123:539–545.

19. Braun JM, Kahn RS, Froehlich TM, Auinger P, Lanphear BP. Exposures to environmental toxicants and attention deficit hyperactivity disorder in U.S. children. *Environ Health Perspect,* 114:1904–1909.

20. Toren P, Karasik A, Eldar S, Wolmer L, Shimon I, Weitz R, Inbar D, Koren S, Pariente C, Reiss A, Weizman R, Laor N. Thyroid function in attention deficit and hyperactivity disorder. *J Psychiatr Res,* 1997; 3e1:359–363.

21. Hauser P, Zametkin AJ, Martinez P et al. Attention deficit-hyperactivity disorder in people with generalized resistance to thyroid hormone. *N Engl J Med,* 1993; 328:997–1001.

22. Refetoff S, Weiss RE, Usala SJ. The syndromes of resistance to thyroid hormone. *Endocrine Rev,* 1993; 14:348–399.

23. Schettler T. Toxic threats to neurologic development of children. *Environ Health Perspect,* 2001; 109(Suppl 6):813–816.

24. Roman GC. Autism: transient in utero hypothyroxinemia related to maternal flavonoid ingestion during pregnancy and to other environmental antithyroid agents. *J Neurol Sci,* 2007; 262:15–26.

25. Doerge DR, Sheehan DM. Goitrogenic and estrogenic activity of soy isoflavones. *Environ Health Perspect,* 2002; 101:349–353.

26. Crinella FM. Does soy-based infant formula cause ADHD? Expert Rev *Neurotherapeutics,* 2003; 3:145–148.

27. Hollowell JG, Staehling NW, Hannon WH, Flanders DW, Gunter EW, Maberly GF et al. Iodine nutrition in the United States. Trends and public health implications: Iodine excretion data from National Health and Nutrition Examination Surveys I and III (1971–1974 and 1988–1994). *J Clin Endocrin and Metab,* 1998; 83:3401–3408.

28. Lee SL. Iodine deficiency. Emedicine 2006. Accessed on April 8, 2008 from: http://www.emedicine.com/med/TOPIC1187.HTM.

29. Simopoulos AP. Evolutionary aspects of diet, the omega-6/omega-3 ratio and genetic variation: nutritional implications for chronic diseases. *Biomed & Pharmacotherapy,* 2006; 60:502–507.

30. Kidd PM. Attention deficit/hyperactivity disorder (ADHD) in children: rationale for its integrative management. *Altern Med Rev,* 2000; 5:401, 402–428.

31. Harding KL, Judah RD, Gant C. Outcome-based comparison of Ritalin versus food-supplement treated children with AD/HD. *Altern Med Rev,* 2003; 8:319–330.

32. National Institutes of Health. NIH Consensus Development Conference: Defined Diets and Childhood Hyperactivity. NIH Consensus Statement. *Clinical Pediatrics,* 1982; 21; 627.

33. Jacobson MF, Schardt MS. Diet, ADHD & Behavior: A Quarter-Century Review. Center for Science in the Public Interest. Accessed February 8, 2007, at: www.cspinet.org.

34. Stare FJ, Whelan EM, Sheridan M. Diet and hyperactivity: is there a relationship? *Pediatrics,* 1980; 66:521–525.

35. Bateman B, Warner JO, Hutchinson E, Dean T, Rowlandson P, Gant C, Grundy J, Fitzgerald C, Stevenson J. The effects of a double blind, placebo controlled, artificial food colourings and benzoate preservative challenge on hyperactivity in a general population sample of preschool children. *Arch Dis Child,* 2004; 89:506–511.

36. Schab DW, Trinh N-HT. Do artificial food colors promote hyperactivity in children with hyperactive syndromes? A meta-analysis of double-blind placebo-controlled trials. *Dev Behav Peds,* 2004; 25: 423–434.

37. Kavale KA, Forness SR. Hyperactivity and diet treatment: a meta-analysis of the Feingold hypothesis. *J Learn Disabil,* 1983; 16:3324–3330.

38. Boris M, Mandel FS. Foods and additives are common causes of the attention deficit hyperactive disorder in children. *Ann Allergy,* 1994; 72:462–468.

39. Rowe KS, Rowe JK. Synthetic food coloring and behavior: a dose response effect in a double-blind, placebo-controlled, repeated-measures study. *J Pediatrics,* 1994; 125:691–698.

40. Feingold BF. *Why your child is hyperactive.* 1975. New York: Random House.

41. Feingold BF. Hyperkinesis and learning disabilities linked to artificial food flavors and colors. *Am J Nurs,* 1975; 75:797.

42. Feingold BF. Hyperkinesis and learning disabilities linked to the ingestion of artificial food colors and flavors. *J Learn Disabil,* 1976; 9:19.

43. Klassen AF, Miller A, Fine S. Health-related quality of life in children and adolescents who have a diagnosis of attention-deficit/hyperactivity disorder. *Pediatrics,* 2004; 114:e541–547.

44. Crook WG. Diet and hyperactivity. *Pediatrics,* 1981; 68:300–301.

45. Egger J, Carter CM, Graham PJ, Gumley D, Soothill. Controlled trial of oligoantigenic treatment in the hyperkinetic syndrome. *Lancet,* 1985; 540–545.

46. Carter CM, Urbanowicz M, Hemsley R, Mantilla L, Strobel S, Graham PJ, Taylor E. Effects of a few food diet in attention deficit disorder. *Arch Dis Child,* 1993; 69:564–568.

47. Schulte-Korne G, Deimel W, Gutenbrunner C, Hennighausen K, Blank R, Rieger C, Remschmidt H. Effect of an oligo-antigen diet on the behavior of hyperkinetic children. *Zeitschrift fur Kinder-und Jugendpsychiatrie und Psychotherapie,* 1996; 24:176–183.

48. Pelsser LM, Buitelaar JK. Favourable effect of a standard elimination diet on the behavior of young children with attention deficit hyperactivity disorder (ADHD): a pilot study. *Nederlands Tijdschrift voor Geneeskunde,* 2002; 146:2543–2547.

49. Wender EH, Solanto MV. Effects of sugar on aggressive and inattentive behavior in children with attention deficit disorder with hyperactivity and normal children. *Pediatrics,* 1991; 88:960–966.

50. Rapp DJ. Does diet affect hyperactivity? *J Learn Disabil,* 1978; 11:383–389.

51. Prinz RJ, Roberts WA, Hantman E. Dietary correlates of hyperactive behavior in children. *J Consult Clin Psychol,* 1980; 48:760–769.

52. Rosen LA, Booth SR, Bender ME, McGrath ML, Sorrell S, Drabman R. Effects of sugar (sucrose) on children's behavior. *J Consult Clin Psychol,* 1988; 56:583–589.

53. Goldman JA, Lerman RH, Contois JH, et al. Behavioral effects of sucrose on preschool children. *J Abnorm Child Psychol,* 1986; 14:565–577.

54. Prinz RJ, Riddle DB. Association between nutrition and behavior. *Nutr Rev,* 1986; 44(Suppl):151–158.

55. Conners CK, Glasgow A, Raiten D, et al. Hyperactives differ from normals in blood sugar and hormonal response to sucrose. Presented at Annual Meeting, American Psychological Association; August 1987; New York, NY.

56. Wesnes KA, Pincock C, Richardson D, Helm G, Hails S. Breakfast reduces declines in attention and memory over the morning in schoolchildren. *Appetite,* 2003; 41:329–331.

57. Wolraich M, Stumbo P, Milich R, Chenard C, Schultz F. Dietary characteristics of hyperactive and controls boys and their behavioural correlates. *J Am Diet Assoc,* 1986; 84:500–504.

58. Arnold LE, Nemzer E. New evidence on diet in hyperkinesis. *Pediatrics,* 1982; 69:250.

59. Benton D. The impact of the supply of glucose to the brain on mood and memory. *Nutr Rev,* 2001; 59: S20–21.

60. Wolraich M, Milich R, Stumbo P, Schultz F. Effects of sucrose ingestion on the behavior of hyperactive boys. *J Pediatr,* 1985; 106:675.

61. Ferguson HB, Stoddart C, Simeon PG. Double blind challenge studies of behavioural and cognitive effects of sucrose-aspartame ingestion in normal children. *Nutr Rev,* 1986; 44(Suppl):144–150.

62. Roshon MS, Hagen RL. Sugar consumption, locomotion, task orientation, and learning in preschool children. *J Abnorm Child Psychol,* 1989; 17:349–357.

63. Mahan LK, Chase M, Furukawa CT, Sulzacher S, Shapiro GG, Pierson W, Bierman CW. Sugar "allergy" and children's behavior. *Ann Allergy,* 1988; 61:453–458.

64. Behar D, Rapoport JL, Adams AA, Berg CK, Cornblath M. Sugar challenge testing with children considered behaviorally "sugar reactive." *Nutr Behav,* 1984; 1:277–288.

65. Saravis S, Schachar R, Zlotkin S, Leiber LA, Anderson GH. Aspartame: effects on learning, behavior and mood. *Pediatrics,* 1990; 86:75–80.
66. Garriga MM, Metcalfe DD. Aspartame intolerance. *Ann Allergy,* 1988; 61:63–69.
67. Maher TJ, Wurtman RJ. Possible neurologic effects of aspartame, a widely used food additive. *Environ Health Perspect,* 1987; 75:53–57.
68. Coulombe RA, Sharma RP. Neurobiological alterations induced by the artificial sweetener aspartame (NutraSweet). *Toxicol Appl Pharmacol,* 1986; 83:79–85.
69. Craig ML, Hollis KL, Dess NK. The bitter truth: sensitivity to saccharin's bitterness predicts overactivity in highly arousable female dieters. *Int J Eat Disord,* 2003; 34:71–82.
70. Richardson AJ, Puri BK. The potential role of fatty acids in attention-deficit hyperactivity disorder. *Prostaglandins Leukot Essent Fatty Acids,* 2000; 63:79–87.
71. Yehuda S, Rabinovitz S, Mostofsky DI. Essential fatty acids and the brain: from infancy to aging. *Neurobio of Aging,* 2005; 26S:S98–102.
72. Yehuda S, Rabonivitz S, Mostofsky DI. Essential fatty acids are mediators of brain biochemistry and cognitive functions. *J Neurosci Re,* 1999; 56:565–570.
73. Attar-Bashi NM, Frydenberg M, Li D, Sinclair AJ. Docosahexaenoic acid (DHA) accumulation is regulated by the polyunsaturated fat content of the diet. *Asia Pac J Clin Nutr,* 2004; 13(Suppl):S78.
74. Richardson AJ. Long-chain polyunsaturated fatty acids in childhood developmental and psychiatric disorders. *Lipids,* 2004; 39:1215–1222.
75. Simopoulos AP. The importance of the ratio of omega-6/omega-3 essential fatty acids. *Biomed Pharmacother,* 2002; 56:365–379.
76. Colquhoun I, Bunday S. A lack of essential fatty acids as a possible cause of hyperactivity in children. *Med Hypotheses,* 1981; 7:673–679.
77. Mitchell EA, Aman MG, Turbott SH, Manku M. Clinical characteristics and serum fatty acid levels in hyperactive children. *Clin Pediatr,* 1987; 26:406–411.
78. Stevens LJ, Zental SS, Deck JL, Abate ML, Lipp SR, Burgess JR. Essential fatty acid metabolism in boys with attention-deficit hyperactivity disorder. *Am J Clin Nutr,* 1995; 62:761–768.
79. Chen JR, Hsu SF, Hsu CD, Hwang LH, Yang SC. Dietary patterns and blood fatty acid composition in children with attention-deficit hyperactivity disorder in Taiwan. *J Nutr Biochem,* 2004; 15:467–472.
80. Young GS, Maharaj NJ, Conquer JA. Blood phospholipids fatty acid analysis of adults with and without attention deficit/hyperactivity disorder. *Lipids,* 2004; 39:117–123.
81. Ross BM, McKEnzie I, Glen I, Bennett CP. Increased levels of ethane, a non-invasive marker of n-3 fatty acid oxidation, in breath of children with attention deficit hyperactivity disorder. *Nutr Neurosci,* 2003; 6:277–281.
82. Brookes KJ, Chen W, Xu X, Taylor E, Asherson P. Association of fatty acid desaturase genes with attention-deficit/hyperactivity disorder. *Biol Psychiatry,* 2006; 60:1053–1061.
83. Yehuda S. n-6/n-3 ratio and brain-related functions. *World Rev Nutr Diet,* 2003; 92:37–56.
84. Aman MG, Mitchell EA, Turbott SH. The effects of essential fatty acid supplementation by Efamol in hyperactive children. *J Abnorm Child Psychol,* 1987; 15:75–90.
85. Arnold LE, Kleykamp D, Votolato NA, Taylor WA, Kontras SB, Tobin K. Gamma-linolenic acid for attention-deficit hyperactivity disorder: placebo-controlled comparison to D-amphetamine. *Biol Psychiatry,* 1989; 25:222–228.
86. Voigt RG, Llorente A, Jensen CL, Fraley JK, Berretta MC, Heird WC. A randomized, double-blind, placebo-controlled trial of docosahexaenoic acid supplementation in children with attention-deficit/hyperactivity disorder. *J Pediat,* 2001; 139:189–196.
87. Hirayama S, Hamazaki T, Terasawa K. Effect of docosahexaenoic acid-containing food administration on symptoms of attention-deficit/hyperactivity disorder—a placebo-controlled double-blind study. *Eur J Clin Nutr,* 2004; 58:467–473.
88. Sinn N, Bryan J. Effect of supplementation with polyunsaturated fatty acids and micronutrients on learning and behavior problems associated with child ADHD. *J Dev Behav Pediatr,* 2007; 28:82–91.
89. Joshi K, Lad S, Kale M, Patwardhan B, Mahadik SP, Patni B, Chaudhary A, Bhave S, Pandit A. Supplementation with flax oil and vitamin C improves the outcome of attention deficit hyperactivity disorder (ADHD). *Prostaglandins Leukot Essent Fatty Acids,* 2006; 74:17–21.
90. Stevens L, Zhang W, Peck L, Kuczek T, Grevstad N, Mahon A, Zentall SS, Arnold LE, Burgess JR. EFA supplementation in children with inattention, hyperactivity, and other disruptive behaviors. *Lipids,* 2003; 38:1007–1021.
91. Virmani A, Binienda Z. Role of carnitine esters in brain neuropathology. *Mol Aspects Med,* 2004; 25:533–549.

92. Van Oudheusden LJ, Scholte HR. Efficacy of carnitine in the treatment of children with attention-deficit hyperactivity disorder. *Prostaglandins Leukot Essent Fatty Acids,* 2002; 67:33–38.

93. Youdim MB, Ben-Shachar D, Yehuda S. Putative biological mechanisms of the effect of iron deficiency on brain biochemistry and behavior. *Am J Clin Nutr,* 1989; 50(3 Suppl):607–615.

94. Konofal E, Cortese S, Marchand M, Mouren M-C, Arnulf I, Lecendreux M. Impact of restless legs syndrome and iron deficiency on attention-deficit/hyperactivity disorder in children. *Sleep Medicine,* 2007; 8:711–715.

95. Konofal E, Lecendreux M, Arnulf I, Mouren MC. Iron deficiency in children with attention-deficit/ hyperactivity disorder. *Arch Pediatr Adolesc Med,* 2004; 158:1113–1115.

96. Oner O, Alkar OY, Oner P. Relation of ferritin levels with symptom ratings and cognitive performance in children with attention deficit-hyperactivity disorder. *Pediatr Int,* 2008; 50:40–44.

97. Sever Y, Ashkenazi A, Tyano S, Weizman A. Iron treatment in children with attention deficit hyperactivity disorder. A preliminary report. *Neuropsychobiology,* 1997; 35:178–180.

98. Konofal E, Lecendreux M, Deron J, Marchand M, Cortese S, Zaïm M, Mouren Mc Arnulf I. Effects of iron supplementation on attention deficit hyperactivity disorder in children. *Pediatr Neurol,* 2008; 38:20–26.

99. Konofal E, Cortese S. Restless legs syndrome and attention-deficit/hyperactivity disorder. *Ann Neurol,* 2005; 58:341–342.

100. Cortese S, Konofal E, Lecendreux M, Arnulf I, Mouren M-C, Darra F et al. Restless legs syndrome and attention-deficit/hyperactivity disorder: a review of the literature. *Sleep,* 2005; 28:1007–1013.

101. Walters AS, Mandelbaum DE, Lewin DS, Kugler S, England SJ, Miller M et al. Dopaminergic therapy in children with restless legs/periodic limb movements in sleep and ADHD. *Pediatric Neurology,* 2000; 22:182–186.

102. Tran TT, Chowanadisai W, Lonnerdal B, Le L, Parker M, Chicz-Demet A, Crinella FM. Effects of neonatal dietary manganese exposure on brain dopamine levels and neurocognitive functions. *Neurotoxicology,* 2002; 23:645–651.

103. Stastny D, Vogel RS, Picciano MF. Manganese intake and serum manganese concentration of human milk-fed and formula-fed infants. *Am J Clin Nutrition,* 1984; 39:972–978.

104. Black MM. Zinc deficiency and child development. *J Clin Nutr,* 1998; 8(suppl):464S–469S.

105. Arnold LE, Pinkham SM, Votolato N. Does zinc moderate essential fatty acid and amphetamine treatment of attention-deficit/hyperactivity disorder? *J Child Adolesc Psychopharmacol,* 2000; 10:111–117.

106. Toren P, Eldar S, Sela BA, Wolmer L, Weitz R, Inbar D, Koren S, Reiss A, Weizman R, Laor N. Zinc deficiency in attention-deficit hyperactivity disorder. *Biol Psychiatry,* 1996; 40:1308–1310.

107. Bekaroglu M, Aslan Y, Gedik Y, Deger O, Mocan H, Erduran E, Karahan C. Relationships between serum free fatty acids and zinc, and attention deficit hyperactivity disorder: a research note. *J Child Psychol Psychiatry,* 1996; 37:225–227.

108. Akhondzadeh S, Mohammadi M-R, Khademi M. Zinc sulfate as an adjunct to methylphenidate for the treatment of attention deficit hyperactivity disorder in children: a double blind and randomized trial. *BMC Psychiatry,* 2004; 4:9.

109. Kozielec T, Starobrat-Hermelin B. Assessment of magnesium levels in children with attention deficit hyperactivity disorder (ADHD). *Magnes Res,* 1997; 10:143–148.

110. Starobrat-Hermelin B. The effect of deficiency of selected bioelements on hyperactivity in children with certain specified mental disorders. *Annales Academiae Medicae Stetinensis,* 1998; 44:297–314.

111. Starobrat-Hermelin B, Kozielec T. The effects of magnesium physiological supplementation on hyperactivity in children with attention deficit hyperactivity disorder (ADHD). Positive response to magnesium oral loading test. *Magnesium Res,* 1997; 10:149–156.

112. Monsain-Bosc M, Roche M, Polge A, Pradal-Prat D, Rapin J, Bali JP. Improvement of neurobehavioral disorders in children supplemented with magnesium-vitamin B6. I. Attention deficit hyperactivity disorders. *Magnesium Res,* 2006; 19:46–52.

113. Wurtman RJ, Fernstrom JD. Control of brain neurotransmitter synthesis by precursor availability. *Biochem Pharmacol,* 1976; 25:1691–1696.

114. Wood D, Reimherr F, Wender PH. Effects of levodopa on attention deficit disorder, residual type. *Psychiatry Res,* 1982; 6:13–20.

115. Wood DR, Reimherr FW, Wender PH. Treatment of attention deficit disorder with dl-phenylalanine. *Psychiatry Res,* 1985; 16:21–26.

116. Reimherr FW, Wender PH, Wood DR, Ward M. An open trial of l-tyrosine in the treatment of attention deficit disorder, residual type. *Am J Psychiatry,* 1987; 144:1071–1073.

117. Neff R. Amino Acids and ADHD—A Retrospective Review (abstract). Accessed on April 10, 2008 from http://www.drrossonline.com/amino-acid-research_a/246.htm.
118. McTavish SF, McPherson MH, Sharp T, Cowen PJ. Attenuation of some subjective effects of amphetamine following tyrosine depletion. *J Psychopharmacol,* 1999; 13:144–147.
119. Coleman M, Steinberg G, Tippett J et al. A preliminary study of the effect of pyridoxine administration in a subgroup of hyperkinetic children: a double-blind crossover comparison with methylphenidate. *Biol Psychiatry,* 1979; 14:741–751.
120. Bellisle F. Effects of diet on behaviour and cognition in children. *British Journal of Nutrition,* 2004; 92(Suppl 2):S227–232.
121. Benton D, Griffiths S, Haller J. Thiamin supplementation, mood and cognitive functioning. *Psychopharmacology,* 1997; 129; 66–71.
122. Dykman KD, Dykman RA. Effect of nutritional supplements on attentional-deficit hyperactivity disorder. *Integr Physiol Behav Sci,* 1998; 33:49–60.
123. Jadad AR, Boyle M, Cunningham C, Kim M, Schachar R. Treatment of attention-deficit/hyperactivity disorder. Evidence report/technology assessment, 1999; 11 (AHCPR Publication No.99-E01). Rockville, MD: Agency for Health Care Policy and Research.
124. Spencer T, Biederman J, Wilens T et al. Pharmacotherapy of attention-deficit hyperactivity disorder across the life cycles. *J Am Acad Child Adolesc Psychiatry,* 1996; 35:409–432.
125. Banaschewski T, Roessner V, Dittmann RW, Santosh PJ, Rothernberger A. Non-stimulant medications in the treatment of ADHD. *Eur Child Adolesc Psychiatry,* 2004; 13, 102–116.
126. DeMaray MK, Elting J, Schaefer K. Assessment of Attention-Deficit/Hyperactivity Disorder (ADHD): A comparative evaluation of five, commonly used, published rating scales. *Psychol Sch,* 2003; 40: 341–361.

26 Migraine Headaches

Food Triggers and Nutrient Therapies

Christina Sun-Edelstein, M.D., and Alexander Mauskop, M.D.

I. INTRODUCTION

Migraine is a common and disabling disorder that affects millions of Americans. It is also one of the most common ailments with which patients present to their primary care providers. Though a wide range of acute and preventive headache medications are now available, most patients will not have a significant improvement in their headaches unless lifestyle modifications are made. These include sleep hygiene, stress management, aerobic exercise, and dietary modification. In this chapter the role of food and nutrients in the treatment and prevention of migraine headaches will be discussed.

II. EPIDEMIOLOGY

Migraine is a common neurological disorder that affects 18% of women and 6% of men in the United States [1], and has an estimated worldwide prevalence of about 10% [2]. The prevalence of migraine rises throughout early adult life and falls after midlife. Population-based studies have reported that migraine is inherited, with a relative risk of migraine headache in a first-degree family member ranging from 1.4 to 1.9 [3, 4]. In monozygotic twins the concordance rates for migraine range from 37% to 52%, and 15% to 21% for dizygotic twins [5, 6]. These figures indicate that environmental factors play a significant role in migraine.

Of the migraine sufferers who consult a physician, about two-thirds visit primary care physicians. Only 16% consult neurologists or headache specialists. These observations emphasize the importance of continuously improving the ability of primary care physicians to accurately diagnose migraine in their patients [7].

III. PATHOPHYSIOLOGY

Though the understanding of migraine pathophysiology has increased dramatically in recent years, the exact etiology remains to be defined. The current prevailing theory is based on a hyperexcitable "trigeminovascular complex" in patients who are genetically predisposed to migraine. In these people, there is a lowered threshold for migraine attacks and a vulnerability to environmental triggers. The theory proposes that in susceptible individuals, the trigeminovascular neurons release neurotransmitters, such as calcitonin gene-related peptide (CGRP) and Substance P, when headache triggers are encountered. This leads to vasodilation, mast cell degranulation, increased vascular permeability, and meningeal edema, resulting in neurogenic inflammation. This nociceptive information is transmitted from the trigeminal nerve to brainstem nuclei, thalamic nuclei, and the cortex, where migraine pain is ultimately perceived [8]. The locus coeruleus, which comprises noradrenergic neurons, the dorsal raphe, which consists of serotoninergic neurons, and the periaqueductal gray also play modulatory roles in the transmission of pain [9].

Mitochondrial dysfunction, which leads to impaired oxygen metabolism, has been speculated to play a role in migraine pathophysiology [10–12], as migraineurs have been shown to have a reduction in mitochondrial phosphorylation potential in intervals between headaches [13, 14]. This theory is the basis for the use of supplements that enhance mitochondrial function in the treatment of migraine, such as riboflavin, coenzyme Q10 (CoQ10), and alpha lipoic acid.

IV. THE ROLE OF FOOD AND NUTRIENTS IN MIGRAINE

GLUCOSE DYSREGULATION

The importance of eating regularly cannot be overemphasized, as skipping meals can trigger headaches [15]. Skipped meals and fasting were reported migraine triggers in up to 57% of subjects in clinic and population-based studies [16–19]. While the mechanism by which fasting and skipping meals triggers headaches is unknown, several theories have been proposed. Alterations in serotonin and norepinephrine in brainstem pathways could precipitate headache onset [20], as could the release of stress hormones such as cortisol. Hypoglycemia could potentially bring on a headache [9]. In one study [21] three-quarters of participants with migraine headaches demonstrated 5-hour glucose tolerance tests consistent with reactive hypoglycemia. Micronutrients involved in glucose regulation include chromium, biotin, magnesium, zinc, copper, vitamin E, and l-carnitine [22].

FOOD TRIGGERS

The recognition of dietary migraine triggers is important because it helps not only in reducing the frequency of migraine, but also in giving migraineurs a sense of control over a condition that can render them helpless and debilitated [9]. Although the scientific basis for many of these triggers remains controversial, it appears that subsets of migraineurs may be sensitive to them [9]. Patients should therefore be aware that the foods and substances listed in Table 26.1 [9, 17, 23–38] are potential migraine triggers. Caffeine and alcohol are discussed in detail because of their complex relationship to headache. Not all of the foods listed will trigger a migraine in any one individual. Headaches are generally triggered by a combination of substances, during a time of particular vulnerability such as menses or emotional stress. Food diaries are helpful in sorting out which substances or circumstances are problematic for each patient.

Alcohol

Alcohol, in particular red wine, is frequently cited as a migraine trigger. Wine contains tyramine, sulfites, histamine, and the phenolic flavonoids, all of which can theoretically precipitate migraines [9]. Histamine may trigger headache via the release of nitric oxide from the vascular endothelium, resulting in vasodilation [35]. Phenolic flavonoids in red wine have been shown to cause the release of serotonin from platelets, which may occur in parallel with the release of serotonin in the central nervous system, potentially leading to headache [36].

Alcohol hangover headache (AHH) is a common occurrence that generally occurs after ingesting large amounts of alcohol. In addition to headache, AHH comprises a constellation of physical, cognitive, and psychological symptoms including anorexia, tremulousness, dizziness, nausea, tachycardia, and irritability [39]. The headache usually occurs the morning after alcohol consumption, when the blood alcohol concentration is falling [40], and can continue for 24 hours after the blood alcohol concentration reaches zero. AHH is not always dose related and in fact occurs more commonly in

TABLE 26.1
Potential Food Triggers in Migraine

Trigger	Food	Mechanism	Prevalence	Reference(s)
Phenylethamine	Chocolate, cacao.	Releases vasoactive amines such as serotonin and catecholamines in migraineurs with MAO-B deficiency.	19–50%	17, 23–26
Tyramine	Aged cheese, smoked fish, cured meats, yeast extract, beer, fermented foods.	May trigger migraines via the release of norepinephrine and its agonist effect at alpha-adrenergic receptors.	9–18%	9, 17, 25
Aspartame	NutraSweet®	Possibly via an alteration of serotonergic metabolism in the brain.	—	27–29
Monosodium glutamate (MSG) Also known as hydrolyzed vegetable protein (HVP), autolyzed yeast, sodium caseinate, yeast extract, hydrolyzed oat flour, texturized protein, and calcium casinate	Chinese food, meat tenderizer, many canned and prepared foods	Possibly via a direct vasoconstrictor effect or by activation of a neurotransmission pathway in which nitric oxide is released in endothelial cells, inducing vasodilation.	13%	17, 25, 30–31
Nitrates and Nitrites	Sausages, cured meats and fish such as hot dogs, bacon, ham, salami, pepperoni, corned beef, pastrami, lox	Probably via the release of nitric oxide and subsequent vasodilation, although the interaction of nitrites with blood pigment to produce methemglobin may also play a role.	—	9, 26, 32–34
Alcohol	Red and white wine, beer, darker colored beverages such as bourbon and whiskey	Tyramine, histamine, phenolic flavenoids and sulfites in wine may precipitate migraines (see discussion in text).	29–35%	9, 17, 25, 35–36
Caffeine	Coffee, tea, soda, medications such as Excedrin®, Fiorinal®, and Fioricet®	Via the blockade of inhibitory and excitatory adenosine receptors in the brain and vasculature, resulting in vasoconstriction and the release of excitatory neurotransmitters.	14%	17, 25, 37–38

light or moderate drinkers than regular heavy drinkers [41–42]. In migraineurs, a migraine can be triggered the day after moderate alcohol ingestion, while nonmigraineurs usually need to consume large amounts in order to develop AHH.

Darker colored alcoholic beverages, such as red wine, bourbon, and beer contain congeners, which are natural byproducts of alcohol fermentation. These drinks are more likely to induce AHH as compared to clear alcoholic beverages such as gin or vodka. The pathophysiology of AHH may involve a vasodilatory effect in the intracranial vasculature, alteration of sleep patterns, or an inflammatory mechanism via an alteration of cytokine pathways and prostaglandin release [43–45]. Magnesium depletion may also play a role. Patients who are prone to AHH should be advised to drink in moderation and stay well-hydrated. Eating greasy food prior to alcohol consumption may help to slow or delay alcohol absorption, and consuming foods naturally rich in fructose, such as honey and tomato juice, allows for more effective alcohol metabolism.

Caffeine

Caffeine is a common dietary substance found in coffee, tea, soda, and chocolate. It is also included in various prescription (Fioricet®, Fiorinal®, Esgic®) and over-the-counter headache medications (Excedrin®). Caffeine works via the blockade of inhibitory and excitatory adenosine receptors in the brain and vasculature, resulting in vasoconstriction and the release of excitatory neurotransmitters. Some of the involved pathways are important in pain perception [37–38].

Caffeine's effect on the central nervous system varies with the dose and frequency of use. In general, one serving of brewed coffee has 115 mg caffeine, while a serving of Pepsi has 38 mg. Excedrin contains 65 mg caffeine per tablet. At low to moderate doses (50 to 300 mg), caffeine causes increased alertness, concentration, and energy. At doses greater than 300 mg, anxiety, insomnia, and irritability can occur [9, 46]. Caffeine's effect on headaches is paradoxical in that it can worsen or alleviate headaches, depending on dosage and frequency. When used infrequently, caffeine is effective in headache treatment because it has a mild, direct analgesic effect [47] and also assists in the absorption of other analgesics. It also crosses the blood-brain barrier quickly, and reaches therapeutic levels in the brain within 20 minutes. These characteristics make caffeine a useful component of combination analgesics (i.e., Fiorinal, Fioricet). High doses (>300 mg/day) consumed on a regular basis are associated with headache. Regular use of caffeine-containing analgesics is associated with medication-overuse headaches [48–50].

Headaches also occur with abrupt withdrawal of caffeine. The higher the level of baseline caffeine ingestion, the greater the likelihood of caffeine withdrawal headache, although these headaches can occur in patients consuming moderate amounts of caffeine [51], and when patients consuming 100 mg caffeine daily stop abruptly [52]. Caffeine withdrawal is also associated with depression, drowsiness, and impaired concentration. Patients with headaches who wish to continue drinking caffeinated beverages should limit their daily intake to less than 200 mg. Patients who use caffeine-containing analgesics should limit intake to 2 to 3 days per week to avoid medication-overuse headache. Those who wish to cease caffeine consumption should gradually taper their intake over several weeks [9]. Patients should also be aware that drinking grapefruit juice increases the time for caffeine metabolism, since it occupies the same enzyme. This may modify the effects of caffeine during periods of consumption and withdrawal.

NUTRIENTS

For many migraine sufferers, traditional acute and preventative medications such as triptans, anti-inflammatories, antiepileptics, blood pressure medications, and antidepressants are contraindicated, or have side effects that limit their use. Over-the-counter medications such as acetaminophen or ibuprofen tend to become less effective in alleviating headaches over time, and can lead to medication-overuse headache. For these reasons, migraineurs often seek alternative treatment options. In recent years there has been an increasing demand for natural therapies for common ailments such as headache.

Magnesium

Magnesium is an essential cation that plays a vital role in multiple physiological processes, regulating tissue and cell functions. Deficits in magnesium can be seen in any chronic medical illness, including cardiovascular disease, diabetes, pre-eclampsia, eclampsia, sickle cell disease, and chronic alcoholism [53]. Symptoms of magnesium deficiency include premenstrual syndrome, leg muscle cramps, coldness of extremities, weakness, anorexia, nausea, digestive disorders, lack of coordination, and confusion. Magnesium may be involved in migraine pathogenesis by counteracting vasospasm, inhibiting platelet aggregation, and stabilizing of cell membranes [54]. Its concentration influences serotonin receptors, nitric oxide synthesis and release, inflammatory mediators, and various other migraine-related receptors and neurotransmitters [55]. Magnesium also plays a role in the control of vascular tone and reactivity to endogenous hormones and neurotransmitters, via its relationship with the N-methyl D-aspartate (NMDA) receptor [56–57]. In the brain, a deficiency of magnesium results in contraction and potentiation of vasoconstrictors [58].

Studies have shown that migraineurs have low brain magnesium during migraine attacks [59] and may also have a systemic magnesium deficiency [60, 61]. Furthermore, a deficiency of magnesium may play a particularly important role in menstrual migraine [62]. There have been two double-blind, placebo-controlled trials that have shown that oral magnesium supplementation is effective in headache prevention [63–64]. A third study [65] was negative, but this result has been attributed to the use of a poorly absorbed magnesium salt, since diarrhea occurred in almost half of patients in the treatment group. Intravenous magnesium has been shown to be an effective migraine abortive agent in patients with low ionized magnesium levels, but not in those with normal levels [66]. The most commonly reported adverse effect of magnesium supplementation is diarrhea.

A potential nutrient-nutrient interaction occurs between magnesium and calcium supplements. Women of childbearing age are advised to take calcium supplements for bone health. Calcium supplements that do not also contain magnesium can reduce the absorption of magnesium since the two minerals compete for absorption. Often women who take calcium without magnesium experience constipation, which should alert physicians to the presence of supplement-induced low magnesium.

Riboflavin

Riboflavin, also known as vitamin B2, is a precursor for flavin mononucleotides that are cofactors in the Krebs cycle. It is essential for membrane stability and the maintenance of energy-related cellular functions [67]. A randomized controlled trial evaluating the use of riboflavin (400 mg) as a migraine prophylactic agent with a total of 128 subjects was positive [68]. Minor adverse reactions included diarrhea and polyuria.

CoQ10

CoQ10 is an endogenous enzyme cofactor made by all cells in the body, functioning to promote mitochondrial proton-electron translocation. It has been used in the treatment of mitochondriopathies and mitochondrial encephalomyopathies such as Kearns-Sayre syndrome, and is being investigated for use in neurodegenerative disorders, cancer, and blood pressure management.

In an open label study [69] in which 31 patients with migraine, with and without aura, used 150 mg daily of CoQ10 for 3 months, 61% had at least a 50% reduction in migraine days without significant adverse events. Supplementation was effective within the first month of therapy. Later, a small randomized controlled trial [70] was conducted over 3 months with 42 patients. CoQ10, in a dose of 100 mg three times daily, significantly decreased attack frequency, headache days, and days with nausea. Nausea, anorexia, dyspepsia, diarrhea, and cutaneous allergy were reported, but at a low rate [69–70].

Alpha Lipoic Acid

Like riboflavin and CoQ10, alpha lipoic acid, also known as thioctic acid, is a nutrient that enhances mitochondrial oxygen metabolism and adenosine triphosphate (ATP) production [71], with very few adverse effects. Supplementation has resulted in clinical and biochemical improvement in several mitochondriopathies [71–73]. Its use in migraine prevention has been evaluated in one open pilot study [unpublished data, discussed in reference 74] and one randomized placebo-controlled trial (RCT) [74] to date.

Although there was a clear trend for reduction of migraine frequency after treatment with 600 mg alpha lipoic acid in the RCT, the result was not significant. The authors attributed the equivocal result to the fact that the study was underpowered. Within-group analyses did show a significant reduction in attack frequency, headache days, and headache severity in patients in the treatment group.

HERBAL SUPPLEMENTS

Feverfew *(Tanacetum parthenium)*

Feverfew is an herbal preparation that is available as the dried leaves of the weed plant *Tanacetum parthenium*. It was used to treat headache, inflammation, and fever several centuries ago, and was rediscovered in the late 20th century. The mechanism by which it works in migraine prophylaxis may be related to the parthenolides within the leaves. These may inhibit serotonin release from platelets and white blood cells, and inhibit platelet aggregation. Feverfew may also have anti-inflammatory action through the inhibition of prostaglandin synthesis and phospholipase A [75–78].

Randomized controlled studies conducted over the past few decades have yielded conflicting results [79–83]. Inconsistencies in these results were possibility related to the fact that different preparations have been found to vary more than 400% in the strength of the active ingredient, parthenolide [84], and different methods of feverfew extraction have resulted in differences in extract stability [85]. Taking into account these variables, a new, more stable feverfew extract (MIG-99) was evaluated in a three-arm randomized controlled trial (2.08 mg, 6.25 mg, 18.75 mg TID versus placebo) [86]. Although none of the doses were significant for the primary endpoint, a subset of patients with high frequency of migraine attacks did seem to benefit. In a follow-up study, investigators evaluated 6.25 mg TID of MIG-99 versus placebo, and reported a statistically significant and clinically relevant reduction in migraine frequency in the MIG-99 group. While MIG-99 may be mildly effective, there are no known commercially available preparations [67]. Side effects reported in the RCTs include gastrointestinal disturbances, mouth ulcers, and a "post-feverfew syndrome" of joint aches.

Butterbur *(Petasites hybridus)*

In recent years, *Petasites hybridus* root extract, also known as butterbur, has emerged as a potential new treatment in the prevention of migraine. The butterbur plant is a perennial shrub that was used in ancient times for its medicinal properties. It was rediscovered in the middle of the 20th century and used as an analgesic and antispasmodic agent for migraine, asthma, urinary tract spasm, and back pain [87–91]. *Petasites* is thought to act through calcium channel regulation and inhibition of peptide-leukotriene biosynthesis. Leukotrienes and other inflammatory mediators may have a role in the inflammatory cascade associated with migraine [92–94]. *Petasites* is also used to ameliorate allergic rhinitis, which has a similar pathophysiology. In the United States, the *Petasites* extract is marketed as a food supplement called Petadolex, which contains 50 mg of *Petasites* per capsule.

Several studies have been conducted to evaluate the efficacy of *Petasites hybridus* in migraine prevention. A randomized, double-blind, placebo-controlled trial [87] using 50 mg of Petadolex twice daily showed a significantly reduced number of migraine attacks and migraine days per month. Lipton and colleagues [95] compared *Petasites* extract 75 mg twice daily, *Petasites* extract 50 mg twice daily, and placebo twice daily in a randomized trial of 245 patients and found that the higher dose of *Petasites* extract was more effective than placebo in decreasing the number of monthly migraine attacks. A multicenter prospective open-label study [96] of Petadolex in 109 children and adolescents with migraine resulted in 77% of all patients reporting a reduction in migraine frequency of at least 50%. In all three studies, Petadolex was well-tolerated and no serious adverse events occurred. The most frequently reported adverse reactions were mild gastrointestinal symptoms, predominantly eructation (burping).

Other

Ginger has been used for its medicinal qualities in China for centuries, in the treatment of pain, inflammation, and musculoskeletal symptoms. It has anti-inflammatory qualities that could be related to the reduction of platelet aggregation and the inhibition of prostaglandin and leukotriene biosynthesis [97]. There are anecdotal and folkloric descriptions of its efficacy in relieving headache.

Valerian root is a perennial herb that is used for its sedative and hypnotic qualities, especially in insomniacs [98]. The effective dose for insomnia is 300 to 600 mg, which is equivalent to 2 to 3 g of dried herbal valerian root soaked in one cup of hot water for 10 to 15 minutes [99]. In migraine patients with anxiety, it may be preferable to benzodiazepines as it is not associated with sleepiness on awakening. At high doses, it is associated with headaches and muscle spasm.

DIETARY FAT COMPOSITION

Eicosapentaenoic acid (EPA), an unsaturated fatty acid that is one of the body's natural omega-3 fatty acids, may also be useful in headache prevention. Small studies [100] have suggested that headache severity and frequency can be reduced by adding EPA to the diet, possibly by lowering prostaglandin levels and serotonin activity. A dose of 600 mg/day in three divided doses has been suggested for headache prevention [101–102]. Foods richest in EPA are fish that inhabit cold deep water, such as salmon, tuna, mackerel, and herring. A high disproportion of dietary omega-6 fats, consumption of *trans* fats, and an impairment in the conversion of dietary omega-3 fats into EPA all suggest a deficit in EPA. Dietary changes can reduce or obviate the need for EPA supplementation long-term.

V.   MIGRAINE AND COMORBID CONDITIONS

GENERAL INFORMATION

Migraine is comorbid with numerous medical conditions, some of which are well-defined medical disorders (stroke, hypertension, hypothyroidism, asthma, allergies, and endometriosis), and others of which are idiopathic symptomatic medical conditions (irritable bowel syndrome, fibromyalgia, chronic fatigue syndrome, interstitial cystitis, and pelvic pain) [103–111]. Psychiatric comorbidities have been described as well [112–113]. A putative neurobiological link has been suggested [114] because of the bidirectional link between migraine and many of these disorders.

A recent retrospective chart review of 223 patients seen at a university headache clinic [115] showed that among patients presenting for evaluation at a specialty headache center, there are two groups of migraine comorbid conditions, in addition to a group characterized by a lack of comorbidities. One of the groups had a strong association with metabolic disorders such as diabetes mellitus (DM), hypertension (HTN), and hypercholesterolemia, while the other group was defined by a link with fibromyalgia, depression, and anxiety.

MOOD DISORDERS, MIGRAINE, AND OBESITY

Migraine has been linked to mood disorders in both community and clinic-based studies [116]. While the association between migraine and depression has been most widely reported, migraine is also linked to anxiety disorders and bipolar disorder [116]. Large-scale population studies [117–120] have shown that migraineurs are 2.2 to 4.0 times more likely to have depression, and other studies have reported that the relationship between the two disorders is bidirectional, with each disorder increasing the risk for the other [112, 121–122].

Depression and anxiety are also strongly associated with obesity [123–129], and obesity is associated with migraine. Longitudinal population-based studies have shown that obesity is a risk factor for developing chronic daily headache [130], and, in people with episodic migraine, body mass index (BMI) is associated with migraine attack frequency and severity [131]. A recent cross-sectional multicenter study [132] on comorbid conditions in headache clinic patients showed that both depression and anxiety were more common in obese subjects, and both depression and anxiety modified the strength of the relationship of obesity with migraine frequency and disability.

The above relationships between obesity, depression, anxiety, and chronic, disabling migraine are suggestive of a common pathogenetic pathway among the disorders [132]. A proinflammatory mechanism has been proposed to explain the relationship between obesity and migraine [130–133], and a neurobiological link mediated by common brain monoamines and peptides has been proposed as the connection between mood disorders, migraine, and the regulation of body weight [132, 134–135]. Alterations in the hypothalamic-pituitary-adrenal system may also be involved [132, 136–139].

MIGRAINE, VASCULAR AND RELATED METABOLIC DISORDERS

Migraine has been associated with a constellation of metabolic disorders (DM, HTN, hypercholesterolemia) [115], all of which are risk factors for cardiac and cerebrovascular disease. While migraine with aura had not been associated with early-onset coronary heart disease in large cohort studies [140–143], two recent large-scale prospective cohort studies [144–145] found positive relationships between migraine and ischemic heart disease. Women who reported a history of migraine without aura did not have an increased risk for any ischemic vascular events.

The link between migraine and ischemic stroke has been well-described in both clinic and population-based studies. Recently, two large-scale prospective cohort studies [146–147] were published. The Women's Health Study [146], with over 39,000 participants, found a 1.7-fold increased risk for ischemic stroke in women with migraine with aura as compared to women without migraine, with the risk being strongest in women ages 45 to 55 years. This risk was not seen in older women or those with migraine without aura. The Atherosclerosis Risk in Communities Study [147] with over 12,000 subjects over age 55 found that migraineurs with aura had a 1.8-fold increased risk of ischemic stroke compared to those without migraine or other headache. This result did not reach statistical significance, which may be explained by vague diagnostic terminology used in the study. The evidence is most convincing for younger women with migraine with aura, although the migraine and stroke relationship may also apply to older individuals. Stroke risk is significantly increased by smoking and the use of oral contraceptives [148–150].

MIGRAINE, IRRITABLE BOWEL SYNDROME, AND CELIAC DISEASE

Irritable bowel syndrome (IBS) is a chronic, functional gastrointestinal disorder in which episodic attacks are marked by abdominal discomfort and alterations in bowel movements (constipation, diarrhea, or alternating periods of both) [151]. IBS patients tend to have a higher likelihood of comorbid "affective spectrum disorders" or "functional somatic syndromes," which include migraine, fibromyalgia, and depression [152–153] and a familial association among patients with IBS, migraine, depression, and fibromyalgia has also been noted [154]. More recently, a prevalence study [155] of migraine, fibromyalgia, and depression in people with IBS showed that for migraine, subjects in the IBS cohort had a 60% higher odds compared to non-IBS subjects.

Celiac disease is a gluten-sensitive enteropathy characterized by malabsorption and weight loss, which can be reversed with a gluten-free diet. Gluten is a component of foods with wheat, barley, and rye [156]. While there have been several studies [157–159] evaluating the association between migraine and celiac disease, the evidence is inconclusive. However, in migraine patients with prominent gastrointestinal features, IBS and celiac disease should be considered.

MIGRAINE AND RESTLESS LEG SYNDROME

Restless Leg Syndrome (RLS) is a disorder characterized by sensory symptoms and motor disturbances of the limbs, usually when at rest. These features include: a desire to move the limbs, often associated with paresthesia or dysesthesia, exacerbation of symptoms at rest and relief with activity, motor restlessness, and nocturnal worsening of symptoms [160]. While most cases are idiopathic, RLS may be secondary to iron deficiency, peripheral neuropathy, and renal disease, especially in patients with later onset of symptoms [161–163]. Iron deficiency should therefore be ruled out with serum ferritin levels in patients presenting with RLS.

A recent case-control study [164] showed that RLS occurs more frequently in patients with migraine than those without, and older age and longer duration of migraine may raise the risk of RLS. Age and duration of migraine merit special consideration when evaluating those patients because the RLS may be secondary to iron deficiency, as noted above, or renal insufficiency resulting from long-time use of headache medications.

A dysfunctional dopaminergic system might explain the relationship between migraine and RLS, and a common genetic factor for both disorders may be established with future studies.

VI. TREATMENT RECOMMENDATIONS

Reactive hypoglycemia should be suspected in migraineurs who crave sweets, or develop headaches after fasting. Those patients should be advised to avoid refined sugar and eat frequent meals. Increasing protein, complex carbohydrates, and fiber in the diet may also be beneficial in preventing hypoglycemia [22].

Given the data discussed above, the most effective supplements for headache prevention are magnesium and *Petasites hybridus*. Second-line supplements in migraine prevention include feverfew, CoQ10, riboflavin, and alpha lipoic acid. Though gastrointestinal side effects have been reported with these supplements, they are generally well-tolerated and appeal to patients who prefer natural therapies to traditional prescription medications. In addition, some of the supplements may be especially beneficial in patients who have relevant comorbid conditions. For example, riboflavin may provide an added benefit in patients with cheilosis.

Oral magnesium supplementation may be beneficial for many migraineurs with frequent headaches, especially those with menstrual migraine. Magnesium oxide, chelated magnesium, and slow-release magnesium are the recommended formulations as they are likely to be the best absorbed. Daily supplementation with 400 mg should be used for at least 3 months. Diarrhea may be a limiting adverse effect in some patients.

Intravenous magnesium (1 g magnesium sulfate in 10 mL normal saline), given within 1 week of menstruation, is an option for women with menstrual migraines who do not respond to oral supplementation. Patients with nonmenstrual migraines can also be given magnesium infusions on an as-needed or monthly basis if they do not respond to oral magnesium or have gastrointestinal side effects from oral dosing.

The relationship between migraine, vascular, and metabolic disorders emphasizes the importance of addressing and treating modifiable risk factors such as obesity, hypertension, high cholesterol, and diabetes mellitus early, and with a multidisciplinary approach that includes nutritional recommendations. RLS, irritable bowel syndrome, and celiac disease are other potential comorbid conditions with nutritional implications.

VII. SPECIAL CONSIDERATIONS

Pediatric Migraine

Migraine headaches are not limited to the adult population. Childhood migraine can be severe and debilitating, and is associated with missed days of school, anxiety, and depression [165–166]. Among children, the prevalence of migraine has been increasing over the past few decades, much more so than that in adults [167–168]. Although the cause of this increase is not known, dietary trends of increased caffeine consumption, aspartame in diet drinks, and underage drinking are likely to play a role [169].

Pediatric migraine differs from adult migraine in that attacks tend to be shorter in duration [170]. Anorexia, abdominal pain, and vomiting are prominent features, occurring in 90% of patients [171–172]. These features affect treatment options in that gastroparesis from nausea and vomiting may limit the use of oral analgesics, and the shorter headache duration means that symptoms may resolve even before oral analgesics reach therapeutic levels. Furthermore, the cognitive side effects of migraine-preventive drugs are particularly problematic in children. For these reasons dietary modification in this population cannot be overemphasized.

As with adult migraineurs, pediatric migraineurs and their parents should be counseled regarding potential food triggers. In addition to the triggers described earlier in this chapter, food dyes and frozen foods or snacks may be particularly relevant to the pediatric population. Food diaries should be kept for these patients, and a well-balanced diet without fasting or skipping meals is strongly advised [169]. Other nonpharmacologic therapies such as biofeedback are also indicated in the treatment of pediatric migraine. For those children who continue to have frequent debilitating headaches, the supplements described above may be a more palatable option than prescription medications.

PREGNANCY

Pregnancy also warrants special consideration in the treatment of the migraineur. While migraines generally improve during pregnancy, headaches may worsen or remain the same in some women [173]. In particular, women may experience an increase in headaches during the first trimester, triggered by wide fluctuations in estrogen levels. After the first trimester, headaches generally improve due to a stabilization in estrogen levels.

VIII. SUMMARY

Reactive hypoglycemia is a poorly recognized but important migraine trigger. This is a challenge since excess weight predisposes to migraines and losing the weight often involves eating less to the point that blood glucose dips. Patients are advised to eat smaller, more frequent meals, with more protein, complex carbohydrates, and fiber. Glucose tolerance testing may be warranted in those who continue to have symptoms.

Food allergies are addressed as per the protocol outlined in Chapter 15, "Food Reactivities." Migraineurs should be aware of potential food triggers, and advised to avoid the foods and food components listed in Table 26.1.

Of the herbal supplements, we most commonly use magnesium oxide, chelated or slow-release magnesium in a dose of 400 mg daily, and butterbur in a dose of 50 mg three times daily for migraine prevention. Feverfew, CoQ10, and riboflavin are other options for migraine prophylaxis. While we do use magnesium during pregnancy, butterbur and most other herbal preparations should be avoided in pregnant women.

Nonpharmacologic measures are particularly important in pediatric migraine, given the shorter headache duration in children and prominent nausea and vomiting. We emphasize the avoidance of food triggers and skipped meals, and recommend magnesium, CoQ10, feverfew, as well as biofeedback in these patients.

REFERENCES

1. Lipton RB, Stewart WF, Diamond S et al. Prevalence and burden of migraine in the United States: data from the American Migraine Study II. *Headache* 2001; 41:646–657.
2. Sheffield RE. Migraine prevalence: a literature review. *Headache* 1998; 38:595–601.
3. Russel MB, Iselius L, Olesen J. Migraine without and migraine with aura are inherited disorders. *Cephalalgia* 1997; 16:305–309.

4. Stewart WF, Staffa J, Lipton RB, et al. Familial risk of migraine: a population-based study. *Ann Neurol* 1997; 41:166–172.
5. Larsson B, Billie B, Pedersen NL. Genetic influence in headache: a Swedish twin study. *Headache* 1995; 3:513–519.
6. Merikangas K, Tierney C, Martin N, et al. Genetics of migraine in the Australian twin registry. In: Rose C (ed). *New advances in headache research 4.* London: Smith-Gordon & Company, 1994; 27–28.
7. Lipton RB, Stewart WF, Simon D. Medical consultation for migraine: results from the American Migraine Study. *Headache* 1998; 38:87–96.
8. Moskowitz MA. The neurobiology of vascular head pain. *Ann Neurol* 1984; 16:157–168.
9. Martin VT, Behbehani MM. Toward a rational understanding of migraine trigger factors. *Medical Clinics of North America* 2001; 85:911–941.
10. Lanteri-Minet M, Desnuelle C. Migraine and mitochondrial dysfunction. *Rev Neurol* 1996; 152:234–238.
11. Koo, B, Becker LE, Chuang S, et al. Mitochondrial encephalomyopathy, lactic acidosis, stroke-like episodes (MELAS): clinical, radiological, pathological, and genetic observations. *Ann Neurol* 1993; 34:25–32.
12. Bresolin N, Martineeli P, Barbiroli B, et al. Muscle mitochondrial DNA deletion and 31P-NMR spectroscopy alterations in a migraine patient. *J Neurol* 1991; 104:182–189.
13. Montagna P, Cortell P, Barbiroli B. Magnetic resonance spectroscopy studies in migraine. *Cephalalgia* 1994; 14:184–193.
14. Schoenen J, Lenaerts M, Bastings E. High dose riboflavin as a prophylactic treatment of migraine: results of an open pilot study. *Cephalalgia* 1994; 14:328–329.
15. Tfelt-Hansen P, Mathew NT. General approach to treatment. In: Olesen J, Tfelt-Hansen P, Welch KMA (eds). *The headaches. 2nd ed.* Philadelphia: Lippincott, Williams & Wilkins, 1999; 367–369.
16. Kelman L. The triggers or precipitants of the acute migraine attack. *Cephalalgia* 2007; 27:394–402.
17. Scharff L, Turk DC, Marcus DA. Triggers of headache episodes and coping response of headache diagnostic groups. *Headache* 1995; 35:397–403.
18. Turner LC, Molgaard CA, Gardner CH, et al. Migraine trigger factors in non-clinical Mexican-American population in San Diego county: implications for etiology. *Cephalalgia* 1995; 15:523–530.
19. Robbins L. Precipitating factors in migraine: a retrospective review of 494 patients. *Headache* 1994; 34:214–216.
20. Fuenmayor LD, Garcia S. The effect of fasting on 5-hydroxytryptamine metabolism in brain regions of the albino rat. *Br J Pharmacol* 1984; 83:357–362.
21. Dexter JD, et al. The five-hour glucose tolerance test and effect of low sucrose diet in migraine. *Headache* 1978; 18:91–94.
22. Gaby AR. Literature review and commentary. *Townsend Letter* 2007; 292:54–56.
23. Sandler M, Youdim MBH, Hannington E. A phenylethylamine oxidizing defect in migraine. *Nature* 1974; 250:335–337.
24. Moffet AM, Swash M, Scott DR. Effect of chocolate in migraine: a double-blind study. *J Neurol Neurosurg Psychiatry* 1974; 37:445–448.
25. Peatfield RC, Glover V, Littlewood JT, et al. The prevalence of diet-induced migraine. *Cephalalgia* 1984; 4:179–183.
26. Pereira Monteiro JM, Dahlof CG. Single use of substances. In: Olesen J, Tfelt-Hansen P, Welch KMA (eds). *The headaches. 2nd ed.* Philadelphia: Lippincott, Williams & Wilkins, 1999; 861–869.
27. Van den Eeden SK, Koepsell TD, Longstreth WT, Jr, Van Belle G, Daling JR, McKnight B. Aspartame ingestion and headaches: a randomized crossover trial. *Neurology* 1994; 44:1787–1793.
28. Loehler SM, Glaros A. The effect of aspartame on migraine headache. *Headache* 1988; 28:10–14.
29. Labra-Ruiz N, Calderon-Guzman D, Vences-Mejia A, et al. Effect of aspartame on the biogenic amines in rat brain. *Epidemiology* 2007; 18(Suppl 1):S90–91.
30. Merrit JE, Williams PB. Vasospasm contributes to monosodium glutamate-induced headache. *Headache* 1990; 30:575–580.
31. Scher W, Scher BM. A possible role for nitric oxide in glutamate (MSG)-induced Chinese restaurant syndrome, glutamate induced asthma, "hot-dog headache," pugilistic Alzheimer's disease, and other disorders. *Med Hypotheses* 1992; 38:185–188.
32. Henderson WR, Raskin NH. Hot-dog headache: individual susceptibility to nitrite. *Lancet* 1972; 2:1162–1163.
33. Askew GI, Finelli L, Genese CA, Sorhage FE, Sosin DM, Spitalny HC. Bouillabaisse: an outbreak of methemoglobinemia in New Jersey in 1992. *Pediatrics* 1994; 94:381–384.

34. Mauskop A, Fox B. *What your doctor may not tell you about migraines. The breakthrough program that can help end your pain.* New York: Warner Books, Inc. 2001.
35. Lassen LH, Thomsen LL, Olesen J. Histamine induces migraine via the H1-receptor: support for the NO hypothesis of migraine. *Neuroreport* 1995; 6:1475–1479.
36. Pattichis K, Louca LL, Jarman J, et al. 5-Hydroxytryptamine release from platelets by different red wines: implications for migraine. *Eur J Pharmacol* 1995; 292:173–177.
37. Mathew RJ, Barr DL, Weinman ML. Caffeine and cerebral blood flow. *Br J Psychiatry* 1983; 143: 604–608.
38. Sawynok J. Adenosine receptor activation and nociception. *Cur J Pharmacol* 1998; 347:1–11.
39. Evans RW, Sun C, Lay C. Expert opinion: alcohol hangover headache. *Headache* 2007; 47:277–279.
40. Swift R, Davidson D. Alcohol hangover: mechanisms and mediators. *Alcohol Health Res World* 1998; 22:54–60.
41. Harburg E, David, Cummings KM, Gunn R. Negative affect, alcohol consumption and hangover symptoms among normal drinkers in a small community. *J Stud Alcohol* 1981; 42:998–1012.
42. Gunn R. Hangovers and attitudes towards drinking. *Q J Studies Alcohol* 1973; 34:194–198.
43. Wiese JG, Shlipak MG, Browner WS. The alcohol hangover. *Ann Intern Med* 2000; 132:897–902.
44. Kangasaho M, Hillbom M, Kaste M, Vigatalo H. Effects of ethanol intoxication and hangover on plasma levels of thromboxane B2 and 6-ketoprostaglandin F1 alpha and on thromboxane B2 formation by platelets in man. *Thromb Haemost* 1982; 48:232–234.
45. Calder I. Hangovers. *BMJ* 1997; 314:2–3.
46. Nehlig A. Are we dependent upon coffee and caffeine? A review on human and animal data. *Neurosci Biobehav Rev* 1999; 23:563–576.
47. Ward N, Whitney C, Avery D, Dunner D. The analgesic effects of caffeine in headache. *Pain* 1991; 44: 151–155.
48. Mathew NT, Reuveni U, Perez F. Transformed or evolutive migraine. *Headache* 1987; 27:102–106.
49. Mathew NT, Stubits E, Higam MP. Transformation of episodic migraine into daily headache: analysis of factors. *Headache* 1982; 22:66–68.
50. Rapoport A, Stang P, Gutterman DL, et al. Analgesic rebound headache in clinical practice: data from a physician survey. *Headache* 1996; 36:14–19.
51. Silverman K, Evans SM, Strain EC, Griffiths RR. Withdrawal syndrome after the double-blind cessation of caffeine consumption. *NEJM* 1992; 327:1160–1161.
52. Evans SM, Griffiths RR. Caffeine withdrawal: a parametric analysis of caffeine dosing conditions. *J Pharmacol Exp Ther* 1999; 289:285–294.
53. Laires MJ, Monteiro CP, Bicho M. Role of cellular magnesium in health and human disease. *Front Biosci* 2004; 1:262–276.
54. McCarty MF. Magnesium taurate and fish oil for prevention of migraine. *Med Hypotheses* 1996; 47: 461–466.
55. Bianchi A, Salomone S, Caraci F, et al. Role of magnesium, coenzyme Q10, riboflavin, and vitamin B12 in migraine prophylaxis. *Vitamins and Hormones* 2004; 69:297–312.
56. Turlapaty PDMV, Altura BM. Magnesium deficiency produces spasms of coronary arteries: relationship to etiology of sudden death ischemic heart disease. *Science* 1980; 208:198–200.
57. Altura BM, Altura BT, Carella A, Gebrewold A, Murakawa T, Nishio A. Mg2+- Ca2+ interaction in contractility of vascular smooth muscle: Mg2+ versus organic calcium channel blockers on myogenic tone and agonist-induced responsiveness of blood vessels. *Can J Physiol Pharmacol* 1987; 65:729–745.
58. Altura BT, Altura BM. Withdrawal of magnesium causes vasospasm while elevated magnesium produces relaxation of tone in cerebral arteries. *Neuroscience Lett* 1980; 20:323–327.
59. Ramadan NM, Halvorson H, Vande-Linde A. Low brain magnesium in migraine. *Headache* 1989; 29: 590–593.
60. Trauinger A, Pfund Z, Koszegi T, Czopf J. Oral magnesium load test in patients with migraine. *Headache* 2002; 42:114–119.
61. Mauskop A, Altura BM. Role of magnesium in the pathogenesis and treatment of migraine. *Clin Neurosci* 998; 5:24–27.
62. Mauskop A, Altura BT, Altura BM. Serum ionized magnesium in serum ionized calcium/ionized magnesium ratios in women with menstrual migraine. *Headache* 2001; 42:242–248.
63. Facchinetti F, Sances G, Borella P, Genazzani AR, Nappi G. Magnesium prophylaxis of menstrual migraine: effects on intracellular magnesium. *Headache* 1991; 31:298–301.
64. Peikert A, Wilimzig C, Kohne-Volland R. Prophylaxis of migraine with oral magnesium: results from a prospective, multicenter, placebo-controlled and double-blind randomized study. *Cephalalgia* 1996; 16:257–263.

65. Pfaffenrath V, Wessely P, Meyer C, et al. Magnesium in the prophylaxis of migraine—a double-blind placebo-controlled study. *Cephalalgia* 1996; 16:436–440.
66. Mauskop A, Altura BT, Cracco RQ, Altura BM. Intravenous magnesium sulfate relieves migraine attacks in patients with low serum ionized magnesium levels; a pilot study. *Clinical Science* 1995; 89:633–636.
67. Evans RW, Taylor FR. Expert opinion: "natural" or alternative medications for migraine prevention. *Headache* 2006; 46:1012–1018.
68. Schoenen J, Jacquy J, Lanaerts M. Effectiveness of high-dose riboflavin in migraine prophylaxis. *Neurology* 1998; 50:466–470.
69. Rozen TD, Oshinsky ML, Gebeline CA, Bradley KC, Young WB, Schechter AL, Silberstein SD. Open label trial of coenzyme Q10 as a migraine preventive. *Cephalalgia* 2002; 22:137–141.
70. Sandor PS, DiClemente L, Coppola G, Saenger U, Fumal A, Magis D, Seidel L, Agosti RM, Schoenen J. Efficacy of coenzyme Q10 in migraine prophylaxis: a randomized controlled trial. *Neurology* 2005; 64: 713–715.
71. Matalon R, Tumpf DA, Kimberlee M, et al. Lipoamide dehydrogenase deficiency with primary lactic acidosis: favorable response to treatment with oral lipoic acid. *J Pediatr* 1984; 104:65–69.
72. Clayton BE, Dobbs RH, Parick AD. Leigh's subacute necrotizing encephalopathy: clinical and biochemical study with special reference to therapy with lipoate. *Arch Dis Child* 1967; 42:467–472.
73. Maesaka H, Komiya K, Misugi K, Tada K. Hyperalaninemia, hyperpyruvicemia, and lactic acidosis due to pyruvate carboxylase deficiency of the liver: treatment with thiamine and lipoic acid. *Eur J Peiatr* 1976; 122:159–168.
74. Magis D, Ambrosini A, Sandor P, et al. A randomized double-blind placebo-controlled trial of thioctic acid in migraine prophylaxis. *Headache* 2007; 47:52–57.
75. Heptinstall S, White A, Williamson L, Mitchell JRA. Extracts of feverfew inhibit granule secretion in blood platelets and polymorphonuclear leukocytes. *Lancet* 1985; 1:1071–1074.
76. Heptinstall S, Goenewegen WA, Spangenberg P, Loesche W. Extracts of feverfew may inhibit platelet behaviour via neutralisation of suphydryl groups. *J Pharm Pharmacol* 1987; 39:459–465.
77. Pugh WH, Sambo K. Prostaglandin synthetase inhibitors in feverfew. *J Pharm Pharmacol* 1988; 40:743–745.
78. Makheja AM, Bailey JM. A platelet phospholipase inhibitor from the medicinal herb feverfew (Tanacetum parthenium). *Prostaglandins Leukotrienes Med* 1982; 8:653–660.
79. Johnson ES, Kadam NP, Hylands DM, Hylands PJ. Efficacy of feverfew as prophylactic treatment of migraine. *Br Med J* 1985; 291:569–573.
80. Murphy JJ, Heptinstall S, Mitchell JR. Randomised double-blind placebo-controlled trial of feverfew in migraine prevention. *Lancet* 1988; 2:189–192.
81. Kuritzky A, Elhacham Y, Yerushalmi Z, Hering R. Feverfew in the treatment of migraine: its effect on serotonin uptake and platelet activity. *Neurology* 1994; 44(suppl):293P.
82. De Weerdt CJ, Bootsma HPR, Hendricks H. Herbal medicines in migraine prevention: randomized double-blind placebo-controlled crossover trial of feverfew preparation. *Phytomoedicine* 1996; 3: 225–230.
83. Palevitch D, Earon G, Carasso R. Feverfew (*Tanacetum parthenium*) as a prophylactic treatment for migraine: a placebo-controlled double-blind study. *Phytother Res* 1997; 11:508–511.
84. Draves AH, Walker SE. Parthenolide content of Canadian commercial feverfew preparations: label claims are misleading in most cases. *Can Pharm J* (RPC) 2003; 136:23–30.
85. Willigmann I, Freudenstein J. Production of a stable feverfew (Tanadetum parthenium) extract as an active substance for a pharmaceutical product. Poster Symposiu. Vienna: Society for Medicinal Plant Research, 1998.
86. Pfaffenrath V, Diener HC, Fisher M, Friede M, Henneicke-von Zepelin HH. The efficacy and safety of Tanacetum parthenium (feverfew) in migraine prophylaxis—a double-blind, multicentre, randomized placebo-controlled dose-response study. *Cephalalgia* 2002; 22:523–532.
87. Grossman M, Schmidrams H. An extract of Petasites hybridus is effective in the prophylaxis of migraine. *Int J Clin Pharmacol Ther* 2000; 38:430–435.
88. Ziolo G, Samochewiec L. Study on clinical properties and mechanism of action of Petasites in bronchial asthma and chronic obstructive bronchitis. *Pharm Acta Helv* 1998; 72:359–380.
89. Barsom S. Behandlung von Koliken und Spasmen in der Urologie mit einem pflanzlichen Spasmolytikum [Treatment of colics and spasms in urology with an herbal spasmolytic]. *Erfahrungsheilkunde* 1986; 35:1–11.
90. Gruia FS. Phlanzliche Analgetika-Therapie bei WS-Syndrom [Therapy with an herbal analgesic for back pain]. *Biol Med* 1987; 3:454.

91. Bucher K. Uber ein antispastisches Prinzip in Petasites officinalis Moench [A spasmolytic principle in petasites officinalis Moench]. *Arch Exper Path Pkarmakol* 1951; 213:69–71.
92. Eaton J. Butterbur: herbal help for migraine. *Natural Pharmacother* 1998; 2:23–24.
93. Sheftell F, Rapoport A, Weeks R, Walker B, Gammerman I, Baskin S. Montelukast in the prophylaxis of migraine: a potential role for leukotriene modifiers. *Headache* 2000; 40:158–163.
94. Pearlman EM, Fisher S. Preventive treatment for childhood and adolescent headache: role of once-daily montelukast sodium. *Cephalalgia* 2001; 21:461.
95. Lipton RB, Gobel H, Einhaupl KM, Wilks K, Mauskop A. Petsites hybridus root (butterbur) is an effective preventive treatment for migraine. *Neurology* 2004; 63:2240–2244.
96. Pothmann R, Danesch U. Migraine prevention in children and adolescents: results of an open study with a special butterbur root extract. *Headache* 2005; 45:196–203.
97. Srivastava KC, Mustafa T. Ginger (*Zingziber officinale*) in rheumatism and musculoskeletal disorder. *Med Hypotheses* 1992; 33:342–348.
98. Hadley S, Petry JJ. Valerian. *Am Fam Physician* 2003; 67:1755–1758.
99. Schulz V, Hansel R, Tyler VE. *Rational phytotherapy: a physician's guide to herbal medicine.* Berlin: Springer, 1998; 81.
100. Werbach MR. Headache. In: *Nutritional influence on illness: a sourcebook of clinical research.* Tarzana, CA: Third Line Press, Inc; 1988.
101. Dupois S. A comprehensive approach to treatment of intractable headaches. *Townsend Letter for Doctors*, 1990:740–744.
102. Mauskop A, Brill MA. *The headache alternative: a neurologist's guide to drug-free relief.* New York: Dell Publishing, 1997.
103. Scher AI, Terwindt GM, Picavet HS, Verschuren WM, Ferrari MD, Launer LJ. Cardiovascular risk factors and migraine: the GEM population-based study. *Neurology* 2005; 64:614–620.
104. Williams FM, Cherkas LF, Spector TD, MacGregor AJ. A common genetic factor underlies hypertension and other cardiovascular disorders. *BMC Cardiovasc Disord* 2004; 4:20.
105. Moreau T, Manceau E, Giroud-Baleydier F, Dumas R, Giroud M. Headache in hypothyroidism. Prevalence and outcome under thyroid hormone therapy. *Cephalalgia* 1998; 18:687–689.
106. Bigal ME, Shertell FD, Rapoport AM, Tepper SJ, Lipton RB. Chronic daily headache: identification of factors associated with induction and transformation. *Headache* 2002; 42:575–581.
107. Tietjen GE, Conway F, Utley C, Herial HA. Migraine is associated with menorrhagia and endometriosis. *Headache* 2006; 46:422–428.
108. Peres MF, Young WB, Kaup AO, Zukerman E, Silberstein SD. Fibromyalgia is common in patients with transformed migraine. *Neurology* 2001; 57:1326–1328.
109. Peres MF, Zukerman E, Young WB, Silberstein SD. Fatigue in chronic migraine patients. *Cephalalgia* 2002; 22:720–724.
110. Aaron LA, Burke MM, Buchwald D. Overlapping conditions among patients with chronic fatigue syndrome, fibromyalgia, and temporomandibular disorder. *Arch Intern Med* 2000; 160:221–227.
111. Cohen RI. The treatment of "interstitial cystitis" as a migraine equivalent: report of four cases. *Compr Psychiatry* 1963; 4:58–61.
112. Breslau N, Lipton RB, Stewart WF, Schultz LR, Welch MD. Comorbidity of migraine and depression: investigating potential etiology and prognosis. *Neurology* 2003; 60:1308–1312.
113. Stewart W, Breslau N, Keck PE Jr. Comorbidity of migraine and panic disorder. *Neurology* 1994; 44: S23–27.
114. Warnock JK, Clayton AH. Chronic episodic disorders in women. *Psychiatr Clin North Am* 2003; 26: 725–740.
115. Tietjen GE, Herial NA, Hardgrove J, Utley C, White L. Migraine comorbidity constellations. *Headache* 2007; 47:857–865.
116. Hamelsky SW, Lipton RB. Psychiatric comorbidity of migraine. *Headache* 2006; 46:1327–1333.
117. Swartz KL, Pratt LA, Amerian HK, Lee LC, Eaton WW. Mental disorders and the incidence of migraine headaches in a community sample. *Arch Gen Psychiatry* 2000; 57:945–950.
118. Zwart JA, Dyb G, Hagen K, et al. Depression and anxiety disorders associated with headache frequency. The Nord-Trondelag Study. *Eur J Neurol* 2003; 10:147–152.
119. McWilliams LA, Goodwin RD, Cox BJ. Depression and anxiety associated with three pain conditions: results from a nationally representative sample. *Pain* 2004; 111:77–83.
120. Patel NV, Bigal ME, Kolodner KB, et al. Prevalence and impact of migraine and probable migraine in a health plan. *Neurology* 2004; 63:1432–1438.
121. Breslau N, Davis GC, Schultz LR, Peterson EL. Migraine and major depression: a longitudinal study. *Headache* 1994; 34:387–393.

122. Breslau N, Schultz LR, Stewart WF, Lipton RB, Lucia VC, Welch KMA. Headache and major depression: is the association specific to migraine? *Neurology* 2000; 54:308–313.

123. Roberts RE, Deleger S, Strawbridge WJ, Kaplan GA. Prospective association between obesity and depression: evidence from the Alameda County study. *Int J Obes Relat Metab Disord* 2003; 27:514–521.

124. Sjoberg RL, Nilsson KW, Leppert J. Obesity, shame, and depression in school-aged children: a population-based study. *Pediatrics* 2005; 116:e389–392.

125. Onyike CU, Crum RM, Lee HB, Lyketsos CG, Eaton WW. Is obesity associated with major depression? Results from the Third National Health and Nutrition Examination Survey. *Am J Epidemiol* 2003; 158:1139–1147.

126. Simon EG, Von Korff M, Saunders K, et al. Association between obesity and psychiatric disorders in the US adult population. *Arch Gen Psychiatry* 2006; 64:824–830.

127. Herva A, Laitenen J, Miettunen J, et al. Obesity and depression: results from the longitudinal Northern Finland 1966 Birth Cohort Study. *Int J Obes* 2006; 30:520–527.

128. Pine DS, Goldstein RB, Wolk S, Weissman MM. The association between childhood depression and adulthood body mass index. *Pediatrics* 2001; 107:1049–1056.

129. Kress AM, Peterson MR, Hartzell MC. Association between obesity and depressive symptoms among US Military active duty service personnel, 2002. *J Psychosom Res* 2006; 60:263–271.

130. Scher AI, Stewart WF, Ricci JA, Lipton RB. Factors associated with the onset and remission of chronic daily headache in a population-based study. *Pain* 2003; 106:81–89.

131. Bigal MED, Liberman JN, Lipton RB. Obesity and migraine: a population study. *Neurology* 2006; 66:545–550.

132. Tietjen GE, Peterlin BL, Brandes JL, et al. Depression and anxiety: effect on the migraine-obesity relationship. *Headache* 2007; 47:866–875.

133. Bigal ME, Lipton RB. Obesity is a risk factor for transformed migraine but not chronic tension-type headache. *Neurology* 2006; 67:252–257.

134. Hasler G, Pine DS, Kleinbaum DG, et al. Depressive symptoms during childhood and adult obesity: the Zurich Cohort Study. *Mol Psychiatry* 2005; 10:842–850.

135. Meguid MM, Fetissov SO, Varma M, et al. Hypothalamic dopamine and serotonin in the regulation of food intake. *Nutrition* 2000; 16:843–857.

136. Pariante CM. Depression, stress and the adrenal axis. *J Neurendocrinol* 2003; 15:811–812.

137. Arborelius L, Owen MJ, Plotsky PM, Nemeroff CB. The role of corticotropin-releasing factor in depression and anxiety disorders. *J Endocrinol* 1999; 160:1–12.

138. Peres MF, Sanchez DR, Seabra ML, et al. Hypothalamic involvement in chronic migraine. *J Neurol Neurosurg Psychiatry* 2001; 71:747–751.

139. Gordon ML, Brown SL, Lipton RB, et al. Serotonergic parallels in migraine, depression, and anxiety. In: Nappi G, Bono G, Sandrini G, Marignoni E, Micieli G, eds. *Headache and depression: serotonin pathways as a common clue*. New York: Raven Press, 1991; 21–40.

140. Cook NR, Bensenor IM, Lotufo PA, et al. Migraine and coronary heart disease in women and men. *Headache* 2002; 42:715–727.

141. Rose KM, Carson AP, Sanford CP, et al. Migraine and other headache: associations with Rose angina and coronary heart disease. *Neurology* 2004; 63:2233–2239.

142. Sternfeld B, Stang P, Sidney S. Relationship of migraine headaches to experience of chest pain and subsequent risk for myocardial infarction. *Neurology* 1995; 45:2135–2142.

143. Waters WE, Campbell MJ, Elwood PC. Migraine, headache, and survival in women. *Br Med J Clin Res Ed* 1983; 287:1442–1443.

144. Kurth T, Gaziano JM, Cook NR, et al. Migraine and risk of cardiovascular disease in women. *JAMA* 2006; 296:283–291.

145. Kurth T, Gaziano JM, Cook NR, et al. Migraine and risk of cardiovascular disease in men. *Arch Intern Med* 2007; 167:795–801.

146. Kurth T, Slomke MA, Kase CS, et al. Migraine, headache, and the risk of stroke in women: a prospective study. *Neurology* 2005; 64:1020–1026.

147. Stang PE, Carson AO, Rose KM, et al. Headache, cerebrovascular symptoms, and stroke: the Atherosclerosis Risk in Communities Study. *Neurology* 2005; 64:1573–1577.

148. Kurth T. Migraine and ischaemic vascular events. *Cephalalgia* 2007; 27:967–975.

149. Tzourio C, Tehindrazanarivelo A, Iglesias S, et al. Case-control study of migraine and risk of ischaemic stroke in young women. *Br Med J* 1995; 310:830–833.

150. Chang CL, Donaghy M, Pulter N. Migraine and stroke in young women: case-control study. The World Health Organisation Collaborative Study of Cardiovascular Disease and Steroid Hormone Contraception. *Br Med J* 1999; 318:13–18.

151. Hahn BA, Yan S, Strassels S. Impact of irritable bowel syndrome on quality of life and resource use in the United States and United Kingdom. *Digestion* 1999; 60:77–81.
152. Hudson JI, Pope HG. Affective spectrum disorder: does antidepressant response identify a family of disorders with a common pathophysiology? *Am J Psychiatry* 1990; 147:552–564.
153. Wessely S, Nimnuan C, Sharpe M. Functional somatic syndromes: one or many? *Lancet* 1999; 354: 936–939.
154. Hudson JI, Mangweth B, Pope HGJ, DeCol C, Hausmann A, Gutweniger S et al. Family study of affective spectrum disorder. *Arch Gen Psychiatry* 2003; 60:170–177.
155. Cole JA, Rothman KJ, Cabral HJ, Zhang Y, Farraye F. Migraine, fibromyalgia, and depression among people with IBS: a prevalence study. *BMC Gastroenterology* 2006; 6:26–33.
156. Wills AJ, Unsworth DJ. The neurology of gluten sensitivity: separating the wheat from the chaff. *Curr Opinion Neurol* 2002; 15:519–23.
157. Hadjivassiliou M, Brunewald RA, Lawden M, et al. *Headache* and CNS white matter abnormalities associated with gluten sensitivity. *Neurology* 2001; 56:385–388.
158. Schlesinger I, Hering R. Antigliadin antibodies in migraine patients. *Cephalalgia* 1997; 17:712 {Letter}.
159. Gasbarrini A, Gabrielli M, Fiore G, et al. Association between Helicobacter pylori cytotoxic type I CagA-positive strains and migraine with aura. *Cephalalgia* 2000; 20:561–565.
160. Walters AS, for the International Restless Legs Syndrome Study Group. Toward a better definition of the restless legs syndrome. *Mov Disord* 1995; 10:634–642.
161. O'Keeffe ST. Secondary causes of restless legs syndrome in older people. *Age and Ageing* 2005; 34: 349–352.
162. O'Keeffe S, Noel J, Lavan J. Restless legs syndrome in the elderly. *Postgrad Med J* 1993; 69:701–703.
163. Sun ER, Chen CA, Ho G, et al. Iron and the restless legs syndrome. *Sleep* 1998; 21:371–7.
164. Rhode AM, Hosing VG, Happe S, Biehl K, Young P, Evers S. Comorbidity of migraine and restless legs syndrome-a case-control study. *Cephalalgia* 2007; 27:1255–1260.
165. Laurell K, Larsson B, Eeg-Olofsson O. Headache in schoolchildren: association with other pain, family history, and psychosocial factors. *Pain* 2005; 119:150–158.
166. Karwautz A, Wober C, Lang T, et al. Psychosocial factors in children and adolescents with migraine and tension-type headache: a controlled study and review of the literature. *Cephalalgia* 1999; 19:32–43.
167. Maytal J. Overview of recent advances in migraine and other headaches. In: Millichap JG (ed). *Progress in pediatric neurology III*. Chicago: PNB Publishers, 1997; 163–168.
168. Sillanpaa M, Anttila P. Increasing prevalence of headache in 7-year-old schoolchildren. *Headache* 1996; 36:466–470.
169. Millichap JG, Yee MM. The diet factor in pediatric and adolescent migraine. *Pediatr Neurol* 2003; 28:9–15.
170. Rothner AD, Winner P. *Headaches* in children and adolescents. In: Silberstein SD, Lipton RB, Dalessio DJ (eds). *Wolff's headache and other head pain. 7th ed*. New York: Oxford University Press, Inc, 2001; 539–561.
171. Jones J, Sklar D, Dougherty J, et al. Randomized double-blind trial of intravenous prochlorpherazine for the treatment of acute headache. *JAMA* 1989; 261:1174–1176.
172. Tek DS, McClellan JS, Olshaker JS, et al. A prospective, double-blind study of metoclopramide hydrochloride for the control of migraine in the emergency department. *Ann Emerg Med* 1990; 19:1083–1087.
173. Loder E. Migraine in pregnancy. *Semin Neurol* 2007; 27:425–433.

27 Alzheimer's Disease

Delaying Onset Through Nutrition

*Heidi Wengreen, R.D., Ph.D., Payam Mohassel, M.D.,
Chailyn Nelson, R.D., and Majid Fotuhi, M.D., Ph.D.*

I. INTRODUCTION

Primary care physicians are often asked by their baby boomer patients as to what food or supplements may best prevent their risk of developing Alzheimer's disease (AD). Some arrive with bags filled with different bottles containing anything from Chinese herbs to vitamins and minerals, and would like to know which can best keep their brain healthy and ward off cognitive deterioration that comes with aging. This chapter presents food and nutrients that hold promise in the prevention of AD.

II. EPIDEMIOLOGY

Currently 5 million Americans suffer from AD. Many of the 78 million baby boomers in the United States have concerns about developing memory loss and AD. With the aging population, AD has become a concern not only in the United States, but also all across the world. By the year 2050, the number of patients with AD will be five times higher than it is now; approximately 106 million will suffer from it. As the number of elderly who live into their 80s and 90s increases, the resources for caring for patients with dementia diminishes. The growing epidemic of AD poses a major public health challenge in the world, and may be considered like a slow-growing tsunami, with the potential to destroy many health care systems. In the meantime, governments and individuals are seeking natural and safe remedies to ward off dementia.

III. PATHOPHYSIOLOGY

With the increasing interest in the prevention of AD, thousands of scientists around the world are focused on understanding why some individuals live to their 80s and 90s and remain sharp while others develop disabling memory loss in their 60s and 70s. A few general pictures have emerged.

ACQUISITION OF PLAQUES AND TANGLES

Aggregation of amyloid peptide into plaques and phosphorylated tau in tangles in axons are major cornerstones of AD research. In animal studies, genetic manipulations that lead to accumulation of excessive amounts of amyloid lead to dementia and difficulty with memory. Axonal damage with

445

accumulation of phosphorylated tau equally leads to loss of cognitive function. The combination of amyloid plaques and tau tangles is commonly seen in patients with AD.

Vascular Risk Factors and Insulin Resistance

Recent evidence suggests that plaques and tangles are not the only factors leading to AD. Many patients can harbor large amounts of plaques and tangles in their brain and yet have no cognitive limitation and complain of only mild memory problems. Others may have few plaques and tangles in their brain and yet lose their memory and cognitive abilities in their 60s and 70s. The factor that explains the discrepancy in the relationship between AD pathology and routine performance on daily tasks appears to be vascular issues. Patients who have high blood pressure, diabetes, and obesity are far more likely to become demented with small amounts of plaques and tangles. Those who have AD pathology in their brain, but who do not have significant numbers of vascular risk factors, function well for a longer period of time before they show symptoms of dementia.

Diabetes may affect the brain in ways other than narrowing the blood vessels with atherosclerotic plaques. Insulin in the brain has two separate functions. It helps with uptake of glucose into neurons, and also helps to break down amyloid peptide. In type 2 diabetes, when insulin levels rise, insulin resistance takes place in all organs including the brain, in part as a result of compensatory changes in the blood-brain barrier. This means that less glucose becomes available to neurons and more amyloid builds up into plaques, thus causing more injury and inflammation inside the brain.

More recently, epidemiological studies have indicated that presence of congestive heart failure, renal failure, or liver disease contributes to a decline in cognitive abilities. Patients who have multiple chronic diseases are far more likely to experience memory loss earlier in life. Those who remain healthy and fit, those who take very few medications, and those who exercise regularly seem to ward off AD well into their late 80s and 90s.

Oxidation and Inflammation

Several lines of evidence implicate oxidative stress as a primary event in the development and progression of AD. Beta-amyloid and tau proteins, pathological hallmarks of AD, may induce oxidative stress known to contribute to damage and degeneration of neuronal cells [1]. Antioxidants may reduce neuronal damage from oxidative stress by inhibiting the generation of reactive oxygen species, lipid peroxidation and aggregation, damage to cell membranes and DNA, apoptosis, and beta-amyloid toxicity. Dozens of studies have shown that markers for inflammations are elevated in patients with dementia. Patients with rheumatoid arthritis who take NSAIDs on a regular basis are less likely to develop AD than are patients with similar profiles who do not take anti-inflammatory medications. These observations have fueled research into finding food ingredients that would reduce inflammation.

IV. EVIDENCE FOR FOOD AND NUTRIENT TREATMENTS

Now that the pathophysiology of AD points to vascular risk factors, ischemia, accumulation of plaques and tangles, and high degrees of inflammation, scientists have asked whether food can play a role in prevention of dementia. It appears that diets that reduce coronary artery disease are likely to keep the blood vessels in the brain healthy as well. Foods that are known to have antioxidant components may indeed prove to be beneficial in reducing the inflammatory response in the brains of patients who have memory loss. In this chapter, we will focus on diet and supplements that have the strongest evidence for prevention of dementia.

Fish, Omega-3 Fatty Acids, and DHA

A great body of evidence suggests a role for omega-3 fatty acids in neuronal function and development, neurodegeneration, and neuroprotection. Omega-3 fatty acids, including docosahexaenoic acid (DHA), are essential for neuronal growth, help in development of synapses between neurons, regulate gene expression and neurotransmission, and modulate ion channels [2–5]. In addition, animal studies suggest that omega-3 fatty acids are essential for normal brain development in the fetal and early postnatal period [6, 7]. With aging, DHA levels in the brain tend to decrease [8, 9], suggesting that this change may be associated with age-related changes in cognition and central nervous system function. Animal studies have confirmed this hypothesis. Animals with low DHA diets show significant deficits in cognitive function compared to their counterparts with high DHA diets [10, 11].

Several proposed mechanisms support omega-3 fatty acids' role in prevention of dementia. First, cardiovascular disease is highly associated with dementia and populations with high omega-3 fatty acid diets, such as the Inuit population, have significantly decreased rates of cardiovascular disease. Omega-3 fatty acids may protect against dementia by reducing cardiovascular disease [12]. Second, increased inflammation and pro-inflammatory factors are also highly associated with dementia. Omega-3 fatty acids attenuate inflammation by inhibiting the arachidonic acid conversion to pro-inflammatory factors and may protect against dementia because of these anti-inflammatory properties [13]. Third, omega-3 fatty acids reduce production of beta-amyloid, a compound whose abnormal accumulation in plaques is a pathologic hallmark of AD, and increase its clearance in mouse models of AD [14].

Epidemiologic studies suggest that higher DHA intake is associated with a reduced risk of cognitive impairment [15–20]. In the Chicago Health and Aging Project, a large prospective cohort study with almost 4 years of follow-up, participants who consumed fish at least once a week had 60% reduction in risk of developing AD by the end of the follow-up period (p-value = <0.05) [18]. In the Framingham Heart Study, increased plasma levels of DHA-containing phospholipids was associated with a 47% reduction in the risk of developing all-cause dementia (p = 0.04) [19]. Being observational in nature, such studies cannot fully control for the effects of other potentially confounding factors. However, when taken together, results of these studies provide evidence for a possible benefit from DHA in the form of food or supplements in late-life cognitive health.

A randomized controlled trial of DHA supplementation among 174 participants with cognitive decline in Sweden [21] showed no change in rate of cognitive decline assessed by the modified mini-mental state examination (MMSE) or cognitive portion of the AD Assessment Scale between those who received DHA supplementation and those who received placebo. This randomized study had well-defined outcomes, was double blind, and monitored compliance effectively with serum DHA level measurements. However, it was a relatively small study, had a short duration of therapy (6 months), and suffered from a referral bias due to the different environment and diet of patients in Sweden. However, a subgroup (n = 32) of patients with AD and MMSE scores >27 who received DHA had statistically significant reduction in MMSE decline when compared with those taking the placebo. This result suggests that DHA supplementation or diet intake of approximately 1.5 to 2.0 g of DHA per day in patients with mild cognitive impairment or very mild AD may reduce the rate of progression of AD.

Larger scale clinical trials examining the effects of DHA supplementation in preventing AD and its progression are needed. Three randomized trials, the OPAL (Older People And n-3 Long chain polyunsaturated fatty acids [22]), MEMO (Mental health in Elderly Maintained with Omega-3 [23]), and DHA in Slowing the Progression of AD [24], are ongoing or near completion. These trials will ascertain the efficacy of DHA supplementation in primary or secondary prevention of AD. Given the potential benefit of attenuating cognitive decline, especially in patients with mild cognitive impairment or very mild AD, and the favorable safety profile of DHA supplementation [20, 25] clinicians may consider recommending DHA, while awaiting the results of the ongoing clinical trials.

ANTIOXIDANTS INCLUDING VITAMIN E, VITAMIN C, AND SELENIUM

Antioxidants are more likely to be beneficial in combinations, as found naturally in a balanced diet that contains ample fruits and vegetables. It is of interest to note that doses of dietary supplements often far exceed the highest levels achieved by usual dietary intake, and that such high doses may be associated with increased risk of adverse health outcomes among at-risk subgroups.

Fruits and vegetables are a rich source of many antioxidants including vitamin C and beta-carotene, along with other essential nutrients likely beneficial for cognitive health. Few adults consume the recommended amounts of fruits and vegetables. The current More Matters campaign emphasizes the need of most Americans to consume more fruits and vegetables for optimal health. *Dietary Guidelines for Americans*, a 2005 publication, recommends 2.5 cups of vegetables and 2 cups of fruit per day based on a 2000 calorie diet.

Although fruits and vegetables are nutrient-dense sources of most antioxidants, they are, for the most part, not a rich source of vitamin E, a potent fat-soluble antioxidant that exists in eight different forms including 4 (alpha, beta, gamma, and delta) tocopherols and 4 tocotrienols. The most nutrient-dense food sources of vitamin E include minimally processed vegetable oils, nuts, whole grains, and green leafy vegetables. Natural whole foods provide a good source of all forms of vitamin E. However, supplements and foods enriched or fortified with vitamin E typically contain only the alpha tocopherol form of the vitamin, often in a form (all racemic alpha-tocopherol) that is less bioavailable than its natural counterpart.

Antioxidant nutrients such as vitamin E (mixed tocopherols and tocotrienols), vitamin C, and vitamin A in the form of beta-carotene work to protect neural cells from oxidative damage by donating a lone electron and thereby neutralizing reactive oxygen species. Alternatively, minerals such as selenium are said to have antioxidant function because they serve as cofactors for important antioxidant enzymes. Biological evidence supports synergistic relationships between multiple antioxidants. The following example illustrates this point. Vitamin E, a fat-soluble nutrient, readily donates electrons to neutralize reactive oxygen species and may be especially important in protecting lipid membranes in the oxygen-rich environment of the brain. In the process of neutralizing free radicals, vitamin E becomes oxidized, itself losing its oxidative ability; vitamin C, a water-soluble nutrient, readily donates electrons to vitamin E to restore its oxidative ability. Selenium is essential for the activity of glutathione peroxidase, the enzyme responsible for the catabolism of hydrogen peroxide and other organic peroxides that contribute to oxidative stress.

Despite the biological plausibility and vast amount of experimental evidence that antioxidants protect neurons from oxidative stress and reduce markers of AD, evidence from human observational studies is less clear. Several groups have examined associations between both food and supplemental sources of antioxidants and risk of AD or other dementias among large population-based cohorts. At least seven studies have examined supplemental intake of antioxidants on risk of dementia, with three of the seven [26–28] finding beneficial effects of antioxidant supplements. However, even these findings are somewhat inconsistent in that one study observed protective effects for only high dose vitamin E and C combined [28], and another found protective effects for vascular dementia but not AD [27]. Methodological differences of observational studies, such as what dose, form of nutrient, and frequency of intake defines the supplemented group, make it difficult to compare results across studies.

Four large prospective studies have examined associations between food sources of antioxidants and risk of dementia [26, 29, 30, 31]. One study among a cohort of elderly men and women residing in a biracial community who reported high intake of vitamin E from food was associated with reduced risk of AD [26]. In a follow-up study of this same cohort, Morris et al. [32] examined the effect of different tocopherol forms from food sources and found total vitamin E as well as alpha tocopherol and gamma tocopherol were independently associated with a reduced risk of AD (26%, 34%, and 40% reduction in risk, respectively). A second study conducted in the Netherlands found high dietary intake of vitamin C and vitamin E was associated with reduced risk of AD, although no association was observed for other antioxidants including beta-carotene and flavonoids [29]. Although some have argued that midlife exposures may better predict risk of later-life dementia, no association was found between midlife intake of beta-carotene, flavonoids, or vitamins E and C and risk of late-life dementia or AD among a cohort of Japanese American men [31].

There is little prospective observational evidence regarding associations between other antioxidants, including selenium, zinc, flavonoids, and other carotenoids, and risk of dementia. However, several epidemiologic studies provide evidence supporting a beneficial effect of selenium on prevention of cognitive decline during late life [33]. In addition, the PREADVISE trial of vitamin E and selenium supplementation and prevention of AD among over 10,000 men over the age of 60 is ongoing. One published trial of zinc supplementation showed 6 months of moderate dose zinc supplementation among healthy 55- to 70-year-old Europeans had no effect on in vitro copper-induced LDL oxidation levels [34].

Imbalances of trace elements, including iron, zinc, copper, and mercury, have been implicated in free-radical-induced oxidative stress in neurodegenerative disease. Abnormal interactions of copper, zinc, and iron with metal-binding proteins including amyoid-beta peptide (A-beta) have been associated with A-beta precipitation and toxicity [35]. Epidemiologic evidence suggests that elevated levels of these metals in the brain may be linked to the development of AD [36] although less is known about how dietary intake of such metals is associated with development of AD.

A high level of mercury, the main dietary exposure of which is from fish, is known to induce potent toxic effects on the central nervous system. However, selenium status should be considered when assessing mercury exposure due to the strong interactions between these two elements. Selenium may protect against mercury exposure but just as likely, the mercury exposure may reduce the activity of selenium-dependent antioxidant enzymes including glutathione peroxidase.

Few clinical trials have been conducted on antioxidant supplements and primary or secondary prevention of AD. There have been no published clinical trials on the effects of beta-carotene, vitamin C, or selenium and prevention or progression of AD; there have been two published randomized controlled trials on vitamin E (as solely alpha tocopherol) and AD. Large doses of alpha tocopherol (2000 IU/day) slowed the progression of AD among patients with preexisting disease of moderate severity in one well-designed multicenter randomized trial [37]. A more recent trial conducted by the same research group examined the ability of alpha tocopherol and donepezil, current standard therapies for AD, to prevent progression of cognitive impairment earlier in the course of disease progression. Results of this long-awaited trial showed no benefit of alpha tocopherol supplementation on progression of cognitive impairment [38].

Recent meta-analyses of available trials have identified increased risk of mortality among participants taking antioxidant supplements including beta-carotene, vitamin A, and vitamin E of unspecified form [39]. One such meta-analysis of vitamin E trials found a dose-response relationship such that doses of greater than 150 IU/day were associated with increased mortality; authors of this study concluded that high-dose supplements of vitamin E greater than or equal to 400 IU/day should be avoided [39]. Further exploration of this association using evidence from a population-based observational study identified differential vitamin E related risk in mortality by existence of cardiovascular disease such that alpha tocopherol increased risk of mortality only among those with preexisting cardiovascular disease [40].

Although alpha tocopherol and selenium are generally considered as safe, the Food and Nutrition Board (FNB) has set upper limits (UL) for them. Upper limits are defined as the highest level of a nutrient likely to pose no risk of adverse health to 98% of the population. The current UL for alpha tocopherol is 1500 IU/day and the UL for selenium is 400 μg/day. No upper limit has been set for vitamin C although doses greater than 2 g (2000 mg/day) have been associated with gastrointestinal distress and in vitro evidence suggests high levels of vitamin C may act as a pro-oxidant under certain conditions such as the presence of metal ions or without other co-antioxidants. Beta-carotene is not considered an essential nutrient and so no reference values for beta-carotene are provided by the FNB, although supplementation with 20 to 30 mg/day of beta-carotene was associated with increased risk of lung cancer among former smokers [41].

Dietary supplements of vitamin E in the form of alpha tocopherol remain widely used as both a preventive measure and treatment for AD. The safety of high-dose alpha tocopherol has been appropriately called into question. Vitamin E supplements of mixed tocopherols and the corresponding tocotrienols are more expensive than alpha tocopherol forms and clinical trials have not been conducted. However since supplements containing all eight forms of vitamin E simulate the vitamin E found in foods, their safety and efficacy hold promise.

Folate and Other B-Vitamins

Interest in folate and other B-vitamins in relation to dementia is mechanistically based on the role these nutrients play in methylation reactions. Deficiencies of folate and B-vitamins including vitamin B12 and vitamin B6 have been identified as a cause of elevated total homocysteine (thcy) [42]. Hyperhomocysteinemia has been widely studied as a possible independent risk factor for cognitive decline and AD. Researchers studying such associations have yet to conclude whether the observed relationships between elevated thcy and cognition is causal [42] or if abnormal thcy is a marker of the disease (perhaps as a secondary product resulting from poor diet in cognitively impaired individuals). Both folate and vitamin B12 are essential for the production of S-adenosyl-methionine (SAM), the major methyl donor for important methylation reactions of protein, nucleotides, and neurotransmitters. Deficiency of folate and/or vitamin B12, by impacting synthesis of SAM, may seriously alter normal methylation reactions in the brain. Research exploring observed relationships between folate, B-vitamins, and dementia results is inconsistent. Some studies have indicated negative associations, some no association, and others have even observed positive associations [33].

In the Normative Aging Study of 321 aging men, dietary folate was associated with less of a decline in verbal fluency, and hyperhomocysteinemia was associated with greater decline in recall memory [43]. Conversely, a prospective study among 3718 biracial elders (65 years and older) living in the Chicago area found no relationship between dietary intakes of folate, vitamins B12 or B6, and AD incidence [44]. However, higher intake of folate was associated with rates of cognitive decline twice that of the group with the lowest dietary intake in a secondary analysis involving the same participants [45]. No studies have examined associations between supplemental intake of B vitamins, independent of dietary intake, and risk of cognitive decline or AD.

A study by Kado and colleagues involving 499 high-functioning participants (ages 70 to 79), found those in the lowest quintile of serum folic acid had significantly increased risk for cognitive decline over 7 years [33] and found no significant association between serum homocysteine, folic acid, or vitamin B12 and cognitive decline [33]. Another study observed plasma elevated homocysteine and low folic acid to be independently related to increased risk for incident dementia and AD in 816 dementia-free elders [33]. In addition, a study of 1092 participants from the Framingham cohort discovered those with homocysteine levels greater than 14 μmol/L had almost twice the risk of incident AD. A study including 370 nondemented persons, ages 75 years and older by Wang and colleauges found low folic acid and/or vitamin B12 was also related to almost twice the risk for AD [33].

There is a small amount of evidence from clinical trials that directly indicates B-vitamin supplementation is a protective measure for cognitive outcome. From the FACIT trial, 818 participants taking 800 μg of folic acid per day (200% DRI) for 3 years had 576% higher serum folate, 26% lower homocysteine levels, and significantly less decline in memory after 3 years when compared to the placebo [46]. Bryon and colleagues found improvements in memory and other cognitive measures with supplementation of 750 μg of folic acid, 15 μg vitamin B12, and 75 mg vitamin B6 [33]. Durga and colleagues found similar results using folic acid (800 μg daily) supplementation alone [33]. On the other hand, a study done by McMahon and colleagues found no effect of supplementation with B-vitamins including 1000 μg of folic acid, 500 μg B12, and 10 mg B6 on cognitive function.

The prevalence of micronutrient deficiencies including deficiencies of vitamin B12 and folate generally increase with age. Vitamin B12 is one nutrient of particular interest among the elderly because many have problems absorbing vitamin B12 from food. Some estimate that as many as 5% to 10% of those over the age of 65 are deficient in vitamin B12 [47]. Common reasons for malabsorption of vitamin B12 include decreased levels of gastric acid secretion, either due to the effect of medications or simply related to age, as well as the conditions of pernicious anemia, gastric resection, and inflammatory bowel disorders. Also less consumption of meat, a major source of vitamin B12, occurs with poor dentition. High folate intake, primarily from highly fortified food sources, may have the potential to mask vitamin B12 deficiency, which may result in irreversible neurological damage that includes memory impairments [48].

Supplementing with B-vitamins appears to be safe, although food sources are preferred. Adequate dietary intake of vitamin B12 may be difficult or impossible to obtain among people with problems of malabsorption. Blanket recommendations regarding supplementation with high folic acid in the current era of folic acid fortification, even in response to elevated homocysteine, are controversial. Effects of folate may be modified by vitamin B12 status. In an analysis of the National Health and Nutrition Examination Survey (1999 to 2002), high serum folate was associated with a more than two-fold higher risk of cognitive decline among those with low vitamin B12 status as compared to those with normal status of both folate and vitamin B12, although high serum folate was associated with lower risk of cognitive decline among those with normal vitamin B12 status [45]. Given this evidence, practitioners should closely monitor status of both vitamin B12 and folate, and recommend supplements according to individual need [49, 50].

Recent publications have argued that the biomarkers methylmalonic acid and holotranscobalamin are better indicators of vitamin B12 status than is serum B12 [35, 36]. The acceptable serum methylmalonic acid range is stated to be less than 376 nmol/L and levels above this indicate deficiency. Serum concentrations of holotranscobalamin 45 pmol/L or greater are considered normal and indicate adequate vitamin B12 status. The holotranscobalamin measurement is thought to detect early B12 imbalance [51]. It should also be noted that a gap between adequacy and optimal levels appears to exist and so absence of deficiency should not be interpreted as optimal. Elderly patients with gastritis, taking antacids, with a history of gastric resection, who are vegetarian or consume only small amounts of meat, or who exhibit signs of anemia should be carefully screened for B12 deficiency. Food sources high in vitamin B12 (fortified foods, shellfish, meat, poultry, dairy products, eggs) should be recommended as should supplements in the case of suspected malabsorption. Elderly patients should be encouraged to eat foods high in folate and B-vitamins. The best sources for folate include leafy green vegetables, fruits, dried beans, and fortified cereal grains.

Supplementation with folic acid should be reserved for obvious cases of folate deficiency, not in response to hyperhomocysteinemia or macrocytic anemia. Currently, there is not enough evidence to suggest supplementation with folic acid or vitamins B12 or B6 as a protective measure against or treatment for cognitive decline or AD. Elderly people taking folic acid supplements should be screened for vitamin B12 deficiency to prevent the irreversible damage that may result from the masking of such deficiency by folic acid.

CURCUMIN AS A NOVEL SOURCE OF FLAVONOID

Curcumin and curcuminoid compounds have potent anti-inflammatory and antioxidant properties; they prevent neuronal death [52] and reduce oxidative damage [53] in mouse models for AD. Curcumin attenuates the inflammatory response in the brain [54, 55] and inhibits the formation of inflammatory factors [56], most of which have been implicated as a cause for AD. Curcumin can reduce or reverse some of the main pathologic features of AD, namely the formation of amyloid plaques [57, 58], by clearing or reducing the size of senile plaques and reversing the structural changes in dystrophic dendrites [59]. Like omega-3 fatty acids, curcumin can be considered a natural NSAID, which may be in part the cause for their protective properties against AD. Several studies have shown that NSAIDs used for more than 2 years during midlife are associated with substantially less chance of AD later in life [60, 61].

Some epidemiologic studies suggest that curcumin could be beneficial in the prevention of AD. Incidence of AD in India, where turmeric and curcumin are used frequently in the diet, is estimated at 4.7 per 1000 person-years, substantially lower than the corresponding rate of 17.5 per 1000 person-years in the United States [62]. In addition, a cohort study conducted in Singapore among 1010 elderly men and women investigated the role of curcumin in prevention of cognitive decline. Compared with those who had never or rarely consumed curry, participants with higher levels of curry consumption showed higher mean MMSE scores ($p = 0.023$), when controlled for potential confounding by known and putative correlates of MMSE performance [63].

One pilot, randomized, placebo-controlled trial has investigated the role of curcumin in patients with AD. Patients diagnosed with AD (n = 34) were randomized to placebo, 1 g curcumin, or 4 g curcumin daily for 6 months. This study showed no statistically significant improvement in MMSE of patients on placebo, 1 g curcumin, or 4 g curcumin (p = 0.43). However, the trial had several shortcomings: (1) seven patients dropped out, (2) it was underpowered, and (3) it failed to detect decline in MMSE in the placebo arm, suggesting inadequate length of study [64]. Curcumin in Patients With Mild to Moderate AD is an ongoing trial that may help determine the efficacy of curcumin for treatment of mild to moderate AD [65].

Turmeric, which contains curcumin, is generally recognized as safe (GRAS) by the United States Food and Drug Administration (FDA). Widespread use of curcumin in food without known adverse effects supports its safety. Also, curcumin has been used at high doses in some studies and is generally well tolerated. Doses of up to 1200 mg/day did not cause any major side effects [66–69]. In another study doses of up to 8000 mg/day were tolerated well except for the large volume of the treatment [70]. Some patients with peptic ulcer disease reported gastric irritation when treated with curcumin [71] and nausea and diarrhea bothered some with colon cancer [72]. However, in the randomized controlled trial discussed above, curcumin did not seem to cause side effects in AD patients. There was a tendency toward fewer adverse events among participants taking 4 g/day [64]. Curcumin may be safely administered even at higher doses with possibly increasing clinical results.

It is likely that the multiple essential nutrients found in such a dietary pattern work together to impact multiple mechanisms associated with the etiology of AD and other dementias and that this synergistic effect is far more beneficial than is the effect of any single nutrient. Foods including spices and herbs are indeed a multinutrient package.

Vitamin D

Cholecalciferol, vitamin D3, is made in the skin in response to sunlight exposure and is obtained in the diet. Cholecalciferol is converted by two hydroxylation reactions to the biologically active metabolite known as calcitriol (1,25-dihydroxyvitamin D). Calcitriol binds to nuclear vitamin D receptors, identified in more than 50 types of human tissue including the brain, and mediates the expression of a broad array of genes. Vitamin D has been shown to alter the expression of several genes with probable brain function including neurotrophins, proteins that support the survival and differentiation of neurons, and choline acetyltransferase, the enzyme responsible for the synthesis of the important neurotransmitter acetylcholine [73]. Treatment with calcitriol, known to inhibit nitric oxide synthetase, has been found to offer neuroprotection in rodent models and may serve to protect the brain from free-radical–induced damage. In addition, calcitriol is important for the immune system and both in vitro and in vivo evidence supports a role of calcitriol in modulation of pro-inflammatory cytokines [73].

There has been little work on the direct effect of vitamin D status and cognition in humans. There are no large-scale prospective randomized studies of vitamin D supplementation to treat memory loss or neurodegenerative disease. However, low vitamin D status has been identified among patients with AD [74] and at least one retrospective study has identified a significant positive correlation between vitamin D status and cognitive function among older adults with memory problems [75].

Circulating levels of calcidiol (25-hydroxyvitamin D), not calcitriol, are generally used as a functional marker of vitamin D and respond to both sun exposure and dietary intake. The current adequate intake (AI) as set by the Food and Nutrition Board for vitamin D (400 to 600 IU for adults 50+ years of age) was set to maintain serum levels of calcidiol at 37 nmol/L; a level known to prevent bone-related diseases associated with vitamin D deficiency. However, many experts in the field agree that higher levels are needed to support the noncalcitropic functions of vitamin D and that levels of 80 to 120 nmol/L are more likely to support optimal health [76].

The major dietary sources of vitamin D are fortified dairy products, oily fish, and meat, although diet alone is usually insufficient to maintain adequate serum levels. Elderly people are at increased risk for vitamin D deficiency because of reduced sun exposure in addition to decreased skin production of cholecalciferol and reduced ability to convert the inactive forms to the fully functional calcitriol. Supplementation of vitamin D at levels of 800 to 1000 IU/day, an amount greater than the current AI of 400 to 600 IU/day, is likely necessary to maintain optimal levels of calcidiol (80 to 120 nmol/L) especially among those who cannot rely on sun exposure for synthesis [76, 77].

OTHER SUPPLEMENTS

Nutrition stores have several rows of supplement with claims for stronger memory and sharper brains. One such supplement, *Gingko biloba,* was subjected to two double-blind placebo-controlled studies and failed to show any significant improvement in memory [78, 79]. As such, none of these supplements can be recommended to the general public for delaying onset of AD or for memory loss more broadly. This chapter does not strive to inventory all supplements that claim sharper memory. Rather it is set in the context of many other chapters that treat other medical conditions. Strategic use of nutrients to treat other diseases may concurrently forestall dementia, especially if the supplements reduce inflammation, oxidative stress, and atherosclerosis.

SUMMARY

Dementia is a multifactorial condition that is brought on by not only plaques and tangles of AD, but also by vascular risk factors, inflammation, and poor health. Patient education regarding healthy lifestyle, including recommendations regarding a healthy dietary pattern, is extremely important in helping them prevent memory loss and AD. Obesity needs to be confronted and treated aggressively. Much comorbidity brought on by obesity contributes to the frailness of the brain and subsequent dementia.

Eating four or five pieces of fruits and vegetables daily, consuming fish two to three times weekly, and maintaining a healthy body below the neck are cornerstones of keeping the brain healthy and sharp. People who find it difficult to consume three to four daily servings of fruits and vegetables should be reminded of the health benefits of spicing it up. Herbs and spices in general confer health benefits similar to fruits and vegetables. This chapter highlights recent research on the curcumin-containing spices (turmeric, curry, and zedoary). Nuts, seeds, and minimally processed cooking oils such as extra virgin olive oil are sources of all eight forms of vitamin E and fat-soluble phytonutrients. Avoidance of processed fats may be equally important.

Physicians will find there is a basis in the medical literature for vitamin B12 screening and optimization, use of fish oil supplements, and attention to the quality of vitamin E supplements. Vitamin E containing mixed tocopherols and tocotrienols most closely resembles the vitamin E found in food and should be recommended over supplemental dosing of alpha tocopherol, which is but one of the eight forms of vitamin E. Safe doses of vitamin C, vitamin E in mixed form, curcumin, and DHA, as well as supplemental nutrients recommended for treatment of other medical conditions (vitamin D and calcium for osteoporosis) may be additionally beneficial for prevention of dementia.

REFERENCES

1. Lethem, R., and Orrell, M. *Antioxidants and dementia.* Lancet, 1997. 349(9060): p. 1189–90.
2. Grossfield, A., Feller, S.E., and Pitman, M.C. *A role for direct interactions in modulation of rhodopsin by omega-3 polyunsaturated lipids.* Proc Natl Acad Sci USA, 2006. 103: p. 4888–93.
3. Stillwell, W., et al. *Docosahexadonic acid affects cell signaling by altering lipid rafts.* Reprod Nutr Dev, 2005. 43: p. 559–79.
4. Chalon, S. *Omega-3 fatty acids and monoamine neurotransmission.* Prostaglandins Leukot Essent Fatty Acids, 2006. 75: p. 259–69.
5. Bazan, N. *Cell survival matters: docosahexanaenoic acid signaling, neuroprotection and photoreceptors.* Trends Neurosci, 2006. 29: p. 263–71.

6. Coti, B., O'Kusky, J., and Innis, S.M. *Maternal dietary n-3 fatty acid deficiency alters neurogenesis in the embryonic rat brain.* J Nutr, 2006. 36: p. 1570–75.

7. Innis, S.M. *Dietary (n-3) fatty acids and brain development.* J Nutr, 2007. 137(4): p. 855–59.

8. Uauy, R., and Dangour, A. *Nutrition in brain development and aging: role of essential fatty acids.* Nutr Rev, 2006. 64: p. S24–S33.

9. Giusto, N.M., et al. *Age-associated changes in central nervous system glycerophospholipids composition and metabolism.* Neurochem Res, 2002. 27: p. 1513–23.

10. Connor, W., Neuringer, M., and Lin, D.S. *Dietary effects on brain fatty acid composition: the reversibility of n-3 fatty acid deficiency and turnover of docosahexaenoic acid in the brain, erythrocytes, and plasma of rhesus monkeys.* J Lipid Res, 1990. 31: p. 237–47.

11. Gamoh, S., et al. *Chronic administration of docosahexaenoic acid improves reference memory-related learning ability in young rats.* Neuroscience, 1999. 93: p. 237–41.

12. Tully, A.M., et al. *Low serum cholesteryl ester-docosahexaenoic acid levels in Alzheimer's disease: a case control study.* British Journal of Nutrition, 2003. 89: p. 483–89.

13. Akiyama, H., et al. *Inflammation and Alzheimer's disease.* Neurobiology of Aging, 2000: p. 383–421.

14. Friedland, R. *Fish consumption and the risk of Alzheimer disease.* Archives of Neurology, 2003. 60: p. 923–24.

15. Huang, T.L., et al. *Benefits of fatty fish on dementia risk are stronger for those without APOE epsilon-4.* Neurology, 2005. 65: p. 1409–14.

16. Kalmijn, S., et al. *Dietary fat intake and the risk of incident dementia in the Rotterdam Study.* Annals of Neurology 1997. 42: p. 776–82.

17. Barberger-Gateau, P., et al. *Fish, meat and risk of dementia: cohort study.* British Medical Journal 2002. 325: p. 932–33.

18. Morris, M.C., et al. *Dietary fish and the risk of incident Alzheimer Disease.* Archives of Neurology, 2003a. 60: p. 194–200.

19. Schaefer, E.J., et al. *Plasma phosphatidylcholine docosahexaenoic acid content and risk of dementia and Alzheimer disease: the Framingham Heart Study.* Arch Neurol, 2006. 63(11): p. 1545–55.

20. Lim, W.S., et al. *Omega 3 fatty acid for the prevention of dementia.* Cochrane Database Syst Rev, 2006(1).

21. Freund-Levi, Y., et al. *Omega-3 fatty acid treatment in 174 patients with mild to moderate Alzheimer disease: OmegAD study: a randomized double-blind trial.* Arch Neurol, 2006. 63(10): p. 1402–8.

22. Dangour, A.D., et al. *A randomised controlled trial investigating the effect of n-3 long-chain polyunsaturated fatty acid supplementation on cognitive and retinal function in cognitively healthy older people: the Older People And n-3 Long-chain polyunsaturated fatty acids (OPAL) study protocol [ISRCTN72331636].* Nutr J, 2006: p. 20.

23. Van de Rest, O. *The MEMO study: Mental Health in Elderly Maintained with Omega-3.* Current controlled trials. http://www.controlled-trials.com/ISRCTN46249783.

24. Quinn, J. *DHA (Docosahexaenoic Acid), an Omega 3 Fatty Acid, in Slowing the Progression of Alzheimer's Disease.* Current clinical trials http://clinicaltrials.gov/ct2/show/NCT00440050.

25. Hooper, L., et al. *Omega 3 fatty acids for prevention and treatment of cardiovascular disease.* Cochrane Database Syst Rev, 2004(4).

26. Morris, M.C., et al. *Dietary intake of antioxidant nutrients and the risk of incident Alzheimer disease in a biracial community study.* JAMA, 2002. 287(24): p. 3230–37.

27. Masaki, K.H., et al. *Association of vitamin E and C supplement use with cognitive function and dementia in elderly men.* Neurology, 2000. 54(6): p. 1265–72.

28. Zandi, P.P., et al. *Reduced risk of Alzheimer disease in users of antioxidant vitamin supplements: the Cache County Study.* Arch Neurol, 2004. 61(1): p. 82–88.

29. Engelhart, M.J., et al. *Dietary intake of antioxidants and risk of Alzheimer disease.* JAMA, 2002. 287(24): p. 3223–29.

30. Luchsinger, J.A., et al. *Antioxidant vitamin intake and risk of Alzheimer disease.* Arch Neurol, 2003. 60(2): p. 203–8.

31. Laurin, D., et al. *Midlife dietary intake of antioxidants and risk of late-life incident dementia: the Honolulu-Asia Aging Study.* Am J Epidemiol, 2004. 159(10): p. 959–67.

32. Morris, M.C., et al. *Relation of the tocopherol forms to incident Alzheimer disease and to cognitive change.* Am J Clin Nutr, 2005. 81(2): p. 508–14.

33. Gillette Guyonnet, S., et al. *IANA task force on nutrition and cognitive decline with aging.* J Nutr Health Aging, 2007. 11(2): p. 132–52.

34. Feillet-Coudray, C., et al. *Effect of zinc supplementation on in vitro copper-induced oxidation of low-density lipoproteins in healthy French subjects aged 55–70 years: the Zenith Study.* Br J Nutr, 2006. 95(6): p. 1134–42.

35. Doraiswamy, P.M., and Finefrock, A.E. *Metals in our minds: therapeutic implications for neurodegenerative disorders.* Lancet Neurol, 2004. 3(7): p. 431–34.

36. Shcherbatykh, I., and Carpenter, D.O. *The role of metals in the etiology of Alzheimer's disease.* J Alzheimers Dis, 2007. 11(2): p. 191–205.

37. Sano, M., et al. *A controlled trial of selegiline, alpha-tocopherol, or both as treatment for Alzheimer's disease. The Alzheimer's Disease Cooperative Study.* N Engl J Med, 1997. 336(17): p. 1216–22.

38. Petersen, R.C., et al. *Vitamin E and donepezil for the treatment of mild cognitive impairment.* N Engl J Med, 2005. 352(23): p. 2379–88.

39. Miller, E.R., III, et al. *Meta-analysis: high-dosage vitamin E supplementation may increase all-cause mortality.* Ann Intern Med, 2005. 142(1): p. 37–46.

40. Hayden, K.M., et al. *Risk of mortality with vitamin E supplements: the Cache County study.* Am J Med, 2007. 120(2): p. 180–84.

41. Vainio, H., and Rautalahti, M. *An international evaluation of the cancer preventive potential of carotenoids.* Cancer Epidemiol Biomarkers Prev, 1998. 7(8): p. 725–28.

42. Morris, M.S. *Folate, homocysteine, and neurological function.* Nutr Clin Care, 2002. 5(3): p. 124–32.

43. Tucker, K.L., et al. *High homocysteine and low B vitamins predict cognitive decline in aging men: the Veterans Affairs Normative Aging Study.* Am J Clin Nutr, 2005. 82(3): p. 627–35.

44. Morris, M.C., et al. *Dietary folate and vitamins B-12 and B-6 not associated with incident Alzheimer's disease.* J Alzheimers Dis, 2006. 9(4): p. 435–43.

45. Morris, M.C., et al. *Dietary folate and vitamin B12 intake and cognitive decline among community-dwelling older persons.* Arch Neurol, 2005. 62(4): p. 641–45.

46. Durga, J., et al. *Effect of 3-year folic acid supplementation on cognitive function in older adults in the FACIT trial: a randomised, double blind, controlled trial.* Lancet, 2007. 369(9557): p. 208–16.

47. Clarke, R., et al. *Vitamin B12 and folate deficiency in later life.* Age Ageing, 2004. 33(1): p. 34–41.

48. Choumenkovitch, S.F., et al. *Folic acid fortification increases red blood cell folate concentrations in the Framingham study.* J Nutr, 2001. 131(12): p. 3277–80.

49. Morris, M.C., Schneider, J.A., and Tangney, C.C. *Thoughts on B-vitamins and dementia.* J Alzheimers Dis, 2006. 9(4): p. 429–33.

50. Refsum, H., and Smith, A.D. *Low vitamin B-12 status in confirmed Alzheimer's disease as revealed by serum holotranscobalamin.* J Neurol Neurosurg Psychiatry, 2003. 74(7): p. 959–61.

51. Sauberlich, H.E. *Laboratory Tests for the Assessment of Nutritional Status.* 1999. p. 143–48.

52. Shukla, P.K., et al. *Protective effect of curcumin against lead neurotoxicity in rat.* Hum Exp Toxicol, 2003. 22: p. 653–58.

53. Lim, G.P., et al. *The curry spice curcumin reduces oxidative damage and amyloid pathology in an Alzheimer transgenic mouse.* J Neurosci, 2001. 21: p. 8370–77.

54. Kim, H.Y., et al. *Curcumin suppresses Janus kinase-STAT inflammatory signaling through activation of Src homology 2 domain-containing tyrosine phosphatase 2 in brain microglia.* J Immunol, 2003. 171: p. 6072–79.

55. Jung, K.K., et al. *Inhibitory effect of curcumin on nitric oxide production from lipopolysaccharide-activated primary microglia.* Life Sci, 2006. 79: p. 2022–31.

56. Ammon, H.P., et al. *Mechanism of antiinflammatory actions of curcumine and boswellic acids.* J Ethnopharmacol, 1993. 38(2–3): p. 113–19.

57. Yang, F., et al. *Curcumin inhibits formation of amyloid beta oligomers and fibrils, binds plaques, and reduces amyloid in vivo.* J Biol Chem, 2005. 280: p. 5892–5901.

58. Ono, K., et al. *Curcumin has potent anti-amyloidogenic effects for Alzheimer's beta-amyloid fibrils in vitro.* J Neurosci Res, 2004. 75: p. 742–50.

59. Garcia-Alloza, M., et al. *Curcumin labels amyloid pathology in vivo, disrupts existing plaques, and partially restores distorted neurites in an Alzheimer mouse model.* J of Neurochem, 2007. 102(4): p. 1095–1104.

60. Hayden, K.M., et al. *Does NSAID use modify cognitive trajectories in the elderly? The Cache County study.* Neurology, 2007. 69(3): p. 275–82.

61. in t' Veld, B.A., et al. *Nonsteroidal antiinflammatory drugs and the risk of Alzheimer's disease.* N Engl J Med, 2001. 345(21): p. 1515–21.

62. Chandra, V., et al. *Incidence of Alzheimer's disease in a rural community in India: the Indo-US study.* Neurology, 2001. 57(6): p. 985–89.

63. Ng, T.P., et al. *Curry consumption and cognitive function in the elderly.* Am J Epidemiol, 2006. 164: p. 898–906.

64. Baum, L., et al. *Six-Month Randomized, Placebo-Controlled, Double-Blind, Pilot Clinical Trial of Curcumin in Patients With Alzheimer Disease.* J Clin Psychopharmacol, 2008. 28(1): p. 110–13.

65. Ringman, J. *Curcumin in Patients With Mild to Moderate Alzheimer's Disease.* Current clinical trials. http://clinicaltrials.gov/ct2/show/NCT00099710.

66. Deodhar, S.D., Sethi, R., and Srimal, R.C. *Preliminary study on antirheumatic activity of curcumin (diferuloyl methane).* Indian J Med Res, 1980. 71: p. 632–34.

67. Satoskar, R.R., Shah, S.J., and Shenoy, S.G. *Evaluation of anti-inflammatory property of curcumin (diferuloyl methane) in patients with postoperative inflammation.* Int J Clin Pharmacol Ther Toxicol, 1986. 24(12): p. 651–54.

68. Lal, B., et al. *Role of curcumin in idiopathic inflammatory orbital pseudotumours.* Phytother Res, 2000. 14(6): p. 443–47.

69. Ringman, J.M., et al. *A potential role of the curry spice curcumin in Alzheimer's disease.* Curr Alzheimer Res, 2005. 2(2): p. 131–36.

70. Cheng, A.L., et al. *Phase I clinical trial of curcumin, a chemopreventive agent, in patients with high-risk or pre-malignant lesions.* Anticancer Res, 2001. 21(4B): p. 2895–2900.

71. Chainani-Wu, N. *Safety and anti-inflammatory activity of curcumin: a component of tumeric (Curcuma longa).* J Altern Complement Med, 2003. 9(1): p. 161–68.

72. Sharma, R.A., et al. *Pharmacodynamic and pharmacokinetic study of oral Curcuma extract in patients with colorectal cancer.* Clin Cancer Res, 2001. 7(7): p. 1894–1900.

73. McCann, J. *Is there convincing biological or behavioral evidence linking vitamin D deficiency to brain dysfunction?* FSEB Journal, 2008. 22: p. 1–20.

74. Sato, Y., et al. *Amelioration of osteoporosis and hypovitaminosis D by sunlight exposure in hospitalized, elderly women with Alzheimer's disease: a randomized controlled trial.* J Bone Miner Res, 2005. 20(8): p. 1327–33.

75. Przybelski, R.J., and Binkley, N.C. *Is vitamin D important for preserving cognition? A positive correlation of serum 25-hydroxyvitamin D concentration with cognitive function.* Arch Biochem Biophys, 2007. 460(2): p. 202–5.

76. Holick, M.F. *Vitamin D deficiency.* N Engl J Med, 2007. 357(3): p. 266–81.

77. Bischoff-Ferrari, H.A., et al. *Estimation of optimal serum concentrations of 25-hydroxyvitamin D for multiple health outcomes.* Am J Clin Nutr, 2006. 84(1): p. 18–28.

78. Solomon, P.R., et al. *Ginkgo for memory enhancement: a randomized controlled trial.* JAMA, 2002. 288(7): p. 835–40.

79. Carlson J.J., et al. *Safety and efficacy of a ginkgo biloba-containing dietary supplement on cognitive function, quality of life, and platelet function in healthy, cognitively intact older adults.* J Am Diet Assoc, 2007. 107(3): p. 422–32.

28 Parkinson's Disease

Nutrient Interventions Targeting Disease Progression

David Perlmutter, M.D.

I. INTRODUCTION

Most authoritative texts attribute the first description of Parkinson's disease to James Parkinson who described the disease in 1817 in his "Essay on the Shaking Palsy." However, exploring medical literature beyond those of Western cultures reveals descriptions of this disease predating that of James Parkinson's by more than 2000 years, in the *Yellow Emperor's Internal Classic*, considered the first Chinese medical classic, written around 425–221 BC:

> A person appears with crouching of the head and with staring eyes, bending the trunk with shoulders drooped, with difficulty turning and rocking the low back, inability of the knees to flex and extend, with the back bowed, failure to stand for long periods, and tremor while walking.[1]

This description most certainly represents what would more than 2000 years later be called Parkinson's disease.

Even more prescient, however, is that the text describes Parkinson's disease as a consequence of liver dysfunction. Western science is only recently recognizing the association of genetic polymorphisms related to hepatic detoxification and Parkinson's risk.[2] It is the disease link with the body's ability to decrease toxicant burden that is salient to disease treatment and the critical role of food and nutrients.

II. EPIDEMIOLOGY

Parkinson's disease is the second most common neurodegenerative disorder after Alzheimer's disease.[3] In the United States, Parkinson's afflicts approximately 1 million people with more than 50,000 new cases being diagnosed each year.[3] The incidence of the disease increases steadily with age, possibly as a consequence of progressive decline in antioxidant functionality leading to an overall increasing prevalence of the disease as our population ages.

III. PHARMACOLOGY

The physical manifestations of Parkinson's disease, including tremor, bradykinesia, rigidity, loss of automatic movements, and impaired balance, are thought to represent downstream effects of a primary brain biochemical abnormality—loss of dopamine production as a consequence of neuronal degeneration in the pars compacta of the substantia nigra. Projection of dopamine from the substantia nigra to other brain centers including the caudate nucleus and the putamen plays a pivotal role in initiating and coordinating motor activity. With compromise of dopaminergic transmission, these motor activities deteriorate.

For the most part, pharmaceutical approaches to the treatment of Parkinson's disease target this dopaminergic deficiency in an attempt to ameliorate the various motor manifestations described above. These approaches include the use of dopamine-based preparations designed to directly stimulate the dopaminergic receptor, including Sinemet®, Sinemet CR®, Stalevo®, and Parcopa®, as well as a newer group of nondopamine-based agents that nevertheless also stimulate the dopamine receptor—the dopamine agonists including Mirapex® and Requip®. Other agents including anticholinergics (used for controlling tremor) and medications designed to enhance the activity of the dopaminergic drugs are also commonly prescribed.

When patients have exhausted the benefits of pharmacotherapy, an increasing number of surgical options are becoming available. These procedures include ablative surgery targeting inhibitory brain centers as well as deep brain stimulator (DBS) implantation technology designed to activate deep brain structures rendered dormant by dopamine deficiency.[5]

The horizon holds promise for surgical interventions that do more than treat symptoms. Future restorative treatment modalities include gene therapy and neural transplantation.[6]

Important to underscore is that food and nutrient interventions have also been shown to be more than palliative. They restore function and delay disease progression, possibly long enough for patients to benefit from surgical restorative treatments as they become available. In other words, nutrition focuses on the fire, not just the smoke.

Further, pharmaceutical interventions may compromise health as a consequence of specific nutritional deficiencies they induce. For example, the metabolism of levodopa consumes pyridoxine (vitamin B6), which may lead to a functional deficiency of this nutrient and may enhance the risk for homocysteine elevation. Laboratory assessments of pyridoxine and homocysteine levels are available in standard clinical laboratories and should be routinely performed when patients are treated with levodopa. Other nutritional considerations include decreased absorption of Mirapex® when taken with food, while it is recommended that Requip® be taken with a meal to reduce the risk of nausea.

IV. PATHOPHYSIOLOGY

Treating the fire, the underlying predisposing conditions, requires addressing oxidative damage to mitochondria and whole body inflammation. Out of this pathophysiology meaningful clinical interventions emerge.

MITOCHONDRIAL DYSFUNCTION AND OXIDATIVE STRESS

Mitochondrial dysfunction of dopaminergic neurons in the substantia nigra is now looked upon as having a pivotal role in the pathogenesis of Parkinson's disease.[7] Specifically, complex I of the electron transport chain involved in the process of oxidative phosphorylation has been demonstrated to be compromised in Parkinson's patients.[8] Interestingly, this deficiency is not confined to the substantia nigra, or even to the brain, having been observed systemically in platelets, fibroblasts, and muscle cells. The impairment of complex I activity ranges from 16% to 54%, with the degree of impairment correlating with the severity of the disease.[9,10] A fundamental consequence of impaired mitochondrial energy production is an increase in endogenous oxidative burden. That is, as mitochondrial function is compromised there is a consequent increase in the production of damaging oxyradicals. This heightened condition of increased oxidative stress damages neurons and is thought to underlie the progressive decline in dopamine production from substantia nigra neurons in Parkinson's disease.

The specific initiating factor leading to mitochondrial function in Parkinson's disease remains unclear. Multiple studies have demonstrated a strong epidemiological relationship between exposure to various environmental mitochondrial toxins, including herbicides, pesticides, industrial chemicals, and heavy metals, and Parkinson's disease risk.[11–14] Further, specific genetic polymorphisms are now identified that may enhance susceptibility of an individual to Parkinson's disease by conferring deficiency of detoxification or antioxidant function, emphasizing the potential significance of gene-environment interactions.[15] Genetic susceptibility testing for hepatic detoxification flaws that may predispose an individual to the development of Parkinson's disease is now widely available.[16] Beyond family members of Parkinson's patients who could be at increased risk for carrying these genetic polymorphisms, screening all individuals for this predisposition represents a new threshold in preventive medicine.

Ultimately, a feed-forward cycle is produced whereby excessive oxyradicals produced as a consequence of mitochondrial complex I dysfunction further damage mitochondrial function, enhancing oxyradical production. This situation is exacerbated by a deficiency of antioxidant protection of substantia nigra neurons. Multiple studies have described a dramatic deficiency of neuron protective reduced glutathione in the substantia nigra of Parkinson's disease patients and the degree of glutathione depletion correlates directly with disease severity.[17–19] Based upon the understanding of the protective role of glutathione as a neuronal antioxidant, its pivotal role in detoxification processes related to potentially neurotoxic environmental exposures, and the finding of deficiency in the Parkinson's brain, Sechi and colleagues at the University of Sassari, Italy, administered reduced glutathione intravenously to a group of Parkinson's patients twice daily for 30 days. The subjects were then evaluated at 1-month intervals for the following 6 months. Their published report indicated, "All patients improved significantly with a 42% decline in disability. Once glutathione was stopped, the therapeutic effect lasted 2–4 months." They concluded that "glutathione has symptomatic efficacy and possibly retards the progression of the disease."[20] Our experience with intravenous reduced glutathione has been similar and we are currently concluding a double-blind, placebo-controlled trial using 1400 mg of reduced glutathione given intravenously three times weekly.

Coenzyme Q10 (CoQ10) serves a critical role as an electron acceptor for complex I in oxidative phosphorylation. In addition, it also has potent antioxidant activity.[21] And like glutathione, deficiency of CoQ10 is also noted in the mitochondria of platelets from Parkinson's when compared to controls.[22] These attributes have placed CoQ10 in the spotlight as a candidate to affect disease progression in Parkinson's patients.

In a landmark study, Dr. Clifford Shults and coworkers at the University of California–San Diego, evaluated the effectiveness of mitochondrial therapy on the progression of Parkinson's disease using CoQ10. Their large, multicenter randomized, placebo-controlled double-blind study demonstrated that high-dosage CoQ10 (1200 mg/day) slowed the functional decline in Parkinson's patients by a remarkable 44% when compared to the placebo group as measured by the Unified Parkinson's Disease Rating Scale (UPDRS). The effect on total UPDRS was due to slowed decline in all three components of this widely used scale—mental function, activities of daily living, and motor function.[23]

Oxidative stress plays a central role in the progression and possibly the initiation of nigral metabolic compromise ultimately manifesting in the clinical picture of Parkinson's disease, prompting in-depth investigation of the role of antioxidants.[24] Studies evaluating risk for the disease as well as disease progression in relation to dietary intake of antioxidants date back at least two decades. These reports have included both retrospective epidemiological studies correlating dietary habits with risk for the disease as well as actual interventional studies wherein the administration of one or more specific antioxidant(s) is evaluated in terms of effectiveness on disease progression. In 1988 the report, "Case-Control Study of Early Life Dietary Factors in Parkinson's Disease," was published in *Archives of Neurology*. This early report paved the way to the current understanding that dietary choices may offer protection against a neurodegenerative condition. The researchers found that simple dietary sources of vitamin E profoundly reduced the risk of Parkinson's disease. Risk was reduced to 39% in those reporting the highest consumption of nuts, while consumers of seed-based salad dressing had a risk of 30%, and those who regularly consumed plums, a rich source of water-soluble antioxidants, demonstrated risk for the disease of only 24% in comparison to those not engaged in this dietary preference.[25]

More recently, German researchers published a report evaluating the retrospective specific micronutrient and macronutrient intake of 342 Parkinson's patients in comparison to 342 control individuals from the same neighborhood or region.[26] This study provides strong evidence that dietary choices play a meaningful role in risk determination for the disease. Risk for Parkinson's disease was markedly reduced in those individuals whose dietary choices provided the highest levels of certain antioxidants. Disease risk was reduced by 33% in those having the highest consumption of beta-carotene with those consuming the most vitamin C having a risk 40% less than those reporting the least consumption. High levels of monosaccharide as well as total energy consumption were very strongly associated with disease risk. While the authors didn't specifically comment on this finding, research published subsequent to their report may help explain this relationship. Increased caloric consumption of total calories, especially monosaccharides, favors the formation of advanced glycosylation end products (AGEs). AGEs are formed when monosaccharides react non-enzymatically with the terminal amino group of proteins. This posttranslational change imparts pathophysiological activity, stimulating inflammation and its many downstream effects. As a consequence, AGEs are thought to play an important role in neurodegeneration and aging.[27] Risk for Parkinson's disease was reduced by 51% in those with the highest riboflavin consumption compared to the lowest quartile. In human metabolism, riboflavin plays a role in diverse redox reactions through the coenzyme electron carriers flavin adenine dinucleotide (FAD) and flavin mononucleotide (FMN).[28] FAD is part of the electron transport chain, and as such it is a requisite participant in mitochondrial function. Further, glutathione reductase is an FAD-dependent enzyme that participates in the regeneration of glutathione, a fundamentally important brain-protective antioxidant that is deficient in Parkinson's patients (see previous discussion). Perhaps because of the role of riboflavin in glutathione production, deficiency of riboflavin is associated with increased oxidative stress.[29] In an interventional trial, researchers at the University of Sao Paulo provided oral riboflavin 30 mg every 8 hours to a group of 31 advanced-stage Parkinson's patients. Interestingly, blood levels of riboflavin were depressed in all participants. After 6 months, motor capacity improved from 44% to 71% (Hoehn and Yahr scale) with improvements noted in nighttime sleep, reasoning, motivation, as well as reduced depression. These improvements were correlated with increased blood levels of riboflavin.[30] The highest quartile of folic acid consumption showed a reduced risk for Parkinson's disease of 49% compared to the lowest. Folate coenzymes are required for the metabolism of several important amino acids including the synthesis of methionine from homocysteine. Thus, folate deficiency is strongly associated with elevation of homocysteine, and elevation of homocysteine levels are common in Parkinson's patients.[31] Germane to the previously described pathophysiological model of Parkinson's disease, homocysteine enhances oxidative stress, compromises mitochondrial function, and ultimately leads to neuronal apoptosis.[32] (See Table 28.1.)

INFLAMMATION

Indeed, a fundamental pathophysiological feature of this disease is the finding of enhanced parameters of inflammation.[33] Areas of maximal degeneration within the substantia nigra demonstrate robust increases in the number of activated immune-mediating microglial cells along with elevated levels of cytokines including interleukin-1β, tumor necrosis factor-alpha and interferon-γ, which are increased by 7- to 15-fold in the substantia nigra of Parkinson's patients.[34,35] Cyclooxygenase-2 (COX-2) is also significantly elevated in the Parkinson's brain. COX-2 converts arachidonic acid to pro-inflammatory prostanoid prostaglandin E2, with research by Dr. Peter Teismann and coworkers demonstrating "a critical role for COX-2 in both the pathogenesis and selectivity of the Parkinson's disease neurodegenerative process."[36]

Epidemiological studies also support the relationship between Parkinson's disease and inflammation with research demonstrating an overall risk reduction for the disease by 45% in regular users of over-the-counter nonsteroidal anti-inflammatory medications (NSAIDs).[37] Further, glial cell mediated inflammation is not unique to Parkinson's disease and is implicated in a variety of

TABLE 28.1

Adjusted Odds Ratios for Parkinson's Disease by Quartiles of Macronutrient and Micronutrient Intakes With "1" Representing the Lowest Quartile and "4" the Highest

Variable	Quartile	Adjusted Odds Ratio
Beta-carotene	1	1.00
	2	1.13
	3	0.85
	4	0.67
Ascorbic acid	1	1.00
	2	1.19
	3	0.97
	4	0.60
Riboflavin	1	1.00
	2	0.65
	3	0.67
	4	0.49
Folic acid	1	1.00
	2	0.86
	3	0.62
	4	0.51
Monosaccharides	1	1.00
	2	1.67
	3	1.57
	4	2.59
Total energy intake	1	1.00
	2	2.19
	3	2.91
	4	3.25

Source: [26].

other common neurodegenerative conditions including Alzheimer's disease and amyotrophic lateral sclerosis.[38,39]

One important mechanism by which NSAIDs suppress inflammation is by activation of peroxisome proliferator-activated receptor-γ (PPARγ). This finding has led researchers to explore more fully the role of PPARγ in reducing inflammation in neurodegenerative disorders including Parkinson's disease.[40] In what has now become the standard animal model of Parkinson's disease, researchers are able to mimic human neuropathological changes in animals treated with the neurotoxin 1-methyl-4-phenyl-1,2,3,6-tetrahydropyridine (MPTP). MPTP-treated mice demonstrate mitochondrial dysfunction and consequent dramatic enhancement in the generation of reactive oxygen species, excitotoxicity, and apoptosis specifically in dopaminergic cells of the pars compacta of the substantia nigra. Further, these changes are accompanied by marked neuroinflammatory changes including microglial activation.[41]

To more fully elucidate the role of PPARγ in the Parkinson's disease animal model, Dr. Tilo Breidert and colleagues evaluated the neuroprotective effects of specific PPARγ ligands in MPTP-treated mice. Their research demonstrated significant reduction of neuronal death in substantia nigra dopaminergic neurons in animals treated with the PPARγ ligand pioglitazone (Actos®).[42]

The profound activity of PPARγ ligand mediated activation in terms of modulating inflammation is now a major focus of research in several important neurodegenerative conditions, including

Alzheimer's disease, multiple sclerosis, amyotrophic lateral sclerosis, and cerebral ischemia.[43] One would anticipate that the outcome of the basic science and ultimately interventional trials would be focused on development of an effective and pharmaceutical agent. This could provide meaningful interventions for these and other devastating neurological conditions, but many years hence. Further, pharmaceutical manipulation of PPARγ is not without risk as has been noted with the recent finding of a marked increase in risk of cardiovascular death in individuals using the diabetes medication rosiglitazone (Avandia®).[44]

What naturally serves as a ligand for PPARγ? How can biochemistry, perhaps the body's own biochemistry made from food and nutrients, affect the role of PPARγ in modulating inflammation?

Docosahaexaenoic acid (DHA) is known to have beneficial effects in a variety of human diseases including atherosclerosis, asthma, cardiovascular disease, cancer, and depression.[45] These benefits are presumably derived from the anti-inflammatory activity of this fatty acid, which demonstrates potent inhibition of COX-2.[46] In a recent publication, "Identification of Putative Metabolites of Docosahaexaenoic Acid as Potent PPARγ Agonists and Antidiabetic Agents," Japanese researchers discovered potent PPARγ ligand activity from several metabolites of DHA, with one metabolite demonstrating almost twice the potency compared to pioglitazone (Actos®).[47] This new information adds to the understanding of the mechanisms underlying the potent anti-inflammatory effects of DHA and further helps explain why, for example, people with the highest blood levels of DHA have been shown to have a 47% lower risk of developing dementia and a 39% lower risk of developing Alzheimer's disease, compared with those with lower DHA levels.[48]

While no study has as yet been undertaken to assess risk for Parkinson's disease in relation to DHA levels, based upon the understanding of its role in PPARγ-mediated inflammation modulation it seems reasonable to consider adequate dietary supplementation of this important nutrient. Further, with the unique sensitivity of dopaminergic neurons in genetically sensitive individuals to neurotoxins, which may concentrate higher in the food chain, nonfish-derived vegetarian sources of DHA may seem more appropriate. Indeed, vegetarian-sourced DHA derived from marine algae is now widely available as a nutritional supplement as well as being used to fortify various food products including infant formula, eggs, beverages, cereals, and yogurt.

While the concept of preventive medicine has taken root in such disciplines as cardiology and women's health, precious little attention is paid to applying evidence-based information to health recommendations related to neurodegenerative conditions. Clearly, a large body of science supports the contention that modifiable lifestyle factors are important considerations in relation to risk and progression of conditions like Parkinson's disease. Understanding the central roles of oxidative stress and inflammation in this disease should serve as motivation for dietary changes enhancing antioxidant protection while reducing the propensity for inflammation. With respect to the former, recommendations for higher consumption of whole fruits and vegetables, nuts and seeds, with judicious use of oral antioxidant supplements, seems clearly justified. As for the latter, these same dietary recommendations form the basis of the Mediterranean diet, now well described as having a marked effect in terms of reducing inflammation.[49] Key components of the Mediterranean diet[50] include:

- Eating generous amount of fruits and vegetables
- Consuming healthy fats such as olive oil and canola oil
- Eating small portions of nuts
- Drinking red wine, in moderation, for some
- Consuming very little red meat
- Eating fish on a regular basis

Further, specific supplementation with DHA provides a powerful nonpharmaceutical approach to inflammation as mediated through both COX-2 inhibition as well as through PPARγ. In our clinic we generally recommend a daily consumption of DHA as a supplement in a dosage of 800 mg for Parkinson's disease.

V. COMORBID CONDITIONS

Obesity is a cause of mitochondrial dysfunction that is readily modifiable and shows strong relationship to Parkinson's disease risk. In the study Midlife Adiposity and the Future Risk of Parkinson's Disease, researchers determined adiposity using measurement of triceps skinfold thickness in a group of 7990 men ages 45 to 68 years between the years 1965 and 1968. Surviving participants were then examined an average of 30 years later. Comparing the incidence of Parkinson's disease in those originally in the highest quartile of triceps skinfold thickness to those with the lowest found an increased risk of developing Parkinson's disease of 300% associated with the thickest triceps skinfold.[51]

Body fat may act as a reservoir for lipid-soluble neurotoxins that selectively damage dopamine-producing neurons in the substantia nigra. Several persistent organic pollutants such as pesticides are lipid soluble and act as neurotoxins as a consequence of their ability to disrupt mitochondrial function. In addition, excessive body fat is associated with up-regulation of inflammatory cytokines, which in turn act to increase the production of mitochondria-damaging oxyradicals.

VI. CONCLUSION

Modern therapeutic interventions for Parkinson's disease are clearly effective in symptom management, but provide very little in terms of modulating disease progression. However, food and nutrient interventions have been shown to treat the underlying pathophysiology. The following interventions and studies can be incorporated into medical practice:

- Understanding and correcting nutrient-drug interactions
- Optimizing antioxidant function to include CoQ10, 200 mg/day; vitamin C 1000 mg/day; vitamin E 400 IU/day; alpha lipoic acid 200 mg/day; N-acetyl cysteine 800 mg/day; acetyl-l-carnitine 800 mg/day; vitamin D 400 IU/day; beta-carotene 25,000 IU/day
- Blood tests for nutrient optimizations to include measurements of antioxidant function (lipid peroxide profile) as well as levels of specific nutrients including pyridoxine, beta-carotene, riboflavin, folate, vitamin B12, and CoQ10
- Reducing inflammation with DHA 800 mg/day as a supplement
- Attention to lifestyle issues including exercise and weight management

REFERENCES

1. Zhang Z, Dong Z, Román GC. Early Descriptions of Parkinson Disease in Ancient China. *Arch Neurol* 2006; 63:782–784.
2. Elbaz A, Levecque C, Clavel J, Vidal JS, Richard F, Amouyel P, Alpérovitch A, Chartier-Harlin MC, Tzourio C. CYP2D6 polymorphism, pesticide exposure, and Parkinson's disease. *Ann Neurol* 2004 Mar; 55(3):430–434.
3. Saunders CD. *Parkinson's Disease: A New Hope.* Boston, MA: Harvard Health Publications; 2000.
4. Removed at proofs.
5. Krack P, Poepping M, Weinert D, et al. Thalamic, pallidal, or subthalamic surgery for Parkinson's disease? *J Neurol* 2000; 247 Suppl. 2:122–134.
6. Erlick AC, et al. Surgical insights into Parkinson's disease. *J R Soc Med* 2006; 99:238–244.
7. Reichmann H, Janetsky B. Mitochondrial dysfunction—a pathogenetic factor in Parkinson's disease. *J Neurol* 2000; 247 Suppl. 2:63–68.
8. Haas RH, Nasirian F, Nakano K, et al. Low platelet mitochondrial complex I and complex II/III activity in early untreated Parkinson's disease. *Ann Neurol* 1995; 37:714–722.
9. Reichmann H, Janetsky B. Mitochondrial dysfunction—a pathogenetic factor in Parkinson's disease. *J Neurol* 2000; 247 Suppl. 2:63–68.
10. Swerdlow RH, Parks JK, Miller SW, et al. Origin and functional consequences of the complex I defect in Parkinson's disease. *Ann Neurol* 1996; 40:663–671.

11. Hirsch EC, Brandel JP, Galle P, et al. Iron and aluminum increase in the substantia nigra of patients with Parkinson's disease: an X-ray microanalysis. *J Neurochem* 1991; 56:446–451.
12. Bocchetta A, Corsini GU. Parkinson's disease and pesticides. *Lancet* 1986; 2:1163.
13. Tanner CM, Langston JW. Do environmental toxins cause Parkinson's disease? A critical review. *Neurology* 1990; 40 Suppl. 3:17–31.
14. Stephenson J. Exposure to home pesticides linked to Parkinson's disease. JAMA 2000; 283:3055–3056.
15. Checkoway H, Farin FM, Costa-Mallen P, Kirchner SC, Costa LG. Genetic polymorphisms in Parkinson's disease. *Neurotoxicology.* 1998 Aug–Oct; 19(4–5):635–643.
16. Genovations™ Genova Diagnostics, 63 Zillicoa Street, Asheville, NC 28801-1074 Tel. 800-522-4762.
17. Perry TL, Godin DV, Hansen S. Parkinson's disease: a disorder due to nigral glutathione deficiency? *Neurosci Lett* 1982; 33:305–310.
18. Jenner P. Oxidative mechanisms in nigral cell death in Parkinson's disease. *Mov Disord* 1998; 13:S24–S34.
19. Riederer P, Sofic E, Rausch W, et al. Transition metals, ferritin, glutathione, and ascorbic acid in parkinsonian brains. *J Neurochem* 1989; 52:515–520.
20. Sechi G, Deledda MG, Bua G, et al. Reduced intravenous glutathione in the treatment of early Parkinson's disease. *Progr Neuropsychopharmacol Biol Psychiatry* 1996; 20:1159–1170.
21. Shults, CW. Effects of coenzyme Q10 in early Parkinson's disease—evidence of slowing of the functional decline. *Arch Neurol* 2002; 59:1541–1550.
22. Matsubara TA, et al. Serum coenzyme Q10 level in Parkinson syndrome. In: Folkers K., et al eds. *Biomedical and Clinical Aspects of Coenzyme Q10.* New York: Elsevier Science Publishers, 1991: 159–166.
23. Shults CW, et al. Effects of coenzyme Q10 in early Parkinson's disease – evidence of slowing of the functional decline. *Arch Neurol* 2002; 59:1541–1550.
24. Hellenbrand W, Seidler A, Boeing H, Robra B-P, Vieregge P, Nischan P, Joerg J, Oertel WH, Schneider E, Ulm G. Diet and Parkinson's disease I: A possible role for the past intake of specific foods and food groups: results from a self-administered food-frequency questionnaire in a case-control study. *Neurology* 1996; 47:636–643.
25. Golbe LI, Farrell TM, David PH. Case-controlled study of early life dietary factors in Parkinson's disease. *Arch Neurol* 1988; 45(12):1350–1353.
26. Hellenbrand W, Boeing H, Robra B-P, Seidler A, Vieregge P, Nischan P, Joerg J, Oertel WH, Schneider E, Ulm G. Diet and Parkinson's disease 11: A possible role for the past intake of specific nutrients: results from a self-administered food-frequency questionnaire in a case-control study. *Neurology* 1996; 47:644–650.
27. Ramasamy R, Vannucci SJ, Yan SSD, Herold K, Yan SF, Schmidt AM. Advanced glycation end products and RAGE: a common thread in aging, diabetes, neurodegeneration, and inflammation. *Glycobiology* July 1, 2005; 15(7):16R–28R.
28. McCormick DB, Innis WSA, Merrill AH, Jr, Bowers-Komro DM, Oka M, Chastain JL. An update on flavin metabolism in rats and humans. In: Edmondson DE, McCormick DB, eds. *Flavin and flavoproteins.* New York: Walter de Gruyter, 1988: 459–471.
29. Powers HJ. Current knowledge concerning optimum nutritional status of riboflavin, niacin and pyridoxine. *Proc Nutr Soc* 1999; 58(2):435–440.
30. Coimbra CG, Junqueira VBC. High doses of riboflavin and the elimination of dietary red meat promote the recovery of some motor functions in Parkinson's disease patients. *Brazilian J of Med & Bio Res* 2003; 36:1409–1417.
31. Religa D, Czyzewski K, Styczynska M, Peplonska B, Lokk J, Chodakowska-Zebrowska M, Stepien K, Winblad B, Barcikowska M. Hyperhomocysteinemia and methylenetetrahydrofolate reductase polymorphism in patients with Parkinson's disease. *Neurosci Lett* 2006 Aug 14; 404(1–2):56–60.
32. Mattson MP, Kruman II, Duan W. Folic acid and homocysteine in age-related disease. *Ageing Research Reviews* 2002; 1:95–111.
33. Hirsch EC, Hunot S, Damier P, Brugg B, Faucheux BA, Michel PP, Ruberg M, Muriel MP, Mouatt-Prigent A, Agid Y. Glia cells and inflammation in Parkinson's disease: a role in neurodegeneration. *Ann Neurol* 1990; 44 Suppl. 1:S115–S120.
34. Mogi M, Harada M, Narabayashi H, Inogaki H, Minami M. Nagatsu T. Interleukin (IL)-1 beta, IL-2, IL-4, IL-6 and transforming growth factor-alpha levels are elevated in ventricular cerebrospinal fluid in juvenile parkinsonism and Parkinson's disease. *Neurosci Lett* 1996; 211:13–16.
35. Hirsch EC, Hunot S, Damier P, Brugg B, Faucheux BA, Michel PP, Ruberg M, Muriel MP, Mouatt-Prigent A, Agid Y. Glia cells and inflammation in Parkinson's disease: a role in neurodegeneration. *Ann Neurol* 1998; 44 Suppl. 1:S115–S120.

36. Teismann P, Tieu K, Choi DK, Wu DC, Naini A, Hunot S, Vila M, Jackson-Lewis V, Przedborski S. Cyclooxygenase-2 is instrumental in Parkinson's disease neurodegeneration. *Proc Natl Acad Sci USA* 2003 Apr 29; 100(9):5473–5478.

37. Chen H, Zhang SM, Hernán MA, Schwarzschild MA, Willett WC, Colditz GA, Speizer FE, Ascherio A. Nonsteroidal anti-inflammatory drugs and the risk of Parkinson disease. *Arch Neurol* 2003; 60: 1059–1064.

38. Klegeris A, McGeer PL. Cyclooxygenase and 3-lipoxygenase inhibitors protect against mononuclear phagocyte neurotoxicity. *Neurobiol Aging* 2002; 23:787–794.

39. In t' Veld BA, Ruitenberg A, Hofman A, et al. Nonsteroidal antiinflammatory drugs and the risk of Alzheimer's disease. *N Engl J Med* 2001; 345:1515–1521.

40. Heneka MT, Landreth GE, Hüll M. Drug insight: effects mediated by peroxisome proliferator-activated receptor-gamma in CNS disorders. *Nat Clin Pract Neurol* 2007 Sep; 3(9):496–504.

41. Liberatore GT et al. Inducible nitric oxide synthase stimulates dopaminergic neurodegeneration in the MPTP model of Parkinson disease. *Nat Med* 1999; 5:1403–1409.

42. Breidert T et al. Protective action of the peroxisome proliferator-activated receptor-gamma agonist pioglitazone in a mouse model of Parkinson's disease. *J Neurochem* 2002; 82:615–624.

43. Heneka MT, Landreth GE, Hüll M. Drug insight: effects mediated by peroxisome proliferator-activated receptor-gamma in CNS disorders. *Nat Clin Pract Neurol* 2007 Sep; 3(9):496–504.

44. Nissen SE, Wolski K. Effect of rosiglitazone on the risk of myocardial infarction and death from cardiovascular causes. *N Engl J Med* 2007; 356:2457–2471.

45. Horrocks LA, Yeo YK. Health benefits of docosahexaenoic acid (DHA). *Pharmacol Res* 1999 Sep; 40(3): 211–225.

46. Massaro M, Habib A, Lubrano L, Del Turco S, Lazzerini G, Bourcier T, Weksler BB, De Caterina R. The omega-3 fatty acid docosahexaenoate attenuates endothelial cyclooxygenase-2 induction through both NADP(H) oxidase and PKCε inhibition. *Proc Natl Acad Sci USA* 2006; 103:15184–15189.

47. Yamamoto K, Itoh T, Abe D, Shimizu M, Kanda T, Koyama T, Nishikawa M, Tamai T, Ooizumi H, Yamada S. Identification of putative metabolites of docosahexaenoic acid as potent PPARγ agonists and antidiabetic agents. *Bioorganic & Medicinal Chemistry Letters* 2005; 15:517–522.

48. Schaefer EJ, Bongard V, Beiser AS, Lamon-Fava S, Robins SJ, Au R, Tucker KL, Kyle DJ, Wilson PWF, Wolf PA. Plasma Phosphatidylcholine Docosahexaenoic Acid Content and Risk of Dementia and Alzheimer Disease—The Framingham Heart Study. *Arch Neurol* 2006; 63:1545–1550.

49. Trichopoulou A, Costacou T, Bamia C, Trichopoulos D. Adherence to a Mediterranean diet and survival in a Greek population. *NEJM* 2003; 348:2600–2608.

50. Mediterranean diet for heart health. MayoClinic.com. www.mayoclinic.com/health/mediterranean-diet/CL00011.

51. Abbott RD, Ross GW, White LR, et al. Midlife adiposity and the future risk of Parkinson's disease. *Neurology* 59; 1051–1057:2002.

29 Depression

Marty Hinz, M.D.

I. INTRODUCTION

Since amino acids obtained from dietary sources are the precursors of mood-regulating neurotransmitters such as serotonin and dopamine, amino acids are considered to hold potential in treating depression. Neurotransmitter precursors are the subject of ongoing research.

So why is this topic relevant to primary care medicine? Patients have taken matters into their own hands. Patients are self-treating their depression with amino acid supplements and appear to be motivated by a perceived benefit in their mood and overall health. The amino acid precursors tryptophan, tyrosine, 5-hydroxytryptophan, and L-dopa are readily available as supplements at doses that exceed feasible dietary intake. Amino acid supplements have less potential for harm and larger therapeutic effect when their use is physician-guided.

This chapter presents the bundle damage theory of depression to probe the biologic basis of amino acid therapy. It offers primary care physicians a treatment protocol that implements laboratory testing to guide dosing; explains the potential side effects and how these can be minimized; offers quality regulation in product selection; and presents a protocol for simultaneous use of medication and nutrients in the treatment of clinical depression.

II. EPIDEMIOLOGY

Depression is a global problem. The World Health Organization notes:[32]

> Nearly 5–10% of persons in a community at a given time are in need of help for depression. As much as 8–20% of persons carry the risk of developing depression during their lifetime. The average age of the onset for major depression is between 20 and 40 years. Women have higher rates of depression than men. Race or ethnicity does not influence the prevalence of depression. World wide depression is the fourth leading cause of disease burden, accounting for 4.4% of total Disability-Adjusted Life-Years (DALYs) in the year 2000. It causes the largest amount of non-fatal burden. Disability from depression world wide is increasing. In 1990, the total years lived with disability (YLD) was 10.7%. By 2000, the YLD had increased to 12.1% worldwide.[33] Mental health conditions have a tendency to move upwards in ranking, while ranked as the fourth leading cause of disease burden in 2000, it is expected that depression will move to second place by 2020, second only to heart disease.[34]

Population surveys suggest that while the incidence of depression is higher in the developed countries of North America and Europe than in other regions, it is nonetheless a common condition throughout the world.[38] The rate difference is often attributed to underdiagnosis, but newer data suggest that the Western diet, stressful lifestyle, and higher toxicant exposures contribute to the prevailing high rates in Westernized countries.[32]

The monoamine theory fails to explain why the incidences of depression are increasing on a worldwide basis and are more prevalent in developed countries.[1]

III. PATHOPHYSIOLOGY

THE MONOAMINE THEORY

The monoamine theory of depression has long been the major framework against which the treatment of depression has been examined and developed, due to the fact that the theory attempts to provide a pathophysiologic explanation for depression and the actions of antidepressants. The central premise of the monoamine theory states that it may be possible to restore normal function in depressed patients by targeting the catecholamine and/or serotonin systems with antidepressants. This theory is based on evidence that depression symptoms can be improved by administering compounds that are capable of increasing monoamine concentrations in the nerve synapses. Early research focused on deficits in the catecholamine system with specific emphasis on noradrenalin as a potential cause for depression. With further research, the theory was expanded to include the serotonin system as a cause for depression. This research has led to treating depression with drugs that affect changes in monoamine uptake and enzymatic metabolism.[1]

While many of the depression treatments based on the monoamine theory appear to be initially useful, many of them lack the short-term and long-term efficacy needed for relief of symptoms in most patients. In several studies of reuptake inhibitors administered, only 8% to 13% of subjects obtained relief of symptoms greater than placebo. Remission rates for escitalopram compared to placebo in adults were studied (48.7% vs. 37.6%, P = 0.003). Here, 11.1% of subjects obtained relief greater than placebo.[35] Remission rates for citalopram versus placebo in another study were studied (52.8% vs. 43.5%, P = 0.003). Here, 9.4% of patients obtained relief greater than placebo.[35] Venlafaxine-XR was similar to escitralopram and citalopram (P = 0.03).[35]

Treatment of the elderly in the primary care setting under the monoamine theory reveals no relief of symptoms versus placebo. In the elderly (79.6 years, SD = 4.4, N = 174), it was concluded that citalopram, "was not more effective than placebo for the treatment of depression."[27] In treatment of depression in patients over 60 years of age with a mean age of 68 years, "Escitalopram treatment was not significantly different from placebo treatment" (N = 264).[29]

Depression treatment of children and adolescents ages 7 to 17 (N = 174) with citalopram, under a double-blind 20 mg/day, 40 mg/day option, found 24% of patients treated with placebo showed improvement versus 36% of patients taking citalopram.[28]

Other studies of other reuptake inhibitors revealed similar results.[50–55]

Reuptake inhibitors are effective in treating other disorders than those for which they were initially developed, such as obesity, panic disorder, anxiety, migraine headaches, ADHD/ADD, premenstrual syndrome, dementia, fibromyalgia, psychotic illness, insomnia, obsessive-compulsive disorder, and bulimia/anorexia; yet not all drugs that increase serotonin or catecholamine transmission are effective when treating depression.[1]

Treatment with reuptake inhibitors is based on the monoamine theory, which does not explain why most subjects studied achieve results no better than placebo and why treatment is much less efficacious in the elderly. Neither does it explain the efficacy of treating other conditions. In sum, the mechanism and corresponding medication for the treatment of depression suggest there may be more to the underlying pathophysiology.

PARKINSONISM MODEL

Insights into the pathophysiology of depression can be gained from understanding another monoamine neurotransmitter disease, Parkinson's disease. Parkinsonism is caused by damage to the dopamine postsynaptic neurons of the substantia nigra at levels that result in clinical compromise of fine motor movement.

Parkinson's disease has a study model of neurotoxin damage.[49] A great deal of understanding about Parkinson's disease has resulted from research and case studies involving the neurotoxin MPTP (1-methyl 4-phenyl 1,2,3,6-tetrahydropyridine). In 1982, the first writings on MPTP appeared in the medical literature after several heroin addicts administered synthetic heroin (MPPP) that contained the byproduct of synthesis, MPTP.[9] Since that time, the MPTP mechanism of action has become the prototype in the study of Parkinson's disease. At present, most medical school students study the ability of MPTP to quickly induce advanced Parkinson's symptoms in patients without prior history of the disease.

MPTP is a free radical neurotoxin, which interferes with mitochondrial metabolism and leads to cell death (apoptosis). It freely crosses the blood-brain barrier and has an affinity for the post-synaptic dopamine neurons of the substantia nigra, which it destroys. MPTP is chemically similar to MPPP (synthetic heroin) and may be produced as a byproduct during the illegal manufacturing of MPPP and other narcotics.[9] The MPTP model of Parkinson's disease has taught us a lot about the dopamine neurons of the substantia nigra. The main point is that if enough dopamine neurons are damaged, the flow of electrical impulses is compromised and Parkinson's symptoms will occur. The way to compensate for neurotoxin-induced damage is to increase neurotransmitter levels higher than is normally found in the system.[9]

Consistent with the findings of the MPTP model, the pharmacologic treatment is dopamine agonists, which raise the existing levels of this neurotransmitter above population norms in order to boost damaged neurons. Dopamine agonists, such as bromocriptine, pergolide, ropinirole, pramipex-ole, and cabergoline, can be used as a monotherapy or in combination with L-dopa. L-dopa crosses the blood-brain barrier and is freely synthesized into dopamine without biochemical regulation.[3] The elevation of dopamine in the central nervous system stimulates the remaining viable dopamine neurons of the substantia nigra by increasing the electrical flow, which results in restoration of the regulator function of the dopamine bundles and improvement of disease symptoms.[7] The shortcom-ing is tachyphylaxis, where the dopamine agonist and/or L-dopa become ineffective.

With Parkinson's patients, establishing dopamine levels in the reference range reported by the laboratory does not provide relief of symptoms. For example, the reference range of urinary dop-amine reported by the laboratory is 40 to 390 micrograms of dopamine per gram of creatinine (the neurotransmitter-creatinine ratio compensates for dilution of the urine). In our years of research, we have not observed a patient with Parkinson's who was able to achieve relief of symptoms with dopamine levels in this range. For treatment of patients with Parkinson's, the therapeutic range of urinary dopamine is 6000 to 8000 micrograms of dopamine per gram of creatinine. Dopamine levels of this magnitude can be achieved by administration of the amino acid precursor, L-dopa. Amino acid supplementation can reduce the tachyphylaxis generally associated with pharmacologic interventions. Once the synaptic levels of dopamine are high enough and the flow of electricity is once again adequate to regulate fine motor control, clinical resolution of the Parkinsonian tremor and other symptoms are seen.[40]

As with Parkinsonism, the damage to other neuron bundles of the serotonin/catecholamine path-ways as seen in depression can be dealt with effectively by increasing the neurotransmitter levels higher than is normally found in the system. This has led our group to propose the bundle damage theory of depression.

THE BUNDLE DAMAGE THEORY

The bundle damage theory states:

> Neurotransmitter dysfunction disease symptoms, such as symptoms of depression, develop when the electrical flow through the neuron bundles that regulate function is compromised by damage to the individual neurons or the neuron components composing the neuron bundle which conducts electricity to regulate or control function. In order to optimally restore neuron bundle regulatory function, synap-tic neurotransmitter levels of the remaining viable neurons must be increased to levels higher than is normally found in the system, which restores adequate electrical outflow resulting in relief of symptoms and optimal regulatory function.

Bundles of neurons convey electricity that regulates numerous functions in the body. If enough of the individual neurons of a bundle become damaged, the flow of electricity through the bundle is diminished. Decreased function causes symptoms of disease to develop. Technically synaptic neurotransmitter levels prior to treatment in patients with disease due to neuron bundle damage are in the normal range for the population.

The bundle damage theory and the monoamine theory are not mutually exclusive of each other. Instead these two theories can be viewed as complementary in that they address different mechanisms of action leading to neurotransmitter dysfunction and compromised electrical flow out of the postsynaptic neuron. The monoamine theory addresses low levels of neurotransmitters in the synapse as the etiology of impedance of electrical flow needed to regulate function and keep disease symptoms under control. The bundle damage theory addresses damage to the primarily postsynaptic neuron structures that impede the flow of electricity needed to regulate function and keep disease symptoms under control. With the monoamine theory and the bundle damage theory the flow of electrical energy needed to regulate function is not adequate. Differentiation of the two theories lies in the etiology of the dysfunction. Under monoamine theory returning neurotransmitter levels to normal will relieve disease symptoms. Under the bundle damage theory synaptic neurotransmitter levels need to be established that are higher than the reference range of the population.

It is the mechanical damage to the postsynaptic neurons as suggested by the bundle damage theory and not the synaptic neurotransmitter levels that is the primary cause of monoamine disease. This subset is composed of about 88% of adult patients and 100% of the elderly patients with depressive symptoms—the nonresponders from the depression studies above.

Neurons are intended to function for life. Loss of a neuron to apoptosis is permanent, although in limited areas of the brain neurons may regenerate to replace the neurons that have undergone apoptosis.[58] As neurons go into apoptosis in the postsynaptic neuron and become completely nonfunctional they tend to go through an agonizing death where the electrical brilliance with which they function slowly fades until the electrical flow through the neuron regulating function decreases and stops over time.

The only way to increase neurotransmitter levels in the central nervous system is to administer amino acid precursors that cross the blood-brain barrier and are then synthesized into neurotransmitters. Increasing neurotransmitter levels in the synapse is analogous to increasing the voltage in an electrical wire, where by turning up the voltage you get more electricity out of the other end of the wire. Turning up the voltage increases the electrical potential (pressure) of the electrons entering a partially damaged wiring connection, leading to more electrons (electricity) flowing out of the other end. In the case of neurotransmitter disease where the neurons of the neuron bundles are damaged to the point that the electricity flowing out of the neuron bundles is diminished disease develops. Increasing neurotransmitter levels will effectively increase voltage in the remaining viable neurons in the bundle, causing electrical flow out of the damaged neuron bundles to increase to the point that normal regulation and/or control is once again observed. In this state, from a clinical standpoint, the symptoms of disease are under control.

ETIOLOGY OF BUNDLE DAMAGE

Bundles of monoamine neurons can be impaired from neurotoxin exposures, trauma, or biological insult.[56] Neurotoxin exposures are poorly defined and ongoing exposures are in contrast to the MPTP study model of Parkinsonism. The most comprehensive listing located reveals 1179 known neurotoxins.[39] Susceptibility of individuals based on genetic predisposition, environmental influences, synergy between chemicals, or other predisposing factors suggests that some individuals may experience neurotoxicity from many unlisted substances and at lower than threshold doses of known neurotoxins, and needs to be considered. Under the bundle damage theory it is assumed that neurotoxins are the leading cause of monoamine bundle damage leading to the following speculation:

The bundle damage's theory of repeated insult during a lifetime can explain the lack of efficacy seen in the treatment of elderly with reuptake inhibitors who presumably have greater cumulative lifetime effects from neurotoxins and other events that cause neuron damage. In the end these patients need to have neurotransmitter levels established that are much higher than can be achieved with reuptake inhibitors alone.

With repeated insult more damage occurs, which is cumulative. When the damage is at the point where the neurotransmitter levels needed to control disease symptoms cannot be achieved with the use of reuptake inhibitors alone, from a clinical standpoint it appears that the drug is not working. This may explain why about 90% of adults treated with reuptake inhibitors achieve results no better than placebo.

The bundle damage theory may also explain why developed countries have a higher rate of depression as the population is exposed at a higher rate to neurotoxins.

Since insult exposure may be ongoing in patients with depression, optimizing nutritional status is important. Improving neuronal ability to minimize and recover from toxic insult forms the basis of the antioxidant nutrients in Chapter 28, "Parkinson's Disease," and the membrane-stabilizing nutrients in Chapter 24, "Seizures."

IV. PHARMACOLOGY

AMINO ACIDS

Treatment of depression, as well as any other monoamine neurotransmitter diseases, is not possible through the direct administration of monoamine neurotransmitters. This is due to the fact that monoamine neurotransmitters do not cross the blood-brain barrier, as depicted in Figure 29.1.[2–5] The only way to increase the levels of central nervous system monoamine neurotransmitter molecules is to provide amino acid precursors, which cross the blood-brain barrier and are synthesized into their respective neurotransmitters by presynaptic neurons.[6,7]

REUPTAKE INHIBITOR DEPLETION OF MONOAMINE

The National Institute of Drug Abuse presents a detailed discussion on its website on how reuptake inhibitors deplete neurotransmitters.[22] Medicines used to treat depression are not the only drugs that block reuptake; cocaine and amphetamines block reuptake as well.[22] Reuptake inhibitors block

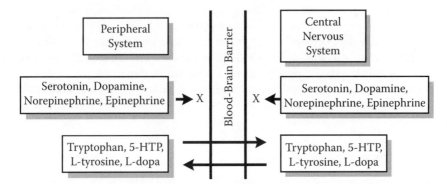

FIGURE 29.1 The monoamine neurotransmitters serotonin, dopamine, norepinephrine, and epinephrine do not cross the blood-brain barrier; therefore, peripheral administration of these neurotransmitters will not increase central nervous system neurotransmitter levels. The amino acid precursors of these neurotransmitters do cross the blood-brain barrier. The way to increase central nervous system neurotransmitter levels is through administration of amino acid precursors.

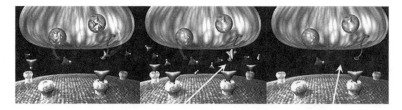

FIGURE 29.2 The effects of reuptake inhibitors on neurotransmitter levels, reuptake inhibition may deplete neurotransmitters. In the left picture, prior to treatment, neurotransmitter levels are not high enough to prevent symptoms of disease. In the center picture, reuptake is blocked, neurotransmitters move from the vesicles of the presynaptic neuron to the synapse. In the right picture, the neurotransmitters are depleted, the increase in synaptic neurotransmitter levels results in an increase in MAO and COMT metabolism. (From [22].)

the uptake of neurotransmitters back into the presynaptic neuron. In doing so, synaptic levels are increased. As synaptic neurotransmitter levels rise, relief of symptoms is observed.

Monoamine Oxidase (MAO) and the Catecholamine O-Methyl Transferase (COMT) enzymes metabolize serotonin, dopamine, norepinephrine, and epinephrine. The monoamine neurotransmitters are relatively stable and are not metabolized until they come in contact with the MAO and COMT enzymes. When neurotransmitters are in the vesicles of the presynaptic neuron, they are not exposed to metabolism by the MAO and COMT enzymes; they are safe and stable. When neurotransmitters are in the synapse between the presynaptic and postsynaptic neuron, they are exposed to enzymatic metabolism, which leads to the depletion of neurotransmitters if proper levels of amino acid precursors are not administered to compensate for this process.[24]

In depressed patients, synaptic neurotransmitter levels are not high enough to prevent disease symptoms, as illustrated in Figure 29.2. Treatment with reuptake inhibitors leads to a decrease in presynaptic neurotransmitter levels (where they are safe from enzymatic metabolism) and an increase in the number of neurotransmitters in the synapse. The blocking of neurotransmitter reuptake increases synaptic levels and the probability that neurotransmitters will experience enzymatic metabolism.

With regard to Figure 29.2, the net effect of enzymatic metabolism is the depletion of neurotransmitter levels in the central nervous system. Neurotransmitters do not cross the blood-brain barrier. Therefore, the only way to increase central nervous system levels or to prevent the overall depletion of neurotransmitters when administering prescription drugs that block reuptake is to provide amino acid precursors, which are then synthesized into neurotransmitters. Administering L-tyrosine (not phenylalanine or n-acetyl-tyrosine) or L-dopa is the only way to predictably raise dopamine, norepinephrine, and epinephrine. Administering tryptophan or 5-hydroxytryptophan (5-HTP) is the only way to predictably raise serotonin levels in the central nervous system. It is noted that 5-HTP, L-dopa, and tyrosine are available in the United States without a prescription. The ability of tryptophan to raise serotonin levels is limited because it is a rate-limited reaction.

The effects of neurotransmitter depletion by drugs may have far-ranging implications. It has been found in studies that depletion of serotonin by drugs may also lead to a reduction in the number of serotonin synapses in the hippocampus.[43]

Monoamine Synthesis From Amino Acids

The synthesis of serotonin and the catecholamines is illustrated in Figure 29.3. Peripheral administration of only 5-HTP (serotonin system) or only L-dopa (dopamine system) will decrease the synthesis of the other system (dopamine or serotonin respectively).[57] With administration of only one amino acid precursor, the administered amino acid precursor dominates the enzyme and compromises proper synthesis of the other system's neurotransmitters. This is due to the fact that the same enzyme catalyzes the conversion of 5-HTP to serotonin and L-dopa to dopamine everywhere in the body.

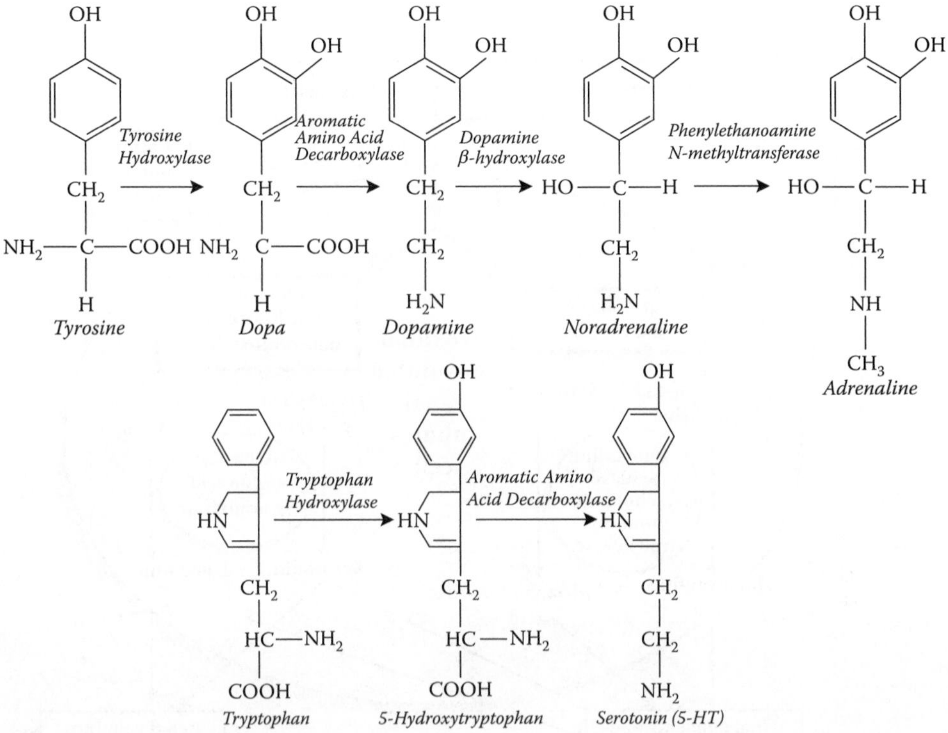

FIGURE 29.3 The synthesis of serotonin, dopamine, norepinephrine, and epinephrine from amino acid precursors.

The aromatic L-amino acid decarboxylase enzyme is also known as 5-HTP decarboxylase, L-dopa decarboxylase, and the general decarboxylase enzyme. Its function is illustrated in a kidney in Figure 29.4 (bottom right). The implications of this fact are profound.[10] The administration of only 5-HTP or L-dopa will compete with and inhibit the synthesis of the opposite precursor (dopamine and serotonin, respectively) at the enzyme.

In patients with Parkinson's, the long-term administration of L-dopa with insufficient serotonin precursors will result in depression. The literature is very clear that this depression is a serotonin-dependent depression, which responds optimally to the most serotonin specific reuptake inhibitor, citalopram.[11]

AMINO ACIDS AND MONOAMINE METABOLISM

The MAO and COMT enzymes metabolize serotonin and the catecholamines, as illustrated in the kidney in Figure 29.4 (bottom left).[12] The implications are that the levels of these two enzyme systems are not static; they fluctuate in response to changing neurotransmitter levels. When neurotransmitter levels are increased, enzymatic activity also increases.[14,23-26]

If you administer L-dopa or 5-HTP, the activity of MAO and COMT increases due to the increase in dopamine and serotonin levels, respectively. When L-dopa is administered without 5-HTP; both dopamine and serotonin will be subjected to increases in metabolism by these two enzyme systems. However, serotonin will not experience an increase in production, which leads to further depletion. The same rule is true of 5-HTP administered without the use of dopamine precursors. In sum, the administration of 5-HTP or L-dopa that is improperly balanced with the amino acid precursors of the other system will deplete the other system due to the increased metabolism of MAO and COMT, decreased synthesis, and uptake competition (as covered in the next section).

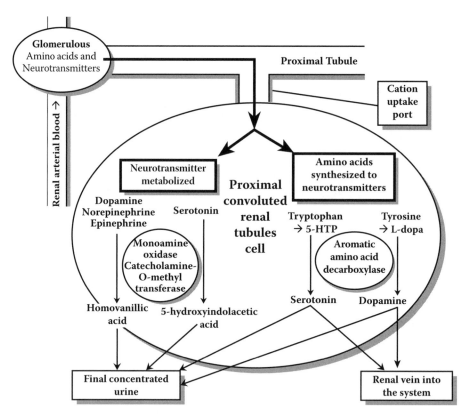

FIGURE 29.4 The neurotransmitters and amino acids are filtered at the glomerulous are uptaked in the proximal renal tubules by the cation ports of the proximal convoluted renal tubule cells. The proximal convoluted renal tubule cells then further filter the neurotransmitters and amino acids into separate areas where the neurotransmitters are metabolized and the amino acids are synthesized into new neurotransmitters that are then either excreted into the urine or secreted into the system via the renal veins.

AMINO ACID UPTAKE

In order for the synthesis of monoamine neurotransmitters to occur, the amino acid precursors must undergo uptake into the cells performing synthesis. This process occurs in numerous places throughout the body including the central nervous system, kidneys, liver, gastrointestinal tract, mesentery, lungs, and peripheral nerves. The "cation uptake ports" found in the proximal convoluted renal tubule cells are a prototype for amino acid uptake (see Figure 29.4 at the top center).[16]

Neurotransmitters synthesized by the kidneys are the source of urinary serotonin and catecholamines.[16–19] Serotonin and the catecholamines are synthesized by the kidneys, then excreted into the urine or secreted into the system via the renal veins.[20] Competition occurs for the uptake of amino acids. Administration of only L-dopa inhibits uptake of 5-HTP.[44] Administration of only 5-HTP has the same effect on L-dopa uptake.

V. TREATMENT

It is not possible to design a diet where the patient can obtain enough amino acids to affect even level 1 amino acid dosing (see Table 29.1), since the amino acid dosing requirement is higher than can be achieved with diet alone. Amino acid precursors of serotonin and dopamine have two primary applications. First, proper use of amino acid precursors will keep drugs that work with neurotransmitters

TABLE 29.1
Amino Acid Dosing Protocol (milligrams of 5-HTP/milligrams of tyrosine)

LEVEL	AM	NOON	4 PM	7 PM
1	150/1500		150/1500	
2	150/1500	150/1500	300/1500	
3	150/1500	150/1500	300/1500	300/1500

Note: If relief of symptoms is not obtained with level 3 dosing, obtain urinary neurotransmitter testing. Use of proper levels of cofactors and sulfur amino acids is required for optimal results.

from depleting neurotransmitters, thus allowing the drugs to keep functioning and functioning optimally. Second, proper use of amino acids can also serve as the treatment modality.

The generic protocol developed for treatment of neurotransmitter dysfunction disease relating to the catecholamine system and/or serotonin system involves the use of tyrosine, 5-HTP, and cofactors. Results do not appear to be dependent on taking the amino acids with or without food. The following cofactors need to be used along with the amino acid precursors:

- Vitamin C 1000 mg/day
- Vitamin B6 75 mg/day
- Calcium 500 mg/day

In addition:

- Cysteine 4500 mg/day in equally divided doses
- Selenium 400 μg/day
- Folic acid 2000 to 3000 μg/day

should also be used to prevent depletion of the methionine-homocysteine cycle (Figure 29.5) by L-dopa and presumably by L-tyrosine from which L-dopa is synthesized. Administration of L-dopa leads to depletion of S-adenosyl-methionine (SAMe), a component of the methionine-homocysteine cycle that is the one carbon methyl donor of the body; proper levels of SAMe are needed in order for norepinephrine to be methylated to epinephrine. Long-term use of L-dopa without proper administration of amino acids of the methionine-homocysteine cycle leads to depletion of epinephrine.[37]

There is a "total loss" of sulfur amino acid associated with treatment of Parkinsonism with L-dopa as evidenced by the loss of total glutathione that occurs.[41]

Glutathione is synthesized in a side chain reaction off the methionine-homocysteine cycle (see Figure 29.5). The loss of total glutathione leads to a state where the body's most powerful detoxifying agent (glutathione) is no longer functioning properly and is unable to neutralize further toxic insult, leaving the patient in a state where more toxic damage is facilitated. All patients taking L-dopa and/or L-tyrosine need to be supplemented with adequate levels of sulfur amino acid to prevent depletion of the methionine-homocysteine cycle, depletion of glutathione, depletion of epinephrine, and the other components dependent on the methionine-homocysteine cycle. While administration of any of the sulfur amino acids in the cycle is adequate if the dosing is high enough, cysteine is chosen since it costs only about 11 cents per day wholesale.

Selenium 400 μg/day needs to be administered with cysteine to prevent cysteine (sulfur amino acids) from creating an environment that contributes to central nervous system neurotoxicity from methylmercury. Administration of cysteine can potentially facilitate concentration of methylmercury

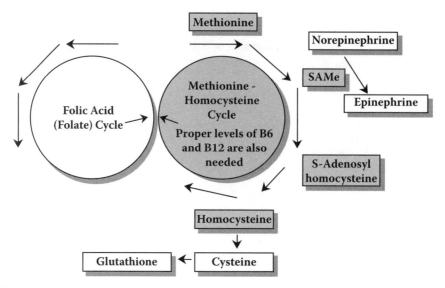

FIGURE 29.5 The methionine–homocysteine cycle.

into the central nervous system.[46] Selenium binds irreversibly to methylmercury in the central nervous system, rendering the methylmercury biologically inactive and nontoxic.[47]

Folic acid is required in order to provide optimal function of the folic acid cycle, which in turn prevents hyperhomocysteinemia from preventing the methionine-homocysteine cycle from functioning properly. As noted previously, without proper administration of amino acids of the methionine-homocysteine cycle there will be depletion of epinephrine. It would appear the second factor driving epinephrine levels beyond methionine-homocysteine cycle depletion is hyperhomocysteinemia. It can take 3 to 6 months for hyperhomocysteinemia to return to normal when proper levels of folate, vitamin B6, and vitamin B12 are provided for. It appears to be no coincidence that it can take 3 to 6 months for epinephrine levels to return to normal—a fact that appears to parallel homocysteine improvement.

When the goal of treatment is to prevent depletion of neurotransmitters by prescription drugs or in associated situations where prescription drugs are no longer working effectively during treatment due to the neurotransmitter levels falling too low from depletion due to circumstance set up by the drug,[45] the patient should be placed on the level 1 amino acid dosing (see Table 29.1) along with the prescription drug, cysteine, selenium, and folate. While amino acid precursors when used alone and properly are highly effective, a drug/amino acid combination may be desirable with severe disease, such as the suicidal patient, the catatonic patient, or the patient unable to take part in normal day-to-day functions such as work. Supplementing with amino acid precursors allows reuptake inhibitors to continue to function optimally without tachyphylaxis.

When amino acids are used as the initial therapy, start all patients on the level 1 dosing protocol of Table 29.1 along with cofactors and proper methionine-homocysteine cycle support at the first visit. Patients should return in 1 week, at which time focus on how the patient's symptoms were the previous day. Asking about the previous day's symptoms is more indicative of changes in the system brought about by amino acid therapy since it takes 3 to 5 days for the full effects of starting or changing an amino acid dosing to be displayed.

If symptoms are not fully under control in 1 week, increase to the level 2 dosing along with cofactors and proper sulfur amino acid support and instruct the patient to return in 1 week. At the third visit, if symptoms are not under control, increase to the level 3 dosing along with cofactors and proper sulfur amino acid support and have the patient return to the clinic in 1 week. If in 1 week symptoms are not under control, continue the level 3 dosing and obtain a urinary neurotransmitter test of the caliber provided by a laboratory under the direction of a hospital-based laboratory pathologist.[40] Follow the amino acid dosing recommendations generated after review of testing preformed under the supervision of a board-certified laboratory pathologist. Patients should return in 1 week to discuss results and amino acid dosing changes that may be needed. Any time an amino acid dosing change occurs, patients should return in 1 week to evaluate the results. Over 60% of patients tested needed only one neurotransmitter test. This is consistent with complete resolution of symptoms after adjusting the amino acid dosing in accordance with the consultant recommendations on the test.

When treating depression, if amino acid dosing changes establish both the serotonin and dopamine in the phase 3 therapeutic range (see urinary neurotransmitter testing in the following) and no relief of symptoms is achieved, consider the possibility of depressive bipolar disorder. Under treatment with the amino acid protocol approximately 2% of patients are found to suffer from depressive bipolar disorder that has not been previously diagnosed. The primary care physician at this point should continue the amino acids and initiate a psychiatric referral in order to affect starting of a mood-stabilizing bipolar drug. It is noted that as long as the amino acids are continued, over 99% of patients started on mood-stabilizing drugs such as lithium, Depakote, or Lamictil find complete resolution of depression on the standard starting dose.

VI. SAFETY

The following is a side effect profile developed from approximately 50 patient-years of databased treatment in hand at NeuroResearch Clinics, Inc. The following results were obtained from patients taking only amino acids with no prescription drugs:

Dry mouth	34 (2.1%)
Insomnia	14 (0.9%)
Headache	12 (0.7%)
Nausea	10 (0.6%)
Dizziness	6 (0.4%)
Constipation	6 (0.4%)

All other side effects were reported at a rate of less than 1 in 500 visits (0.02%). No irreversible side effects were noted.

Amino acid precursors are safe to administer with any prescription drug, but amino acid precursors can also cause the side effects of the prescription drugs to be displayed. Any side effect associated with the drug can be triggered. For example, a patient was taking an SSRI with the side effect of malignant neuroleptic syndrome listed. As the amino acids were started, the patient developed new onset malignant neuroleptic syndrome. When drug side effects occur, it is necessary to manage the situation as you would with any other prescription drug side effect, which in general means decreasing or stopping the drug, not the amino acid.

With regards to pregnancy there is nothing in the literature indicating that the amino acid precursors are a problem. Nor is there anything in the literature indicating studies have been performed indicating they are safe. In this light it is recommended that amino acid precursors not be used in the first trimester of pregnancy.

VII. SYSTEMS PRIORITY

The serotonin and/or catecholamine system has a role, either directly or indirectly, in controlling most of the other systems and functions in the body. For example, cortisol synthesis is controlled in part by norepinephrine. Hormone synthesis is dependent on norepinephrine. The sympathetic nervous system is controlled by norepinephrine. Other neurotransmitter systems are partially controlled by the serotonin and/or catecholamine systems. For example, the gamma aminobutyric acid

(GABA) neurotransmitter system is associated with control of anxiety and panic attacks. Yet when the serotonin and/or catecholamine neurotransmitter levels are brought to proper levels, as confirmed by lab testing, these diseases may be fully under control. This would indicate control of GABA by the serotonin/catecholamine system even though at this time we have been unable to identify a chemical pathway for such in the literature.

VIII. PATIENT EVALUATION: URINARY NEUROTRANSMITTER TESTING MONOAMINES IN THE KIDNEYS

There is no correlation between baseline urinary neurotransmitter testing and urinary neurotransmitter phases once the patient is taking amino acid precursors. It is not necessary or even useful to measure baseline urinary neurotransmitters in treatment.[40]

Urinary monoamine neurotransmitters do not cross the blood-brain barrier.[2-5] Urinary monoamine neurotransmitters are not neurotransmitters filtered by the glomerulous of the kidneys and excreted into the urine. They are neurotransmitters that are synthesized by the kidneys and excreted into the urine or secreted into the system via the renal veins.[20] With simultaneous administration of serotonin and dopamine amino acid precursors, three phases of urinary neurotransmitter response have been identified on laboratory assay of the urine (see Figures 29.6 and 29.7). The three phases of response apply to both serotonin and dopamine. In all the life forms tested that have kidneys along with serotonin and catecholamine systems, the three phases of urinary neurotransmitter response exist.[40] In reviewing the literature it would appear that the three phases of urinary response to neurotransmitters were present in previous writings but were not identified as such. For example, a 1999 article notes that administration of L-dopa can increase urinary dopamine levels (phase 3) and decrease urinary serotonin levels (phase 1).[42]

The goal of treatment is to establish both urinary serotonin and dopamine levels in the phase 3 therapeutic range. To determine the phase of serotonin and dopamine with certainty requires two urinary neurotransmitter tests to be performed with the patient simultaneously taking a different amino acid dosing of dopamine and serotonin amino acid precursors on each test and comparing the results. Not all patients will need to have the urinary serotonin and dopamine levels in the phase 3 therapeutic range for relief of symptoms. In many cases, adjusting the amino acids so that the patient moves closer to the phase 3 therapeutic range of urinary serotonin and dopamine induces relief of symptoms. Then, no further amino acid adjustments or testing are needed unless disease symptoms return. If the patient misses one or more amino acid doses in the week prior to testing, wait until 1 week has passed with the patient properly taking all of their amino acids.

In phase 1, neurotransmitters synthesized by the kidneys are inappropriately excreted into the urine instead of being secreted into the system via the renal vein where they are needed (see Figures 29.6 and 29.7). Increasing the amino acid dose in phase 1 will correct the problem of inappropriate neurotransmitter excretion. The amino acid precursor dosing of serotonin and dopamine, where the individual patient is in phase 1, varies widely in the population. The level at which the urinary serotonin is no longer in phase 1 ranges from 37.5 mg of 5-HTP per day to 3000 mg of 5-HTP per day. The level at which the urinary dopamine is no longer in phase 1 ranges from no L-dopa (with the use of L-tyrosine only in some patients) to 5400 mg of L-dopa per day in the patients not under treatment for Parkinsonism or restless leg syndrome.

Administration of proper levels of tyrosine with L-dopa is known as a "tyrosine base." Proper use of the tyrosine base greatly reduces wild fluctuations in dopamine levels found with administration of L-dopa alone and greatly decreases the need for L-dopa. It is postulated that the tyrosine hydroxylase enzyme is not completely shut down with the administration of L-dopa, leading to fluctuations in the L-dopa produced from tyrosine synthesized to L-dopa then dopamine, which ultimately causes fluctuations of dopamine. By providing ample tyrosine with administration of L-dopa, these fluctuations of dopamine cease and the overall dosing needs of L-dopa decrease.

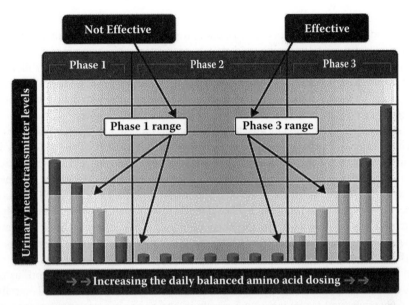

FIGURE 29.6 The three phases of urinary neurotransmitter excretion in response to amino acid dosing. The horizontal axis is not labeled with specific amounts; it reflects the general trend seen in the population. Amino acid dosing needs are highly individualized. The dosing level needed to inflect into the next level varies greatly throughout the general population. For example, some patients inflect into phase 3 on 37.5 mg of 5-HTP per day, while others need as high as 3000 mg/day. (From [40].)

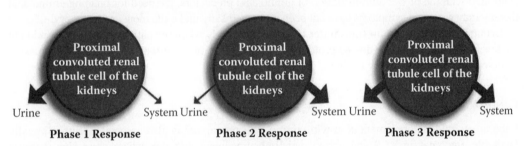

FIGURE 29.7 The three phases of urinary response to amino acid dosing. Two urinary neurotransmitter tests are required to determine the phase with certainty. PHASE 1: In phase 1, as the amino acid dosing increases or decreases the urinary serotonin or dopamine decreases or increases respectively. In phase 1, there is inappropriate excretion of neurotransmitters into the urine instead of the system where they are needed. PHASE 2: In phase 2, as the amino acid dosing increases or decreases the urinary serotonin or dopamine is low (<800 μgr/gr creatinine for serotonin or <300 μgr/gr creatinine for dopamine). In phase 2, there is no inappropriate excretion of neurotransmitters into the urine. The neurotransmitters are being excreted appropriately into the system and the urine. PHASE 3: In phase 3, as the amino acid dosing increases or decreases the urinary serotonin or dopamine increases or decreases respectively. In phase 3, there are adequate systemic serotonin and dopamine levels. The excess serotonin and dopamine are appropriately excreted into the urine.

By increasing the amino acid dosing of serotonin and dopamine precursors above the dosing of phase 1, the phase 2 response is observed (see Figures 29.6 and 29.7). In phase 2, urinary neurotransmitter levels are low (<475 micrograms dopamine per gram of creatinine or <800 micrograms serotonin per gram of creatinine; the neurotransmitter-creatinine ratio compensates for dilution of the urine) and the inappropriate excretion of neurotransmitters into the urine has ceased. When in phase 2, neurotransmitters are being appropriately secreted into the system and not into the urine.

The model used to explain phase 2 is, "inappropriate excretion of neurotransmitters has now ceased as the amino acid precursor dosing is increased and the system is now filling up appropriately."

As serotonin and dopamine amino acid precursors are increased above phase 1 and phase 2 levels, all patients enter the phase 3 response (see Figures 29.6 and 29.7). Further increases in the amino acid dosing lead to increases in urinary dopamine and serotonin neurotransmitter levels if they are in phase 3. Phase 3 represents appropriate secretion into the system and appropriate excretion of excess neurotransmitters synthesized by the kidneys into the urine.

In the case of chronic depression, research has shown neurotransmitter levels need to be established at levels that are in phase 3 and higher than the reference range reported by the laboratory in order to achieve optimal relief of group symptoms.[40] In the case of serotonin, the reference range reported by the research lab is 48.9 to 194.9 micrograms of serotonin per gram of creatinine. The therapeutic range of urinary serotonin for the treatment of chronic depression is defined as 800 to 2400 micrograms of serotonin per gram of creatinine in phase 3. The reference range reported by the research lab of urinary dopamine reported by the laboratory is 40 to 390 micrograms of dopamine per gram of creatinine. The therapeutic range of urinary dopamine for the treatment of chronic depression is defined as 475 to 775 micrograms of dopamine per gram of creatinine in phase 3.

It would appear that in depression, the same mechanism of action may be at work as is found in Parkinson's disease. There is damage to dopamine and/or serotonin neuron bundles controlling affect, which can be compensated for by increasing serotonin and dopamine neurotransmitter levels higher than is normally found in the system. Just as with Parkinson's disease, the bundle damage in chronic depression is permanent. In most patients simply returning neurotransmitter levels to normal or the reference range reported by the lab, as suggested by the monoamine theory, will not lead to relief of symptoms. As with Parkinsonism, treatment of depression may require long-term use of amino acids to control symptoms. After symptoms associated with monoamine neurotransmitter diseases are controlled with the proper administration of amino acid precursors, the need for ongoing amino acid therapy may present if symptoms have not been addressed fully under the monoamine theory.

Urinary monoamine neurotransmitter testing is used only when the patient has not responded to the levels 1 through 3 of the dosing protocol. Over 80% of patients will achieve relief of depression symptoms without laboratory testing.

Generalizability

Laboratory-guided supplementation with amino acid precursors is also associated with clinically favorable outcomes in RLS and peroxismal limb movement disorder, where dopamine agonists are also the first line of therapy and clinical response is readily observable by patients and documented with sleep studies. The dosing level of L-dopa at which dopamine is no longer in phase 1, in patients not suffering from RLS, ranges from 0 milligrams of L-dopa per day to 6000 mg of L-dopa per day. With a proper "tyrosine base" in place, L-dopa dosing in these patients ranges from 10 to 1040 mg/day.

IX. CONCLUSIONS

The bundle damage theory creates a framework by which to offer patients new treatments for clinical depression. The theory underscores the importance of minimizing toxic exposures, through avoidance where possible, through diminished uptake, and through adequate nutrients. Similarly patients who have inadequate substrate for neurotransmitter synthesis may need cofactors, nutrients involved in sulfur pathways, and amino acid precursors. Patients may also receive benefit from amino acid precursors beyond what can be obtained from diet alone.

There are three primary considerations in the use of amino acids for treating depression. First, proper levels of amino acids should be administered with the drugs to prevent depletion of neurotransmitters. Second, proper use of amino acids will keep the drug functioning properly, avoiding tachyphylaxis. Third, the use of amino acids may cause a drug side effect to become active. In summary, amino acids hold more therapeutic potential and less potential for harm when administration is physician guided.

REFERENCES

1. Hirschfeld RM. History and evolution of the monoamine hypothesis of depression. *J Clin Psychiatry.* 2000; 61 Suppl 6:4–6.
2. Pyle AC, Argyropoulos SV, Nutt DJ. The role of serotonin in panic: evidence from tryptophan depletion studies. *Acta Neuropsychiatrica.* 2004; 16:79–84.
3. Verde G, Oppizzi G, Colussi G, Cremascoli G, Botalla L, Muller EE, Silvestrini F, Chiodini PG, Liuzzi A. Effect of dopamine infusion on plasma levels of growth hormone in normal subjects and in agromegalic patients. *Clin Endocrinol (Oxf).* 1976 Jul; 5(4):419–423.
4. Gozzi A, Ceolin L, Schwarz A, Reese T, Bertani S, Crestan V, Bifone A. A multimodality investigation of cerebral hemodynamics and autoregulation in pharmacological MRI. *Magn Reson Imaging.* 2007 Apr; 25:826–833.
5. Ziegler MG, Aung M, Kennedy B. Sources of human urinary epinephrine. *Kidney Int.* 1997; 51: 324–327.
6. Birdsall TC. 5-Hydroxytryptophan: a clinically-effective serotonin precursor. *Altern Med Rev.* 1998 Aug; 3(4):271–280.
7. Barker R. Adrenal grafting for Parkinson's disease: a role for substance P. *Int J Neurosci.* 1989 May; 46(1–2):47–51.
8. Matsubara K, Aoyama K, Suno M, Awaya T. N-methylation underlying Parkinson's disease. *Neurotoxicol Teratol.* 2002 Sep–Oct; 24(5):593.
9. Nicotra A, Parvez S. Apoptotic molecules and MPTP-induced cell death. *Neurotoxicol Teratol.* 2002 Sep–Oct; 24(5):599.
10. Verbeek MM, Geurtz PB, Willemsen MA, Wevers RA. Aromatic L-amino acid decarboxylase enzyme activity in deficient patients and heterozygotes. *Mol Genet Metab.* 2007 Apr; 90(4):363–369. Epub 2007 Jan 19.
11. Menza M, Marin H, Kaufman K, Mark M, Lauritano M. Citalopram treatment of depression in Parkinson's disease: the impact on anxiety, disability, and cognition. *J Neuropsychiatry Clin Neurosci.* 2004 Summer; 16(3):315–319.
12. Wang Y, Berndt TJ, Gross JM, Peterson MA, So MJ, Knox FG. Effect of inhibition of MAO and COMT on intrarenal dopamine and serotonin and on renal function. *Am J Physiol Regul Integr Comp Physiol.* 2001 Jan; 280(1):R248–254.
13. Davis TL, Brughitta G, Baronti F, Mouradian MM. Acute effects of pulsatile levodopa administration on central dopamine pharmacodynamics. *Neurology.* 1991 May; 41(5):630–633.
14. Sakumoto T, Sakai K, Jouvet M, Kimura H, Maeda T. 5-HT immunoreactive hypothalamic neurons in rat and cat after 5-HTP administration. *Brain Res Bull.* 1984 Jun; 12(6):721–733.
15. Gründemann D, Köster S, Kiefer N, Breidert T, Engelhardt M, Spitzenberger F, Obermüller N, Schömig E. Transport of monoamine transmitters by the organic cation transporter Type 2, OCT2 *J Biol Chem.* 1998 Nov 20; 273(47):30915–30920.
16. Wa TC, Burns NJ, Williams BC, Freestone S, Lee MR. Blood and urine 5-hydroxytryptophan and 5-hydroxytryptamine levels after administration of two 5-hydroxytryptamine precursors in normal man. *Br J Clin Pharmacol.* 1995 Mar; 39(3):327–329.
17. Zimlichman R, Levinson PD, Kelly G, Stull R, Keiser HR, Goldstein DS. Derivation of urinary dopamine from plasma dopa. *Clin Sci (Lond).* 1988 Nov; 75(5):515–520.
18. Buu NT, Duhaime J, Kuchel O. Handling of dopamine and dopamine sulfate by isolated perfused rat kidney. *Am J Physiol.* 1986 Jun; 250(6 Pt 2):F975–979.
19. Ziegler MG, Aung M, Kennedy B. Sources of human urinary epinephrine. *Kidney Int.* 1997 Jan; 51(1):324–327.
20. Ball SG, Gunn IG, Douglas IH. Renal handling of dopa, dopamine, norepinephrine, and epinephrine in the dog. *Am J Physiol.* 1982 Jan; 242(1):F56–62.
21. Druml W, Hübl W, Roth E, Lochs H. Utilization of tyrosine-containing dipeptides and N-acetyl-tyrosine in hepatic failure. *Hepatology.* 1995 Apr; 21(4):923–928.
22. The Neurobiology of Ecstasy (MDMA) National Institute of Drug Abuse (NIDA), slides 9 through 11. http://www.nida.nih.gov/pubs/teaching/Teaching4/Teaching.html.

23. Meszaros Z, Borcsiczky D, Mate M, Tarcali J, Szombathy T, Tekes K, Magyar K. Platelet MAO-B activity and serotonin content in patients with dementia: effect of age, medication, and disease. *Neurochemical Research.* June 1998:863–868.

24. Lundquist I, Panagiotidis G, Stenstrom A. Effect of L-dopa administration on islet monoamine oxidase activity and glucose-induced insulin release in the mouse. *Pancreas.* 1991 Sep; 6(5):522–527.

25. Robinson DS, Sourkes TL, Nies A, Harris LS, Spector S, Bartlett DL, Kaye IS. Monoamine metabolism in human brain. *Arch Gen Psychiatry.* 1977 Jan; 34(1):89–92.

26. Tunbridge EM, Bannerman DM, Sharp T, Harrison PJ. Catechol-O-Methyltransferase inhibition improves set-shifting performance and elevates stimulated dopamine release in the rat prefrontal cortex. *J of Neuroscience.* 2004 June 9; 24(23):5331–5335.

27. Roose SP, Sackeim HA, Krishnan KR, Pollock BG, Alexopoulos G, Lavretsky H, Katz IR, Hakkarainen H; Old-Old Depression Study Group. Antidepressant pharmacotherapy in the treatment of depression in the very old: a randomized, placebo-controlled trial. *Am J Psychiatry.* 2004 Nov; 161(11):2050–2059.

28. Wagner KD, Robb AS, Findling RL, Jin J, Gutierrez MM, Heydorn WE. A Randomized, Placebo-Controlled Trial of Citalopram for the Treatment of Major Depression in Children and Adolescents. *Am J Psychiatry.* 2004 June; 161:1079–1083.

29. Bose A, Li D, Gandhi C. Escitalopram in the acute treatment of depressed patients aged 60 years or older. *Am J Geriatr Psychiatry* 2008 Jan; 16:14–20.

30. Schneider LS, Nelson JC, Clary CM, Newhouse P, Krishnan KR, Shiovitz T, Weihs K; Sertraline Elderly Depression Study Group. An 8-week multicenter, parallel-group, double-blind, placebo-controlled study of sertraline in elderly outpatients with major depression. *Am J Psychiatry.* 2003 Jul; 160(7):1277–1285.

31. Posternak MA, Zimmerman M. Dual reuptake inhibitors incur lower rates of tachyphylaxis than selective serotonin reuptake inhibitors: a retrospective study. *J Clin Psychiatry.* 2005; 66(6):705–707.

32. *Mental Health and Substance Abuse Facts and Figures: Conquering Depression.* World Health Organization 2008.

33. Ustün TB, Ayuso-Mateos JL, Chatterji S, Mathers C, Murray CJ. Global burden of depressive disorders in the year 2000. *Br J Psychiatry.* 2004 May; 184:386–392.

34. *Mental Health.* Pan American Health Organization World Health Organization 43rd Directing Council July 20, 2001.

35. Einarson, TR. Evidence based review of escitalopram in treating major depressive disorder in primary care. *Int Clin Psychopharmacol.* 2004 Sep; 19(5):305–310.

36. Meyer JH, Ginovart N, Boovariwala A, Sagrati S, Hussey D, Garcia A, Young T, Praschak-Rieder N, Wilson AA, Houle S. Elevated Monoamine oxidase A levels in the brain. *Arch Gen Psychiatry.* 2006; 63:1209–1216.

37. Lo CM, Kwok ML, Wurtman RJ. O-methylation and decarboxylation of alpha-methyldopa in brain and spinal cord: depletion of S-adenosylmethionine and accumulation of metabolites in catecholaminergic neurons. *Neuropharmacology.* 1976 Jul; 15(7):395–402.

38. Crawford MJ. Depression: international intervention for a global problem. *Br J Psychiatry.* 2004; 184:379–380.

39. *Polluting Our future: Chemical Pollution in the U.S. That Affects Child Development and Learning.* In September of 2000 under the joint efforts of The National Environmental Trust, Physicians for Social Responsibility, The Learning Disabilities Association of America.

40. DBS Labs neurotransmitter data base, Tom Uncini, MD hospital base dual board certified laboratory pathologist, medical director 8723 Falcon St. Duluth, MN 55808.

41. Zeevalk GD, Manzino L, Sonsalla PK, Bernard LP. Characterization of intracellular elevation of glutathione (GSH) with glutathione monoethyl ester and GSH in brain and neuronal cultures: relevance to Parkinson's disease. *Exp Neurol.* 2007 Feb; 203(2):512–520. Epub 2006 Oct 17.

42. Garcia NH, Berndt TJ, Tyce GM, Knox FG. Chronic oral L-DOPA increases dopamine and decreases serotonin excretions. *Am J Physiol.* 1999 Nov; 277(5 Pt 2):R1476–1480.

43. Matsukawa M, Ogawa M, Nakadate K, Maeshima T, Ichitani Y, Kawai N, Okadoa N. Serotonin and acetylcholine are crucial to maintain hippocampal synapses and memory acquisition in rats. *Neuroscience Letters.* 1997; 230:13–16.

44. Soares-da-Silva P, Pinto-do-O PC. Antagonistic actions of renal dopamine and 5-hydroxytryptamine: effects of amine precursors on the cell inward transfer and decarboxylation. *Br J Pharmacol.* 1996 Mar; 117(6):1187–1192.

45. Delgado PL, Moreno FA. Role of norepinephrine in depression. *J Clin Psychiatry.* 2000; 61 Suppl 1:5–12.

46. Aschner M. Brain, kidney and liver 203Hg-methyl mercury uptake in the rat: relationship to the neutral amino acid carrier. *Pharmacol Toxicol.* 1989 Jul; 65(1):17–20.
47. Cavalli S, Cardellicchio N. Direct determination of seleno-amino acids in biological tissues by anion-exchange separation and electrochemical detection. *J Chromatogr A.* 1995 Jul 7; 706(1–2):429–436.
48. Lew M. Overview of Parkinson's disease. *Pharmacotherapy.* 2007 Dec; 27(12 Pt 2):155S–160S.
49. Langston JW, Ballard P. Parkinsonism induced by 1-methyl-4-phenyl-1,2,3,6-tetrahydropyridine (MPTP): implications for treatment and the pathogenesis of Parkinson's disease. *Can J Neurol Sci.* 1984 Feb; 11(1 Suppl):160–165.
50. Kasper S, de Swart H, Friis Andersen H. Escitalopram in the treatment of depressed elderly patients. *Am J Geriatr Psychiatry.* 2005 Oct; 13(10):884–891.
51. Schneider LS, Nelson JC, Clary CM, Newhouse P, Krishnan KR, Shiovitz T, Weihs K; Sertraline Elderly Depression Study Group. An 8-week multicenter, parallel-group, double-blind, placebo-controlled study of sertraline in elderly outpatients with major depression. *Am J Psychiatry.* 2003 Jul; 160(7):1277–1285.
52. Roose SP, Sackeim HA, Krishnan KR, Pollock BG, Alexopoulos G, Lavretsky H, Katz IR, Hakkarainen H; Old-Old Depression Study Group. Antidepressant pharmacotherapy in the treatment of depression in the very old: a randomized, placebo-controlled trial. *Am J Psychiatry.* 2004 Nov; 161(11):2050–2059.
53. Nemeroff CB, Thase ME; EPIC 014 Study Group. A double-blind, placebo-controlled comparison of venlafaxine and fluoxetine treatment in depressed outpatients. *J Psychiatr Res.* 2007 Apr–Jun; 41(3–4): 351–9. Epub 2005 Sep 12.
54. Donnelly CL, Wagner KD, Rynn M, Ambrosini P, Landau P, Yang R, Wohlberg CJ. Sertraline in children and adolescents with major depressive disorder. *J Am Acad Child Adolesc Psychiatry.* 2006 Oct; 45(10):1162–1170.
55. Lépine JP, Caillard V, Bisserbe JC, Troy S, Hotton JM, Boyer P. A randomized, placebo-controlled trial of sertraline for prophylactic treatment of highly recurrent major depressive disorder. *Am J Psychiatry.* 2004 May; 161(5):836–842.
56. Takahashi M, Yamada T. Viral etiology for Parkinson's disease—a possible role of influenza A virus infection. *Jpn J Infect Dis.* 1999 Jun; 52(3):89–98.
57. Anupom Borah Æ Kochupurackal P. Mohanakumar. Long-Term L-DOPA Treatment Causes Indiscriminate Increase in Dopamine Levels at the Cost of Serotonin Synthesis in Discrete Brain Regions of Rats. *Cell Mol Neurobiol.* (2007) 27:985–996.
58. Nadareishvili Z, Hallenbeck J. Neuronal regeneration after stroke. *N Engl J Med.* 2003 Jun 5; 348(23): 2355–2356.

30 Sleep Disturbance

Jyotsna Sahni, M.D.

I. INTRODUCTION

Fifty to 70 million Americans have chronic problems with sleep. Adequate, quality sleep is crucial to good health yet there are many medical barriers to achieving it. Only 60% of physicians ask their patients about the quality of their sleep and only 20% of patients initiate a conversation about their sleep problems with their physicians.[1] The biologic basis of these disturbances may be influenced by nutrition. This chapter presents diet, food, and nutrient strategies as adjunct interventions in a primary care setting.

II. PHYSIOLOGY OF SLEEP

Sleep has five stages known as sleep architecture. Each stage lasts roughly 90 minutes. Stages 1 and 2 are light, while stages 3 and 4 are deep and restorative. During deep sleep the body synthesizes growth hormone, testosterone, thyroid hormone, and immune mediators. Stages 1 through 4 are followed by the fifth stage known as rapid eye movement (REM) sleep. REM accounts for approximately 25% of sleep. It is the dream cycle, the lightest sleep, during which time we consolidate memories.[2]

III. NUTRITION-RELATED CONSEQUENCES OF POOR SLEEP

Sleep deprivation is associated with weight gain. In a study of 924 participants between the ages of 18 and 91, researchers found that people who slept the least weighed the most.[3] Sleep deprivation may also lead to poor food choices that affect weight gain. In a study of 1203 individuals in the rural Midwest, the participants with less sleep ate more, chose fewer fruits and vegetables, and were less physically active.[4] The Wisconsin Sleep Cohort Study showed that participants with less sleep had reduced leptin and elevated ghrelin.[5] Since leptin signals satiety and ghrelin mediates hunger, the higher rates of obesity were attributed to excess caloric intake. In an epidemiological study of 2494 individuals born from 1981 to 1983 in Australia, sleeping problems at ages 2 to 4 years increased the odds of being obese in young adulthood by 90%.[6] A 13-year prospective trial of young adults in the United States also showed an association of short sleep duration and obesity.[7] The association between less sleep and body weight spans age groups but the underlying mechanisms remain poorly characterized.

Sleep duration and quality have emerged as predictors of levels of *Hemoglobin A1c*.[8] The Massachusetts Male Aging Study, a large prospective trial of 1564 men followed for 16 years, reported that those whose sleep duration was less than or equal to 5 and 6 hours were twice as likely to develop diabetes. Men reporting sleep duration greater than 8 hours were more than three times as likely to develop diabetes. Since this was a self-report, overall sleep time in this latter group is likely to represent duration in bed and could have represented men with Obstructive Sleep Apnea (OSA) who may spend more time in bed sleeping poorly. The authors suggest that the effects of sleep on diabetes could be mediated via changes in endogenous testosterone levels. The relative ratios of risk remained significant when adjusted for testosterone levels.[9] Short and long duration sleep times were associated with type 2 diabetes and impaired glucose tolerance in both men and women.[10] Collectively these studies suggest a novel approach to optimizing glycemic control: optimize sleep quantity and quality.

IV. MEDICAL CONDITIONS THAT DISRUPT SLEEP

INSOMNIA

Trouble sleeping is a common complaint of patients and is often a symptom of another medical problem. By working on the root problem, the insomnia is usually improved. There are two main kinds of insomnia. The first is called *sleep onset insomnia* where the onset of sleep is delayed beyond the average 5 to 20 minute sleep latency. Behavioral evaluation and techniques are often successful in treating sleep onset insomnia. The second form of insomnia, *maintenance insomnia*, involves difficulty staying asleep. Frequent awakenings usually require medical evaluation and treatment. Many patients suffer from both types of insomnia. Women have more trouble with insomnia than men.

There are multiple reasons for both types of insomnia. Many medications, prescribed or OTC, affect sleep. Avoiding these drugs, using them sparingly, or finding substitutes that do not have sleep side effects can help. The treatments throughout this book can decrease or eliminate the need for many medications (see Table 30.1).

ANXIETY AND DEPRESSION

Sleep, diet, and anxiety affect one another. Anxiety makes restful sleep difficult to achieve while difficulty sleeping can increase anxiety. Increased anxiety can lead to food cravings that can

---

TABLE 30.1

Substances That Keep People Awake

Alcohol

Nicotine

Cocaine

Caffeine

Decongestants like Sudafed™ (pseudophedrine)

Ritalin™ (methylphenidate), diet pills, or other stimulants

Ginkgo

Guarana

Siberian ginseng

Ephedrine, ephedra, and ma huang

Bitter orange

Yohimbe

Kola nut

Beta-blockers

Albuterol

Theophylline

Wellbutrin™ (bupropion)

Selective serotonin reuptake inhibitors

Prednisone and other steroids

---

interfere with sleep. Stimulants including foods with caffeine and high glycemic index carbohydrates should be avoided. Psychological and/or nutritional counseling can help many people reduce anxiety. Natural mind-body relaxation techniques such as meditation, yoga, and yogic breathing are shown to be effective at reducing anxiety.[11–13]

Depression and poor sleep are linked, but it is not always clear which comes first. It is interesting to note that sad mood, irritability, difficulty making decisions, and a sense of hopelessness and helplessness can be part of a diagnosis of clinical depression as well as of sleep deprivation. While early morning awakening can signal depression, insomnia itself can cause depression. Common antidepressants such as Prozac or Wellbutrin may have a negative impact on sleep. A study in patients with obstructive sleep apnea showed that treatment with continuous positive airway pressure (CPAP) caused symptoms of depression to abate.[14] Nutritional strategies for treating depression including vitamin D, omega-3 fats, and neurotransmitter precursors such as L-tryptophan may also improve sleep quality.[15]

Pain

Pain from arthritis, headaches, GERD, and fibromyalgia can make it hard to fall asleep and stay asleep. Sleep deprivation exacerbates pain.[16] Medications and nutritional therapies targeted at the cause of pain can be employed to reduce pain and maximize good sleep.

Bladder Problems

Patients commonly complain that frequent trips to the bathroom during the night disturb their sleep. A multiple sclerosis patient may have a neurogenic bladder. A urinary tract infection may cause urinary frequency, urgency, and dysuria. Prostatic hypertrophy can cause urinary frequency. Taking prescription diuretics before bed such as hydrochlorothiazide or Lasix for blood pressure or heart issues, or drinking a diuretic "dieter's" tea such as dandelion root may cause a patient to have urinary urgency during the night. Simply overdoing fluids before going to bed will result in a necessary and appropriate diuresis. Caffeinated beverages exacerbate this problem because the caffeine acts as a stimulant and also a mild diuretic. However, most patients misperceive that they're getting up to urinate when in fact they are awakening for another reason. It is therefore important for a physician to consider alternative explanations and treatable diagnoses.

Gastroesophageal Reflux

Consuming too much food close to bedtime can disturb sleep. Symptoms of gastroesophageal reflux disease (GERD) can significantly diminish sleep quality and quantity.[17,18] Shorter dinner-to-bed time has been associated with an increased risk of GERD. Ideally, a gap of 4 hours between eating and sleeping is recommended.[19]

Food Reactivities

Infants with cow milk intolerance may present with a disturbed sleep pattern, along with the more usual cutaneous, gastrointestinal, and respiratory problems.[20] Sleep disturbance secondary to food allergies has a broad biologic basis, but its prevalence and pathophysiology are understudied.

Menopausal Symptoms

The classic sleep disturbance of menopause involves falling asleep easily, but then being troubled with multiple awakenings throughout the night. The arousals may occur in isolation or be followed by a hot flash.[21] These multiple arousals can set the stage for sleep maintenance insomnia and depression. The frequent disturbances make other sleep problems such as restless leg syndrome worse. Treatment with isoflavones from soy foods and supplemental use of the herb black cohosh may help.[22,23] Sometimes hormone replacement therapy is necessary. Sleep disturbances in menopausal women should not be assumed to be a consequence of falling levels of hormones. There is a three-fold increase in obstructive sleep apnea in women immediately following the onset of menopause, and diagnostic evaluation with polysomnogram may be warranted.

OBSTRUCTIVE SLEEP APNEA (OSA)

OSA is characterized by disordered breathing during sleep. To make the diagnosis, apnea must last for at least 10 seconds five times in 1 hour of sleep. Patients may be unaware of their frequent arousals or may awake with an obvious "resuscitative" snort. Although 5% of the population has OSA, both physicians and patients alike are poorly aware of this common disorder. People with OSA are at higher risk for hypertension, heart attacks, arrhythmias, diabetes,[24] strokes,[25] and motor vehicle accidents. Most of the time, OSA is easy to identify and to treat. The most frequent symptom is excessive daytime sleepiness, the severity of which can be determined by the Epworth Sleepiness Scale, a simple questionnaire that can be administered to the patient in the waiting room before the doctor appointment (see Figure 30.1). A score greater than 10 is associated with significant disability and should prompt referral to a sleep specialist or directly to a polysomnogram.

The diagnosis of OSA is made by taking a good history of the patient's sleepiness and snoring. A bed partner can be interviewed or patients can videotape themselves sleeping. Physical exam may identify obesity, neck girth greater than 17 inches in men or 16 inches in women, a small chin, and large tonsils. Patients with risk factors can be referred for a polysomnogram. This entails an overnight stay at a hospital or sleep lab where a patient can be monitored for abnormalities in respiration, EKG, EEG, and limb movement. CPAP, which blows air into the nose and/or oral cavity to keep the soft tissues from collapsing, can be adjusted during the sleep study. Diagnosis and treatment can be accomplished on the same visit.

Weight loss is usually necessary to improve, if not cure, OSA. This has prompted some physicians to emphasize weight reduction without diagnosing and treating OSA. However, for many

Use the following scale to choose the most appropriate number for each situation:

- *0 = no chance of dozing*
- *1 = slight chance of dozing*
- *2 = moderate chance of dozing*
- *3 = high chance of dozing*

Situation	Chance of Dozing
Sitting and reading	
Watching TV	
Sitting inactive in a public place (e.g a theater or a meeting)	
As a passenger in a car for an hour without a break	
Lying down to rest in the afternoon when circumstances permit	
Sitting and talking to someone	
Sitting quietly after a lunch without alcohol	
In a car, while stopped for a few minutes in traffic	

The practitioner adds the values for the final score. A score of 10 or above is usually associated with significant disability and warrants further evaluation.

FIGURE 30.1   Epworth Sleepiness Scale.

patients, weight loss can only be achieved once the OSA is appropriately treated with CPAP.[26] OSA promotes insulin resistance and sleep deprivation, creating a vicious cycle of weight gain and worsening OSA. CPAP should therefore be viewed as a primary care intervention for obesity as well as a treatment for OSA.

RESTLESS LEG SYNDROME

Restless leg syndrome (RLS) is a disorder that is characterized by an uncomfortable, creepy, crawling feeling in the legs, feet, or thighs that is temporarily relieved by movement. Sometimes patients describe a pins-and-needles sensation and try to rub their legs or walk it off to relieve the discomfort. It can make falling asleep and staying asleep difficult. It can also occur during the day when one has to sit still at a desk or in a movie. Afflicting about 10% of the population, it tends to begin in the third decade of life and get worse over time. It is about 60% genetic and occurs more in women than men. RLS is thought to be due to abnormal iron metabolism and dopaminergic systems in the brain. It can be a primary disorder or secondary to iron deficiency. Of individuals with conditions associated with iron-deficiency states, including pregnancy, renal failure, and anemia, 25% to 30% may develop RLS.[27] Caffeine, nicotine, saccharine,[28] several prescription medications, fatigue, and extreme temperatures of either hot or cold can exacerbate this condition. RLS can cause periodic limb movements, insomnia, sleepiness, and phase delay. It is associated with attention deficit hyperactivity disorder and depression. RLS is underdiagnosed.

Adequate doses of iron may help treat restless leg syndrome and give relief to the patients who suffer from it.[29] Iron repletion improved sleep disturbance in children with autism.[30] Iron-rich foods, cooking in iron pots, and iron supplements have been shown to be effective in normalizing serum ferritin levels to at least 40 ng/mL. Minerals influence the central nervous system in poorly understood ways. Food cravings stemming from iron deficiency were identified in the 1950s and given the name pica, although the mechanism is still not understood. Folate[31] and magnesium supplements[32] may help. Nutritional analysis using RBC levels are available to quantify deficiencies of these and other minerals. Typically these tests give a retrospective look at the 3 months prior to testing as that is the lifespan of the typical red cell. As nutritional deficits are identified, specific diet and supplement recommendations can be made by the clinician. Sedating herbs such as kava kava, valerian, and hops also have a helpful role in promotion of sleep.

Gamma aminobutyric acid (GABA) is the most abundant inhibitory neurotransmitter in the mammalian brain. Barbiturates, benzodiazepines, nonbenzodiazepine hypnotics, and alcohol all affect the GABA receptor.[33] GABA is produced from glutamate with the aid of vitamin B6. GABA is available as an over-the-counter supplement. It has shown efficacy as a relaxant and anxiolytic.[34] Dopamine agonists such as Mirapex (pramipexole) and Requip (ropinirole) are considered first-line pharmacologic treatments for RLS; however gabapentin and opioids do have a role in refractory cases.[35] L-tryptophan has also been shown to increase dopamine levels and may be beneficial in symptomatic relief of RLS.

PERIODIC LIMB MOVEMENT DISORDER

Periodic limb movement disorder (PLMD) causes the legs to twitch during the night, causing a brief awakening. The twitching typically occurs every 20 to 40 seconds and lasts between half a second to 5 seconds. PLMD can involve the big toe, ankle, knee, or hip. It can occur in one leg, both, or alternate legs and occasionally the arms. Since PLMD usually occurs during light sleep, stages 1 and 2, it may be difficult to fall asleep. Some patients are unaware of their kicking, but know they have trouble falling asleep; others feel that their feet are extremely cold; some report excessive daytime sleepiness. Bed partners are often aware of the kicking behavior and may sleep elsewhere to avoid being kicked all night. The diagnosis is made by a polysomnogram and is defined by five or more kicks in each hour of sleep that cause an awakening. The underlying cause of periodic limb movement disorder is not well understood, but it does seem to have a genetic component and worsens with age. Similar to RLS, iron supplementation may improve severity of symptoms[36] and dopaminergic medications are the first line of pharmacologic treatment. Medications that interfere with neurotransmitter balance such as selective serotonin reuptake inhibitors, most antipsychotic drugs, and anti-dopaminergics like metoclopramide can precipitate PLMD. The amino acid neurotransmitter precursors presented in Chapter 29, "Depression," have not been studied for PLMD and RLS.

DESYNCHRONOSIS

There are differences in circadian rhythms based on stage of life and also among individuals. Teenagers prefer going to bed late and waking up late. They also need closer to 9 hours of sleep, a little more than the typical adult. This tendency is known as delayed phase disorder. While most outgrow this pattern eventually, many continue to prefer the night when they are most alert and energetic. With age, many shift to an early-to-bed, early-to-rise routine. If bedtime has become unreasonably early (i.e., 7 p.m.), this is known as advanced phase disorder. Treatment for both delayed and advanced phase disorders includes consistency of wake and bedtimes, phototherapy, and possibly melatonin replacement.

Abnormal patterns and production of cortisol can be seen in disorders of desynchronosis. Cortisol levels are easily and reliably measured by saliva testing at intervals throughout the day.[37] In a normal individual, cortisol levels are high in the morning, upon awakening, giving alertness and energy during the day. Levels should wane in the evening, allowing for sleep. At times, this pattern is reversed, resulting in both sleep onset and/or sleep maintenance insomnia. If cortisol levels are abnormally high suggesting some degree of adrenal hyperreactivity, dietary intervention with high-potency multivitamins with extra vitamin C, vitamin B5, vitamin B6, zinc, and phosphatidyl serine may be beneficial. Conversely, low cortisol levels suggest some degree of adrenal insufficiency and may lead to nonrestorative sleep and daytime fatigue. This situation may be served by a higher protein, balanced blood sugar with lower carbohydrate diet[38] with ample fiber and complex carbohydrates along with the above-mentioned supplements. In both hyper or hypocortisolemia, herbs, glandular formulas, and hormone replacement may be helpful. If cortisol patterns are significantly disturbed, this may prompt investigation into the diurnal variation of melatonin levels, which may also be abnormal. Hypercortisolemia is associated with decreased melatonin levels, disrupting circadian rhythms (Figure 30.2).[39] It is the tendency for patients with desynchronosis from whatever cause to choose stimulant foods high in sugar, fat,[40] salt, and caffeine. In addition to poor food choices, patients may also time their meals poorly. Abnormal cortisol production may be both a cause and consequence of poor sleep as well as excess weight. In a British study, blunted cortisol profiles were associated with significantly poorer sleep quality and significantly greater waist-hip ratio as well as a tendency to exhibit a less favorable metabolic profile.[41]

According to the National Sleep Foundation, 17% of Americans are shift workers and their sleep problems are compounded. As a group, they tend to be more sleep deprived than people working traditional hours. It's very difficult to reset internal circadian clocks. The body's urge to sleep is strongest between 12 midnight and 6 a.m. This is why 10% to 20% of shift workers report falling asleep on the job, especially on the second half of the shift. This also accounts for why it may be hard for shift workers to sleep during the day despite being tired. Sleep deprivation increases the probability of having other health problems, particularly indigestion, colds, flu, weight gain, cardiac problems, and higher blood pressure. Female shift workers also suffer irregular menstrual cycles, difficulty getting pregnant, higher rates of miscarriages, premature births, and low-birthweight babies. The risk of workplace accidents and automobile crashes rises for shift workers, especially on the drive to and from work.

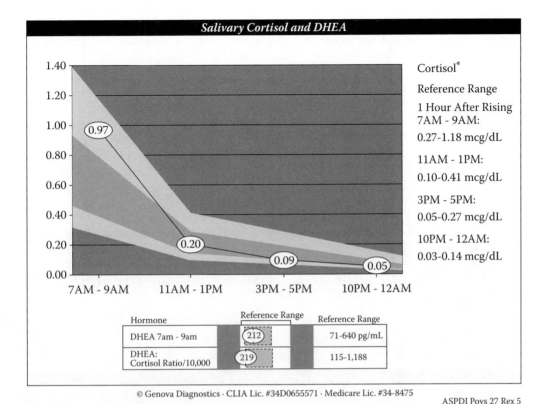

FIGURE 30.2 Salivary cortisol and DHEA sample lab report. (From Genova Diagnostics Labs. With permission.)

To combat jet lag, a few days before traveling, a gradual shift to the sleep and wake times of the destination will help. Upon arriving at the destination, adopting the prevailing sleep/wake time as soon as possible also is beneficial. In the morning, natural light in the eyes sends messages to the pineal gland, the area of the brain that makes melatonin. Melatonin is a chronobiotic hormone that is synthesized from tryptophan. It affects the circadian rhythm, duping the brain into thinking it is dark and therefore time to go to sleep. This resets the internal clock and has sleep-promoting effects, both shortening sleep latency and lengthening sleep duration. Levels of melatonin are highest prior to bedtime. When traveling west to east, melatonin supplements, which are sold over the counter, may diminish sleep latency and reduce the number of days necessary to establish a normal sleep pattern, improve alertness, and reduce daytime sleepiness.[42–44] Melatonin supplementation should be started on the day of travel (close to the target bedtime at the destination) and continued for several days.[45] Doses range from 0.5 to 5 mg; above 5 mg there seems to be no added benefit. In one study, the smaller and larger doses had similar efficacy, although the larger dose did afford an earlier sleep onset.[46] In a study of 100 children with sleep problems, over 80% benefited from supplementation with melatonin, which proved to be effective, inexpensive, and safe.[47] Ramelteon is a prescription agonist that works only on melatonin MT(1) and MT(2) receptors and decreases sleep latency and increases total sleep time and sleep efficiency, without causing hangover, addiction, or withdrawal, at least for short-term application.[48] Conversely, if traveling east to west, taking Benadryl (diphenhydramine), which tends to prolong the night and allows longer sleep, is a better choice. In general, it is easier to travel east to west because this lengthens the day.

Independent of travel and shift work, melatonin production may be abnormal, resulting in poor sleep. Melatonin can be accurately measured by saliva measurement with specimens obtained in the morning, at noon, at midnight, over a complete dark-light cycle. Since melatonin is a key hormone in regulating the HPA and supplementation is safe, evaluation is valuable (Figure 30.3).

V.   NUTRITIONAL INTERVENTIONS

NEW FINDINGS IN CAFFEINE

Caffeine worsens most sleep disorders. It increases both adrenocorticotropin (ACTH) and cortisol secretion in humans.[49] Caffeine's effect on glucocorticoid regulation therefore has the potential both to alter circadian rhythms and diet, causing a vicious cycle of poor sleep, increased hunger, and poor dietary choices.[50]

1. Caffeine is often hidden (Table 30.2).
2. What we eat up-regulates or down-regulates caffeine metabolism by acting on the same hepatic enzymes. Grapefruit juice delays the clearance of caffeine while smoking can double the rate of clearance. Alcohol is widely consumed throughout the world and is a known inducer of P450 (CYP2E1). Like smoking, chronic alcohol use may lead to increased clearance of caffeine.[51]

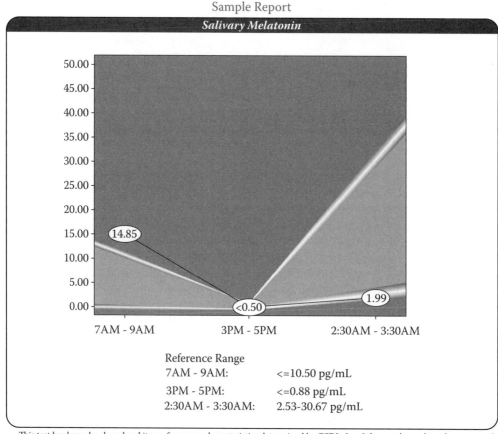

This test has been developed and its performance characteristics determined by GSDL, Inc. It has not been cleared or approved by the U.S. Food and Drug Administration.

FIGURE 30.3   Salivary melatonin sample lab report. (From Genova Diagnostics Labs. With permission.)

3. Many common drugs interfere with the metabolism of caffeine. This may result both in an increase in caffeine blood levels and also may enhance caffeine's diuretic effect. Unlike the other fluoroquinolones, ciprofloxacin inhibits the metabolism of caffeine, resulting in increased effects of caffeine. Cimetidine also increases caffeine levels, thereby a different H_2 antagonist (e.g., ranitidine, famotidine) should be administered to chronic caffeine users. Oral contraceptives and prednisone also increase caffeine levels due to the inhibition of caffeine metabolism.[52] Conversely, caffeine inhibits the metabolism of theophylline, which shares a similar chemical structure with caffeine, and can increase the serum concentrations of theophylline.[53] A synergistic effect of increased stimulation can occur in patients taking theophylline and caffeine-containing foods and beverages.

4. Caffeine metabolism varies widely based on genetics. That means medications that are hepatically metabolized influence people differently. Medication can make one person more sensitive to their daily cup of coffee and not affect someone else's metabolism of three cups of coffee. If a patient notices difficulty in sleep at the time they began a medication, they may want to reevaluate their caffeine intake even if it hasn't changed because their metabolism did change.

FOOD AS A SOURCE OF NEUROTRANSMITTER PRECURSORS

Going to bed hungry interrupts sleep. Hypoglycemia can cause multiple awakenings. Later in the night, hormonal counter-regulatory mechanisms are less effective.[54]

Nutritional rehabilitation of infants with protein-energy malnutrition measurably improved sleep quality. Disturbed serotonin levels were postulated to affect the sleep-wake cycle.[55] Protein malnutrition is an extreme situation with inadequate substrate to synthesize the neurotransmitters required to mediate sleep. The principle, however, appears more broadly applicable. In a cross-over design study, healthy infants given milk enhanced with tryptophan, a serotonin precursor, showed improvements in sleep parameters compared to when they were given standard milk.[56] A study of Horlicks,™ a malted milk hot drink popular in the United Kingdom, was shown to promote sleep and reduce bodily movements when drunk at bedtime.[57] A diet low in carbohydrates and high in dairy intake intended to generate ketosis in children with epilepsy improved sleep quality.[58] In a small study of elderly Japanese men and women given 100 g of fermented milk that contained *Lactobacillus helveticus*, there were significant improvements in both sleep efficiency and number of wakening episodes.[59] Here's another reason "breast is best." Parents of infants who were breast-fed in the evening and/or at night slept an average of 40 to 45 minutes more than parents of infants given formula. This held true for fathers as well as mothers, so it was not due to the extra rest needed for breastfeeding. Rather the parental sleep was a marker for the infant's sleep.[60]

FOOD AS A SOURCE OF MICRONUTRIENTS

Information that treating iron deficiency improves sleep is likely to be one of many findings on how nutrient-components of food influence brain function. Neuroimaging techniques are just now becoming available to study this. An interesting study that points to upcoming research is that dietary patterns influence our dreams. Choices of food intake before bed may influence dream content, as seen in a small study showing differing effects of micronutrient-rich organic food versus nutrient-poor "junk" foods.[63]

ALCOHOL

Alcohol is a commonly used soporific because of its effect as a central nervous system depressant. After an initial disinhibition, one becomes sleepy. But for each drink, this early sedation is then

TABLE 30.2
Caffeine Content of Food & Drugs

Coffees	Serving Size (oz)	Caffeine (mg)
Coffee, generic brewed	8	133 (range: 102–200)
	16	266
Starbucks™ Brewed Coffee (Grande)	16	320
Einstein Bros.™ regular coffee	16	300
Dunkin' Donuts™ regular coffee	16	206
Starbucks™ Vanilla Latte (Grande)	16	150
Coffee, generic instant	8	93 (range: 27–173)
Coffee, generic decaffeinated	8	5 (range: 3–12)
Starbucks™ Espresso, doppio	6.5	150
Starbucks™ Frappuccino™ blended coffee beverages, average	9.5	115
Starbucks™ Espresso, solo	1	75
Einstein Bros.™ Espresso	1	75
Espresso, generic	1	40 (range: 30–90)
Starbucks™ Espresso decaffeinated	1	4

Teas	Serving Size (oz)	Caffeine (mg)
Tea, brewed	8	53 (range: 40–120)
Starbucks™ Tazo Chai Tea Latte (Grande)	16	100
Snapple™ Lemon (and diet version)	16	42
Snapple™ Peach (and diet version)	16	42
Snapple™ Raspberry (and diet version)	16	42
Arizona Iced Tea™ black	16	32
Nestea™	12	26
Snapple,™ Just Plain Unsweetened	16	18
Arizona Iced Tea,™ green	16	15
Snapple, Kiwi Teawi™	16	10

Soft Drinks	Serving Size (oz)	Caffeine (mg)
FDA official limit for cola and pepper soft drinks	*12*	*71*
Vault™	12	71 (20 = 118)
Jolt Cola™	12	72
Mountain Dew MDX,™ regular or diet	12	71 (20 = 118)
Coke Black™	12	69 (20 = 115)
Coke Red™ regular or diet	12	54 (20 = 90)
Mountain Dew™ regular or diet	12	54 (20 = 90)
Pepsi One™	12	54 (20 = 90)
Mello Yellow™	12	53
Diet Coke™	12	47 (20 = 78)
Diet Coke Lime™	12	47 (20 = 78)
Tab™	12	46.5
Pibb Xtra, Diet Mr. Pibb, Pibb Zero™	12	41 (20 = 68)
Dr. Pepper™	12	42 (20 = 68)
Dr. Pepper diet™	12	44 (20 = 68)
Pepsi™	12	38 (20 = 63)
Pepsi Lime, regular or diet™	12	38 (20 = 63)
Pepsi Vanilla™	12	37
Pepsi Twist™	12	38 (20 = 63)
Pepsi Wild Cherry, regular or diet™	12	38 (20 = 63)
Diet Pepsi™	12	36 (20 = 60)

TABLE 30.2 *(continued)*

Soft Drinks	Serving Size (oz)	Caffeine (mg)
Pepsi Twist diet™	12	36 (20 = 60)
Coca-Cola Classic™	12	35 (20 = 58)
Coke Black Cherry Vanilla,™ regular/diet	12	35 (20 = 58)
Coke C2™	12	35 (20 = 58)
Coke Cherry,™ regular/diet	12	35 (20 = 58)
Coke Lime™	12	35 (20 = 58)
Coke Vanilla™	12	35 (20 = 58)
Coke Zero™	12	35 (20 = 58)
Barq's Diet Root Beer™	12	23 (20 = 38)
Barq's Root Beer™	12	23 (20 = 38)
7-Up,™ regular/diet	12	0
Fanta,™ all flavors	12	0
Fresca,™ all flavors	12	0
Mug Root Beer,™ regular/diet	12	0
Sierra Mist,™ regular or Free	12	0
Sprite,™ regular/diet	12	0

Energy Drinks	Serving Size (oz)	Caffeine (mg)
Spike Shooter™	8.4	300
Cocaine™	8.4	280
Monster Energy™	16	160
Full Throttle™	16	144
Rip It,™ all varieties	8	100
Enviga™	12	100
Tab Energy™	10.5	95
SoBe No Fear™	8	83
Red Bull™	8.3	80
Red Bull Sugarfree™	8.3	80
Rockstar Energy Drink™	8	80
SoBe Adrenaline Rush™	8.3	79
Amp™	8.4	74
Glaceau Vitamin Water Energy Citrus™	20	50
SoBe Essential Energy,™ Berry/Orange	8	48

Frozen Desserts	Serving Size (fl. oz)	Caffeine (mg)
Ben & Jerry's™ Coffee Heath Bar Crunch	8	84
Ben & Jerry's™ Coffee Flavored Ice Cream	8	68
Haagen-Dazs™ Coffee Ice Cream	8	58
Haagen-Dazs™ Coffee Light Ice Cream	8	58
Haagen-Dazs™ Coffee Frozen Yogurt	8	58
Haagen-Dazs™ Coffee & Almond Crunch Bar	8	58
Starbucks™ Coffee Ice Cream	8	50–60

Chocolates/Candies/Other	Serving Size	Caffeine (mg)
Jolt Caffeinated Gum™	1 stick	33
Hershey's™ Special Dark Chocolate Bar	1.45 oz	31
Hershey's™ Chocolate Bar	1.55 oz	9
Hershey's Kisses™	41g (9 pieces)	9
Hot cocoa	8 oz	9 (range: 3–13)

continued

TABLE 30.2   *(continued)*

Over-the-Counter Drugs	Serving Size	Caffeine (mg)
NoDoz™ (Maximum Strength)	1 tablet	200
Vivarin™	1 tablet	200
Excedrin™ (Extra Strength)	2 tablets	130
Anacin™ (Maximum Strength)	2 tablets	64

Source: From [61]. Most information was obtained from company websites or direct inquiries. Additional information from [62].

Note: Serving sizes are based on commonly eaten portions, pharmaceutical instructions, or the amount of the leading-selling container size. For example, beverages sold in 16-ounce or 20-ounce bottles were counted as one serving.

followed by an equal amount of arousal. The sedation lasts roughly 1 hour and the hyperadrenergic stimulation lasts for roughly 1 hour. Therefore, it takes the liver about 2 hours to clear each drink. Excess alcohol intake leads to a restless sleep, night sweats, and headaches.[64,65] Restricting quantity of alcohol, drinking it earlier in the evening, and slowing its absorption by eating food will help reduce the deleterious effects on sleep. Adequate hydration can also help. Alcohol, like any sedating drug, can worsen snoring and OSA.[66]

VI.   CONCLUSION

Sleep disturbance is exceedingly common and is associated with many medical problems such as obesity, diabetes, cognitive challenges, pain, hypertension, and mood disorders. Primary care physicians should be able to diagnose common sleep disorders, understand their clinical consequences, and prescribe appropriate interventions that include diet and nutrient recommendations.

REFERENCES

1. National Sleep Foundation. Survey: *Sleep in America*. Washington, DC. National Sleep Foundation: 2000.
2. Ancoli-Israel S. *All I Want Is a Good Night's Sleep*. St. Louis: Mosby-Year Book. 1996.
3. Vorona RD, Winn MP, Babineau TW et al. *Overweight and Obese Patients in a Primary Care Population Report Less Sleep Than Patients With a Normal Body Mass Index*. Arch Intern Med. 2005; 165:25–30.
4. Stamatakis KA, Brownson RC. *Sleep duration and obesity-related risk factors in the rural midwest*. Prev Med. 2007 Nov 22 [Epub ahead of print].
5. Taheri S, Lin L, Austin D et al. *Short sleep duration is associated with reduced leptin, elevated ghrelin, and increased body mass index*. PLoS Med. 2004 Dec; 1(3):e62.
6. Al Mamun A, Lawlor DA, Cramb S et al. *Do Childhood Sleeping Problems Predict Obesity in Young Adulthood? Evidence from a Prospective Birth Cohort Study*. Am. J. Epidemiol. 2007; 166:1368–1373.
7. Hasler G, Buysse DJ, Klaghofer R et al. *The association between short sleep duration and obesity in young adults: a 13-year prospective study*. Sleep. 2004 Jun 15; 27(4):661–666.
8. Knutson KL, Ryden AM, Mander VA, Van Cauter E. *Role of sleep duration and quality in the risk and severity of type 2 diabetes mellitus*. Arch Intern Med. 2006; 166:1768–1764.
9. Yaggi HK, Araujo AB, McKinlay JB. *Sleep duration as a risk factor for the development of type 2 diabetes*. Diabetes Care. 2006 Mar; 29(3):657–661.
10. Chaput JP, Després JP, Bouchard C, Tremblay A. *Association of sleep duration with type 2 diabetes and impaired glucose tolerance*. Diabetologia. 2007 Nov; 50(11):2298–2304.
11. Brown RP, Gerbarg PL, and Muskin PR. *Complementary and Alternative Treatments in Psychiatry*. In Tosman A, Kay J, Lieberman J (Eds.), *Psychiatry*, 2nd ed. (Chapter 104). New York: Wiley, 2003.

12. Jerath R, Edry JW, Barnes VA, Jerath V. *Physiology of long pranayamic breathing.* Medical Hypotheses. 2006; 67: 566–571.

13. Naga Venkatesha Murthy PJ, Janakiramaiah N, Gangadhar BN, Subbakrishna DK. *P300 amplitude and antidepressant response to Sudarshan Kriya Yoga (SKY).* J Affect Disord. 1998 Jul; 50(1):45–48.

14. Schwartz DJ, Kohler WC, Karatinos G. *Symptoms of depression in individuals with obstructive sleep apnea may be amenable to treatment with continuous positive airway pressure.* Chest. 2005; 128:1304–1306.

15. Conklin SM, Manuck SB et al. *High omega-6 and low omega-3 fatty acids are associated with depressive symptoms and neuroticism.* Psychosom Med. 2007 Dec; 69(9):932–934.

16. Roth T, Krystal AD, Lieberman JA 3rd. *Long-term issues in the treatment of sleep disorders.* CNS Spectr. 2007 Jul; 12(7 Suppl 10):1–13.

17. Dickman R, Green C et al. *Relationships between sleep quality and pH monitoring findings in persons with gastroesophageal reflux disease.* J Clin Sleep Med. 2007 Aug 15; 3(5):505–513.

18. Chen CL, Robert JJ et al. *Sleep symptoms and gastroesophageal reflux.* J Clin Gastroenterol. 2008 Jan; 42(1):13–17.

19. Fujiwara Y, Machida A, Watanabe Y et al. *Association between dinner-to-bed time and gastro-esophageal reflux disease.* Am J Gastroenterol. 2005 Dec; 100(12):2633–2636.

20. Jamison JR, Davie NJ. *Chiropractic management of cow's milk protein intolerance in infants with sleep dysfunction syndrome: a therapeutic trial.* J Manipulative Physiol Ther. 2006 Jul–Aug; 29(6):469–474.

21. Eichling PS, Sahni, J. *Menopause Related Sleep Disorders.* Journal of Clinical Sleep Medicine. 2005; 1(3):291–300.

22. Jacobson JS, Troxel AB, Evans J et al. *Randomized trial of black cohosh for the treatment of hot flashes among women with a history of breast cancer.* J Clin Oncol. 2001; 19:2739–2745.

23. Tice JA, Ettinger B, Ensrud K, et al. *Phytoestrogen supplements for the treatment of hot flashes: the Isoflavone Clove Extract Study: a randomized controlled trial.* JAMA 2003; 290:207–214.

24. Punjabi NM, Polotsky VY. *Disorders of glucose metabolism in sleep apnea.* J Appl Physiol. 2005; 99(5):1998–2007.

25. Kasasbeh E, Chi DS, Krishnaswamy G. *Inflammatory aspects of sleep apnea and their cardiovascular consequences.* South Med J. 2006; 99:58–67.

26. Trenell, MI et al. *Influence of constant positive airway pressure therapy on lipid storage, muscle metabolism and insulin action in obese patients with severe obstructive sleep apnoea syndrome.* Diabes Obes Metab. 2007; 9(5):679–687.

27. Ryan M, Slevin JT. *Restless Leg Syndrome.* Am J Health Syst Pharm. 2006 Sept; 1p63(17): 1599–1612.

28. Tijdschr Tandheelkd N. *Restless legs due to ingestion of 'light' beverages containing saccharine. Results of an N-of-1 trial.* 2007 Jun; 114(6):263–266.

29. Earley CJ, Connor JR, et al. *Abnormalities in CSF concentrations of ferritin and transferrin in restless legs syndrome.* Neurology. 2000; 54:1698–1700.

30. Dosman CF, Brian JA, Drmic IE, Senthilselvan A, Harford MM, Smith RW, Sharieff W, Zlotkin SH, Moldofsky H, Roberts SW. *Children with autism: effect of iron supplementation on sleep and ferritin.* Pediatr Neurol. 2007 Mar; 36(3):152–158.

31. Patrick LR. *Restless legs syndrome: pathophysiology and the role of iron and folate.* Altern Med Rev. 2007 Jun; 12(2):101–112.

32. Bartell S, Zallek S. *Intravenous magnesium sulfate may relieve restless legs syndrome in pregnancy.* J Clin Sleep Med. 2006; 2:187–188.

33. Harrison NL. *Mechanisms of sleep induction by GABA(A) receptor agonists.* J Clin Psychiatry. 2007; 68 Suppl 5:6–12.

34. Abdou AM, Higashiguchi S, Horie K, Kim M, Hatta H, Yokogoshi H. *Relaxation and immunity enhancement effects of gamma-aminobutyric acid (GABA) administration in humans.* Biofactors. 2006; 26(3):201–208.

35. Winkelman JW, Allen RP, Tenzer P, Hening W. *Restless legs syndrome: nonpharmacologic and pharmacologic treatments.* Geriatrics. 2007 Oct; 62(10):13–16.

36. Simakajornboon N, Gozal D et al. *Periodic limb movements in sleep and iron status in children.* Sleep. 2003 Sep; 26(6):735–738.

37. Gozansky WS, Lynn JS, Laudenslager ML, Kohrt WM. *Salivary cortisol determined by enzyme immunoassay is preferable to serum total cortisol for assessment of dynamic hypothalamic—pituitary—adrenal axis activity.* Clin Endocrinol (Oxf). 2005 Sep; 63(3):336–341.

38. Anderson KE, Rosner W, Khan MS et al. *Diet-hormone interactions: protein-carbohydrate ratio alters reciprocally the plasma levels of testosterone and cortisol and their respective binding globulins in man.* Life Sci. 1987; 40:1761–1768.

39. Soszyinski P, Stowinsk-Stednicka J, Kasperlik-Zatuska A et al. *Decreased melatonin in Cushing Sydrome.* Horm Metab Res. 1989; 21:673–674.

40. Torres SJ, Nowson CA. *Relationship between stress, eating behavior, and obesity.* Nutrition. 2007 Nov–Dec; 23(11–12):887–894.

41. Lasikiewicz N, Hendrickx et al. *Exploration of basal diurnal salivary cortisol profiles in middle-aged adults: associations with sleep quality and metabolic parameters.* Psychoneuroendocrinology. 2008 Feb; 33(2):143–151.

42. Mishima K, Satoh K, Shimizu T et al. *Hypnotic and hypothermic action of daytime-administered melatonin.* Psychopharmacology (Berl). 1997; 133:168–171.

43. Haimov I, Lavie P, Laudon M et al. *Melatonin replacement therapy of elderly insomniacs.* Sleep. 1995; 18:598–603.

44. Hughes RJ, Sack RL, Lewy AJ. *The role of melatonin and circadian phase in age-related sleep-maintenance insomnia: assessment in a clinical trial of melatonin replacement.* Sleep. 1998; 21:52–68.

45. Almeida Montes LG, Ontiveros Uribe MP, Cortes Sotres J et al. *Treatment of primary insomnia with melatonin: a double-blind, placebo-controlled, crossover study.* J Psychiatry Neurosci. 2003; 28(3):191–196.

46. Herxheimer A, Petrie KJ. *Melatonin for the prevention and treatment of jet lag.* Cochrane Database Syst Rev. 2002; (2):CD001520.

47. Jan EJ, O'Donnell ME. *Use of melatonin in the treatment of paediatric sleep disorders.* J Pineal Res. 1996; (21):193–199.

48. Pandi-Perumal SR, Srinivasan V et al. *Insight: the use of melatonergic agonists for the treatment of insomnia-focus on ramelteon.* Nat Clin Pract Neurol. 2007 Apr; 3(4):221–228.

49. Lovallo WR, al'Absi M et al. *Stress-like adrenocorticotropin responses to caffeine in young healthy men.* Pharmacol Biochem Behav. 1996; 55:365–369.

50. Lovallo, WR, Whitsett, TL et al. *Caffeine Stimulation of Cortisol Secretion Across the Waking Hours in Relation to Caffeine Intake Levels.* Psychosomatic Medicine. 2005; 67:734–739.

51. Djordjević D, Nikolić J, Stefanović V. *Ethanol interactions with other cytochrome P450 substrates including drugs, xenobiotics, and carcinogens.* Pathol Biol (Paris). 1998 Dec; 46(10):760–770.

52. Lacy CF, Armstrong LL, Goldman MP, Lance LL. *Lexi-Drugs Comprehensive and specialty fields.* Hudson, OH: Lexi-Comp, Inc; 2006.

53. Leibovich ER, Deamer RL, Sanserson LA. *Food-drug interactions: careful drug selection and patient counseling can reduce the risk in older patients.* Geriatrics. 2004; 59:19–33.

54. Jauch-Chara K, Hallschmid M et al. *Awakening and counter regulatory response to hypoglycemia during early and late sleep.* Diabetes. 2007 Jul; 56(7):1938–1942.

55. Shaaban SY, Ei-Saved HL, Nassar MF et al. *Sleep-wake cycle disturbances in protein-energy malnutrion: effect of nutritional rehabilitation.* East Mediterr Health J. 2007 May–June; 13(3): 633–645.

56. Aparicio S, Garau C, Esteban S et al. *Chrononutrition: use of dissociated day/night infant milk formulas to improve the development of the wake-sleep rhythms. Effects of tryptophan.* Nutr Neurosci. 2007 Jun–Aug; 10(3–4):137–143.

57. Southwell PR, Evans CR et al. *Effect of a Hot Milk Drink on Movements During Sleep.* Br Med J. 1972 May 20; 2(5811):429–431.

58. Hallböök T, Lundgren J, Rosén I. *Ketogenic diet improves sleep quality in children with therapy-resistant epilepsy.* Epilepsia. 2007 Jan; 48(1):59–65.

59. Yamamura S, Morishima H, Kumano-Go T et al. *The effect of Lactobacillus helveticus fermented milk on sleep and health perception in elderly subjects.* Eur J Clin Nutr. 2007 Sep 12 [Epub ahead of print].

60. Doan T, Gardiner A, Gay CL, Lee KA. *Breast-feeding increases sleep duration of new parents.* J Perinat Neonatal Nurs. 2007 Jul–Sep; 21(3):200–206.

61. Center for Science in the Public Interest. Nutrition Action Health Letter. September 2007. Available: www.cspinet.org.

62. Juliano LM, Griffiths RR. Caffeine. In Lowinson, JH, Ruiz, P, Millman, RB, Langrod, JG. (Eds.). *Substance Abuse: A Comprehensive Textbook*, 4th ed. (pp.403–421). Baltimore: Lippincott, Williams, & Wilkins, 2005.

63. Kroth J, Briggs A, Cummings M, Rodriguez G, Martin E. *Retrospective reports of dream characteristics and preferences for organic vs. junk foods.* 2007 Aug; 101(1):335–338.

64. Yules RB, Lippman ME, Freedman DX. *Alcohol administration prior to sleep; the effect on EEG sleep stages*. Arch Gen Psychiatry. 1967; 16; 94–97.
65. Madsen BW, Rossi L. *Sleep and Michaelis-Menten elimination of ethanol*. Clin Pharmacol Ther. 1980; 27:114–119.
66. Scanlan MF, Roebuck T, Little PJ et al. *Effect of moderate alcohol upon obstructive sleep apnea*. Eur Respir J. 2000; 16:909–913.

Section VII

Musculoskeletal and Soft Tissue Disorders

31 Osteoporosis

The Scientific Basis of the Alkaline Diet

Lynda Frassetto, M.D., and Shoma Berkemeyer, Ph.D.

I. INTRODUCTION

Osteoporosis, or bone thinning, is typically a disease common in older age. Many factors including genetics and environment interact in bone growth and maintenance of adequate bone architecture. One such factor is the acid-base balance, which recent data suggest may be linked to osteoporosis. The chemical definition of an acid is a substance that generates hydrogen ions [H^+] in solution, and a base or alkali is a substance that generates hydroxide ions [OH^-] in solution. The measure of the balance between the acids and the bases in the blood is called the pH. Normal blood pH is alkaline, at about 7.4 with a normal range from 7.35 to 7.45. Hence, a pH of 7.3 is chemically alkaline, since it is above 7.0, but physiologically acidic. This balance between acids and bases is typically affected by the body's internal metabolic conditions and diet. A diet is considered to be acid forming if the balance between the acids and bases from dietary intake tips the balance toward the acid side.

Bone is one of the body's endogenous reserves of base, since one major component is alkaline mineral salts such as calcium carbonate. As we will discuss in detail later on, exposing the bones to the excess acids from the diet [1] could potentially hasten bone demineralization and be associated with development of osteoporosis in later years. The kidney's ability to excrete excess acid declines with age [2, 3]. The combination of high dietary acid intake and reduced renal acid excretion tends to produce higher net acid balances, especially in the age groups most at risk for osteoporosis [4]. To maintain electrical neutrality and buffer excess acid, the body must make a "trade-off," using endogenous buffers such as bone alkali, and may have to accept a slightly higher net acid balance, which manifests as a slightly lower blood pH and plasma bicarbonate, although still within the range considered to be "normal" [5]. Eating a diet that does not produce a high diet acid load can reduce bone catabolism. The premise of this chapter is that modern-day diets in industrialized countries, which tend to be net acid forming due to the high intake of grains and animal food products and the relatively low intake of fruits and vegetables, may be one of the important factors in osteoporosis.

II. EPIDEMIOLOGY

The Rancho Bernardo and the Studies of Osteoporotic Fractures groups in California, and the Framingham cohort in Massachusetts each closely examined osteoporosis risk factors [6–8]. The epidemiology indicates that the nonmodifiable risk factors of race, gender, and age explain less of the disease than previously thought:

- Currently over 75 million people in the United States, Europe, and Japan may have osteoporosis [9].
- Although osteoporosis is more prevalent among women, elderly men are at moderate risk of developing hip fractures [10] and about 20% to 25% of all hip fractures occur in men. Men over 50 yrs have an estimated lifetime risk of experiencing osteoporotic fracture of 30%, which is the same as that of developing prostate cancer [11].
- Osteoporosis can occur in childhood. Juvenile osteoporosis has an average age of onset between 8 and 14 yrs and is observed especially during growth spurts [12, 13]. Children who experience their first fracture in early life (<4 yrs) are vulnerable to further fractures [14]. Prevention of osteoporosis implies optimal bone growth from childhood to adulthood, so that the bones achieve the individual peak bone mass and, thereafter, the maintenance of the adult bone mass. A nonoptimal achievement of adult bone mass implies a compromised start to the normal aging process.
- Osteoporosis can be secondary to other diseases such as hyperthyroidism, diabetes mellitus, Cushing's syndrome, malabsorption syndromes, and medications, such as corticosteroids, immunosuppressives, or anti-convulsants. These risk factors interact with the nonmodifiable risk factors.
- Nutrition, lifestyle, and hormones such as testosterone, estrogen, and growth hormone all contribute to the development of strong bones. Adequate protein, calcium, and vitamin D intake with regular physical exercise are usually recommended for optimal bone growth.

At least in modern Western societies, epidemiologic data support the hypothesis that modern diets [15–17] accompanied by a largely sedentary lifestyle [12] predispose people to osteoporosis. Dietary protein intake and the dietary ratio of animal foods to plant foods are the two primary factors in determining dietary acid or base load. Diet analyses from both the NHANES database and European database suggest that 60% to 70% of calories in the typical Western diet come from meat and dairy products, grains, and energy-rich, nutrient-poor food items. This is in contrast to poorer nations and regions with diets grossly characterized by higher intake of plant foods compared with animal foods where osteoporosis is much less prevalent [1, 18].

Adequate dietary protein intake is vital for bone health [18]. Several large cohort studies have demonstrated the relationship between increased dietary protein intake and increased bone mineral density (BMD) [7, 8]. In contrast, Sellmeyer and colleagues demonstrated in a prospective cohort of elderly Caucasian women in the United States that high intake of animal protein was independently associated with lower BMD and a greater risk of fracture [6] (Figure 31.1). New and colleagues, evaluating an elderly population in the United Kingdom, also found a correlation between increased intake of animal foods and lower BMD [19]. A very recent study may resolve the apparent discrepancies between these studies. Thorpe and colleagues demonstrated that after adjusting for the sulfate (nonvolatile fixed acid) content in protein, increased protein intake does correlate with increased BMD [20].

People in poorer nations and many preagricultural societies eat a higher proportion of vegetables [1, 17]. Vegetables generally contain limited amounts of protein and large amounts of alkali salts.

Renal function in the elderly is generally worse than in younger people [2, 3]. Declining renal function means lower blood flow to the kidneys, decreases in the amount of fluid filtered through the glomerulus, and decreased ability to excrete an acid load in the urine [21]. Since the kidneys are responsible for managing the body's net acid balance, the elderly will tend to have higher levels of blood acidity than younger population groups [4]. Studies from the Rancho Bernardo cohort of older adults have demonstrated that hip BMD is lowest in those with the greatest degree of renal failure [22].

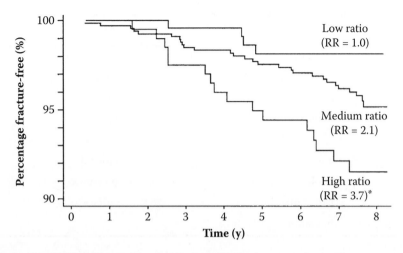

*p<0.04, RR = relative risk by proportional hazards modeling

FIGURE 31.1 Hip fracture-free survival in 1035 women by ratio of animal to vegetable protein intake after multivariate adjustment. (From [6].)

III. SOURCES OF ENDOGENOUS AND DIETARY ACIDS AND ACID EFFECTS ON BONE IN IN VITRO STUDIES

Physiologically metabolic acidosis is defined as blood pH less than 7.35. Bone cells that dissolve bone mineral are more active in an acid environment. We will discuss how dietary factors contribute to the acid-base balance of the body. Western diets in particular lead to increased acid levels in the body, so that metabolic acidosis [4] or a long-term subclinical latent acidosis [23] prevails. Aging exacerbates this phenomenon [3, 4]. So, eating a Westernized diet may promote bone breakdown, and over a lifetime, predispose to osteoporosis.

Biochemistry of Acid Production

Dietary acids are produced from metabolism of the sulfur-containing amino acids cysteine and methionine, which are present in diet proteins. This process results in the endogenous production of sulfuric acid from organic acids formed as intermediate metabolites:

$$Glucose \Rightarrow 2 \; lactate^- + 2H^+$$
$$Triglycerides \Rightarrow acetate^- + H^+$$
$$Nucleoproteins \Rightarrow urate^- + H^+$$

and from phosphoric acid produced by hydrolysis and metabolism of phosphoproteins [24]. Dietary base is thought to be produced from the potassium salts of organic anions metabolized to bicarbonate, such as potassium citrate or malate (see Figure 31.2). There is a difference in foods that are chemically acidic but physiologically alkaline. For example, citric acid, which is found in most citrus fruits, is an acid based on physical chemistry. However, inside the body at a pH of 7.4, citric acid forms citrate, an excellent supplier of base equivalents that can be metabolized to bicarbonate. One of the main methods the body uses to excrete excess acid is by adding hydrogen ions to bicarbonate, forming the unstable carbonic acid intermediate, and excreting the carbon dioxide (CO_2) in the lungs as a volatile acid.

$$CO_2 + H_2O \leftrightarrow H_2CO_3 \leftrightarrow H^+ + HCO_3$$
$$\text{volatile} \quad \text{carbonic acid} \quad \text{nonvolatile}$$
$$\text{intermediate}$$

	Cations		Anions
Mineral	sodium	Organic	bicarbonate
	potassium		citrate
	calcium		malate
	magnesium		urate
Organic	amines	Mineral	chloride
	choline		phosphate
	catecholamines		sulfate
	histamine		

FIGURE 31.2 The body's electrical neutrality is maintained by balancing the cations and anions, many of which contribute to acid-base balance.

This rapid interchange between carbon-dioxide and bicarbonate contributes to the difficulty esti-mating their contribution to the net acid load [25]: Organic acids are thus an important contributor to the body's net acid load [24, 26], and its net excretion is thought to be more or less a constant, after accounting for body size, even on Westernized diets (50 to 100 milliequivalents per day [mEq/d]*) [26, 27]. Mineral acids, such as sulfates and phosphates, are stronger acids and remain highly disso-ciated and thus reactive at the normal blood pH. Metabolic acids are excreted by the kidneys, which is the major reason renal failure leads to a metabolic acidosis.

The gold standard for evaluating dietary net acid loads is considered to be 24-hour urine collec-tions for net acid excretion (NAE); that is, all of the acids that can be titrated, including the organic acids, minus the urine bicarbonate content. Because these studies require a research laboratory to analyze the urine contents, a simpler methodology, namely estimating the diet net acid load from dietary intake, exists.

METABOLIC ACIDOSIS EFFECTS ON BONE IN IN VITRO STUDIES

In vitro studies by David Bushinsky, Thomas Arnett, and their colleagues on metabolic acido-sis on bone health in mouse calvaria have demonstrated that as the acid levels in the medium increase, the amount of calcium released from bone increases, as well as phosphates and carbon-ates, with greater release of phosphates than bicarbonates [28]. Higher acid levels decrease both gene activation and bone mineralization activities of osteoblasts, the cells that build up bone [29, 30] and induce osteoblast production of prostaglandins that activate osteoclasts, the bone cells that increase bone breakdown [31–35]. In these studies, at a higher, more alkaline, pH, the bone loses less mineral content and is less likely to break down when exposed to hormones such as parathyroid hormone and vitamin D, which normally increase bone calcium release.

In vivo studies on metabolic acidosis on bone health in animals and humans have demonstrated that acidosis is negatively associated with growth. In animals, metabolic acidosis produces distur-bances in normal growth hormone secretion patterns leading to growth retardation [36]. Human

---

* Milliequivalents (mEq) are useful units because the body is electrically neutral, so the positive ions must equal the nega-tive ions. To calculate milliequivalents from milligrams, divide the milligrams by the molecular weight of the compound [to get millimoles (mmol)] and multiply that by the charge on the ion.

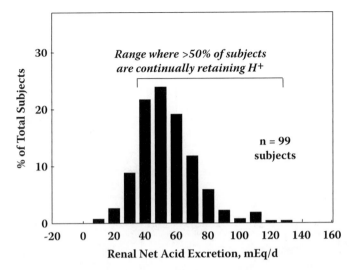

FIGURE 31.3   Proportion of subjects on typical American diets whose total body acid levels are increased. (From [39].)

studies have demonstrated stunted growth in children [37, 38] due to metabolic acidosis, with increases in growth after alkali administration [37].

ACIDOGENIC OR ALKALINIZING CONTRIBUTION OF DIET INTAKES: PROTEIN, FRUITS, AND VEGETABLES

In typical diets in industrialized countries, the average person excretes acidic urine, indicative of the high acid intake in the diet (Figure 31.3) [39]. At higher diet acid intakes, the body's ability to excrete the total acid load produced seems to be insufficient, and may lead to net acid retention. This was observed with diet acid loads greater than approximately 1 mEq/kilogram (kg) body weight [40].

The preagricultural human diet, however, was reported to be net basic [15, 17], despite a relatively high protein consumption. One explanation for this is a greater intake of fruits and vegetables than meats and grains. Further, the nutritional density and net base producing potential of vegetables in earlier eras is proposed to have been higher than that of today's agricultural produce [15].

Natural foods are low in sodium and chloride, while processed foods use table salt as both a preservative and a taste enhancer. Salt itself is an independent factor leading to higher acid loads [41]. Taken together, the present-day consumption of cereals (acidogenic), simple sugars (acidogenic when partially metabolized), non-neutralized protein consumption (acidogenic), and salt intake (acidogenic) leads to a daily net acid load, principally of dietary origin, to the extent of 50 to 100 mEq/d [16, 17, 42], as observable in Figure 31.3.

One consequence may be a corresponding decrease in plasma bicarbonate. As the body's free acid (hydrogen ion) levels are very tightly controlled, this means the body must use its endogenous stores of buffers in order to render the acid load in vivo harmless. Such endogenous buffers include the basic salts found in the bones, as well as intracellular buffers in the erythrocytes and muscles.

Dietary protein is an important factor in increasing diet acid load. To what extent this is true varies on the protein molecules, which are metabolized differently based on their amino acid content. Studies by Lennon, Lemann, and Relman clearly demonstrate higher urinary sulfate excretion in patients fed a high egg-white diet compared with those fed a soy protein diet [43]. This group of investigators, however, also demonstrated that soy protein is high in phosphoproteins, actually increasing total urinary acid excretion to a greater extent than an equivalent amount of protein

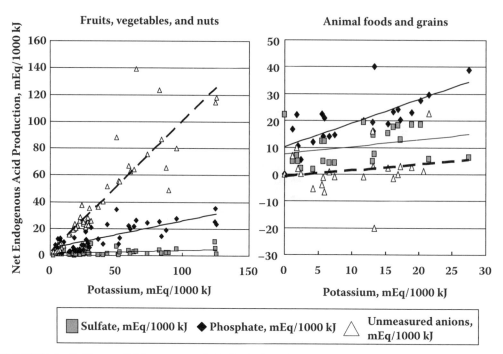

FIGURE 31.4 Evidence of higher content of alkali salts in fruits and vegetables compared with animal foods and grains.

nitrogen fed as beefsteak [44]. Thus, different sources of dietary protein can contribute differing amounts of acid precursors. The majority of protein in typical Western diets comes from animal foods, which tend to be very low in alkalinizing compounds (see Figure 31.4) and therefore contribute mainly to the acid load of the diet.

To further evaluate the potential alkalinizing effects of fruits and vegetables, the authors analyzed data from the U.S. Department of Agriculture nutrient database[*] to determine the calculated net acid or base load for individual foods [17], the median content of phosphates and sulfates in fruits and vegetables, which are significantly lower than in animal foods, and the potassium and organic anion, which is significantly higher than in animal foods. Figure 31.4 demonstrates that plant foods contain significantly higher potassium than animal foods. It further illustrates differences in the factors used to calculate NEAP between animal foods and plant foods. In general, fruits and vegetables are higher in alkali, and increased ingestion should help balance the high acid loads found in the animal-food and grain-based diets most prevalent in industrialized countries.

It is important to recognize that not all plant foods may be equally healthy. For example, children who eat a macrobiotic diet with a high percent of calories from grains have lower bone mass as adolescents than children not following a macrobiotic diet [45].

Estimating the Net Endogenous Acid Production (NEAP) From Diet Intakes

The acid or alkaline load of the diet or even food groups can be estimated by means of various published formulae that estimate the "net endogenous acid production" (NEAP), that is, the difference between the total amount of acid produced and the total amount of acid excreted by the body. Such analyses require access to a detailed food database. Acid production stems from metabolism of both the exogenous diet and the body's endogenous substrates. One such diet-based estimate of NEAP is

---

[*] http://www.nal.usda.gov/fnic/foodcomp/search/.

derived from the Remer-Manz model [46]. A detailed estimate of NEAP is calculated by summing a diet-based net acid load component called the potential renal acid load (PRAL) [46], and a non-diet-based organic acid component called the anthropometric organic acid (OA_{anthro}) [26, 27]. PRAL itself is a net summation of the diet cations and anions, taking their gastrointestinal absorptions into account. The sulfate anion of PRAL is calculated using the average sulfur content per gram protein across all foods containing sulfurated amino acids. The formula for NEAP estimated according to this method is as follows.

$$NEAP = PRAL + OA_{anthro} \tag{1}$$

where

$$PRAL = [(0.04 \times Na) + (0.02 \times K) + (0.01 \times Ca) + (0.03 \times Mg)]$$
$$- [(0.03 \times Cl) + (0.04 \times PO4) + (0.0005 \times SO4)]$$
$$OA_{anthro} = \text{individual body surface area} \times [41/1.73]$$

A simplified model to estimate NEAP has been put forward by Frassetto and colleagues [16]. Similar to Remer-Manz's model, this method estimates the diet acid load using total diet protein intake (Pro) and the diet alkali load from the total diet potassium intake (K), and assumes that organic acid production is relatively constant between food groups. Unadjusted for energy intake, the formula is

$$NEAP = -10.2 + 54.5 \text{ [Protein (Pro, gms)/Potassium (K, mEq)]} \tag{2}$$

The main advantage of this model is that only two dietary components need to be known. The main disadvantage is that it was derived from mainly acid-producing diets, and can only estimate NEAP (or rather, net base production) down to –10 mEq/day when the term $54.5 \times (Pro/K)$ goes to zero.

A third model has been developed by Sebastian and colleagues [17]:

$$NEAP = \text{Dietary unmeasured anion (DUA)} + OA_{diet} + \text{Sulfate} \tag{3}$$

This model estimates sulfate intake from dietary cysteine and methionine* rather than as a fixed percentage of protein intake. It estimates organic acid intake from the diet as a function of the urine organic anion excretion using empirical data obtained from studies by Lemann and Kleinman [43]:

$$DUA = (Na + K + Ca + Mg) - (Cl + P)$$

The organic anion component is estimated as

$$OA_{diet} = 32.9 + (0.15 \times DUA)$$

Calculations of potential acid or base food items are shown in Table 31.1 [17].

To test whether or not these models accurately reflect the diet acid intake requires studies where diet net acid loads are both estimated from formulas and then measured by 24-hour urine NAE. Only a few such studies have been done [35–37, 40, 42, 44, 46].

IV. DIET THERAPY

General treatment considerations when developing an alkaline diet are the adequacy of protein intake, the adequacy of fruit and vegetable intake, and the balance between the acid load from protein and the base load from fruit and vegetable intake.

---

* To calculate milliequivalents for methionine and cystine, calculate the millimoles of sulfur (methionine contains one S and cystine 2) and multiple that number by two to get milliequivalents.

TABLE 31.1
Acid and Alkaline Loads of Selected Foods

Food Group	# Items	Net Acid Load mEq/100 kcal	Net Acid Load [17] mEq/2500 kcal	Potassium mEq/100 kcal	Protein g/100 kcal	Protein [16] g/100 mEq Potassium
Acid-Producing Foods						
Fish	8	+14.6	+398	8.1	16.8	207
Meat	3	+12.4	+342	7.6	18.4	242
Poultry	2	+7.8	+227	4.7	13.4	287
Egg	1	+7.3	+215	2.4	8.3	339
Shellfish	3	+7.3	+215	18.4	18.0	159
Cheese	9	+3.3	+115	0.8	7.1	982
Milk	4	+1.3	+64	6.4	5.7	90
Cereal Grains	7	+1.1	+60	2.6	3.2	153
Near-Neutral Foods						
Legumes	6	−0.4	+24	12.6	10.6	100
Base-Producing Foods						
Nut	6	−1.1	+6	3.8	2.5	86
Fresh Fruit	11	−5.2	−98	9.4	1.6	16
Tuber	2	−5.4	−102	11.8	2.2	18
Mushroom	1	−11.2	−247	62.3	25.7	41
Root Vegetable	5	−17.1	−395	34.3	6.8	21
Vegetable/Fruit	1	−17.5	−404	35.5	5.6	15
Leafy Greens	6	−23.4	−553	43.5	10.0	24
Plant Stalks	1	−24.9	−590	54.8	4.6	8

Source: [17].

1. Adequate protein intake. As mentioned, dietary protein is very important to bone health [18]. Some proteins contain a higher content of acid precursors than others, and animal foods, which supply the majority of dietary protein, are very low in alkalinizing compounds. Typically then, dietary protein contributes mainly to the acid load of the diet.
2. Adequate fruits and vegetables. Some fruits and vegetables are higher in base content than others, and some contain a high content of acid precursors. However, in general the net balance of precursors in fruits and vegetables is base (see Figure 31.4).
3. Adequate vitamin and mineral intake. This topic will not be covered in this chapter, except to say that adequate vitamin D, vitamin B12, calcium, magnesium, and phosphate are necessary for bone health.

Balancing Acid and Base Intake in the Diet

Although correct food combinations can keep the body's net acid load low, or even net alkaline, only a few studies have directly measured changes in renal acid excretion from specific food items. These will be described in some detail here.

The first such studies were done by Nathan Blatherwick in 1914 [47]. He fed so-called "basal diets," which approximately reproduce the acid loads of the Western diet. The Blatherwick basal diet 1 consisted of graham crackers, butter, and milk at each meal, plus one egg and one apple at dinnertime, and had an average acid load of 36.6 mEq/d. This diet could be neutralized by the consumption of 2.3 kg apples/day. This large intake of apples is, quantitatively speaking, difficult to maintain on a daily basis. A total of 750 g/day baked potato consumption provided a more feasible alternative to alkalize the system. Supplement of sodium bicarbonate, in dosages varying from 5 to 15 g, also resulted in a net alkali excretion on a Western diet. The Blatherwick basal diet 2 consisted of graham crackers, butter, milk, and peanut butter at each meal, plus one egg and one apple at dinnertime, and had an average acid load of 81.5 mEq/d. This diet could only be neutralized with the supplement of 15 g of sodium bicarbonate. Thus, regular Western diets leading to a net diet acid load of 50 to 100 mEq/d, can be partially or completely neutralized using large quantities of alkaline food items or alkaline supplements such as sodium bicarbonate.

Fruits and vegetables, with the exception of cranberries, prunes, and plums, reduce the total acid load from the outgoing, original basal acid load [48]. Another of the Blatherwick studies [49] reported on the acidogenic properties of adding 300 g of cranberries and prunes to the diet. Such foods contain chlorogenic and phenolic acids, which are metabolized to benzoic acid and ultimately excreted from the body as hippuric acid [50]. A similar, more recent study showed a significant decrease in urinary pH after consumption of 330 mL of cranberry juice for 5 days whereas 330 mL of blackcurrant juice significantly increased urinary pH and citrate excretion, and plum juice did not have any significant effect [51]. Black teas (Table 31.2) are also mildly acidogenic. As with cranberries, black tea phenols are metabolized to benzoic acid [50].

Plant species may also contain varying quantities of benzoic acid. For example, the native sweet potatoes of the highlands of Papua New Guinea have a very high content of benzoic acid and, hence, are net acidogenic [52]. In contrast, consumption of the sweet potato species available in Western markets resulted in a decrease of the renal net acid excretion with increases in urine pH [42]. Thus, the sweet potato found in Western markets is not as acidogenic as the sweet potato species of the highlands of Papua New Guinea.

Coffee has been reported to be acidic (Table 31.2), but a more recent intervention study suggests otherwise. A single person was put on a basal diet for 6 days with an intervention of 1 L of espresso coffee on the last 3 days. Urine collected on days 3 and 6 of the experiment showed no change in the net acid excreted (67 mEq/d and 61.5 mEq/d, respectively). This one study suggested that espresso coffee is actually a neutral substance [53].

Similarly divergent data exist from studies of cereal grains. In Table 31.2, which reports a composite of data gathered from the authors as well as from the literature, white rice is noted to be mildly acid producing whereas wild rice is mildly alkali producing. Blatherwick showed all rice to be mildly acid producing. As noted earlier for sweet potatoes, different varieties of the same food or different processing of the same food may affect the net acidogenic properties of the food. In a more recent study by Jajoo and colleagues [54], addition of cereal grains to a basal diet of 0.75 g protein/kg/day increased NAE from 39 ± 23 to 56 ± 23 mmol/day. Cereals in this study consisted of couscous, pasta, rice, granola, and Pop Tarts™.

In addition to being acidic, commercial breads contain table salt (NaCl). Sodium chloride is known to cause metabolic acidosis by increasing the blood proton concentration [41], that is, a decrease in blood pH. This was also demonstrated by Blatherwick [46]. In general, it can be inferred that an excess of the anionic chloride over the cationic component would add to the acid load. In case reports, other halides have also been associated with metabolic acidosis, including iodide ingestion [55], bromide infusion [56], and fluoride injection [57]. General nutritional recommendations follow to keep table salt consumption low and to enhance food flavors with use of herbs and spices instead.

Other studies have looked at how mineral waters affect net acid excretion and bone health. A 6-month double-blind placebo-controlled trial of 152 postmenopausal women showed that a daily intervention of 1 liter of high-calcium mineral water decreased serum parathyroid hormone, osteocalcin, bone alkaline phosphatase, and serum and urinary type-1 collagen C-telopeptide compared with the placebo group [58]. Buclin and colleagues [59] showed in a four-period double-crossover study that an acid-forming diet increased urinary calcium excretion by 74% compared with a base-forming diet, both at baseline and after oral calcium load. C-telopeptide excretion also increased by 19%, confirming the skeletal origin of the urinary calcium. Another study compared two

TABLE 31.2A
Food & Chemical Effects on Acid Chemical Balance™

Food Category	Most Alkaline	More Alkaline	Low Alkaline	Lowest Alkaline
Spice/Herb	Baking Soda	Spices (most): Cinnamon • Valerian Licorice • Black Cohosh Agave	• Herbs (most): Arnica, Bergamot, Echinacea Chrysanthemum, Ephedra, Feverfew, Goldenseal, Lemongrass, Aloe Vera, Nettle	• White Willow Bark • Slippery Elm • Artemesia Annua
Preservative	Sea Salt			*Sulfite*
Beverage	Mineral Water	• Kambucha	• Green or Mu Tea	Ginger Tea
Sweetener		Molasses	Rice Syrup	• Sucanat
Vinegar		Soy Sauce	Apple Cider Vinegar	• Umeboshi Vinegar
Therapeutic	• Umeboshi Plum		• Sake	• Algae, Blue Green
Processed Dairy				• Ghee (Clarified Butter)
Cow/Human				Human Breast Milk
Egg			• Quail Egg	• Duck Egg
Grain/ Cereal/ Grass				Oat • Quinoa Wild Rice/Amaranth/ Japonica Rice
Oil/Seeds/Nuts	Pumpkin Seed	Poppy Seed Cashew Chestnut Peppercorn	Primrose Oil Sesame Seed Cod Liver Oil Almond	Avocado Oil Seeds (most) Coconut Oil Olive/Macadamia Oil Linseed/Flax Oil
Bean/Vegetable/ Legume/ Pulse/ Root	Lentil Seaweed Onion/Miso • Daikon/Taro Root Dandelion Greens • Burdock/• Lotus Root Sweet Potato/Yam	Kohlrabi Parsnip/Taro Garlic Asparagus Kale/Parsley Endive/Arugula Mustard Greens Jerusalem Artichoke Ginger Root Broccoli	Potato/Bell Pepper Mushroom/Fungi Cauliflower Cabbage Rutabaga • Salsify/Ginseng Eggplant Pumpkin Collard Greens	Brussel Sprout Beet Chive/Cilantro Celery/Scallion Okra/Cucumber Turnip Greens Squash Artichoke Lettuce Jicama
Fruit	Lime Nectarine Persimmon Raspberry Watermelon Tangerine Pineapple	Grapefruit Canteloupe Honeydew Citrus Olive • Dewberry Loganberry Mango	Lemon Pear Avocado Apple Blackberry Cherry Peach Papaya	Orange Apricot Banana Blueberry Pineapple Juice Raisin, Currant Grape Strawberry

• Gourmet or exotic items   *Italicized items are NOT recommended*

TABLE 31.2B
Food & Chemical Effects on Acid Chemical Balance™

Food Category	Lowest Acid	Low Acid	More Acid	Most Acid
Spice/Herb	Curry	Vanilla/Stevia	Nutmeg	*Pudding/Jam/Jelly*
Preservative	*MSG*	*Benzoate*	*Aspartame*	*Table Salt (NaCL)*
Beverage	*Kona Coffee*	*Alcohol*	*Coffee*	*Beer, 'Soda'*
		Black Tea		*Yeast/Hops/Malt*
Sweetener	Honey/Maple Syrup		*Saccharin*	*Sugar*/Cocoa
Vinegar	Rice Vinegar	Balsamic Vinegar	Red Wine Vinegar	White/Acetic Vinegar
Therapeutic		*Antihistamines*	*Psychotropics*	*Antibiotics*
Processed Dairy	Cream/Butter	Cow Milk	• Casein, Milk Protein, Cottage Cheese	*Processed Cheese*
Cow/Human	Yogurt	Aged Cheese	New Cheese	Ice Cream
Soy		Soy Cheese	Soy Milk	
Goat/Sheep	Goat/Sheep Cheese	Goat Milk		
Egg	Chicken Egg			
Meat	Gelatin/Organs	Lamb/Mutton	Pork/Veal	Beef
Game	• Venison	• Boar/Elk	• Bear	
Fish/Shell Fish	Fish	Mollusks	• Mussel/Squid	Shell Fish (Processed)
		Shell Fish (Whole)		• Lobster
Fowl	Wild Duck	Goose/Turkey	Chicken	Pheasant
Grain/ Cereal/	• Triticale	Buckwheat	Maize	Barley
Grass	Millet	Wheat	Barley Groat	Processed Flour
	Kasha	• Spelt/Teff/Kamut	Corn	
	Brown Rice	Farina/Semolina	Rye	
		White Rice	Oat Bran	
Oil/Seeds/Nuts	Pumpkin Seed Oil	Almond Oil	Pistachio Seed	*Cottonseed Oil/Meal*
	Grape Seed Oil	Sesame Oil	Chestnut Oil	Hazelnut
	Sunflower Oil	Safflower Oil	*Lard*	Walnut
	Pine Nut	Tapioca	Pecan	Brazil Nut
	Canola Oil	• Seitan or Tofu	Palm Kernel Oil	*Fried Food*
Bean/ Vegetable/	Spinach	Split Pea	Green Pea	Soybean
Legume/ Pulse/	Fava Bean	Pinto Bean	Peanut	Carob
Root	Kidney Bean	White Bean	Snow Pea	
	Black-eyed Pea	Navy/Red Bean		
	String/Wax Bean	Aduki Bean	Legumes (other)	
	Zucchini	Lima or Mung Bean	Carrot	
	Chutney	Chard	Chickpea/Garbanzo	
	Rhubarb			
Fruit	Coconut			
	Guava	Plum	Cranberry	
	• Pickled Fruit	Prune	Pomegranate	
	Dry Fruit	Tomato		
	Fig			
	Persimmon Juice			
	• Cherimoya			
	Date			

• Gourmet or exotic items   *Italicized items are NOT recommended*

Sources: [73].   Prepared by Dr. Russell Jaffe, Fellow, Health Studies Collegium. Reprints available from Health Studies Collegium, 2 Pidgeon Hill Drive, #410, Sterling, VA 20165, 703-788-5126. Sources include USDA food data base (Rev 9 & 10), Food & Nutrition Encyclopedia; Nutrition Applied Personally, by M. Walczak; Acid & Alkaline by H. Aihara. Food growth, transport, storage, processing, preparation, combination, and assimilation influence affect intensity. Thanks to Hank Liers for his original work. [Rev 7/07]

Note: Prescription medications are to be administered under medical supervision.

different drinking waters containing the same amount of calcium to analyze the effects of the anions in mineral water on bone health. Water with a high bicarbonate content produced a greater increase in urinary pH, and a corresponding greater decrease in urine titratable acid (minus bicarbonate), ammonium, and urinary bone resorption markers compared with baseline, than did high sulfate water [60]. Although studies on drinking water are few to date, they indicate that mineral waters, like food, affect net acid-base balance and bone health and should not be ignored when considering diet modification of acid load. Presently, what can be said is that if the acidic anions in water (chloride, sulfate, phosphate) exceed the basic (potassium, sodium, magnesium, and calcium), then water will tend to be net acidic. Bicarbonate in water would increase its alkali load.*

As is apparent from the findings described above, there is as yet no foolproof method of determining whether any specific food item is actually net acid or net base producing without testing it, and only a small fraction of foods have actually been tested. By far, this is the biggest unknown in trying to determine whether and to what extent a diet is net acid or net base producing, without using dietary alkali supplements.

The few studies that report neutralization of the acidic Western diet and changes in bone markers or BMD used either sodium or potassium bicarbonate or citrate [61–63] to neutralize diet net acid load. Therefore we are unable to itemize how individual foods can prevent osteoporosis.

V. PHARMACOLOGY

Research has probed the possibility of giving pharmacologic alkali supplements as an osteoporosis treatment. Several clinical studies have administered alkali supplements and reported the effects on diet net acid load and bone turnover.

Sebastian and colleagues demonstrated that in older otherwise healthy women, potassium bicarbonate had a dose-dependent effect on lowering blood levels of hydrogen ion (acid) content and decreasing amount of acid excreted by the kidneys [62]. Importantly at the higher dose of 2 mEq of potassium bicarbonate per kilogram body weight per day, the women's plasma bicarbonate levels remained within the range considered to be normal. Associated with this decrease in net acid load was an improvement in both calcium and phosphate balance and a decline in the urinary excretion of one of the biomarkers of bone breakdown, hydroxyproline.

Krapf and colleagues [61] demonstrated a decrease in other biomarkers of bone breakdown— pyridinoline, deoxypyridinoline, and N-telopeptide—in young healthy subjects given 1.1 mEq/kg body weight of potassium and sodium bicarbonate as a replacement for an equal amount of the chloride salts, and a lower rate of decline in both hip and spine BMD in older women with osteopenia or osteoporosis treated for 12 months with approximately 0.5 mEq/kg body weight [64].

Sellmeyer and colleagues [63] demonstrated that potassium citrate at a dose of approximately 1.5 mEq/kg body weight lowered urine calcium excretion in women randomized to a high sodium chloride diet compared with those on a low salt diet. Associated with this lower urine calcium excretion was a decrease in urinary N-telopeptide excretion, suggesting a decrease in bone breakdown and concomitant urinary losses of both calcium and collagen matrix.

Other dietary alkali supplements also are available. Some contain a mixture of calcium, potassium, and magnesium; others contain a mixture of trace minerals, and often use hydroxide, citrate, acetate, or other organic anions as the base (e.g., calcium citrate would be an alkali salt). Small uncontrolled studies by these supplement makers suggest that taking them daily can help decrease dietary acid intake [65] and improve bone density. The amounts of alkali per dose vary, and since these are dietary supplements, these claims are not reviewed by the FDA.

Thus, pharmacologic replacement of alkali salts has been shown in studies of small groups of patients to help decrease bone breakdown and the rate of decline of BMD.

---

* Readers are referred to www.mineralwaters.org, a website detailing mineral water content on thousands of mineral waters from around the world, though readers are cautioned to validate claims for themselves.

VI. PATIENT EVALUATION AND TREATMENT

MONITORING RESPONSES TO THERAPY

Evaluating the response to alkaline diet therapy is difficult as many of the tests mentioned previously (e.g., 24-hour urine collection for net acid excretion and bone biomarkers) are conducted in research laboratories. In search of clinically applicable diagnostics some authors recommend measuring urine pH to determine whether the diet is sufficiently alkaline [48]. For example, one dietary alkali supplement guide suggests that an optimal first morning void urine pH is between 6.5 and 7.5. The authors of that guide recommend using the first morning void to estimate the body's average 24-hour net excretion of acid (NAE). One major problem with this approach is that first morning void urine pH has been shown to correlate only to overnight NAE when the subjects are fasting overnight, and not to the entire 24-hour NAE when the subject is eating and therefore taking in more acid or base [66]. Twenty-four-hour urine pH does correlate with 24-hour urine NAE [67], but doing 24-hour urine collections can be tedious. Urine pH has also been shown to decrease with insulin resistance and markers of the metabolic syndrome [68]. So, while urine pH may be the easiest test to do, there are quite a few caveats in how to interpret the results.

USING AN ALKALI DIET TO TREAT OTHER MEDICAL PROBLEMS

One study has reported that both magnesium-enriched water and natural mineral water increased urinary excretion of magnesium in hypertensive subjects with low baseline excretion of magnesium and calcium, along with a significant decrease in blood pressure in those subjects consuming mineral water after 2 and 4 weeks of intervention [69].

Various types of kidney stones may be less likely to form or grow in acid or alkaline urine, depending on the type of kidney stone. Since cranberry juice lowers urine pH and lowers the relative supersaturation for brushite and struvite, cranberry juice may be useful in the treatment of brushite or struvite stones [51]. Blackcurrant, orange, and apple juice can increase urine pH and citrate and oxalate excretion, and help in the treatment of uric acid and calcium oxalate stones, which are the most common [51, 70].

Plant phenols and benzoic acid, such as in cranberries, prunes, black teas, and so on, while being acidogenic, may also be antimicrobial in nature. These and other beneficial effects of acidogenic foods need be considered, along with the effect of these foods on acid-base balance. Cranberry juice has also been used as an initial treatment for urinary tract infections.

Very low food consumption as in starvation or anorexia nervosa automatically promotes endogenous production of ketonic acids. Very low calorie diets can exert a similar effect. Alkalinizing diets can potentially counteract bone loss during weight reduction and potentially preserve other lean tissue as well.

CONTRAINDICATIONS AND PRECAUTIONS OF THE ALKALINE DIET

Anyone currently diagnosed with low bone mass or at risk for developing osteoporosis is a potential candidate for alkali diet therapy. Evaluation should begin with a thorough history, including risk factors for osteoporosis, risk factors for vascular disease, history of renal disease such as recurrent infections, nephrolithiasis, and family history of renal disease, medication review, and physical examination. Subjects who already have osteoporosis or osteoporotic fractures should discuss other therapy options with their physicians. Unlike this kind of diet therapy, therapies with estrogenic compounds or bisphosphonates have been shown to increase BMD, and have been proven to decrease the chances of new osteoporotic fractures.

Advanced renal failure and diseases such as renal tubular acidosis (RTA) or diabetes may be contraindications to eating an alkaline diet as such a diet, also contains a high potassium content, which can raise blood potassium content to abnormally high levels. Very high potassium blood levels can lead to cardiac arrhythmias and death. A history of renal disease, and laboratory tests including blood urea nitrogen (BUN), creatinine, electrolytes, and urinalysis may be appropriate to screen for renal disease.

In several renal diseases, the kidneys are unable to excrete all of the acids in the body. One such disease process, RTA, may be either genetic; related to damage to the renal tubules from diabetes mellitus, kidney stones, or recurrent infections; or from several kinds of medications. A detailed discussion of renal tubular acidosis is beyond the scope of this chapter; the reader is referred to reference [71]. Much more common is the progressive worsening of renal function with aging, and often associated or worsened by concomitant high blood pressure, diabetes mellitus, and/or the metabolic syndrome [2, 21]. Since both bone mass and renal function decline with aging, the majority of older people are at risk for these problems.

Very high potassium alkali diets should be used cautiously, if at all, in patients with advanced chronic kidney diseases, where potassium restriction is recommended; in patients with lung disease and CO_2 retention; in patients who are on medications that tend to raise serum potassium levels such as angiotensin-enzyme inhibitors, angiotensin receptor blockers, or sodium channel blockers such as spironolactone; or in patients with specific diseases that inhibit urinary potassium excretion, such as diabetes with Type 4 RTA.

Another important consideration is that diets very high in fruits and vegetables can also be very high in fiber. In extremely large quantities, fiber can cause the intestines to feel bloated and can actually cause constipation. People with "sensitive" intestinal systems, or who have had multiple surgeries for intestinal obstruction, may not be good candidates for this therapy. To habituate the intestines to large vegetable intake (high fiber), we recommend starting slowly, spreading the meals out during the day, and gradually increasing the fruits and vegetables intake, along with large quantities of water or other fluids. In this manner, we have managed to avoid intestinal complaints (constipation, bloating, feeling full) among research subjects in our studies.

People with autonomic neuropathy, however, are among those likely to be symptomatic. Among these would be people with multiple complications from poorly controlled diabetes mellitus, spinal cord injuries or diseases, or perhaps strokes.

High dietary intake of protein, such as occurs with the Atkin's diet, increases dietary acid load, as does the accidental or intentional ingestion of toxic substances such as ethylene glycol or methanol, which are metabolized to oxalic and formic acid, respectively. Other disease states that can increase the formation of endogenous metabolic acids are diabetic ketoacidosis, or lactic acidosis from overwhelming infection or tissue hypoperfusion.

One final special case is in children with seizures treated with a ketogenic diet, which is high in fat. Although intensive acid-base studies of ketogenesis have not been done on these patients, in one study of 76 children treated for 6 months with ketogenic diets, BMD decreased in 12 patients and 2 patients developed kidney stones [72], problems also seen with the ketosis that develops using the Atkins diet, which has been shown to increase diet net acid load. Further studies on the long-term effects of such a diet in relation to acid-base balance are needed.

VII. SUMMARY

Diet influences osteoporosis risk and disease progression. A diet that lowers a patient's current acid load, shifting it toward an alkalinizing diet, is a potential therapeutic intervention. This is not due to a single nutrient, to specific foods, or to supplements, but requires a rather marked degree of dietary intervention. The shift in dietary pattern can to some extent be adjusted to a patient's preferences. One such approach is demonstrated in Figure 31.5, where the calories from energy-dense, nutrient-poor foods, beans, and grains are replaced by an equal amount of calories from fruits and vegetables. Diet acid production decreased from about 50 mEq/d to –50 mEq/d (that is, the diet became highly net base producing). The optimal degree of change in diet acid production needed to affect bone metabolism and osteoporosis risk is unknown and is likely to vary among individuals.

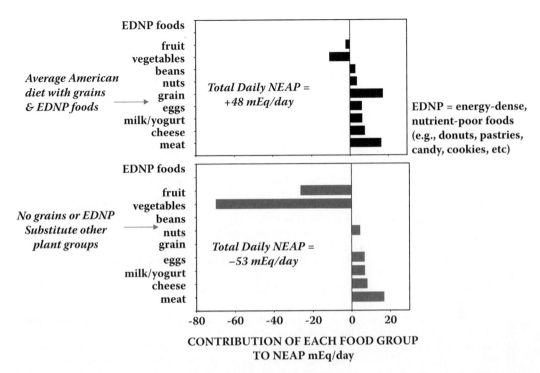

FIGURE 31.5 When transitioning to a net base producing diet, substitute nongrain plant foods for energy-dense, nutrient-poor foods.

This dietary modification presumably should be sustained to prevent osteoporosis, and the degree of benefit derived from only short-term dietary interventions are not known. It is best implemented as a physician-guided treatment:

- There are contraindications to an alkalinizing diet, which would be best recognized by a physician.
- Patients may experience side effects of the diet, which may require adjusting not only the diet but patient medications as well.
- The patient may benefit from diagnostic testing since osteoporosis screening is best performed in the setting of optimized bone-building nutrients and periodic bone density testing.

A patient who is unwilling or unable to follow this diet may benefit from alkali supplements; this is an area of ongoing research. There are also no clear dosage guidelines, but approximately 1 mEq/kg body weight is a reasonable starting dose, which can be followed by evaluating 24-hour urine pH 1 to 2 weeks after starting therapy. Diet remains first-line therapy.

REFERENCES

1. Frassetto LA, Todd KM, Morris RC, Jr., Sebastian A. Worldwide incidence of hip fracture in elderly women: relation to consumption of animal and vegetable foods. *J Gerontol A Biol Sci Med Sci* 2000;55:M585–92.
2. Shock NW, Andres R, Norris AH, Tobin JD. Patterns of longitudinal changes in renal function. In: Orimo H, Maeda D, eds. *Recent Advances in Gerontology XI International Congress*. Amsterdam: Exceprta Medica, 1979:384–686.
3. Berkemeyer S, Vormann J, Günther ALB, Rylander R, Frassetto LA, Remer T. Renal net acid excretion capacity is comparable in prepubescence, adolescence and young adulthood, but is reduced with aging. *J Am Geriatr Soc*, in submission.

4. Frassetto LA, Morris RCJ, Sebastian A. Effect of age on blood acid-base composition in adult humans: role of age-related renal functional decline. *Am J Physiol* 1996;271:F1114–22.
5. Alpern RJ. Trade-offs in the adaptation to acidosis. *Kidney Int* 1995;47:1205–15.
6. Sellmeyer DE, Stone KL, Sebastian A, Cummings SR. A high ratio of dietary animal to vegetable protein increases the rate of bone loss and the risk of fracture in postmenopausal women. Study of Osteoporotic Fractures Research Group. *Am J Clin Nutr* 2001;73:118–22.
7. Tucker KL, Chen H, Hannan MT, et al. Bone mineral density and dietary patterns in older adults: the Framingham Osteoporosis Study. *Am J Clin Nutr* 2002;76:245–52.
8. Promislow JH, Goodman-Gruen D, Slymen DJ, Barrett-Connor E. Protein consumption and bone mineral density in the elderly: the Rancho Bernardo Study. *Am J Epidemiol* 2002;155:636–44.
9. Who are candidates for prevention and treatment for osteoporosis? *Osteoporos Int* 1997;7:1–6.
10. Szulc P, Munoz F, Duboeuf F, Marchand F, Delmas PD. Bone mineral density predicts osteoporotic fractures in elderly men: the MINOS study. *Osteoporos Int* 2005;16:1184–92.
11. Merrill RM, Weed DL, Feuer EJ. The lifetime risk of developing prostate cancer in white and black men. *Cancer Epidemiol Biomarkers Prev* 1997;6:763–68.
12. Bass SL, Saxon L, Daly RM, et al. The effect of mechanical loading on the size and shape of bone in pre-, peri-, and postpubertal girls: a study in tennis players. *J Bone Miner Res* 2002;17:2274–80.
13. Semler O, Vezyroglou K, Fricke O, Schoenau E. Osteoporosis in childhood [Osteoporose im Kindesalter]. *Paediat Prax* 2007;70:667–80.
14. Yeh FJ, Grant AM, Williams SM, Goulding A. Children who experience their first fracture at a young age have high rates of fracture. *Osteoporos Int* 2006;17:267–72.
15. Cordain L, Eaton SB, Sebastian A, et al. Origins and evolution of the Western diet: health implications for the 21st century. *Am J Clin Nutr* 2005;81:341–54.
16. Frassetto LA, Todd KM, Morris RC, Jr., Sebastian A. Estimation of net endogenous noncarbonic acid production in humans from diet potassium and protein contents. *Am J Clin Nutr* 1998;68:576–83.
17. Sebastian A, Frassetto LA, Sellmeyer DE, Merriam RL, Morris RC, Jr. Estimation of the net acid load of the diet of ancestral preagricultural Homo sapiens and their hominid ancestors. *Am J Clin Nutr* 2002;76:1308–16.
18. Bonjour JP. Dietary Protein: an essential nutrient for bone health. *J Am Coll Nutr* 2005; 24:526S–536S.
19. New SA, Robins SP, Campbell MK, et al. Dietary influences on bone mass and bone metabolism: further evidence of a positive link between fruit and vegetable consumption and bone health? *Am J Clin Nutr* 2000;71:142–51.
20. Thorpe M, Mojtahedi MC, Chapman-Novakofski K, McAuley E, Evans EM. A positive association of lumbar spine bone mineral density with dietary protein is suppressed by a negative association with protein sulfur. *J Nutr* 2008;138:80–85.
21. Lindeman RD. Overview: renal physiology and pathophysiology of aging. *Am J Kidney Dis* 1990;16:275–82.
22. Jassal SK, von Muhlen D, Barrett-Connor E. Measures of renal function, BMD, bone loss, and osteoporotic fracture in older adults: the Rancho Bernardo study. *J Bone Miner Res* 2007;22:203–10.
23. Vormann J, Goedeke T. Latent acidosis: acidity as a cause for chronic diseases [Latente Azidose: Übersäuerung als Ursache chronischer Erkrankungen]. *Schewiz Zschr Ganszheits Medizin* 2002; 2:90–96.
24. Relman AS, Lennon EJ, Lemann J, Jr. Endogenous production of fixed acid and the measurement of the net acid balance in normal subjects. *J Clin Invest* 1961;40:1621–30.
25. Berkemeyer S. PhD thesis. Dietary and renal acid loads across various age-groups. Landwirtschaftliche Fakultät. Bonn: Rheinische Friedrich-Wilhelms-Universität, 2007:140.
26. Berkemeyer S, Remer T. Anthropometrics provide a better estimate of urinary organic acid anion excretion than a dietary mineral intake-based estimate in children, adolescents, and young adults. *J Nutr* 2006;136:1203–8.
27. Manz F, Vecsei P, Wesch H. [Renal acid excretion and renal molar load in healthy children and adults]. *Monatsschr Kinderheilkd* 1984;132:163–67.
28. Bushinsky DA, Smith SB, Gavrilov KL, Gavrilov LF, Li J, Levi-Setti R. Chronic acidosis-induced alteration in bone bicarbonate and phosphate. *Am J Physiol Renal Physiol* 2003;285:F532–39.
29. Frick KK, Bushinsky DA. Chronic metabolic acidosis reversibly inhibits extracellular matrix gene expression in mouse osteoblasts. *Am J Physiol* 1998;275:F840–47.
30. Brandao-Burch A, Utting JC, Orriss IR, Arnett TR. Acidosis inhibits bone formation by osteoblasts in vitro by preventing mineralization. *Calcif Tissue Int* 2005;77:167–74.

31. Arnett TR, Dempster DW. Effect of pH on bone resorption by rat osteoclasts in vitro. *Endocrinology* 1986;119:119–24.
32. Bushinsky DA. Acid-base imbalance and the skeleton. *Eur J Nutr* 2001;40:238–44.
33. Krieger NS, Frick KK, Bushinsky DA. Mechanism of acid-induced bone resorption. *Curr Opin Nephrol Hypertens* 2004;13:423–36.
34. Arnett TR, Spowage M. Modulation of the resorptive activity of rat osteoclasts by small changes in extracellular pH near the physiological range. *Bone* 1996;18:277–79.
35. Meghji S, Morrison MS, Henderson B, Arnett TR. pH dependence of bone resorption: mouse calvarial osteoclasts are activated by acidosis. *Am J Physiol Endocrinol Metab* 2001;280:E112–19.
36. Challa A, Krieg RJ, Jr., Thabet MA, Veldhuis JD, Chan JC. Metabolic acidosis inhibits growth hormone secretion in rats: mechanism of growth retardation. *Am J Physiol* 1993;265:E547–53.
37. McSherry E, Morris RC, Jr. Attainment and maintenance of normal stature with alkali therapy in infants and children with classic renal tubular acidosis. *J Clin Invest* 1978;61:509–27.
38. Sharma AP, Sharma RK, Kapoor R, Kornecki A, Sural S, Filler G. Incomplete distal renal tubular acidosis affects growth in children. *Nephrol Dial Transplant* 2007;22:2879–85.
39. Lemann J, Jr. Relationship between urinary calcium and net acid excretion as determined by dietary protein and potassium: a review. *Nephron* 1999;81 Suppl 1:18–25.
40. Kurtz I, Maher T, Hulter HN, Schambelan M, Sebastian A. Effect of diet on plasma acid-base composition in normal humans. *Kidney Int* 1983;24:670–80.
41. Frassetto LA, Morris RC, Jr., Sebastian A. Dietary sodium chloride intake independently predicts the degree of hyperchloremic metabolic acidosis in healthy humans consuming a net acid-producing diet. *Am J Physiol Renal Physiol* 2007;293;293.
42. Remer T, Manz F. Estimation of the renal net acid excretion by adults consuming diets containing variable amounts of protein. *Am J Clin Nutr* 1994;59:1356–61.
43. Kleinmann JG, Lemann JJ. Acid production. In: Maxwell MH, Kleeman CR, Narins RG, eds. *Clinical Disorders of Fluid and Electrolyte Metabolism*. New York: McGraw-Hill, 1987:159–73.
44. Lennon EJ, Lemann J, Jr., Relman AS. The effects of phosphoproteins on acid balance in normal subjects. *J Clin Invest* 1962;41:637–45.
45. Parsons TJ, van Dusseldorp M, van der Vliet M, van de Werken K, Schaafsma G, van Staveren WA. Reduced bone mass in Dutch adolescents fed a macrobiotic diet in early life. *J Bone Miner Res* 1997;12:1486–94.
46. Remer T, Manz F. Potential renal acid load of foods and its influence on urine pH. *J Am Diet Assoc* 1995;95:791–97.
47. Blatherwick NR. The specific role of foods in relation to the composition of the urine. *Arch Intern Med* 1914;14:409–50.
48. Brown SE, Trivieri L. *The Acid Alkaline Food Guide*. New York: Square One Publishers, 2006:79–161.
49. Blatherwick NR, Long ML. Studies of urine acidity II. The increased acidity produced by eating prunes and cranberries. *J Biol Chem* 1923;57:815–18.
50. Olthof MR, Hollman PC, Buijsman MN, van Amelsvoort JM, Katan MB. Chlorogenic acid, quercetin-3-rutinoside and black tea phenols are extensively metabolized in humans. *J Nutr* 2003;133:1806–14.
51. Kessler T, Jansen B, Hesse A. Effect of blackcurrant-, cranberry- and plum-juice consumption on risk factors associated with kidney stone formation. *Eur J Clin Nutr* 2002;56:1020–23.
52. Oomen HA. Nitrogen compounds and electrolytes in the urine of New Guinean sweet potato eaters. A study of normal values. *Trop Geogr Med* 1967;19:31–47.
53. Frassetto LA. Personal communication.
54. Jajoo R, Song L, Rasmussen H, Harris SS, Dawson-Hughes B. Dietary acid-base balance, bone resorption, and calcium excretion. *J Am Coll Nutr* 2006;25:224–30.
55. Dyck RF, Bear RA, Goldstein MB, Halperin ML. Iodine/iodide toxic reaction: case report with emphasis on the nature of the metabolic acidosis. *Can Med Assoc J* 1979;120:704–6.
56. Momblano P, Pradere B, Jarrige N, Concina D, Bloom E. Metabolic acidosis induced by cetrimonium bromide. *Lancet* 1984;2:1045.
57. Adachi K, Dote T, Dote E, Mitsui G, Kono K. Strong acute toxicity, severe hepatic damage, renal injury and abnormal serum electrolytes after intravenous administration of cadmium fluoride in rats. *J Occup Health* 2007;49:235–41.
58. Meunier PJ, Jenvrin C, Munoz F, de la Gueronniere V, Garnero P, Menz M. Consumption of a high calcium mineral water lowers biochemical indices of bone remodeling in postmenopausal women with low calcium intake. *Osteoporos Int* 2005;16:1203–9.

59. Buclin T, Cosma M, Appenzeller M, et al. Diet acids and alkalis influence calcium retention in bone. *Osteoporos Int* 2001;12:493–99.
60. Roux S, Baudoin C, Boute D, Brazier M, De La Gueronniere V, De Vernejoul MC. Biological effects of drinking-water mineral composition on calcium balance and bone remodeling markers. *J Nutr Health Aging* 2004;8:380–84.
61. Maurer M, Riesen W, Muser J, Hulter HN, Krapf R. Neutralization of Western diet inhibits bone resorption independently of K intake and reduces cortisol secretion in humans. *Am J Physiol Renal Physiol* 2003;284:F32–40.
62. Sebastian A, Morris RC, Jr. Improved mineral balance and skeletal metabolism in postmenopausal women treated with potassium bicarbonate. *N Engl J Med* 1994;331:279.
63. Sellmeyer DE, Schloetter M, Sebastian A. Potassium citrate prevents increased urine calcium excretion and bone resorption induced by a high sodium chloride diet. *J Clin Endocrinol Metab* 2002;87:2008–12.
64. Jehle S, Zanetti A, Muser J, Hulter HN, Krapf R. Partial neutralization of the acidogenic Western diet with potassium citrate increases bone mass in postmenopausal women with osteopenia. *J Am Soc Nephrol* 2006;17:3213–22.
65. www.erque.com. 2008.
66. Whiting SJ, Muirhead JA. Measurement of net acid excretion by use of paper strips. *Nutrition* 2005;21:961–63.
67. Frassetto LA. Unpublished data.
68. Maalouf NM, Cameron MA, Moe OW, Adams-Huet B, Sakhaee K. Low urine pH: a novel feature of the metabolic syndrome. *Clin J Am Soc Nephrol* 2007;2:883–88.
69. Rylander R, Arnaud MJ. Mineral water intake reduces blood pressure among subjects with low urinary magnesium and calcium levels. *BMC Public Health* 2004;4:56.
70. Honow R, Laube N, Schneider A, Kessler T, Hesse A. Influence of grapefruit-, orange- and apple-juice consumption on urinary variables and risk of crystallization. *Br J Nutr* 2003;90:295–300.
71. Rodriguez Soriano J. Renal tubular acidosis: the clinical entity. *J Am Soc Nephrol* 2002;13:2160–70.
72. Seo JH, Lee YM, Lee JS, Kang HC, Kim HD. Efficacy and tolerability of the ketogenic diet according to lipid:nonlipid ratios—comparison of 3:1 with 4:1 diet. *Epilepsia* 2007;48:801–5.
73. Jaffe R. *Food Effects on Body Chemistry*. Sterling, VA, 2007.

32 Metabolic Bone Disease

Nutrient, Drug, and Disease Interactions

Joseph J. Lamb, M.D., and Susan E. Williams, M.D., M.S., R.D.

I. INTRODUCTION

Osteoporosis, literally "porous bone," is defined as a reduction in the mass and quality of bone and/ or the presence of a fragility fracture. Osteoporosis is common, preventable, serious, diagnosable, and treatable. Osteoporosis is a clinically silent systemic skeletal disease characterized by compromised bone strength predisposing to an increased risk of fracture. It can occur as a primary disease or secondary to underlying chronic disease or use of certain medications (Table 32.1). Osteoporosis can be prevented or ameliorated by lifestyle interventions. This chapter imparts a science-based understanding of the etiology and pathophysiology, which enables an interested clinician to diagnose osteoporosis and apply nutritional interventions.

II. EPIDEMIOLOGY

Osteoporosis poses a major health threat for more than 44 million U.S. adults ages 50 and older, and it is estimated that an additional 18 million people have undiagnosed low bone mass. About 1.3 million osteoporotic fractures occur each year in the United States, and of those patients who suffer a hip fracture, only 40% fully regain their pre-fracture level of independence, leaving 60% who will experience chronic pain, disability, and a 10% to 20% excess mortality within 1 year.[1] It is therefore essential that early diagnosis and treatment strategies be designed and implemented in all patients at risk.

III. PHYSIOLOGY

Bone mineralization is regulated primarily by the activity of the three cell types, osteoblasts, osteoclasts, and osteocytes, which are under both local and systemic control. These bone cells respond to changing environmental stimuli such as nutrient availability, inflammation, and physiological demands.

Mechanical loading is one such physiologic demand, modulated by the osteocyte through a complex array of cell signaling pathways. The mechanical message is transformed into altered gene expression, resulting in proliferation and matrix synthesis. This message leads to up-regulation of growth factors including insulin-like growth factors (IGF), vascular endothelial growth factors, and bone morphogenetic protein (BMP) 2 and 4.[2]

TABLE 32.1
Secondary Causes of Bone Loss

SYSTEM	ETIOLOGY
Endocrine	Hyperparathyroidism, thyrotoxicosis, insulin-dependent diabetes mellitus, acromegaly, hyperprolactinemia, Cushing's disease, perimenopause/menopause, amenorrhea, anorexia nervosa, pregnancy and lactation, and other estrogen-deficient states.
Nutrition and gastroenterology	Low body weight, low calcium intake, protein-calorie malnutrition; parenteral nutrition; gastric or small bowel resection; malabsorption syndromes; end-stage liver disease including biliary cirrhosis.
Orthopedics & rheumatology	Rheumatoid arthritis, ankylosing spondylitis, scoliosis, history of paralytic poliomyelitis.
Hematology & oncology	Pernicious anemia; multiple myeloma; lymphoma, leukemia, parathyroid hormone-related protein production due to underlying malignancy; mastocytosis; hemophilia, thalassemia major.
Genetic predisposition & genetically determined diseases	Caucasian or Asian race; positive family history; inherited hypogonadal states (Turner's and Klinefelter's syndromes); osteogenesis imperfecta, Marfan's syndrome, hemochromatosis, hypophosphatasia, glycogen storage disease, homocystinuria, Ehlers-Danlos syndrome, and porphyria.
Pharmacology	Excessive thyroxine, glucocorticoids, anticonvulsants, heparin, lithium, cyclosporine, aluminum, cytotoxic drugs, proton pump inhibitors, gonadotrophin-releasing hormone agonists.
Miscellaneous	Short stature and short bones, immobilization, paralysis, chronic obstructive pulmonary disease, multiple sclerosis, sarcoidosis, amyloidosis, endogenous (hypermetabolic) stress response.

Source: [119–127].

Many structures are intimately involved in the regulation of matrix secretion and mineralization: cell surface receptors, extracellular matrix structure and integrins, cadherins, and $Ca+^2$ channels in the cellular cytoskeleton, intracellular signaling kinases, prostaglandins, and nitric oxide.[3] Messengers involved in mediating bone growth are often intimately involved in inflammatory signaling pathways. The interplay of these messages is complex and bidirectional. Many growth factors influence osteoblast formation. Core binding Factor A1 (CBFA1) is a transcription factor expressed in osteoblast progenitors and stromal support cells that has been shown to be important in the control of osteoblast development. It regulates the expression of several osteoblast-specific genes including type 1 collagen, receptor-activator of NFκB (RANK) ligand also called osteoclast differentiation factor, osteocalcin, osteopontin, and bone sialoprotein. Osteoblasts, through secretion of RANK ligand (RANKL), actually promote differentiation and maturation of osteoclasts. Interestingly, when responding to different environmental signals, osteoblasts secrete osteoprotegerin, also called osteoclastogenesis inhibitory factor, which binds RANKL and acts as a receptor decoy to inhibit differentiation of osteoclasts.[4] Stromal support cells secrete macrophage colony stimulating factor and RANKL to promote osteoclast differentiation and maturation. Macrophages and adipocytes, residents of the bone marrow, play a role in this complex interplay releasing locally produced growth factors and cytokines including gamma interferon, interleukins 1, 6, and 11 (IL-1, IL-6, IL-11), and tumor necrosis factor-α (TNFα). These cytokines play an important role in the osteoclast maturation process by stimulating secretion of RANKL.

In addition to the cell-mediated local control, several hormones provide systemwide oversight of bone metabolism. Both parathyroid hormone (PTH) and 1,25-dihydroxyvitamin D3 directly modulate osteoclastic activity to maintain appropriate serum calcium and phosphorus levels. Estrogen influences bone metabolism. Deficiency increases bone remodeling intensity, which exacerbates propensity to bone resorption in functionally challenged bone and contributes to the development of primary osteoporosis in perimenopausal women. Testosterone has also been shown to be associated with osteoporosis.[5] Intervention trials have demonstrated that supplementation with estrogen in women, DHEA in men and women,[6] and testosterone in hypogonadal men[7] are effective.

This interaction of local cells, communicating by growth factors and cytokines and modulated by systemic hormones, is the healthy norm of bone metabolism. Osteoporosis is the pathophysiologic disturbance of this process.

IV. PATHOPHYSIOLOGY

As we explore the pathophysiology of osteoporosis, we find that mechanisms rather than broad organ system classifications may cast more light on the underlying causes of osteoporosis. Mechanistic categories include diminished achievement of peak bone mass, decreased mineral availability, decreased osteoblast activity, increased osteoclast activity, abnormal protein metabolism, and systemic inflammation.

In a clinical setting osteoporosis is often defined as primary or secondary. In a postmenopausal woman, estrogen deficiency results in a diagnosis of primary osteoporosis whereas suppressed estrogen levels due to an adolescent girl receiving a GnRH agonist as contraception or a premenopausal woman receiving chemotherapy for breast cancer often lead to a diagnosis of secondary osteoporosis.

Secondary osteoporosis occurs in patients who are less likely to be screened for the disease because they may not present as a prototypic osteoporosis patient. The pathophysiology of secondary osteoporosis is presented with the goal of increasing "clinical suspicion" (Table 32.1).

PEAK BONE MASS

Bone mass acquisition is largely genetically determined, with greater than 50% being attained during adolescence and peak mass typically achieved by the early 20s.[8–10] Before adulthood, bone forms by two separate mechanisms. Endochondral bone formation is the restructuring and replacing of previously calcified cartilage. Intermembranous bone formation is *de novo* development without a calcified matrix.[11] After adolescence, endochondral formation ceases. Emphasis needs to be placed on maximizing peak bone mass during adolescence or future BMD will be compromised as even relatively small incremental losses will have a proportionately greater affect on a lower peak bone mass. Acquisitional osteopenia is the failure to achieve the genetically determined peak bone mass and can be the result of chronic illness, use of certain medications, malnutrition, malabsorption, or disruption of key metabolic pathways.[12–14]

Radioisotope studies have demonstrated turnovers of up to 18% of the calcium in adult bone per year—an indication of the significant persistent metabolic activity in postadolescent bone. Despite this, bone remodeling is a much slower process in adulthood than during adolescence. The primary purpose of adult bone remodeling is homeostasis during the ever-present processes of microdamage repairs, and skeletal strength maintenance.

Failure to attain peak bone mass occurs from the following:

- Adolescent eating disorders, including both anorexia and bulimia, are conditions associated with failure to achieve peak bone mass. In addition to decreased mineral and protein availability because of insufficient intake, contributing factors to osteoporosis include amenorrhea, calcium and vitamin D deficiency, increased endogenous steroid production, and low levels of growth factors including IGF. In these patients, nutritional rehabilitation with weight gain, adequate calcium and vitamin D intake, moderate weight-bearing exercise, and resumption of normal menses have been shown to improve but not normalize bone mineral density.[15,16]
- Use of Depo-Provera as contraception produces estrogen deficiency. Adolescent females who use Depo-Provera are at risk for low bone mass due to failure to achieve peak bone mass.[17] With calcium supplementation in adolescents, some of the potential loss, but apparently not all, can be ameliorated.

- Lead exposure. A study in children with high lead exposure revealed significantly increased bone mineral density compared to normal controls. Despite the potential for heavy metals creating a false negative result in DXA scanning because of x-ray absorption by lead and not calcium, the investigators postulated that lead exposure may actually accelerate boney maturation by inhibition of PTH. However, they concluded that the accelerated bone maturation results in a shorter period of mineralization and growth, resulting in decreased peak bone mass.[18]

Decreased Mineral Availability

Conditions that decrease mineral uptake from the gastrointestinal tract include malabsorption syndromes.

- Inflammatory bowel disease (IBD) activity strongly correlates with the severity of bone loss; therefore effective disease management including calcium and vitamin D supplementation, risk factor reduction, and avoidance of glucocorticoids are equally important aspects of treatment.[19] And although appropriate diagnostic and therapeutic regimens addressing BMD in IBD patients are essential, a standard treatment strategy has yet to be defined.[20,21] Celiac enteropathy causes marked mineral and calorie malabsorption (see more in the following).
- Primary biliary cirrhosis (PBC) with its resultant underlying fat malabsorption has been shown to contribute to insufficiencies of fat-soluble vitamins, specifically vitamin D and vitamin K.[22] Additionally, PBC patients have attenuation of the liver's ability to adequately hydroxylate vitamin D.
- Lactase deficiency. Several studies have demonstrated a strong correlation with adult lactase deficiency and the development of osteoporosis. Patient avoidance of milk and other dairy products resulted in an increased incidence of osteoporosis and bone fracture.[23] Though it was once believed that lactose was essential for optimal calcium absorption, it is now known that calcium absorption from various dairy products is equivalent, regardless of the lactose content or the chemical form of calcium.
- Gastrectomy. Essentially all post-gastrectomy patients have an increased risk of fracture and should be routinely evaluated for the presence of metabolic bone disease (MBD). The incidence of osteomalacia in this population is estimated to be 10% to 20%, and although the incidence of osteoporosis in this patient population is unknown it is estimated to be as high as 32% to 42%.[24]
- Bariatric surgery. Morbid obesity has historically been viewed as having a protective effect against the development of MBD. However, recent research has revealed that many obese individuals have inadequate nutrition status, vitamin D deficiency, elevated parathyroid hormone levels, and are at risk for low bone mass.[25,26] Studies attempting to define the presurgical prevalence of vitamin D deficiency have identified rates in excess of 60% among patients selected to undergo weight loss surgery.[27,28] Similarly, the prevalence of preoperative elevated intact parathyroid hormone (PTH) in this population ranged from 25% to 48%.[29] Postsurgically, significant weight loss, severely restricted oral intake, calcium malabsorption, and concomitant vitamin D deficiency places these patients at extremely high risk for the development of MBD. Several factors are likely involved. Primarily, malabsorption plays a critical role with malabsorption of calcium, magnesium, fat-soluble vitamins including vitamin D, protein, B12, and folic acid all being reported.
- Gastric hypoacidity because of atrophy, proton pump inhibitors, and H_2 blockers. Gastroesophageal reflux disease (GERD) does not share a causal relationship with MBD. Yet, chronic

overuse of antacids containing aluminum hydroxide can lead to phosphorus deficiency and osteomalacia.[30,31] Hypophosphatemia results in increased levels of $1,25(OH)_2D_3$, increased calcium absorption, hypercalciuria, and increased bone resorption. Known as antacid-induced osteomalacia, symptomatic patients experience diffuse bone pain, proximal muscle weakness, and difficulty climbing stairs and rising from a chair.

Calcium must be ionized to be optimally absorbed, and ionization of calcium requires an acidic environment. Reduced gastric acidity contributes to the failure to ionize calcium in the small intestine and decreases the bioavailability of calcium. Calcium carbonate is much more vulnerable to being malabsorbed as opposed to other forms of calcium including citrate, lactate, and gluconate, as it is not already ionized. Although the effects of achlorhydria on the bioavailability of calcium are well documented, the relationship to MBD remains unclear. Advancing age combined with the growing use of H_2 blockers and proton pump inhibitors now available over the counter for dyspepsia contribute to the magnitude of the problem. Adequate calcium absorption can be achieved by instructing the patient to take calcium supplements with meals, or by switching to calcium citrate.

- High sodium diets and acid load diets. The evidence of a detrimental effect of high salt intake on bone health is primarily limited to short-term effects of sodium on calcium metabolism. There is strong evidence in support of the fact that high salt intake produces a calciuretic effect but investigations attempting to define the association of sodium with bone loss and BMD have produced conflicting results.[32] The typical Western diet contains sodium far above evolutionary norms and potassium far below those norms. These changes associated with a decrease in fruit and vegetable intake create a net acid producing load. As a result of a need to excrete this acid load, renal calcium losses are increased.[33]

- Caffeine use. Caffeine is known to increase urinary calcium losses and may have harmful effects on bone. A recent prospective study demonstrated that bone loss occurred in those women who had both low calcium intake and high caffeine intakes.[34] The deleterious effects of caffeine on bone can be negated by consuming adequate calcium.[35,36]

- High protein diets despite their potential to contain high amounts of calcium. Dietary protein is required to maintain bone structure; however, studies have shown a positive association between excess protein intake and urinary excretion of calcium, contributing to a negative calcium balance.[37] A link between high protein intake and an increased risk of fracture has also been demonstrated, regardless of whether it was of animal or vegetable origin.[38,39] However, when high protein intake is coupled with adequate calcium intake, the potentially harmful effects of protein appear to be ameliorated.[40-42]

- Phosphorus is plentiful in the food supply predominantly due to the increased use of phosphate salts in food additives and cola beverages. And although phosphorus is an essential nutrient, the current literature notes that both phosphorus deficiency and excess intake interfere with calcium absorption and lead to bone loss.[43] A large study examining carbonated beverages and incidence of fractures in schoolgirls found a statistically significant increase in fractures in those girls who regularly consumed carbonated beverages; however, it appeared that the fracture risk was the consequence of consuming less milk.[44]

- Hypovitaminosis D interferes with absorption of calcium. Vitamin D plays a role both in intestinal adsorption of calcium as well as modifying the speed of bone turnover. Vitamin D is essential for calcium and phosphate absorption in the gut, stimulation of osteoblast activity, calcium reabsorption in the renal tubules, and normal bone mineralization throughout the lifespan. Absorption of vitamin D occurs mainly by passive diffusion in the proximal and mid small intestine and is highly dependent on bile salts.[45]

DECREASED OSTEOBLAST ACTIVITY

Conditions that decrease osteoblast activity resulting in less bone formation include:

- Diabetes mellitus. Type 1 diabetes mellitus (DM) has been implicated as a cause of osteoporosis, but the causal relationship is still being defined. Reports on causal connections in type 2 DM are inconsistent as well, although some oral agents (PPARγ agonists, specifically the thiazolidinediones)[46] commonly prescribed to treat type 2 DM have also been implicated. Please see the section below on inflammation for a discussion of the connection between insulin resistance and inflammation. Given the prevalence of DM, surveillance for osteoporosis in diabetics is of great importance.[47]
- Tobacco abuse. Tobacco has direct toxic effects on osteoblasts and also acts indirectly by modifying estrogen metabolism. Cigarette smokers on average reach menopause approximately 1 to 2 years earlier than nonsmokers. Tobacco abuse also leads to an increase in illnesses and earlier frailty by decreasing exercise capacity and increasing the likelihood of requiring corticosteroids for treatment of pulmonary diseases.[48]
- Alcohol abuse. Excessive alcohol has been shown to decrease osteoblast activity.[49] And yet several studies have shown that moderate consumption has positive impact on bone health.[50] Higher consumption, especially in men, however, increased the rate of fracture, perhaps related to increased falls or nutritional compromise related to alcohol abuse. Daily alcohol consumption of 50 grams (approximately three standard drinks) results in a dose dependent decrease in osteoblast activity; daily consumption of greater than 100 grams eventually results in an osteopenic skeleton and increased risk for the development of osteoporosis.[51] One drink per day for women and two drinks per day for men is the recommended safe upper limit for consumption.
- Corticosteroid excess, whether exogenous or endogenous, can result in deleterious effects on healthy bone primarily due to decreasing osteoblast activity.[52] The profound effect of steroid excess is demonstrated by noting that it is the most common cause of secondary osteoporosis and is second only to menopause as a cause of overall osteoporosis. Glucocorticoid-induced bone loss occurs following the administration of pharmacologic doses of glucocorticoids for greater than a few days, and is the result of uncoupling of the normal relationship between the resorption and formation phases of bone remodeling.[53] Glucocorticoids suppress 1-hydroxylase activity and function as a 1,25(OH)D antagonist thereby blunting calcium absorption.[54,55] Fifty percent of patients on chronic corticosteroid administration for 6 months or longer develop osteoporosis. In fact, a daily dose of 2.5 to 5.0 mg of prednisone may be sufficient to cause osteoporosis.[56] There is also evidence that potent inhaled glucocorticoids may have deleterious effects on the skeleton.[57] The cumulative dose of glucocorticoids correlates with the severity of the bone disease and the incidence of fracture. Of note, patients maintained on corticosteroid replacement due to adrenal insufficiency do not appear to be at increased risk.[58]

  The diagnosis of osteoporosis can also be the presenting symptom of Cushing's disease. Subclinical hypercortisolism may be more common than generally recognized with an 11% prevalence among patients with low BMD and vertebral fractures.[59]
- Persistent physical and psychological stress can induce endogenous corticosteroids excess and increase BMD losses. Depression has been associated with elevated cortisol levels. Daily usage of selective serotonin reuptake inhibitors in adults over 50 has been associated with a two-fold increased risk of clinical fragility fracture and decreased bone mineral density in the hip.[60]

INCREASED OSTEOCLAST ACTIVITY

The following contribute to an increase in osteoclastic activity:

- Hyperparathyroidism. An increase in osteoclast activity is the primary effect of PTH to maintain calcium and phosphorus in a narrow physiologic range. It does so by increasing activation of 25-hydroxyvitamin D3 to 1,25-dihydroxyvitamin D3 to increase bone resorption. Secondary hyperparathyroidism is the response to a lowered serum calcium level resulting in an increase in PTH levels and increased bone resorption. Interestingly, intermittent exposure to PTH actually leads to increases in BMD by favoring formation over resorption.[61]
- Postmenopausal estrogen deficiency and other hypogonadal states, both primary and secondary. Estrogen deficiency increases the population of pre-B cells, a subset of bone marrow stromal cells, which in turn increases production of IL-1 and TNFα. These cytokines induce cyclo-oxygenase 2 activity increasing prostaglandin E_2 production by osteoblasts and subsequent increase in RANKL expression and resultant osteoclastogenesis.[62] Many cancer therapies for breast, ovarian, and prostate cancer patients produce hypogonadal states. Tamoxifen has been shown to produce osteoporosis in premenopausal women. And both aromatase inhibitors and GnRH agonists produce estrogen deficiency. Estrogen deficiency may also be associated with the genetic hypogonadal states such as Turner's syndrome and Klinefelter's syndrome.

  Several recent papers point to the need for appropriate balance of the metabolites of estrone and estradiol. Normal ratios of 2-hydroxy to 16α-hydroxy estrogens are associated with optimal bone health, while imbalances marked by either an excess of 2-hydroxy or 16α-hydroxy estrogens is associated with osteoporosis.[63,64]
- Heparin, a potent anticoagulant, stimulates both osteoclastic bone resorption as well as suppressing osteoblastic activity. Heparin doses of 15,000 units or greater daily for 6 months have been shown to increase the risk for osteoporosis.[65]
- Inactivity, immobilization, paraplegia, and sarcopenia. Mature osteocytes, by sensing the mechanical forces exerted on bone by physical activity, directly influence bone remodeling. Any condition that decreases these forces will have a negative effect on bone strength. Physical immobilization after trauma, or neural damage due to cerebrovascular accident, poliomyelitis, or multiple sclerosis has been associated with osteoporosis. A reduction in compressive mechanical forces because of immobilization reduces the canalicular fluid flow in bone with resultant osteocyte hypoxemia and death leading to increased osteoclast activity.[66]
- Hyperthyroidism is associated with both increased osteoblastic and osteoclastic activities. Resorption is favored overall, however, as increased formation cannot keep pace with increased resorption. Treatment of thyrotoxicosis has been shown to increase bone density, but fails to restore BMD to healthy norms. The effect of exogenous subclinical hyperthyroidism on BMD in women is unclear, with mixed reports of normal and decreased BMD.[67] However, a small uncontrolled case series, following women treated for thyroid hormone resistance with the development of exogenous subclinical hyperthyroidism manifested by modest suppression of TSH, revealed increased BMD with thyroid hormone supplementation.[68]
- Cadmium exposure. Low levels of chronic cadmium exposure have been associated with the development of osteoporosis.[69]
- The term "methotrexate osteopathy" was first used to name a syndrome of bone pain, fragility fractures, and radiographic osteopenia first reported predominantly in children placed on long-term treatment for acute lymphoblastic leukemia in the 1970s. The negative effects of high-dose MTX on bone appear to be due to increased bone resorption in the presence of inhibited bone formation[70] while lower dose MTX does not appear to cause accelerated bone loss.[71]

Impaired Protein Metabolism

The following conditions affecting protein metabolism have a very important role in the pathogenesis of osteoporosis as well:

- Protein-calorie malnutrition. Protein-calorie malnutrition (PCM) occurs as a result of many chronic diseases and, left uncorrected, results in MBD. In the NHANES 1 study, hip fractures were associated with low energy intake, low serum albumin, and decreased muscle strength, all reflecting protein and caloric deficit.[72] A 10% decrease in body weight typically results in a 1% to 2% bone loss, and more severe weight loss and malnutrition are considered risk factors for osteoporosis which is likely due to low protein intake.[73]

  High-protein diets have been shown to increase urinary calcium losses. However, there is growing evidence that a low-protein diet has a detrimental effect on bone. In two interventional trials examining graded levels of protein intake on calcium homeostasis, decreased calcium absorption and an acute rise in PTH was noted by day four of the 0.7 and 0.8 g/kg diets but not during the 0.9 or 1.0 g/kg diets.[74,75] This is particularly worrisome, in that these studies suggest the current RDA of 0.8 g protein/kg is inadequate to promote calcium homeostasis.
- Cushing's syndrome, whether primary or secondary to exogenous long-term administration of glucocorticoids, can cause decreased deposition of protein throughout the body in addition to increasing protein catabolism.
- Increasing age is marked by decreasing levels of growth hormones and decreased protein anabolic activity.
- Deficiency of vitamin C, which is necessary for secretion of intercellular protein, interferes with formation of the matrix by osteoblasts.[76]
- Lead exposure. Osteocalcin in bone matrix preferentially binds lead resulting in decreased calcium binding and failure to bind hydroxyapatite, resulting in decreased bone formation.[77] Serum lead levels increase by 25% to 30% due to mobilization as bone is resorbed in postmenopausal women with osteoporosis[78] contributing to lead toxicity and resultant illnesses late in life.
- Liver disease. Cholestatic disease, autoimmune hepatitis, chronic viral hepatitis, and alcoholic liver disease can result in osteoporosis. Vitamin D levels are typically low in patients with alcoholic liver disease, autoimmune hepatitis treated with glucocorticoids, and primary biliary cirrhosis, thereby increasing the risk of osteoporosis as well as osteomalacia.[79,80] In fact, osteoporosis can be one of the first clinical manifestations of cholestatic disease.[81] Advanced chronic cholestatic disorders such as primary sclerosing cholangitis also place the patient at significant risk of developing low bone mass.[82]

Inflammation

Given the role of inflammatory messengers and cytokines in the cell-to-cell communication vital to the balanced remodeling process, systemic inflammatory diseases with resultant increases in proinflammatory messengers have direct effects on bone leading to increased risk for the development of osteoporosis. These cytokines have been associated with increased osteoclastogenesis in multiple conditions including rheumatoid arthritis, periodontal disease, and multiple myeloma for example. Falling estrogen levels are associated with increased proinflammatory cytokines, and RANKL gene expression is increased during postmenopause compared to premenopause.[83]

- Insulin resistance. Much research has recently focused on the close connection between insulin resistance, inflammatory adipocyte function, and the development of osteoporosis. RANKL and its downstream cytokines have important roles in bone, metabolic, and vascular disease.[84] Several single nucleotide polymorphisms of RANKL have been associated with obesity.[85] Abnormal development of the skeleton associated with suppressed osteomaturation rates was noted in the db/db and ob/ob mouse models of diabetes and obesity.[86] Advanced glycation end products have been implicated in the up-regulation of RANKL (inducing increased osteoclastogenesis) and down-regulation of alkaline phosphatase and osteocalcin (impairing matrix mineralization).[87] Leptin administration in the ob/ob mouse model has been shown to induce adipocyte apoptosis and increase bone formation.[88] This work has led certain authors to question whether "osteoporosis is the obesity of bone."[89]

- Inflammatory bowel disease. Patients with inflammatory bowel disease (IBD) have a high prevalence of decreased bone mineral density and an increased rate of vertebral fractures. Circulating proinflammatory cytokines increase osteoclast activity. Indeed, TNFα decreases differentiation of osteoblasts, increases differentiation of osteoclasts, and increases osteoclast survival by decreasing apoptosis. High levels of IL-6 have been found in osteoporotic patients suffering from Crohn's disease compared to non-osteoporotic patients.[90]
- Gluten-sensitive enteropathy (celiac disease). Celiac disease is an autoimmune disorder of varying severity characterized by small bowel enteropathy resulting from exposure to wheat gluten in genetically susceptible individuals, and is frequently diagnosed in patients presenting with osteoporosis.[91] It is estimated that celiac disease affects 1% of the population and of those affected, approximately 50% of patients will not have clinically significant diarrhea.[92]
- Calcineurin inhibitors (CI). Cyclosporine A and tacrolimus are potent immunomodulators used in transplant patients who are frequently in poor health and have osteoporosis prior to their surgery. Calcineurin inhibitors have multiple effects on bone including decreased bone formation, but the more important mechanism appears to be their effect on T-lymphocytes, which then produce osteoclast stimulatory cytokines. The overall loss in BMD in these patients is exacerbated by the frequent concurrent use with corticosteroids.[93]
- Several chronic diseases of aging have been noted to be comorbid conditions with osteoporosis. These conditions, including atherosclerosis, osteoarthritis, and periodontal disease, share inflammation[94] as an underlying pathophysiological derangement.

UNCLEAR ETIOLOGIES

- Antiepileptic drugs (AEDs) have been associated with bone disease. Early reports on institutionalized patients were primarily of rickets and osteomalacia. But more recent reports, particularly in outpatients, have demonstrated evidence of osteoporosis. Mechanisms proposed include increased catabolism of vitamin D by the cytochrome P450 enzyme system, impairment of calcium absorption, impaired bone resorption and formation, and poor vitamin K status.[95]
- Parenteral nutrition support. Osteoporosis has been recognized as a complication of parenteral nutrition (PN) for more than 25 years and appears to be multifactorial. Early studies found intravenous nutrition solutions to contain excess aluminum, but despite newer formulations that limit this element, osteoporosis continues to occur.[96] A longitudinal study conducted in Denmark noted an absence of accelerated bone lost but found the BMD of many long-term PN patients substantially reduced, making them susceptible to fragility fractures and in need of preventive strategies.[97]
- Vitamin A (retinol) taken in excess can result in osteoporosis and can also lead to hypercalcemia. This noted toxic effect occurs in smaller doses as well and has been identified as a risk factor for hip fractures. Vitamin A as beta carotene does not appear to be associated with increased fracture risk; however, this fact is still being argued.[98,99]

V. PATIENT EVALUATION

Bone strength is an integration of bone density and bone quality.[100] Central dual-energy x-ray absorptiometry (DEXA) is the most common study used to determine bone density and from that data, current bone status and risk stratification for future fractures can be determined. The World Health Organization (WHO) has defined normal bone density, osteopenia, and osteoporosis based on the T score. DXA results also quantify the standard deviation from that of an age- and gender-matched control, reported as the Z score. If bone loss is exclusively due to the normal process of aging, the Z score will be near zero; therefore secondary disease should be suspected when there is a negative deviation of greater than –1.5.[101,102]

There is still no substitute for a thorough history and physical. And ideally, the risk factors for osteoporosis would be identified in all susceptible patients prior to any disease manifestations. A vigilant physician can clinically identify individuals at high risk for osteoporosis by using a stadiometer to measure height and monitor for height changes. When height is discordant with prior measured height or the patient's stated height by greater than 1 inch, this should prompt further evaluation.

Celiac disease is also a silent, nutritionally treatable disease and it predisposes to malabsorption and inflammation. Celiac disease is estimated to be 5- to 10-fold more common among those with osteoporosis. (See Chapter 15, "Food Reactivities.")

Screening for hypovitaminosis D by checking a serum 25-hydroxyvitamin D (25(OH)D) is indicated in the evaluation of osteoporosis and osteomalacia. Osteomalacia, an abnormal mineralization of cartilage and bone, is most commonly caused by vitamin D deficiency. Vitamin D deficiency can occur as a result of inadequate intake of vitamin D, inadequate exposure to sunlight, or malabsorption syndromes, and is frequently found in patients following gastrectomy, small bowel resection, and bariatric procedures.[103–105] Unlike osteoporosis, osteomalacia affects primarily cortical bone; therefore bone densitometry testing is unlikely to confirm the diagnosis. Clinically, these patients can present with bone pain and proximal muscle weakness; however, distinguishing osteomalacia from osteoporosis can be difficult. Diagnosis can be guided by clinical presentation and treatment can be guided by biochemical indices including 25(OH)D, calcium, phosphate, bone-specific alkaline phosphatase, parathyroid hormone, and urine calcium and phosphate.[106,107]

VI. TREATMENT

OVERVIEW

The first step in treatment is prompt diagnosis. Often the underlying pathophysiology can point to individualized food and nutrient interventions. For example, patients with vitamin D deficiency require immediate and aggressive therapy. Repletion can be achieved by giving oral pharmacological doses (50,000 IU of vitamin D2 or 15,000 IU of vitamin D3) once weekly for 8 weeks. Efficacy of the treatment should be determined by repeat serum levels, and an additional 8-week course prescribed if needed. For patients who are chronically deficient, after the initial 8-week course, twice-per-month maintenance dosing is recommended. And for patients who are unable to tolerate or adequately absorb oral supplements, exposure to sunlight (UVB radiation) is still the best source of vitamin D and is an effective alternative.[108]

DIETARY PATTERN

Diet as a first-line treatment cannot be overemphasized. (See Chapter 31, "Osteoporosis.") Eating five to nine servings of fruits and vegetables rich in potassium daily produces a net alkaline load and offsets the net calcium loss induced by the typical American diet's high sodium and acid load.[109] Fiber is an important component of the alkaline diet. Some forms of fiber can impair mineral

TABLE 32.2
Key Bone-Building Nutrients

Nutrient	Adult RDA or AI	Common Therapeutic Range for Bone Health	Dietary Considerations
Calcium	800–1200 mg	1000–1500 mg	Typical diet is inadequate, averages 500–600 mg.[128,129]
Phosphorus	700 mg	700–1200 mg	Inadequate intake is rare except in elderly and malnourished; excessive intake common with use of processed foods and soft drinks.
Magnesium	420 mg men; 320 mg women	400–800 mg	Intake generally inadequate: All ages, sexes, classes, except children less than 5, fail to consume this RDA. 40% of population, 50% of adolescents consume less than 2/3 the RDA.[129–132]
Fluoride	4.0 mg men; 3.0 mg women	—	Fluoride overdose has occurred through ingestion of fluoride toothpaste and high fluoride waters.[130]
Silica	No values yet set	5–20 mg	Intake is unknown. Silica is removed in food processing; current intake is suspected to be low.
Zinc	11 mg men; 8 mg women	20–30 mg	Marginal zinc deficiency is common, especially among children.[130] Average intake was 46 to 63% of the RDA.[132]
Manganese	2.3 mg men; 1.8 mg women	10–25 mg	Intakes are generally inadequate, 1.76 mg adolescent girls, 2.05 mg women, 2.5 males.[133]
Copper	900 µg men and women	2–3 mg	75% of diets fail to contain the RDA.[132,134] Average intake is below the RDA.[130]
Boron	No RDA established	3–4 mg	1/4 mg intake is common[135] to perhaps optimum of 3 mg.
Potassium	4700 mg men and women	4700–5000	Adult intake averages 2300 mg for women and 3100 mg for men.[136]
Vitamin D	400 until age 70; then 600 IU, men and women	800–2000 IU & up as needed	Deficiency is common especially among the elderly, dark skinned, and those with little UV sunlight exposure.
Vitamin C	90 mg men; 75 mg women	Oral 500 mg–to bowel tolerance as needed	Average daily intake is about 95 mg for women and 107 for men.[137]
Vitamin A	2997 IU men; 2331 IU adult women	5000 IU or less	31% consume less than 70% of the RDA.[138] Current intake for women is about 2373 µg/day.[139]
Vitamin B6	1.7 mg men; 1.5 mg women	25–50 mg	Studies indicate widespread inadequate vitamin B6 consumption among all sectors of the population.[140]
Folic acid	400 µg men and women	800–1000 µg	Inadequate intake was common among all age groups, but is improving with food fortification.[130]
Vitamin K	120 µg men; 90 µg women	1000 µg	Averages 45 to 150 µg, which is well below the recommendation AI.[141]
Vitamin B12	2.4 mg men and women	100–1000 µg	12% consume less than 70% RDA.[138] Older people and vegans are especially at risk.[130]
Fats	Should comprise 7% of calories minimum; general recommendation is not to exceed 30% of calories	20% to 30% of total calories is perhaps more ideal	The average American consumes 33% of calories in fat. The consumption of essential fatty acids, however, is frequently inadequate (26).[130]

absorption, but this is not uniformly the case and a diet high in fiber is recommended. One specific type of fiber found in fruits and vegetables is the inulin-type fructans, a subclass of fructooligosaccharides, which have been shown to improve calcium absorption in adolescents and adults.[110]

Food Selection

Treatment can extend to individual food choices. For example, a single food, dried plums, has been shown to have a positive effect in animal models on bone density and a positive effect on bone formation biomarkers in human studies.[111]

Coffee or tea? Tea drinkers have higher bone density compared to nondrinkers. Research demonstrates that the flavonoids found in tea may offset caffeine's effect and actually increase bone density. A recent prospective study demonstrated that bone loss occurred in those women who had both low calcium intake and high caffeine intakes.[112] The deleterious effects of caffeine on bone can be negated by consuming adequate calcium.[113,114] Carbonated beverages, particularly in children, may be troublesome primarily because they displace calcium-containing beverages from the diet.[115]

Isoflavones, found in soy and red clover, have attracted the most research interest to date for the prevention and treatment of osteoporosis. Dose-dependent beneficial effects have been identified in premenopausal and perimenopausal women, but not in postmenopausal women. Despite these findings, soy isoflavones have been marketed in relatively high doses with resultant concerns regarding their safety, particularly their procarcinogenic and goitrogenic effects. One serving of soy food per day had no demonstrable negative effects across a broad range of hormonal parameters including thyroid function tests, follicle stimulating hormone and luteinizing hormone levels, and total estrogen levels.[116,117]

Nutrient Supplementation

Nutrient interventions are also available, with much ongoing research extending beyond calcium for bone mineralization. Bone nutrients are detailed in Table 32.2. Bone nutrients are best supplemented together. In general, chelated minerals, which are bound to organic acids, may be better absorbed than inorganic forms. Chelating minerals with citrate may offer additional advantages. Calcium citrate has been shown to attenuate the risk of calcium nephrolithiasis, is alkalinizing, is soluble in the presence of achlorhydria, and is absorbed as both ionic calcium and a calcium citrate complex.[118]

VII. SUMMARY

In sum, early detection of metabolic bone disease allows for timely treatment interventions. Treatment for osteoporosis involves addressing the underlying contributing factors, many of which involve food and nutrients. A comprehensive treatment approach extends beyond calcium supplementation. It involves dietary patterns, food selection, and attention to individualized nutrients.

REFERENCES

1. Lamb JJ. Osteoporosis. In: Kohlstadt I (ed) *Scientific Evidence for Musculoskeletal, Bariatric and Sports Nutrition*. Boca Raton: CRC Press—Taylor and Francis Group, 2006; pp. 473–490.
2. Liedert et al. Signal transduction pathways involved in mechanotransduction in bone cells. *Biochemical and Biophysiological Research Communications* 2006; 349:1–5.
3. Liedert et al. Signal transduction pathways involved in mechanotransduction in bone cells. *Biochemical and Biophysiological Research Communications* 2006; 349:1–5.
4. Jilka RL. Biology of the basic multicellular unit and the pathophysiology of osteoporosis. *Medical and Pediatric Oncology* 2003; 41:182–185.

5. Meier C, Nguyen TV, Handelsman DJ, Schindler C, Kushnir MM, Rockwood Al, Meikle AW, Center JR, Eisman JA, Seibel MJ. Endogenous sex hormones and incident fracture risk in older men: the Dubbo Osteoporosis Epidemiology Study. *Arch Intern Med* 2008; 168(1):47–54.

6. von Muhlen D, Laughlin GA, Kritz-Silveerstein D, Bergstrom J, Bettencourt R. Effect of dehydroepi-androsterone supplementation on bone mineral density, bone markers, and body composition in older adults: the DAWN Study. *Osteoporosis Int* 2008; 19(5):699–707.

7. Armory JK, Watts NB, Easley KA et al. Exogenous testosterone or testosterone with finasteride increases bone mineral density in older men with low serum testosterone. *J Clin Endocrinol Metab* 2004; 89:503–510.

8. Shoback D, Marcus R, Bilke, D. Metabolic bone disease. In: Greenspan FS, Gardner DG (eds) *Basic and Clinical Endocrinology* (7th ed.). New York: McGraw-Hill, 2004; pp. 295–361.

9. Styne D. Puberty. In: Greenspan FS, Gardner DG (eds) *Basic and Clinical Endocrinology* (7th ed.). New York: McGraw Hill, 2004; pp. 608–636.

10. National Osteoporosis Foundation. Osteoporosis Clinical Updates: Osteoporosis in children and adolescents. http://www.nof.org. Washington D.C. Fall, 2005.

11. Russell G. Pathogenesis of osteoporosis. In: Hochberg MC, Silman AJ, Smolen JS, Weinblatt ME, Weisman MH (eds) *Rheumatology* (3rd ed.). Edinburgh: Mosby, 2003, pp. 2075–2080.

12. Shoback D, Marcus R, Bilke D. Metabolic bone disease. In: Greenspan FS, Gardner DG (eds) *Basic and Clinical Endocrinology* (7th ed.). New York: McGraw-Hill, 2004; pp. 295–361.

13. Dennisson E. Osteoporosis. In: Pinchera A, Bertagna X, Fischer J (eds) *Endocrinology and Metabolism*. London: McGraw-Hill International (UK) Ltd., 2001; pp. 271–282.

14. Fiore CE, Pennisi P, Ferro G, et al. Altered osteoprotegerin/RANKL ratio and low bone mineral density in celiac patients on long-term treatment with gluten-free diet. *Horm Metab Res* 2006; 38:417–422.

15. National Osteoporosis Foundation. Osteoporosis Clinical Updates: Osteoporosis in children and adolescents. http://www.nof.org. Washington D.C. Fall, 2005.

16. Stein E, Shane E. Secondary osteoporosis. *Endocrinology and Metabolism Clinics of North America* 2003; 32:115–134.

17. Stein E, Shane E. Secondary osteoporosis. *Endocrinology and Metabolism Clinics of North America* 2003; 32:115–134.

18. Campbell JR, Rosier RN, Novotry L, Puzas JE. The association between environmental lead exposure and bone density in children. *Environmental Health Perspectives* 2004; 112:1200–1203.

19. Lichtenstein GR, Sands BE, Paziansa M. Prevention and treatment of osteoporosis in inflammatory bowel disease. *Inflamm Bowel Dis* 2006; 12(8):797–813.

20. von Tirpitz C, Reinshagen M. Management of osteoporosis in patients with gastrointestinal diseases. *Eur J Gastroenterol Hepatol* 2003; 15(8):869–876.

21. Klaus J, Brueckel J, Steinkamp M, et al. High prevalence of vertebral fractures in patients with Crohn's disease. *Gut* 2002; 51:654–658.

22. Levy C, Lindor KD. Management of primary biliary cirrhosis. *Current Treatment and Opinions in Gastroenterology* 2003; 6:497–498.

23. Obermayer-Pietsch BM, Bonelli CM, Walter DE, et al. Genetic predisposition for adult lactose intolerance and relation to diet, bone density, and bone fractures. *J Bone Miner Res* 2004; 19(1):42–47.

24. Bernstein CN, Leslie WD, Leboff M. AGA Technical Review: Osteoporosis in gastrointestinal diseases. *Gastroenterology* 2003; 124(3):795–841.

25. Carlin AM, Rao DS, Meslemani AM, et al. Prevalence of vitamin D depletion among morbidly obese patients seeking gastric bypass surgery. *Surg Obes Rel Dis* 2006; 2(2):98–103.

26. Hamoui N, Anthone G, Crookes F. Calcium metabolism in the morbidly obese. *Obes Surg* 2004; 14(1):9–12.

27. Mason EM, Jalagani H, Vinik AI. Metabolic complications of bariatric surgery: diagnosis and management issues. *Gastroenterol Clin N Am* 2006; 34:25–33.

28. Carlin AM, Rao DS, Meslemani AM, et al. Prevalence of vitamin D depletion among morbidly obese patients seeking gastric bypass surgery. *Surg Obes Rel Dis* 2006; 2(2):98–103.

29. Carlin AM, Rao DS, Meslemani AM, et al. Prevalence of vitamin D depletion among morbidly obese patients seeking gastric bypass surgery. *Surg Obes Rel Dis* 2006; 2(2):98–103.

30. Chines A, Pacifici R. Antacid and sucralfate-induced hypophosphatemic osteomalacia: a case report and review of the literature. *Calcif Tissue Int* 1990; 47(5):291–295.

31. Neumann L, Jensen BG. Osteomalacia from Al and Mg antacids. Report of a case of bilateral hip fracture. *Acta Orthop Scand* 1989; 60(3):361–362.

32. Teucher B, Fairweather-Tait S. Dietary sodium as a risk factor for osteoporosis: where is the evidence? *Proceedings of the Nutrition Society* 2003; 62:859–866.

33. Frasseto LA et al. Adverse effects of sodium chloride on bone in the aging human population resulting from habitual consumption of typical American diets. *J Nutr* 2008; 138:419S–422S.

34. Massey LK. Is caffeine a risk factor for bone loss in the elderly? *Am J Clin Nutr* 2001; 74:569–570.

35. National Osteoporosis Foundation. Osteoporosis Clinical Updates: Over-the-counter products & osteoporosis: Case discussions. 2002; 3(2). Washington D.C.

36. Massey LK. Is caffeine a risk factor for bone loss in the elderly? *Am J Clin Nutr* 2001; 74:569–570.

37. Munger RG, Cerhan JR, Chiu BC. Prospective study of dietary protein intake and risk of hip fracture in postmenopausal women. *Am J Clin Nutr* 1999; 69:147–152.

38. Munger RG, Cerhan JR, Chiu BC. Prospective study of dietary protein intake and risk of hip fracture in postmenopausal women. *Am J Clin Nutr* 1999; 69:147–152.

39. Rizzoli R, Ammann P, Chevalley T, et al. Protein intake and bone disorders in the elderly. *Joint Bone Spine* 2001; 68:383–392.

40. Weikert C, Walter D, Hoffmann K, et al. The relation between dietary protein, calcium and bone health in women: results from the EPIC-Potsdam cohort. *Ann Nutr Metab* 2005; 49:312–318.

41. Whiting SJ, Boyle JL, Thompson A. Dietary protein, phosphorus and potassium are beneficial to bone mineral density in adult men consuming adequate dietary calcium. *J Am Col Nutr* 2002; 21:402–409.

42. Teegarden D, Lyle RM, McCabe GP, et al. Dietary calcium, protein, and phosphorus are related to bone mineral density and content in young women. *Am J Clin Nutr* 1998; 68:749–754.

43. Ilich JZ, Kerstetter JE. Nutrition in bone health revisited: a story beyond calcium. *J Am Coll Nutr* 2000; 19(6):715–737.

44. Burckhardt P. Mineral waters: effects on bone and bone metabolism. In: Burckhardt P, Dawson-Hughes B, Heaney RP (eds) *Nutritional Aspects of Osteoporosis* (2nd ed.). Boston: Elsevier, 2004; pp. 439–447.

45. Shoback D, Marcus R, Bilke, D. Metabolic bone disease. In: Greenspan FS, Gardner DG (eds) *Basic and Clinical Endocrinology* (7th ed.). New York: McGraw-Hill, 2004; pp. 295–361.

46. Wan Y et al. PPAR-γ regulates osteoclastogenesis in mice. *Nature Med* 2007; 13(12):1496–1503.

47. Stein E, Shane E. Secondary osteoporosis. *Endocrinology and Metabolism Clinics of North America* 2003; 32:115–134.

48. Lindsay R, Cosman F. Osteoporosis. In: Braunwald E, Fauci AS, Kasper DL, Hauser SL, Longo DL, Jameson JL (eds) *Harrison's Principles of Internal Medicine* (15th ed.). New York: McGraw-Hill, 2001; pp. 2226–2237.

49. Shepherd AJ. A review of osteoporosis. *Alternative Therapies in Health and Medicine* 2004; 10:26–33.

50. Shepherd AJ. A review of osteoporosis. *Alternative Therapies in Health and Medicine* 2004; 10:26–33.

51. Chakkalakal DA. Alcohol-induced bone loss and deficient bone repair. *Alcohol Clin Exp Res* 2005; 29(12):2077–2090.

52. Saag KG. Glucocorticoid-induced osteoporosis. *Endocrinology and Metabolism Clinics of North America* 2003; 32:115–134.

53. Shoback D, Marcus R, Bilke D. Metabolic bone disease. In: Greenspan FS, Gardner DG (eds) *Basic and Clinical Endocrinology* (7th ed.). New York: McGraw-Hill, 2004; pp. 295–361.

54. Shoback D, Marcus R, Bilke, D. Metabolic bone disease. In: Greenspan FS, Gardner DG (eds) *Basic and Clinical Endocrinology* (7th ed.). New York: McGraw-Hill, 2004; pp. 295–361.

55. National Osteoporosis Foundation. Osteoporosis Clinical Updates: The many faces of secondary osteoporosis. 2002; 3(3). Washington D.C.

56. Epstein S, Inzerillo AM, Caminis J, Zaidi M. Disorders associated with acute rapid and severe bone loss. *Journal of Bone and Mineral Research* 2003; 18:2083–2094.

57. Lipworth BJ. Systemic adverse effects of inhaled corticosteroid therapy: a systematic review and meta analysis. *Arch Intern Med* 1999; 159:941–955.

58. Shoback D, Marcus R, Bilke, D. Metabolic bone disease. In: Greenspan FS, Gardner DG (eds) *Basic and Clinical Endocrinology* (7th ed.). New York: McGraw-Hill, 2004; pp. 295–361.

59. Chiodini I et al. Subclinical hypercortisolism among outpatients referred for osteoporosis. *Ann Intern Med* 2007; 147:541–548.

60. Richards JB et al. Effect of selective serotonin reuptake inhibitors on the risk of fracture. *Arch Intern Med* 2007; 167(2):188–194.

61. Potts JT, Jr. Diseases of the parathyroid gland and other hyper- and hypocalcemic disorders. In: Braunwald E, Fauci AS, Kasper DL, Hauser SL, Longo DL, Jameson JL (eds) *Harrison's Principles of Internal Medicine* (15th ed.). New York: McGraw-Hill, 2001; 2205–2226.

62. Theriault RL. Pathophysiology and implications of cancer treatment—induced bone loss. *Oncology* 2004; 18:11–15.
63. Napoli N et al. Increased 2-hydroxylation of estrogen in women with a family history of osteoporosis. *J Clin Endocrinol Metab* 2005; 90:2035–2041.
64. Armamento-Villareal RC et al. The oxidative metabolism of estrogen modulates response to ERT/HRT in postmenopausal women. *Bone* 2004; 35:682–688.
65. Stein E, Shane E. Secondary osteoporosis. *Endocrinology and Metabolism Clinics of North America* 2003; 32:115–134.
66. Epstein S, Inzerillo AM, Caminis J, Zaidi M. Disorders associated with acute rapid and severe bone loss. *Journal of Bone and Mineral Research* 2003; 18:2083–2094.
67. Stein E, Shane E. Secondary osteoporosis. *Endocrinology and Metabolism Clinics of North America* 2003; 32:115–134.
68. Hurlock, DG. Personal communication.
69. Altuer T, Elinder CG, Carlsson MD, Grubb A, Hellstrom L, Persson B, Patterson C, Spang G, Schultz A, Jarup L. Low level chronic cadmium exposure and osteoporosis. *Journal of Bone and Mineral Research* 2000; 5:1579–1586.
70. Pfeilschifter J, Diel IJ. Osteoporosis due to cancer treatment: pathogenesis and management. *J Clin Oncology* 2000; 28:1570–1593.
71. Di Munno O, Mazzantini M, Sinigaglia L, et al. Effect of low dose Methotrexate on bone density in women with rheumatoid arthritis: results from a multicenter cross-sectional study. *J Rheum* 2004; 31:1305–1309.
72. Huang Z, Himes JH, McGovern PG. Nutrition and subsequent hip fracture risk among a national cohort of white women. *Am J Epidemiol* 1996; 144:124–234.
73. Ilich JZ, Kerstetter JE. Nutrition in bone health revisited: A story beyond calcium. *J Am Coll Nutr* 2000; 19(6):715–737.
74. Kerstetter J, Svastisalee C, Caseria D, et al. A threshold for low-protein-diet-induced elevations in parathyroid hormone. *Am J Clin Nutr* 2000; 72:168–173.
75. Giannini S, Nobile M, Sartori L, et al. Acute effects of moderate dietary protein restriction in patients with idiopathic hypercalciuria and calcium nephrolithiasis. *Am J Clin Nutr* 1999; 69:267–271.
76. Guyton AC, Hall JE. Parathyroid hormone, calcitonin, calcium and phosphate metabolism, vitamin D, bone, and teeth. In: *Textbook of Medical Physiology* (10th ed.). Philadelphia: W.B. Saunders Company, 2000; pp. 899–914.
77. Dowd TL, Rosen JF, Mirts L, Gundberg CM. The effect of Pb(2+) on the structure and hydroxyapatite binding properties of osteocalcin. *Biochimica Biophysica Acta* 2001; 1535:153–163.
78. Nash D, Magder LS, Sherwin R, Rubin RT, Silbergeld EK. Bone density related predictors of blood lead levels among peri- and post-menopausal women in the United States, 3rd National Health Nutritional Examination Survey 1988–1994. *American Journal of Epidemiology* 2004; 160:901–911.
79. Cijevschi C, Mihai C, Zbranca E, et al. Osteoporosis in liver cirrhosis. *Rom J Gastroenterol* 2005; 14(4):337–341.
80. Sanchez AJ, Aranda-Michel J. Liver disease and osteoporosis. *Nutr Clin Prac* 2006; 21:273–278.
81. Bernstein CN, Leslie WD, Leboff M. AGA Technical Review: osteoporosis in gastrointestinal diseases. *Gastroenterology* 2003; 124(3):795–841.
82. Sanchez AJ, Aranda-Michel J. Liver disease and osteoporosis. *Nutr Clin Prac* 2006; 21:273–278.
83. Mundy GR. Osteoporosis and inflammation. *Nutrition reviews* 2007(II); 65(12):S147–S151.
84. Hofbauer LC et al. Clinical implications of the Osteoprotegerin/RANKL/RANK System for Bone and Vascular Disease. *JAMA* 2004; 292:490–495.
85. Zhao LJ et al. Is a gene important for bone resorption a candidate for obesity? An association and linkage study on the RANK gene in a large Caucasian sample. *Hum Genet* 2006; 120:561–570.
86. Burkemper KM et al. Influences of obese (ob/ob) and diabetes (db/db) genotype mutations on lumbar vertebral radiological and morphometric indices: skeletal deformation associated with dysregulated system glucometabolism. *BMC Musculoskeletal Disorders* 2006; 7(10):1–7.
87. Franke S et al. Advanced glycation endproducts influence the mRNA expression of RAGE, RANKL, and various osteoblastic genes in human osteoblasts. *Arch Physiol Biochem* 2007; 113(3):154–161.
88. Hamrick MW et al. Leptin treatment induces loss of bone marrow adipocytes and increase bone formation in leptin deficient ob/ob mice. *J Bone Miner Res* 2005; 20(6):994–1001.
89. Rosen CJ et al. Mechanisms of disease: is osteoporosis the obesity of bone? *Nature Clinical Practice Rheumatology* 2006; 2(1):35–43.

90. Siffledeen JS, Fedorak RN, Siminoski K, Jen H, Vaudan E, Abraham N, Seinhart H, Greenberg G. Bones and Crohn's: risk factors associated with low bone mineral density in patient's with Crohn's disease. *Inflammatory Bowel Disease* 2004; 10:220–228.

91. Fiore CE, Pennisi P, Ferro G, et al. Altered osteoprotegerin/RANKL ratio and low bone mineral density in celiac patients on long-term treatment with gluten-free diet. *Horm Metab Res* 2006; 38:417–422.

92. Lee SK, Green PHR. Celiac sprue (the great modern-day imposter). *Curr Opin Rheumatol* 2006; 18:101–107.

93. Stein E, Ebeling P, Shane E. Post-transplantation osteoporosis. *Endocrinol Metab Clin North Am* 2007; 34(4):937–963.

94. Serhan CN. Clues for new therapeutics in osteoporosis and periodontal disease: a new role for lipoxygenase. *Expert Opinion and Therapeutic Targets* 2004; 8:643–654.

95. Pack AM, Gidal B, Vasquez B. Bone disease associated with antiepileptic drugs. *Cleveland Clinic Journal of Medicine* 2004; 71:s42–s48.

96. Seidner DL, Licata AA. Parenteral nutrition-associated metabolic bone disease: pathophysiology, evaluation, and treatment. *Nutr Clin Prac* 2000; 15:163–170.

97. Haderslev KV, Tjellesen L, Haderslev PH, et al. Assessment of the longitudinal changes in bone mineral density in patients receiving home parenteral nutrition. *JPEN* 2004; 28(5):289–294.

98. Maggio D, Polidori MC, Barabani M. Low levels of carotenoids and retinol in involutional osteoporosis. *Bone* 2006; 38:244–248.

99. National Osteoporosis Foundation. Osteoporosis Clinical Updates: Over-the-counter products & osteoporosis: Case discussions. 2002; 3(2). Washington D.C.

100. National Institutes of Health Consensus Conference: Osteoporosis prevention, diagnosis and therapy. *JAMA* 2001; 285(6):785–795.

101. Dennisson E. Osteoporosis. In: Pinchera A, Bertagna X, Fischer J (eds) *Endocrinology and metabolism.* London: McGraw-Hill International (UK) Ltd., 2001; pp. 271–282.

102. National Osteoporosis Foundation. Physician's Guide to Prevention and Treatment of Osteoporosis. http://www.nof.org/physguide. Washington D.C. 1998.

103. Shoback D, Marcus R, Bilke D. Metabolic bone disease. In: Greenspan FS, Gardner DG (eds) *Basic and Clinical Endocrinology* (7th ed.). New York: McGraw-Hill, 2004; pp. 295–361.

104. Bernstein CN, Leslie WD, Leboff M. AGA Technical Review: osteoporosis in gastrointestinal diseases. *Gastroenterology* 2003; 124(3):795–841.

105. Mason EM, Jalagani H, Vinik AI. Metabolic complications of bariatric surgery: diagnosis and management issues. *Gastroenterol Clin N Am* 2006; 34:25–33.

106. Shoback D, Marcus R, Bilke D. Metabolic bone disease. In: Greenspan FS, Gardner DG (eds) *Basic and Clinical Endocrinology* (7th ed.). New York: McGraw-Hill, 2004; pp. 295–361.

107. Cijevschi C, Mihai C, Zbranca E, et al. Osteoporosis in liver cirrhosis. *Rom J Gastroenterol* 2005; 14(4):337–341.

108. Rosen CJ. Vitamin D and bone health in adults and the elderly. In: Holick MF. *Vitamin D: Physiology, Molecular Biology, and Clinical Applications.* New Jersey: Humana Press, 1999; pp. 287–306.

109. New SA. Intake of fruits and vegetables: implications for bone health. *Proc Nutr Soc* 2003; 62(4): 889–899.

110. Coxam V. Current data with inulin-type fructans and calcium, targeting bone health in adults. *J Nutr* 2007; 137:2527S–2533S.

111. Shepherd AJ. A review of osteoporosis. *Alternative Therapies in Health and Medicine* 2004; 10:26–33.

112. Massey LK. Is caffeine a risk factor for bone loss in the elderly? *Am J Clin Nutr* 2001; 74:569–570.

113. National Osteoporosis Foundation. Osteoporosis Clinical Updates: Over-the-counter products & osteoporosis: Case discussions. 2002; 3(2). Washington D.C.

114. Massey LK. Is caffeine a risk factor for bone loss in the elderly? *Am J Clin Nutr* 2001; 74:569–570.

115. Murray MT, Pizzorno JE, Jr. Osteoporosis. In: Murray MT, Pizzorno JE, Jr. (eds) *Textbook of Natural Medicine* (2nd ed.). Edinburgh: Churchill Livingston, 1999; pp. 1453–1461.

116. Kurzer MS. Hormonal effects of soy in premenopausal women and men. *J Nutr* 2003; 132(3):570S–573S.

117. Persky VW, Turyk ME, Wang L, Freek S, Chatterton R Jr, Barmes S, Erdman J Jr, Sepkovic DW, Bradlow HL, Potter S. Effect of soy protein on endogenous hormone in postmenopausal women. *Am J Clin Nutr* 2002; 75(1):145–153.

118. Pak CY. Citrate and renal calculi: an update. *Miner Electrolyte Metab* 1994; 20(6):371–377.

119. Shoback D, Marcus R, Bilke D. Metabolic bone disease. In: Greenspan FS, Gardner DG (eds) *Basic and Clinical Endocrinology* (7th ed.). New York: McGraw-Hill, 2004; pp. 295–361.

120. Obermayer-Pietsch BM, Bonelli CM, Walter DE, et al. Genetic predisposition for adult lactose intolerance and relation to diet, bone density, and bone fractures. *J Bone Miner Res* 2004; 19(1):42–47.
121. Bernstein CN, Leslie WD, Leboff M. AGA technical review: osteoporosis in gastrointestinal diseases. *Gastroenterology* 2003; 124(3):795–841.
122. National Osteoporosis Foundation. Osteoporosis Clinical Updates: The many faces of secondary osteoporosis. 2002; 3(3). Washington D.C.
123. Sanchez AJ, Aranda-Michel J. Liver disease and osteoporosis. *Nutr Clin Prac* 2006; 21:273–278.
124. Weaver CM, Heaney RP. Calcium. In: Shils ME, Olsen JA, Shine M, et al (eds) *Modern Nutrition in Health and Disease* (9th ed.). Philadelphia: Lippincott Williams & Wilkins, 1999; pp. 141–155.
125. Cohen A, Ebeling P, Sprague S, et al. Transplantation osteoporosis. In: Favus M (ed) *Primer on the Metabolic Bone Diseases and Disorders of Mineral Metabolism* (6th ed.). Washington D.C.: American Society for Bone and Mineral Research, 2006; pp. 302–309.
126. Fryer JP. Intestinal transplant: an update. *Curr Opin Gastroenterol* 2005; 21(2):162–168.
127. Licata AA. Osteoporosis in men: suspect secondary disease first. *Cleveland Clin J Med* 2003; 70(3): 247–254.
128. U.S. Department of Health and Human Services. Bone Health and Osteoporosis: A Report of the Surgeon General. Rockville, MD: U.S. Department of Health and Human Services, Office of the Surgeon General, 2004.
129. Morgan K. Magnesium and calcium. *J American College Nutrition* 1985; 4(2):195–206.
130. Brown JE. *Nutrition Now* (4th ed.). Belmont, CA: Thomson Wadsworth, 2005.
131. Lakshmanan F. Magnesium intakes, balances and blood levels of adults consuming self-selected diets. *Amer Jrnl of Clinical Nutrition* 1984; 40(Dec):1380–1389.
132. Pennington J, Young B, Wilson D, Johnson R, Vanderveen J. Mineral content of food and total diets: The Selected Minerals in Foods Survey, 1982 to 1984. *J Am Diet Assoc* 1986; 86:876–891.
133. Freeland-Graves J. Manganese: an essential nutrient for humans. *Nutrition Today* 1988 (Nov/Dec):13–19.
134. Klevay L. Evidence of dietary copper and zinc deficiencies. *JAMA* 1979; 241:1917–1918.
135. Nielsen F, Hunt C, Mullen L. Effect of dietary boron on mineral, estrogen, and testosterone metabolism in postmenopausal women. *FASEB J* 1987; 1:394–397.
136. Hajjar IM, Grim CE, George V, Kotchen TA. Impact of diet on blood pressure and age-related changes in blood pressure in the US population: analysis of NHANES III. *Arch Intern Med* 2001; 161(4):589–593.
137. http://www.pdrhealth.com/drug_info/nmdrugprofiles/nutsupdrugs/vit_0264.shtml.
138. Pao E, Mickle S. Problem nutrients in the United States. *Food Technology* 1981:58–64.
139. Feskanich D, Singh V, Willett WC, Colditz GA. Vitamin A intake and hip fractures among postmenopausal women. *JAMA* 2002; 287(1):47–54.
140. Serfontein WJ, De Villiers LS, Ubbink J, Pitout MJ. Vitamin B6 revisited. Evidence of subclinical deficiencies in various segments of the population and possible consequences thereof. *S Afr Med J* 1984; 66(12):437–441.
141. Booth SL, Suttie JW. Dietary intake and adequacy of vitamin K. *J Nutr* 1998; 128(5):785–788.

33 Osteoarthritis

David Musnick, M.D.

I. INTRODUCTION

Physicians in primary care practices have a significant number of patient visits in which the patient has complaints of musculoskeletal pain or joint dysfunction. A significant percent of these patient visits involve joints that are compromised by osteoarthritis (OA). Visits for OA-related pain are even more common in specialty practices such as physiatry, orthopedic surgery, rheumatology, and sports medicine. The usual approach of prescribing nonsteroidal anti-inflammatory drugs (NSAIDs) and pain medications does not adequately address the problems that most patients have in regard to dysfunction of their joints. It may also not adequately slow the breakdown of cartilage. NSAIDs and pain medication can have significant side effect profiles. Nutritional approaches to OA can decrease pain and improve function. There is also evidence that the use of nutritional therapies may slow progression of OA. This chapter will provide a clinical approach to this highly prevalent condition.

II. EPIDEMIOLOGY

OA is the most common type of arthritis. It can affect any joint of the body but most commonly involves the knees, hips, neck, low back, and hands. In early 2008 a study was published that estimated the prevalence of OA in the U.S. adult population to be approximately 27 million having clinically significant OA [1].

This estimate has increased by 6 million from the 2005 figures, which shows a significant increase in the disease. The data are likely to underestimate the actual number of people with symptomatic OA in any one joint, because the data were related to symptomatic OA of the knee, hand, or hip and did not include data on OA of the neck or low back, for example.

III. PATHOPHYSIOLOGY

OA is characterized by progressive degeneration of articular cartilage with resultant joint space narrowing, cysts, and osteophyte formation. In addition there can be subchondral bone changes. In the spine, OA is also characterized by disc dehydration, decreased disc space height and dysfunction as well as facet joint hypertrophy and narrowing of the neuroforamen. OA of the knee may involve the articular cartilage of the patellofemoral joint, proximal tibia fibula joint as well as the tibia femur joint. OA of the knee commonly involves degeneration and tearing of meniscal cartilage on the medial or lateral meniscus, which increases risk of degeneration of the articular cartilage.

OA progresses when tissue regeneration cannot keep pace with the rate of cartilage loss. Joint damage may occur when the biomaterial properties of the articular cartilage are inadequate or the load on the joint is excessive [2, 3]. Contributing factors related to the development or progression of OA in a particular joint are: traumatic injury including sprains and contusion, malalignment including myofascial tightness and ligament laxity, prolonged muscle weakness in muscles stabilizing

539

or moving the joint, genetic predisposition, aging, and nutritional factors. Additional insult on the total joint load can come from the extra weight burden associated with obesity and certain physical activities such as high-impact sports.

OA is characterized initially by irregularities of the articular cartilage surface, a thickening of subchondral bone, and formation of marginal osteophytes. Eventually changes include cartilage softening, ulceration, and focal disintegration within the joint with the most striking changes usually seen in load-bearing areas of the articular cartilage.

Chondrocytes comprise the entire cellular matrix of the joint capsule whereas the substrate of the extracellular matrix is comprised of collagen and polysaccharides known as glucosaminoglycans (GAGs). Substantial GAGs in the extracellular matrix include hyaluronic acid, chondroitin-4-sulfate, chondroitin-6-sulfate, dermatan sulfate, and keratan sulfate. The primary roles of the extracellular matrix include absorbing shock, maintaining viscosity, and nourishing chondrocytes. The primary role of the chondrocytes is the ongoing synthesis of matrix components. In short, the health of the joint is dependent on the function and quality of the chondrocyte and the extracellular matrix.

Early in the course of the disease there is evidence of enhanced chondrocyte replication, suggestive of attempts at repair. In spite of accelerated metabolism within the chondrocyte, the synthesis of matrix substrates is insufficient and results in a decreased concentration of sulfur-containing proteoglycans within the extracellular space. The failure of chondrocytes to compensate for the proteoglycan loss results in a net loss of major matrix contents, including chondrocytes [4].

The loss of proteoglycan density causes an influx of water into the matrix. The influx of water weakens the chemical bonds within the matrix, decreasing the matrix viscosity as well as its capacity to absorb shock and nourish the chondrocytes. The hypertrophy and subsequent death of the chondrocytes cause hyaline cartilage to degenerate and the matrix begins to calcify [5, 6].

The progressive depletion of sulfated proteoglycans from the extracellular matrix of articular cartilage, one of the earliest manifestations of OA, is thought to be due to enhanced activity of the lysosomal enzymes arylsulfatases A and B [7].

There are inflammatory mediators in OA. Interleukin-1 (IL-1) is the prototypical inflammatory cytokine implicated in signaling the degradation of cartilage matrix in OA. IL-1 is synthesized by chondrocytes and mononuclear cells lining the synovium, and it suppresses the synthesis of type 2 (articular) cartilage and promotes formation of type 1 (fibrous) cartilage. IL-1 induces catabolic enzymes such as stromelysin and collagenase, and IL-1 upregulates the production of aggrecanases, which cleave proteoglycan. Intra-articular injection of IL-1 induces proteoglycan loss and an IL-1 receptor antagonist slows progression of cartilage loss in animal models of OA [8]. Given the role of IL-1 in promoting cartilage degradation, IL-1 inhibition is a logical treatment target in OA.

In addition to the production of aggrecanases, IL-1 triggers an entire cascade of proinflammatory and catabolic cytokines, including tumor necrosis factor-α (TNFα), IL-6, IL-8, and PGE$_2$, which act synergistically with IL-1 to perpetuate the proinflammatory cascade [8]. TNFα induces cartilage degeneration by both sustaining cytokine production and increasing expression of collagenases and aggrecanases [9].

In response to IL-1, chondrocytes secrete neutral metalloproteinases (MMP) and active oxygen species that are directly implicated in the destruction of cartilage matrix. IL-1 is a potent inhibitor of proteoglycan and collagen synthesis [10].

There are other cytokines that may play a role in OA and these include IGF 1, transforming growth factor beta and osteopontin. These cytokines may be primarily anabolic for cartilage.

A number of proteases including metalloproteinases can lead to degeneration of cartilage. These include collagenases, which are a family of enzymes known to cleave helical type 2 cartilage and have activity against type X cartilage. Connective tissue cells produce tissue inhibitors of metalloproteinases (TIMPs). There is likely an imbalance between the level of TIMPs and the metalloproteases that may lead to a catabolic effect and subsequent cartilage degradation [11].

Age is the risk factor most strongly correlated with OA, and some studies suggest that more than 80% of individuals over the age of 75 are affected [12, 13]. Age-related tissue changes are believed to be due to a decrease in the repair mechanisms of chondrocytes. With age, chondrocytes are unable to maintain synthetic activity, exhibit decreased responsiveness to anabolic growth factors, synthesize smaller and less uniform proteoglycans and express fewer functional link proteins [13].

IV. PATIENT EVALUATION

In general, severe degenerative joint disease (DJD) is associated with significant pain and disability. A patient may have mild to moderate OA of the knee and hip and not be very symptomatic. Patients can progress to becoming symptomatic and having significant dysfunction with progress of OA of the involved joint. OA appears to progress in perimenopause and menopause in women. Given the vulnerability of aging joints to OA it is advisable to include in a yearly physical exam visit a preventative history and physical examination directed at the knee and hip joints.

In this exam, evaluate lower extremity joint mechanics and alignment, looking especially for varus or valgus knee alignment and excessive pronation or supination of the feet. Evaluate and make suggestions on gait and footwear as many people, especially women, have footwear that does not support their feet well especially against the pronation forces of gait, and this could place abnormal forces on their knees and hips. Evaluate and make suggestions to help patients sit in neutral spine posture to slow or prevent neck and low back OA. Evaluate and treat muscle weakness, muscle tightness, and age-related sarcopenia.

Assessing dysfunctional biomechanics of the knee and hip is essential for a complete treatment approach for OA. OA occurs more commonly in a number of areas of the body: the C5-7 areas of the cervical spine, the L4-S1 areas of the lumbar spine, the knees, the hips, and the interphalangeal (IP) and distal interphalangeal (DIP) joints of the hands as well as the carpometacarpal (CMP) joint of the thumb. The hips and knees are weight-bearing joints and excessive or abnormal loads can contribute to the development and progression of OA. Dysfunctional mechanics at a joint can create excessive shearing and abnormal forces on articular cartilage contributing to the progression of DJD. Dysfunctional mechanics can result from alignment dysfunction from tight muscles (myofascial factors), loss of cartilage, gait dysfunction, weak muscles, poor posture, lax ligaments, and nonsupportive footwear. It is important to evaluate a patient that has OA for these factors and to suggest treatment. Biomechanical assessment also forms the basis of exercise recommendations to avoid excessive impact on the effected joints and to maximize the safe exercise in which patients will engage.

A clinical exam can also evaluate the comorbidities discussed below.

OVERWEIGHT AND OBESITY

Greater body mass index (BMI) in both women and men has been associated with an increased risk of knee OA. Obesity leads to abnormal alignment and loads at weight-bearing joints, especially the knee and hip. It may lead to altered posture (in standing, sitting, and sleeping), altered biomechanics of gait, and less physical activity, any or all of which may further contribute to altered joint biomechanics [14].

Obesity may also contribute to OA because of the contribution of adipose cells of inflammatory cytokines. In any patient that has OA and is overweight or obese it is important to have a treatment plan to include weight loss that is concurrent with other OA recommendations. Obesity is an important comorbid condition to treat because of the increased relative risk of OA in obese patients [15]. There is an increased relative risk of OA of the contralateral knee within 2 years of the onset of OA of a knee [16].

HYPERMOBILITY SYNDROMES

Patients who have ligament laxity in a single joint have a higher risk of developing OA in that joint. Patients who have joint laxity in numerous joints have a higher risk of developing OA in lower and upper extremity joints.

This is more common in patients who have the Benign Hypermobile Joint Syndrome (BHJS) [17]. Patients should be screened on history and physical exam for evidence of hypermobility. Patients with hypermobility of their hands are at higher risk of thumb OA at the first CMC joint. Patients with ligament laxity in the knee are at higher risk of progression of knee OA. Patients with BHJS should be given information regarding how to protect each hypermobile joint. They should be seen by a physical therapist trained in this disorder. It is also advisable for the patient to be on daily joint support such as glucosamine sulfate. Extraarticular ligament injections (prolotherapy) may be appropriate to stabilize hypermobile joints.

HEMOCHROMATOSIS

An iron storage disease, hemochromatosis is a comorbid condition as it can predispose to OA, especially of the metacarpophalangeal (MCP) joints of the hand. Serum ferritin, iron, and transferrin saturation should be checked in any patient with widespread OA or OA at an early age to rule out hemachromatoses.

IV. TREATMENT

The primary treatment targets for OA include the reduction of pain and inflammation, improvement of joint function and joint biomechanical alignment, halting or slowing degeneration, and encouraging regeneration of cartilage. Nutritional therapies may be especially useful in the treatment of OA because they can provide the substrate for cartilage regeneration and have demonstrated efficacy in controlling pain and inflammation. Nutritional therapies are outlined in Table 33.1.

NUTRITIONAL THERAPY CAN REDUCE THE SIDE EFFECTS OF MEDICATIONS

NSAIDs, both over the counter (OTC) and prescription, have been the primary treatment of OA. They appear to be moderately effective for pain control and in improving function. They are, unfortunately, associated with a significant side-effect profile. These side effects include stomach and duodenal ulcers and decreased renal blood flow along with potential decline in renal function.

While NSAIDs are effective in the reduction of pain, the long-term use of NSAIDs is not recommended in OA [18] due to the tremendous side-effect profile of these agents. Each year, as many as 7600 deaths and 76,000 hospitalizations in the United States, 2000 deaths in the United Kingdom, and 365 deaths and 3900 hospitalizations in Canada may be attributable to NSAIDs [19]. In addition to the inherent side effects of NSAIDs, there is evidence, both in animals with experimental OA and in humans, that administration of NSAIDs may actually accelerate joint destruction [20–23] but this is still debated in the literature [24]. Due to the high incidence of side effects from NSAIDS, clinicians are advised to avoid or minimize their use when possible and use on a short-term basis when necessary.

NSAIDs may lead to defects in the mucous lining of the gastric mucosa, or the small or large intestine. They can lead to damage of the wall of the intestine. The former may be treated with nutritional support to improve the mucous lining. NSAIDs may also lead to an iron deficiency anemia, which may be treated with supplemental iron. Prolonged NSAID use may increase the permeability of the small intestine and may predispose an individual to food allergies, which may further aggravate joint pain.

Narcotic pain-relieving medications are less frequently used for OA pain. These can slow intestinal motility and lead to constipation. These drugs may upset sleep and can even lead to pain sensitization.

Several nutritional supplements have been shown to be as effective as NSAIDs in reducing pain and improving functional limitation in patients with OA without adverse effects common to NSAIDs. These include glucosamine sulfate, lyprinol, and SAMe. A 2004 study demonstrated SAMe (1200 mg/day) was as effective as a commonly prescribed COX-2 inhibitor, but with a slower onset of action and a lower incidence of side effects [25].

TABLE 33.1
Mechanism of Action by Which Nutrients Protect Against OA

Nutrient	Mechanism of Action	Reference
Analgesic		
Avocado/Soybean Unsaponifiable Residues (ASU)	Analgesic	Lequesne, Maheu et al. 2002
Chondroitin sulfate	Analgesic	Morreale, Manopulo et al. 1996
Glucosamine sulfate	Analgesic	Matheson and Perry 2003; Bruyere, Pavelka et al. 2004
SAMe	Analgesic	Najm, Reinsch et al. 2004
Modulate Inflammation		
Avocado/Soybean Unsaponifiable Residues (ASU)	Modulate inflammation by suppressing IL-1, PGE-2, IL-6, IL-8	Hauselmann 2001
Omega-3 Fatty Acids	Modulate inflammation by suppressing IL-1, TNFα, PGE-2, 5-LOX, FLAP, COX-2	Curtis 2000
SAMe	Modulate inflammation by suppressing IL-1, TNFα	Gloystein, Gillespie et al. 2003
Glucoasamine	Modulate inflammation by suppressing PGE-2	Nakamura, Shibakawa, et al. 2004
Cartilage Regeneration		
Chondroitin sulfate	Increase proteoglycan synthesis	Reginster 2003
Glucosamine sulfate	Increase proteoglycan synthesis, Increase chondrocyte matrix gene expression	Matheson and Perry 2003; Poustie, Carran et al. 2004
SAMe	Increase proteoglycan synthesis	Gloystein, Gillespie et al. 2003; Bottiglieri 2002
Vitamin C	Increase proteoglycan synthesis	Schwartz & Adamy 1977
Avocado/Soybean Unsaponifiable Residues (ASU)	Increase collagen synthesis, Stimulate TGF-beta1, Stimulate plasminogen activator inhibitor-1 expression	Boumediene, Felisaz et al. 1999; Hauselmann 2001
Vitamin C	Increase collagen synthesis, Stabilization of the mature collagen fibril	Spanheimer, Bird et al. 1986; Peterkofsky 1991
Decrease Degradation		
Glucosamine sulfate	Decrease collagen degradation	Christgau, Henrotin et al. 2004
n-3 PUFA	Decreases degradation by inhibiting ADAMTS-4, MMP-3, MMP-13, aggrecanase	Curtis 2000
Vitamin C	Decrease degradation by inhibiting aggrecanase	Schwartz & Adamy 1977
Avocado/Soybean Unsaponifiable Residues (ASU)	Decrease degradation by inhibiting metalloproteinase activity and collagenase synthesis	Henrotin, Labasse et al. 1998; Ernst 2003; Hauselmann 2001

Source: Reprinted from [26]. With permission.

NUTRITIONAL THERAPIES CAN REDUCE INFLAMMATION

Inflammatory mediators are integral in the pathogenesis of OA. Human OA cartilage expresses modulators of inflammation (COX-2, 5-LOX, FLAP, IL-1α, TNFα) [27] that normal human cartilage does not.

Inhibition of inflammatory mediators may slow disease progression and has long been a target for treatment. The past decade has elucidated the mechanism by which several nutritional supplements reduce inflammation. Table 33.1 summarizes the mechanism by which avocado/soybean unsaponifiable residues, omega-3 fatty acids, SAMe, and glucosamine interfere with the inflammatory cascade. The clinician should also consider placing a patient on an anti-inflammatory, low-toxin diet rich in food-based antioxidants as part of a long-term treatment program to reduce inflammatory mediators.

NUTRITIONAL THERAPIES CAN PROVIDE SUBSTRATES FOR CARTILAGE REPAIR AND REGENERATION

The regeneration of cartilage must be an emphasis of treatment to minimize disease progression. Substantial evidence, in vitro and in vivo, attests to the ability of nutritional agents to enhance proteoglycan synthesis, increase strength of collagen network, decrease proteinases that degrade collagen and proteoglycans (aggrecanase), and decrease IL-1 and subsequent proinflammatory cytokines that further perpetuate cartilage degradation.

Nourishment of the joint is complicated in that articular cartilage is neither vascularized nor supplied with nerves or lymphatic vessels. The outer third of the knee meniscus has a reasonable blood supply. Chondrocytes receive their nourishment from synovial fluid. The use of nutritional supplements to support joints with osteoarthritic changes makes sense primarily if there is cartilage surface remaining as opposed to bone-on-bone anatomy. It also makes sense as prevention for other joints in the setting of a joint that has minimal cartilage remaining or in one that has been replaced. Most of the studies regarding nutraceutical support have been done regarding OA of the knee, but it is very reasonable to consider their use in other joints with OA.

JOINT SUPPORT NUTRIENTS

Glucosamine

The vast majority of published clinical research studies have demonstrated that glucosamine is effective for decreasing pain, improving range of motion, and improving function. N-acetyl-D-glucosamine is a naturally occurring amino sugar found in all human tissues. It functions as a building block in the synthesis of structural substrates such as glycoproteins, glycolipids, GAGs, hyaluronate, and proteoglycans and is required to manufacture joint lubricants and protective agents such as mucin and mucous secretions [28].

Although glucosamine is not generally found in the human diet, it is easily obtained from the exoskeletons of shrimp, crabs, and lobsters for use in medical applications. As a supplement glucosamine is available as glucosamine sulfate, glucosamine hydrochloride, and N-acetyl glucosamine. Thus far, the majority of clinical research demonstrating efficacy in OA has been conducted with the sulfate form. Glucosamine sulfate is the recommended form at this time.

When administered orally, the absorption rate for glucosamine sulfate (GS) in the human GI tract is approximately 87% [29]. In recent years, a topical cream containing glucosamine and chondroitin sulfate has shown efficacy in relieving pain in OA of the knee [30]. Topical GS is reasonable to use for peripheral meniscus tears in patients with reasonable knee function, chondromalacia patella, and OA of the great toe, thumb, and fingers. It should be applied 2 to 3 times per day over the joint line areas.

Glucosamine sulfate has been shown in a number of studies to slow progression of joint space narrowing in the knee. One study compared GS 1500 mg/day versus placebo and followed the patients for 3 years. It demonstrated a mean joint space narrowing of 0.04 mm in the GS group versus 0.19 mm in the placebo group [31]. These results were similar to another 3-year study of GS versus placebo published in *Lancet* in 2001 [32].

In 2004, a study was published documenting that GS had the ability to reduce joint space narrowing in postmenopausal women with OA of the knee [33]. The mechanism of action is purported to be the increased availability of substrate for proteoglycan synthesis as well as anti-inflammatory actions [23, 27].

All of the above studies used a single daily dose of GS of 1500 mg. It is reasonable for the clinician to recommend that their patient use this dose and a dosing method as a minimum dose to achieve structure-modifying effects.

While studies of glucosamine and OA are largely positive, there are a few negative studies that raise several interesting questions about whether or not glucosamine may be more effective in OA subtypes. In a 2004 study, Christgau and colleagues used specific markers of collagen turnover to help classify patients at baseline. Using these markers, they were able to demonstrate that those patients who initially had high cartilage turnover were particularly responsive to glucosamine therapy [34]. Another question remaining for clinical investigation is the generalizability to glucosamine to treating OA of all joints, since the knee has been the most widely studied.

The one constant found in all studies reported in the medical literature is that glucosamine appears to be remarkably safe and well tolerated at 1500 mg/day given either once daily or in divided doses. Side effects are significantly less common with glucosamine than either NSAIDs or placebo [35]. Recent studies have addressed concerns that glucosamine, a sugar, can have adverse effects on levels of plasma glucose and insulin but further research has found these concerns to be unfounded [35–38].

Glucosamine is often derived from shellfish and several authors have expressed concern that the supplement may cause allergic reactions in people who are sensitive to shellfish. Glucosamine is derived from the exoskeletons of shellfish but antibodies in individuals allergic to shellfish are targeted at antigens in the meat, not the shell. Thus far, there have been no documented reports of allergic reactions to glucosamine among shellfish-sensitive patients, but it is prudent to recommend the synthetically derived, generally corn-based, form of the supplement be used in this population [39].

Most studies have concluded that patients taking glucosamine do not seem to notice much effect for at least 6 weeks. Patients need to be educated in regard to the duration of supplementation and how long it may take to notice an effect. Guidelines will be given at the end of this chapter for the duration of joint support supplementation.

Chondroitin Sulfate

Chondroitin sulfate (CS), a mucopolysaccharide, is a proteoglycan component that functions in the maintenance of cartilage elasticity, strength, and mass. In humans, CS is made from GS derivatives. CS, like glucosamine, is not present in significant amounts in the human diet. It is extracted from either bovine trachea or marine shell sources for use in OA.

The medical literature contains numerous studies, of varying quality, pertaining to the use of chondroitin as a therapy for OA. Many early studies have shown efficacy in relieving pain and improving function whereas some later studies and meta-analyses have not [40]. Chondroitin studies have often used combinations of chondroitin with glucosamine (often in the HCL form). CS has been shown in many studies to alleviate pain, decrease NSAID use, and improve joint mobility. A number of studies have shown that CS may be able to slow the progression of joint space narrowing with OA of the knee [41–43]. A recent study demonstrated reduction in joint space narrowing of 0.1 mm compared to 0.24 mm in the placebo group [44].

Results of chondroitin supplementation typically take 8 to 12 weeks to become apparent as in the glucosamine studies. The recommended dosage is 800 to 1200 mg/day given orally in 1 or 2–3 divided doses. Studies showing a reduction in joint space narrowing have evaluated single dosing at 800 mg/day [45, 46].

There is not enough evidence to suggest an additive benefit of chondroitin when GS is already being used in therapeutic doses, but CS is generally relatively inexpensive and without side effects. Because of this it is recommended that the clinician recommend GS as a first-line agent and make sure the patient is using GS because of the research to support that formulation. One could then add 1200 mg/day of CS after a minimum of 12 weeks on GS to see if the patient improves in pain and function. It would also be reasonable to choose a different second agent other than CS based on the recent meta-analysis.

An important controversy in the medical literature as it pertains to the efficacy of chondroitin is whether or not clinically significant amounts are available to the body via oral dosing given the large size of the molecule. During the past few years, several studies have demonstrated a low oral absorption of CS and have shown absorption estimates across the gut mucosa range from 10% to 70% [47, 48]. Low-molecular-weight CS was developed to improve absorption of CS.

Other than mild gastrointestinal distress, the incidence of adverse effects with CS is extremely low. Chondroitin is typically extracted from bovine trachea and concern has been expressed about the potential risk of contamination by animals infected with bovine spongiform encephalopathy (BSE, mad cow disease). There are currently no documented cases of such contamination and risk of transmission is thought to be low. Low-molecular-weight CS is made from shellfish sources. Vegetarian patients should be informed of the bovine origin of chondroitin products.

SAMe (S-Adenosyl Methionine)

SAMe is synthesized endogenously from methionine and adenosine triphosphate (ATP). It is a methyl donor to numerous acceptor molecules and plays an essential role in many biochemical reactions involving enzymatic transmethylation. In addition it has proved efficacious in treatment of OA in regard to treatment of inflammation and cartilage regeneration, and its use is primarily limited by quality and cost factors.

SAMe has been shown to inhibit the synthesis and activity of IL-1 and TNFα at multiple locations in its signal transduction pathways. SAMe has demonstrated the ability to up-regulate the proteoglycan synthesis and proliferation rate of chondrocytes, thereby promoting cartilage formation and repair. SAMe is an alternative to NSAIDs for treatment of joint inflammation and pain caused by trauma and disease states such as OA. It is a proven therapy for OA and has a low side-effect profile. The consensus among several published reviews is that SAMe appears to be of equivalent effectiveness to NSAIDs in reducing pain and improving functional limitations, with fewer side effects. One study suggested SAMe has a slower onset of action than NSAIDs with equivalent results at 4 weeks [49].

B12 and folate aid the body in using SAMe, and it may be useful to supplement with these nutrients as well. The amounts in a good multiple vitamin would usually be sufficient. SAMe can interact with tramadol as well as serotonergic antidepressants. One should try and use other agents when these drugs are prescribed or use SAMe with caution and monitor patients for a serotonergic syndrome. There appears to be some efficacy of SAMe in patients with fibromyalgia; therefore, it would be a good choice in a patient with OA and fibromyalgia [50].

SAMe is efficacious in depression so that its use would be indicated in a patient with OA and comorbid depression. One would then evaluate its efficacy on mood as well as its effect on pain.

There are a number of forms of SAMe available. Patients should be encouraged to use enteric-coated SAMe. Most of the SAMe products available are in the tosylate form. The butanedisulfonate is more bioavailable and more stable although it is more expensive. The dosage of SAMe is typically 200 mg three times per day for OA and 800 mg/day if treating OA and fibromyalgia.

Methylsulfonylmethane (MSM)

MSM is a source of sulfur as well as a methyl donor. In one study MSM and GS were used alone and in combination. Both agents were found to be efficacious in OA but the combination of 500 mg of MSM and 500 mg of GS were found to be more efficacious than the use of one of them alone. Also in this study patients reported improvement in symptoms with less lag time than with the individual agents alone [51]. MSM has been shown at doses of 3 g two times per day in a placebo-controlled trial to decrease pain and improve function in activities of daily living [52]. MSM appears to have a minimal side-effect profile. Although there have only been two studies MSM appears to show efficacy. Doses of 3000 mg twice a day are recommend if used alone or 500 mg three times a day if used concurrently with GS.

Hyaluronic Acid (HA)

HA is the main component of the extracellular matrix within the joint. It is a hydrophilic polysaccharide varying in length from 250 to 25,000 disaccharide units. The large size of this molecule and the water it holds give the matrix solution remarkable viscosity, tensile, and shock absorption properties. The oral form of HA is not well absorbed.

It is important to note that oral cartilage support supplements do not appear to have much effect in joints with little surface or meniscus cartilage remaining. Intra-articular hyaluronans (viscosupplementation) have been used extensively to treat pain and mechanical dysfunction associated with OA of the knee. Many controlled clinical studies have demonstrated their efficacy and a low side-effect profile for this indication and application [53–56].

Intra-articular injections of the knee are indicated if the patient has very little cartilage surface and wishes to avoid surgery. They are done one time per week for 3 to 5 weeks (depending on the viscosupplementation formulation used). An improvement in pain levels and in function appears to have clinical benefit lasting from 6 to 9 months. The treatment often needs to be repeated after 6 to 9 months. Side effects are minimal and may include swelling. It is of note that this treatment is usually given to patients in whom there is little cartilage and joint space remaining. It can in fact be very beneficial in patients with mild to moderate joint space narrowing and in patients with chondromalacia patella.

Omega-3 Fatty Acids

Osteoarthritic cartilage expresses markers of inflammation that contribute to the dysregulation of chondrocyte function and the progressive degradation of the cartilage matrix. In vitro, when human OA cartilage explants are exposed to omega-3 polyunsaturated fatty acids, the molecular modulators of inflammation are inhibited. Curtis and colleagues cultured human OA articular cartilage with various fatty acids and concluded omega-3 fatty acids, but not other fats, have the capacity to improve late-stage OA chondrocyte function. They found culture for 24 hours with omega-3 fatty acids resulted in a decreased loss of GAGs, reduced collagenase cleavage of type II collagen, and a dose-dependent reduction in aggrecanases, and all studied modulators of inflammation (COX-2, 5-LOX, FLAP, IL-1α) and joint destruction (ADAMTS-4, MMP-3, MMP-13) were abrogated or reduced [57].

The concentration and distribution of fatty acids in the diet have long been known to exert influence over the inflammatory cascade. While no large-scale clinical studies have yet been done on the influence of omega-3 fatty acids on the symptoms or progression of OA, several clinical studies have demonstrated dietary supplementation with omega-3 fatty acids reduces the inflammatory symptoms of rheumatoid arthritis [58, 59].

When treating patients with omega-3 fatty acids it is reasonable to use fish oil products consisting of EPA and DHA. It is reasonable to choose products that have been tested for purity and that are extremely low in contaminants of pesticides, mercury, and PCBs. It is reasonable to use approximately 2 to 4 g of high-EPA fish oil per day. In patients with sluggish delta-6-desaturase enzymes, the omega-6 equivalent GLA may also need to be taken even though it is omega-6. This would be recommended for patients who are obese as well as for patients who have metabolic syndrome. Side effects of fish oil are minimal but caution should be used if a patient is on a medication such as Coumadin because of the platelet effects of fish oil.

Lyprinol is a patented extraction of New Zealand green-lipped mussel powder derived from *Perna canaliculus*. It has been shown to provide significant pain relief and improvement in joint function in 80% of subjects after 8 weeks of treatment without adverse effect. The therapeutic value of Lyprinol has been attributed, in part, to its high concentration of omega-3 fatty acids [60].

There have been variable results in efficacy of trials using Lyprinol in patients with OA at the current starting dose of 900 to 1200 mg/day. It would not be a first-line approach and EPA/DHA capsules or oil should be used first for its anti-inflammatory effect because of extensive research on safety and beneficial effects in joints and nonjoint systems. It appears that Lyprinol does not have the same adverse GI side-effect profile as NSAIDs and therefore could be used as a safe anti-inflammatory for patients with OA.

Cetylated Fatty Acids (CFAs)

CFAs have been used in studies both orally and topically. CFAs have been marketed under the name of Celadrin and Cetyl Myristoleate and have minimal side effects. They have been demonstrated in short-term studies to improve range of motion and function of patients with knee OA [61, 62]. A single short-term study has demonstrated efficacy of topical CFAs on wrist and elbow function and endurance during exercise [63]. CFAs may be taken orally in a dose of 350 mg or used topically to improve pain and function in OA of the knee, elbow, and wrist. One could extend this use to the thumb at the CMC joint.

Vitamin C/Ascorbic Acid

Ascorbic acid plays a role in the synthesis of joint components, encourages cartilage synthesis in vitro, and epidemiologic data suggest dietary intake of ascorbic acid is associated with a reduction of OA progression. Vitamin C is necessary for the synthesis of collagen and GAGs within the joint capsule. In collagen synthesis, ascorbic acid is a cofactor for enzymes essential for stabilization of the mature collagen fibril [64, 65].

The role of vitamin C as a carrier of sulfate groups also makes it a requirement for GAG synthesis [7].

In vitro, addition of ascorbic acid to OA cultures results in a decreased level of aggrecanase, the primary enzyme responsible for the degradation of proteoglycan. Vitamin C has been shown to significantly increase the biosynthesis of proteoglycan in both normal and osteoarthritic tissues, suggesting it may be helpful in joint repair [7].

In the Framingham OA Cohort Study, a moderate intake of vitamin C (120 to 200 mg/day) was associated with a three-fold lower risk of OA progression. The association was strong and highly significant and was consistent between sexes and among individuals with different severities of OA. The higher vitamin C intake also reduced the likelihood of development of knee pain [66].

Avocado/Soybean Unsaponifiable Residues (ASU)

ASU is a manufactured product, distributed in France as Piascledine, consisting of 1/3 avocado oil and 2/3 soybean unsaponifiables [67]. Three of four rigorous clinical trials suggest that ASU is an effective symptomatic treatment of OA. A dose of 300 mg ASU per day has demonstrated efficacy in both knee and hip OA but appears to have been studied more extensively for hip OA. Outcome measures have included a reduction in NSAID and analgesic intake, a reduction in pain, and an increase in function. ASU has been shown to have structure-modifying effects in the hip [68]. No serious side effects were reported in any of the published studies.

Based on in vitro research, the apparent mechanism of effect of ASU is via the attenuation of inflammatory mediators and the stimulation of anabolic processes within the cartilage. The anti-inflammatory effects of ASU include the inhibition of IL-1 and the inhibition of IL-1-stimulated PGE_2 and proinflammatory cytokines IL-6 and IL-8 in vitro, and prevented the deleterious action of IL-1 on synovial cells and on articular chondrocytes of rabbits in vivo [10, 69].

Several in vitro studies on cultured chondrocytes have demonstrated these unsaponifiable residues have an inhibitory action on collagenase synthesis, metalloproteinases, proinflammatory cytokines, IL-6 and IL-8, the inducible form of nitric oxide synthase, and PGE_2, all of which decrease inflammation [16, 70]. The anabolic effects of ASU include the in vitro stimulation of collagen synthesis and transforming growth factor-$\beta 1$ in articular chondrocyte cultures and the expression of plasminogen activator inhibitor-1 by articular chondrocytes [69]. ASU has also been found in a lab model to promote tissue inhibitors of metalloproteinases and limit MMP-3 production [71].

Niacinamide/Vitamin B3

Niacin, or vitamin B3, occurs in two forms, nicotinic acid (usually referred to as niacin) and nicotinamide (typically referred to as niacinamide). While both forms have many functions in the body and are crucial to cellular energy production as precursors of NAD and NADP, their therapeutic uses differ considerably.

Niacinamide has been in use as a therapy for OA since the 1940s based on preliminary work by Kaufman [72, 73]. In office clinical research, reported by Kaufman on 455 patients receiving 1500 to 4000 mg/day, niacinamide compared against untreated age-matched controls suggested an increase in joint range index and subsequent reduction in pain in 4 to 8 weeks. Recently investigators have examined efficacy and potential mechanism of action of niacinamide in OA more closely. Jonas and colleagues demonstrated in a 12-week randomized double-blind placebo-controlled trial (N = 72) that patients who took niacinamide (3000 mg daily) experienced an improvement in the global impact of their OA, increased joint flexibility, reduced inflammation, and decreased use of anti-inflammatory medication, compared to controls [74].

While the mechanism of action of niacinamide in OA has yet to be fully elucidated, current theories suggest that niacinamide acts on chondrocytes to decrease cytokine-mediated inhibition of aggrecan and type II collagen synthesis. In addition, reduction in either production or effect of IL-1 on chondrocytes has been suggested as a plausible mechanism [75].

Adverse affects have not been widely reported with pharmaceutical-grade niacinamide [76]; however, nausea, heartburn, flatulence, and diarrhea have been reported. Elevated liver enzymes have been reported with the administration of niacinamide [77] and for this reason it is advisable to ensure niacinamide supplement quality and evaluate baseline liver function tests prior to, and periodically after, niacinamide administration. While large-scale safety, efficacy, and dosing studies are clearly lacking for the general recommendation of niacinamide treatment for OA, preliminary research suggests the nutrient has therapeutic value and warrants further investigation.

Strontium

Strontium ranelate is a nutrient that is being used in some European countries for the treatment of postmenopausal osteoporosis. A number of formulations of strontium have been used in the United States for the same purpose. Studies have provided a preclinical basis for the use of strontium ranelate in OA. In OA and normal chondrocytes that are treated with or without interleukin 1β (IL-1β), strontium ranelate has been shown to stimulate the synthesis of type II collagen and proteoglycan [78]. In a 3-year post-hoc analysis of the pool of Spinal Osteoporosis Therapeutic Intervention (SOTI) and Treatment of Peripheral Osteoporosis studies, strontium ranelate was shown to significantly decrease the levels of urinary C-terminal telopeptides of type II collagen (u-CTX-II), a cartilage degradation biomarker, compared with placebo [79].

A post-hoc analysis was done of pooled data on 1105 women with osteoporosis and OA of the spine [80]. The data were from the Spinal Osteoporosis Therapeutic Intervention (SOTI) and Treatment of Peripheral Osteoporosis (TROPOS) trials. In this study one group of women took 2 g of strontium ranelate daily for 3 years and they were compared to a placebo group. The admission criteria for these studies were women age 50 and older who had been postmenopausal for at least 5 years and had osteoporosis documented by DEXA scan. The conclusions of the post-hoc study were, "The proportion of patients with worsening overall spinal OA score was reduced by 42% in the strontium ranelate group compared to a placebo group." [80] There appears to be a symptom and structure-modifying effect of strontium in the spine. Studies have not looked at other joints. This study appears to indicate a role for strontium in patients that have spinal OA and osteoporosis. Because of the mechanism of action of strontium, it is highly likely that it would be efficacious in women with osteoporosis and OA who were perimenopausal and or immediately postmenopausal as well as for women who were quite far out from the onset of menopause. Strontium ranelate at 2 g/day would be the preferred form and delivers 680 mg of elemental strontium. Strontium chloride has not been adequately studied. Strontium ranelate appears to have interactions with calcium and vitamin D. There also may be a slight increased risk of venous thrombosis. The clinician should follow vitamin D levels and augment as necessary and consider using strontium in patients with combined osteoporosis and OA of the spine.

Vitamin D

Vitamin D has been used for many years for prevention of rickets and in the treatment of osteoporosis. Recently vitamin D has been recommended for cancer prevention and for reduction in all-cause mortality.

The expression of vitamin D receptors is up-regulated in human OA chondrocytes [81]. The Framingham Study found a three-fold increase in risk of OA progression for patients in the middle and lowest tertiles of serum levels of 25-hydroxyvitamin D. Low serum levels of vitamin D also predicted osteophyte growth and loss of joint space [82]. Low vitamin D levels have been associated with an increased risk of falls in the elderly population [83]. Vitamin D receptors have been found in muscle. It is recommended that clinicians check serum 25-hydroxyvitamin D levels in their patients with OA. It is recommended based on the physiology and clinical research that clinicians use supplemental vitamin D3 to increase the serum level of vitamin D to well within the normal range (above 32 ng/mL). Preliminary results of a study that is ongoing at Tufts University on the relationship of vitamin D deficiency and symptoms of knee OA were presented in the Fall 2007 Meeting of the American College of Rheumatology. Having a low vitamin D level was associated with more knee pain and greater functional limitations. The above information is convincing enough to support serum testing and supplementation of vitamin D in patients with OA.

Selenium

Low selenium levels have been reported as a risk factor for OA [84]. The primary organic forms of selenium are the amino-acid-based selenocysteine and selenomethionine. Selenium is used in the body in a number of enzyme systems. Selenium can be obtained from dietary sources although the soils are deficient in selenium in many countries. 100 μg per day is usually recommended either in dietary or supplement sources.

Devil's Claw (*Harpagophytum procumbens*)

There have been a number of studies assessing the effectiveness of supplementing with Devil's Claw for low back pain or for OA. These studies have been reviewed recently [85]. Most of the studies are short term or lack controls. A recent study of patients with hip or knee OA using an aqueous extract of Devil's Claw used 2400 mg of extract daily, corresponding to 50 mg of harpagoside, showed efficacy in pain reduction and improvement in function but was carried out for only 12 weeks [86]. The long-term safety of Devil's Claw needs more investigation before it can be recommended for long-term use.

Taking Devil's Claw orally alone or in conjunction with nonsteroidal anti-inflammatory drugs (NSAIDs) seems to help decrease OA-related pain.

Hydration

It is important to recommend to patients that they remain well hydrated. There is evidence that chronic low-grade dehydration may contribute to OA of the knee and low back. The clinician can recommend a minimum intake of fluid with most of it in the form of filtered water. Water may also be obtained from juices low in sugar and in higher-water-content fruits and vegetables. Figure 33.1 demonstrates in visual form some of the effects of dehydration on the joint.

DURATION OF JOINT SUPPORT SUPPLEMENTATION

The duration of supplementation depends on the pathology that the clinician is treating. If you are treating an acutely injured joint (knee, hip, or spinal joint), it is reasonable to start supplementation

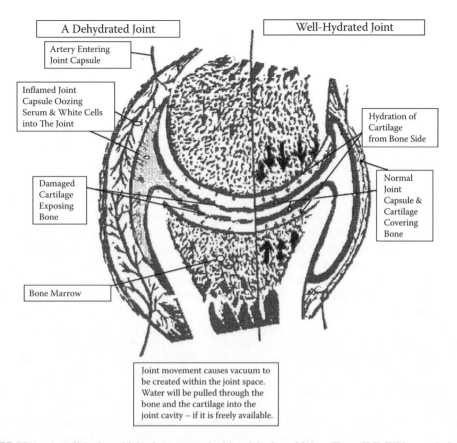

A Dehydrated Joint

Artery Entering
Joint Capsule

Inflamed Joint
Capsule Oozing
Serum & White Cells
into The Joint

Damaged
Cartilage
Exposing
Bone

Bone Marrow

Well-Hydrated Joint

Hydration of
Cartilage
from Bone Side

Normal
Joint
Capsule &
Cartilage
Covering
Bone

Joint movement causes vacuum to
be created within the joint space.
Water will be pulled through the
bone and the cartilage into the
joint cavity – if it is freely available.

FIGURE 33.1   A well-hydrated joint is contrasted with a dehydrated joint. (From [26]. With permission.)

immediately upon diagnosis and continue treatment for approximately 12 weeks. It is also reasonable to consider an X-ray of the joint 6 months after the original injury to make sure that no significant OA changes have occurred. If OA has developed, consider the guidelines in the following. If you are treating a joint with OA that has articular cartilage remaining, you will need to make a long-term plan for nutritional joint support.

CHOICE AND TIMING OF NUTRITIONAL SUPPLEMENTS FOR OA

The choice of nutritional support for patients with OA can be based on a number of factors including the monthly cost of an individual supplement, the efficacy of each nutritional intervention, current clinical studies, and side-effect profiles. It is also related to the pathology and clinical progression of OA in the joint or joints being treated. The clinician should always make recommendations for exercise, posture, stable shoe wear, physical therapy, ligament laxity, and manipulative therapies when appropriate to normalize joint mechanics and forces. Although most of the research has been in regard to OA of the knee and hip, one can use the following nutritional approach with OA of any joint, including the spine.

The patient with OA should also be started on a balanced and well-formulated multivitamin mineral formula because of the information on selenium, vitamin D, and vitamin C. This formula should contain at least 100 µg of selenium, at least 200 mg of vitamin C, and at least 600 to 800 IU of vitamin D3. Vitamin D levels should be tested, and patients should be supplemented appropriately to bring their level up to at least 32 ng/mL.

Nutritional approaches can block proteases and inflammatory cytokines and also augment sulfur and chondrocyte nutrients and anabolic agents. When starting or adding any supplement for joint support, it is important to inform the patient that they should monitor their pain level and functional abilities in a journal, wait at least 8 weeks before starting any new supplement, and compare pain and function to just before they started the new product.

Start a patient on GS at the 1500 mg/day dose for a minimum of 10 weeks. A second dose of 500 to 1500 mg may be considered depending on the patient's body weight and number of osteoarthritic joints. At approximately 10 weeks assess the patient's functional abilities and pain level. At this point the clinician has a number of options on what to add. The clinician can consider adding CS (unless the patient is vegetarian) at the 1200 mg dose to see if there is an added benefit in symptoms and function after 8 to 12 weeks. It would be reasonable to use the low molecular weight form for better absorption. If there is no significant additive effect after 10 weeks, it is not reasonable to continue CS (unless they come to you already on a CS product and they feel that it is working well for them). For control of the inflammation component consider adding a purified fish oil product with about 2 to 4 g/day but it would not be recommended as an isolated treatment. It would be especially useful if there were other comorbidities such as depression, hypertriglyceridemia, and ulcerative colitis or signs of inflammation. If fish oil was not helpful enough for inflammation-related symptoms, a patient could try Lyprinol.

ASU would be a reasonable next agent because of the research regarding its utility in blocking cytokines as well as blocking metalloproteinases. One could use 300 mg of ASU per day. If this agent was too costly or not efficacious, niacinamide could be used in doses of 1500 to 4000 mg/day. One should monitor liver enzymes if this agent is added. SAMe at a dose of 200 mg three times a day can be considered if there is not enough benefit with the above or as an additional nutraceutical. SAMe has proved quite efficacious, but it is costly and there are issues with quality and stability.

Intra-articular hyaluronic acid should be considered for advanced knee and hip OA. This would be added to nutritional support, and if it is efficacious can be repeated approximately every 9 months. It is reasonable to consider it for moderate OA as well as chondromalacia patella. Long-term use of glucosamine, chondroitin, SAMe, and vitamin D appear safe and patients can be maintained on any combination of these for long periods of time. ASU has not been used long term but it should be safe unless there is an allergy to soy.

Nutritional Support for Sprains and OA Prevention

There is a rationale for the use of joint support nutrients after traumatic injury that involves meniscus or articular cartilage including moderate to severe sprains or contusions to a joint. This would include motor vehicle injuries to the facets of the neck, thoracic and lumbar spine, contusions to the patella, ankle, knee meniscus, and other extremity sprains. No long-term studies document the prevention of OA with joint support nutrients after traumatic injury, but the rationale of nutritionally supporting the healing and biochemical substrates of cartilage healing are very sound. GS with or without CS may be started at the time of diagnosis and continued for a minimum of 8 weeks and preferably for 12 weeks after the sprain. There is a definite preventative indication here with low chance of side effects. In addition to traumatic injuries there appears to be good clinical response to the use of GS in problems involving the articular cartilage of the patella in both patellofemoral tracking syndrome and chondromalacia. The clinician can recommend starting joint support nutrients 6 to 8 weeks before high use of the knee in sports. If the problem and use of the knee are ongoing, then nutritional support should be continuous.

Limit higher risk activities such as contact sports and sports with a high risk of falling. Limit running in patients with moderate OA of the knee or hip. Encourage cross training for exercise. Limit work and household-related activities of squatting, kneeling, and excessive stair climbing.

V. SUMMARY

A nutritional approach to OA is theoretically justified and has been overwhelmingly validated in laboratory and clinical trials. Whereas conventional therapeutics may offer the most effective short-term pain relief in OA, long-term pain relief, improvement in function, and regeneration of the joint are better accomplished with nutritional therapies with fewer side effects. Nutritional support when combined with assessment and optimization of biomechanics, strength, and balance can offer both immediate and long-term improvements in function and in pain relief of OA. It may also offer a slowing or stopping of joint surface loss.

REFERENCES

1. Lawrence RC, Felson DT, Helmick CG, Arnold LM, Choi H, Deyo RA, Gabriel S, Hirsch R, Hochberg MC, Hunder GG, Jordan JM, Katz JN, Kremers HM, Wolfe F; National Arthritis Data Workgroup. Estimates of the prevalence of arthritis and other rheumatic conditions in the United States. Part II *Arthritis Rheum* 2008 Jan; 58(1):26–35.
2. Felson DT, Schurman DJ. Risk factors for OA: understanding joint vulnerability. *Clin Orthop* 2004(427 Suppl): S16–21.
3. Brandt KD. OA, in *Harrison's Principles of Internal Medicine*, A.S. Fauci, et al., Editors, McGraw-Hill: New York. 1935–1941.
4. Hungin AP, Kean WF. Nonsteroidal anti-inflammatory drugs: overused or underused in OA? *Am J Med* 2001; 110(1A): 8S–11S.
5. Gartner L, Hiatt J. Cartilage and bone, in *Color Textbook of Histology*. 1997, W.B. Saunders Company. 112.
6. Lorenzo P, Bayliss MT, Heinegard D. Altered patterns and synthesis of extracellular matrix macromolecules in early OA. *Matrix Biol* 2004; 23(6): 381–391.
7. Schwartz ER, Adamy L. Effect of ascorbic acid on arylsulfatase activities and sulfated proteoglycan metabolism in chondrocyte cultures. *J Clin Invest* 1977; 60(1): 96–106.
8. Goldring SR, Goldring MB, Buckwalter J. The role of cytokines in cartilage matrix degeneration in OA. *Clin Orthop* 2004(427 Suppl): S27–36.
9. Dozin B, et al. Response of young, aged and osteoarthritic human articular chondrocytes to inflammatory cytokines: molecular and cellular aspects. *Matrix Biol* 2002; 21(5): 449–459.
10. Henrotin YE, et al. Effects of three avocado/soybean unsaponifiable mixtures on metalloproteinases, cytokines and prostaglandin E2 production by human articular chondrocytes. *Clin Rheumatol* 1998; 17(1): 31–39.
11. Dean DD, Martel-Pelletier J, Pelletier JP, Howell DS, Woessner JF Jr. Evidence for metalloproteinase and metalloproteinase inhibitor imbalance in human osteoarthritic cartilage. *J Clin Invest* 1989 Aug; 84(2):678–685.
12. Badley EM. The effect of OA on disability and health care use in Canada. J *Rheumatol Suppl* 1995; 43: 19–22.
13. Di Cesare P, Abramson S. Pathogenesis of osteoarthritis, in *Harris: Kelly's Textbook of Rheumatology*, E.J. Harris, et al., Editor. 2005, Elsevier. 1493–1537.
14. Jadelis K, et al. Strength, balance, and the modifying effects of obesity and knee pain: results from the Observational Arthritis Study in Seniors (oasis). *J Am Geriatr Soc* 2001; 49(7): 884–891.
15. Hart DJ, Spector TD. The relationship of obesity, fat distribution and OA in women in the general population: The Chingford study. *J Rheumatol* 1993; 20:331.
16. Spector TD, Hart DJ, Doyle DV. Incidence and progression of OA in women with unilateral knee disease in the general population: the effect of obesity. *Ann Rheum Dis* 1994; 53:565.
17. Bridges AJ, Smith E. Joint hypermobility in adults referred to rheumatology clinics. *Ann Rheum Dis* 1992 Jun; 51(6):793–796.
18. Bjordal JM, et al. Non-steroidal anti-inflammatory drugs, including cyclo-oxygenase-2 inhibitors, in osteoarthritic knee pain: meta-analysis of randomized placebo controlled trials. *BMJ* 2004; 329(7478):1317.
19. Hungin AP, Kean WF. Nonsteroidal anti-inflammatory drugs: overused or underused in OA? *Am J Med* 2001; 110(1A):8S–11S.
20. Brandt KD. Effects of nonsteroidal anti-inflammatory drugs on chondrocyte metabolism in vitro and in vivo. *Am J Med* 1987; 83(5A):29–34.

21. Brandt KD. Nonsteroidal antiinflammatory drugs and articular cartilage. *J Rheumatol* 1987; 14 Spec No:132–133.

22. Brandt KD, Slowman-Kovacs S. Nonsteroidal antiinflammatory drugs in treatment of OA. *Clin Orthop* 1986; 213:84–91.

23. Rashad S, et al. Effect of non-steroidal anti-inflammatory drugs on the course of OA. *Lancet* 1989; 2(8662):519–522.

24. El Hajjaji H, et al. Celecoxib has a positive effect on the overall metabolism of hyaluronan and proteo-glycans in human osteoarthritic cartilage. *J Rheumatol* 2003; 30(11):2444–2451.

25. Soeken KL, et al. Safety and efficacy of S-adenosylmethionine (SAMe) for OA. *J Fam Pract* 2002; 51(5):425–430.

26. Kohlstadt I (Ed.). *Scientific Evidence for Musculoskeletal, Bariatric, and Sports Nutrition.* Boca Raton, FL: CRC Press, Taylor & Francis, 2006.

27. Curtis CL, et al. Pathologic indicators of degradation and inflammation in human osteoarthritic cartilage are abrogated by exposure to n-3 fatty acids. *Arthritis Rheum* 2002; 46(6):1544–1553.

28. Matheson AJ, Perry CM. Glucosamine: a review of its use in the management of OA. *Drugs Aging* 2003; 20(14):1041–1060.

29. Setnikar I, et al. Pharmacokinetics of glucosamine in man. *Arzneimittelforschung* 1993; 43(10): 1109–1113.

30. Cohen M, et al. A randomized, double blind, placebo controlled trial of a topical cream contain-ing glucosamine sulfate, chondroitin sulfate, and camphor for OA of the knee. *J Rheumatol* 2003; 30(3):523–528.

31. Pavelka K, Gatterova J, Olejarova M, et al. Glucosamine sulfate use and delay of progression of knee OA: a 3-year, randomized, placebo-controlled, double-blind study. *Arch Intern Med* 2002; 162:2113–2123.

32. Reginster JY, Deroisy R, Rovati LC, et al. Long-term effects of glucosamine sulfate on OA progression: a randomized, placebo-controlled trial. *Lancet* 2001; 357:251–256.

33. Bruyere O, et al. Glucosamine sulfate reduces OA progression in postmenopausal women with knee OA: evidence from two 3-year studies. *Menopause* 2004; 11(2): 138–143.

34. Christgau S, et al. Osteoarthritic patients with high cartilage turnover show increased responsiveness to the cartilage protecting effects of glucosamine sulphate. *Clin Exp Rheumatol* 2004; 22(1):36–42.

35. Anderson JW, Nicolosi RJ, Borzelleca JF. Glucosamine effects in humans: a review of effects on glucose metabolism, side effects, safety considerations and efficacy. *Food Chem Toxicol* 2005; 43(2):187–201.

36. Scroggie DA, Albright A, Harris MD. The effect of glucosamine-chondroitin supplementation on glyco-sylated hemoglobin levels in patients with type 2 diabetes mellitus: a placebo-controlled, double-blinded, randomized clinical trial. *Arch Intern Med* 2003; 163(13):1587–1590.

37. Tannis AJ, Barban J, Conquer JA. Effect of glucosamine supplementation on fasting and non-fasting plasma glucose and serum insulin concentrations in healthy individuals. *OA Cartilage* 2004; 12(6):506–511.

38. Virkamaki A, et al. Activation of the hexosamine pathway by glucosamine in vivo induces insulin resis-tance in multiple insulin sensitive tissues. *Endocrinology* 1997; 138(6):2501–2507.

39. Gray HC, Hutcheson PS, Slavin RG. Is glucosamine safe in patients with seafood allergy? *J Allergy Clin Immunol* 2004; 114(2):459–460.

40. Reichenbach S, Sterchi R, Scherer M, et al. Meta-analysis: chondroitin for OA of the knee or hip. *Ann Intern Med* 2007; 146:580–590.

41. Morreale P, et al. Comparison of the antiinflammatory efficacy of chondroitin sulfate and diclofenac sodium in patients with knee OA. *J Rheumatol* 1996; 23(8):1385–1391.

42. Rovetta G, et al. Chondroitin sulfate in erosive OA of the hands. *Int J Tissue React* 2002; 24(1):29–32.

43. Reginster JY, et al. Naturocetic (glucosamine and chondroitin sulfate) compounds as structure-modifying drugs in the treatment of OA. *Curr Opin Rheumatol* 2003; 15(5):651–655.

44. Kahan A. STOPP (STudy on OA Progression Prevention): a new two-year trial with chondroitin 4&6 sulfate (CS). Available at: www.ibsa-ch.com/eular_2006_amsterdam_vignon-2.pdf

45. Uebelhart D, Thonar EJ, Delmas PD, et al. Effects of oral chondroitin sulfate on the progression of knee OA: a pilot study. *OA Cartilage* 1998; 6:39–46.

46. Uebelhart D, Malaise M, Marcolongo R, et al. Intermittent treatment of knee OA with oral chondroitin sulfate: a one-year, randomized, double-blind, multicenter study versus placebo. *OA Cartilage* 2004; 12:269–276.

47. Barthe L, et al. In vitro intestinal degradation and absorption of chondroitin sulfate, a glycosaminoglycan drug. *Arzneimittelforschung* 2004; 54(5):286–292.

48. Conte A, et al. Biochemical and pharmacokinetic aspects of oral treatment with chondroitin sulfate. *Arzneimittelforschung* 1995; 45(8):918–925.

49. Najm WI, et al. S-adenosyl methionine (SAMe) versus celecoxib for the treatment of OA symptoms: a double-blind cross-over trial. [ISRCTN36233495]. *BMC Musculoskelet Disord* 2004; 5(1):6.

50. Jacobsen S, Danneskiold-Samsoe B, Andersen RB. Oral S-adenosylmethionine in primary fibromyalgia. Double-blind clinical evaluation. *Scand J Rheumatol* 1991; 20:294–302.

51. Usha PR, Naidu MUR. Randomised, double-blind, parallel, placebo-controlled study of oral glucosamine, methylsulfonylmethane and their combinations. *Clin Drug Invest* 2004; 24:353–363.

52. Kim LS, Axelrod LJ, Howard P, Buratovich N, Waters RF. Efficacy of methylsulfonylmethane (MSM) in OA pain of the knee: a pilot clinical trial. *OA Cartilage* 2006; 14:286–294.

53. Kelly MA, Kurzweil PR, Moskowitz RW. Intra-articular hyaluronans in knee OA: rationale and practical considerations. *Am J Orthop* 2004; 33(2 Suppl):15–22.

54. Aggarwal A, Sempowski IP. Hyaluronic acid injections for knee OA. Systematic review of the literature. *Can Fam Physician* 2004; 50:249–256.

55. Kelly MA, et al. OA and beyond: a consensus on the past, present, and future of hyaluronans in orthopedics. *Orthopedics* 2003; 26(10):1064–1079; quiz 1080–1081.

56. Hammesfahr JF, Knopf AB, Stitik T. Safety of intra-articular hyaluronates for pain associated with OA of the knee. *Am J Orthop* 2003; 32(6):277–283.

57. Curtis CL, et al. Pathologic indicators of degradation and inflammation in human osteoarthritic cartilage are abrogated by exposure to n-3 fatty acids. *Arthritis Rheum* 2002; 46(6):1544–1553.

58. Kremer JM. Effects of modulation of inflammatory and immune parameters in patients with rheumatic and inflammatory disease receiving dietary supplementation of n-3 and n-6 fatty acids. *Lipids* 1996; 31 Suppl:S243–247.

59. Ariza-Ariza R, Mestanza-Peralta M, Cardiel MH. Omega-3 fatty acids in rheumatoid arthritis: an overview. *Semin Arthritis Rheum* 1998; 27(6):366–370.

60. Cho SH, et al. Clinical efficacy and safety of Lyprinol, a patented extract from New Zealand green-lipped mussel (Perna Canaliculus) in patients with OA of the hip and knee: a multicenter 2-month clinical trial. *Allerg Immunol* (Paris), 2003; 35(6):212–216.

61. Hesslink R Jr, Armstrong D 3rd, Nagendran MV, Sreevatsan S, Barathur R. Cetylated fatty acids improve knee function in patients with OA. *J Rheumatol* 2002 Aug; 29(8):1708–1712.

62. Kraemer WJ, Ratamess NA, Anderson JM, Maresh CM, Tiberio DP, Joyce ME, Messinger BN, French DN, Rubin MR, Gómez AL, Volek JS, Hesslink R Jr. Effect of a cetylated fatty acid topical cream on functional mobility and quality of life of patients with OA. *J Rheumatol* 2004 Apr; 31(4):767–774.

63. Kraemer WJ, Ratamess NA, Maresh CM, Anderson JA, Volek JS, Tiberio DP, Joyce ME, Messinger BN, French DN, Sharman MJ, Rubin MR, Gómez AL, Silvestre R, Hesslink RL Jr. A cetylated fatty acid topical cream with menthol reduces pain and improves functional performance in individuals with arthritis. *J Strength Cond Res* 2005 May; 19(2):475–480.

64. Peterkofsky B. Ascorbate requirement for hydroxylation and secretion of procollagen: relationship to inhibition of collagen synthesis in scurvy. *Am J Clin Nutr* 1991; 54(6 Suppl):1135S–1140S.

65. Spanheimer RG, Bird TA, Peterkofsky B. Regulation of collagen synthesis and mRNA levels in articular cartilage of scorbutic guinea pigs. *Arch Biochem Biophys* 1986; 246(1):33–41.

66. McAlindon TE, et al. Do antioxidant micronutrients protect against the development and progression of knee OA? *Arthritis Rheum* 1996; 39(4):648–656.

67. Hauselmann HJ. Nutripharmaceuticals for OA. *Best Pract Res Clin Rheumatol* 2001; 15(4):595–607.

68. Lequesne M, et al. Structural effect of avocado/soybean unsaponifiables on joint space loss in OA of the hip. *Arthritis Rheum* 2002; 47(1):50–58.

69. Boumediene K, et al. Avocado/soya unsaponifiables enhance the expression of transforming growth factor beta1 and beta2 in cultured articular chondrocytes. *Arthritis Rheum* 1999; 42(1):148–156.

70. Ernst E. Avocado-soybean unsaponifiables (ASU) for OA—a systematic review. *Clin Rheumatol* 2003; 22(4–5):285–288.

71. Henrotin YE, Sanchez C, Deberg MA, et al. Avocado/soybean unsaponifiables increase aggrecan synthesis and reduce catabolic and proinflammatory mediator production by human osteoarthritic chondrocytes. *J Rheumatol* 2003; 30:1825–1834.

72. Kaufman W. The use of vitamin therapy to reverse certain concomitants of aging. *J Am Geriatr Soc* 1955; 3:927.

73. Kaufman W. Niacinamide: a most neglected vitamin. *J Int Acad Prev Med* 1983 (Winter): 5–25.

74. Jonas WB, Rapoza CP, Blair WF. The effect of niacinamide on OA: a pilot study. *Inflamm Res* 1996; 45(7):330–334.

75. McCarty MF, Russell AL. Niacinamide therapy for OA—does it inhibit nitric oxide synthase induction by interleukin 1 in chondrocytes? *Med Hypotheses* 1999; 53(4):350–360.

76. Lampeter EF, Scherbaum KA. The Deutsche Nicotinamide Intervention Study: an attempt to prevent type 1 diabetes. *Diabetes* 1998; 47:980–984.

77. Knip M, et al. Safety of high-dose nicotinamide: a review. *Diabetologia* 2000; 43(11):1337–1345.

78. Henrotin Y, Labasse A, Zheng SX, Galais P, Tsouderos Y, Crielaard JM, et al. Strontium ranelate increases cartilage matrix formation. *J Bone Miner Res* 2001; 16:299–308.

79. Alexanderson P, Karsdal M, Qvist P, Reginster JY, Christiansen C. Strontium ranelate reduces the urinary level of cartilage degradation biomarker CTX-II in postmenopausal women. *Bone* 2007; 40:218–222.

80. Bruyere O, Delferriere D, Roux C, Wark JD, Spector T, Devogelaer J-P, Brixen K, Adami S, Fechtenbaum J, Kolta S, Reginster J-Y. Effects of strontium ranelate on spinal OA progression. *Annals of the Rheumatic Diseases* 2008; 67:335–339.

81. Tetlow LC, Woolley DE. Expression of vitamin D receptors and matrix metalloproteinases in osteoarthritic cartilage and human articular chondrocytes in vitro. *OA Cartilage* 2001; 9:423–431.

82. McAlindon TE, Felson DT, Zhang Y, Hannan MT, Aliabadi P, Weissman B, Rush D, Wilson PW, Jacques P. Relation of dietary intake and serum levels of vitamin D to progression of OA of the knee among participants in the Framingham Study. *Ann Intern Med* 1996; 125:353–359.

83. Flicker L, Mead K, MacInnis RJ, et al. Serum vitamin D and falls in older women in residential care in Australia. *J Am Geriatr Soc* 2003; 51:1533–1538.

84. Jordan JM, Fang F, Arab L, et al. Low selenium levels are associated with increased risk for OA of the knee. American College of Rheumatology Annual Meeting. San Diego November 12–17, 2005. Abstract 1189.

85. Brien S, Lewith GT, McGregor G. Devil's Claw (Harpagophytum procumbens) as a treatment for OA: a review of efficacy and safety. *J Altern Complement Med* 2006 Dec; 12(10):981–993.

86. Wegener T, Lüpke NP. Treatment of patients with arthrosis of hip or knee with an aqueous extract of devil's claw. *Phytother Res* 2003 Dec; 17(10):1165–1172.

34 Fibromyalgia and Chronic Fatigue Syndrome

Jacob Teitelbaum, M.D.

I. INTRODUCTION

Fibromyalgia (FMS) and chronic fatigue syndrome (CFS) are two common names for an overlapping spectrum of disabling syndromes. It is estimated that FMS alone affects 6 to 12 million Americans, causing more disability than rheumatoid arthritis.[1] The prevalence of CFS/FMS is rapidly increasing, likely having increased by 200% to 400% in the last 10 years alone,[2-5] reflecting the stress placed on our systems as our diets worsen and chemical exposures in the environment increase. Fortunately, although we still have much to learn, effective treatment is now available for the large majority of these patients.[6,7]

II. PATHOPHYSIOLOGY

CFS/FMS represents a syndrome, a spectrum of processes with a common end point. Because the syndromes affect major control systems in the body, there are myriad symptoms that initially do not seem to be related. Recent research has implicated mitochondrial and hypothalamic dysfunction as common denominators in these syndromes.[8-11] Dysfunction of hormonal, sleep, and autonomic control (all centered in the hypothalamus) and energy production centers can explain the large number of symptoms and why most patients have a similar set of complaints.

Research in genetic mitochondrial diseases shows not simply myopathic changes, but also marked hypothalamic disruption. As the hypothalamus controls sleep, the hormonal and autonomic systems, and temperature regulation, it has higher energy needs for its size than other areas of our body. Because of this, as energy stores are depleted, hypothalamic dysfunction occurs early on, resulting in the disordered sleep, autonomic dysfunction, low body temperatures, and hormonal dysfunctions commonly seen in these syndromes. In addition, inadequate energy stores in a muscle results in muscle shortening and pain, which is further accentuated by the loss of deep sleep. Reductions in stages 3–4 of deep sleep result in secondary drops in growth hormone and tissue repair. Disrupted sleep then contributes to pain and immune dysfunction.

Anything that results in inadequate energy production or energy needs greater than the body's production ability can trigger hypothalamic dysfunction. This includes nutritional deficiencies, infections, disrupted sleep, pregnancy, hormonal deficiencies, and other physical or situational stresses. Although still controversial, a large body of research also strongly suggests mitochondrial dysfunction as a unifying theory in CFS/FMS.[11] Some viral infections have been shown to suppress both mitochondrial and hypothalamic function. As noted, in several genetic mitochondrial diseases, severe hypothalamic dysfunction is seen. This is likely because the hypothalamus has high energy needs.

TABLE 34.1
Comorbid Conditions Associated With FMS and CFS

Spastic colon/irritable bowel syndrome	Treat bowel infections and restore mucosal integrity of bowels.
Migraines	Acute migraines are responsive to IV magnesium.[12–14] This will eliminate most attacks within 15 minutes, but gets little attention because the medication costs ~5 cents/dose. Vitamin B2 (riboflavin) 100–400 mg/day will decrease the frequency of migraine headaches by ~67% in placebo controlled studies.[15, 16] Eliminating food allergies is also very helpful.
Myofascial pain syndrome	Pain caused by muscle shortening shares many of the same underlying causes as FMS and responds excellently to the treatments discussed.
Chronic sinusitis	This usually resolves with antifungal therapies, especially Diflucan 200 mg/d × 6 weeks. Candida overgrowth triggers an immune reaction in nasal tissues, causing swelling, obstruction, and secondary bacterial infections. Antibiotics increase yeast overgrowth, resulting in the sinusitis becoming chronic.
Pelvic pain syndromes, vulvodynia, proctalgia fugax, and prostadynia	Treatment—treating the candida, and the overall process with the S.H.I.N.E protocol can help, as can the medications Elavil 10–25 mg plus Neurontin at bedtime.
Food reactivities	These often resolve with eliminating yeast and other bowel infections and giving adrenal support.
Restless leg syndrome (RLS)	Commonly triggered by iron deficiency, as iron is critical for dopamine production and RLS is triggered by dopamine deficiency. Keep ferritin levels >50 ng/mL and iron percent saturation >22% in these patients.
Obstructive sleep apnea and upper airway resistance syndrome	Weight loss (for apnea) and concurrent continuous positive airway pressure.

III. DIAGNOSIS AND PATIENT EVALUATION

The Centers for Disease Control and Prevention designed diagnostic criteria for CFS, and the American College of Rheumatology has created them for FMS. An important clinical feature is the paradox of severe fatigue combined with insomnia (if one is exhausted, sleep should occur all night). If these symptoms do not go away with vacation, the patient likely will have a CFS-related process. If the patient also has widespread pain, FMS is probably present as well. CFS and FMS respond well to proper treatment as discussed below regardless of whether or not the patient meets the exact diagnostic criteria.

These are complex patients who usually have dozens of symptoms and need a thorough history to determine the underlying processes that need to be treated. Using questionnaires that the patient can fill out at home facilitates the patient history.

Evaluation should also include identifying comorbid conditions. Because energy depletion causes widespread problems throughout the body, and many problems cause energy depletion, there are numerous comorbid conditions, many of which resolve with treatment. Table 34.1 presents common associated problems, which often have nutrient-related strategies to ameliorate them.

IV. TREATMENT OVERVIEW

Restoring adequate energy production through nutritional, hormonal, and sleep support and eliminating the stresses that over-utilize energy restores function in the hypothalamic "circuit breaker" and also allows muscles to release, thus allowing pain to resolve. Our pilot and placebo-controlled study showed that when this is done, 91% of patients improve, with an average 90% improvement in quality of life, and the majority of patients no longer qualified as having FMS by the end of 3 months (p < .0001 vs. placebo).[6,7]

Let's discuss the protocol, which includes treating *S*leep, *H*ormonal dysfunction, *I*nfections, optimizing *N*utritional support, and *E*xercise as able—referred to as the S.H.I.N.E. protocol.

DISORDERED SLEEP

For patients to get well, it is critical that they take enough of the correct sleep treatments to get 8 to 9 hours sleep at night! When one recognizes that CFS/FMS is a hypothalamic sleep disorder—not poor sleep hygiene—this approach makes sense. Helpful medications include Ambien, Desyrel, Klonopin, and, if they don't have restless leg syndrome, Flexeril and/or Elavil.

Look for and treat restless leg syndrome, sleep apnea, and upper airway resistance syndrome if clinically suspected.

HORMONAL DEFICIENCIES

The hypothalamus is the main control center for most of the glands in our body, through the hypothalamic-pituitary axis. When the hypothalamus is not able to efficiently regulate hormone balance, medical management can do so until hypothalamic function is restored. When focusing on achieving hormonal balance, the standard laboratory testing is not reliable for many reasons. For example, increased hormone binding to carrier proteins is often present in CFS/FMS. Because of this, total hormone levels are often normal while the active hormone levels are low. This creates a functional deficiency in the patient. Also, most blood tests use two standard deviations to define blood test norms. By definition, only the lowest or highest 2.5% of the population is in the abnormal (treatment) range. This does not work well if over 2.5 % of the population has a problem. For example, it is estimated that as many as 20% of women over 60 have positive anti-TPO antibodies and may be hypothyroid. Other tests use late signs of deficiency such as anemia for iron or B12 levels to define an abnormal lab value. The goal in CFS/FMS management is to restore optimal function while keeping labs in the normal range for safety.

1. Thyroid
   Almost all of these patients require support with natural prescription Armour Thyroid. In addition, correcting iodine deficiency, which is increasing because there is less added to wheat than in the past, and selenium deficiency (as selenium is critical for conversion of inactive T4 to active T3) is also important. Making sure the patient does not have excessive amounts of soy in the diet (e.g., vegans who use it as a meat/milk substitute) is also important as this can result in decreased thyroid hormone function.
2. Adrenal
   Adrenal support is also important in many of these patients. Bioidentical ultra-low-dose cortisol (Cortef by prescription) can be very safe and helpful. Natural support is also helpful. The needed natural therapies include:
   • Adrenal glandulars, which contain most of the "building blocks" needed for adrenal repair.
   • Licorice extract, which contains glycyrrhizin, a compound that raises adrenal hormone levels.
   • Pantothenic acid, vitamin C, vitamin B6, betaine and tyrosine are critical for adrenal function and energy, and high doses are often needed.
3. Sex hormones
   Bioidentical estriol, estradiol, progesterone, and testosterone are also helpful in many cases.

UNUSUAL INFECTIONS

Many studies have shown immune system dysfunction in FMS/CFS. The immune dysfunction can result in many unusual infections. These include viral infections (e.g., HHV-6, CMV, and EBV), parasites and other bowel infections, infections sensitive to long-term treatment with the antibiotics Cipro and Doxycycline (e.g., mycoplasma, chlamydia, Lyme's, etc.) and fungal infections. Although the latter is controversial, both our study and extensive clinical experience have found treating with an antifungal to be very helpful with the symptoms seen in these syndromes. Avoiding sweets (stevia is okay) and taking acidophilus pearls (healthy milk bacteria, two pearls twice a day for 5 months) can be very helpful. It is also very helpful to add Diflucan, a prescription antifungal, at a dose of 200 mg/day for 6 weeks. A new antiviral (Valcyte) has also been extremely beneficial in those whose testing suggests HHV-6 or CMV viral infections.

NUTRITION AND DIET

Nutrition and diet are discussed below.

EXERCISE AS TOLERATED

Instruct patients to not push to the point of crashing the next day. Start by walking as long as they comfortably can, even if that is only 2 minutes. After 10 weeks on treatment, they can increase their walks by up to 1 minute more each day as able. When they are up to an hour of walking, they can increase intensity.

V. DIET AND FOOD-BASED TREATMENT APPROACHES

I recommend that patients eat those things that leave them feeling the best. I caution them that what makes them feel best can be and often is different from what they crave.

The majority of CFS patients find that they do best with a high-protein, low-carbohydrate diet. The most critical advice is that the patient should avoid sugar, excessive caffeine, and excess alcohol. Warn the patient that there may be a 7- to 10-day withdrawal period when coming off sugar and caffeine. When I tell them to avoid sugar, I do add "Except for chocolate." Dark chocolate contains little sugar and is high in antioxidants and mood-elevating compounds. It has actually been shown in a randomized controlled study that 45 g/day of an 85% cocoa dark chocolate helped improve symptoms in CFS.[17] In addition, when eliminating something pleasurable, always add in a healthy substitute. Stevia is a sweetener substitute as is ribose, discussed later in this chapter. Ribose is heat stable, and can be added to hot liquids and used in cooking.

If the patient has low blood pressure and/or orthostatic dizziness, increasing salt intake markedly should also be considered. Sea salt is preferable. Because of the low antidiuretic hormone production, these patients are often dehydrated despite drinking far more than most people. Do not have the patient counting glasses of water all day. Rather, have them keep a bottle or glass of water on hand and avoid dry mouth and lips.

VI. NUTRIENT-BASED TREATMENT

CFS/FMS patients are often nutritionally deficient because of malabsorption, increased physiologic demand, and inadequate diet. Multiple nutrients are critical. B-vitamins, ribose, magnesium, iron, coenzyme Q_{10}, malic acid, and carnitine are essential for mitochondrial function. These nutrients are also critical for many other processes. Although blood testing is not reliable or necessary for most nutrients, I do recommend checking B12, iron (Fe), total iron binding capacity (TIBC), and ferritin levels.

I begin patients with CFS/FMS on the following nutritional regimen.

MULTIVITAMIN OF HIGH QUALITY

A multivitamin should contain at least a 50 mg B complex, 150 mg of magnesium glycinate, 900 mg of malic acid, 600 IU of vitamin D, 500 mg of vitamin C, zinc 15 to 20 mg, selenium 200 µg, chromium 200 μg, and amino acids. A powdered vitamin is generally better tolerated, better absorbed, and less expensive. A powdered vitamin can be a good-tasting drink that can replace what might otherwise be dozens of tablets. A multivitamin should be taken long term.

IRON

If the iron percent saturation is under 22% or the ferritin is under 40 mg/mL, supplement with iron. I recommend Chromagen FA, one every other day for 4 to 8 months. It should be taken on an empty stomach, since food decreases iron absorption by over 60%. It should not be taken within 6 hours of thyroid hormone, since iron blocks thyroid absorption. As daily iron can cause decreased absorption, taking it 3 weeks each month or every other day is preferable to daily dosing. Continue treatment until the iron percent saturation is over 22% and ferritin is over 50 mg/mL or over 100 mg/mL if the patient has had hair loss with illness. If ferritin levels are elevated initially, rule out hemochromatosis, which can also cause FMS.

VITAMIN B12

If the B12 level is under 540 pg/mL, I recommend B12 injections, 3000 μg IM three times a week for 15 weeks, then as needed based on the patient's clinical response. Although controversial, this treatment is both very helpful and very safe. Studies on CFS are showing absent or near-absent CSF B12 levels despite normal serum B12 levels.[18] Metabolic evidence of B12 deficiency is seen even at levels of 540 pg/mL or more.[19] Severe neuropsychiatric changes are also seen from B12 deficiency even at levels of 300 pg/mL (a level over 209 is technically normal).[20] As an editorial in *The New England Journal of Medicine* suggests, the old-time doctors may have been right about giving B12 shots.[21] Compounding pharmacies can make B12 at 3000 μg/cc concentrations. I use hydroxycobalmin, although methylcobalmin may be more effective, though also more expensive. Use multivitamins that contain at least 500 μg of B12 daily for ongoing use.

COENZYME Q10

Coenzyme Q_{10} is a conditionally essential nutrient that improves energy production in patients with CFS/FMS. A daily supplemental dose of 200 mg is especially critical in patients on Mevacor-family cholesterol treatments,[22] which can actually cause FMS pain. Quality control is especially important with this nutrient.[23]

ACETYL-L-CARNITINE

Carnitine plays many roles in the body. It has the critical function of preventing the mitochondria from being shut down when the system backs up. It does this by keeping a substance called acetyl coenzyme A from building up and shutting down the tricyclic acid cycle and the electron transport system, the cell's effective energy burning systems. Also, without sufficient carnitine, the body cannot burn fat and often makes excess fat, potentially resulting in large weight gains.

Acetyl-l-carnitine at 500 mg twice daily for 4 months is strongly recommended to help restore energy function. Muscle biopsies show CFS patients' intracellular levels to routinely be low.[24,25] I recommend the acetyl form of carnitine, as it is clinically more effective, and has stronger antioxidant activity than L-carnitine.[26]

D-RIBOSE

D-ribose should be administered 5 gm three time a day for 3 weeks, then twice a day. D-ribose alone increased energy an average of 45% in FMS and CFS patients after 3 weeks.[27] It also decreased pain.

A seldom-seen side effect is a mild drop in blood sugar as ribose gets energy production moving. If the patient feels dizzy or hungry upon taking ribose, have him take it with a meal or lower the dose. The only significant side effects in our studies were that two people felt too energized and anxious on the ribose. The side effect resolved by lowering the dose and/or taking ribose with food.

Since CFS/FMS represents an energy crisis, it is critical that the patients have what is needed for optimal mitochondrial function. In some patients ribose availability may be a rate-limiting step in energy production. Adenosine triphosphate (ATP), nicotinamide adenine dinucleotide (NADH), and the reduced form of flavin adenine dinucleotide (FADH) represent the energy currency of the body, and are like the paper that money is printed on. A person can have all the fuel they want, but if it cannot be converted to these molecules, it is useless. In particular, ATP is important because the amount of ATP people have in their tissues determines whether they will be fatigued or have the energy needed to live vital, active lives.

D-ribose is a simple, 5-carbon (pentose) sugar, generally preserved for ATP synthesis and the production of DNA and RNA. CFS/FMS causes the body to dump key energy molecules such as acetyl-l-carnitine and ribose. Our study included 41 patients with a diagnosis of CFS or FMS and was intended to determine whether or not ribose would be effective in relieving the overwhelming fatigue, pain, soreness, and stiffness suffered by patients having these debilitating conditions. During the study, patients were given ribose at a dose of 5 g three times per day for 3 weeks.

We found the ribose treatment led to significant improvement in energy levels, sleep patterns, mental clarity, pain intensity, and overall well-being. Of the patients participating in the study, 65.7% experienced significant improvement while on ribose (improvement began at 12 days), with an average increase in energy of 44.7% and overall well-being of 30%, remarkable results from a single nutrient.[27]

One important study involved healthy athletes participating in high-intensity, endurance exercise over the course of 1 week. After exercise, the energy level in the athlete's muscle was reduced by almost 30%. Giving 10 g of ribose per day for 3 days following exercise restored muscle energy levels to normal in contrast to the control group.[28] After 3 days of rest, muscle that was not treated with ribose remained energy starved and fatigued.

Two very interesting animal studies conducted by Ron Terjung, M.D., showed how dramatic the effect of ribose could be on energy recovery in fatigued muscle. Ribose administration in fatigued muscle increased the rate of energy recovery by 340% to 430%, depending on which type of muscle was tested.[29] It was also found that even very small amounts of ribose had the effect of helping the muscle cell preserve energy, a process known as energy salvage, and the higher the ribose dose, the more dramatic the effect on energy preservation.[30]

A compelling case study of a veterinarian diagnosed with FMS was published in *Pharmacotherapy* in 2004.[31] This case study told the story of a veterinary surgeon diagnosed with FMS whose condition resolved with supplemental ribose, relapsed without the ribose, and was again fully recovered when the ribose was resumed.

Another line of evidence supporting the use of ribose in fatigue of muscles is the responsiveness to ribose demonstrated in patients with congestive heart failure, fatigued cardiac muscle. (See Chapter 6, "Congestive Heart Failure and Cardiomyopathy.") Dr. Paul Cheney's research has demonstrated an association between heart muscle dysfunction and CFS.

VII. SUMMARY

CFS and FMS reflect an energy crisis in the body. It is similar to blowing a fuse in a house. There can be many causes, it protects the body from further harm, but it dramatically reduces function. Causes include nutritional deficiencies, infections, disrupted sleep, pregnancy, hormonal deficiencies, toxins, and other physical or situational stresses. The "blown fuse" is the hypothalamus short circuit resulting in poor sleep, and hormonal, autonomic, and temperature dysregulation. Energy depletion also causes muscle shortening and widespread pain.

Two studies including our RCT showed an average 90% improvement rate in CFS/FMS when using the S.H.I.N.E. protocol: *S*leep, *H*ormonal support, *I*nfections, *N*utritional support, and *E*xercise as able.

Widespread nutritional deficiencies are common, and no single tablet will take care of them all. I recommend the following:

1. The Energy Revitalization System* powder contains over 50 key nutrients, replacing over 35 tablets of supplements daily with one drink and should be used long term.
2. Ribose (Corvalen) 5 gm three times a day for 3 weeks, then twice a day. D-ribose alone can increase energy an average of 45% in these patients. It also can help decrease the pain.
3. Coenzyme Q_{10} at 200 mg/day.
4. Acetyl-l-carnitine 1000 mg daily for approximately 4 months.
5. Drinking a lot of water and avoiding sugar (except for chocolate) is important as well.
6. Increasing salt intake if low blood pressure and orthostatic dizziness are issues.
7. A high-protein, low-carbohydrate diet usually works best, but patients should eat what leaves them feeling the best.
8. Keep ferritin levels over 40 ng/mL and keep vitamin B12 levels over 540 pg/mL.

These are complex patients who usually have dozens of symptoms and need a thorough history to determine the underlying processes that need to be treated. This is best done by using questionnaires that the patient can fill out at home.** I thank you for caring enough to help these patients.

REFERENCES

1. F. Wolfe, K. Ross, J. Anderson, et al. The Prevalence and Characteristics of FMS in the General Population. *Arthritis and Rheumatism* 1995 Jan; 38(1):19–28.
2. C. Schmitt, M. Spaeth, E. André, J. Caubere and C. Taieb. FMS Syndrome: A German Epidemiological Survey. *Annals of the Rheumatic Diseases* 2006; 65(Suppl 2):554.
3. M. Matucci Cerinic, M. Zoppi, C. Taieb, J. Caubere, G. Hamelin and C. Schmitt. Prevalence of FMS in Italy: Updated Results. *Annals of the Rheumatic Diseases* 2006; 65(Suppl 2):555.
4. M. Guermazi, S. Ghroubi, M. Sellami, M. Elleuch, E. André, C. Schmitt, C. Taieb, J. Damak and M. Elleuch. Epidemiology of FMS in Tunisia. *Annals of the Rheumatic Diseases* 2006; 65(Suppl 2):553.
5. V. Cobankara, Ö. Ünal, M. Öztürk and A. Bozkurt. The Prevalence of FMS among Textile Workers in the City of Denizli in Turkey. *Annals of the Rheumatic Diseases* 2006; 65(Suppl 2):554.
6. J. Teitelbaum and B. Bird. Effective Treatment of Severe Chronic Fatigue: A Report of a Series of 64 Patients. *Journal of Musculoskeletal Pain* 1995; 3(4):91–110.
7. J.E. Teitelbaum, B. Bird, R.M. Greenfield, et al. Effective Treatment of CFS and FMS: A Randomized, Double-Blind Placebo Controlled Study. *Journal of CFS* 2001; 8(2). The full text of the study can be found at www.Vitality101.com
8. M.A. Demitrack, K. Dale, S.E. Straus, et al. Evidence for Impaired Activation of the Hypothalamic-Pituitary-Adrenal Axis in Patients with CFS. *Journal of Clinical Endocrinology and Metabolism* 1991 Dec; 73(6):1223–1234.
9. J. Teitelbaum. Estrogen and Testosterone in CFIDS/FMS. *From Fatigued To Fantastic Newsletter* 1997 Feb.
10. P.O. Behan. Post-Viral Fatigue Syndrome Research, in *The Clinical and Scientific Basis of Myalgic Encephalitis and CFS,* ed. Byron Hyde, Jay Goldstein, and Paul Levine (Ottawa, Ontario, Canada: Nightingale Research Foundation, 1992), p. 238.
11. J. Teitelbaum. Mitochondrial Dysfunction [in CFS/FMS]. *From Fatigued to Fantastic Newsletter* 1997; 1(2). Contains numerous references on this topic.

---

* The multivitamin I use in my practice for almost all of my patients is called the Energy Revitalization System by Integrative Therapeutics.

** I will be happy to e-mail you a free file containing long and short form patient questionnaires and treatment checklists that you can modify for use in your office. E-mail me through the Q&A section at www.Vitality101.com Web site to request the file.

12. S. Demirkaya, et al. Efficacy of Intravenous Magnesium Sulfate in the Treatment of Acute Migraine Attacks. *Headache* 2001; 41:171–177.
13. Mausop A, Altura BT, Cracco RQ, Altura BM. Intravenous Magnesium Sulphate Relieves Migraine Attacks in Patients with Low Serum Ionized Magnesium Levels: A Pilot Study. *Clinical Science* 1995; 89:633–636.
14. B. Dora. Migraine Headache and Magnesium Sulfate. *Clinical Pearls News* 2002 Apr.
15. J. Schoenen, et al. High-dose Riboflavin as a Prophylactic Treatment of Migraine: Results of an Open Pilot Study. *Cephalgia* 1994 Oct; 14(5):328–329.
16. J. Schoenen, et al. Effectiveness of High-dose Riboflavin in Migraine Prophylaxis. A Randomized Controlled Trial. *Neurology* 1998 Febr; 50(2):466–470.
17. http://www.thesun.co.uk/article/0,,2-2006580423,00.html
18. B. Regland, M. Andersson, L. Abrahamsson, et al. Increased Concentrations of Homocysteine in the Cerebrospinal Fluid in Patients with FMS and CFS. *Scandinavian Journal of Rheumatology* 1997; 26(4):301–307.
19. J. Lindenbaum, I.H. Rosenberg, P.W. Wilson, et al. Prevalence of Cobalamin Deficiency in the Framingham Elderly Population. *American Journal of Clinical Nutrition* 1994 Jul; 60(1):2–11.
20. J. Lindenbaum, E.B. Healton, D.G. Savage, et al. Neuropsychiatric Disorders Caused by Cobalamin Deficiency in the Absence of Anemia or Macrocytoses. *New England Journal of Medicine* 1988 Jun 30; 318(26):1720–1728.
21. W.S. Beck. Cobalmin and the Nervous System. Editorial. *New England Journal of Medicine* 1988 June 30; 318(26):1752–1754.
22. http://www.healthy-heart-guide.com/statin-side-effects.html
23. http://www.pubmedcentral.nih.gov/articlerender.fcgi?artid=2170950
24. A.V. Plioplys, S. Plioplys. Amantadine and L-Carnitine Treatment of CFS. *Neuropsychobiology* 1997; 35(1):16–23.
25. H. Kuratsune, K. Yamaguti, M. Takahashi, et al. Acylcarnitine Deficiency in CFS. *Clinical Infectious Disease* 1994 Jan; 18(3 Supplement 1): S62–S67.
26. http://www.freeradicalscience.com/showabstract.php?pmid=15591009
27. J.E. Teitelbaum, J.A. St. Cyr, C. Johnson. The Use of D-ribose in Chronic Fatigue Syndrome and Fibromyalgia: A Pilot Study. *J Alternative and Complementary Medicine* 2006; 12(9):857–862.
28. Y. Hellsten, L. Skadgauge, J. Bangsbo. Effect of Ribose Supplementation on Resynthesis of Adenine Nucleotides after Intense Intermittent Training in Humans. *American Journal of Physiology* 2004; 286(1):R182–R188.
29. P.C. Tullson, R.L. Terjung. Adenine Nucleotide Synthesis in Exercising and Endurance-trained Skeletal Muscle. *American Journal of Physiology* 1991; 261:C342–C347.
30. J.J. Brault, R.L. Terjung. Purine Salvage to Adenine Nucleotides in Different Skeletal Muscle Fiber Types. *Journal of Applied Physiology* 2001; 91:231–238.
31. B. Gebhart, J.A. Jorgenson. Benefit of Ribose in a Patient with Fibromyalgia. *Pharmacotherapy* 2004; 24(11):1146–1648.

35 Orthopedic Surgery

Nutrients to Optimize Outcomes

Frederick T. Sutter, M.D., M.B.A.

I. INTRODUCTION

This chapter provides the primary care physician with specific strategies to support patients who have chosen to proceed with elective or nonemergent orthopedic surgery. This would include patients undergoing arthroscopy, spinal surgery, or total joint arthroplasty, among others. Elective orthopedic procedures allow for a more generous preoperative interval to prepare a willing patient to achieve the best result possible. The following offers a concise combination of current science and clinical experience outlining how busy physicians can effectively guide patients to improved outcomes with the use of nutrients, even if there are no overt risk factors for negative outcomes. With this facilitation, the patient and the surgeon can then team up to achieve optimal results.

II. EPIDEMIOLOGY

The current scientific literature has made increasingly clear the interrelationship of nutrient intake and general health status. Physicians have had little training or continuing education about the use of nutrient therapies and the identification and treatment of sarcopenia and obesity. They get questions almost daily about the use of dietary supplements and must routinely advise their patients to lose weight and exercise more. This combination of patient interest and an impending procedure creates a superb opportunity for the treating physician to spark meaningful patient cooperation in a preoperative program.

   The prevalence of obesity has more than doubled in the last 30 years, with an increase in total calories consumed primarily in the form of carbohydrates and a slight decrease in the amount of protein calories.[1] Obesity has increased the incidence of arthritic conditions requiring orthopedic procedures in younger adults, with greater complication rates of wound infection, deep venous thrombosis, cardiac events, and anesthesia risks.[2-5] Sarcopenic obesity increases these risks.[6]

III. PATHOPHYSIOLOGY

The perioperative period creates many risks for the patient. Even anticipation of the procedure increases stress, can interfere with sleep, and can prompt misguided attempts to lose weight. Mobility restriction frequently promotes chronic deconditioning and loss of appetite with secondary loss of lean body mass. A homebound patient generally has limited sun exposure with an associated decline in vitamin D status. Restricting calories decreases lean body mass and creates additional risk in the form of sarcopenia, which is associated with unfavorable outcomes.[7] Joint disease and subsequent surgery increases demand on the contralateral limb, thereby increasing risk of additional surgery.[8] The restriction of nutrients during the NPO period prior to surgery initiates catabolism of lean tissue and dehydration. Rapid elimination of caffeine can induce severe withdrawal headaches, complicating postoperative care and pain management. Eliminating anti-inflammatory medications and supplements to avoid bleeding and anesthesia complications can increase pain, immobility, and the need for additional narcotic analgesics.

After surgery, postanesthesia nausea and vomiting and immobilization can advance catabolic wasting and limit nutrient intake. Wound healing and blood loss increase demand for many nutrients in excess of normal dietary intake. The physiology of orthopedic surgical wound healing is not unlike that of general surgery, with emphasis on bone metabolism, the impact of immobility, and loss of muscle mass and function. In this setting, for most elderly and sarcopenic surgical patients, consuming a "regular diet" is very unlikely to meet the metabolic demands for optimal healing.

IV. PHARMACOLOGY

The use of NSAIDs, COX-2 inhibitors, DMARDs, and biological response modifiers in the perioperative period needs some consideration given their impact on how inflammation contributes to the wound healing process. Potential complications include wound dehiscence, infection, and impaired collagen synthesis. There is no current consensus on the optimum time for withholding drug therapy prior to surgery other than that regarding antiplatelet effects.[9] Prudent limitation of NSAIDs in patients with proven stress fractures has been recommended in a more recent article.[10] For many of these medications, there are no human studies and some only have animal studies. The practitioner will need to consider disease severity, risk of exacerbation, and other risk factors in the context of the drug pharmacokinetics prior to making recommendations for cessation of therapy. In some cases, this would require a period of 4 weeks. Treatment options for exacerbation of disease can combine alternative therapies for pain management that might include prescription analgesics and medical food products, supportive nutrients, specific diets for weight loss[11] and dysinflammation, acupuncture, and physical therapy, among other integrative approaches. Using a baseline symptom questionnaire can be very useful in the complex patient to monitor response to changes in therapy (e.g., MOS SF-36). Rakel's *Integrative Medicine* is an excellent reference source, with handheld software for managing patients in this setting.[12]

The orthopedic patient with months of chronic pain has challenges with sleeping. Frequently, the patient has a myofascial pain disorder, in which several studies have found significantly reduced sleep quality. Even without chronic pain, normal individuals who are sleep deprived or have disrupted sleep for a period of time will experience a lowered pain threshold and an increase in musculoskeletal discomfort and fatigue.[13] The majority of addictive, prescription sleep medications actually decrease time spent in the deep stages 3 and 4, except for clonazepam and alprazolam.

V. PATIENT EVALUATION

Physical Exam

The definition and significance of sarcopenia have been reviewed by Kohlstadt.[6] In general, sarcopenia can be defined as the age- or disuse-related loss of muscle and fat-free body mass, reducing muscle metabolism, strength, and mobility in older adults. Skeletal muscle mass is quantified as being less than or equal to two standard deviations (SD) below the mean. Incidence in otherwise healthy individuals over the age of 60 years varies in reports from 8% to 25% and increases dramatically in the very old, with a large increase over 80 years of 43% to 60%. Associated risk factors for sarcopenia are cigarette smoking, chronic illnesses, underweight, physical inactivity, and poorer sense of psychosocial well-being.[14,15]

Waist and hip circumference used alone or in combination with BMI is an anthropometric indicator of health risk and is easily performed. The combination of both is a very sensitive metric to predict health risk. The National Institutes of Health[16] suggest abdominal obesity as a significant risk factor can be identified with waist circumference (measured at the umbilicus) in men ≥ 102 cm (40 inches) and in women ≥ 88 cm (35 inches). These individuals would be identified as having "high" abdominal fat, and therefore a "very high" health risk. The waist-to-hip ratio (WHR) is calculated by measuring the unclothed waist at the narrowest point between ribs and hips after exhaling when viewed from the front. The hip measurement is performed over light clothing at the level of the widest diameter around the buttocks. It is the preferred clinical measure of central obesity for predicting mortality, even in those regarded as very lean (BMI <20), normal, and overweight (BMI >25). Risk starts to rise significantly for cardiovascular mortality when the WHR goes beyond 0.8 for women and 0.9 for men.[17,18]

Clinical identification of sarcopenic obesity is more challenging. Features more suggestive of poor fat-free mass (FFM) in obese individuals can be appreciated as pendulous adiposity in the arms, abdomen, and even the thighs and legs. Gentle palpation over the triceps area, as if performing a fat skin-fold measurement and observing the remaining muscle, can also be revealing. This presentation would be opposed to the more stout or "solid" individual with considerable muscle mass, despite being identified as obese with a BMI in the Class I range of 30 to 34.9.

Individuals without sarcopenia have higher intakes of protein and antioxidant micronutrients than healthy individuals with sarcopenia.[19] Despite good nutrition, one would think that the anabolic response to increased protein intake would be impaired in the elderly; however, recent research has shown evidence to the contrary.[20] This supports bench research on age-related sarcopenia and fatigability in rats that demonstrated the presence of enhanced reactive oxygen species (ROS), or free radical production, apoptotic susceptibility, and reduced mitochondrial biogenesis.[21] Therefore, consuming an antioxidant-rich diet or taking supplemental antioxidants may protect the individual who is exercising and consuming adequate protein from progression of sarcopenia.

Sarcopenic obesity in the frail elderly presents a great challenge. Simple interventions with nutrition, exercise, and weight loss have been demonstrated in recent literature to ameliorate these risk factors over longer periods of time, such as 6 months. However, these results are likely to require a team approach for consistent success.[22,23]

RISK AND NUTRITION-SPECIFIC PREOPERATIVE LABORATORY EVALUATION

With the usual preoperative lab studies, several additional laboratory studies can be very useful in assessing potential nutritional deficiencies or surgical risks (see Table 35.1). Supplementing a low normal nutrient value prepares the patient for the catabolic stress of healing. Scientific literature has described "metabolic therapy" as that which involves the administration of a substance normally found in the body to enhance a metabolic reaction. This can be achieved in two ways: one, by giving a substance to achieve greater than normal levels in the body to drive a biochemical reaction in the desired direction; two, by using a substance to correct relative or absolute deficiency of a cellular component. This concept is useful in the context of prescribing nutrients to promote orthopedic surgery outcomes.

TABLE 35.1

Nutrition-Specific Preoperative Laboratory Assessment

Lab	Optimal range	Indicator	Note	References
Albumin	3.9 g/dL or greater	↑ length of stay (LOS) and complication rates when low, associated with low muscle mass in limbs	↑ dietary intake 0.8–1.4 g protein/kg body wt/day; best at midday meal	26
High Sensitivity CRP	<3 mg/L	If >3 mg/L, associated with ↑ complication and LOS for orthopedic pts	Treat with anti-inflammatory diet; see Table 35.2	27
DEXA	BMD <1SD above young adult mean	Instrumented procedures for ↑ risk osteoporosis pts	Vitamin D, minerals	
DHEA-Sulfate	Women 150–180 μg/dL, men 350–400 μg/dL	Sarcopenia, precursor of testosterone	Monitor DHEA-S levels monthly with treatment	28
Folate	>5.4 ng/mL	Lowers Hcy	See Table 35.3	
Iron, Ferritin	Support if low	Supports blood element formation	See Table 35.3	29
Homocysteine (Hcy)	4–8 μM/L	↑ levels associated with ↑ risk of stroke, CAD, DVT, osteoporosis	↑ risk 9–17 μM/L ↑↑ risk >17 μM/L; see Table 35.2	30–33
Magnesium	High normal	Bone healing, ↓ in obesity, chronic pain	Rx depletion in combination with low intake in typical diet	34
Vitamin B6	>50 nmol/L	↑ DVT <23 nmol/L	See Table 35.3	35
Vitamin B12	>500 pg/mL	10% to 15% over 60 years are deficient	IM injection typically not covered by insurances; pts usually willing to pay minor cost	34
Vitamin D (25-OH D3)	50–70 ng/dL	Bone healing, ↓ in obesity, chronic pain	See Table 35.3	36

High-sensitivity C-reactive protein has been associated with higher complications and greater length of stay for orthopedic patients. To address this, removing sugar, consuming low arachidonic acid food groups, targeting protein intake, and taking antioxidants are best (see Table 35.2). Patients with low albumin were twice as likely to require prolonged hospitalization (>15 days) for elective total hip replacement, compared with those in whom the albumin level was 3.9 g/dl or greater.[24] Following transferrin and albumin levels perioperatively has also been used to predict delayed wound healing after total hip arthroplasty.[24]

Homocysteine (Hcy) is a cholesterol-independent risk factor for stroke, heart, bone, and thromboembolic disease.[25] Homocysteinemia is less common since fortification of grain products with folic acid began in 1998. B vitamins can safely lower elevation of Hcy. High Hcy levels have been associated with higher bone turnover, poor physical performance, and lower bone mineral density.

Bone health can be assessed by DEXA screening or follow-up study. More specific information can be obtained about lean body mass, or appendicular muscle mass with DEXA scanning that can assist in the determination of sarcopenia; however, this type of assessment is primarily being used at research institutions.

TABLE 35.2A
Dietary Guidelines for the Management of Inflammation

Food Category	Serving Size	Svg/day	Cal/Svg	Choices*
Concentrated Protein	3.5 oz (after cooking)	Aim to consume no more than 60 mg arachidonic acid (AA) daily.	150	Poultry (remove all skin): turkey breast and chicken. Lean meats: sliced boiled ham, pork tenderloin, beef flank steak, ground beef (5% fat). Fish (avoid farmed fish). (Table 35.2B) Dairy: cottage cheese: 1%, 3/4 cup; ricotta: reduced fat, 1/2 cup. Tofu products: tofu, 1 cup; tempeh, 1/2 cup; soy burger, 4 oz.
Vegetables	1/2 cup	5 to 7	10 to 25	All vegetables are allowed except white potato, turnip, parsnip, rutabaga, and corn. Fresh vegetable juice or green beverages are allowed.
Fruits	Approximately 1 medium	3 to 4	80	All whole fruits except banana, pineapple, and papaya. Fruit juice not recommended.
Dairy	6 oz.	1–2 (if tolerated)	80 to 100	Plain yogurt (low fat or nonfat), milk (nonfat, 1%, 2%), buttermilk, milk substitutes (soy, rice, nut).
Legumes	1/2 to 1 cup	1 to 2	100 to 200	All peas and beans, hummus, bean soups.
Grains	1/2 cup	1 to 3	75 to 100	Whole grains such as 100% whole wheat bread and pasta, brown rice, whole oats, rye crackers, and pearled barley with at least 3 grams or more of fiber per serving.
Nuts/Seeds	1 small handful	1 serving per day	150 to 200	All nuts except cashews and macadamias, 1–2 tbsp of nut butter.
Oils	1 tsp	4 to 6	40	Olive and canola oils for cooking, flax seed (refrigerate) and walnut oils for salads, mayonnaise from canola oil (no egg or sugar added), avocado (1/8 of whole), green or black olives (8–10).
Beverages	Unlimited	Water intake recommended at 1/2 body weight in ounces.	0	Water, herbal tea, decaffeinated coffee or tea, mineral water, club soda, or seltzer, plain or flavored (no added artificial sweeteners).
Condiments	Unlimited, except salt	As desired	0	Cinnamon, carob, mustard, horseradish, vinegar, lemon, lime, flavored extracts, herbs/spices, stevia. No refined sugars or artificial sweeteners are allowed.

*These items should be avoided in patients with food reactivities.

continued

TABLE 35.2B *(continued)*
Arachidonic Acid Calculator

Concentrated Protein Food	Arachidonic Acid Content
Meat and Poultry:	(mg/3.5 oz)
Ham, sliced boiled	0
Pork tenderloin	30
Turkey breast, roast	40
Beef, flank steak	40
Ground beef, 5% fat	50
Chicken breast	60
Fish:	
Mahi mahi	0
Pacific mackerel	10
Pink salmon	10
Pacific cod	20
Sockeye salmon	30
Atlantic cod	30
Haddock	30
Snapper	40
Yellowfin tuna	40
White tuna, canned in water	50
Flounder	50
Atlantic mackerel	50
Grouper	60
Dairy	negligible
Soy	negligible

Source: Adapted from [37].

VI. TREATMENT RECOMMENDATIONS

DIET

Adequate caloric intake is essential, especially in the form of protein. It is a key macronutrient in wound healing and managing complications related to sarcopenia, along with exercise.[38] Instruct the patient to target at least the RDA of 0.8 g/kg body wt of protein intake, provided there is no concomitant liver or renal disease, or a history of gout. Protein sources in the form of seafood and organ meats can be high in purines, usually restricted in gout. However, consumption of these in the presence of caffeinated or alcoholic beverages (especially beer) is more likely to precipitate a gouty attack at the RDA level for protein.[39] Higher dietary intakes (up to 1.6 g protein/kg/day) may enhance response to resistance exercise in the elderly.[40,41] Protein intake will be metabolized best if consumed with the midday meal or in the form of an afternoon protein shake. Advise the patient to continue targeted protein intake as close to NPO status as possible.

General dietary guidelines to redirect the inflammatory cascade focus on fat content, arachidonic acid, refined carbohydrates, and simple sugars. Arachidonic acid is the physiologic precursor of pro-inflammatory eicosanoids such as prostaglandins and leukotrienes. These molecules can then go on to produce superoxide, which can play a role in a feed-forward, or propagated lipid peroxidation chain reaction, increasing antioxidant demand for the body. Many times, appreciable results occur within 10 days, although the first 5 to 7 days are more challenging if considerable sugar consumption has been habitual prior to initiating dietary changes. In this case, the initial period of withdrawal can be associated with significant cravings, diuresis, cramps, and irritability for the first 2 to 4 days. Preparing the patient for this possibility is the most effective strategy for compliance and will help them pass through this period quickly and with greater ease.

If the patient is consuming large amounts of caffeinated beverages, these should be tapered over 2 weeks prior to surgery. This can be done with minimal withdrawal headaches by reducing consumption of one serving every 3 to 4 days and replacing that serving with an equal volume of clean water; for example, if consuming four caffeinated beverages daily, day one of a taper would be three servings plus one serving of water, and so on until the last serving, which is cut in half and then eliminated in 2 to 3 days.

Table 35.2 outlines specific dietary recommendations to optimize nutrition in the perioperative period.

NUTRIENTS TO OPTIMIZE ORTHOPEDIC SURGICAL OUTCOMES

Over the last 2 decades, multiple studies and market surveys have shown an increase in the self-directed use of supplemental nutrients, frequently unbeknownst to the individual's physician. A national study on the reasons patients use supplemental nutrients (considered by the study to be alternative medicine) concluded patients are choosing supplemental nutrients not because they are dissatisfied with conventional medicine, but because these "alternatives" are more congruent with their own values, beliefs, and philosophical orientations toward health and life.[42,43] Multiple publications have effectively addressed many of the risks associated with the use of supplements in the preoperative period, and various surgical societies have recommended eliminating all supplements for some defined period prior to surgery.

Two possible exceptions appear to be the withdrawal of the beneficial effects of fish oils on the risk of venous thrombosis[44] and the therapeutic use of ginger oil for the treatment of postoperative nausea and vomiting.[45] Both of these nutrients have demonstrated clinical efficacy and no proven impact on platelet aggregation. Clinical trials have shown high-dose omega-3 fatty acid consumption to be safe, even when concurrently used with other agents that may increase bleeding, including aspirin and warfarin, and in fact have been used up until the day of aortocoronary bypass surgery (dosage 3 gm/day) and for 1 month after surgery with no bleeding complications.[46]

Ginger oil can be applied topically in children and with inhalations from the cupped palms over the nose and mouth in adults. Applied in this way, ginger oil can be 80% effective for high risk, postanesthesia nausea patients when used with multimodal intravenous medication therapy. Ginger has been used safely and effectively for years to treat motion sickness and nausea and vomiting of pregnancy. Nutrients listed in Table 35.3 can be used safely and effectively in conjunction with the surgical guidelines.

Discussion regarding the general classes of nutrients listed in Table 35.3 is worthwhile, as many of these applications pertain to the previously described "metabolic therapy" which uses nutrient substances to achieve greater than normal levels in the body to drive a desired biochemical response, or to meet a conditionally specific nutrient demand. Research is moving beyond the notion of treating or preventing deficiency disease states to study safe and economical nutrient applications in specific environments, to promote a desired, measurable result.

The simple recommendation of a high-quality multivitamin is the first step in optimizing surgical outcomes because it will enhance a broad spectrum of micronutrients with little effort. See Table 35.4 for guidelines in choosing quality supplemental nutrients.

AMINO ACIDS

Arginine and glutamine are "semi-essential" or conditionally indispensible amino acids during critical illness and severe trauma. Arginine is considered to be a direct nitric oxide (NO) precursor. It induces nitric oxide release, which inhibits smooth muscle contraction, increases blood flow, and

TABLE 35.3
Nutrients to Optimize Orthopedic Surgical Outcomes

Nutrient	Dose	Support	Notes	Food Sources	Adult DRI	References
N-Acetyl Cysteine	500–600 mg bid	Antioxidant, ↓ LOS/pain mgmt for tourniquet surgery	Well tolerated	Precursor to glutathione	ND	
L-Arginine	3–6 g bid, powder or time-release tabs	Collagen formation, supports synthesis of protein and mitochondria	Start at lower doses in diabetes and HTN, HSV infections	Dairy, beef, pork, nuts	ND	47–49
Calcium	1200–1500 mg Ca carbonate; 800–1000 mg chelated MCHC products	Typical diet 500–600 mg day, supports bone healing	Monitor for constipation; citrate, malate best form Balance 2Ca:1Mg	Dairy, kale, broccoli	1000–2500 mg	
L-Carnitine	0.5–2 g bid	Sarcopenia, muscle/cardiac support, ↑ mitochondrial efficiency	Low in vegans	Red meats	ND	50–52
Chondroitin Sulfate	400–600 mg bid	Chondroprotectant, pain mgmt	Typically synergistic with glucosamine sulfate	Limited	ND	12,53
Coenzyme Q10	50–1200 mg/day	Antioxidant, higher doses with CHF; monitor prothrombin time for warfarin pts	Reduced by statins, helps fatigue and muscle recovery	Insignificant amount in food	ND	54–56
Copper	1–4 mg/day	Collagen cross-linking	Use with zinc, dietary intake is low	Organ meats, seafood, nuts and seeds	0.9–10 mg	57,58
Creatine	3–5 g after exercise	Sarcopenia in elderly		n/a	ND	59
DHEA	10–15 mg/day women, 15–25 mg/day men	Declines in elderly	Monitor levels q8 wks	n/a	ND	52,60
EFAs: EPA/DHA	2000–2500 mg EPA+DHA	Reduces inflammation, prevents sarcopenia	Take with food, refrigeration helps "fish repeats," anticoagulant effect controversial	Coldwater fish	ND	61
Folate	0.8–5 mg/day	Supports ↑ Hcy	Use with B6, B12	Dark greens, grains, beans	0.4–1 mg	

	Dose	Uses	Cautions	Food Source	RDA	Ref
Flavocoxid	250–500 mg q 12 h	Pain mgmt, "medical food," anti-inflammatory, helps muscle recovery	Rx only. Can use with warfarin, monitor prothrombin time	Colored vegetables	ND	
Ginger Oil	10% essential oil of Ginger	Postop nausea	Vaporized nasal and transdermal application	Zingiber officinale root	ND	45
Glucosamine Sulfate	750 mg bid	Pain mgmt joint disease			ND	62
Glutamine	5 g bid	Supports GI integrity, prevents loss of muscle mass	Avoid with shellfish allergy Constipation	"Conditionally essential" amino acid	ND	
Iron	Iron Glycinate™, Chromagen FA	Use gluconate, bis-glycinate chelate, vit C ↑↑ absorption	GI upset	Meats, fish, poultry, and dark greens	8–45 mg	
Lipoic Acid	300–600 mg bid	Diabetic neuropathy, ↓ damage ischemic reperfusion	May lower blood glucose levels, monitor diabetics	Kidney, heart, liver, broccoli, spinach, potatoes	ND	
Magnesium	400–800 mg/day	Bone healing, use 2:1, Ca:Mg, intake is generally inadequate	Can loosen stools	Leafy greens, grains, nuts	310–420 mg †	
Manganese	5–10 mg/day	Bone healing, enzyme and protein metabolism	Limit with liver disease/cholestasis	Grains, tea, greens	1.8–11 mg	63
Melatonin	0.5–3 mg 30 min before bedtime	Sleep and pain support	Studies done with lower doses, avoid in leukemia, Hodgkin's disease	Tart cherries	ND	64
MSM	1000–3000 mg bid	Pain mgmt joint disease	GI intolerance		ND	65
Probiotics	1–10 B CFUs/day, L.acidophilus, B. bifidum, S. boulardii	Supports GI integrity, post-abx diarrhea	Flatulence	Yogurt	ND	66
Protein	0.8–1.6 g/kg/day	Poorly digested in hypochlohydric elderly, essential for wound healing, common deficiency worldwide	Use hydrolyzed protein shakes	Meat, poultry, fish, eggs, milk, yogurt, nuts, legumes, seeds	0.66–1.52 g/kd/day	
S-Adenosyl Methionine	400–600 mg bid	Pain mgmt joint disease	GI intolerance May activate bipolar patients	Occurs naturally in the body	ND	67–69

continued

TABLE 35.3 *(continued)*

Nutrient	Dose	Support	Notes	Food Sources	Adult DRI	References
Selenium	50–400 µg/day	Antioxidant, supports healing, ↓ intake associated with sarcopenia	Hair loss, brittle nails in doses > 1 mg/day	Meat, seafood, grains, vegetables	55–400 µg/day	19,58
Silicon		Deficiency leads to bone defects	Use caution in renal lithiasis	Cereal and unrefined grain products	ND	70,71
L-Theanine	50–200 mg	Improves mood and helps sleep	Well tolerated	Green tea (*Camellia sinensis*)	ND	72
L-Tryptophan	500 mg–3 g hs	Precursor of serotonin, supports sleep	Theoretical risk of serotonin syndrome if given with SSRI Rx	Chocolate, oats, dried dates, turkey	ND	73
Vitamin A (preformed retinol or carotenoids)	15,000–25,000 IU/day	Antioxidant, wound healing, osteoporosis, sarcopenia	Use combination of mixed carotenoids and retinol	Retinol animal based foods, carotenoids vegetables, fruits	2310–9900 IU	74
Vitamin B2 (Riboflavin)	10–100 mg/day	↑ intake - ↓ hip fx	Sensitive to light exposure	Fortified cereals, organ meats	1.1–1.3 mg/day	75
Vitamin B5 (Pantothenate)	500–750 mg bid	Wound healing	No toxicity	Chicken, beef, potatoes	5 mg/day	63
Vitamin B6	10–100 mg/day	Supports ↑ Hcy, low serum B6 assoc. w/ DVT	Makes urine bright yellow	Cereals, beef liver, organ meats	1.1–100 mg	75
Vitamin B12	500–5000 µg/day	Lowers ↑ Hcy, best form methylcobalamin, can help with sleep disruption	Well tolerated	Shellfish, organ meats, sardines	2.0–2.4 µg	
Vitamin C	1–2 g bid	Wound/bone healing, prevents sarcopenia, ↑ need in smokers	If GI intolerance, use buffered or ester C	Citrus fruits, vegetables, tomatoes	75–2000 mg	76
Vitamin D3	800 IU daily to 50,000 IU weekly	Bone metabolism, low in chronic pain, may influence seasonal affective disorder	Well tolerated, hypercalcemia at 160–500 ng/dL, monitor levels q8–12 wks	Enriched food sources likely inadequate for surgical patients	200–2000 IU	

Vitamin E	100–200 IU/day mixed tocopherols	Prevents sarcopenia, supports high PUFA intakes (EFAs)	Use caution in warfarin therapy or vitamin K deficiency	Vegetable oils, grains, vegetables, meats	12–15 mg (8–10 IU)	
Zinc	30–50 mg/day	Essential in wound healing	Take with copper, can cause GI upset	Seafood (oysters and sardines), organ meats, sunflower seeds	6.8–40 mg	77,78

Note: All DRIs were obtained from Dietary Reference Intakes. Institute of Medicine.[34]
DRI = Dietary Reference Intakes, AI = Adequate Intakes, UL = Upper Limit, ND = Not Determined, CFU = Colony Forming Units. Adult = 19 years and older. DRI presented as a range from RDA (Recommended Daily Allowance = average daily dietary nutrient intake level sufficient to meet requirements of 97% to 98% healthy individuals), or AI (Adequate Intake = recommended daily intake estimates when RDA cannot be determined) to UL (Tolerable Upper Limit = highest daily intake that is likely to pose no risk of adverse health effects to almost all individuals in the general population).

†UL of 350 mg based on diarrhea as endpoint. RDA is stated here. Higher levels tolerated clinically.

TABLE 35.4
Better Quality Supplements

The product demonstrates:

Chelated minerals

Independent lab testing

Fish oils: package states free of heavy metals, PCBs

No artificial colors and limited fillers, e.g., glycols, sucrose, etc.

Manufacturing guidelines:

cGMP (Current Good Manufacturing Practices)

NSF™ (NSF International, The Public Health and Safety Company™)

ISO 9000 or ISO 9001:2000 (International Organization for Standardization)

---

results in increased nutrient uptake and glucose utilization into muscle, particularly during exercise. Arginine stimulates collagen deposition in wound healing and dramatically increases strength in trained men compared with controls.[79] A time-released product is available, which adds to convenience for individuals that do not prefer powders. Use with caution and at lower starting doses if the individual is diabetic, on blood pressure medicine, or has a history of herpes simplex virus (HSV) infections. The precaution with HSV and arginine is because arginine shares transport proteins with lysine, and relative deficiencies of lysine can be a trigger for an outbreak of cold sores. High arginine foods such as cashews, peanuts, chocolate, and coffee can also limit lysine availability enough to induce HSV symptoms.

N-acetylcysteine (NAC) has been studied with attention to ischemia/reperfusion of orthopedically operated limbs. It appears to lessen the need for postoperative analgesics, and can decrease hospital stay.[80] Along other dietary amino acids such as glutamine and glycine, antioxidants such as vitamins C and E, selenium, phytonutrients, and lipoic acid, NAC provides cysteine as a substrate for the recycling of glutathione, which is frequently depleted in the presence of oxidative stress. Glutathione is recognized as the final pathway for the reduction of oxidants produced by reactive oxygen species. L-Carnitine is important for vegetarians, or those with metabolic syndrome and has been shown to enhance cardiac performance and increase exercise tolerance in humans with ischemic heart and peripheral vascular disease.[81–83]

Creatine can be useful in the frail elderly as an adjunctive support to increase muscle strength and mass with an exercise program. It can be mixed with the patient's favorite juice or nonalcoholic beverage and consumed 1 to 2 times per day. When taken along with caffeinated beverages, a stimulating effect may be experienced, so it is best taken earlier in the day.

SAMe is a naturally occurring byproduct of the amino acid methionine. It is a methyl donor and inhibits synthesis of proinflammatory interleukens and TNF-alpha. It up-regulates proteoglycan synthesis and the proliferation rate of chondrocytes, promoting cartilage formation and repair in doses ranging from 400 to 1600 mg/day in divided doses. In a double-blind crossover study at 1200 mg/day compared with celecoxib (200 mg), it had the same efficacy and a lower incidence of side effects over a 2-month period. It can also elevate mood and help with anxiety.

ANTIOXIDANTS

Recent research has demonstrated the role of ROS in aseptic loosening of hip prostheses.[84] This alone suggests the rational use of antioxidants perioperatively. Coenzyme Q10 (CoQ10) has been safely prescribed for individuals with CHF and severe neurological conditions in doses of 400 to 1200 mg. In times of severe oxidative stress, CoQ10 along with lipoic acid can be viewed as conditionally essential nutrients, because the body cannot make enough of them. There has been one case report of reduced effectiveness of warfarin drugs with CoQ10 use. In over 15 years, this author has only twice seen increases in prothrombin after introducing CoQ10 in anticoagulated patients. More frequent testing is indicated when initiating CoQ10 therapy in this patient group. This coenzyme produces a favorable response in treating fatigue on a very consistent basis. For individuals taking statin prescription medications (as well as red yeast rice, the natural form of lovastatin), myopathy and the more common myalgias may be supported by the use of CoQ10.[55,85]

Alpha lipoic acid is a potent, multifunctional antioxidant that improves tissue glutathione levels, reduces lipid peroxides, increases insulin sensitivity, and helps regenerate vitamins C and E. It has been used effectively in Germany for over 30 years orally and intravenously for the treatment of diabetic polyneuropathy.[86] It can be a useful adjunct for improving insulin sensitivity and surgical recovery involving neural structures, especially in patients with diabetes. Alpha lipoic acid was used in combination with CoQ10, magnesium, and omega-3 fatty acids preoperatively, up until the day of surgery and for 1 month thereafter, and was demonstrated to enhance several recovery parameters.[46]

MINERALS

Minerals in the form of inorganic mineral salts such as carbonates, oxides, phosphates, and sulfates compete with one another for absorption. When minerals are provided as inorganic salts they can also be blocked by the intake of natural fiber found in cereals and fruits.[87] While there are several implications to absorption and alterations to absorption when patients are taking one mineral such as iron preoperatively, an important aspect is to supplement calcium and magnesium together. Generally a ratio of two parts calcium to one part magnesium is recommended. Apart from any pain medications that alter bowel motility, patients may find calcium to be constipating and magnesium to have a laxative effect. Calcium citrate and magnesium citrate may be better absorbed in patients with hypochlorhydria and can also confer an alkalinizing effect. Microcrystalline hydroxyapatite is a blend of minerals found in bone.

Silicon can be helpful with bone healing and in addressing osteoporosis in men and premenopausal women. It is best absorbed as orthosilicic acid and is available in multivitamin preparations, usually in the form of silicon dioxide or magnesium trisilicate at about 2 mg. It has been shown to stimulate collagen synthesis. Silica is often removed from food during processing.

Zinc carnosine is a preparation that has been helpful with relieving mild gastric upset, while supporting zinc levels. Dosage is 75 mg bid and provides 32 mg of zinc.[78]

HORMONES

Melatonin in combination with L-tryptophan can be very effective in supporting patients with disrupted sleep patterns.[64] L-tryptophan has recently been cleared once again by the FDA for use after a decades-long ban related to contamination with an industrial chemical by one manufacturer, which resulted in hundreds of illnesses. 5-hydoxytryptophan is available and is a suitable substitute. There is a theoretical risk of serotonin syndrome with nausea, vomiting, and excessive drowsiness if either is given in conjunction with selective serotonin reuptake inhibitors, so it is recommended to avoid this combination until further studies have been completed.

Dehydroepiandrosterone (DHEA) therapy by supporting low DHEA-sulfate levels in the elderly can be helpful with sarcopenia. Limit use to 3 to 6 months while following serum levels. Occasional activation can occur, and the dosage may be adjusted downward with this side effect.

VITAMINS

B12 absorption is inadequate in approximately 15% population over 65 due to lack of gastric acidity, decreased intrinsic factor, and in *Helicobacter pylori* infections.[34] For individuals with low serum B12 levels and intramuscular dosing is not an option, doses of 5000 μg/day are available

TABLE 35.5
Perioperative Treatment Guidelines for Low 25-Hydroxy Vitamin D3

Starting 25-OH D3 Levels (ng/mL)	Starting Dose	Testing Interval*	Next Dose	Retest	Maintenance
<20	5000–10,000 IU/day	6–8 wks	3000–5000 IU/day	q 8–12 wks until level maintained	As indicated by lab values
20–32	5000 IU	6–8 wks	2000–5000 IU	16 wks	2000 IU
32–50	2000–5000 IU	q 3–4 mos until stable	2000 IU	q 6 mos	
50–75	800–2000 IU	Annually in winter			

*Retest 25-OH D3 and serum calcium.

in sublingual form of methylcobalamin for shorter term use. Low serum B6 is associated with an increased risk of DVT[35,88] and is best supplemented in its activated form of pyridoxal-5'-phosphate. B5 (pantothenic acid) enhanced wound healing in a human study with a dosage of 200 to 900 mg/day.[63] In individuals with rheumatoid arthritis treated with methotrexate, which inhibits B6 metabolism, there is a much higher incidence of heart disease and elevated Hcy levels than in healthy controls. B6 therapy is frequently prescribed; however, when associated with elevated Hcy, the addition of B12 and folate is indicated.

Guidelines for treatment of low 25-hydroxyvitamin D levels to optimize physiologic levels in the perioperative setting are included in Table 35.5. The recommended form for treatment is vitamin D3, which has been shown in one calculation to have a relative potency of D3:D2 of 9.5:1; in another calculation, D2 was one-third that of D3.[89] The guide is intentionally accelerated for achieving results in the near term and to minimize the expense of retesting,[90–93] and represents this author's approach based on recent publications. The targeted serum level for individuals with osteoporosis/-penia and sarcopenia is 50 to 70 ng/mL. If these levels appear alarming, it is best to know that levels of 54 to 90 ng/mL have been measured in "normals" in sunny countries. Because of the findings of these more recent studies, the current guidelines are being revised upwards.

MACRONUTRIENTS

One fish oil study raises the possibility that the anti-inflammatory actions of omega-3 fatty acids may play a role in the prevention of sarcopenia.[61] Essential fatty acids in the form of eicosapentaenoic acid (EPA) and docoxahexaenoic acid (DHA) at 1 g/day has been recommended by the American Heart Association in patients with documented atherosclerosis based on their anti-atherothrombotic effects. Recent review of the literature by Bays[44] demonstrated that clinical trials have shown high-dose omega-3 fatty acid consumption to be safe, even when concurrently administered with other agents that may increase bleeding, such as aspirin and warfarin. For the management of preoperative pain, particularly after withdrawal of NSAIDs or other prescription drugs, this author suggests that patients use 2000 to 2500 mg of EPA and DHA (combined dose) for about 3 to 4 weeks prior to withdrawal of the prescription drugs.

VII. SUMMARY AND CLINICAL RECOMMENDATIONS

Elective orthopedic surgery has potential complications that are willingly assumed in order to improve the quality of life for patients. Many orthopedic patients have inadequate levels of nutrients, which may have impaired various metabolic pathways and contributed to the development of their orthopedic condition. The additional catabolic stressors of the perioperative period create further depletion of multiple nutrients that are essential for optimal recovery. The scientific literature demonstrates improved outcomes with targeted, metabolic nutrient therapies using isolated nutrient interventions, particularly with antioxidants. There is great opportunity for rational, complex, and balanced nutrient therapy interventions to improve outcomes. Many patients have already seized this opportunity using little professional advice, and are eager to find knowledgeable physician guidance. Primary care physicians are well positioned to initiate effective nutrient therapies to optimize orthopedic surgical outcomes through targeted diet, exercise, and nutrient therapies. The key points are:

- Nutrient therapy is safe and can measurably improve outcomes.
- The distinctive circumstance of impending surgical threat, combined with patient interest in nutrient therapy, creates a superb opportunity for the physician to spark motivated patient compliance in a preoperative program.
- The nutrient status of many orthopedic patients is surprisingly poor, particularly the obese elderly.
- Sarcopenia is underdiagnosed and treatable with professionally guided exercise and nutrient support. A first step to nutrient support is recommending unrefined, whole foods and high-quality nutrients, starting with a multivitamin. Practitioners or their staff should become familiar with three or four preparations and where to direct patients to find them.
- Three-day food diaries to measure protein content demonstrate inadequate protein intake with surprising frequency. Increase protein intake for 6 weeks before and after surgery, and maintain intake as close as possible to the time the patient must be NPO for surgery. Protein shakes and amino acid formulas are convenient supplements and medical foods to support poor food intake.
- Limit negative pharmaceutical and dietary influences on healing.
- Jump start bone metabolism with focused treatment of vitamin D insufficiency, and supplement with balanced, chelated minerals.
- Perioperative antioxidant therapy has shown great promise to improve surgical outcomes in multiple studies.
- Invite all, work with the willing, and meet the rest with an invitation by sharing previous good outcomes.
- For the nutrient neophyte, advice can be as simple as just eat right (no to "white stuff," yes to lean meats, five half-cup servings of vegetables/day), drink only clean water, and take a good quality multivitamin.
- For complex patients, establish a baseline symptom reference to ease follow-up assessment such as the validated MOS SF-36[94] or the clinically useful Medical Symptoms Questionnaire.[95]

REFERENCES

1. Wright, J.D., et al., *Trends in intake of energy and macronutrients-United States, 1971-2000.* MMWR Feb 6, 2004;53(4):80–82.
2. Patel, N., et al., *Obesity and spine surgery: relation to perioperative complications.* J Neruosurg Spine 2007 Apr;6(4):291–297.
3. Harms, S., et al., *Obesity increases the likelihood of total joint replacement surgery among younger adults.* Int Orthop 2007 Feb;31(1):23–26 Epub 2006 May 11.
4. Liu, B., et al., *Relationship of height, weight and body mass index to the risk of hip and knee replacements in middle-aged women.* Rheumatology (Oxford). 2007 May;46(5):861–867 Epub 2007 Feb 4.
5. Stürmer, T., et al., *Obesity, overweight and patterns of osteoarthritis: the Ulm Osteoarthritis Study.* J Clin Epidemiol 2000 Mar 1;53(3):307–313.
6. Kohlstadt, I., *Scientific Evidence for Musculoskeletal, Bariatric, and Sports Nutrition.* 2006, Boca Raton: CRC Taylor & Francis.

7. Cosqueric, G., et al., *Sarcopenia is predictive of nosocomial infection in care of the elderly.* Br J Nutr 2006 Nov;96(5):895–901.

8. McMahon, M. and J.A. Block, *The risk of contralateral total knee arthroplasty after knee replacement for osteoarthritis.* J Rheumatol 2003 Aug;30(8):1822–1824.

9. Busti, A.J., et al., *Effects of perioperative anti-inflammatory and immunomodulating therapy on surgical wound healing.* Pharmacotherapy 2005 Nov;25(11):1566–1591.

10. Wheeler, P., *Do non-steroidal anti-inflammatory drugs adversely affect stress fracture healing?* Br J Sports Med 2005;39:65–69.

11. Christensen, R., et al., *Effect of weight reduction in obese patients diagnosed with knee osteoarthritis: a systematic review and meta-analysis.* Ann Rheum Dis 2007;66:433–439.

12. Rakel, D., *Integrative medicine*, 2nd Edition. 2007, Philadelphia: Saunders, 1238p.

13. Lentz, M.J., et al., *Effects of selective slow wave sleep disruption on musculoskeletal pain and fatigue in middle aged women.* J Rheumatol 1999;26:1586–1592.

14. Petersen, A.M., et al, *Smoking impairs muscle protein synthesis and increases the expression of myostatin and MAFbx in muscle.* Am J Physiol Endocrinol Metab 2007 Sep;293(3):E943–948. Epub 2007 Jul 3.

15. Lee, J.S., et al., *Associated factors and health impact of sarcopenia in older Chinese men and women: a cross-sectional study.* Gerontol 2007 Aug 16;53(6):166–172.

16. National Institutes of Health National Heart Lung and Blood Institute, Clinical guidelines on the identification, evaluation, and treatment of overweight and obesity in adults: the evidence report. Obes Res 6, S51–S210, 1998.

17. Welborn, T.A., Dhaliwal, S.S., *Preferred clinical measures of central obesity for predicting mortality.*

18. Yusuf, S., et al., *Obesity and the risk of myocardial infarction in 27,000 participants from 52 countries: a case-control study.* Lancet 2005;366:1640–1649.

19. Chaput, J.P., et al., *Relationship between antioxidant intakes and class I sarcopenia in elderly men and women.* J Nutr Health Aging 2007 Jul–Aug;11(4):363–369.

20. Symons T.B., et al., *Aging does not impair the anabolic response to a protein-rich meal.* Am J Clin Nutr 2007 Aug;86(2):451–456.

21. Chabi, B., et al., *Mitochondrial function and apoptotic susceptibility in aging skeletal muscle.* Aging Cell 2007 Nov 19 [Epub ahead of print].

22. Kyle, U.G., et al., *Total body mass, fat mass, fat-free mass, and skeletal muscle on older people: cross-sectional differences in 60-year-old persons.* J Am Geriatr Soc 2001 Dec;49(12):1633–1640.

23. Villareal, D.T., et al., *Effect of weight loss and exercise on frailty in obese older adults.* Arch Int Med 2006;166:860–866.

24. Gherini, S., et al., *Delayed wound healing and nutritional deficiencies after total hip arthroplasty.* Clin Orthop Relat Res 1993;293:188–195.

25. Cattaneo, M., *Hyperhomocysteinemia and venous thromboembolism.* Semin Thromb Hemost 2006 Oct;32(7):716–723.

26. Del Savio, G.C., et al., *Preoperative nutritional status and outcome of elective total hip replacement.* Clin Orthop Relat Res 1996 May;(326):153–161.

27. Ackland, G.L., et al., *Pre-operative high sensitivity C-reactive protein and postoperative outcome in patients undergoing elective orthopaedic surgery.* Anaesthesia 2007 Sep;62(9):888–894.

28. Teitelbaum, J. Fibromyalgia. In: Kohlstadt, I. (ed.), *Scientific evidence for Musculoskeletal, Bariatric, and Sports Nutrition.* 2006, Boca Raton, FL: CRC, Taylor & Francis, p. 416.

29. Theusinger, O., et al., *Treatment of Iron Deficiency Anemia in Orthopedic Surgery with Intravenous Iron: Efficacy and Limits: A Prospective Study.* Anesthesiology 2007 Dec;107(6):923–927.

30. McCully, K., *Homocysteine, vitamins, and vascular disease prevention.* Am J Clin Nutr 2007;86(suppl):1563S–1568S.

31. Gerdhem, P., et al., *Associations between homocysteine, bone turnover, BMD, mortality and fracture risk in elderly women.* J Bone Miner Res 2007 Jan;22(1):127–134.

32. Selhub, J., et al., *Vitamin status and intake as primary determinants of homocysteinemia in an elderly population.* JAMA 1993;270:2693–2698.

33. Spence, J.D., *Homocysteine-lowering therapy: a tale in stroke prevention?* Lancet Neurol 2007;6:830–838.

34. Institute of Medicine, *Dietary Reference Intakes.* 2006 The National Academies Press, Washington, D.C. 343p

35. Hron, G., et al., *Low vitamin B6 levels and the risk of recurrent venous thromboembolism.* Haematologica 2007 Sep;92(9):1250–1253 Epub 2007 Aug 1.

36. Bischoff-Ferrari, H.A., et al., *Higher 25-hydroxyvitamin D concentrations are associated with better lower-extremity function in both active and inactive persons aged=60 y.* Am J Clin Nutr 2004;80:752–758.

37. www.metagenics.com
38. Campbell, W.W., *Synergistic use of higher-protein diets or nutritional supplements with resistance training to counter sarcopenia.* Nutr Rev 2007 Sep;65(9):416–422.
39. Helman, T. Gout. In: Kohlstadt, I. (ed.), *Scientific Evidence for Musculoskeletal, Bariatric, and Sports Nutrition.* 2006, Boca Raton, FL: CRC, Taylor & Francis, p. 427.
40. Evans, W.J., *Protein nutrition, exercise and aging.* J Am Coll Nutr. 2004 Dec;23(6Suppl):601S–609S.
41. Campbell, W.W., *Synergistic use of higher-protein diets or nutritional supplements with resistance training to counter sarcopenia.* Nutr Rev 2007 Sep;(65):416–422.
42. Astin, J.A., *Why patients use alternative medicine.* JAMA 1998;279(19):1548–1553.
43. Eisenberg, D.M., et al., *Unconventional medicine in the United States-prevalence, cost and patterns of use.* N Engl J Med 1993 Jan;328(4):246–252.
44. Bays, H., *Safety considerations with omerga-3 fatty acid therapy.* Am J Card 2007;99(6A):35C–43C.
45. Geiger, J.L., *The essential oil of ginger, Zingiber officinale, and anesthesia.* International Journal of Aromatherapy 2005;15:7–14.
46. Hadj, A., et al., *Pre-operative preparation for cardiac surgery utilizing a combination of metabolic, physical and mental therapy.* Heart Lung Circ 2006 Jun;15(3):172–181. Epub 2006 May 19.
47. Preli, R.B., et al., *Vascular effects of dietary L-arginine supplementation.* Atherosclerosis 2002; 162:1–15.
48. Nicoli, E., et al., *Effects of nitric oxide on proliferation and differentiation of rat brown adipocytes in primary cultures.* Br J Pharmacol Oct 1998;125(4):888–894.
49. Barbul, A, et al., *Arginine enhances wound healing and lymphocyte immune response in humans.* Surgery 1990;108:331–337.
50. *L-carnitine.* Monograph. *Alter Med Rev* 2005;10:42–50.
51. Short, K.R. Muscle Atrophy During Aging. In: Kohlstadt, I.(ed.), *Scientific Evidence for Musculoskeletal, Bariatric, and Sports Nutrition.* 2006, Boca Raton, FL: CRC, Taylor & Francis, p. 317.
52. Joseph, V.A., Kohlstadt, I. Preparing for Orthopedic Surgery. In: Kohlstadt, I. (ed.), *Scientific Evidence for Musculoskeletal, Bariatric, and Sports Nutrition.* 2006, Boca Raton, FL: CRC, Taylor & Franics, pp. 517–518.
53. Mischley, L., Musnick, D. Osteoarthritis. In: Kohlstadt, I. (ed.), *Scientific Evidence for Musculoskeletal, Bariatric, and Sports Nutrition.* 2006, Boca Raton, FL: CRC, Taylor & Francis, pp. 398–399.
54. Spigset, O., *Reduced effect of warfarin caused by ubidecarenone.* Lancet 1994;344:1372–1373.
55. Rosenson, R.S., *Current overview of statin-induced myopathy,* Am JM Med 2004;116:408–416.
56. Kohlstadt, I., Schweitzer, E., Mutter, K, Godwin, L.B. Muscle Strain. In: Kohlstadt, I. (ed.), *Scientific Evidence for Musculoskeletal, Bariatric, and Sports Nutrition.* 2006, Boca Raton, FL: CRC, Taylor & Francis, p. 354.
57. Brown S.E. Bone Nutrition. In: Kohlstadt, I. (ed.), *Scientific Evidence for Musculoskeletal, Bariatric, and Sports Nutrition.* 2006, Boca Raton, FL: CRC, Taylor & Franics, p. 454.
58. Berger, M.M., Shenkin, A., *Trace element requirements in critically ill burned patients.* J Trace Elem Med Biol 2007;21 Suppl 1:44–48. Epub 2007 Oct 31.
59. Candow, D.G., Chilibeck, P.D. *Effect of creatine supplementation during resistance training on muscle accretion in the elderly.* J Nutr Health Aging 2007 Mar–Apr;11(2):185–188.
60. Valenti, G., et al., *Effect of DHEAS on skeletal muscle over the life span: the InCHIANTI study.* J Gerontol A Biol Sci Med Sci 2004 May;59(5):466–472.
61. Robinson, S.M., et al., *Diet and its relationship with grip strength in community dwelling older men and women: The Hertfordshire Cohort study.* J Am Geriatr Soc 2007 Nov 15 [Epub ahead of print].
62. Reginster, J.Y., et al., *Current role of glucosamine in the treatment of osteoarthritis.* Rheumatology 2007;46:731–735.
63. Vaxman, F., et al., *Can the wound healing process be improved by vitamin supplementations? Experimental study on humans.* Eur Surg Res 1996 Jul–Aug;28(4):306–314.
64. Brzezinski, A., et al., *Effects of exogenous melatonin on sleep; a meta-analysis.* Sleep Med Rev 2005 Feb;9(1):41–50.
65. Jacobs, S., *MSM.* The Arthritis Foundation's Guide to Alternative Therapies. Atlanta, Arthritis Foundation, 1999: p. 223.
66. Gionchetti, P., et al., *Probiotics in infective diarrhea and inflammatory bowel diseases.* J Gastroenterol Hepatol 2000 May;15(5):489–493. Review
67. Najm, W.I., et al., *S-Adenosyl-L-methionine (SAMe) versus celecoxib for the treatment of osteoarthritis symptoms: a double-blind cross-over trial [ISRCTN36233495],* BMC Musculoskelet Disord 2004 Feb 26;5:6.

68. Muller-Fassbender, H., *Double-blind clinical trial of S-adenosylmethionine versus ibuprofen in the treatment of osteoarthritis.* Am J Med 1987;83(Suppl 5A):S81–S83.

69. Vetter, G., *Double blind clinical trial with S-adenosylmethionine and indomethacin in the treatment of osteoarthritis.* Am J Med 1987;83(Suppl 5A):S78–S80.

70. Reffitt, D.M., et al., *Orthosilicic acid stimulates collagen type 1 synthesis and osteoblastic differentiation in human osteoblast-like cells in vitro.* Bone 2003 Feb;32(2):127–135.

71. Jugdaohsingh, R., et al., *Dietary silicon intake is positively associated with bone mineral density in men and premenopausal women of the Framingham Offspring cohort.* Bone 2003 May;32:S192.

72. Juneja, L.R., et al., *L-Theanine-a unique amino acid of green tea and its relaxation effect in humans.* Trends Food Sci Tech 1999;10:199–204.

73. *L-Tryptophan.* Monograph. Altern Med Rev 2006 Mar;11(1):52–56.

74. Wicke, C., et al., *Effects of steroids and retinoids on wound healing.* Arch Surg 2000;135(11):1265–1270.

75. Yazdanpanah, N., et al., *Effect of dietary B vitamins on BMD and risk of fracture in elderly men and women: The Rotterdam Study.* Bone 2007;41:987–994.

76. Alcantara-Martos, T., et al., *Effect of vitamin C on fracture healing in elderly osteogenic disorder Shionogi rats.* J Bone Joint Surg Br 2007 Mar;89(3):402–407.

77. Williams, J.Z., Barbul, A., *Nutrition and wound healing,* Surg Clin N Am 2003;83:571–596.

78. Mahmood, A., et al., *Zinc carnosine, a health food supplement that stabilises small bowel integrity and stimulates gut repair processes.* Gut 2007 Feb;56(2):168–175. Epub 2006 Jun 15.

79. Campbell, B., et al., *Pharmacokinetics, safety, and effects on exercise performance of l-arginine alpha-ketoglutarate in trained adult men.* Nutrition 2006 Sep;22(9):872–881.

80. Orban, J.C., et al., *Effects of acetylcysteine and ischaemic preconditioning on muscular function and postoperative pain after orthopaedic surgery using a pneumatic tourniquet.* Eur J Anaesthesiol 2006 Dec;23(12):1025–1030. Epub 2006 Jun 19.

81. Cherchi, A., et al., *Effects of L-carnitine on exercise tolerance in chronic stable angina: a multicenter, double-blind, randomized, placebo controlled crossover study.* Int J Clin Pharmacol Ther Toxicol 1985;23:569–572.

82. Brevetti, G., et al., *Increases in walking distance in patients with peripheral vascular disease treated with L-carnitine: a double-blind, cross-over study.* Circulation 1988;77:767–783.

83. Jeejeebhoy, F., et al., *Nutritional supplementation with Myo Vive repletes essential cardiac myocyte nutrients and reduces left ventricular size in patients with left ventricular dysfunction.* Am Heart J 2002;143:1092–1100.

84. Kinov, P., et al., *Role of free radicals in aseptic loosening of hip arthroplasty.* J Orthop Res 2006 Jan;24(1):55–62.

85. Rundek, T., et al., *Atorvastatin decreases the coenzyme Q10 level in the blood of patients at risk for cardiovascular disease and stroke.* Arch Neurol 2004;61:889–892.

86. Ziegler, D., *Thioctic acid for patients with symptomatic diabetic polyneuropathy: a critical review.* Treat Endocrinol 2004;3(3):173–189.

87. Knudsen E, et al., *Zinc, copper and magnesium absorption from a fiber-rich diet.* J Trace Elem Med Biol 1996;2(10):68–76.

88. Cattaneo, M., et al., *Low plasma levels of vitamin B(6) are independently associated with a heightened risk of deep-vein thrombosis.* Circulation 2001 Nov 13;104(20):2442–2446.

89. Armas, L.A., et al., *Vitamin D2 is much less effective than vitamin D3 in humans.* J Clin Endoncrinol Metab 2004 Nov:89(11):5387–5391.

90. Cannell, J.J., et al., *Diagnosis and treatment of vitamin D deficiency.* Expert Opin Pharmacother 2008 Jan;9(1):107–118.

91. Hollis, B.W., et al., *Circulating 25-hydroxyvitamin D levels indicative of vitamin D sufficiency: implications for establishing a new effective dietary intake recommendation for vitamin D,* In *Symposium: Vitamin D Insufficiency: a significant risk factor in chronic diseases and potential disease-specific biomarkers of vitamin D sufficiency.* J Nutr 2005 Feb;135(2):317–322.

92. Adams, J.S., et al., *Resolution of vitamin D insufficiency in osteopenic patients results in rapid recovery of bone mineral density.* J Clin Endocrinol Metab 1999 Aug;84(8):2729–2730.

93. Grant, W.B., Holick, M.F., *Benefits and requirements of vitamin D for optimal health: a review.* Altern Med Rev 2005 Jun;10(2):94–111.

94. www.sf-36.org.

95. Bland, J.S., Brailey, A. Medical Symptoms Questionnaire. Unpublished.

36 Wound Healing

Addressing Nutrient Needs with Diet

Joseph A. Molnar, M.D., Ph.D., and
Paula Stuart, M.M.S., P.A.-C., R.D.

I. INTRODUCTION

The process of wound healing is complex. Like any construction project, wound healing requires adequate blood flow as a supply line, and nutrients as the building blocks of the reparative process. The general health status of the patient can also influence the outcome of the healing process as it may alter the ability of the individual to respond to the injury and redistribute the ingested nutrients. Wound repair depends upon sufficient ingestion, absorption, and metabolic distribution of macronutrients (carbohydrates, protein, fat) and micronutrients (vitamins and trace elements). Imbalance due to inadequate supply or excessive demand may lead to an inability to heal wounds. While small wounds mend in healthy people without special attention, the metabolic demands of large wounds may outstrip the resources of even the well-nourished patient, making wound care most challenging.

This chapter describes the value of providing both macronutrients and micronutrients for wound healing. We will discuss the particular circumstances that may be nutritionally challenging in wound repair. Guidelines will be made for nutrients and foods in proper amounts for the patient with a healing wound.

II. EPIDEMIOLOGY

Nutrition for wound healing is a widening health challenge. Protein deficiency impairs wound healing, and it is a widespread problem in adults and children.[1] Protein-energy malnutrition is the most common nutritional deficiency in the hospital. It has been found in 44% to 50% of hospitalized patients.[2] Regrettably 25% to 30% of hospitalized patients are well-nourished initially but will become malnourished at some point in their stay.[2]

Malnutrition in the elderly is a global dilemma. It is estimated that up to 60% of institutionalized or nursing home patients are malnourished.[3] Pressure ulcers are challenging in the elderly, and are more commonly found with malnourished elderly patients, especially those in nursing homes or those receiving home health care. Pressure ulcers have a reported prevalence of 2.7% to 29.5% in hospitalized patients.[4] It is estimated that as many as 10% of hospitalized aged patients will acquire pressure ulcers at some stage in their hospital visit.[5]

Patients with diabetes often have wounds that are difficult to heal due to hyperglycemia and peripheral vascular and small vessel disease. As stated by the Centers for Disease Control and

Prevention, in the United States approximately 60% of all lower extremity amputations occur among persons with diabetes; of these, approximately 85% are preceded by a foot ulcer.[6]

Nutritional status influences susceptibility of wounds to infection. Surgical site infections are problematic in the clinical setting. The Centers for Disease Control and Prevention estimates a 2.8% incidence of surgical site infections, approximately 500,000 per year. Surgical site infections are connected with increased morbidity and mortality, and lengthen hospital stay resulting in increased hospital costs. Staggeringly, 77% of the deaths of surgical patients were associated with surgical wound infection.[7] A relative risk of death of 2.2-fold has been shown to be due to surgical site infections.[8]

Burn injury and trauma represent the largest wounds treated in the clinical setting. Such patients have their own set of nutritional challenges due to severe metabolic demands and inflammatory disturbances. National Hospital Ambulatory Medical Care Survey data collected between 1993 and 2004 determined that emergency department visits of patients with burns are declining, but rates remain elevated in men, African American patients, and children, occurring in the first and third decades of life.[9] Data gathered by the National Burn Registry from January 1996 through June 2006 showed that out of 142,318 patients with burns, 58% were Caucasian, 17.4% African American, 12.8% Hispanic, 2% Asian, and 0.6% Native American; 69.7% were male and 30.3% were female.[10]

Other sources of trauma such as motor vehicle accidents, sports-related injuries, and war-related injuries create large wounds, usually in young individuals in the first decades of life. Despite the overall healthy premorbid conditions, the metabolic demands of such large injury may outstrip the endogenous metabolic stores of the individuals involved.[11]

III. PATHOPHYSIOLOGY OF WOUND HEALING

STAGES OF HEALING

The understanding of the physiological processes of the stages of wound healing is constantly improving and ever-changing. It is also important to note that not all wounds heal in the same way and the various stages may actually overlap in time. The type of wound, existence or lack of infection, and nutritional, medical, or surgical interventions can affect the healing process.[12] The mechanism of wound healing helps us to understand the nutritional demands of the process.

Metabolic activity is dramatically increased to meet the demands of the reparative process. Stages of wound healing, as described in detail in Table 36.1, include hemostasis, inflammation, proliferation, contraction, and remodeling. Each stage requires macronutrients and micronutrients. Disturbance of one or more of these stages with nutrient deficiency will impede the healing process.[12]

Hemostasis

Immediately upon injury, blood is released into the wound, while reflexive vasoconstriction minimizes blood loss. The blood present in the wound provides substrate for Hageman Factor (XII) to begin the clotting cascade. Collagen, which is present in all tissues, becomes exposed and stimulates the alternate complement pathway to aid in clotting. Subsequent platelet adherence leads to degranulation and the release of numerous cytokines such as platelet-derived growth factor (PDGF). Fibrinogen converts to fibrin, which, with platelets, forms a scab offering a short-term protective barrier.[12]

Inflammation

Leukocytes travel into the wound during this period to fight infection and set the stage for proliferation. Prostaglandins, nitric oxide, and other inflammatory mediators promote vasodilation, which prevents blood loss. Plasma containing enzymes, antibodies, and nutrients seeps out into the interstitial area due to a resultant capillary leak. Monocytes help eradicate debris and harmful bacteria from the wound.[12]

TABLE 36.1
Stages of Wound Healing

Stage	Course
Hemostasis	• May take minutes to occur.
	• Stops exsanguination.
	• Begins process of healing by creating a protective layer to minimize infection risk, supplying a biochemical environment and structure for upcoming stages.
	• Vasoconstriction occurs, reducing blood loss. Blood released in the wound quickens Hageman Factor (XII) to initiate clotting cascade.
	• Collagen exposed in the wound stimulates alternate complement pathway, platelet adherence, and degranulation.
	• Fibrinogen converts to fibrin, along with platelets, forming a scab offering a temporary protective barrier.
	• Platelets quickly aggregate and degranulate in the wound.
	• Numerous cytokines are released.
Inflammation	• May last several days and overlap hemostasis.
	• Leukocytes are going into the wound.
	• Vasoconstriction replaced by vasodilation; clotted vessels prevent persistent blood loss.
	• Release of bradykinin, histamines, and free radicals from leukocytes leads to amplified vascular permeability.
	• Enzymes, antibodies, and nutrients flux into interstitial space.
	• Glucose and oxygen crucial for this stage. Arginine into the wound site may serve as precursor for nitric oxide. Lipids in the wound may be altered by free radicals in the wound to create isoprostane, stimulating important cascade of events in the wound.
	• Monocytes become phagocytic macrophages taking away debris and bacteria. They exude proteases, producing interferon and prostaglandins and cytokines, which are chemoattractants for mesenchymal cells, which differentiate into fibroblasts that are involved in proliferative phase and connective tissue formation.
Proliferation	• May take weeks.
	• Dominates several days after injury. May correspond chronologically to the flow or hypermetabolic phase of metabolic response to injury.
	• Debris may be removed during this stage surgically by wound care or whirlpool. Crucial intervention is closing the wound.
	• Optimal support to help with tissue perfusion and optimizing immune response by providing substrate for energy or protein synthesis is necessary for this stage for most favorable outcomes.
	• Fibroblasts proliferate rapidly, responsible for key extracellular structural components of healing wound.
	• Scar formation is made from collagen, one of the most complex proteins in the body. Lacking available amino acids and cofactors such as vitamin C there would be insufficient collagen. Without enough collagen wounds would leak, leading to dehiscence.
	• This stage involves influx of endothelial cells and neovascularization. Epithelialization occurs.
	• Cells proceed across a newly produced collagen matrix, producing a new basement membrane essential to normal epithelial cell activity.
Contraction	• Wound shrinks by recruiting adjacent tissue and pulling it into the wound.
Remodeling	• May persist for months or years. The balance of synthesis and degradation is vital to maintain a healed wound still years after initial injury.
	• Nutritional requirements of wound healing will be diminishing.
	• Scar is transformed to the final mature healed wound.

Source: Adapted from [12].

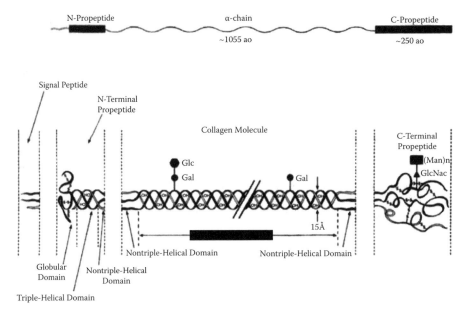

FIGURE 36.1   The synthesis of collagen is the cornerstone of scar production to give strength to the healing wound. Not only does this require the amino acid building blocks, but it also requires micronutrients such as vitamin C and iron for the hydroxylation of lysine and proline. (From Pesciotta, D.M. and Olsen, B.R., *The Cell Biology of Collagen Secretion* in H. Furthmayr, *Immunochemistry of the Extracellular Matrix*, Vol. 2, CRC Press, Boca Raton, FL, 1982. With permission.)

Proliferation

Proliferation becomes the governing stage a few days after the initial injury. Fibroblasts, which help produce essential structural elements of the healing wound such as collagen, advance forward in the wound and proliferate. During this phase collagen becomes an essential component in the scar formed during the reparative process, since collagen provides a fibrous matrix to provide wound strength. With insufficient collagen wounds would be frail, resulting in dehiscence. Such processes of proliferation require large amounts of energy as carbohydrate for mobility of the cells as well as manufacture of the essential building blocks of the wound. Amino acids are necessary for all the protein and enzyme synthesis of this stage. Collagen production not only requires energy and amino acids but also micronutrients such as vitamin C and iron for the post-translational hydroxylation of proline and lysine (Figure 36.1).[12] Without vitamin C, the collagen production will be inadequate, resulting in the clinical manifestations of scurvy with the breakdown of wounds.[13]

During the proliferative stage, endothelial cells also flood the area and neovascularization occurs, which also necessitates energy input as well as amino acids and micronutrients for protein synthesis. This course takes over during healing by secondary intention, and red vascular tissue called granulation tissue is the result. Epithelialization also occurs and may dominate the process in wounds such as superficial burns. Cytokines regulate epithelial cells, which travel across the wound periphery, generating a fresh basement membrane crucial for normal epithelial cell activity.[12]

Contraction

During this stage the wound reduces in size by essentially pulling in neighboring tissue. Myofibroblasts are the cells responsible for this movement that pulls the edges of the wound toward the center in another energy-requiring process. Collagen enhances this activity by facilitating fibroblast stabilization.[12]

Remodeling

The nutritional requirements decrease during this phase, as the wound now has increased tensile strength approaching undamaged tissue. This stage can carry on for several weeks to years. Rather than amplified collagen production, there is a fine balance of collagen synthesis and degradation. The wound is transformed to chiefly Type I collagen instead of Type I and Type III. During this stage the collagen cross-linking increases.[12]

IV. STRESS RESPONSE TO INJURY

Patients who have large burns and who are critically ill have modifications in digestion, absorption, and metabolism, which in turn ultimately increases protein needs. Patients who experience trauma have increased protein turnover, and during critical illness digestion in the gut is compromised. Consequently, the body may need modifications in administration of dietary protein as well as the composition and quantities of food. The metabolic response to injury is aimed at healing rather than conserving the lean body mass, ultimately altering amino acid requirements (Figure 36.2).[12]

Hypermetabolism takes place during stress from a large burn or traumatic injury. The lean body mass, comprised of muscle, skin collagen, bone, and visceral protein, is swiftly depleted during the metabolic response to injury.[14–20] The body essentially "eats itself" in order to meet the demands of injury (Figure 36.2). Appropriate nutritional intervention can lessen protein catabolism during the hypermetabolic state.[16] Throughout the stress response to injury, protein catabolism exceeds protein synthesis, resulting in an enhanced excretion of urinary nitrogen. Glucocorticoids aid the movement of amino acids from the skeletal muscle to the liver.[17]

V. COMORBID CONDITIONS

Adipose tissue is inadequately perfused, leading to decreased nutrient delivery to the wound. Obesity increases the incidence of infections and overall delayed wound repair and wound

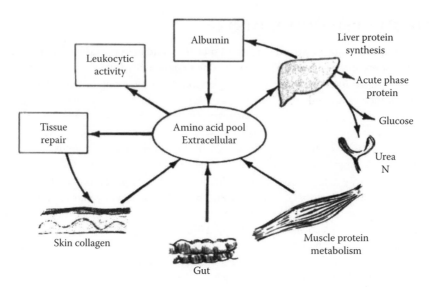

FIGURE 36.2 In periods of metabolic stress such as injury, the body undergoes an effective catabolism of the "carcass" to support visceral protein synthesis. Providing appropriate nutritional support, especially protein, may minimize the peripheral catabolism to some extent but it cannot be totally eliminated. (From [20]. With permission.)

dehiscence. Patients with diabetes (frequently also obese) need to be particularly vigilant with their regulation of carbohydrate intake, and close monitoring of fingerstick blood sugar levels. Hyperglycemia increases the risk of infection and delayed wound healing.[21] Hypothyroidism, adrenal insufficiency, chronic kidney disease, and hepatic failure also impair the nutrient utilization required for wound healing. Alcoholism, drug addiction, poverty, and old age are all associated with protein, protein-calorie, and micronutrient deficiencies. Care must be taken to provide appropriate evaluation.

Individuals with cancer may have delayed wound healing as the malignancy can complicate every step of the wound healing process. Radiation therapy can alter the healing of wounds by slowing the inflammatory response of healing. Dose, timing of therapy, and area of therapy can complicate healing. Chemotherapy can also alter the inflammatory response to injury.

VI. PATIENT EVALUATION

To assess for malnutrition one must determine the percentage of unintentional weight loss that the patient has suffered by disease or comorbidities. An unintentional weight loss of 10% or more of premorbid weight has been shown to cause impaired physiologic functions and decreased morbidity and mortality.[22]

Anthropometric measurements of nutritional status, which include height, weight, and skin fold measurements, can be performed. Skin fold analysis is operator dependant and varies with conditions creating edema. Weights fluctuate, depending upon fluid status, and if edema or ascites are present. Biochemical tests including albumin, prealbumin, and transferrin may give some indication of current nutritional status by assessing visceral protein status. Unfortunately, such tests can be affected by fluid status and metabolic stress, making them also inconsistently reliable.

In the clinical management of wound healing, one does not routinely assess for micronutrient deficiency. While it is possible to measure tissue and serum levels of micronutrients, they are unreliable during metabolic stress such as trauma.[23] Fluid shifts and changes in production of carrier protein may give falsely low values. Consequently, treatment with micronutrients is often empiric.

VII. TREATMENT RECOMMENDATIONS

Nutrients have myriad roles in wound healing (Table 36.2) and are generally obtained through food (Table 36.3). The presence of wounds is associated with deficiency states of these nutrients required for healing. Additional food and sometimes supplemental dosing are an important adjunct to surgical and medical interventions.

MACRONUTRIENTS

Carbohydrates

Glucose provides energy to skin cells in wound healing. During wound repair carbohydrates are utilized as energy for inflammatory cells and fibroblasts.[12] Glucose is a key nutrient for patients with a traumatic injury since it is needed for cellular expansion, leukocyte function, and fibroblastic mobility. If a patient with increased metabolic demands has a carbohydrate intake that is inadequate, there may be more conversion of amino acids to glucose, which in turn may deplete lean body mass. Alternatively, excessive intake of carbohydrates or glucose could lead to hyperglycemia, which will also have a detrimental effect on wound repair.[12]

Resting metabolic rates in the critically ill are generally higher than healthy patients. Numerous formulae are available to predict resting energy expenditure in patients.[23–26] The amounts of carbohydrate required by a patient with wounds vary from patient to patient, and may not necessarily be related to wound size alone.

TABLE 36.2
Function of Some Key Nutrients Involved in Wound Healing

Nutrient Class	Specific Nutrient	Contribution to Wound Healing
Proteins	Amino acids	Needed for platelet function, neovascularization, lymphocyte formation, fibroblast proliferation, collagen synthesis, and wound remodeling.
		Required for certain cell-mediated responses, including phagocytosis and intracellular killing of bacteria.
		Gluconeogenic precursors.
Carbohydrates	Glucose	Energy substrate of leukocytes and fibroblasts.
Fats	Fatty acids	Serve as building blocks for prostaglandins, isoprostanes that are inflammatory mediators; energy source for some cell types.
	Cholesterol	Are constituents of triglycerides and fatty acids contained in cellular and subcellular membranes.
Vitamins	Vitamin C	Hydroxylates proline and lysine in collagen synthesis.
		Free radical scavenger.
		Is a necessary component of complement that functions in immune reactions and increases defenses to infection.
	Vitamin B Complex	Serves as a cofactor of enzyme systems.
		Required for antibody formation and white blood cell function, essential for nucleic acid metabolism.
	Vitamin A	Enhances epithelialization of cell membranes.
		Enhances rate of collagen synthesis and cross-linking of newly formed collagen.
		Antagonizes the inhibitory effects of glucocorticoids on cell membranes.
	Vitamin D	Necessary for absorption, transport, and metabolism of calcium.
		Indirectly affects phosphorus metabolism.
	Vitamin E	Free radical scavenger.
	Vitamin K	Needed for synthesis of prothrombin and clotting factors VII, IX, and X.
Minerals	Zinc	Stabilizes cell membranes; enzyme cofactor.
		Needed for cell mitosis and cell proliferation in wound repair.
	Iron	Needed for hydroxylation of praline and lysine in collagen synthesis.
		Enhances bactericidal activity of leukocytes.
		Hemoglobin oxygen transport to wound.
	Copper	Integral part of the enzyme lysyloxidase, which catalyzes formation of stable collagen cross-links.

Source: From [12]. With permission.

An indirect calorimeter may be helpful for predicting energy expenditure for the critically ill patient. This particular device measures oxygen consumed to determine metabolic rate. When compared to carbon dioxide produced during respiration (RQ or Respiratory Quotient) one can estimate the metabolic blend of nutrients consumed for energy production. This technique is particularly useful as respiratory quotients greater than 1.0 indicate that the patient is receiving too much carbohydrate and is now converting the excess to fat.[27]

The balance between adequate calories for healing and avoiding overconsumption of nutrients is sometimes best guided by calculation of energy needs, even among ambulatory patients who are not critically ill. Previous energy expenditure studies have not centered on outpatients. Two

TABLE 36.3
Food Sources of Micronutrients Involved in Wound Healing

Nutrient Class	Specific Nutrient	Food Sources
Vitamins	Vitamin C	Citrus fruit, strawberries, red peppers, kiwi fruit, oranges, orange juice, green peppers, grapefruit juice, vegetable juice cocktail, Brussels sprouts, cantaloupe, papaya, kohlrabi, broccoli, edible pod peas, sweet potato, tomato juice, cauliflower, pineapple, kale, mango, dark green leafy vegetables, fortified bread and cereals
	Vitamin B Complex	Ready-to-eat cereal, potato, banana, garbanzo beans, chicken, oatmeal, pork, roast beef, trout, sunflower seeds, spinach, tomato juice, avocado, salmon, tuna, wheat bran, peanut butter, walnuts, soybeans, lima beans
	Vitamin A	Organ meats, carrot juice, sweet potato, pumpkin, carrots, spinach, collards, kale, mixed vegetables, turnip greens, instant fortified cereals, beet greens, winter squash, dandelion greens, cantaloupe, mustard greens, pickled herring, red sweet pepper, Chinese cabbage
	Vitamin D	Cod liver oil, salmon, mackerel, tuna fish, sardines, milk, margarine, ready-to-eat cereal, egg, liver, beef, cheese
	Vitamin E	Fortified ready-to-eat cereals, sunflower seeds, almonds, sunflower oil, cottonseed oil, safflower oil, hazelnuts, mixed nuts, turnip greens, tomato paste, pine nuts, peanut butter, tomato puree, tomato sauce, canola oil, wheat germ, peanuts, avocado, carrot juice, peanut oil, corn oil, olive oil, spinach, dandelion greens, sardines, Brazil nuts, herring
	Vitamin K	Swiss chard, kale, parsley, Brussels sprouts, spinach, purslane, broccoli, turnip greens, watercress, endive, lettuce leaves, spring onions, mustard greens, cabbage, lettuce, coleslaw
Minerals	Zinc	Oysters, red meat, poultry, beans, nuts, certain seafood, whole grains, fortified breakfast cereals, dairy products
	Iron	Clams, fortified cereals, oysters, organ meats, soybeans, pumpkin, white beans, molasses, lentils, spinach, beef, kidney beans, sardines, chickpeas, duck, lamb, prune juice, shrimp, cowpeas, ground beef, tomato puree, lima beans, soybeans, navy beans, refried beans, tomato paste
	Copper	Oysters, shellfish, whole grains, beans, nuts, potatoes, kidney, liver, dark leafy greens, dried fruits, prunes, cocoa, black pepper, yeast

Source: [61].

equations are suggested (Table 36.4). For obese patients, actual body weight should be used for these equations.[25,26]

The type of carbohydrate used may also influence wound healing. Avoiding sweetened beverages and high glycemic index foods can help patients adhere to caloric balance.[28]

Protein

Protein requirements are increased for patients with large wounds. During the inflammatory and proliferative stages of wound healing, the amino acid requirements in the injury will be high due to the elevated level of enzymatic activity and the soaring rate of cell turnover.[29] Protein needs can rise up to 1.5 to 2.0 g/kg body weight of protein.[30] Calculations are based upon actual body weight or weight prior to illness.[31] Dietary intake of protein can be calculated (Table 36.5) and adjusted for the type of wound (Table 36.6).

TABLE 36.4
Energy Expenditure Equations for Healthy Patients

Ireton-Jones*
IJEE (s) = 629 – 11 (A) + 25 (W) – 609 (O)
IJEE = kcals/day
A = age (years)
W = actual weight (kg)
O = obesity (if present = 1, absent = 0)
No activity or injury factor is added

Mifflin**
Male: Resting Metabolic Rate (kcal/day) = 10 (W) + 6.25 (H) – 5 (A) + 5
Female: Resting Metabolic Rate (kcal/day) = 10 (W) + 6.25 (H) – 5 (A) – 161
H = height (cm)
W = actual weight (kg)
A = age (years)
Use with activity factors:
Moderate: Resting Metabolic Rate × 1.2–1.3
Intense: Resting Metabolic Rate × 1.4–1.5

Source: Adapted from [12, 20].
* From Ireton-Jones C, Jone J. Improved equations for estimating energy expenditure in patients: the Ireton-Jones equations. *Nutr Clin Prac* 2002;17(4):236–239.
** From Mifflin MD, St. Jeor ST, Hill LA, et al. A new predictive equation for resting energy expenditure in healthy individuals. *Am J Clin Nutr* 1990;51:241–247.

Certain amino acids can become conditionally essential during periods of metabolic stress with large wounds. Arginine and glutamine have been found to have special requirements in wound healing that sometimes require specific supplementation.[32]

Arginine

Arginine, normally a nonessential amino acid, is found in protein-rich foods. It is valuable for wound healing because it is the only substrate for nitric oxide synthesis.[33–35] In a rat wound healing model, supplemental arginine restored nitric oxide levels to near-normal and significantly increased wound-breaking strength, a marker of wound healing and collagen synthesis.

Arginine supplementation can assist in improving endothelial dysfunction and enhancing immune function, thus aiding wound healing.[35] Arginine and glutamine supplementation has been shown to boost collagen synthesis in healthy elderly volunteers and is a safe way of hastening wound repair.[36]

Thirty-six hospitalized patients with pressure sores and severe cognitive impairment were studied.[37] The patients who drank high-calorie, high-protein supplements had quicker progress in pressure ulcer repair than those patients who did not consume an oral supplement. The fastest healing was observed in the group supplemented with arginine, zinc, and antioxidants.

Thirty grams of arginine supplemented daily for at least 3 days increased peripheral blood lymphocyte blastogenic responses to mitogens, and natural killer lymphokine-activated killer cells increased.[38] Collagen synthesis was enhanced in healthy aging patients when given supplemental arginine, HMB (beta hydroxy-methyburate), and glutamine.[36]

Supplemental arginine has been shown to be well tolerated in less than 2 week duration. Thirty grams of arginine ingested per day for at least 3 days was well tolerated and appears to be safe for the promotion of wound healing and stimulation of immune response and may benefit patients at risk of infection.[35,38]

TABLE 36.5
Food Sources of Protein

Food	Serving	Protein Grams
Duck, meat only, cooked	½ duck	52
Chicken, stewed, meat only	1 cup	43
Fish, halibut	½ fillet	42
Turkey, meat only, roasted	1 cup	41
Fast food hamburger, double	1 sandwich	34
Tuna salad	1 cup	33
Taco	1 large	32
Cottage cheese	1 cup	31
Beef, braised	3 oz	29
Soybeans, boiled	1 cup	29
Crab, canned	1 cup	27
Pork, cooked	3 oz	27
Chili con carne	1 cup	25
Chicken fillet sandwich	1 sandwich	24
Dry couscous	1 cup	22
Trail mix	1 cup	21
Pinto beans, cooked	1 cup	15
Enriched rice	1 cup	13
Pizza, pepperoni, slice from 14-inch pizza	1 slice	13
Chicken pot pie	1 small pie	13
Yogurt, skim milk	8 oz container	13
Soup, bean and ham	1 cup	13
Milkshake	11 fl oz	12
Milk, 1%	1 cup	8
Cheese	1 oz	7
Egg, whole, raw	1 extra large	7
Peanuts	1 oz (28 nuts)	7
Soy milk	1 cup	7

Source: [61].

TABLE 36.6
Suggested Protein Intake for Wound Healing

Type of Wound	Protein Recommended (grams/kg/day)
Pressure Ulcers	
Stage I	1.0–1.2
Stage II	1.2
Stage III	1.3–1.4
Stage IV	1.5–1.6
Burns	
< 20% TBSA	1.5–1.8
> 20% TBSA	2.0–2.5

TBSA = Total body surface area

Dietary sources of arginine include walnuts, hazelnuts, pecans, Brazil nuts, sesame and sunflower seeds, brown rice, raisins, coconut, gelatin, buckwheat, almonds, barley, cashews, cereal, chicken, chocolate, corn, dairy products, meats, oats, and peanuts.[39–41]

Commercial powders are available that contain approximately 4.5 g of l-arginine per serving. Ready-to-serve liquids containing l-arginine, zinc, and vitamins C and E are also on the market.

Glutamine

Glutamine has many diverse roles. It is the most plentiful free amino acid in the body, and it is conditionally essential in times of stress. It helps sustain barrier function of the intestines, and it functions as a fuel source for the cells of the intestinal mucosa and gut-associated lymphoid tissue. Additionally it preserves immune cell function, serving as a key fuel source for lymphocytes, macrophages, neutrophils, and natural killer cells.[42]

It is known that there is a quick decline in plasma and muscle glutamine levels after injury.[43] However, supplemental glutamine has not yet been confirmed to have any clear effect on wound healing.[44] Glutamine does appear to help improve gut permeability of injured patients, facilitate protein synthesis, and decrease hospital length of stay.[45,46]

The recommended dose of glutamine is debatable because no large studies are available at this time defining the most favorable prescribed amount. Twenty to 40 g of glutamine each day could be required in catabolic states. Most research studies do illustrate a benefit from consuming doses of 0.6 g/kg or less.[47] Glutamine should be used with care in those with liver failure or kidney failure because it may lead to excess ammonia production in these patients.[48]

Food sources of glutamine include beef, chicken, fish, eggs, milk, dairy products, cabbage, beets, beans, spinach, and parsley.[41]

Selections of glutamine supplements are available on the market. Some products come as a single-dose packet of powder that is mixed with juice or soda. Most can also be used in enteral feedings. Some of the powders contain 10 to 15 g of glutamine, 75 to 90 Kcal, 20 mg of zinc, 500 mg of vitamin C, 5000 IU of vitamin A, and 140 mg of arginine.

Collagen hydrolysate protein supplement helps heal pressure ulcers. Benefit has been demonstrated from the ready-to-use liquid concentrated fortified form. This product contains 15 g protein per 30 mL. It contains the arginine, glycine, proline, and hydroxyproline that helps with tissue healing, and helps preserve lean body mass.[49]

Fat

Fat serves as an energy source and as a substrate for inflammatory mediators (prostaglandins, isoprostanes) that influence metabolism in the wound. Fats also function as building blocks for the cell membrane and organelles, which are lipid bilayers.[12]

Research shows that glucose and fatty acids are the chief energy providers for those who are wounded or stressed, even when carbohydrates are available.[50,51] Dietary fat and fatty acids freed from adipose tissue are swiftly employed during wound healing and are potential inflammatory modulators of the healing response.[14] Fat malabsorption can lead to inadequate fat intake, which can negatively affect healing of wounds.[52] Those patients receiving fat-free total parenteral nutrition and those who have had intestinal surgery (especially terminal ileum resection) may be at risk of inadequate intake. It is interesting that fat-free total parenteral nutrition (TPN) is the most frequent cause of essential fatty acid deficiency, which can occur within 10 days of initiation.[53]

Excess fat can result in hepatic steatosis. Excess intake of polyunsaturated fatty acids (PUFA) can influence the immune system, leading to immunosuppression.[54] Overindulgence of saturated or monounsaturated fatty acids is neither unsafe nor advantageous to wound healing. Intake of *trans* fatty acids should be reduced as much as possible. Monounsaturated fatty acids are better as a fat source because they do not have adverse cardiovascular effects.

One study by Albina, Gladden, and Walsh suggested that animals eating diets supplemented with omega-3 fatty acids have wounds of weaker quality because omega-3 fatty acids may modify the fibroblastic or maturational phases of the healing response.[55] The advantage of consuming omega-3 fatty acids may be in their ability to positively modulate the inflammatory and immunological response rather than in wound repair. Studies of persons and guinea pigs with burns after intake of a diet rich in omega-3 fatty acids have shown enhanced immune function, better survival, and decreased infectious complications.[56,57]

MICRONUTRIENTS

B Vitamins

B vitamins serve as coenzymes during the inflammatory phase of wound repair and are vital in the removal of dead tissue and bacteria from a wound. Additionally they are important for antibody formation, leukocyte function, and nucleic acid metabolism, which is essential in the healing wound with rapid cellular proliferation.[12] At certain points in the proliferative and remodeling phases of wound healing, B vitamins help with production and interlinking of collagen. They also facilitate the synthesis of new tissues and blood vessels. B vitamins aid in wound contraction during the final phase of wound healing and help support the resulting scar.[58]

It is important for patients with wounds to consume adequate amounts of B vitamins. If patients consume a variety of foods, usually requirements for B vitamins are met. The RDAs (Recommended Dietary Allowances) are prudent to follow in this regard. Those at risk of deficiency (malnourished, poor, elderly, those with malabsorptive diseases) need to be supplemented.[58] It is important to keep in mind when considering the B vitamins that if vitamin B12 deficiency is suspected folate should be tested due to their metabolic interactions. Those at risk of deficiency are those with alcoholism, limited diets, or limited availability of nutrients or income.

B vitamins can be supplemented in a multivitamin formulation. They should be provided in amounts to at least meet the RDA. Due to the low toxicity of water-soluble vitamins, taking modestly larger amounts is usually safe.[58]

Vitamin C

Insufficient intake of ascorbic acid leads to poor healing of wounds. In the most severe manifestation, the patient will suffer from scurvy and spontaneous breakdown of wounds. While it has long been known that vitamin C helps increase strength of the wound, functioning as a cofactor in collagen synthesis (Figure 36.1), it has become recently accepted that ascorbic acid also functions as a free radical scavenger.[59] Recent studies suggest that pharmacologic doses of vitamin C may decrease the early systemic inflammatory response in burns and trauma.[60]

Nutrient sources of vitamin C include citrus fruits such as oranges, lemons, and limes as well as other fresh fruits and vegetables including strawberries and tomatoes.

Patients at risk of deficiency include hospitalized patients on restricted diets, alcoholics, and the geriatric patient on nominal income with limited intake of fresh fruits and vegetables.[61] Since it is difficult for patients who are ill to consume large quantities of fruit and vegetables, it is suggested that the patient receive supplementation. Patients with small wounds should receive 500 to 1000 mg daily in two divided doses while patients with larger injuries should be given 1 to 2 g/day. Vitamin C should be given in divided doses because large amounts can result in abdominal pain, nausea, and loose stools. Use prudence when recommending supplemental vitamin C with patients who are predisposed to renal colic or have iron excess.[62]

Zinc

Zinc has been employed for the management of dermatologic ailments for years. Zinc is required for protein synthesis and is also a cofactor in enzymatic reactions. Zinc levels can be severely depleted in periods of stress.[63] Zinc deficiency (levels <100 mg/mL) can occur in malnourished patients and in those who are stressed or those receiving steroids for a long period of time,[64,65] which impairs wound healing because of decreased wound strength and delayed epithelialization.[66]

Deficient patients have increased vulnerability to infection and delayed wound repair. This deficiency is swiftly corrected when patients are supplemented with zinc, resulting in the numbers of circulating T-cell lymphocytes rising as well as the capacity of lymphocytes to battle infection.

To date, no studies have demonstrated advancement in wound healing after zinc supplementation to patients who are not deficient in zinc. However, assessment of a patient's dietary intake using a 24-hour or 3-day food record may offer a clinician insight into their patient's zinc status and potential need for supplementation. Some studies suggest that patients with chronic wounds often have low zinc intake.[67,68] Topical zinc ointments have been found to be helpful for those with chronic leg ulcers, pressure ulcers, diabetic ulcers, and burns.[69–72]

Alcoholism predisposes to zinc deficiency because alcohol reduces the absorption of zinc and escalates loss of zinc in urine. Dinsmore and colleagues found lower postprandial serum zinc concentrations in alcoholics after a standardized meal supplemented with 50 mg zinc, which may imply a decreased absorptive capacity of zinc.[73] Patients who have had gastrointestinal surgical procedures, chronic diarrhea, malabsorption, Crohn's disease, celiac sprue, and short gut syndrome are also at greater risk of a zinc deficiency.[74]

The current RDA for zinc is 15 mg. Suggested dietary sources of zinc are beef, liver, oysters, whole wheat products, nuts, cheddar cheese, poultry, lamb, pork, and popcorn.[61]

POTENTIAL SUPPLEMENT AND FOOD INTERACTIONS

Calcium and zinc should be taken at different times during the day because calcium reduces zinc absorption.[75] Vitamin B6 and zinc should be taken together because vitamin B6 increases the absorption of zinc.[76] Too much supplementation of zinc can impair wound healing by inducing a relative copper deficiency.

It is recommended to wait 1 hour after taking vitamins and minerals before drinking tea, since black tea inhibits the absorption of iron. Green tea also inhibits absorption but less than dark tea. Coffee and calcium are also inhibiting factors for iron. Phytates, which are found in whole grain breads, cereals, and legumes, can decrease zinc absorption.[77]

VIII. MEETING NUTRITIONAL REQUIREMENTS FOR WOUND HEALING WITH FOOD

The choice of foods for the patient with healing wounds depends on the patient's overall condition. Clearly, the critically ill patient will be unable to eat and will require supplementation with tube feedings and in some cases with total parenteral nutrition. With such defined formulae, meeting requirements according to the above guidelines is relatively straightforward assuming normal bowel function. Enteral nutrition is preferred when feasible as it helps maintain a healthy gut and allows for the advantages of direct liver metabolic modulation of the nutrients.[78,79]

Patients who are able to consume a normal oral intake present a more interesting challenge for wound care. Hospitalized patients may be directly provided an appropriate diet with the help of a dietician to determine dietary preferences. Generally speaking, adequate caloric intake is met with the diet but some patients' dietary choices leave the diet insufficient in protein and micronutrients. Emphasizing the need to take in protein may resolve this problem. In some patients, oral liquid supplements may be necessary to provide adequate protein. Supplementation with multivitamin preparations and specific nutrients such as vitamin C is usually required to meet micronutrient needs.

When these individuals are outpatients the clinician has little direct control on the patient's diet except through education and providing certain supplements. If the wounds are small, minimal alterations of the diet are likely necessary assuming that the patient is well-nourished at the time of injury. However, many patients are malnourished at the time of injury and need appropriate adjustments.

Like the hospitalized patient, caloric needs are often met in the outpatient, but protein and micronutrients are likely to be inadequate without assistance. The patient should be educated on foods that are high in protein and other essential nutrients. Cost of these food items must also be considered for the patient with a limited income. For example, many people have restricted their intake of eggs due to health concerns of cholesterol. Nonetheless, eggs are an excellent, inexpensive source of high-quality protein and numerous micronutrients. Daily supplementation of the diet with eggs may assist in wound healing with minimal cost. While some may be concerned of the long-term risks of atherosclerosis, albeit controversial, liberalization of diet for a period of time is usually worth the medical risk–benefit ratio.

Tuna may be an excellent alternative source of protein for some people. Individuals such as the senior citizen living alone may find the cost and convenient size of a can of tuna to be an appealing protein source. A single 6 oz can could meet approximately one-half of the protein requirement of some individuals for the whole day.[80]

It is often assumed that micronutrients require pharmacologic supplementation. As mentioned, food sources such as eggs include reasonable quantities of micronutrients, minimizing the need for supplementation. Simply maintaining a diet that is well-balanced with the major food groups may be all that is required for patients with small wounds. In those individuals for whom there are some concerns of the quality of diet, it is reasonable to at least provide a multivitamin for daily supplementation. The cost and physiologic risk are low.

One must be careful to understand the potential problems with pharmacologic supplementation. For example, patients are frequently put on a zinc supplement to help heal their wounds. In some individuals, zinc supplementation creates gastrointestinal discomfort and may interfere with intake of other food. Iron supplementation may also cause constipation and gastrointestinal discomfort that may interfere with the diet.

In addition, the bioavailability of elemental iron is affected by other dietary nutrients. Correcting the pH by drinking orange juice with the iron supplement will change the valence of the iron and improve absorption.[81] Even under the best conditions, the bioavailability of elemental iron in a supplement tablet is only approximately one-tenth the availability of iron bound to the hemoglobin molecule.[82,83] Providing iron through more normal dietary sources may be more effective than pills in some individuals. Liver is an excellent source of iron as is red meat. While there may be some concerns about the intake of this food in some patients with hyperlipidemia, in most patients it would be an acceptable risk for a short period of time. Liver and meat also provide other complex micronutrients and protein.

IX. SUMMARY

Wound healing is a complex process that can place considerable metabolic demands on the host. Processes of hemostasis, inflammation, proliferation, and remodeling require the building blocks of all nutrients. Meeting the nutritional demands with normal food sources is difficult, and with large wounds with associated injury may be impossible. Macronutrient demands are usually met with high-quality protein-rich foods if the gastrointestinal tract is working normally. Specific supplementation of micronutrients, particularly vitamin C, the B vitamins, and zinc, is often required to meet the needs of large wounds.

REFERENCES

1. Stephenson LS, Latham MC, Ottesen EA. Global malnutrition. *Parasitology* 2000;121 Suppl:S5–22. PMID: 11386691.
2. Bistrian BR, Blackburn GL, Vitale J, Cochran D, Naylor J. Prevalence of malnutrition in general medical patients. *JAMA* 1976 Apr 12;235(15):1567–1570. PMID: 814258.
3. Silver AJ, Morley JE, Strome LS. Nutritional status in an academic nursing home. *J Am Geriatr Soc* 1988;36:487–491. Shaver HJ, Loper JA, Lutes RA. Nutritional status of nursing home patients. *J Parenter Enteral Nutr* 1980;4:367–370.
4. Muncie HJ, Carbonetto C. Prevalence of protein-calorie malnutrition in an extended care facility. *J Fam Pract* 1982;14:1061–1064.

5. Thomas DR, Goode PS, Tarquine PH, Allman RM. Hospital—acquired pressure ulcers and risk of death. *J Am Geriatr Soc* 1996;44:1435–1440.
6. History of foot ulcer among persons with diabetes—United States, 2000–2002. Centers for Disease Control and Prevention (CDC).
7. Mangram AJ, Horan TC, Pearson ML. Guideline for prevention of surgical site infection, 1999. Hospital Infection Control Practices Advisory Committee. *Infect Control Hosp Epidemiol* 1999 Apr;20(4):250–278; quiz 279–280.
8. Kirkland KB, Briggs JP, Trivette SL. The impact of surgical-site infections in the 1990s: attributable mortality, excess length of hospitalization, and extra costs. *Infect Control Hosp Epidemiol* 1999 Nov;20(11):725–730.
9. Fagenholz PJ, Sheridan RL, Harris NS, Pelletier AJ, Camargo CA Jr. National study of emergency department visits for burn injuries, 1993 to 2004. Department of Surgery, Massachusetts General Hospital, Harvard Medical School, Boston, Massachusetts 02114, USA.
10. Latenser BA, Miller SF, Bessey PQ, Browning SM, Caruso DM, Gomez M, et al. National Burn Repository 2006: a ten-year review. *J Burn Care Res* 2007 Sep–Oct;28(5):635–658.
11. Clark M, Plank LD, Hill GL. Wound healing associated with severe surgical illness. *World J Surg* 2000;24:648.
12. Molnar JA. Overview of Nutrition and Wound Healing. In J Molnar (Ed.), *Nutrition and Wound Healing*. Boca Raton, FL: CRC Press, 2007, pp. 1–13.
13. Padayatty S, Levine M. New insights into the physiology and pharmacology of vitamin C. *CMAJ* 2001;164:353.
14. Cuthbertson DP. Observations on the disturbance of metabolism produced by injury to the limbs. *Quart J Med* 1932;1:233.
15. Molnar JA, Burke JF. Nutritional aspects of surgical physiology. In JF Burke (Ed.), *Surgical Physiology*. Philadelphia: W.B. Saunders, 1983.
16. Albina JE. Nutrition and wound healing. *JPEN* 1994;18(4):367–376.
17. Clark M, Plank LD, Hill GL. Wound healing associated with severe surgical illness. *World J Surg* 2000;24:648.
18. Cuthbertson DP. The disturbance of metabolism produced by bony and non-bony injury with notes on certain abnormal conditions of bone. *Biochem J* 1930;24:1244.
19. Cuthbertson DP, Tilstone WJ. Nutrition of the injured. *Am J Clin Nutr* 1968;24:911.
20. Molnar JA, Wolfe RR, Burke JF. Burns: metabolism and nutritional therapy in thermal injury. In HA Schneider, CE Anderson, and DB Coursin (Eds.), *Nutritional Support of Medical Practice*, 2nd ed. Philadelphia: Harper & Row, 1983.
21. Gore DC, Chinkes D, Heggers J, Herndon DN, Wolf SE, Desai M. Association of hyperglycemia with increased mortality after severe burn injury. *Trauma* 2001;51(3):540–544.
22. Ryan C, Bryant E, Eleazer P, Rhodes A, Guest K. Unintentional weight loss in long-term care: predictor of mortality in the elderly. *South Med J* 1995;88:721–724.
23. Shenkin A. Trace elements and inflammatory response: implications for nutritional support. *Nutrition* 1995;11:100–105.
24. Ireton-Jones CS. Use of indirect calorimetry in burn care. *J Burn Care Rehabil.* 1988 Sep–Oct;9(5):526–529.
25. Mifflin MD, St Jeor ST, Hill LA, Scott BJ, Daugherty SA, Koh YO. A new predictive equation for resting energy expenditure in healthy individuals. *Am J Clin Nutr.* 1990 Feb;51(2):241–247.
26. Ireton-Jones CS, Turner WW, Liepa GW, et al. Equations for estimating energy expenditure in burn patients with special reference to ventilatory status. *J Burn Care Rehabil* 1992;13:330–333.
27. Flancbaum L, Choban PS, Sambucco S, Verducci J, Burge JC. Comparison of indirect calorimetry, the Fick method, and prediction equations in estimating the energy requirements of critically ill patients. *Am J Clin Nutr* 1999 Mar;69(3):461–466. PMID: 10075331.
28. Ludwig DS, Majzoub JA, Al-Zaharani A, Dallal GE, Blanco I, Roberts SB. High glycemic index foods, overeating, and obesity. *Pediatrics* 1999;103(3):26–40.
29. Soeters PB, van de Poll MCG, van Gemert WG, Dejong CHC. Amino acid adequacy in pathophysiological states. *J Nutr* 2004;134:1575S–1582S.
30. Flancbaum L, Choban PS, Sambucco S, Verducci J, Burge JC. Comparison of indirect calorimetry, the Fick method, and prediction equations in estimating the energy requirements of critically ill patients. *Am J Clin Nutr* 1999 Mar;69(3):461–466. PMID: 10075331.
31. Trujillo EB, Robinson MK, Jacobs DO. Nutritional assessment in the critically ill. *Crit Care Nurse* 1999 Feb;19(1):67–78. PMID: 10401292.

32. Stechmiller JK, Childress B, Cowan L. Arginine supplementation and wound healing. *Nutr Clin Pract* 2005 Feb;20(1):52–61. Review.

33. Kirk SJ, Hurson M, Regan MC, et al. Arginine stimulates wound healing and immune function in elderly human beings. *Surgery* 1993 Aug;114(2):155–159. PMID: 8342121.

34. Witte MB, Thornton FJ, Tantry U, Barbul A. L-Arginine supplementation enhances diabetic wound healing: involvement of the nitric oxide synthase and arginase pathways. *Metabolism* 2002 Oct; 51(10):1269–1273. PMID: 12370845. doi:10.1053/meta.2002.35185.

35. Flynn NE, Meininger CJ, Haynes TE, Wu G. The metabolic basis of arginine nutrition and pharmacotherapy. *Biomed Pharmacother* 2002 Nov;56(9):427–438. PMID: 12481979. doi:10.1016/S0753-3322(02)00273-1.

36. Williams JZ, Abumrad N, Barbul A. Effect of a specialized amino acid mixture on human collagen deposition. *Ann Surg* 2002 Sep;236(3):369–375. PMID: 12192323. doi:10.1097/00000658-200209000-00013.

37. Benati G, Delvecchio S, Cilla D, Pedone V. Impact on pressure ulcer healing of an arginine-enriched nutritional solution in patients with severe cognitive impairment. *Arch Gerontol Geriatr* 2001 Jan;33 Suppl 1:43–47. PMID: 11431045. doi:10.1016/S0167-4943(01)00120-0.

38. Barbul A, Sisto DA, Wasserkrug HL, Efron G. Arginine stimulates lymphocyte immune responses in healthy humans. *Surgery* 1981 Aug;90(2):244–251. PMID: 7020137.

39. Coates AM, Howe PR. Edible nuts and metabolic health. *Curr Opin Lipidol.* 2007 Feb;18(1):25–30.

40. Cooper MPH, Kenneth H. *Advanced Nutritional Therapies.* Nashville: Thomas Nelson, Inc. Publishers, 1996, pp. 87–88, 93, 94.

41. Murray ND, Michael T, Pizzorno J. *Encyclopedia of Natural Medicine.* Rocklin, CA: Prima Publishing, 1991, p. 359.

42. Krebs H. Glutamine metabolism in the animal body. In J. Mora and R. Palacios (Eds.), *Glutamine: Metabolism, Enzymology, and Regulation.* New York: Academic, 1980.

43. Askanazi J, Carpentier YA, Michelsen CB, et al. Muscle and plasma amino acids following injury: influence of intercurrent infection. *Ann Surg* 1980;192:78.

44. McCauley R, Platell C, Hall J, McCulloch R. Effects of glutamine infusion on colonic anastomotic strength in the rat. *JPEN* 1991;15:437.

45. Peng X, Yan H, You Z, Wang P, Wang S. Clinical and protein metabolic efficacy of glutamine granules-supplemented enteral nutrition in severely burned patients. *Burns* 2005;31:342.

46. Zhou YP, Jiang ZM, Sun YH, Wang XR, Ma EL, Wilmore D. The effect of supplemental enteral glutamine on plasma levels, gut function, and outcome in severe burns: a randomized, double-blind, controlled clinical trial. *JPEN* 2003;27:241.

47. Hall JC, Heel K, McCauley R. Glutamine. *Br J Surg* 1996;83(3):305–312.

48. Gottschlich MM (Ed.) *The Science and Practice of Nutrition Support.* Dubuque, IA: Kendall/Hunt Publishing Company, 2001, p. 149.

49. Kwon L, et al. Pressure ulcer healing with a concentrated, fortified, collagen hydrolysate protein supplement: a randomized controlled trial. *Advances in Skin & Wound Care* 2006 Mar;19(2):92, 94–96.

50. Long CL, et al. A physiologic basis for the provision fuel mixtures in normal and stressed patients. *J Trauma* 1990;30:1077.

51. Patel GK. The role of nutrition in the management of lower extremity wounds. *Int J Low Extrem Wounds* 2005;4(1):12–22.

52. Desai HG, Merchant PC, Antia FP. Malabsorption in cirrhosis of liver. Relationship of fecal fat and vitamin B12 excretion. *Indian J Med Sci* 1973;27:673.

53. Wolfram G, Eckart J, Walther B, Zollner N. Factors influencing essential fatty acid requirement in total parenteral nutrition (TPN). *JPEN* 1978;2:634.

54. Meydani SN, et al. Oral (n-3) fatty acid supplementation suppresses cytokine production and lymphocyte proliferation: comparison between young and older women. *J Nutr* 1991;121:547.

55. Albina JE, Gladden P, Walsh WR. Detrimental effects of an omega-3 fatty acid-enriched diet on wound healing. *JPEN* 1993;17:519.

56. Gottschlich MM, Jenkins M, Warden GD, et al. Differential effects of three enteral dietary regimens on selected outcome variables in burn patients. *JPEN* 1990;14:225.

57. Alexander JW, Saito H, Trocki O, Ogle CK. The importance of lipid type in the diet after burn injury. *Ann Surg* 1986;204:1.

58. Liepa GU, Ireton-Jones C, Basu H, Baxter CR, Molnar JA. B Vitamins and Wound Healing. In J Molnar (Ed.), *Nutrition and Wound Healing.* Boca Raton, FL: CRC Press, 2007, pp. 99–116.

59. Jacob RA, Sotoudeh G. Vitamin C function and status in chronic disease. *Nutr Clin Care.* 2002 Mar–Apr;5(2):66–74.
60. Berger MM. Antioxidant micronutrients in major trauma and burns: evidence and practice. *Nutr Clin Pract.* 2006 Oct;21(5):438–449.
61. USDA. Food Sources of Selected Nutrients. Dietary Guidelines for Americans 2005.
62. Tanaka H, Molnar J. Vitamin C and wound healing in nutrition and wound healing. In J Molnar (Ed.), *Nutrition and Wound Healing.* Boca Raton, FL: CRC Press, 2007, pp. 121–148.
63. Prasad AS. Acquired zinc deficiency and immune dysfunction in sickle cell anemia. In S Cunningham-Rundles (Ed.), *Nutrient Modulation of the Immune Response.* New York: Marcel Dekker, 1993, p. 393.
64. Wilkinson EA, Hawke CI. Does oral zinc aid the healing of chronic leg ulcers? A systematic literature review. *Arch Dermatol* 1998;134:1556–1560.
65. Prasad AS. Zinc in growth and development and spectrum of human zinc deficiency. *J Am Coll Nutr* 1988;7:377.
66. Barbul A, Purtill WA. Nutrition in wound healing. *Clin Dermatol* 1994;12:133.
67. Wissing U, Unosson M, Lennernas MA, Ek AC. Nutritional intake and physical activity in leg ulcer patients. *J Adv Nurs* 1997;25:571–578.
68. Raffoul W, Far MS, Cayeux MC, Berger MM. Nutritional status and food intake in nine patients with chronic low-limb ulcers and pressure ulcers: importance of oral supplements. *Nutrition* 2006;22:82–88.
69. Strömberg HE, Ågren MS. Topical zinc oxide treatment improves arterial and venous leg ulcers. *Br J Dermatol* 1984;111:461–468.
70. Apelqvist J, Larsson J, Stenstrom A. Topical treatment of necrotic foot ulcers in diabetic patients: a comparative trial of DuoDerm and MeZinc. *Br J Dermatol* 1990;123:787–792.
71. Moore J. Diabetes watch: can zinc oxide have an impact on wound healing? *Podiatry Today* 2003;16:22–25.
72. Gang RK. Adhesive zinc tape in burns: results of a clinical trial. *Burns* 1980;7:322–325.
73. Dinsmore WW, Callender ME, McMaster D, Love AH. The absorption of zinc from a standardized meal in alcoholics and in normal volunteers. *Am J Clin Nutr.* 1985 Oct;42(4):688–693.
74. Baumgartner TG. Trace elements and wound healing. In J Molnar (Ed.), *Nutrition and Wound Healing.* Boca Raton, FL: CRC Press, 2007, pp. 173–217.
75. Wood RJ, Zheng JJ. High dietary calcium intakes reduce zinc absorption and balance in humans. *Am J Clin Nutr* 1997;65:1803–1809.
76. Rostan EF, DeBuys HV, Madey DL, et al. Evidence supporting zinc as an important antioxidant for skin. *Int J Derm* 2002;41:606–611.
77. Fredlund K, Isaksson M, Rossander-Hulthén L, Almgren A, Sandberg A-S. Absorption of zinc and retention of calcium: dose-dependent inhibition by phytate. *J Trace Elements Med Bioly* 2006 May;20(1):49–5774.
78. Hadley MN, Grahm TW, Harrington T, Schiller WR, McDermott MK, Posillico DB. Nutritional support and neurotrauma: a critical review of early nutrition in forty-five acute head injury patients. *Neurosurgery* 1986;19:367–373.
79. Young B, Ott L, Twyman D, Norton J, Rapp R, et al. The effect of nutritional support on outcome from severe head injury. *J Neurosurg* 1987;67:668–676.
80. http://www.fns.usda.gov/fdd/facts/hhpfacts/FS-ChunkLightTuna.pdf
81. Ballot D, Baynes RD, Bothwell TH, et al. The effects of fruit juices and fruits on the absorption of iron from a rice meal. *Br J Nutr* 1987;57:331–343. [Medline]
82. Cowin I, Emond A, Emmett P. Association between composition of the diet and haemoglobin and ferritin levels in 18-month-old children. *Eur J Clin Nutr* 2001;55:278–286. [Medline]
83. Fleming DJ, Tucker KL, Jacques PF, et al. Dietary factors associated with the risk of high iron stores in the elderly Framingham Heart Study cohort. *Am J Clin Nutr* 2002;76:1375–1384.

Section VIII

Neoplasms

37 Breast Cancer

Nutrition to Promote Recovery and Diminish Recurrence Risk

Keith I. Block, M.D., and Charlotte Gyllenhaal, Ph.D.

I. INTRODUCTION

There are presently over 2 million breast cancer survivors in the United States [1]. These patients undergo intensive surgery, radiation and chemotherapy, and long-term, less-intensive endocrine treatments. During intensive treatment, the breast cancer patient is usually under the care of specialists. However, patients may see their primary care physicians for scheduled checkups, treatment of comorbid conditions, and management of side effects or complications from chemotherapy, surgery, or radiation. During long-term endocrine treatment, the primary care physician may see the patient more regularly, since hormone-blocking or aromatase inhibitor therapies can continue for years, across stages.

Primary care physicians who provide long-term care for breast cancer survivors are well-placed to implement nutritional strategies. Recent research in nutrition is leading toward a consensus that management of weight, energy balance, and dietary patterns may contribute substantially to breast cancer survival, reduce comorbidities, and improve patient well-being.

II. EPIDEMIOLOGY

Research suggests breast cancer is a family of diseases, each of which must be treated distinctively. For example, breast cancers that are estrogen receptor (ER) positive are treated with tamoxifen, while those that are ER negative receive chemotherapy. A further distinction is made for Her2/*neu* positive breast cancer, which is treated with Herceptin®. Treatment guidelines for breast cancer constitute a complex decision tree with very different treatment protocols for different situations. Conventional breast cancer treatment is thus becoming increasingly individualized. Genetic classifications in breast cancer are helpful in the epidemiologic study of nutrition. In the future, nutrition recommendations may be specific to breast cancer subtype, in contrast to the current recommendations, which are more general.

III. PATHOPHYSIOLOGY

While breast cancer treatment has been perceived for many years to be related to nutrition, the relationships have been controversial. Recent advances in research appear to be clarifying the situation. Dietary patterns and caloric intake influence inflammation and insulin responsiveness to ultimately improve breast cancer survival. Fruits and vegetables are phytochemically rich foods and may also influence outcomes.

DIETARY PATTERNS

The evidence for nutritional impacts on breast cancer is growing, although the efficacy of nutritional treatment is by no means proven. Rock and Demark–Wahnefried reviewed studies on nutritional variables and survival after breast cancer, based on cohort studies of breast cancer survivors [68]. The researchers determined that obesity and dietary fat intake predicted lower survival, and that high fruit and vegetable consumption correlated with longer survival. Two large trials of diet and breast cancer have recently reported results: the Women's Healthy Eating and Living (WHEL) randomized trial of a low-fat diet high in vegetables, fruit, and fiber [60, 61], and the Women's Intervention Nutrition Study (WINS) trial of a low-fat diet [15].

The two studies had different outcomes (Table 37.1). In the WINS study, the intervention group had a lower risk of recurrence, most significantly in ER negative patients. In the WHEL study, there was no difference in breast cancer events or in mortality between the two groups. Different implementation of the recommended low-fat (20%) diets may explain these results. In the WINS study, the low-fat and control groups both started out with diets of 29.6% of calories from fat. By the end of the first year, the low-fat group was eating only 20.3% of calories from fat, while the control group continued at 29.2%. The fat intake of the low-fat group was 8 to 9 percentage points lower than the control group throughout the 5 years of the study. The women in the low-fat group were not counseled to decrease calories, but their diet appears to have reduced their caloric intake, since they lost approximately 6 pounds relative to the control group by the end of the study. In the WHEL

TABLE 37.1
Diet Modification Trials in Breast Cancer Patients

Diet Intervention	Cancer Stage	n	Design	Outcomes	Results	Reference
Low-fat, high-fiber, high fruits/ vegetables	Breast, early stage	3088	RCT	Breast cancer event	0.96	[60]
				Mortality	0.91	(WHEL)
Low-fat diet	Breast, early stage	2437	RCT	Relapse events, all diet patients *vs.* controls	0.76	[15] (WINS)
				Estrogen receptor negative pts	0.53	
Diet to support 10-kg weight loss	Breast, stage unclear	54	RCT	Recurrence	4.30	[26]*
				Cancer mortality	0.38	
				All-cause mortality	0.78	
Diet to support 10-kg weight loss	Breast, stage unclear	48	RCT	Recurrence	0.61	[26]*
				Cancer mortality	0.40	
				All-cause mortality	0.28	
Lower calorie, low-fat diet	Breast, stage unclear	110	RCT	Recurrence	0.20	[78]
Protein plus calorie supplement	Breast, stage unclear	47	RCT	Recurrence	6.50	[30]
				Cancer mortality	0.95	
				All-cause mortality	1.33	

Note: Results are hazard ratios; ratios less than 1.0 indicate that diet intervention improves survival or other outcome events, while ratios greater than 1.0 indicate worse outcome for intervention group.

* This study reports separately the results of the same diet intervention given in two populations (Dutch and Polish patients). Recurrence patterns were different in the two populations, but cancer-specific mortality and all-cause mortality were both lowered in the diet weight loss groups.

study the diet intervention group never reached their 15% to 20% fat goal, reaching only 22.7% fat by the end of the first year. By the sixth year, their fat intake rose to 28.9%, approximately the level of the control group. The fat intake of the intervention and control groups never differed by more than 6 percentage points. Although both groups reported reducing their energy intake by over 150 calories per day, neither group in the WHEL study lost weight. Other factors may also contribute to the different results, including a higher proportion of early-stage patients in the WINS study, whose disease may be more easily managed by diet than the later-staged patients of the WHEL study.

Table 37.1 also shows some smaller diet intervention studies [26, 30, 78]. Studies that counseled weight loss or lower caloric intake generally reduced mortality. A study in which patients were given a protein-calorie supplement [30] did not improve survival. Although not a randomized trial, we recently reported a median survival of 38 months for a group of metastatic breast cancer patients (96% with recurrent disease) receiving chemotherapy at our clinic, which emphasizes a low-fat, mostly vegetarian diet along with exercise as part of comprehensive medicine. This suggests that further progress can be made in nutritional treatment of even advanced breast cancer [8].

Obesity and weight gain after diagnosis increase the risk of metastasis and reduce survival in breast cancer, independently of other factors [51, 58]. Experimental studies of diet in breast cancer suggest that controlling weight may improve breast cancer prognosis. Control of weight, however, is not influenced only by the levels of fat, calories, or carbohydrates in the diet. Patients who are overweight or obese, especially if they are undergoing cancer treatment, should be encouraged to consult with a nutritionist for meal planning. They should receive regular follow-up to encourage healthy weight loss to a normal weight.

Exercise has not always been viewed as appropriate for cancer patients, but observational and experimental studies suggest that exercise, along with dietary modification, may be helpful in controlling weight gain, and thus improve breast cancer outcomes [42]. Further, Pierce and colleagues in an analysis of the WHEL control group, found that the patients who ate the most fruits and vegetables, and exercised the most, had half the mortality rate of those who either ate fewer servings of vegetables and fruits, or exercised less [61]. Several studies have shown that weight gain during chemotherapy is associated with poor prognosis, and Demark-Wahnefried has reported a pilot study of a low-fat diet high in fruits and vegetables paired with exercise as a potential way to help prevent weight gain during chemotherapy [25]. With the goal of preventing weight gain coming more into focus, encouraging patients to exercise during and after chemotherapy is becoming acknowledged as part of the nutritional prescription.

Patients who undertake low-fat or low-calorie diets may lose muscle mass (lean body mass) as well as fat, although resistance exercise (strength training) may help to maintain muscle mass [82]. Chemotherapy may also provoke loss of lean body mass and increase of fat mass. This change in body composition is undesirable since it impairs activities of daily living and reduces immune competence. Changes in lean body mass and fat mass can be monitored through body composition analysis [4, 21], a tool used by nutritionists and physical therapists. It is also important to maintain adequate protein in the diet. In the context of a low-fat diet based largely on plant proteins, suitable protein sources include legumes and beans, egg whites, fish, and protein supplements including amino acid or whey supplements. Where appropriate, traditional foods of global cultures can be used, including seitan (wheat gluten) or tempeh (fermented soybeans). Red meat has been associated with breast cancer risk and should be avoided [16, 80].

Hormones, Inflammation, and Insulin

Fats both modulate the hormonal milieu and contribute to the inflammatory potential of the diet. Modification of hormonal levels may require major modification of fat intake. It is primarily saturated fats that modulate the hormonal milieu. Low saturated-fat diets may suppress estrogenic stimulation of breast cancer growth, and some studies of low-fat or high-fiber diets have observed lowering of estradiol levels. Other studies in healthy women observed that low-fat, high-fiber diets lowered serum estrogen, although changes were not always significant, and were not maintained after intervention periods were concluded [34]. Long-term commitment to dietary change may thus be required to alter estrogen levels.

Wallace reviewed the role of nutrition and supplements in modulation of eicosanoid synthesis, especially production of prostaglandin E2 (PGE2), a product of the arachidonic acid cascade [84]. PGE2 promotes cell proliferation, inhibits apoptosis, and increases angiogenesis and invasiveness and may thus contribute to the progression of cancer. Patients with low levels of omega-3 fatty acids tend to have higher proinflammatory markers, indicated by tests such as C-reactive protein (CRP), and lower anti-inflammatory cytokines [32]. This may affect quality of life as well as cancer progression. Both persistent fatigue in breast cancer survivors [18] and chemotherapy-related symptoms such as anorexia, cachexia, sleep disturbance, and depression [86] have been linked to elevated levels of cytokines. However, major dietary changes may be needed to successfully modify levels of these markers [76]. These modifications have not yet been demonstrated in cancer patients, although high intake of *trans* fatty acids was found to be strongly correlated with such inflammatory markers as plasma CRP, interleukin-6, soluble tumor necrosis factor receptors, E-selectin, and soluble cell adhesion molecules in healthy women [49]. Exercise training (stationary bike) has been reported to lower CRP in postmenopausal breast cancer patients [31].

Boyd and Kaaks reviewed the impact of insulin and insulin-like growth factors on cancer [11, 44]. Obesity and type 2 diabetes, both negative prognostic factors in breast cancer, can result in insulin resistance, which leads to hyperinsulinemia [3]. Goodwin et al. and Borugian et al. observed that elevated plasma insulin was associated with increased mortality [37, 10]. Additionally, patients with the highest carbohydrate intakes in these studies had an increased mortality. Patients with very low carbohydrates also had increased mortality, however, possibly due to excessive fat intake with effects described in the previous paragraph. Carbohydrate intake in breast cancer patients should thus be tailored to minimize insulin responses. Whole grain intake has a significant inverse association with the metabolic syndrome and blood glucose [71]. Diets high in fiber are usually recommended in insulin resistance [50], since fiber slows the absorption of dietary carbohydrates. Additionally, insulin resistance is shown in both epidemiological and intervention studies to be aggravated by saturated fat, while monounsaturated fats improve it [66]. Exercise may reduce insulin levels in breast cancer patients [48].

Phytochemicals

Rock and Demark–Wahnefried found that that higher fruit and vegetable intakes are associated with better survival in breast cancer. This suggests that the numerous phytochemicals in plants may improve breast cancer outcomes. Meta-analyses of trials on single antioxidants, however, show that single vitamins or phytochemicals do not improve cancer mortality or recurrence [22, 20]. Trials of diet change that included increasing vegetable and fruit intake or intake of phytochemical-rich foods along with lowering fat also improved outcomes in prostate and skin cancer [6, 24, 59, 73, 79], although not adenoma recurrence [47]. The more complex mixtures of phytochemicals contained in whole plant foods may thus be needed to improve cancer outcomes. Fruits and vegetables are also low in calories, and high consumption can result in lower caloric density in the diet, potentially assisting in weight loss (Chapter 19, "Obesity"). In addition to phytochemical effects, diets high in fruits and vegetables contribute to a more alkaline internal pH, which may help reduce cancer risks.

Phytochemicals in soybeans and flax are of particular interest. The potential impact of soy on breast cancer prognosis was recently summarized by Messina and colleagues [53]. Soy isoflavones have a molecular structure similar to estrogens, and bind to estrogen receptors. They exert estrogen-like effects in some experimental conditions. However, genistein and other isoflavones also have nonestrogenic activities that inhibit cancer cell growth, making them potentially useful in a variety of cancers. There is conflicting evidence regarding isoflavones and breast cancer risk. A protective effect is possible for soy exposure in childhood, but little evidence is available regarding soy consumption and breast cancer recurrence [27]. While a definitive statement on soy and breast cancer is not possible at this time, most experts feel that modest intake of soy foods as part of the diet is reasonable for breast cancer patients [7], but that soy isoflavone supplements need further evaluation in high-risk women and are not recommended for postmenopausal ER positive breast cancer patients [53]. To the extent that soy foods replace higher-calorie meats in the diet, they may contribute to weight maintenance. Several herbal medicines also have phytoestrogenic effects and should not be taken in large amounts by postmenopausal women with ER positive tumors, including licorice, red clover, fennel, fenugreek, hops, yucca, alfalfa, and wild carrot. Black cohosh, used for hot flashes, is not estrogenic but occasional liver damage related to intake has been reported, which may be an idiosyncratic reaction. Data on stimulation of breast cancer cell growth and metastasis are conflicting, but some laboratory studies have shown that extracts or constituents of the plant may inhibit breast cancer growth or potentiate effects of chemotherapy agents [28, 29].

Flax is high in lignans, which are both phytoestrogens and a fiber source that have cancer-suppressive potential. Breast cancer patients who took flax-supplemented muffins before diagnostic surgery had high levels of apoptosis in cancer cells [81]. A study in healthy postmenopausal women examined effects of flax- and soy-supplemented muffins on the ratio of 2-hydroxyestrone, a less cancer-stimulating estrogen metabolite, to 16-alpha hydroxyestrone which is more cancer-stimulating. Flax increased relative amounts of 2-hydroxyestrone significantly whereas soy and placebo did not; serum levels of estradiol and estrone were unchanged by the supplements [12].

Additional phytonutrients are diindolylmethane (DIM), which may increase Taxotere® effects [65], and indole-3-carbinol (I3C), which increases 2-hydroxyestrone relative to 16-alpha-hydroxyestrone [2].

MINERALS AND VITAMINS

Iodine occurs in dietary seaweeds, which are consumed frequently in Asia where breast cancer rates are low, and is attracting attention for its anticarcinogenic effects. Breast cancer patients have been observed to have lower tissue iodine levels than normal controls. Seaweeds, also called sea vegetables, have anticarcinogenic properties and promote apoptosis in cancer cells in laboratory analyses [77]. Optimal thyroid function requires iodine, and is important in maintaining muscle mass and improving body composition. Maintaining normal iodine levels may thus be important for breast cancer patients. Sea vegetables are encouraged in some alternative cancer diets, but not all patients find them palatable. Patients undertaking low-fat vegetarian or vegan diets may inadvertently reduce their iodine intake beyond the Recommended Daily Allowance of 150 µg/day by avoiding seafood, milk, egg yolks, iodized salt and other iodine sources, while eating large amounts of cruciferous vegetables or soy, which can depress iodine absorption. Iodized salt or iodine-containing supplements can optimize iodine status.

Vitamin D is currently of interest in reducing cancer risk and improving prognosis for several cancers, including breast cancer. Studies of vitamin D and breast cancer prevention have been notably inconsistent [70, 5]. Norwegian studies of breast cancer patients, however, reveal interesting relationships of breast cancer prognosis with solar radiation levels. Norway can be divided into regions of different solar radiation levels based on a north–south gradient [63, 67]. One study found a significant geographical gradient in prognosis from areas of low to high solar radiation. Another study observed that patients diagnosed and treated in summer, when sun exposure is highest, have better prognoses than those diagnosed in winter. Low vitamin D levels may be associated with insulin resistance in polycystic ovary syndrome [41], and with a proinflammatory state [56], both of interest in breast cancer.

IV. PHARMACOLOGY

Dietary supplements can both be sources of potential drug interactions with cancer treatments, and, when carefully selected, may present useful adjuncts to cancer treatments. We will discuss these positive and negative interactions by the type of treatment involved. Additionally, some chemotherapy agents deplete important vitamins or minerals; such depletion may be addressed through diet or supplementation in some cases.

Oncologists express concern about the use of dietary supplements concurrently with chemotherapy. Antioxidants in particular are thought to be potentially useful in ameliorating chemotherapy side effects, but there is concern that they may counteract the therapeutic effects of some chemotherapy drugs, which have free-radical-based mechanisms of action. We recently reviewed randomized trials in which various antioxidants were given concurrently with such chemotherapy agents, and did not find evidence for diminished tumor response or survival from such combinations, although the trials involved were small and of lower quality. Antioxidants also appeared to diminish a variety of side effects, suggesting that evidence to date leans toward the use of antioxidants with chemotherapy [9]. A review of antioxidants and radiation therapy found several small trials that showed potential positive effects [57].

A large trial of beta-carotene and vitamin E supplements during radiation therapy for head and neck cancer observed excess recurrence and mortality risks with supplements, but improved side effects. Later analysis, however, showed that excess risks of recurrence and mortality were all among those patients who smoked tobacco during supplementation [54]. Analysis of dietary intakes and plasma beta-carotene showed that patients who had higher dietary beta-carotene intake had lower incidence of adverse radiation effects, and those with higher plasma levels had lower rates of recurrence [55]. An additional complication in this study was that the vitamin E intake was in the form of alpha tocopherol, which is but one of eight forms of vitamin E contained in vitamin-E-rich foods such as nuts, seeds, and cooking oils. Supplemental dosing of alpha tocopherol alone suppresses levels of other vitamin E forms [87]. Supplemental vitamin E should be as mixed tocopherols and tocotrienols in proportion to the ratios in food. In sum, a study using alpha tocopherol as the sole vitamin E form is not applicable to concentrated food sources or quality supplements.

Some chemotherapy agents used in breast cancer deplete critical nutrient stores. Vitamin or mineral supplements may be useful in avoiding deficiencies, although specific evidence is not available in most cases. The most likely potential interactions are the following:

* Adriamycin—riboflavin and possibly iron.
* 5-fluorouracil—niacin and thiamin.
* Cisplatin used in some protocols for relapsed metastatic disease—magnesium, potassium, zinc, l-carnitine. Intravenous magnesium supplementation is commonly used with cisplatin due to the severe deficiencies it causes.
* Methotrexate—folate. Here supplementation should be avoided during treatment unless prescribed by an oncologist, due to the potential to interfere with methotrexate's mechanism of action.

Extended periods of nausea, vomiting, and diarrhea during chemotherapy may cause multinutrient deficiencies. Supplementation or careful dietary adjustments may need to be undertaken during or after chemotherapy for patients who experience poor control of these side effects.

St. John's wort is well known for causing pharmacokinetic herb-drug interactions based on its induction of the cytochrome P450 isoenzyme 3A4, which can cause the many drugs metabolized by this enzyme to drop to subtherapeutic levels in the blood [14]. St. John's wort should be avoided during chemotherapy and related therapies due to the many drugs these protocols involve. Additional herb and food interactions with drugs are shown in Table 37.2 [38–40].

Anticoagulant herbs may affect both patients who have low platelet counts due to chemotherapy and those who are taking warfarin, given to cancer patients to prevent thrombosis. For patients taking warfarin, which has a narrow therapeutic index and is prone to drug interactions, the use of these anticoagulant herbs is problematic, as is the ingestion of foods that contain large amounts of

TABLE 37.2
Supplements and Foods That Induce or Inhibit Cytochrome P450 Isoenzymes Relevant to Drugs Used in Breast Cancer Treatment

Pharmacokinetic Interactions

CYP450 isoenzyme induced or inhibited by foods or supplements	*Breast cancer medications metabolized by CYP450 isoenzyme*
CYP450 3A4	
Goldenseal	Emend®
Grapefruit	Decadron®
Star fruit	Taxol®
St. John's wort	Taxotere®
CYP450 1A2	
Cruciferous vegetables	Zofran®
Char-grilled meat	Warfarin
Echinacea	
CYP450 2D6	
Goldenseal	Zofran®
	Tamoxifen

Source: [33].

Note: Not all potential interactions have been shown to be clinically relevant. Grapefruit interactions apply only to medications taken orally.

vitamin K. This may become clinically relevant for cancer patients who frequently consume leafy green vegetables as part of a low-fat diet or drink beverages based on green vegetables often called "green drinks." If patients take anticoagulant foods and supplements consistently, warfarin dose can be adjusted to account for dietary characteristics, since INR is monitored regularly.

Selected herbs and supplements have the potential to reduce chemotherapy and radiation therapy side effects, as shown in randomized and open-label trials (Table 37.3). The medication Gelclair® combines a licorice phytochemical with hyaluronic acid and a bioadherent gel to assist the two compounds in adhering to the gums as a strategy to decrease mucositis. Milk thistle may be considered as a hepatoprotector in patients with existing liver damage who undergo breast cancer chemotherapy or who experience marked abnormalities in liver function tests [64]. Taxanes, Adriamycin®, and the CMF chemotherapy regimen have some potential to cause hepatotoxicity [46]. High doses of melatonin (20 mg/day at bedtime) have been demonstrated for some chemotherapy protocols to improve survival and decrease chemotherapy side effects, but the protocols in which it is useful for breast cancer are not well-defined.

V. COMORBID CONDITIONS

Obesity, type 2 diabetes, and cardiovascular disease are all important comorbidities in breast cancer. Cardiovascular disease is especially relevant in postmenopausal patients with early stage breast cancer who have completed treatment and are in remission. Dietary patterns that may raise risks of breast cancer recurrence are the same ones that increase cardiovascular risks. Additionally, patients who incur cardiotoxicity from Adriamycin® or Herceptin® will need closer monitoring and perhaps medication.

TABLE 37.3
Supplements With Potential to Relieve Chemotherapy and Radiation Side Effects

Condition	Herb or Nutrient	Contra-indications	Evidence	Dosage	Reference
Delayed nausea and vomiting	Ginger	Low platelet counts; warfarin	RCT	500 mg dried powder every 4 hours	[52]
Fatigue	L-carnitine	None	Open label trials	500 mg/day	[13]
Fatigue	Ginseng (Korean or American)	ER + tumors (though this may depend on extract type); take in AM	Small trials in noncancer patients	1–2 g/day	[45]
Cardiotoxicity from Adriamycin®	Coenzyme Q10	None	Small trials	60–200 mg/day	[19]
Mucositis/ stomatitis	Glutamine	None	RCTs	0.5 g/kg/day "Swish and swallow"	[17]
Mucositis/ stomatitis	Acetyl-l-carnitine	Epilepsy, bipolar disorder	RCTs	500 mg tid	[23, 72]
Radiation skin reaction	Calendula	Allergy to plants in daisy family	RCT	Calendula ointment 1X, 4%	[62]

Cancer treatment can cause bone loss and increase patients' risks for osteoporosis. Chemotherapy or endocrine therapies may cause loss of ovarian function in premenopausal women; therapy with aromatase inhibitors can also raise risks of osteoporosis. The use of an alkaline diet high in fruits and vegetables is relevant to both reducing risk of cancer recurrence and helping to control osteoporosis. Low vitamin D levels, which are widespread in breast cancer patients, may also contribute to excess bone loss, with or without aromatase inhibitor treatment [35].

VI. PATIENT EVALUATION

As part of the physical examination at the primary care visit, weight should be monitored and body mass index (BMI) calculated. Since breast cancer recurrence rates increase markedly at higher BMIs, control of weight is a primary area of intervention. Body composition analysis is particularly important for the patient who loses or gains weight during chemotherapy. Patients may be at risk for loss of muscle mass due to inactivity and loss of appetite from chemotherapy drugs. This can lead to losses of lean muscle and gains in fat mass. Patients should engage in some type of strength exercise to avoid losing muscle mass; loss of fat mass, however, is entirely appropriate for the overweight patient. Advanced cancer patients are at higher risk of weight loss due to cachexia, an inflammatory condition that triggers a loss of muscle tissue. Although cachexia is less common in breast cancer than in gastrointestinal and lung cancers, it can occur in some patients.

Ongoing assessment of inflammation and blood glucose is also recommended and will assist in managing cardiovascular disease risks as well as cancer. C-reactive protein (healthful levels <1.0), erythrocyte sedimentation rate (healthful level 0 to 30 mm/hour), and fibrinogen (healthful level <300 mg/dL) are basic inflammatory measurements. Abnormally high inflammation can be addressed pharmaceutically, or by optimizing the omega-6 to omega-3 ratio and avoiding *trans* fats, and with herbal supplements such as boswellia, curcumin, and bromelain. Elevated fasting blood glucose, or an oral glucose tolerance test, along with hemoglobin A1C, are useful to screen nondiabetic patients for poor glucose tolerance, which could suggest insulin resistance and elevated insulin levels.

VII. SPECIAL CONDITIONS

BONE METASTASES

Recommendations to use diet and exercise to achieve or maintain normal weight apply to patients with bone metastases as well as to other patients. However, referral to a physical therapist may be warranted to help the patient develop safe exercise routines. For instance, high-impact exercises should be avoided, and exercises such as some yoga positions that involve twisting the spine should not be attempted by patients with spinal metastases.

CARDIOMYOPATHY

Patients with cardiomyopathy from Adriamycin® or Herceptin® also need exercise, but should be advised that interval training, in which short periods of exercise alternate with rest, may prevent exhaustion or stress on the heart and are thus preferable to continuous aerobic training. Nutrients involved in ATP production, including ribose, coenzyme Q10, l-carnitine, and magnesium, have been shown to effectively augment pharmacologic management. The herb hawthorn may be used for symptom management [43].

NEUROPATHY

Peripheral neuropathy is a dose-limiting toxicity of taxane treatment, which is commonly used in breast cancer. Up to 88% of Taxol patients may experience mild or moderate neuropathy. Nontraditional therapies for taxane neuropathy are based on those used for diabetic neuropathy. Evening primrose oil and α-lipoic acid have been subjected to trials in diabetes, but only case reports exist to indicate the potential effectiveness of α-lipoic acid in taxane-induced neuropathy [69].

HOT FLASHES

Hot flashes and night sweats are common in breast cancer patients with oophorectomy- or chemotherapy-induced menopause and in those taking tamoxifen. Management of hot flashes in ER positive breast cancer can be perplexing because of the need to avoid hormone therapy. Supplemental doses of black cohosh have yielded mixed results on efficacy and safety [83]. Gold and colleagues analyzed diet composition and hot flashes in women in the WHEL study [36]. Higher severity of symptoms was associated with increased BMI and smoking, while lower severity was associated with high fiber intake.

LYMPHEDEMA

Arm lymphedema following surgical removal of lymph nodes as part of diagnostic assessment is particularly problematic for obese patients. Recent small trials have indicated that weight loss is likely to help manage lymphedema [74, 75].

CACHEXIA

Cachexia is rare in early-stage patients but may occur in late-stage patients. Cachexia is now acknowledged to be in part an inflammatory condition, and supplementation with fish oil as part of an overall anti-inflammatory diet, or use of specific medications may be useful. The diet should contain higher levels of healthful fats, proteins, and other calorie-dense foods.

VIII. SUMMARY

- Intensive chemotherapy treatment or long-term endocrine treatment of breast cancer is now individualized according to disease characteristics and stage.

- Women who adhered to a low-fat diet and mildly reduced caloric intake had a reduced risk of disease recurrence, especially among ER-negative patients in a large recent study (WINS).
- Exercise is safe for breast cancer patients and may be needed in addition to reduction of caloric intake in order to lose or maintain weight and preserve lean mass. Patients with bone metastases and those who have not previously been physically active should be referred to a physical therapist to develop appropriate exercise regimens.
- Combining diet and exercise to maintain normal weight, or to lose weight for patients who are obese or overweight, is likely to improve prognosis. Gaining weight, especially during chemotherapy treatment, worsens prognosis.
- Diets low in saturated, *trans*, and omega-6 fats, and high in fiber such as that from whole grains, are likely to reduce levels of estrogen, inflammation, and insulin resistance, all of which may promote cancer growth.
- Nutrient deficiency states of micronutrients should be evaluated and treated. Two nutrient deficiencies that can potentially exacerbate breast cancer are vitamin D and iodine.
- St. John's wort and a few other herbal supplements and foods listed in Table 37.2 alter the pharmacokinetics of pharmacologic agents used for breast cancer treatment. Clinicians should be aware of potential herb- and food-drug interactions.
- Certain herbs and nutrients taken in supplemental doses may alleviate side effects of cancer treatment (Table 37.3). These include glutamine [85], calendula, l-carnitine, acetyl-l-carnitine, hawthorn, coenzyme Q10, and ginger.
- Obesity, cardiovascular disease, and diabetes are all common comorbid conditions with breast cancer, and should be managed appropriately, especially in light of the cancer-stimulating effects of weight gain and insulin resistance, and the possible cardiac effects of Herceptin® and Adriamycin®.
- Aromatase inhibitors and ovarian ablation (surgical or chemotherapy related) may cause osteoporosis, and patients should receive appropriate dietary counseling to maintain bone health.
- Patient evaluations should include weight, BMI, and referral to a dietitian and/or physical therapist for weight management if needed. C-reactive protein, erythrocyte sedimentation rate, and fibrinogen are appropriate measures for inflammation. Fasting blood glucose, glucose tolerance, and hemoglobin A1c are appropriate measures for detecting risk of insulin resistance.
- A low-fat, plant-based diet can be recommended, emphasizing monounsaturated and omega-3 fats, fiber-rich whole grains, high vegetable and fruit consumption, and protein primarily from plant sources, fish, and egg whites. Fiber intake of approximately 30 g/day can be considered. Soy foods (not supplements) are recommended for use 2 to 3 times per week. Patients should minimize or eliminate refined flours and sugars, low-fiber or high-fat prepared foods. Caloric intake should be commensurate with need to lose, gain, or maintain weight.

REFERENCES

1. American Cancer Society. 2005. Breast cancer facts & figures, 2005–2006. Atlanta: American Cancer Society.
2. Anonymous. 2005. Indole-3-carbinol. *Alternative Medicine Reviews* 10(4):337–342.
3. Bastard JP, Maachi M, Lagathu C, Kim MJ, Caron M, Vidal H, Capeau J and Feve B. 2006. Recent advances in the relationship between obesity, inflammation, and insulin resistance. *European Cytokine Network* 17(1):4–12.
4. Battaglini C, Bottaro M, Dennehy C, Rae L, Shields E, Kirk D and Hackney A. 2007. The effect of an individualized exercise intervention on body composition in breast cancer patients undergoing treatment. *Sao Paulo Medical Journal* 125(1):22–28.

5. Bertone-Johnson ER. 2007. Prospective studies of dietary vitamin D and breast cancer: more questions raised than answered. *Nutrition Reviews* 65(10): 459–466.
6. Black HS, Herd A, Goldberg LJ, Wolf JE, Thornby JI, Rosen T, Bruce S, Tschen JA, Foreyt JP, Scott LW, Jaax S and Andrews K. 1994. Effect of a low-fat diet on the incidence of actinic keratosis. *NEJM* 330:1272–1275.
7. Block KI, Constantinou A, Hilakivi-Clarke L, Hughes C, Tripathy D and Tice JA. 2002. Point-counterpoint: soy intake for breast cancer patients. *Integrative Cancer Therapies* 1(1):90–100.
8. Block KI, Gyllenhaal C, Tripathy D, Freels S, Mead MN, Block PB, Steinmann WC, Newman RA and Shoham J. Survival impact of integrative cancer in advanced metastatic breast cancer. *The Breast Journal*, in press.
9. Block KI, Koch A, Mead MN, Tothy PK, Newman RA and Gyllenhaal C. 2007. Impact of antioxidant supplementation on chemotherapeutic efficacy: a systematic review of the evidence from randomized controlled trials. *Cancer Treatment Reviews* 33(5):407–418.
10. Borugian MJ, Sheps SB, Kim-Sing C, Van Patten C, Potter JD, Dunn B, Gallagher RP and Hislop TG. 2004. Insulin, macronutrient intake, and physical activity: are potential indicators of insulin resistance associated with mortality from breast cancer? *Cancer Epidemiology Biomarkers and Prevention* 13(7):163–172.
11. Boyd DB. 2003. Insulin and cancer. *Integrative Cancer Therapies* 2(4):315–329.
12. Brooks JD, Ward WE, Lewis JE, Hilditch J, Nickell L, Wong E and Thompson LU. 2004. Supplementation with flaxseed alters estrogen metabolism in postmenopausal women to a greater extent than does supplementation with an equal amount of soy. *American Journal of Clinical Nutrition* 79(2):318–325.
13. Carroll JK, Kohli S, Mustian KM, Roscoe JA and Morrow GR. 2007. Pharmacologic treatment of cancer-related fatigue. *The Oncologist* 12 Suppl 1:43–51.
14. Chavez ML, Jordan MA and Chavez PI. 2006. Evidence-based drug—herbal interactions. *Life Sciences* 78(18):2146–2157.
15. Chlebowski RT, Blackburn GL, Thomson CA, Nixon DW, Shapiro A, Hoy MK, Goodman MT, Giuliano AE, Karanja N, McAndrew P, Hudis C, Butler J, Merkel D, Kristal A, Caan B, Michaelson R, Vinciguerra V, Del Prete S, Winkler M, Hall R, Simon M, Winters BL and Elashoff RM. 2006. Dietary fat reduction and breast cancer outcome: interim efficacy results from the Women's Intervention Nutrition Study. *Journal of the National Cancer Institute* 98(24):1767–1776.
16. Cho E, Chen WY, Hunter DJ, Stampfer MJ, Colditz GA, Hankinson SE and Willett WC. 2006. Red meat intake and risk of breast cancer among premenopausal women. *Archives of Internal Medicine* 166(20):2253–2259.
17. Choi K, Lee SS, Oh SJ, Lim SY, Lim SY, Jeon WK, Oh TY and Kim JW. 2007. The effect of oral glutamine on 5-fluorouracil/leucovorin-induced mucositis/stomatitis assessed by intestinal permeability test. *Clinical Nutrition* 26(1):57–62.
18. Collado-Hidalgo A, Bower JE, Ganz PA, Cole SW and Irwin MR. 2006. Inflammatory biomarkers for persistent fatigue in breast cancer survivors. *Clinical Cancer Research* 12(9):2759–2766.
19. Conklin KA. 2005. Coenzyme Q10 for prevention of anthracycline-induced cardiotoxicity. *Integrative Cancer Therapies* 4(2):110–1130.
20. Coulter IA, Hardy ML, Morton SC, Hilton LG, Tu W, Valentine D and Shekelle PG. 2006. Antioxidants vitamin C and vitamin E for the prevention and treatment of cancer. *Journal of General Internal Medicine* 21:735–744.
21. Courneya KS, Segal RJ, Mackey JR, Gelmon K, Reid RD, Friedenreich CM, Ladha AB, Proulx C, Vallance JK, Lane K, Yasui Y and McKenzie DC. 2007. Effects of aerobic and resistance exercise in breast cancer patients receiving adjuvant chemotherapy: a multicenter randomized controlled trial. *Journal of Clinical Oncology* 25(28):4344–4345.
22. Davies AA, Smith GD, Harbord R, Bekkering GE, Stern JAC, Beynon R and Thomas S. 2006. Nutritional interventions and outcomes in patients with cancer or preinvasive lesions: systematic review. *Journal of the National Cancer Institute* 98:961–973.
23. de Grandis D. 2007. Acetyl-L-carnitine for the treatment of chemotherapy-induced peripheral neuropathy: a short review. *CNS Drugs* 21 suppl 1:39–43.
24. Demark-Wahnefried W, Price DT, Polascik TJ, Robertson CN, Anderson EE, Paulson DF, Walther PJ, Gannon M and Vollmer RT. 2001. Pilot study of dietary fat restriction and flaxseed supplementation in men with prostate cancer before surgery: exploring the effects on hormonal levels, prostate-specific antigen, and histopathologic features. *Urology* 58(1):47–52.
25. Demark-Wahnefried W, Kenyon AJ, Eberle P, Skye A and Kraus WE. 2002. Preventing sarcopenic obesity among breast cancer patients who receive adjuvant chemotherapy: results of a feasibility study. *Clinical Exercise Physiology* 4(1):44–49.

26. de Waard F, Ramlau R, Mulders Y, de Vries T, van Waveren S. 1993. A feasibility study on weight reduction in obese postmenopausal breast cancer patients. *European Journal of Cancer Prevention* 12(3):233–238.

27. Duffy C, Perez K and Partridge A. Implications of phytoestrogen intake for breast cancer. *CA. Cancer Journal for Clinicians* 57:260–277.

28. Einbond LS, Shimizu M, Nuntanakorn P, Seter C, Cheng R, Jiang B, Kronenberg F, Kennelly EJ and Weinstein IB. 2006. Actein and a fraction of black cohosh potentiate antiproliferative effects of chemotherapy agents on human breast cancer cells. *Planta Medica* 72(13):1200–1206.

29. Einbond LS, Wen-Cai Y, He K, Wu HA, Cruz E, Roller M and Kronenberg F. 2008. Growth inhibitory activity of extracts and compounds from *Cimicifuga* species on human breast cancer cells. *Phytomedicine* 15(6–7):504–511.

30. Elkort RJ, Baker FL, Vitale JJ, Cordano A. 1981. Long-term nutritional support as an adjunct to chemotherapy for breast cancer. *JPEN* 5(5):385–390.

31. Fairey AS, Courneya KS, Field CJ, Bell GJ, Jones LW, Martin BS and Mackey JR. 2005. Effect of exercise training on C-reactive protein in postmenopausal breast cancer patients: a randomized controlled trial. *Brain Behavior and Immunity* 19(5):381–388.

32. Ferrucci L, Cherubini A, Bandinelli S, Bartali B, Corsi A, Lauretani F, Martin A, Andres-Lacueva C, Senin U and Guralnik JM. 2006. Relationship of plasma polyunsaturated fatty acids to circulating inflammatory markers. *Journal of Clinical Endocrinology and Metabolism* 91(2):439–446.

33. Flockhart D. 2007. Drug Interactions. Version 4, August 2007. Available at: http://medicine.iupui.edu/flockhart/.

34. Forman MR. 2007. Changes in dietary fat and fiber and serum hormone concentrations: nutritional strategies for breast cancer prevention over the life course. *Journal of Nutrition* 137:170S–174S.

35. Geisler J, Lonning PE, Krag LE, Lokkevik E, Risberg T, Hagen AI, Schlichting E, Lien EA, Ofjord ES, Eide GE, Polli A, diSalle E and Paolini J. 2006. Changes in bone and lipid metabolism in postmenopausal women with early breast cancer after terminating 2-year treatment with exemestane: a randomized, placebo-controlled study. *European Journal of Cancer* 42(17):2968–2975.

36. Gold EB, Flatt SW, Pierce JP, Bardwell WA, Hajek RA, Newman VA, Rock CL and Stefanick ML. 2006. Dietary factors and vasomotor symptoms in breast cancer survivors: the WHEL study. *Menopause* 13(3):423–433.

37. Goodwin PJ, Ennis M, Pritchard KI, Trudeau ME, Koo J, Madarnas Y, Hartwick W, Hoffman B and Hood N. 2002. Fasting insulin and outcome in early-stage breast cancer: results of a prospective cohort study. *Journal of Clinical Oncology* 20(1):42–51.

38. Gorski JC, Huang SM, Pinto A, Hamman MA, Hilligoss JK, Zaheer NA, Desai M, Miller M and Hall SD. 2004. The effect of echinacea (*Echinacea purpurea* root) on cytochrome P450 activity in mice. *Clinical Pharmacology and Therapeutics* 75(1):89–100.

39. Gurley BJ, Gardner SF, Hubbard MA, Williams DK, Gentry WB, Carrier J, Khan IA, Edwards DJ and Shah A. 2004. In vivo assessment of botanical supplementation on human cytochrome P450 phenotypes: *Citrus aurantium, Echinacea purpurea*, milk thistle, and saw palmetto. *Clinical Pharmacology and Therapeutics* 76(5):428–440.

40. Gurley BJ, Gardner SF, Hubbard MA, Williams DK, Gentry WB, Khan IA and Shah A. 2005. In vivo effects of goldenseal, kava kava, black cohosh and valerian on human cytochrome P450 1A2, 2D6, 2E1 and 3A4/5 phenotypes. *Clinical Pharmacology and Therapeutics* 77(5):415–426.

41. Hahn S, Haselhorst U, Tan S, Quadbeck B, Schmidt M, Roesler S, Kimmig R, Mann K and Janssen OE. 2006. Low serum 25-hydroxyvitamin D concentrations are associated with insulin resistance and obesity in women with polycystic ovary syndrome. *Experimental and Clinical Endocrinology and Diabetes* 114(10):577–583.

42. Holmes MD, Chen WY, Feskanich D et al. 2005. Physical activity and survival after breast cancer diagnosis. *JAMA* 293:2479–2486.

43. Holubarsch CJF, Colucci WS, Meinertz T, et al. Crataegus extract WS 1442 postpones cardiac death in patients with congestive heart failure class NYHA II-III: a randomized, placebo-controlled, double-blind trial in 2681 patients. American College of Cardiology 2007 Scientific Sessions March 27, 2007; New Orleans, LA. Late breaking clinical trials-3, Session 414-5.

44. Kaaks R. 2004. Nutrition, insulin, IGF-1 metabolism and cancer risk: a summary of epidemiological evidence. *Novartis Foundation Symposium* 262:247–260.

45. King ML, Adler SR and Murphy LL. 2006. Extraction-dependent effects of American ginseng (*Panax quinquefolium*) on human breast cancer cell proliferation and estrogen receptor activation. *Integrative Cancer Therapies* 5(3):236–264.

46. King PD and Perry MC. 2001. Hepatotoxicity of chemotherapy. *Oncologist* 6(2):162–176.

47. Lanza E, Yu B, Murphy G, Albert PS, Caan B, Marshall JR, Lance P, Paskett ED, Weissfeld J, Slattery M, Burt R, Iber F, Shike M, Kikendall JW, Brewer BK, Schatzkin A and Polyp Prevention Trial Study Group. 2007. The Polyp Prevention Trial continued follow-up study: no effect of a low-fat, high-fiber, high-fruit and -vegetable diet on adenoma recurrence eight years after randomization. *Cancer Epidemiology Biomarkers and Prevention* 16(9):1745–1752.

48. Ligibel JA, Campbell N, Partridge A, Chen WY, Salinardi T, Chen H, Adloff K, Keshaviah A and Winer EP. 2008. Impact of a mixed strength and endurance exercise intervention on insulin levels in breast cancer survivors. *Journal of Clinical Oncology* 26(6):907–912.

49. Lopez-Garcia E, Schulze MB, Meigs JB, Manson JE, Rifai N, Stampfer MJ, Willett WC and Hu FB. 2005. Consumption of *trans* fatty acids is related to plasma biomarkers of inflammation and endothelial dysfunction. *Journal of Nutrition* 135(3):562–566.

50. McAuley K and Mann J. 2006. Thematic review series: patient-oriented research. Nutritional determinants of insulin resistance. *Journal of Lipid Research* 47(8):1668–1676.

51. Majed B, Moreau T, Senouci K, Salmon RJ, Fourquet A and Asselain B. 2007. Is obesity an independent prognosis factor in woman breast cancer? *Breast Cancer Research and Treatment* October 16 (Epub ahead of treatment).

52. Manusirivithaya S, Sripramote M, Tangjitgamol S, Sheanakul C, Leelahakorn S, Thavaramara T, Tangcharoenpanich K. 2004. Antiemetic effect of ginger in gynecologic oncology patients receiving cisplatin. *Int J Gynecol Cancer* Nov-Dec;14(6):1063–9.

53. Messina M, McCaskill-Stevens W and Lampe JW. 2006. Addressing the soy and breast cancer relationship: review, commentary and workshop proceedings. *Journal of the National Cancer Institute* 98(18):1275–1284.

54. Meyer F, Bairati I, Fortin A, Gélinas M, Nabid A, Brochet F and Têtu B. 2007a. Interaction between antioxidant vitamin supplementation and cigarette smoking during radiation therapy in relation to long-term effects on recurrence and mortality: a randomized trial among head and neck cancer patients. *International Journal of Cancer* 122(7):1679–1683.

55. Meyer F, Bairati I, Jobin E, Gélinas M, Fortin A, Nabid A and Têtu B. 2007b. Acute adverse effects of radiation therapy and local recurrence in relation to dietary and plasma beta carotene and alpha tocopherol in head and neck cancer patients. *Nutrition and Cancer* 59(1):29–35.

56. Miller RR, Hicks GE, Shardell MD, Cappola AR, Hawkes WG, Yu-Yahiro JA, Keegan A and Magaziner J. 2007. Association of serum vitamin D levels with inflammatory response following hip fracture: the Baltimore Hip Studies. *The Journals of Gerontology. Series A, Biological Sciences and Medical Sciences* 62(12):1402–1406.

57. Moss RW. 2007. Do antioxidants interfere with radiation therapy for cancer? *Integrative Cancer Therapies* 6(3):281–292.

58. Nichols HB, Trentham-Dietz A, Newcomb PA, Titus-Ernstoff L, Holick CN and Egan KM. Post-diagnosis weight change, body mass index, and breast cancer survival. Presented at 6th Annual Conference on Frontiers in Cancer Prevention Research, December 7, 2007. Abstract B95.

59. Ornish D, Weidner G, Fair WR, Marlin R, Pettengill EB, Raisin CJ, Dunn-Emke S, Crutchfield L, Jacobs FN, Barnard RJ, Aronson WJ, McCormac P, McKnight DJ, Fein JD, Dnistrian AM, Weinstein J, Ngo TH, Mendell NR and Carroll PR. 2005. Intensive lifestyle changes may affect the progression of prostate cancer. *Journal of Urology* 174(3):1065–1069.

60. Pierce JP, Natarajan L, Caan BJ et al. 2007a. Influence of a diet very high in vegetables, fruit, and fiber and low in fat on prognosis following treatment for breast cancer. *JAMA* 298(3):289–298.

61. Pierce JP, Stefanick ML, Flatt SW et al. 2007b. Greater survival after breast cancer in physically active women with high vegetable-fruit intake regardless of obesity. *Journal of Clinical Oncology* 28(17):2345–2351.

62. Pommier P, Gomez F, Sunyach MP, D'Hombres A, Carrie C and Montbarbon X. 2004. Phase III randomized trial of *Calendula officinalis* compared with trolamine for the prevention of acute dermatitis during irradiation for breast cancer. *Journal of Clinical Oncology* 22(8):1447–1453.

63. Porojnicu AC, Lagunova Z, Robsahn TE, Berg JP, Dahlback A and Moan J. 2007. Changes in risk of death from breast cancer with season and latitude: sun exposure and breast cancer survival in Norway. *Breast Cancer Research and Treatment* 102(3):323–328.

64. Post-White J, Ladas EJ and Kelly KM. 2007. Advances in the use of milk thistle. *Integrative Cancer Therapies* 6(2):104–109.

65. Rahman KM, Ali S, Aboukameel A, Sarkar SH, Wang Z, Philip PA, Sakr WA and Raz A. 2007. Inactivation of NF-kappaB by 3,3'-diindolylmethane contributes to increased apoptosis induced by chemotherapeutic agent in breast cancer cells. *Molecular Cancer Therapies* 6(10):2757–2765.

66. Riccardi G, Giacco R and Rivellese AA. 2004. Dietary fat, insulin sensitivity and the metabolic syndrome. *Clinical Nutrition* 22(4):447–456.

67. Robsahm TE, Trettli S, Dahlback A and Moan J. 2004. Vitamin D3 from sunlight may improve the prognosis of breast-, colon- and prostate cancer (Norway). *Cancer Causes and Control* 15(2):149–158.

68. Rock CL and Demark-Wahnefried W. 2002. Nutrition and survival after the diagnosis of breast cancer: a review of the evidence. *Journal of Clinical Oncology* 20(15):3302–3316.

69. Rock E and DeMichele A. 2003. Nutritional approaches to late toxicities of adjuvant chemotherapy in breast cancer survivors. *Journal of Nutrition* 133:3785S–3793S.

70. Rohan T. 2007. Epidemiological studies of vitamin D and breast cancer. *Nutrition Reviews* 65(8):S80–S83.

71. Sahyoun NR, Jacques PF, Zhang XL, Juan W and McKeown NM. 2006. Whole-grain intake is inversely associated with the metabolic syndrome and mortality in older adults. *American Journal of Clinical Nutrition* 83(1):124–131.

72. Savarese DM, Savy G, Vahdat L, Wischmeyher PE and Corey B. 2003. Prevention of chemotherapy and radiation toxicity with glutamine. *Cancer Treatment Reviews* 29(6):501–513.

73. Saxe GA, Major JM, Nguyen JU, Freeman KM, Downs TM and Salem CE. 2006. Potential attenuation of disease progression in recurrent prostate cancer with plant-based diet and stress reduction. *Integrative Cancer Therapies* 5(3):206–213.

74. Shaw C, Mortimer P and Judd PA. 2007a. A randomized controlled trial of weight reduction as a treatment for breast cancer-related lymphedema. *Cancer* 110(8):1868–1874.

75. Shaw C, Mortimer P and Judd PA. 2007b. Randomized controlled trial comparing a low-fat diet with a weight-reduction diet in breast cancer-related lymphedema. *Cancer* 109(10):1949–1956.

76. Simopoulos AP. 2002. The importance of the ratio of omega-6/omega-3 essential fatty acids. *Biomedicine and Pharmacotherapy* 56(8):365–379.

77. Smyth PPA. 2003. The thyroid, iodine and breast cancer. *Breast Cancer Research* 5:235–238.

78. Sopotsinskaia EB, Balitskii KP, Tarutinov VI, Zhukova VM, Semenchuk DD, Kozlovskaia SG and Grigorov IG. 1992. Experience with the use of a low-calorie diet in breast cancer patients to prevent metastasis. *Voprosy Onkologii* 38(5):592–599.

79. Spentzos D, Mantzoros C, Regan MM, Morrissey ME, Duggan S, Flickner-Garvey S, McCormick H, DeWolf W, Balk S and Bubley GJ. 2003. Minimal effect of a low-fat/high soy diet for asymptomatic, hormonally naïve prostate cancer patients. *Clinical Cancer Research* 9(9):3282–3287.

80. Taylor EF, Burley VJ, Greenwood DC and Cade JE. 2007. Meat consumption and risk of breast cancer in the UK Women's Cohort Study. *British Journal of Cancer* 96(7):1139–1146.

81. Thompson LU, Chen JM, Strasser-Weippl K and Goss PE. 2005. Dietary flaxseed alters tumor biological markers in postmenopausal breast cancer. *Clinical Cancer Research* 11(10):3828–3835.

82. Visovsky C. 2006. Muscle strength, body composition, and physical activity in women receiving chemotherapy for breast cancer. *Integrative Cancer Therapies* 5(3):183–191.

83. Walji R, Boon H, Guns E, Oneschuck D and Younnus D. 2007. Black cohosh (*Cimicifuga racemosa* [L.] Nutt.): safety and efficacy for cancer patients. *Supportive Care in Cancer* 15(8):913–921.

84. Wallace JM. 2002. Nutritional and botanical modulation of the inflammatory cascade—eicosanoids, cyclooxygenases, and lipoxygenases – as an adjunct in cancer therapy. *Integrative Cancer Therapies* 1(1):7–37.

85. Wischmeyer PE. 2008. Glutamine: role in critical illness and ongoing clinical trials. *Current Opinion in Gastroenterology* 24(2):190–197.

86. Wood LJ, Nail LM, Gilster A, Winters KA and Elsea CR. 2006. Cancer chemotherapy-related symptoms: evidence to suggest a role for proinflammatory cytokines. *Oncology Nursing Forum* 33(3):535–542.

87. Wu JH, Ward NC, Indrawan AP, Almeida CA, Hodgson JM, Proudfoot JM, Puddey IB and Croft KD. 2007. Effects of alpha-tocopherol and mixed tocopherol supplementation on markers of oxidative stress and inflammation in type 2 diabetes. *Clinical Chemistry* 53(3):511–519.

38 Cervical Cancer

Care and Prevention With Nutritional Medicine

Cindy A. Krueger, M.P.H., and Ron N. Shemesh, M.D.

I. INTRODUCTION

No other public health cancer prevention tool has made more of a difference than the PAP smear. Since the introduction of the Papanicoulau (Pap) smear in 1941, this screening tool has reduced the incidence of cervical cancer in the United States by 75% and the death rate continues to decline by 4% a year [1]. Cervical cancer is one of the few cancers with well-defined precancerous stages, allowing for successful treatment with early detection and diagnosis [2–3].

Treatments for cervical cancer include surgery, radiation, and chemotherapy. There is mounting biologic and clinical evidence that another powerful treatment is secondary prevention and cellular therapy through nutrition and lifestyle interventions. This chapter probes the biologic basis of food and nutrient interventions applicable to clinical care for cervical cancer.

II. EPIDEMIOLOGY

Worldwide, cervical cancer ranks fifth for cancer mortality in women [4]. In 2006 an estimated 10,000 women in the United States will have been diagnosed with cervical cancer and nearly 4000 will die from it [5]. Estimated new cases of cervical cancer in 2008 is 11,070 and deaths, 3870 [6].

The major risk factor for the development of pre-invasive or invasive cervical carcinoma is infection with the human papillomavirus (HPV). HPV DNA is detected in virtually all cervical cancers, with HPV subtypes 16, 18, and 31 identified most frequently. Other significant risk factors include oral contraceptive use, smoking, multiple sex partners, and nutritional deficiencies (see Table 38.1) [7–15].

III. PATHOPHYSIOLOGY

HPV has been shown to play a vital role in the development of cervical cancer precursors. While HPV DNA is detected in the majority of cervical cancers, with HPV subtypes 16, 18, and 31 identified most frequently, only a small fraction of those infected eventually develop cancer. It is therefore clear that additional factors contribute to the progression of cervical cancer.

Oncoproteins produced by the HPV virus genes, when integrated into human cell genes, are known to cause a variety of genetic alterations with the most common being changes in the human

617

TABLE 38.1
Risk Factors in Cervical Cancer

Risk Factors in Cervical Cancer	Implications
Age	Risk rises with age; second most common cancer in women under age 35.
Pap smear abnormality	Most widely used preventive screening tool.
Smoking	Risk is twice as likely as nonsmokers.
Multiple sex partners	Sexual intercourse before age 18, multiple sex partners, or bearing a child before age 16 promotes a higher-than-average risk of developing cervical cancer.
Oral contraceptives	Long-term use (over 5–9 years) increases risk, depletes body of folic acid, vitamin B6, and vitamin B12.
Vitamin deficiency	Higher risk for those deficient in beta carotene, lycopene, canthaxanthin, alpha tocopherol, folic acid, and vitamin D3.
Human Papillomavirus infection	Primary risk factor. Only a very small percentage of women infected with untreated HPV will develop cervical cancer.
Immunosuppression	Immune system plays a vital role in destroying cancer cells and slowing their growth to other organs.
Human Immunodeficiency Virus infection	Compromises the immune system. A weakened immune system may cause cervical cancer to develop at a more rapid pace.

p53 tumor suppressor gene. Such genetic alterations can result in uncontrolled progression of the cell cycle. When the genetic alterations are coupled with other epigenetic factors such as environmental, chemical, and other stress factors, they can impact alterations in other cellular functions that enable transformation of benign cells into malignant ones [16]. Epigenetic modifications of cellular DNA can cause changes in gene expression that are potentially reversible molecular events.

Pap smear and HPV testing have been effective as a screening tool because of the frequent lack of any obvious symptoms or clinical features in the early phases of cervical neoplastic disease.

Since food and nutrients provide the substrate for a variety of physiologic processes that include DNA repair, regulation of cell growth, and immune and hormone modulation, nutritional interventions can assist in reversing the impact of epigenetic factors.

Folate, also known as vitamin B9 and folic acid, protects against cervical cancer based on its roles in DNA synthesis and in repair of damaged DNA [17–18]. Folate is involved in DNA methylation, through which it may influence gene stability and expression. Folate utilization increases during pregnancy when required for rapidly growing fetal cell DNA.

The cells that form the cervical epithelium respond to hormonal changes, especially those that would signal pregnancy or an environment nonconducive to pregnancy. Oral contraceptives can send epithelial cells the wrong signal, particularly about DNA methylation and the need for folate. This appears to be the emerging biologic basis for the association between long-term use of oral contraceptives and cancer of the cervix [19].

Since 1973, studies have shown the relationship between folate and pathogenesis of cervical cancer. Some Pap smears reflect folic acid deficiency rather than cervical dysplasia. It has been hypothesized and observed that oral contraceptives block the effects of folic acid within cells. Even though serum levels of folic acid may be normal, the level within the cells of the cervix may be lower than normal [20–21]. Using folic acid reversed megaloblastic changes in the cervical epithelium that were associated with oral contraceptive use [22–23].

There has been a considerable amount of emphasis placed on folate, and folate's role in the synthesis, repair, and methylation of DNA intertwined with the metabolic functions of vitamin B12.

Both are cofactors for methionine synthase, which is the catalyst for the conversion of homocysteine to methionine and also controls the regulator of cellular folate uptake [24–25].

Homocysteine produced during methionine metabolism could be associated with increased risk of cervical cancer. Homocysteine elevation suggests folate and B12 levels inadequate for optimal metabolism since both folic acid and vitamin B12 are inversely associated with homocysteine concentrations, which are a potential marker for cervical cancer and optimal protection against DNA damage [26–27]. Even when serum folate and B12 levels are within the normal range, homocysteine may be elevated and may respond to supplemental dosing of these B vitamins. Normal serum vitamin levels may differ from optimal levels and may not reflect intracellular metabolism.

Deficiency of B vitamins impairs the liver's ability to inactivate excess estrogens and break down xenoestrogens, thereby exposing hormone-responsive cervical epithelial cells to excess estrogen and xenoestrogens.

Women with low dietary intakes of vitamins B1 (thiamine), B2 (riboflavin), B12 (cobalamin), and folic acid may be more at risk of developing cervical dysplasia [28]. The findings suggest that increasing the intake of these vitamins may help prevent the development of cervical cancer. Deficient levels of CoQ10 and vitamin E have also been shown in women with cervical cancer [29].

Phytonutrients, also known as phytochemicals, are natural bioactive compounds found in fruits and vegetables that work together with vitamins, minerals, and fiber to promote good health. They have been shown to help the body contain and eliminate microbial infections. Women whose diets are higher in vegetables containing lycopene and who have higher *cis*-lycopene in the blood were more than 50% less likely to have long-lasting HPV infections. The significant drop in HPV infections would suggest a lower likelihood of developing cervical cancer with a lycopene-rich vegetable diet [30].

Increasing evidence suggests that high intake of Brassica vegetables, better known as cruciferous vegetables, may also help prevent cancer [31, 32]. These vegetables are from the plant family *Brassicaceae* (formerly called *Cruciferae*) and include cabbage, broccoli, bok choy, brussels sprouts, cauliflower, kale, kohlrabi, mustard, rutabaga, and turnips.

One of the anticancer nutrients found in cruciferous vegetables is glucosinolates [33]. Glucosinolates are rich sources of sulfur-containing compounds. When chewed or chopped and digested, these vegetables contain a kind of phytochemical known as isothiocyanate(s) shown to stimulate the body's ability to break down potential carcinogens. They work by preventing the transformation of normal healthy cells into cancerous cells [34, 35].

Another class of nutrients are indole-3-carbinol (I3C) and diindolylmethane (DIM). These are critical components in the chemopreventive effects of crucifers because they affect the action of enzymes within the body, thus influencing the way the body deals with potential carcinogens [36].

Current research suggests that I3C alters the way in which the liver processes hormones, like estrogen, and environmental toxins [37, 38].

The *British Journal of Cancer* reported that genistein (a soy isoflavone) and I3C enhance DNA repair, partially explaining the ability of increased vegetable intake to reduce cancer risk. The study is also among the first to discover a cellular explanation for the correlation between increased vegetable intake and reduced risk of cancer [39].

A Pap smear detects cervical intraepithelial neoplasia (CIN), which is not cancer but the first of the cellular changes that may develop into cancer. In mild dysplasia (CIN I) a "watch and wait" approach is recommended. In a report from Dartmouth Medical School, as many as 60%–80% of mild dysplasia cases will return to normal without further treatment [40].

CIN stage II represents moderate dysplasia and is confined to the basal epithelium. CIN stage III is considered severe dysplasia and is often referred to as cervical carcinoma in situ [41].

In another study researchers treated CIN in stages II and III of its development with a substance extracted from the Brassica family. When this substance was administered during the course of only 12 weeks, between 40% and 50% of cancers disappeared [42, 43].

In a placebo-controlled human trial, 200 mg/day of I3C resulted in complete regression of cervical precancerous growth in four of eight patients, and 400 mg/day resulted in complete regression in four of nine patients. In the placebo group, no patients had complete regression [44].

Indole-3-carbinol appears to work in several ways. It helps to convert estrogen to a less cancer-promoting form, 2-hydroxyestrone, which is less active than estradiol, so when it occupies the estrogen receptor site, it effectively blocks estradiol's strong "grow" signals, and partially blocks the effects of estrogen on cells. It directly kills or inhibits cancer cells, and reduces levels of free radicals, which can promote cancer by damaging DNA [45–48].

Vitamin A as both retinol and beta-carotene have been examined for their role in how they may prevent or reverse cervical dysplasia. Applying *trans*-retinoic acid topically to the cervix resulted in up to a 50% complete reversal of cervical dysplasia in Phase II and Phase III clinical trials. Vaginal and vulvar side effects of this treatment were mild and reversible at the end of treatment. Results like these may suggest this is a viable treatment option for cervical dysplasia. Vitamin A and its natural and synthetic derivatives (retinoids) modulate the growth of cervical cells, slowing growth and enhancing maturation of cells. This can play a vital role in the prevention and reversal of cancers [49].

With the use of an oral application, 30 patients with mild or moderate cervical dysplasia were treated with 30 mg of beta-carotene for up to 6 months. More than 70% of patients showed reversal of their condition by 6 months, but only 3 months were required to realize optimal reversal of this condition as suggested by serum beta-carotene levels and measurement of shed cervicovaginal cells, which were highly correlated [50].

Women at high risk for developing cervical cancer or diagnosed with cervical cancer had significantly decreased levels of the polyphenolic compounds found in foods, namely beta-carotene, lycopene, canthaxanthin, and alpha tocopherol compared to the controls according to one study. Present findings support an association between decreased antioxidant nutrient levels and cervical cancer, according to researchers at Albert Einstein College of Medicine in New York. They hypothesized that the free-radical-fighting ability of these nutrients is responsible for their role in cervical cancer. Researchers suggest that these antioxidants prevent mutational changes to DNA, the basic building blocks of life, that would predispose the body to cancer [51].

IV. PHARMACOLOGY

Several prescription medications have side effects of blocking the uptake, impeding the utilization, and increasing the demand for and promoting the excretion of folate [52–55]. See Table 38.2.

V. PATIENT EVALUATION AND DIAGNOSTICS

In the process of evaluating a patient's cervical health, various indicators of low B vitamin status may present themselves. The clinician familiar with these indicators can follow up with evaluation.

A patient history may include a nutrient-poor diet, medical conditions associated with low B vitamin status, and medications such as those in Table 38.2 that adversely influence B vitamin status. Inadequacies in the folate cycle go beyond cervical dysplasia risk, and include neural tube defects, pediatric developmental problems, psychiatric and neurological problems, and cardiovascular functioning.

Physical exam findings may also point to inadequate B vitamin status. The tongue evaluation is a helpful diagnostic tool. Deficiencies of niacin, riboflavin, pyridoxine, folic acid, or vitamin B12, resulting from poor diet or from the administration of antagonists, may cause a sore, beefy-red tongue without a coat. In the chronic vitamin deficiency state, the tongue may become atrophic and smooth. Riboflavin deficiency can also cause cheilosis or fissuring at the corners of the mouth [56].

A routine complete blood count (CBC) may indicate macrocytic anemia as result of B12 or folate deficiency. Elevated mean cell volume (MCV) and low hemoglobin should also be noted.

TABLE 38.2
Drug/Folate Interactions

Drug Category	Interactions/Side Effects
Analgesics	Increased urinary excretion and reduced blood levels of folate, particularly in rheumatoid patients and those with arthritis; aspirin depletes folic acid by displacing bound serum folate.
Antacids	Inhibits absorption with prolonged intake and may cause low or deficient plasma and erythrocyte levels of folacin.
Beta blockers	Folate is essential for the metabolism of the atherogenic amino acid homocysteine. The reduction of plasma and erythrocyte folate concentrations is also associated with a moderate hyperhomocysteinemia. Moderate hyperhomocysteinaemia is an independent risk factor for cardiovascular disease which may be causal.
Calcium channel blockers	Folic acid lowers levels of homocysteine.
Antidepressant drugs/SSRIs	Folic acid may improve action of the drug or decrease the need entirely.
Antibotic therapy	Disrupts normal gastrointestinal flora, interferring with reabsorption of folic acid.
Oral contraceptives	Impairs folate metabolism and depletes serum levels of vitamin B vitamins, zinc, and magnesium.
Diuretics	Inhibits enzyme necessary for folic acid synthesis, depletes folic acid, and increases homocysteine levels.
Anti-inflammatory	Decreases absorption of folic acid; competitively inhibits the enzymatic synthesis of folic acid.
Anti-seizure	Decreases serum folate and absorption.
Antibacterial	Mild folate antagonist and may create a deficiency with long-term use.
Anti-hyperlipidemia	Depletes folic acid due to poor absorption.

Any of these findings may prompt laboratory evaluation for folate and B12. Serum folic acid can detect folate deficiency, but a normal level of folate does not confirm adequate folate for DNA repair. A B12 serum level is used to eliminate the possibility of a megaloblastic anemia due to B12 deficiency and as a baseline level prior to folic acid supplementation. However, just as in the case of folic acid levels, one may have deficient B12 levels in certain tissues with decreased functioning despite normal serum levels of B12.

Therefore, one can measure methylmalonic acid in the serum, which rises in response to unmet B12 needs, and is therefore considered a most sensitive test of B12 function in the body [57, 58].

Individuals in the early stages of folate deficiency may not show obvious symptoms, but blood levels of homocysteine may increase. Homocysteine is considered to be a crucial marker for measuring adequacy of the tetrahydrofolate cycle with formation of S-adenosyl-metionine (SAM) the active methylating agent for a variety of critical biomolecules including neurotransmitters, steroid hormones, phospholipids, and nucleic acids [59]. Optimal levels range between 5 to 8 micromol per liter. Homocysteine levels can be reduced with B vitamin complex supplementation. In these circumstances homocysteine may serve as a marker of suboptimal folate and B12 even if serum vitamin assays are within the normal ranges. This can occur because the normal range and optimal range differ and because serum levels do not always reflect intracellular processes.

VI. TREATMENT

Precancerous lesions occur at the highest rates among women of childbearing age. Because suboptimal nutrient levels are often associated with neoplasia, the opportunity to implement nutritional interventions in the treatment of neoplasia can have a positive impact on other medical conditions that share associated nutritional deficiencies in this and older age groups. Birth defects, breast cancer, and infections are positively affected by nutritional interventions.

Diet and Lifestyle

The American Institute for Cancer Research (AICR) has become the nation's leading organization pursuing the link between diet/physical activity and cancer and the prevention and treatment of cancer. Because cancer is not restricted to developed and industrialized countries, the AICR is creating partnerships with affiliates around the world to create higher standards of living in order to decrease the incidence of not only cancer but also heart disease and diabetes. A portion of Table 38.3 has been derived from the AICR recommendations.

The following cancer prevention interventions can be incorporated into medical management recommendations [60–62]. See Table 38.3.

Supplemental Nutrients

Correction of nutritional deficiencies with improvement in cellular immune and antioxidant protection using potent nutrients can be obtained from whole foods, fresh vegetables and fruits, and supplements [63].

A supplement protocol can be incorporated based on the level of cervical disease where a more advanced disease would call for inclusion of more supplements with the higher suggested doses [64].

TABLE 38.3
Lifestyle Recommendations for Cancer Prevention

Behaviors	Lifestyle Changes
Be as lean as possible	Maintain a healthy weight based upon BMI recommendations and waist-to-hip ratio.
Exercise	Include aerobic conditioning, strength training, flexibility, and stretching.
Avoid sugary drinks and processed foods	Avoid soft drinks and flavored drinks. Pure water (non-municipal supply) is the best alternative along with natural fruit and vegetable drinks, unsweetened tea and coffee. Avoid boxed and processed foods. Eat plant-based foods.
Eat a variety of vegetables, fruits, whole grains, and beans	A variety of vegetables, fruits, whole grains, and beans contain fiber necessary for normal gastrointestinal function.
Limit consumption of red and processed meats	Avoid processed meats that contain preservatives known to contain cancer causing substances. Limit red meats but consume meats from grass-fed animals.
Consume alcohol in moderation	Modest amounts of alcohol have health protective factors.
Limit high amounts of sodium	Avoid processed foods where most salt in the diet originates.
Use supplements	Begin with a diet of nutrient rich whole foods. Consume supplements not only for deficiency but for optimal health.
Breastfeed exclusively for 6 months	Breastfeeding decreases risk of cancer in mother, protects the child from obesity later in life, and increases antibodies in both.
Avoid environmental toxins	Avoid tobacco, phthalates, plastics, herbicides, pesticides, or any synthetic chemicals.
Avoid *trans* fats/hydrogenated oils	Consume good essential fatty acids, omega-3s, 6s, and 9s in the form of cold-pressed unrefined olive oil and other nut oils, nuts, avocados, and flaxseed.

- Vitamin B complex—50 mg bid. A vitamin B complex should include B6 10 to 50 mg/day, B12 800 to 1000 μg/day, and riboflavin 1.5 mg/day.
- Indole-3-carbinol—200 to 400 mg/day. It is preferable these nutrients are taken at bedtime in order to support the body's circadian rhythm [65].
- Vitamin A—50,000 IU for 3 weeks, then switch to beta-carotene 30,000 IU daily.
- Vitamin C—dose to bowel tolerance (loose stools). While there is no consensus on the dose of vitamin C, it can be recommended as there has been some evidence to suggest that it can play a role in both CIN and cervical cancer [66]. An inverse association was found between dietary vitamin C and CIN in this case-control study of biopsy confirmed CIN patients [67].
- Natural vitamin E—400 IU mixed tococopherols and tocotrienols.
- Folic acid—400 μg to 5 mg daily preferably as folinic acid form, which the body can convert ino any of the more active forms of folate [68]. The dose can be titrated according to serum deficiency levels and cervical disease severity. The use of bioactive forms of the synthetic folic acid is particularly important for approximately 10% to 15% of individuals who have genetic methylene tetrahydrofolate reductase (MTHFR) homozygous polymorphisms, which are associated with lower enzyme activity, lower plasma and red blood cell folate, and elevated plasma homocysteine.

VII. SUMMARY

The slow progression of cervical disease from atypical changes to dysplasia, and on to cancer allows this disease to respond ideally to the integration of a nutritional program that can be followed closely using both current protocols of Pap and/or excisional biopsy monitoring, if necessary, as well as nutritional measurements like serum homocysteine, B12, and folate levels to document the impact on cellular health. Since cellular stress with resultant DNA damage plays a major role in cervical pathology, food and nutrient interventions target the elimination of potential environmental burdens on tissue metabolism, and focus on the replenishment of depleted nutrients crucial for optimal energy for cell turnover and function. There is sufficient evidence to suggest that nutrition and the use of supplements are a vital component of preventing and potentially reversing cervical dysplasia and cervical cancer.

REFERENCES

1. Greenlee RT, Hill-Harmon MB, Murray T, Thun M. Cancer statistics, 2001. *CA Cancer J Clin* 2001;50:7–33.
2. Robbins S, Cotran R. *Pathologic Basis of Disease*, 3rd ed. (Philadelphia: W.B. Saunders, 1984), 1123.
3. Rubin P. *Clinical Oncology*, 6th ed. (Philadelphia: American Cancer Society, 1983), 458–467.
4. American Cancer Society Statistics 2006.
5. World Health Organization Fact Sheet No. 297, February 2006.
6. www.cancer.gov/cancertopics/types/cervical/
7. Casper MJ, Clarke AE. Making the Pap smear into the 'right tool' for the job: cervical cancer screening in the USA, circa 1940–95. *Social Studies of Science* 1998 Apr;28(2):255–290.
8. Women's Cancer Network: www.wcn.org
9. American Cancer Society. *What Are the Risk Factors for Cervical Cancer?* 2006 August 4.
10. Murray MT. *Encyclopedia of Nutritional Supplements* (Rocklin, CA: Prima, 1996), 124.
11. Passwater RA. *Cancer Prevention and Nutritional Therapies* (New Canaan, CT: Keats, 1993), 182.
12. Butterworth CE Jr., et al. Folate-induced regression of cervical intraepithelial neoplasia in users of oral contraceptive agents. *American Journal of Clinical Nutrition* 1980;33:926.
13. Hernandez BY, McDuffie K, Kamemoto L, Goodman MT. Diet and high grade premalignant lesions of the cervix: evidence for a protective role for folate, riboflavin, thiamin and vitamin B12. *Cancer Causes Control* 2003;14(9):859–870.

14. Franceschi S. The IARC commitment to cancer prevention: The example of papillomavirus and cervical cancer. *Cancer Research* 2005;166:277–297.
15. Shiffman M, et al. HPV DNA testing in cervical cancer screening: results from women in a high-risk province of Costa Rica. *Journal of the American Medical Association* 2000.
16. Geisler JP, et al. *Journal of Gynecologic Oncology* 2003;8:286–288.
17 Butterworth CE. Effect of folate on cervical cancer. *Ann NY Acad Sci* 1992;669:293–299.
18. Mason JB, Levesque T. Folate: effects on carcinogenesis and the potential for cancer chemoprevention. *Oncology* (Basel) 1996;10:1727–1742. (Medline)
19. World Health Organization Collaborative Study of Neoplasia and Steroid Contraceptives: Invasive Cervical Cancer and Combined Oral Contraceptives. *Br Med J* 1983;290:961–963.
20. Whitehead N, Reyner F, Lindenbaum J. Megaloblastic changes in the cervical epithelium. Association with oral contraceptive therapy and reversal with folic acid. *Journal of the American Medical Association* 1973 Dec;226(12):1421–1424.
21. Kitay D, Wentz WB. Cervical cytology in folic acid deficiency of pregnancy. *American Journal of Obstetrics and Gynecology* 1969 Aug;104(7):931–938.
22. Whitehead N, Reyner F, Lindenbaum J. Megaloblastic changes in the cervical epithelium. *J Am Med Assoc* 1973;226:1421–1424.
23. Butterworth CE, Hatch KD, Gore H, Mueller H, Krumdieck CL. Improvement in cervical dysplasia associated with folic acid therapy in users of oral contraceptives. *Am J Clin Nutr* 1982;35:73–82.
24. Weir DG, Scott JM. Cobalamins: physiology, dietary sources and requirements. Sadler MJ, Strain JJ, Caballero B, eds. *Encyclopedia of Human Nutrition* (London: Academic Press, 1999), 394–401.
25. McPartlin J, Weir DG, Scott JM. Folic acid: physiology, dietary sources and requirements. Sadler MJ, Strain JJ, Caballero B, eds. *Encyclopedia of Human Nutrition* (London: Academic Press, 1999), 803–811.
26. Flynn MA, Herbert V, Nolph GB, Krause G. Atherogenesis and the homocysteine-folate-cobalamin triad: do we need standardized analyses? *J Am Coll Nutr* 1997;16:258–267. [Abstract]
27. Anthony JA, Selhum J, Shah K, Viscidi RP, Cornstock GW, Helzlsoner KJ. The risk of cervical cancer in relation to serum concentrations of folate, vitamin B12, and homocysteine. *Cancer Epidemiology Biomarkers and Prevention* 2000 Jul 4;9:761–764.
28. Hernandez BY, et al. Diet and premalignant lesions of the cervix: evidence of a protective role for folate, riboflavin, thiamin, and vitamin B12. *Cancer Causes Control* 2003;14(9):859–870.
29. Palan PR, et al. Plasma concentrations of coenzyme Q10 and tocopherols in cervical intraepithelial neoplasia and cervical cancer. *Eur J Cancer Prev* 2003;12(4):321–326.
30. Sedjo RL, et al. Vitamin A, carotenoids, and risk of persistent oncogenic human papillomavirus infection. *Cancer Epidemiol Biomark Prev* 2002;11(9):876–884.
31. Brandi G, et al. Mechanisms of action and antiproliferative properties of Brassica oleracea juice in human breast cancer cell lines. *J Nutr* 2005;135:1503–1509.
32. Auborn KJ, et al. Indole-3-Carbinol is a negative regulator of estrogen. *J Nutr* 2003;133:2470s–2475s.
33. Lampe JW, Peterson S. Brassica, biotransformation and cancer risk: genetic polymorphisms alter the preventive effects of cruciferous vegetables. *J Nutr* 2002;132:2991–2994.
34. American Institute of Cancer Research (AICR). Food, Nutrition, Physical Activity, and the Prevention of Cancer: A Global Perspective, 2008.
35. Fahey JW, Zalcmann AT, Talalay P. The chemical diversity and distribution of glucosinolates and isothiocyanates among plants. *Phytochemistry* 2001;56(1):5–51.
36. Fahey J, et al. Broccoli sprouts: an exceptionally rich source of inducers of enzymes that protect against chemical carcinogens. *Proc Natl Acad Sci* 1997;94:10367–10372.
37. Michnovicz JJ, Bradlow HL. Induction of estradiol metabolism by dietary indole-3-carbinol in humans. *J Natl Cancer Inst* 1990;82:947–9.
38. Michnovicz JJ. Increased estrogen 2-hydroxylation in obese women using oral indole-3-carbinol. *Int J Obes Relat Metab Disord* 1998;22(3):227–229.
39. Fan S, Meng Q, Auborn K, Carter T, Rosen EM. BRCA1 AND BRCA2 as molecular targets for phytochemicals indole-3-carbinol and genistein in breast and prostate cancer cells. *Br J Cancer.* 2006; 94(3):407–26.
40. Currie JL. Treating Pre Invasive Cervical Cancer. Women's Health Resource at the Dartmouth Hitchcock Medical Center, Hanover, New Hampshire, April 2001.
41. Agorastos T, Miliaras D, Lambropoulos A, Chrisafi S, Kotsis A, Manthos A, Bontis J. Detection and typing of human papillomavirus DNA in uterine cervices with coexistent grade I and grade III intraepithelial neoplasia: biologic progression or independent lesions? *Eur J Obstet Gynecol Reprod Biol* 2005;121(1):99–103.

42. Bell MC, Crowley-Nowick P, Bradlow HL, Sepkovic DW, Schmidt Grimminger D, Howell P, Mayeaux EJ, Tucker A, Turbat-Herrera EA, Mathis JM. Department of Obstetrics and Gynecology, Louisiana State University Medical Center-Shreveport, 1501 Kings Highway, Shreveport, Louisiana, 71130-3932, USA. Placebo-controlled trial of indole-3-carbinol in the treatment of CIN. *Gynecol Oncol* 2000 Aug;78(2):123–129.

43. Auborn KJ. Can Indole-3-Carbinol–induced changes in cervical intraepithelial neoplasia be extrapolated to other food components? *Nutr* 2006 Oct;136:2676S–2678S.

44. Snow RR, et al. Estrogen 2-hydroxylase oxidation and menstrual function among elite oarswomen. *J Clin Endocrinol Metab* 1991:69:369–376.

45. Michnovicz JJ. Increased estrogen 2-hydroxylation in obese women using oral indole-3-carbinol. *Int J Obes Relat Metab Disord* 1998;22:227–229.

46. Bradlow HL, Michnovicz JJ, Halper M, et al. Long-term responses of women to indole-3-carbinol or a high fiber diet. *Cancer Epidemiol Biomarkers Prev* 1994;3:591–595.

47. Wong GY, Bradlow L, Sepkovic D, et al. Dose-ranging study of indole-3-carbinol for breast cancer prevention. *J Cell Biochem Suppl* 1997;28–29:111–116.

48. Bradlow HL, Sepkovic DW, Telang NT, et al. Multifunctional aspects of the action of indole-3-carbinol as an antitumor agent. *Ann N Y Acad Sci* 1999;889:204–213.

49. Meyskens FL Jr., Surwit E, Moon TE, et al. Enhancement of regression of cervical intraepithelial neoplasia II (moderate dysplasia) with topical applied all-*trans*-retinoic acid: a randomized trial. *J Natl Cancer Inst* 1994;86:539–543.

50. Butterworth CE Jr., Hatch KD, Soong SJ, et al. Oral folic acid supplementation for cervical dysplasia: a clinical intervention trail. *Am J Obstet Gynecol* 1992;166:803–809.

51. Palan P, et al. Plasma levels of beta-carotene, lycopene, canthaxanthin, retinol, and alpha- and gamma-tocopherol in cervical intraepithelial neoplasia and cancer. *Clinical Cancer Research* 1996;2:181–185.

52. Morrow LE, Grimsley EW. Long-term diuretic therapy in hypertensive patients: effects on serum homocysteine, vitamin B6, vitamin B12, and red blood cell folate concentrations. *South Med J* 1999;92:866–870.

53. Lord RS, Bralley JA. *Laboratory Evaluations for Integrative and Functional Medicine* (Duluth: Metametrix Press, 2008).

54. Landgren F, et al. Plasma homocysteine in acute myocardial infarction: homocysteine-lowering effects of folic acid. *J Intern Med* 1995 Apr;237(4):381–388.

55. Monsen AL, Ueland PM. Homocysteine and methylmalonic acid in diagnosis and risk assessment from infancy to adolescence. *Am J Clin Nutr* 2003;78:7–21.

56. http://www.ncbi.nlm.nih.gov/books/bv.fcgi?rid=cm.chapter.3847

57. Klee GG. Cobalamin and folate evaluation: Measurement of methylmalonic acid and homocysteine vs vitamin B12 and folate. *Clinical Chemistry* 2000;46:1277–1283.

58. Klee GG. Department of Laboratory Medicine and Pathology, Mayo Clinic and Mayo Foundation, 200 First Street SW, Rochester, MN 55905. Fax 507-284-4542; e-mail klee.george@mayo.edu.

59. Stern LL, Bagley PJ, Rosenberg IH, Selhub J. Conversion of 5-formyltetrahydrofolic acid to 5-methyltetrahydrolic acid is unimpaired in folate adequate persons homozygous for the c677T mutation in the methylennetetrahydrofolate reductase gene. *J Nutr* 2000;130:2238–2242.

60. The World Cancer Research Fund International (WCRFI) and the American Institute for Cancer Research (AICR).

61. Hyman M. Paradigm shift: the end of "normal science" in medicine: understanding function in nutrition, health, and disease. *Alternative Therapies* 2004 Sept–Oct;10(5):90–94.

62. Epstein SE. *Cancer-Gate: How to Win the Losing Cancer War* (Amityville, NY: Baywood, 2005).

63. Baker SM. *Detoxification and Healing* (New York: McGraw Hill, 2004).

64. Yardley K. MNIMH. *British Journal of Phytotherapy* 2001;5(4).

65. Baker SM. *Folic Acid* (New Canaan, CT: Keats, 1995).

66. Baker SM. *Detoxification and Healing* (New York: McGraw Hill, 2004).

67. Herrero R, et al. A case-control study of nutrient status and invasive cervical cancer: I. Dietary indicators. *American Journal of Epidemiology* 1991 Dec 1;134(11):1335–1345.

68. VanEenwyk J, et al. Folate, vitamin C, and cervical intraepithelial neoplasia. *Cancer Epidemiol Biomarkers Prevention* 1992 Jan–Feb;1(2):119–124.

39 Colorectal Cancer

Nutrition for Primary and Secondary Prevention

Leah Gramlich, M.D., and Isaac Soo, M.D.

I. INTRODUCTION

Colorectal cancer is increasingly recognized as a condition that may impact longevity. It is a topic commonly discussed between patients and their primary care physician. Patients are increasingly knowledgeable of their health risks and the options available to them, such as various modalities for colorectal cancer screening. Less well known is the association between colorectal cancer risk and diet. Primary care physicians are positioned to counsel patients on diet changes and nutritional interventions that have been shown to affect both colon cancer occurrence and recurrence. This chapter will review what is known about diet and colorectal cancer (CRC) and will attempt to provide the primary care provider with up-to-date knowledge and insights into the role of diet and CRC.

II. EPIDEMIOLOGY

Diet and nutrient choices clearly impact outcome in primary, and possibly secondary, prevention in patients diagnosed with CRC. In a recent review, the working group of the World Cancer Research Fund identified that foods and nutrients have a significant effect on risk for CRC—certain foods and nutrients are associated with risk enhancement and others are associated with risk reduction. Incidence rates of colorectal cancer may relate to changing dietary habits with increased levels of affluence. For example, since the mid-1970s, as Japan, Singapore, and Eastern Europe began the transition from low- to high-income countries, their incidence rates of CRC have doubled.

III. NUTRIENTS AND INCREASED RISK

The vast majority of CRC develops in older individuals over a period of several years through an accumulation of genetic mutations within colonic mucosa. Genomic instability creates a permissive state in which a cell acquires enough mutations to be transformed into a cancer cell. These cumulative effects upon tumor suppressors, oncogenes, and mismatch repair genes manifest as the adenoma to carcinoma sequence. Food and nutrition have a highly important role in the prevention and causation of cancers of the colon and rectum.

RED AND PROCESSED MEATS

Increased red meat/processed meat intake demonstrates the strongest correlation with CRC development. Numerous epidemiological studies have reported this link. Though the risk reduction benefit with decreased meat intake varies between studies, the presence of increased risk with meat intake is consistent. For example, the World Cancer Research Fund (WCRF) reports increases of 50 g of red meat or 50 g of processed meat per day that are associated with 15% and 21% increased risk of CRC, respectively. The National Institute of Environmental Medicine in Stockholm, Sweden, compared individuals with high- and low-meat intake. Those in the highest category of red meat or processed meat had a 28% and 20% increased risk, respectively, of colon and rectal cancer compared to those with the lowest amount of intake.[1] Lastly, the International Agency for Research on Cancer in Lyon, France, determined a reduction of 70 g/week of average meat intake would hypothetically reduce colorectal cancer risk by 11.9% to 25% in men and 7.5% to 17.2% in women from countries where meat consumption is very high.[2]

Precipitants of increased CRC risk from meat intake have been proposed ranging from fat to ammonia content. Among the most well studied include N-nitroso compound exposure, heterocyclic amines, and polycyclic aromatic hydrocarbons. The latter two are byproducts of meat cooked at high temperatures. High temperatures cause reactions between creatinine, creatine, amino acids, and sugars to generate heterocyclic amines (HCAs). As both cooking temperature increases or duration extends, there is correspondent increased production of HCA.[3] Dose-dependent administration of HCA induced colonic tumor formation in rats,[4] and DNA adducts in both animal models and humans.[5] Polycyclic aromatic hydrocarbons (PAH) are related to both the cooking of red meat as well as its processing. When meat is grilled, smoked, or charcoal-broiled, PAH forms and adheres to the surface of the meat. Of the red meats, grilled or well-done steak and hamburgers have been found to possess the highest levels. A group of chemicals not related to preparation method is N-nitroso compounds (NOCs). These have the ability to react with DNA of target tissues and possibly initiate carcinogenesis.[6] Multiple studies have found a dose-response between the amount of meat ingested and increased N-nitroso compound fecal level.[7] The heme content of red meat may also play a role. Heme-fed rats demonstrated destruction of the colonic epithelium with resultant hyperproliferation.[8] Iron itself is unlikely to be a contributing factor as tumors in rats fed beef did not differ significantly from those fed casein, despite having higher serum iron levels.[9]

ALCOHOL

Alcohol ingestion is associated with CRC. The International Agency for Research on Cancer in Lyon, France, analyzed 16 prospective cohort studies including 6300 patients with CRC. A 15% increased risk for colorectal cancer was found per 100 g of alcohol per week. To put this in perspective, the risk of colorectal cancer is increased by 9% for every 10 g ethanol/day. Notably, beverage type has no influence on risk. The pathophysiologic effects of alcohol ingestion are attributable to ethanol content. However, unlike red and processed meats, the impact of alcohol ingestion varied across study cohorts. For example, alcohol has greater effects on CRC risk in people of Asian descent.[10] This likely relates to genetic differences between cohorts.

Carcinogenic mechanisms of alcohol are less well studied than for meat consumption. Central to alcohol's harmful effects are likely the products of ethanol metabolism. Acetaldehyde is generated by alcohol dehydrogenase with ethanol as the enzymatic substrate. Free radicals are also produced, which may bind to cell components and possibly DNA. The potential negative effects of acetaldehyde include suppression of DNA repair mechanisms and methylation of cytosine in DNA, interrupting the cell cycle and producing carcinogenic effects. The importance of acetaldehyde is supported by a study of a Japanese cohort that found possessors of the lesser active aldehyde dehydrogenase (ALDH2) allele had increased acetaldehyde levels and, interestingly, higher risk for colorectal cancer.[11]

There is also a suggestion of increased risk of colorectal cancer with foods containing iron, cheese, animal fats, and sugars. However, studies are limited and further investigation is required.

IV. NUTRIENTS AND PRIMARY PREVENTION

FIBER

One of the most widely studied food products proposed to reduce CRC risk is fiber. Despite several large-scale cohort studies and meta-analyses, findings remain inconclusive. The European Prospective Investigation into Cancer and Nutrition (EPIC) study examined 519,978 individuals from 10 European countries and found dietary intake in fiber protected against development of colon cancer.[12] Similarly, the Prostate, Lung, Colorectal and Ovarian Screening Trial Project Team found reduced risks of distal colonic adenomas were associated with fiber from grains and fruits.[13] However, equally large studies have refuted the benefit of fiber, including prospective studies conducted in Japan[14] and the United States.[15,16] A potential explanation for discordance between these very large epidemiological studies may stem from ingestion of different fiber sources. One of the inherent difficulties with studying the impact of nutrition on cancer risk is differing dietary habits between cohorts. In an attempt to homogenize the definitions of what constitutes grain or fiber, a group from Harvard University conducted a pooled analysis of prospective studies. By doing so, they recategorized original data into new food group classifications for their meta-analysis. In the pooled analysis, grain ingestion, a fiber subgroup, was found to be associated with decreased CRC risk.[13,15] Grain products include barley, oat, rice, and wheat. Similarly, 60,000 women demonstrated a 35% decrease in CRC risk with increased whole grain consumption.[17] There is a possibility that the benefit of grain ingestion is achieved at a baseline level of ingestion. A prospective cohort study of 62,609 men and 70,554 women did not find an association between higher intake of grains and decreased cancer risk, but did identify increased cancer risk among those with very low rates of fiber ingestion.[18] The effect of supplemental fiber has not been found to reduce risk of colorectal adenomas. A systematic review and meta-analysis conducted by the Cochrane database of systematic reviews found intervention with wheat bran fiber, ispaghula husk, or dietary intervention with high-fiber diet to have no effect on the incidence or recurrence of adenomas in a 2- to 4-year span.[19]

Numerous mechanisms have been proposed as the possible protective mechanism of fiber/grains. By increasing stool bulk there may be decreased interaction between fecal carcinogens and the colonic epithelium.[20] Fiber may exert its beneficial effects by attenuating the carcinogenic effect of bile acids. Bile acids have been shown to play an important role in progression of colon cancer. It produces a proliferation-inducing effect on colonic mucosa described by epidemiological studies[21,22] and further confirmed by basic science studies. Deoxycholic acid, a bile acid component, stimulates proteosomal tumor suppressor gene degradation, leading to a tumor-promoting, anti-apoptotic effect.[23] To counter this, once ingested, fiber fermentation may produce short chain fatty acids (SCFA), lowering intestinal pH and reducing bile acid carcinogenic activity. For example, in rats, butyrate has been found to be anti-neoplastic.[24] Chronic inflammation has been linked to CRC development and fiber may exert a beneficial role via anti-inflammatory properties. A colitic mouse model, HLA B27, had attenuation of their inflammatory markers with fiber treatment. Higher levels of SCFA were found in the colitic fiber-treated model and in vitro studies found they possessed a synergistic inhibitory effect on TNFa, a pro-inflammatory cytokine.[25] A small study on humans found fiber supplementation was able to reduce levels of C-reactive protein, a nonspecific marker in inflammation.[26] Whole grains also contain many antioxidants, and may prevent cancer development by preventing oxidative damage.

FRUITS AND VEGETABLES

Diets rich in fruit, yellow and dark green vegetables, and onions were found to be associated with reduced colorectal cancer precursors, adenomas.[27] However, a study involving 45,490 women found no association between fruit and vegetable intake to colorectal cancer risk.[28] Similar findings were identified in Japanese cohorts of 47,605 and 40,106 men and women[29,30] as well as an American study of 36,976 women older than 44 years.[31] There may be benefit with a baseline consumption of fruits and vegetables, and no further benefit conferred with additional ingestion. Five-year follow-up of 488,043 men and women found men with very low intake of vegetables and total fruits and vegetables in fact had increased colorectal cancer risks,[32] as did a study of 62,609 men and 70,554 women in the Cancer Prevention Study II Nutrition Cohort.[18] In the prospective mammography screening study of women in Sweden, individuals with less than 1.5 servings of fruit and vegetables had a relative risk of 1.65 compared to those with more than 2.5 servings.[33]

In addition to its bulk-forming, fiber-like effect, the potential protective effects of vegetables and fruits may stem from a variety of anticarcinogenic substances including carotenoids, vitamins C and E, selenium, fiber, dithiolthiones, glucosinolates, indoles, isothiocyanates, flavonoids, phenols, protease inhibitors, plant sterols, allium compounds, and limonene. The actions of these substances include induction of detoxification enzymes and nitrosamine formation, substrates for antineoplastic agents, alteration of hormone metabolism, and antioxidant effects, among others.[34]

CALCIUM AND VITAMIN D

Calcium and vitamin D are commonly taken for bone health but their beneficial effects may extend to CRC risk reduction. A 5-year study of 60,866 men and 66,883 women found calcium supplementation to reduce risk of colorectal cancer.[35] However, this has been refuted a by randomized controlled trial in which 36,282 postmenopausal women received supplementation with 500 mg elemental calcium with 200 international units of vitamin D twice daily with no effect on colorectal cancer rates.[36] The study authors noted that the study duration may not have been long enough to detect an effect. This is a possibility considering calcium supplementation may benefit in preventing adenoma recurrence as discussed in the following. Often taken with calcium, supplementation with vitamin D 1000 to 2000 IU/day reduces risk by 50% with serum levels >33 ng/mL compared to 12 ng/mL.[37,38]

Similar to fiber, calcium and vitamin D may exert anticarcinogenic effects by binding to bile acids.[39] Calcium may also possess an antiproliferative, apoptotic induction ability on colonic cells. Though the cellular mechanism has not been delineated and what has been described is much more complex than afforded here, study results suggest that calcium has both indirect and direct effects on cellular signaling. In general terms, by activating calcium-sensitive receptors, precancerous cells may be rerouted to produce a well-differentiated cell. Analagously, vitamin D also exerts its anticarcinogenic effects through vitamin D receptors and activation of diverse signaling pathways that include effects on calcium flux and calcium signaling pathways. Vitamin D sufficiency has been associated with apoptosis, and in its absence there is failure of apoptosis and propogation of tumor growth. Vitamin D also prevents angiogenesis, thereby reducing the potential for the malignant cell to survive. In sum, effects on cell differentiation and apoptosis of colonic cells is enhanced by both calcium and vitamin D.[40]

MISCELLANEOUS

Other less well studied food products that may decrease CRC risk include garlic [41] and selenium, but these findings are inconclusive.

TABLE 39.1
Pathophysiologic Mechanisms of Dietary Components on CRC Development

CRC Risk	Food Type	Pathophysiology
Increased	Red and processed meat	• Heterocyclic amines and polycyclic aromatic hydrocarbons generated by grilling, smoking, or charcoal-broiled meat have been found to cause mutations in rats. • Ingestion creates additional N-nitroso compounds, which are alkylating agents with ability to react with DNA or tissue. • Dietary heme iron demonstrates fecal cytotoxicity and induces colonic hyperproliferation in rat studies.
	Ethanol	• Free radical production via acetaldehyde generation via alcohol dehydrogenase.
Decreased	Fiber	• Generates stool bulk to produce decreased interaction between fecal carcinogens and colonocytes. • Short chain fatty acids produced by fiber fermentation may alter pH of the colon and decrease bile acid carcinogenic activity. • Exert anti-inflammatory and antioxidant effects.
	Fruits and vegetables	• Possess an array of chemicals that may have antioxidant, detoxification, and hormone-altering effects.
	Calcium/vitamin D	• Calcium may bind bile acids, preventing their carcinogenic effect. • Both are involved in cellular signaling leading to cell differentiation or apoptosis.

V. NUTRIENTS AND SECONDARY PREVENTION

The impact of diet on colorectal cancer is not limited to primary prevention. A group of 1009 patients with stage III colon cancer without cancer recurrence 3 months following completion of a clinical trial were observed for influence of dietary pattern on recurrence-free survival. Patients with a "Western dietary pattern," including red meat, processed meats, sweets and desserts, French fries, and refined grains had increased colon cancer recurrence and mortality. Patients in the highest quintile of Western dietary pattern were 2.9 times more likely to recur compared to those in the lowest quintile. In contrast, no association between overall survival or recurrence-free survival was seen in patients with a "prudent diet," high in fruit, vegetables, whole grains, legumes, poultry, and fish.[42] Though preliminary, other potentially beneficial dietary changes include calcium supplementation; 1200 mg/day for 3 years resulted in decreased recurrence in patients with a history of colorectal adenoma.[43] This was seen again in a randomized clinical trial of 1200 mg elemental calcium per day,[44,45] though the protective effect may be limited to individuals with adequate vitamin D levels.[46] The beneficial effect of calcium supplementation was seen to last 5 years following discontinuation.[45] Notable food products that have not been found to improve CRC recurrence include dietary supplementation of wheat-bran fiber,[47,48] nor has a low-fat, high-fiber, fruit and vegetable diet.[49]

Nutrient effects on CRC risk and pathophysiological mechanisms are summarized in Table 39.1.

VI. COMORBID CONDITIONS

The risk of developing CRC rises sharply after 40 years of age, with 90% of cancers occurring in persons 50 years or older. The current evidence strongly indicates that the majority of colorectal cancers arise from preexisting adenomas and that risk correlates with number and size of adenomas. Dietary pattern such as Western or prudent may impact whether adenomas undergo transformation to malignant lesions. Individuals who have one carcinoma are at risk for synchronous or metachronous lesions. Family history of colonic polyps or CRC, particularly if they occur at a young age or occur in more than one first-degree relative, is associated with an increased risk for CRC. Correlation of CRC and inflammatory bowel disease relates to the duration of the inflammatory bowel disease and the presence of dysplastic colonic epithelium. In animal studies, diversion of bile to the colon increases the yield of tumor in carcinogen-treated animals. By analogy, cholecystectomy in humans may have the same effect but this has not been seen in human studies.

More recently an impressive body of literature indicates that CRC risk is elevated in those with metabolic syndrome.[8] Underlying risk factors for metabolic syndrome include physical inactivity and obesity, especially abdominal or visceral obesity. The evidence that physical activity is a protective factor for CRC is strong and consistent.[9] This association has been observed in prospective and case-controlled studies, for men and women, for occupational and leisure time activities, and in a wide spectrum of populations. Physical inactivity is becoming widely accepted as a risk factor for CRC.

Increasing body fatness, as measured by Body Mass Index (BMI), is associated with an increased risk for CRC in the majority of studies. The strength of the association between obesity and CRC is generally stronger for men than for women. The World Cancer Research Fund identifies a 15% risk increase for every 5 kg/m^2. In addition, abdominal adiposity, as assessed by waist circumference or increased waist-to-hip ratios, is yet another indicator of increased risk.

Adult onset diabetes has also recently been identified as an independent risk factor for CRC and adenomas and in a recent meta-analysis, the relative risk for CRC in diabetics was 1.43.[17] This strong association has been seen in non-Caucasians, males, and females.

Biologically plausible roles exist for a relationship between CRC and hyperglycemia and hyper-insulinemia, perhaps through insulin-like growth factors, creating an environment that encourages carcinogenesis and discourages apoptosis.

VII. PATIENT EVALUATION

The primary care physician may be seeing a patient who has symptoms of CRC or for consideration of screening for CRC based on risk. Given this presenting history, it may not be intuitive, but it is very important to get a weight history and a diet history as well as a history of activity. Similarly, BMI should be calculated and a waist circumference checked.

Colorectal cancer symptoms include abdominal pain, altering bowel habits, melena/hematochezia, fatigue, and weight loss. A considerable proportion of patients also present with metastatic disease to the liver or lungs, which manifests as dyspnea or right upper quadrant pain. Evidence of iron deficiency anemia is an important red flag, especially in individuals over the age of 50. However, unfortunately, presence of clinical signs and symptoms in CRC manifest in advanced disease with poor prognosis. Lack of early disease detection by physical exam and laboratory findings is one of the reasons the approach to CRC is largely preventative. Early detection of disease is best achieved by adherence to recommendations of colon cancer screening.

The purpose of CRC screening is to detect early disease and identify premalignant conditions such as polyp formation. Numerous modalities are available and the decision of when or who to screen for CRC is influenced by a patient's pretest risk. As above, certain individuals are considered high risk, including those with a history of inflammatory bowel disease, a personal or family history of CRC, an adenomatous polyp, or a genetic predisposition to CRC such as familial adenomatous polyposis (FAP) and hereditary non-polyposis colorectal cancer (HNPCC). These individuals require referral and close follow-up with a gastroenterologist.

For average risk individuals, CRC screening should be initiated at the age of 50. Current modalities include recommendations either for: (1) annual fecal occult blood test (FOBT), (2) flexible sigmoidoscopy every 5 years, (3) annual FOBT and flexible sigmoidoscopy every 5 years, (4) double contrast barium enema (DCBE) every 5 years, or (5) colonoscopy every 10 years. The decision of which test to undergo should be a discussion between the patient and physician. Depending on the findings, positive tests will require follow-up investigations. For a positive FOBT or DCBE, a colonoscopy will be required for diagnosis or possible intervention. In the absence of notable pathology, the suggested intervals for screening are as listed previously.

VIII.   TREATMENT RECOMMENDATIONS

Treatment recommendations for patients interested in primary or secondary prevention of CRC need to include advice regarding goals for weight and physical activity in addition to specific dietary recommendations. Recommendations should be built upon what is known regarding the relationship between CRC and diet (Table 39.2). In an individual concerned about the risk of CRC, there is convincing evidence that physical activity decreases risk and that red meats, processed meat, alcoholic drinks (in men), and body fatness increase risk. Patients should be advised that there is a probable risk reduction from intake of foods containing fiber, garlic, milk, and calcium.

More specific recommendations to patients should include a target BMI between 20 and 25 kg/m^2—patients should strive for leanness without being underweight. In order to help achieve this goal, individuals should avoid sugary, high-energy-dense foods and beverages. With respect to activity, adults should engage in at least moderate physical activity for 30 minutes or more on 5 or more days of the week. Forty-five minutes or more of moderate to vigorous activity on 5 or more days of the week may further enhance the reduction in risk of colorectal cancer.[50] This activity can be undertaken in the context of either work or recreational activity.

The WCRF evaluated 16 cohort and 71 case control studies evaluating the relationship between red meat intake and CRC risk and nearly all the cohort studies showed increased risk with higher intake. Specific recommendations are to limit red meat intake to less than 500 gm cooked (700 to 750 gm uncooked) meat per week and to limit intake of salty or processed meats.

Dietary fiber refers to carbohydrates that cannot be digested. It is present in all plants that are eaten for food, including fruits, vegetables, grains, and legumes. For many years healthcare providers have been suggesting that consumption of a high-fiber diet would reduce the risk of colorectal cancer. More recently, however, larger and better designed studies have failed to show this link. Despite the lack of effect on CRC risk, a diet high in fiber can obviate many of the symptoms that can be confused with symptoms of colorectal cancer such as constipation and symptoms from diverticular disease. In the absence of effect on CRC risk, fiber is an important part of a healthy diet and dietary intakes should be at minimum 25 to 30 g/day for adults. The best sources are whole grains, legumes and nuts, fruits, and vegetables.

There is little or no evidence to support the use of vitamin supplements to reduce CRC risk. A few micronutrients, perhaps, deserve special mention. There is a body of literature that suggests that increases in dietary folate intake may be associated with reduction in CRC risk. There are data from cohort studies with a dose-response relationship but there is some inconsistency in the data. More recently, a randomized controlled trial of folic acid at 1 mg/day for up to 6 years did not reduce the risk of colorectal adenomas, precursors of CRC. Interestingly, this study suggested that there was equivocal evidence for an increase in adenoma risk that requires further investigation, particularly in view of the fortification of the U.S. food supply with folate.[51] Vitamin D is another micronutrient that may be relevant in colorectal cancer prevention. It must be recognized that the effects of calcium and vitamin D are strongly interrelated and that vitamin D status in a given individual is influenced by the latitude at which they reside. People living at higher latitudes are at increased risk for CRC and are more likely to die from the disease than those living at lower latitudes. In addition, the prevalence of vitamin D deficiency is higher at higher latitudes.[52] Given that the evidence supporting the role of vitamin D in reducing the risk of CRC is not robust but that the risk of deficiency is high and that it plays a role in morbidity from other causes, supplementation may be considered.

The previous discussion is relevant for individuals who want to reduce the risk of CRC occurring (primary prevention). In addition, CRC survivors should also follow the guidelines for CRC prevention as this has been found to be associated with reduction in risk of recurrence.

The WCRF guidelines are consistent with the Dietary Guidelines for Americans 2005. Key concepts identified in the most recent Dietary Guidelines (2005) identify maintenance of weight in a healthy range, balancing energy from food and beverages, prevention of gradual weight gain, intake of adequate nutrients within energy needs, physical activity of at least 30 min/day, and adherence

TABLE 39.2
Food Nutrition and Physical Activity and Colorectal Cancer

	Decreases Risk	Increases Risk
Convincing	Physical activity[a,b]	Red meat[c,d]
		Processed meat[d,e]
		Alcoholic drinks (men)[f]
		Body fatness
		Abdominal fatness
Probable	Foods containing dietary fiber[g]	Alcoholic drinks (women)[f]
	Garlic[h]	
	Milk[i,j]	
	Calcium[k]	
Limited	Nonstarch vegetables[h]	Foods containing iron[d,g]
(suggestive)	Fruits[h]	Cheese[i]
	Foods containing folate[g]	Foods containing animal fats[g]
	Foods containing selenium[g]	Foods containing sugars[n]
	Fish	
	Foods containing vitamin D[g,l]	
	Selenium[m]	
Limited	Cereals (grains) and their products; potatoes; poultry; shellfish and other seafood;	
(no conclusion)	other dairy products; total fat; fatty acid composition; cholesterol; sugar	
	(sucrose); coffee; tea; caffeine; total carbohydrate; starch; vitamin A; retinol;	
	vitamin C; vitamin E; multivitamins; nondairy sources of calcium; methionine;	
	beta-carotene; alpha-carotene; lycopene; meal frequency; energy intake	
Substantial effect on risk unlikely	None identified	

Source: [53].

Notes:

[a] Physical activity of all types: occupational, household, transport and recreational.

[b] Much of the evidence reviewed grouped colon cancer and rectal cancer together as "colorectal" cancer. The Panel judges that the evidence is stronger for colon than for rectum.

[c] The term "red meat" refers to beef, pork, lamb, and goat from domesticated animals.

[d] Although red and processed meats contain iron, the general category of "foods containing iron" comprises many other foods, including those of plant origin.

[e] The term "processed meat" refers to meats preserved by smoking, curing, or salting, or addition of chemical preservatives.

[f] The judgments for men and women are different because there are fewer data for women. Increased risk is only apparent about a threshold of 30 g/day of ethanol for both sexes.

[g] Includes both foods naturally containing the constituent and foods that have the constituent added. Dietary fiber is contained in plant foods.

[h] Judgments on vegetables and fruits do not include those preserved by salting and/or pickling.

[i] Although both milk and cheese are included in the general category of dairy products, their different nutritional composition and consumption patterns may result in different findings.

[j] Milk from cows. Most data are from high-income populations, where calcium can be taken to be a marker for milk/dairy consumption. The Panel judges that a higher intake of dietary calcium is one way in which milk could have a protective effect.

[k] The evidence is derived from studies using supplements at a dose of 1200 mg/daily.

[l] Found mostly in fortified foods and animal foods.

[m] The evidence is derived from studies using supplements at a dose of 200 ug/day. Selenium is toxic at high doses.

[n] "Sugars" here mean all "non-milk extrinsic" sugars, including refined and other added sugars, honey, and as contained in fruit juices and syrups. It does not include sugars naturally present in whole foods such as fruits. It also does not include lactose as contained in animal or human milks.

to a diet with less than 35% of energy from fat. The guidelines for meat and alternatives intake suggest 1 to 2 servings (3 oz) meat or poultry (skinless) per day, with a preferred cooking method being either to boil, roast, or broil meat.

Patients who have a diagnosis of cancer are often highly motivated to change behavior. This represents an opportunity for the primary care provider to guide the patient relative to behaviors that can reduce risk of cancer occurrence and recurrence and that may also have an impact on primary and secondary prevention of other chronic diseases.

IX. SUMMARY

Nutrition clearly has an impact on CRC occurrence and recurrence, with nutritional factors playing a role that may increase or decrease risk, based on biologically plausible mechanisms. Data will continue to accumulate that may allow us to refine nutritional recommendations. Currently, based on existing evidence, it is reasonable to suggest the following:

* Limit consumption of red meat.
* If alcohol is consumed, limit to less than 2 drinks/day in men and 1 drink/day in women.
* Increase amount and variety of fruit, vegetables, whole grains, and pulses (beans).
* Be lean without being underweight.
* Be physically active for at least 30 min/day.
* Avoid sugary, energy-dense foods and beverages.
* Limit consumption of salty and prepared foods.
* After treatment, cancer survivors should follow recommendations for cancer prevention.

REFERENCES

1. Larsson SC, Wolk A. Meat consumption and risk of colorectal cancer: a meta-analysis of prospective studies. *International Journal of Cancer* 2006;119(11):2657–64.
2. Norat T, Lukanova A, Ferrari P, et al. Meat consumption and colorectal cancer risk: dose-response meta-analysis of epidemiological studies. *International Journal of Cancer* 2002;98(2):241–56.
3. Lynch AM, Knize MG, Boobis AR, et al. Intra- and interindividual variability in systemic exposure in humans to 2-amino-3,8-dimethylimidazo[4,5-f]quinoxaline and 2-amino-1-methyl- 6-phenylimidazo[4,5-b] pyridine, carcinogens present in cooked beef. *Cancer Research* 1992;52(22):6216–23.
4. Ito N, Hasegawa R, Imaida K, et al. Carcinogenicity of 2-amino-1-methyl-6-phenylimidazo[4,5-b]pyridine (PhIP) in the rat. *Mutation Research* 1997;376(1–2):107–14.
5. Schut HA, Snyderwine EG. DNA adducts of heterocyclic amine food mutagens: implications for mutagenesis and carcinogenesis. *Carcinogenesis* 1999;20(3):353–68.
6. Saffhill R, Margison GP, O'Connor PJ. Mechanisms of carcinogenesis induced by alkylating agents. *Biochimica et Biophysica Acta* 1985;823(2):111–45.
7. Hughes R, Cross AJ, Pollock JR, et al. Dose-dependent effect of dietary meat on endogenous colonic N-nitrosation. *Carcinogenesis* 2001;22(1):199–202.
8. Sesink AL, Termont DS, Kleibeuker JH, et al. Red meat and colon cancer: the cytotoxic and hyperproliferative effects of dietary heme. *Cancer Research* 1999;59(22):5704–9.
9. Lai C, Dunn DM, Miller MF, et al. Non-promoting effects of iron from beef in the rat colon carcinogenesis model. *Cancer Letters* 1997;112(1):87–91.
10. Moskal A, Norat T, Ferrari P, et al. Alcohol intake and colorectal cancer risk: a dose-response meta-analysis of published cohort studies. *International Journal of Cancer* 2007;120(3):664–71.
11. Murata M, Tagawa M, Watanabe S, et al. Genotype difference of aldehyde dehydrogenase 2 gene in alcohol drinkers influences the incidence of Japanese colorectal cancer patients. *Japanese Journal of Cancer Research* 1999;90(7):711–19.
12. Bingham SA, Day NE, Luben R, et al. Dietary fibre in food and protection against colorectal cancer in the European Prospective Investigation into Cancer and Nutrition (EPIC): an observational study. *Lancet* 2003;361(9368):1496–1501.

13. Peters U, Sinha R, Chatterjee N, et al. Dietary fibre and colorectal adenoma in a colorectal cancer early detection programme. *Lancet* 2003;361(9368):1491–95.

14. Otani T, Iwasaki M, Ishihara J, et al. Dietary fiber intake and subsequent risk of colorectal cancer: the Japan Public Health Center-based prospective study. *International Journal of Cancer* 2006;119(6):1475–80.

15. Park Y, Hunter DJ, Spiegelman D, et al. Dietary fiber intake and risk of colorectal cancer: a pooled analysis of prospective cohort studies. *JAMA* 2005;294(22):2849–57.

16. Michels KB, Fuchs CS, Giovannucci E, et al. Fiber intake and incidence of colorectal cancer among 76,947 women and 47,279 men. *Cancer Epidemiology, Biomarkers & Prevention* 2005;14(4):842–49.

17. Larsson SC, Giovannucci E, Bergkvist L, et al. Whole grain consumption and risk of colorectal cancer: a population-based cohort of 60,000 women. *British Journal of Cancer* 2005;92(9):1803–7.

18. McCullough ML, Robertson AS, Chao A, et al. A prospective study of whole grains, fruits, vegetables and colon cancer risk. *Cancer Causes & Control* 2003;14(10):959–70.

19. Asano T, McLeod RS, Asano T, McLeod RS. Dietary fibre for the prevention of colorectal adenomas and carcinomas. *Cochrane Database of Systematic Reviews* 2002;(2):CD003430.

20. Cummings JH, Bingham SA, Heaton KW, et al. Fecal weight, colon cancer risk, and dietary intake of nonstarch polysaccharides (dietary fiber). *Gastroenterology* 1992;103(6):1783–89.

21. Hill MJ, Drasar BS, Williams RE, et al. Faecal bile-acids and clostridia in patients with cancer of the large bowel. *Lancet* 1975;1(7906):535–39.

22. Reddy BS, Wynder EL. Metabolic epidemiology of colon cancer. Fecal bile acids and neutral sterols in colon cancer patients and patients with adenomatous polyps. *Cancer* 1977;39(6):2533–39.

23. Qiao D, Gaitonde SV, Qi W, et al. Deoxycholic acid suppresses p53 by stimulating proteasome-mediated p53 protein degradation. *Carcinogenesis* 2001;22(6):957–64.

24. McIntyre A, Gibson PR, Young GP. Butyrate production from dietary fibre and protection against large bowel cancer in a rat model. *Gut* 1993;34(3):386–91.

25. Rodriguez-Cabezas ME, Galvez J, Camuesco D, et al. Intestinal anti-inflammatory activity of dietary fiber (Plantago ovata seeds) in HLA-B27 transgenic rats. *Clinical Nutrition* 2003;22(5):463–71.

26. King DE, Egan BM, Woolson RF, et al. Effect of a high-fiber diet vs a fiber-supplemented diet on C-reactive protein level. *Archives of Internal Medicine* 2007;167(5):502–6.

27. Millen AE, Subar AF, Graubard BI, et al. Fruit and vegetable intake and prevalence of colorectal adenoma in a cancer screening trial. *American Journal of Clinical Nutrition* 2007;86(6):1754–64.

28. Flood A, Velie EM, Chaterjee N, et al. Fruit and vegetable intakes and the risk of colorectal cancer in the Breast Cancer Detection Demonstration Project follow-up cohort. *American Journal of Clinical Nutrition* 2002;75(5):936–43.

29. Sato Y, Tsubono Y, Nakaya N, et al. Fruit and vegetable consumption and risk of colorectal cancer in Japan: The Miyagi Cohort Study. *Public Health Nutrition* 2005;8(3):309–14.

30. Tsubono Y, Otani T, Kobayashi M, et al. No association between fruit or vegetable consumption and the risk of colorectal cancer in Japan. *British Journal of Cancer* 2005;92(9):1782–84.

31. Lin J, Zhang SM, Cook NR, et al. Dietary intakes of fruit, vegetables, and fiber, and risk of colorectal cancer in a prospective cohort of women (United States). *Cancer Causes & Control* 2005;16(3):225–33.

32. Park Y, Subar AF, Kipnis V, et al. Fruit and vegetable intakes and risk of colorectal cancer in the NIH-AARP diet and health study. *American Journal of Epidemiology* 2007;166(2):170–80.

33. Terry P, Giovannucci E, Michels KB, et al. Fruit, vegetables, dietary fiber, and risk of colorectal cancer. *Journal of the National Cancer Institute* 2001;93(7):525–33.

34. Steinmetz KA, Potter JD. Vegetables, fruit, and cancer. II. Mechanisms. *Cancer Causes & Control* 1991;2(6):427–42.

35. McCullough ML, Robertson AS, Rodriguez C, et al. Calcium, vitamin D, dairy products, and risk of colorectal cancer in the Cancer Prevention Study II Nutrition Cohort (United States). *Cancer Causes & Control* 2003;14(1):1–12.

36. Wactawski-Wende J, Kotchen JM, Anderson GL, et al. Calcium plus vitamin D supplementation and the risk of colorectal cancer. *New England Journal of Medicine* 2006;354(7):684–96.

37. Gorham ED, Garland CF, Garland FC, et al. Optimal vitamin D status for colorectal cancer prevention: a quantitative meta analysis. *American Journal of Preventive Medicine* 2007;32(3):210–16.

38. Gorham ED, Garland CF, Garland FC, et al. Vitamin D and prevention of colorectal cancer. *Journal of Steroid Biochemistry & Molecular Biology* 2005;97(1–2):179–94.

39. Newmark HL, Wargovich MJ, Bruce WR, Newmark HL, Wargovich MJ, Bruce WR. Colon cancer and dietary fat, phosphate, and calcium: a hypothesis. *Journal of the National Cancer Institute* 1984;72(6):1323–25.

40. Lamprecht SA, Lipkin M, Lamprecht SA, Lipkin M. Cellular mechanisms of calcium and vitamin D in the inhibition of colorectal carcinogenesis. *Annals of the New York Academy of Sciences* 2001;952:73–87.

41. Ngo SN, Williams DB, Cobiac L, et al. Does garlic reduce risk of colorectal cancer? A systematic review. *Journal of Nutrition* 2007;137(10):2264–69.

42. Meyerhardt JA, Niedzwiecki D, Hollis D, et al. Association of dietary patterns with cancer recurrence and survival in patients with stage III colon cancer. *JAMA* 2007;298(7):754–64.

43. Bonithon-Kopp C, Kronborg O, Giacosa A, et al. Calcium and fibre supplementation in prevention of colorectal adenoma recurrence: a randomised intervention trial. European Cancer Prevention Organisation Study Group. *Lancet* 2000;356(9238):1300–1306.

44. Baron JA, Beach M, Mandel JS, et al. Calcium supplements for the prevention of colorectal adenomas. Calcium Polyp Prevention Study Group. *New England Journal of Medicine* 1999;340(2):101–7.

45. Grau MV, Baron JA, Sandler RS, et al. Prolonged effect of calcium supplementation on risk of colorectal adenomas in a randomized trial. *Journal of the National Cancer Institute* 2007;99(2):129–36.

46. Grau MV, Baron JA, Sandler RS, et al. Vitamin D, calcium supplementation, and colorectal adenomas: results of a randomized trial. *Journal of the National Cancer Institute* 2003;95(23):1765–71.

47. Alberts DS, Martinez ME, Roe DJ, et al. Lack of effect of a high-fiber cereal supplement on the recurrence of colorectal adenomas. Phoenix Colon Cancer Prevention Physicians' Network. *New England Journal of Medicine* 2000;342(16):1156–62.

48. Jacobs ET, Giuliano AR, Roe DJ, et al. Intake of supplemental and total fiber and risk of colorectal adenoma recurrence in the wheat bran fiber trial. *Cancer Epidemiology, Biomarkers & Prevention* 2002;11(9):906–14.

49. Schatzkin A, Lanza E, Corle D, et al. Lack of effect of a low-fat, high-fiber diet on the recurrence of colorectal adenomas. Polyp Prevention Trial Study Group. *New England Journal of Medicine* 2000;342(16):1149–55.

50. Byers T, Nestle M, McTiernan A, et al. American Cancer Society guidelines on nutrition and physical activity for cancer prevention: reducing the risk of cancer with healthy food choices and physical activity. *CA: A Cancer Journal for Clinicians* 2002;52(2):92–119.

51. Cole BF, Baron JA, Sandler RS, et al. Folic acid for the prevention of colorectal adenomas: a randomized clinical trial. *JAMA* 2007;297(21):2351–59.

52. Holick MF, Holick MF. Vitamin D deficiency. *New England Journal of Medicine* 2007;357(3):266–81.

53. World Cancer Research Fund/American Institute for Cancer Research. *Food, Nutrition, Physical Activity, and the Prevention of Cancer: A Global Perspective*. Washington, DC: WCRF/AICR, 2007.

40 Prostate Cancer

Nutrients That May Slow
Its Progression

Aaron E. Katz, M.D., and
Geovanni Espinosa, N.D., M.S.

I. INTRODUCTION

Prostate cancer (CaP) remains one of the most frequently diagnosed cancers in men in Western countries for the past decade. The number of new cases projected to be diagnosed in the United States alone in 2007 was estimated at 218, 890, with 27,000 deaths expected from the disease [1]. Detection of this disease earlier, as a consequence of introduction of the prostate specific antigen (PSA) blood test, has been acknowledged by the National Cancer Institute (NCI) as one factor contributing to lowering the mortality rate over the past few years [2–5]. In the mid to late-1980s only one-third of prostate cancers were diagnosed at curable stages compared with today when 80% are staged clinically as organ-confined and potentially curable [6–9]. Unfortunately, however, even when the tumor is thought to be localized, up to 25% of men have nonlocalized disease, which declares itself subsequently [10]. Nutrition can possibly slow the rate of disease progression to the point that the disease has no clinical relevance; conversely, poor nutrition may accelerate disease and reduce life and its quality dramatically. This chapter evaluates food, nutrients, and the role of antioxidants in general in delaying cancer of the prostate (CaP).

II. EPIDEMIOLOGY

Although the rates vary widely between countries, it is least common in South and East Asia, more common in Europe, and most common in the United States [11]. In the United States, prostate cancer is least common among Asian American men and most common among Black men, with figures for White men in-between [12, 13]. However, these high rates may be affected by increasing rates of detection [14]. Ecological studies have implicated a Western diet in CaP development. Asian immigrants, who often adopt a Western diet, show an increased incidence of CaP, thought to be related to environmental factors and variations in dietary pattern [15].

The primary risk factor is age. Prostate cancer is uncommon in men less than 45, but becomes more common with advancing age. The average age at the time of diagnosis is 70 [4]. Many men never know they have prostate cancer. Autopsy studies of Chinese, German, Israeli, Jamaican, Swedish, and Ugandan men who died of other causes have found prostate cancer in 30% of men in their 50s, and in 80% of men in their 70s [17]. Nutrition is therefore being considered among the modalities to slow disease progression.

Two genes (BRCA1 and BRCA2) that are important risk factors for ovarian cancer and breast cancer in women have also been implicated in prostate cancer [18]. The possibility of a specific nutrient-gene interaction is intriguing. Meanwhile, men with these genes may wish to use food and nutrients as disease prophylaxis.

The role of nutrition and dietary supplements in CaP is of much interest. However, several unresolved issues that are discussed in this chapter still linger:

- The expected time to achieve an effect is much longer, more variable, and far less well understood, and the progression of disease may be hard to follow.
- The optimal dose and duration needed to test nutritional agents for cancer prevention are largely unidentified, making null findings hard to interpret.
- Baseline nutritional status can be critical [15]. Selenium supplements provided benefit only for those individuals who had lower levels of baseline plasma selenium, whereas subjects with normal or higher levels did not benefit and may have an increased risk for CaP [16].
- Particular nutrients may be effective only in subgroups defined by genotypes or by nutritional status of another nutrient.

III. PATHOPHYSIOLOGY

Well-recognized precursor lesions in the peripheral zones of the prostate, including low-grade or high-grade prostatic intraepithelial neoplasia (PIN), are associated with the development of invasive cancer. Recently, proliferative inflammatory atrophy has been proposed as a precursor to PIN with merging of proliferative inflammatory atrophy and high-grade PIN seen in ~34% of proliferative inflammatory atrophy lesions [19]. Chronic inflammation may damage epithelial cells and result in proliferative lesions, likely precursors of PIN lesions and prostatic carcinomas; prostatitis has therefore been associated with a high risk of CaP [20]. The correlation between organ-specific inflammation and carcinoma is noteworthy. Reduction of inflammation is one likely route by which nutritional interventions influence disease.

IV. FOODS IN PROSTATE CANCER (TABLE 40.1)

Meat

Meat contains high amounts of arachidonic acid. Some byproducts of arachidonic acid have promoted prostate cancer in animals [29]. Preliminary reports have suggested that frequently eating well-done steak [30] or cured meats [31] is a risk factor. Heterocyclic amines (HCAs) and polycyclic aromatic hydrocarbons (PAH) are the carcinogenic chemicals formed from the cooking of muscle meats such as beef, pork, fowl, and fish. HCAs form when amino acids and creatine react at high cooking temperatures. Researchers have identified 17 different HCAs resulting from the cooking of meats that may pose human cancer risk. Cured meats can contain nitrosamines because meats contain amines, and sodium nitrite, a source of nitrosating agents, is added to cured meats as a preservative.

Dietary Fat

When combined with a low-fiber diet, men consuming a high-fat diet have been reported to have higher levels of testosterone, which might increase their risk of prostate cancer. The risk of prostate cancer correlates with dietary fat from country to country [24], a finding supported in some [25, 26], but not all [27], preliminary trials. In one study, prostate cancer patients consuming the most saturated fat (from meat and dairy), and followed for over 5 years, had over three times the risk of dying from prostate cancer compared with men consuming the least amount of saturated fat [28]. Men with higher serum levels of the short-chain omega-6 fatty acid linoleic acid have higher rates

TABLE 40.1
Foods for Prostate Cancer

	Meat/Dairy Source	Vegetable/Fruit Source
Omega-3 fatty acids	Cold water fish (salmon, cod, herring, mackerel, anchovies, sardines), grass-fed beef, fish oils, eggs	Flax seeds and oil, krill oil, walnuts, canola, whole grains, legumes, green leafy vegetables, açai palm fruit, kiwi fruit, black raspberries, wakame (sea vegetable).
Vitamin D	Cod liver oil, salmon, mackeral, sardines, liver, eggs	Green leafy vegetables, fortified cereals.
Vitamin E	Sardines, Atlantic herring, blue crab	Almonds, sunflower seeds, safflower oil, hazelnuts, turnip greens, pine nuts, peanuts, peanut butter, tomato, wheat germ, avocado, carrot juice, olive oil, corn oil, peanut oil, spinach, dandelion greens, Brazil nuts.
Zinc	Grass-fed beef, crabmeat, oysters, lamb, pork, turkey, salmon, chicken, clams, lobster	Brown rice, spinach, beans, rye bread, whole wheat bread, lentils, lima beans, oatmeal, peas, baked potato.
Selenium	Dairy products, liver, cold water fish, shellfish	Asparagus, broccoli, garlic, onions, mushrooms, grains, sea vegetables.
Indole-3-carbinol,5 glucaric acid (calcium D-glucarate)	None	Arugula, broccoli, cauliflower, brussels sprouts, cabbage, watercress, bok choy, turnip greens, mustard greens, collard greens, mizuna, tatsoi, rutabaga, napa or Chinese cabbage, daikon, horseradish, radishes, turnips, kohlrabi, kale.
Lycopene	None	Tomatoes, watermelon, pink grapefruit, pink guava, papaya, red bell pepper, rosehip. Lycopene in tomato paste is four times more bioavailable than in fresh tomatoes.
Genistein, daidzein	None	Soy products—especially fermented soy: miso, natto, Sweet noodle sauce, tamari, tempeh, tofu (pickled), yellow soybean paste.
Cathechins	None	Camellia sinensis: including white tea, green tea, black tea and oolong tea. Catechins are also present in the human diet in chocolate. Most of the EGCG catechin is found in green tea.

of prostate cancer. However, the same series of studies showed that men with elevated levels of long-chain omega-3 (EPA and DHA) had lowered incidence. A long-term study reports that "blood levels of *trans* fatty acids, in particular *trans* fats resulting from the hydrogenation of vegetable oils, are associated with an increased prostate cancer risk" [21].

Alpha-linolenic acid (ALA) is the essential omega-3 amino acid. ALA is associated with increased risk of prostate cancer. Since ALA is the precursor of EPA and DHA known to have anti-inflammatory and possibly anticancer properties, results indicate that people with measurably high ALA would be at increased risk. A significant portion of dietary ALA often does come from meat. Therefore in theory ALA may be a marker for meat consumption. When researchers have adjusted for the intake of meat or saturated fat, a correlation between ALA and prostate cancer risk has remained [31, 32]. Most [26–28], but not all [32], studies have found that high dietary or blood levels of ALA correlate with an increased risk of prostate cancer. Another possible explanation is that the rate-limiting enzyme that converts ALA to DHA and EPA, called delta-6-desaturase, is not functioning optimally. The ALA then accumulates and increased risk of prostate cancer is a result of inadequate enzyme activity. Another mechanism by which a causal pathway could exist is inflammation from a high ratio of omega-6 to omega-3 fats. This is supported by a preliminary study of men with prostate cancer who supplemented 30 g of ground flaxseed per day for approximately 1 month appeared to decrease the rate of tumor growth [26]. Flaxseed is high in both omega-3 and omega-6 fatty acids.

Fish eaters have been reported to have low risk for prostate cancer [33]. The omega-3 fatty acids EPA and DHA found in fish are thought by some researchers to be the components of fish responsible for protection against cancer [34].

CRUCIFEROUS VEGETABLES

Cruciferous vegetables have also been shown to have CaP protective properties. Cabbage, Brussels sprouts, broccoli, and cauliflower belong to the *Brassica* family of vegetables, also known as "cruciferous" vegetables. In test tube and animal studies, these foods were shown to have anticancer activity [35, 36]. A preliminary study of men newly diagnosed with prostate cancer showed a 41% decreased risk of prostate cancer among those eating three or more servings of cruciferous vegetables per week, compared with those eating less than one serving per week [37]. Protective effects of cruciferous vegetables were thought to be due to their high concentration of the carotenoids, lutein, and zeaxanthin, as well as their stimulatory effects on the breakdown of environmental carcinogens associated with prostate cancer [37]. Cruciferous vegetables also contain phytoestrogens.

SOY

Phytoestrogens are fat-soluble nutrients found in a variety of foods, especially vegetables, which modulate the response of fat-soluble hormones, especially estrogen. Phytoestrogens in food have been shown to be protective by helping the body metabolize estrogen-like toxins called xenoestrogens, which can be found in food, food packaging, water, and the environment at large.

Isoflavonoid phytoestrogens, such as genistein, daidzein, and glycitein, act as chemoprotectors by direct inhibition of DNA methyltransferase activity, reversal of DNA hypermethylation, and reactivation of methylation-silenced genes. Phytoestrogens are important regulators of proteins, such as 5α-reductase, tyrosine kinase, topoisomerase, and P450 aromatase, besides exerting an inhibitory effect on vitamin D metabolism in the prostate [38]. Isoflavonoid phytoestrogens show structural similarities with mammalian estrogens and are present in large amounts in soybean and soy products, such as miso and tofu. There is evidence that genistein, equol, and enterolactone inhibit the growth of LNCaP cells and reduce both intracellular and extracellular PSA concentrations. In addition, genistein is an effective inhibitor of angiogenesis and has been reported to decrease PSA levels and prevent metastatic disease in male Lobund-Wistar rats [39]. Studies in animal models showed that rats fed on soy or rye bran exhibited a significant delay in the growth of implanted prostate tumors. Osteopontin, an extracellular matrix protein, may be involved in the transition from clinically insignificant tumors to metastatic CaP. A recent study suggests that dietary genistein improved survival and inhibited progression to advanced CaP in TRAMP mice associated with reduced expression of osteopontin [40].

There is, however, limited data on the effect of oral phytoestrogen supplements in prostate tissue. In one of the three studies conducted thus far, daily oral supplementation of clover phytoestrogen induced a 23-fold and 7-fold increase in prostate tissue concentrations of genistein and daidzein, respectively, when compared with the placebo group [41]. In addition, 90% of the supplemented patients had a detectable plasma equol concentration after the supplementation [41]. However, a definite association with reduced CaP incidence has yet to be established in controlled human trials.

A 16-year-long prospective health study showed that men who consumed more than one glass of soy milk per day had a 70% lower risk of CaP [42].

LYCOPENE

Lycopene is a carotenoid phytonutrient. Most lycopene in our diet comes from tomatoes, and it also gives the red color to watermelons, pink grapefruits, papaya, and guava. Cooked tomatoes and tomato sauce are actually better than raw tomatoes because cooking them releases lycopene from their storage sites, changes the way our bodies absorb it, and affects the growth of prostate cancer cells in other foods. Also as a fat-soluble vitamin, it needs fat in the diet for uptake. V-8 juice or tomatoes in salad should be eaten with a snack or vegetable oil. Lycopene has been reported to inhibit the proliferation of cancer cells in test tube research [43].

There is evidence that lycopene effectively inhibits proliferation of various cancer cell lines with down-regulation of cyclin D1 and consequent cell cycle arrest at the G^0-G^1 phase of the cell cycle. This growth inhibition is extended to the three broadly used CaP cell lines PC-3, DU-145, and LNCaP cells. In addition normal prostate epithelial cells were observed to be even more sensitive to growth inhibition by lycopene than cancer cells. This is important because the pathologic hyperproliferation of prostate cells in men developing benign prostatic hyperplasia may be positively affected by lycopene [44]. Acycloretinoic acid, the oxidative metabolite of lycopene, has been reported to induce apoptosis in PC-3 and DU-145 cells [45]. Lycopene supplementation to rats resulted in decreased IGF-I and IL-6 expression; also a reduction in the expression of 5α-reductase in prostate tumors with subsequent down-regulation of several androgen target genes was noted. Lycopene increased the activity of the phase II enzymes GPx, glutathione-S-transferase, and glutathione reductase, as well as glutathione levels in several animal models, presumably due to antioxidant-response-element–mediated induction of genes [46].

In a preliminary trial, 26 men with prostate cancer were randomly assigned to receive lycopene at 15 mg twice a day or no lycopene for 3 weeks before undergoing prostate surgery. Prostate tissue was then obtained during surgery and examined. Compared with the unsupplemented men, those receiving lycopene were found to have significantly less aggressive growth of cancer cells [47].

In another trial, a 3-week tomato intervention study in CaP patients showed an increase in the apoptotic index of hyperplastic and neoplastic cells in the resected prostate tissue along with lower plasma levels of PSA [48]. Similar results were obtained when lycopene was given to patients undergoing orchidectomy with subsequent decrease in serum PSA level and reduction in the size of primary and secondary tumors [49]. In addition, a phase II study showed that whole-tomato lycopene supplementation had significant results and maintained its effect on PSA over 1 year [50].

However, a more recently concluded phase II trial shows that lycopene-rich tomato supplement was not effective in patients with androgen-independent CaP [51]. In addition, lycopene supplementation in men with biochemically relapsed CaP did not result in any discernible response in serum PSA, and a lack of association between CaP risk and lycopene intake was observed in a multicenter study by Kirsh and colleagues [52]. In view of these seemingly conflicting results, well-designed studies are necessary to establish the role of tomatoes and tomato products in the prevention and therapy of CaP.

Cholesterol-lowering drugs (e.g., probucol) [53], mineral oil, fat substitutes [54], and pectin [55] may decrease the absorption of lycopene; whereas beta carotene [56], medium-chain triglycerides, and dietary oils such as olive oil may enhance the absorption of lycopene [57].

Since tomatoes are a nightshade plant they aren't for everyone. Some patients with psoriasis, for example, may have worsened symptoms with the consumption of tomatoes [58].

GREEN TEA

Evidence from a case-control study conducted in southeast China assessing 130 patients with histologically confirmed incidental prostate cancer and 274 patients without cancer matched by age showed that the prostate cancer risk declined with increasing frequency, duration, and quantity of green tea consumed. The subjects in this trial drank three cups a day. This reduction was statistically significant, suggesting that green tea protects against prostate cancer [59].

However, in a recent phase II trial exploring the antineoplastic effects of green tea in patients with androgen-independent prostate cancer, 42 patients, who were asymptomatic and had progressive PSA increases despite hormone therapy, were instructed to take 6 g of green tea orally per day (the equivalent of six cups a day). The study found no statistically significant reduction in antineoplastic activity (as defined by a decline in PSA levels) among patients with androgen-independent prostate carcinoma. In addition, and of concern, 69% of patients had grade 1–2 toxicity, while there were six episodes of grade 3 and one episode of grade 4 toxicity [60].

In a double-blind trial, men with precancerous changes in the prostate received a green tea extract providing 600 mg of catechins per day or a placebo for 1 year. After 1 year, prostate cancer had developed in 3.3% of the men receiving the green tea extract and in 30% of those given the placebo, a statistically significant difference. These results suggest that drinking green tea or taking green tea catechins may help prevent prostate cancer in men at high risk of developing the disease [62].

Tea, next to water, is the most consumed beverage in the world. Green tea, obtained from the plant *Camellia sinensis*, with its high polyphenolic content has been shown to be an effective chemo-preventive agent against various cancers [63]. The polyphenols present in tea leaves as flavonols, or more commonly known as catechins, are epicatechin, epigallocatechin, epicatechin-3-gallate, and epigallocatechin-3-gallate (EGCG), of which the latter has gained the most attention with respect to its anticarcinogenic activity. EGCG makes up ~10% to 50% of the total catechin content and has a higher antioxidant activity than vitamins C and E. EGCG inhibits cellular proliferation primarily by acting as antioxidants and scavenging the free radicals, by inhibiting the enzymes involved in cell replication and DNA synthesis, along with interfering with cell-to-cell contact adhesion, and inhibiting intracellular communication pathways required for cell division.

Some of the contributing cancer-preventive effects of tea EGCG treatment have been shown to result in the induction of apoptosis in LNCaP, DU145, and PC-3 cells. It is thought to impose an artificial cell cycle checkpoint status in these cells independent of p53 [64].

More recently, Bettuzzi and colleagues reported that EGCG treatment to CaP cells, but not normal cells, resulted in the induction of clusterin with cleavage of both pro–caspase 8 and pro–caspase 3, resulting in apoptosis of cancer cells. Moreover, the chemopreventive action of catechins in the TRAMP mouse model was also accompanied by overexpression of clusterin [65].

EGCG effectively inhibits 5α-reductase in cell-free assays, indicating that it can regulate androgen action in target organs. Replacement of the gallate ester in EGCG with long-chain fatty acids produces potent 5α-reductase inhibitors that are active in both cell-free and whole-cell assay systems [66]. Testosterone mediated induction of ornithine decarboxylase, and an important contributor of CaP development, is inhibited by green tea polyphenols both under in vitro and in vivo situations [67]. Significant inhibition of IGF-I and restoration of IGF-binding protein-3 levels in green-tea-polyphenol–fed mice with marked delay in the progression of CaP and concomitant apoptosis suggest that the autocrine/paracrine loop is a target for CaP chemoprevention by green tea [68]. A more recent study showed that with progression of age and CaP growth, an increase in the expression of S100A4 at mRNA and protein level occurs in dorsolateral prostate of TRAMP, but not in nontransgenic mice. Green tea polyphenol feeding to TRAMP mice resulted in marked inhibition of CaP progression, with reduction of S100A4 and restoration of E-cadherin [59].

Similar results were seen in another clinical trial involving patients with hormone refractory CaP. Green tea extract capsules, prescribed at a dose level of 250 mg twice daily, showed minimal clinical activity against the disease [69]. Both of these studies were conducted in end-stage disease, signifying that green tea may be more effective if used in the early stages of the disease or in patients at high risk.

In this context, Bettuzzi et al. [70] have shown that after a year's p.o. administration of green tea catechins, only one man in a group of 32 with high-grade PIN developed CaP compared with 9 of 30 in the control group; a rate of only 3% in men developing the disease versus the expected rate of 30% in men treated with placebo. Hence, large-scale, prospective, randomized trials are necessary to test the efficacy of green tea for the prevention and treatment of CaP.

Based on all the evidence, green tea can markedly reduce the development of prostate cancer. The evidence also shows that this may be in several different ways and by a multitude of pathways. While the evidence here is restricted to the effects in prostate cancer, there is equally good evidence of protection from developing other types of cancer. Although the evidence for the beneficial effects of green tea is quite compelling, further work needs to be done before this translates to actual treatments for prostate cancer. Meanwhile, perhaps clinicians could encourage patients with an already well-established tea-drinking habit to drink more green tea [61].

POMEGRANATE

Pomegranate is a rich source of polyphenolic compounds, including anthocyanins and hydrolyzable tannins, with a reportedly higher antioxidant activity than green tea and red wine. Recent studies show that anatomically discrete sections of the pomegranate fruit acting synergistically exert antiproliferative and antimetastatic effect against CaP cells.

In a more recent study, pomegranate fruit extract treatment of highly aggressive PC-3 cells resulted in a dose-dependent inhibition of cell growth/cell viability along with induction of apoptosis [71]. A recently concluded 2-year, single center study showed that pomegranate juice increased the mean PSA doubling time coupled with corresponding laboratory effects on CaP in vitro cell proliferation and apoptosis, as well as oxidative stress [71]. No serious adverse effects were reported, and the treatment was well tolerated. These results are being further tested in a randomized, double-blind, three-arm, placebo-controlled study, which began in April 2006, and addresses several limitations of the current study, with the inclusion of two treatment arms in a dose-response design, as well as the use of a placebo control [72].

SAW PALMETTO

Some in vivo studies have reported that saw palmetto may have anti–prostate cancer properties and be useful in prostate cancer patients [122, 123].

Saw palmetto extract reduces the amount of dihydrotestosterone (DHT) (an active form of testosterone) binding in the part of the prostate surrounding the urethra. Test tube studies also suggest that saw palmetto weakly inhibits the action of 5α-reductase, the enzyme responsible for converting testosterone to DHT [124].

There has, however, been no evidence in humans regarding the association with saw palmetto and prostate cancer in a human clinical trial. In one prospective cohort study of 35,171 men aged 50 to 76 years in western Washington State, there was no association with commercial saw palmetto, which varies widely in dose and constituent ratios, with prostate cancer risk [125].

V. VITAMINS AND MINERALS IN PROSTATE CANCER (TABLE 40.2)

VITAMIN D

Ecologic data show that where sun exposure is low, prostate cancer rates increase [73]. In the body, vitamin D is changed into a hormone with great activity. This activated vitamin D causes "cellular differentiation"—essentially the opposite of cancer.

In a preliminary trial, 7 of 16 men who had prostate cancer that had spread to bone and who had been unresponsive to conventional treatment were found to have evidence of vitamin D deficiency [74]. All 16 were given 2000 IU of vitamin D per day for 12 weeks, and levels of pain were recorded for 14 of these men. Vitamin D supplementation led to reduced pain in 4 of the 14 men, and 6 showed evidence of increased strength [74]. Those with vitamin D deficiency were more likely to respond, compared with those who were not deficient [74]. People taking 2000 IU/day of vitamin D should be supervised by a doctor.

TABLE 40.2
Supplemental Nutrients That May Be Beneficial in Prostate Cancer Treatment

Supplement	Dose	Regimen	Interactions	Other
Vitamin D (Cholecalciferol)	2000 IU	Daily	Helpful with patients on docetaxel Corticosteroids reduce active D	25(OH)D in the range of 30-40 ng/mL maximizes intestinal absorption of calcium; interpret keeping seasonal variation in mind
Vitamin E (Mixed tocopherols)	400 IU	Daily	Contraindicated with blood thinning drugs May potentiate chemotherapy	Avoid dl-alpha tocopherol (synthetic). Use mixed tocopherols and tocotrienols
Selenium	200 µg	Daily	None known	Selenomethionine is type with best bioavailability Higher than 400 µg can be toxic—selenosis
Fish oil	1000 mg	2 times a day	High doses can possibly interfere with blood thinning drugs	
Lycopene	15 mg	2 times a day	Statin drugs may lower levels. Fat substitutes like Olestra® may inhibit absorption as can over-the-counter and prescription weight reduction medications.	Lyco-Mato® has been studied
Green tea extract	250 mg	2 times a day	None known	May increase blood pressure in hypertensive patients
Zyflamend: extracts of rosemary, turmeric, ginger, holy basil, green tea, hu zhang, Chinese goldthread, barberry, oregano, and Baikal skullcap.	1 pill	3 times a day	None	Drink with food
Prostabel: *Pao Pereira* and *Rauwolfia vomitoria*	2 pills	2 to 3 times a day	None	Drink on an empty stomach

In another preliminary study, men with prostate cancer that had relapsed after surgery or radiation therapy were treated with 2000 IU of vitamin D per day for 9 months. In approximately half of the men, the prostate-specific antigen (PSA) level decreased, suggesting that the progression of the disease had been halted or reversed; this decrease was sustained for 5 to 17 months [75]. In addition, the study was done in Toronto, Canada, where the amount of sunlight is limited and vitamin D status tends to be low. It is not known whether vitamin D supplementation would be as effective in geographical regions such as the southern United States, where the amount of sunlight is greater.

A normal vitamin D status seems to be an important precondition via the local and autocrine synthesis of calcitriol [1,25(OH)2D] in the target tissues for a lower risk of overall morality due to organ cancer [76]. A plethora of evidence that vitamin D and its synthetic analogues promote differentiation and inhibit the proliferation, invasiveness, and metastasis of human prostatic cancer cells both in in vitro and in vivo models exists [77]. In addition, data from various studies support the concept that adequate exposure to ultraviolet (UV) radiation results in reduced risk of various diseases, including cancer, through a vitamin D–mediated mechanism. A recent analysis of mortality data over a 45-year period (1950 to 1994) by Schwartz and colleagues confirmed their earlier findings that the geographic distribution of CaP mortality is the inverse of that of UV radiation [78].

In addition, recent analysis of the available literature indicates a lack of evidence to support association between vitamin D receptor polymorphisms and risk of CaP [79]. Currently, over 2000 vitamin D analogues have been evaluated, and several have entered phase I or phase II trials in patients with advanced cancer. A variety of drug administration schedules have been tried, including daily or intermittent administration of oral calcitriol, subcutaneous injections, or in combination with other chemotherapeutic agents [80], as the dose-limiting hypercalcemia associated with calcitriol has limited the use of natural vitamin D in cancer prevention. Clinical responses have been seen with the combination of high-dose calcitriol and dexamethasone, and in a large randomized trial in men with an androgen-independent CaP, calcitriol potentiated the antitumor effects of docetaxel [80]. Randomized phase III clinical trials are necessary to determine the optimal dose and preferred vitamin D analogue along with the route and schedule of administration.

It is appropriate to measure 25-hydroxyvitamin D [25(OH)D] in patients to make sure they have adequate levels. Normal ranges are 20 to 56 ng/mL vitamin D level and should not fall below 32 ng/mL. Any levels below 20 ng/mL are considered serious deficiency states [81].

Vitamin E

Vitamin E refers to a group of naturally occurring compounds: the tocopherols, tocotrienols, and their natural and synthetic derivatives. Out of the eight different tocopherols included in the term "vitamin E," alpha tocopherol often exerts specific functions and is the predominant form of vitamin E found in plasma and tissues, whereas gamma tocopherol, and not alpha tocopherol, is the major form present in the diet. Besides its antioxidant function, vitamin E can regulate cell cycle through DNA synthesis arrest in LNCaP, PC-3, and DU-145 CaP cells [82]. Interestingly, tocopherol metabolites have been reported to be as effective as their vitamin precursors in inhibiting PC-3 growth through down-regulation of cyclin expression, with stronger inhibition seen with the gamma forms [83].

Relatively high blood levels of vitamin E have been associated with relatively low levels of hormones linked to prostate cancer [84]. While a relationship between higher blood levels of vitamin E and a reduced risk of prostate cancer has been reported only inconsistently [85, 86], supplemental use of vitamin E has been associated with a reduced risk of prostate cancer in smokers. In a double-blind trial studying smokers, 50 IU of a vitamin E supplementation taken daily for an average of 6 years led to a 32% decrease in prostate cancer incidence and a 41% decrease in prostate cancer deaths [87, 88].

While vitamin E has been demonstrated to be protective, a therapeutic role has not been established [91–94]. An important methodologic consideration is the type and quality of vitamin E used. For example a decrease in CaP risk with alpha-tocopherol occurs through a mechanism that is non-hormonal and independent of IGF-I [89]. Gamma-tocopherol exhibits anti-inflammatory activities by inhibiting cycloxygenase and possibly lipoxygenase-catalyzed formation of prostaglandin E and leukotriene B, respectively [90].

Selenium

Selenium is an essential micronutrient, and part of the body's antioxidant defense system that has been shown to inhibit tumorigenesis in a variety of experimental models. Methylated selenium sensitizes CaP cells to TRAIL-mediated apoptosis, effectively down-regulates the expression of androgen receptor (AR) and PSA in the androgen-responsive LNCaP cells, and inhibits the growth of LNCaP xenografts in nude mice [95, 96].

The double-blind, randomized Nutritional Prevention of Cancer trial, designed to test whether selenized yeast could prevent the recurrence of nonmelanoma skin cancer in 1312 patients, showed a statistically significant increase in nonmelanoma skin cancer, although a secondary end point analysis revealed a striking reduction in CaP incidence in those with low-serum selenium levels. Furthermore, no evidence of selenium toxicity was seen at doses of 400 μg selenium daily in 424 persons for 1220 person-years of observation [97].

Selenium may have a protective effect against mercury and other heavy metal toxicities [98, 99]. Experimental findings have shown that selenium-deficient rodents are more susceptible to the prenatal toxicity of methylmercury. In the neonate, significant alterations of the activities of selenoenzymes, such as glutathione peroxidase and iodothyronine deiodinases, were evident [100].

Selenium appears to antagonize cadmium, especially in acute exposures. In a mouse study, after acute cadmium exposure a significant decrease in cadmium levels was observed in the kidneys and liver following an eight-week daily selenium supplementation [101].

Selenomethionine was selected for the SELECT trial, which tests the effectiveness of dietary supplements of selenium and tocopherol, individually or in combination, in the reduction of clinical incidence of CaP in a population-based cohort of men at risk [94]. The enrollment for SELECT began in 2001, and the final results are anticipated by 2013. SELECT will be analyzed as a four-arm study, with primary analyses consisting of five pair-wise comparisons of CaP incidence, in association with vitamin E versus placebo, selenium versus placebo, vitamin E plus selenium (combination) versus placebo, combination versus vitamin E, and combination versus selenium. The participants are required to take 200 μg/day L-selenomethionine and/or 400 IU/day of alpha-tocopherol supplementation for 7 to 12 years [94].

VI. ANTI-INFLAMMATORY CHEMOPREVENTION

Cyclooxygenese 2 (COX-2) is overexpressed in many cancers, including prostate cancer, and is a well-established and significant target for efforts to forestall cancer growth. Benign prostate tissue in cancerous prostates has been found to have low COX-2, suggesting increased activity of the enzyme with disease progression. COX-2 overexpression is a predictor of worse prostate cancer outcome [102].

Other studies have suggested that angiogenesis is orchestrated in part by increased COX-2 activity and ensuing prostaglandin production—a hypothesis supported by the effects of some COX-2 inhibitor drugs on the biochemical measures of apoptosis. COX-2 inhibitor drug celecoxib (Celebrex) has been found to be a promising chemotherapy. Inhibition of COX-2 in animals suppresses angiogenesis and prostate cancer growth and enhances sensitivity to radiation therapy.

Thus, the anti-inflammatory aspect of chemoprevention appears to be a pivotal one, particularly in cases of prostatic intrarepithelial neoplasia (PIN). PIN, which can appear up to 10 years before diagnosable cancer and which coexists with cancer in more than 85% of cases, offers investigators the opportunity to apply chemopreventive measures when dysplasia is present—the point at which prostate carcinogenesis may be at its earliest stages.

Manipulation of pro-inflammatory eicosanoids can be achieved through two approaches: (1) with manipulation of fatty acid intake, providing the body with increased substrate for the production of anti-inflammatory eicosanoids, which then competitively inhibits formation of pro-inflammatory eicosanoids; and (2) with manipulation of COX and LO enzyme isoforms, inhibiting those that promote the inflammation found to encourage prostate carcinogenesis. So far, it appears that fatty acid intake is a safe and effective intervention in this regard. Manipulating COX and LO with pharmaceutical agents, however, has proven to be a less promising avenue for chemoprevention. Recent case-control studies have found significant risks with long-term COX-2 inhibitor therapy, with increases in mortality and risk of heart failure and gastrointestinal bleeding.

Herbal anti-inflammatory agents have a broader, less specific effect. As herbs are increasingly subjected to the rigors of modern studies, the research community is beginning to recognize their therapeutic value.

Many researchers have explored a variety of natural plant extracts and other natural products to elucidate their specific and nonspecific effects on COX and LO. Curcumin (turmeric), ginger, holy basil, resveratrol (concentrated in grape skins), and berberine (from barberry and Chinese goldthread) are among the most promising candidates in the burgeoning field of herbal anti-inflammatories.

A novel compound that we have studied, Zyflamend, is comprised of these and a few other herbs, most of which have nonselective COX-inhibitory effect. Each of the mixture's components has been found to have anti-inflammatory, antioxidant, and/or antiproliferative effects. Some are anti-angiogenic.

In 2005, Bemis and colleagues published the results of an analysis of Zyflamend's effects on LNCaP cells. The supplement brought about a dramatic drop in both COX-1 and COX-2 activity; increased p21 expression; attenuated cell growth; and induced apoptosis. Interestingly, the effect of the supplement on LNCaP cells appeared to be due to COX-independent mechanisms, including enhanced expression of p21 and reduced expression of AR, pStat3, and PKC alpha and beta [103].

A phase I clinical trial has been recently completed at Columbia in men with PIN to determine whether Zyflamend can influence the progression of biopsy-proven high-grade PIN to prostate cancer [126]. Of the 15 patients that finished the trial, 60% (8/15) had all benign tissue, 36% (5/15) had HGPIN in one core, and 14.3% (2/15) developed prostate cancer at the final 18-month biopsy. A statistically significant reduction in serum C-reactive protein was also observed ($p = 0.045$). Immunoreactive staining for NFκB, COX-2, IL-6, and thromboxane A-2 were determined and a significant reduction in NFκB staining was observed in the 18-month tissue samples (95% CI: 0.8 to 3.0, $p = 0.017$).

Curcumin has also been found to be a potent radiosensitizer that enhances radiation-induced clonogenic inhibition in tumor cells [104]. At Columbia, Dorai and colleagues found that curcumin modulates proteins that suppress apoptosis and interferes with growth factors that promote cancer progression [105].

Ginger root flavors many cuisines, and has been an herbal medicine since antiquity, used to treat nausea, motion sickness, upper respiratory infection, and intestinal parasites. Modern investigators have discovered in this rhizome more than 20 phytochemicals that inhibit COX-2 and 5-LO. Ginger constituents have potent antioxidant and anti-inflammatory activities; some, particularly shogaols and vallinoids [6]-gingerol and [6]-paradol, exhibit cancer-preventive activity in experimental carcinogenesis. This herb's chemopreventive effects have been illustrated in a variety of experimental models [106].

Prostabel, an herbal combination containing extracts of *Pao pereira* (an Amazonian tree) and *Rauwolfia vomitoria* (from the bark of a sub-Saharan plant), was created by the late molecular biologist Mirko Beljanski. These plants have been used in indigenous medical traditions for hundreds of years; Beljanski found that they had anticancer activities in various cancer cell lines, including prostate cancer. Investigations at Columbia have revealed that both *Rauwolfia* and *Pao* extracts suppress prostate tumor cell growth in culture and in vivo. Katz and colleagues of Columbia are enrolling patients with elevated PSA and negative biopsy results for a phase I study of Prostabel; seven regimens are being employed, with subjects taking from two to eight capsules daily of this herbal medicine [107].

The herbs listed here are relatively free of interactions with prescription drugs. Turmeric may potentiate antiplatelet activity in patients on antiplatelet agents; ginger and turmeric may potentiate the effects of blood thinners. Patients should be advised that herbs and drugs can interact in harmful ways, and that they should reveal the use of all medications and supplements to their medical team so that these kinds of interactions can be avoided.

VII. NUTRIENT-DRUG INTERACTIONS

Some in the oncology community contend that patients undergoing chemotherapy and/or radiation therapy should not use food supplement antioxidants and other nutrients. Although there are few studies observing the interactions between antioxidants and chemotherapy and/or radiation with prostate cancer patients, Simone and colleagues researched concomitant nutrient use with chemotherapy and/or radiation therapy (280 peer-reviewed articles including 62 in vitro and 218 in vivo) among different cancer patients from MEDLINE® and CANCERLIT® databases from 1965 to November 2003 [87]. These studies show that vitamin A, beta-carotene, and vitamin E do not interfere with and actually can enhance the killing capabilities of therapeutic modalities for cancer, decrease their side effects, protect normal tissues, and, in some studies, prolong survival.

Antioxidants increase cancer cell differentiation and/or apoptosis, and growth inhibition. Antioxidants selectively inhibit repair of radiation damage of cancer cells but protect normal cells when antioxidants are used before, during, and after radiation. There are no published studies that show antioxidants protect cancer cells against radiation. Vitamin E reduces the expression of vascular endothelial growth factor and thus acts as an anti-angiogenic factor.

Five early studies showed that N-acetylcysteine, an antioxidant, protects the heart from the cardiac toxicity of adriamycin without interfering with the tumor-killing capability of adriamycin [111]. Cellular animal studies [112, 113] and human studies [114–121] have demonstrated that vitamins A, E, C, and K, as well as beta-carotene and selenium—as single agents or in combination—all protect against the toxicity of adriamycin and actually enhance its cancer-killing effects.

Cancer patients suffer from caloric and nutritional malnutrition and have vitamin deficiencies, particularly of folic acid, vitamin C, pyridoxine, and other nutrients because of poor nutrition and treatment [108]. Chemotherapy and radiation therapy reduce serum levels of antioxidant vitamins and minerals due to lipid peroxidation and thus produce higher levels of oxidative stress [22]. Iron could be the intermediate cause of this oxidative stress [109, 110]. Therefore, supplemental iron should not be recommended to cancer patients who have anemia unless it is an iron-deficiency anemia.

VIII.   SUMMARY

In sum, we encourage patients to have diets rich in the foods found in Table 40.1. Equally important is to avoid certain foods: char-grilled meats, *trans* fats, excess omega-6 fats beyond the ratio with omega-3 fats, rancid fats, well-cooked meats, and simple carbohydrates. Nutrient interventions can be synergistic with medical treatment of prostate cancer. Supplemental nutrients with the strongest evidence are listed in Table 40.2.

REFERENCES

1. American Cancer Society. Cancer facts and figures. 2007; www.cancer.org.
2. Bartsch G, Horninger W, Klocker H, Reissigl A, Oberaigner W, Schonitzer D, Severi G, Robertson C, Boyle P. Tyrol Prostate Cancer Screening Group. Decrease in prostate cancer mortality following introduction of prostate specific antigen screening in the federal state of Tyrol, Austria. *J Urol* 2000;163[4]:88.
3. Etzioni R, Legler JM, Feuer EJ, Merrill RM, Cronin KA, Hankey BF. Cancer surveillance series: interpreting trends in prostate cancer—part III: Quantifying the link between population prostate-specific antigen testing and recent declines in prostate cancer mortality. *J Natl Cancer Inst* 1999;91[12]:1033.
4. Hankey BF et al. Cancer surveillance series: "Interpreting trends in prostate cancer—part I: evidence of the effects of screening in recent prostate cancer incidence, morbidity, and survival rates. *J Natl Cancer Inst* 1999;91(12):1017–1024.
5. Schröeder FH Kranse R. Verification bias and the prostate-specific antigen test—is there a case for lower threshold for biopsy? *N Engl J Med* 2003;349(4):393–395.
6. Gann PH, Hennekens CH, Sampfer MJ. A prospective evaluation of plasma prostate specific antigen for detection of prostatic cancer. *JAMA* 1995;273:289–294.
7. Smith DS, Catalona WJ. The nature of prostate cancer detected through prostate specific antigen based screening. *J Urol* 1994;152:1732–1736.
8. Hoedemaeker RF, Rietbergen JB, Kranse R, Schröder FH, van der Kwast TH. Histopathological prostate cancer characteristics at radical prostatectomy after population based screening. *J Urol* 2000;164:411–415.

9. Luboldt HJ, Bex A, Swoboda A, Husing J, Rubben H. Early detection of prostate cancer in Germany: a study using digital rectal examination and 4.0 ng/mL prostate-specific antigen as cutoff. *Eur Urol* 2001;39:131–137.

10. Carter HB, Pearson JD. Prostate-specific antigen testing for early diagnosis of prostate cancer: formulation of guidelines. *Urology* 1999;54[5]:780.

11. IARC Worldwide Cancer Incidence Statistics—Prostate. *JNCI Cancer Spectrum.* Oxford University Press (December 19, 2001]. Retrieved on 2007-04-05 through the Internet Archive.

12. Overview: Prostate Cancer—What Causes Prostate Cancer? American Cancer Society [2006-05-02]. Retrieved on 2007-04-05.

13. Prostate Cancer FAQs. State University of New York School of Medicine Department of Urology [2006-08-31]. Retrieved on 2007-04-05.

14. Potosky A, Miller B, Albertsen P, Kramer B. The role of increasing detection in the rising incidence of prostate cancer. *JAMA* 1995;273[7]:548–552. PMID 7530782.

15. Moyad MA, Carroll PR. Lifestyle recommendations to prevent CaP: I. time to redirect our attention? *Urol Clin North Am* 2004;31:289–300.

16. Moyad MA. Selenium and vitamin E supplements for CaP: evidence or embellishment? *Urology* 2002;59:9–19. [Medline]

17. Breslow N, Chan CW, Dhom G, Drury RA, Franks LM, Gellei B, Lee YS, Lundberg S, Sparke B, Sternby NH, Tulinius H. Latent carcinoma of prostate at autopsy in seven areas. The International Agency for Research on Cancer, Lyons, France. *Int J Cancer* 1977 Nov 15;20[5]: 680–688. PMID 924691.

18. Lorenzo Bermejo J, Hemminki K. Risk of cancer at sites other than the breast in Swedish families eligible for BRCA1 or BRCA2 mutation testing. *Ann Oncol* 2004;15[12]:1834–1841.

19. Nelson WG, De Marzo AM, DeWeese TL, Isaacs WB. The role of inflammation in the pathogenesis of CaP. *J Urol* 2004;172:S6–11. [CrossRef] [Medline]

20. Gann PH, Giovannucci [2005]. Prostate Cancer and Nutrition. Retrieved on February 20, 2006 in PDF format.

21. Chavarro et al. A prospective study of blood *trans* fatty acid levels and risk of prostate cancer. *Proc Amer Assoc Cancer Res* 2006;47:1. See also Ledesma 2004 Nutrition & prostate cancer.

22. McLaughlin AP, Saltzstein SL, McCullough DL, Gittes RF. Prostatic carcinoma: incidence and location of unsuspected lymphatic metastases. *J Urol* 1976;115[1]:89.

23. McNeal JE, Villers AA, Redwine EA, Freiha FS, Stamey TA. Histologic differentiation, cancer volume, and pelvic lymph node metastasis in adenocarcinoma of the prostate. *Cancer* 1990;66[6]:1225.

24. Dorgan JF, Judd JT, Longcope C, et al. Effects of dietary fat and fiber on plasma and urine androgens and estrogens in men: a controlled feeding study. *Am J Clin Nutr* 1996;64:850–855.

25. Peinta KJ, Esper PS. Is dietary fat a risk factor for prostate cancer? *J Natl Cancer Inst* 1993;85:1538–1539 [editorial/review].

26. Giovannucci E, Rimm EB, Colditz GA, et al. A prospective study of dietary fat and risk of prostate cancer. *J Natl Cancer Inst* 1993;85:1571–1579.

27. Le Marchand L, Kolonel LN, Wilkens LR, et al. Animal fat consumption and prostate cancer: a prospective study in Hawaii. *Epidemiology* 1994;5:276–282.

28. Meyer F, Bairati I, Shadmani R, et al. Dietary fat and prostate cancer survival. *Cancer Causes Control* 1999;10:245–251.

29. Ghosh J, Myers C Jr. Arachidonic acid metabolism and cancer of the prostate. *Nutrition* 1998;14:48–57 [editorial].

30. Norrish AE, Ferguson LR, Knize MG, et al. Heterocyclic amine content of cooked meat and risk of prostate cancer. *J Natl Cancer Inst* 1999;91:2038–2044.

31. Schuurman AG, van den Brandt PA, Dorant E, Goldohm RA. Animal products, calcium and protein and prostate cancer risk in the Netherlands Cohort Study. *Br J Cancer* 1999;80:1107–1113.

32. Gann PH, Hennekens CH, Sacks FM, et al. Prospective study of plasma fatty acids and risk of prostate cancer. *J Natl Cancer Inst* 1994;86:281–286.

33. Kune GA. Eating fish protects against some cancers: epidemiological and experimental evidence for a hypothesis. *J Nutr Med* 1990;1:139–144 [review].

34. Rose DP, Connolley JM. Omega-3 fatty acids as cancer chemopreventive agents. *Pharmacol Ther* 1999;83:217–244.

35. Beecher CW. Cancer preventive properties of varieties of Brassica oleracea: a review. *Am J Clin Nutr* 1994;59(suppl):1166–1170S.

36. Zhang Y, Kensler TW, Cho CG, et al. Anticarcinogenic activities of sulforaphane and structurally related synthetic norbornyl isothiocyanates. *Proc Natl Acad Sci USA* 1994;91:3147–3150.

37. Cohen JH, Kristal AR, Stanford JL. Fruit and vegetable intakes and prostate cancer risk. *J Natl Cancer Inst* 2000;92[1]:61–68.
38. Fang MZ, Chen D, Sun Y, Jin Z, Christman JK, Yang CS. Reversal of hypermethylation and reactivation of p16INK4a, RARß, and MGMT genes by genistein and other isoflavones from soy. *Clin Cancer Res* 2005;11:7033–7041.
39. Schleicher RL, Lamartiniere CA, Zheng M, Zhang M. The inhibitory effect of genistein on the growth and metastasis of a transplantable rat accessory sex gland carcinoma. *Cancer Lett* 1999;136:195–201.
40. Adlercreutz H, Heinonen SM, Penalvo-Garcia J. Dietary genistein improves survival and reduces expression of osteopontin in the prostate of transgenic mice with prostatic adenocarcinoma (TRAMP). *J Nutr* 2005;135:989–995.
41. Rannikko A, Petas A, Rannikko S, Adlercreutz H. Plasma and prostate phytoestrogen concentrations in CaP patients after oral phytoestogen supplementation. *Prostate* 2006;66:82–87.
42. Jacobsen BK, Knutsen SF, Fraser GE. Does high soy milk intake reduce CaP incidence? The Adventist Health Study. *Cancer Causes Control* 1998;9:553–557.
43. Levy J, Bosin E, Feldman B, et al. Lycopene is a more potent inhibitor of human cancer cell proliferation than either α-carotene or β-carotene. *Nutr Cancer* 1995;24:257–266.
44. Obermuller-Jevic UC, Olano-Martin E, Corbacho AM, et al. Lycopene inhibits the growth of normal human prostate epithelial cells in vitro. *J Nutr* 2003;133:3356–3360.
45. Kotake-Nara E, Kim SJ, Kobori M, Miyashita K, Nagao A. Acyclo-retinoic acid induces apoptosis in human CaP cells. *Anticancer Res* 2002;22:689–695.
46. Herzog A, Siler U, Spitzer V, et al. Lycopene reduced gene expression of steroid targets and inflammatory markers in normal rat prostate. *FASEB J* 2005;19:272–274. [Abstract/Free Full Text]
47. Kucuk O, Sarkar FH, Sakr W, et al. Phase II randomized clinical trial of lycopene supplementation before radical prostatectomy. *Cancer Epidemiol Biomarkers Prev* 2001;10:861–868.
48. Kucuk O, Sarkar FH, Djuric Z, Sakr et al. Effects of lycopene supplementation in patients with localized CaP. *Exp Biol Med* (Maywood) 2002;227:881–885.
49. Ansari MS, Sgupta NP. A comparison of lycopene and orchidectomy vs orchidectomy alone in the management of advanced CaP. *BJU Int* 2005;95:453.
50. Barber NJ, Zhang X, Zhu G, et al. Lycopene inhibits DNA synthesis in primary prostate epithelial cells in vitro and its administration is associated with a reduced prostate-specific antigen velocity in a phase II clinical study. *Prostate Cancer Prostatic Dis* 2006;9:407–413.
51. Clark PE, Hall MC, Borden LS, Jr., et al. Phase I-II prospective dose-escalating trial of lycopene in patients with biochemical relapse of prostate cancer after definitive local therapy. *Urology* 2006;67:1257–1261.
52. Kirsh VA, Mayne ST, Peters U, et al. A prospective study of lycopene and tomato product intake and risk of prostate cancer. *Cancer Epidemiol Biomarkers Prev* 2006;15:92–98.
53. Elinder LS, Hadell K, Johansson J, et al. Probucol treatment decreases serum concentrations of diet-derived antioxidants. *Arterioscler Thromb Vase Biol* 1995;15:1057–1063.
54. Weststrate JA, Meijer GW. Plant sterol enriched margarines and reduction of plasma total and LDL-cholesterol concentrations in normocholesterolaemic and mildly hypercholesterolaemic subjects. *Fur J Clin Nutr* 1998;52:334–343.
55. Riedl J, Linseisen J, Hoffmann J, Wolfram G. Some dietary fibers reduce the absorption of carotenoids in women. *J Nutr* 1999;129:2170–2176.
56. Johnson EJ, Qin J, Krinsky NI, Russell RM. Ingestion by men of a combined dose of beta-carotene and lycopene does not affect the absorption of beta-carotene but improves that of lycopene. *J Nutr* 1997;127:1833–1837.
57. Clark RM, Yao L, She I, Furr HC. A comparison of lycopene and astaxanthin absorption from corn oil and olive oil emulsions. *Lipids* 2000;35:803–806.
58. Naldi L, Parazzini F, Peli L, Chatenoud L, Cainelli T. Dietary factors and the risk of psoriasis. Results of an Italian case-control study. *Br J Dermatol* 1996 Jan;134[1]:101–106.
59. Jian L, Xie LP, Lee AH, Binns CW. Protective effect of green tea against prostate cancer: a case-control study in southeast China. *Int J Cancer* 2004;108:130–135.
60. Jatoi A, Ellison N, Burch PA, et al. A phase II trial of green tea in the treatment of patients with androgen independent prostate carcinoma. *Cancer* 2003;97:1442–1446.
61. Patel SP, Hotston M, Kommu S, Persad RA. The protective effects of green tea in prostate cancer. *BJU Int* 2005;96[9]:1212–1214.
62. Bettuzzi S, Brausi M, Rizzi F, et al. Chemoprevention of human prostate cancer by oral administration of green tea catechins in volunteers with high-grade prostate intraepithelial neoplasia: a preliminary report from a one-year proof-of-principle study. *Cancer Res* 2006;66:1234–1240.

63. Adhami VM, Ahmad N, Mukhtar H. Molecular targets for green tea in CaP prevention. *J Nutr* 2003;133:2417–2424S.

64. Umeda D, Tachibana H, Yamada K. Epigallocatechin-3-O-gallate disrupts stress fibers and the contractile ring by reducing myosin regulatory light chain phosphorylation mediated through the target molecule 67 kDa laminin receptor. *Biochem Biophys Res Commun* 2005;333:628–635.

65. Caporali A, Davalli P, Astancolle S, et al. The chemopreventive action of catechins in the TRAMP mouse model of prostate carcinogenesis is accompanied by clusterin over-expression. *Carcinogenesis* 2004;25:2217–2224.

66. Liao S, Hiipakka RA. Selective inhibition of steroid 5 {alpha}-reductase isozymes by tea epicatechin-3-gallate and epigallocatechin-3-gallate. *Biochem Biophys Res Commun* 1995;214:833–838.

67. Gupta S, Ahmad N, Mohan RR, Husain MM, Mukhtar H. CaP chemoprevention by green tea: in vitro and in vivo inhibition of testosterone-mediated induction of ornithine decarboxylase. *Cancer Res* 1999;59:2115–2120.

68. Adhami VM, Siddiqui IA, Ahmad N, Gupta S, Mukhtar H. Oral consumption of green tea polyphenols inhibits insulin-like growth factor-I-induced signaling in an autochthonous mouse model of CaP. *Cancer Res* 2004;64:8715–8722.

69. Choan E, Segal R, Jonker D, et al. A prospective clinical trial of green tea for hormone refractory CaP: an evaluation of the complementary/alternative therapy approach. *Urol Oncol* 2005;23:108–113. [Medline]

70. Bettuzzi S, Brausi M, Rizzi F, Castagnetti G, Peracchia G, Corti A. Chemoprevention of human prostate cancer by oral administration of green tea catechins in volunteers with high-grade prostate intra-epithelial neoplasia: a preliminary report from a one-year proof-of-principle study. *Cancer Res* 2006;66:1234–1240.

71. Malik A, Afaq F, Sarfaraz S, Adhami VM, Syed DN, Mukhtar H. Pomegranate fruit juice for chemoprevention and chemotherapy of CaP. *Proc Natl Acad Sci USA* 2005;102:14813–14818.

72. Pantuck AJ, Leppert JT, Zomorodian N, et al. Phase II study of pomegranate juice for men with rising prostate-specific antigen following surgery or radiation for prostate cancer. *Clin Cancer Res* 2006;12:4018–4026.

73. John EM, Koo J, Schwartz GG. Sun exposure and prostate cancer risk: evidence for a protective effect of early-life exposure. *Cancer Epidemiol Biomarkers Prev* 2007;16:1283–1286.

74. Van Veldhuizen PJ, Taylor SA, Williamson S, Drees BM. Treatment of vitamin D deficiency in patients with metastatic prostate cancer may improve bone pain and muscle strength. *J Urol* 2000;163:187–190.

75. Woo TCS, Choo R, Jamieson M, et al. Pilot study: potential role of vitamin D (cholecalciferol) in patients with PSA relapse after definitive therapy. *Nutr Cancer* 2005;51:32–36.

76. Peehl DM, Krishnan AV, Feldman D. Pathways mediating the growth-inhibitory actions of vitamin D in CaP. *J Nutr* 2003;133:2461–2469S.

77. Kubota T, Koshizuka K, Koike M, Uskokovic M, Miyoshi I, Koeffler HP. 19-nor-26,27-bishomo-vitamin D3 analogs: a unique class of potent inhibitors of proliferation of prostate, breast, and hematopoietic cancer cells. *Cancer Res* 1998;58:3370–3375.

78. Schwartz GG, Hanchette CL. UV, latitude, and spatial trends in prostate cancer mortality: all sunlight is not the same (United States). *Cancer Causes Control* 2006;17:1091–1101.

79. Mikhak B, Hunter DJ, Spiegelman D, Platz EA, Hollis BW, Giovannucci E. Vitamin D receptor (VDR) gene polymorphisms and haplotypes, interactions with plasma 25-hydroxyvitamin D and 1,25-dihydroxyvitamin D, and prostate cancer risk. *Prostate* 2007;67:911–923.

80. Beer TM, Myrthue A. Calcitriol in cancer treatment: from the lab to the clinic. *Mol Cancer Ther* 2004;3:373–381.

81. Holick MF. Calcium and vitamin D. Diagnostics and Therapeutics. *Clin Lab Med* 2000 Sep;20[3]:569–590.

82. Basu A, Imrhan V. Vitamin E and CaP: is vitamin E succinate a superior chemopreventive agent? *Nutr Rev* 2005;63:247–251.

83. Hartman TJ, Dorgan JF, Virtamo J, et al. Association between serum α-tocopherol and serum androgens and estrogens in older men. *Nutr Cancer* 1999;35:10–15.

84. Eichholzer M, Stähelin H, Lüdin E, Bernasconi F. Smoking, plasma vitamins C, E, retinol, and carotene, and fatal prostate cancer: seventeen-year follow-up of the Prospective Basel Study. *Prostate* 1999;38:189–198.

85. Hartman TJ, Albanes D, Pietinen P, et al. The association between baseline vitamin E, selenium, and prostate cancer in the alpha-tocopherol, beta-carotene cancer prevention study. *Cancer Epidemiol Biomarkers Prev* 1998;7:335–340.

86. Chan JM, Stampfer MJ, Ma J, et al. Supplemental vitamin E intake and prostate cancer risk in a large cohort of men in the United States. *Cancer Epidemiol Biomarkers Prev* 1999;8:893–899.

87. Simone CB, II, Simone NL, Simone V, Simone CB. Antioxidants and other nutrients do not interface with chemotherapy or radiation therapy and can increase kill and increase survival, part 1. *Altern Ther Health Med* 2007;13[1]:22–28.

88. Heinonen OP, Albanes D, Virtamo J, et al. Prostate cancer and supplementation with alpha-tocopherol and beta-carotene: incidence and mortality in a controlled trial. *J Natl Cancer Inst* 1998;90:440–446.

89. Hernaandez J, Syed S, Weiss G, et al. The modulation of CaP risk with {alpha}-tocopherol: a pilot randomized, controlled clinical trial. *J Urol* 2005;174:519–522.

90. Jiang Q, Wong J, Fyrst H, Saba JD, Ames BN. {gamma}-Tocopherol or combinations of vitamin E forms induce cell death in human CaP cells by interrupting sphingolipid synthesis. *Proc Natl Acad Sci USA* 2004;101:17825–17830.

91. Meyer F, Galan P, Douville P, et al. Antioxidant vitamin and mineral supplementation and CaP prevention in the SU.VI.MAX trial. *Int J Cancer* 2005;116:182–186. [CrossRef] [Medline]

92. Hsing AW, Comstock GW, Abbey H, Polk BF. Serologic precursors of cancer. Retinol, carotenoids and tocopherol and risk of CaP. *J Natl Cancer Inst* 1990;82:941–946.

93. Miller ER, Pastor-Barriuso R, Dalal D, Riemersma RA, Appel LJ, Guallar E. Meta-analysis: high-dosage vitamin E supplementation may increase all-cause mortality. *Ann Intern Med* 2005;142:37–46.

94. Lippman SM, Goodman PJ, Klein EA, et al. Designing the selenium and vitamin E cancer prevention trial (SELECT). *J Natl Cancer Inst* 2005;97:94–102.

95. Yamaguchi K, Uzzo RG, Pimkina J, et al. Methylseleninic acid sensitizes CaP cells to TRAIL-mediated apoptosis. *Oncogene* 2005;24:5868–5877.

96. Lee SO, Yeon Chun J, Nadiminty N, et al. Monomethylated selenium inhibits growth of LNCaP human CaP xenograft accompanied by a decrease in the expression of androgen receptor and prostate-specific antigen (PSA). *Prostate* 2006;66:1070–1075.

97. Duffield-Lillico AJ, Dalkin BL, Reid ME, Clark LC. Selenium supplementation, baseline plasma selenium status and incidence of CaP: an analysis of the complete treatment period of the Nutritional Prevention of Cancer Trial. *BJU Int* 2003;91:608–612.

98. Whanger PD. Selenium and heavy metal toxicity. In: Spallholz JE, Martin JL, Ganther HE, eds. *Selenium in Biology and Medicine*. Westport, CT: AVI; 1981:230–255.

99. Diplock AT, Watkins WJ, Hewison M. Selenium and heavy metals. *Ann Clin Res* 1986;18:55–60.

100. Watanabe C. Selenium deficiency and brain functions: the significance for methylmercury toxicity. *Nippon Eiseigaku Zasshi* 2001;55:581–589. [Article in Japanese]

101. Jamba L, Nehru B, Bansal MP. Selenium supplementation during cadmium exposure: changes in antioxidant enzymes and the ultrastructure of the kidney. *J Trace Elem Exp Med* 1997;10:233–242.

102. Study first: over-expression of COX-2 can predict prostate cancer outcome. Medical News Today, www.medicalnewstoday.com/medicalnews.php?newsid=56224, accessed 11/28/06.

103. Bemis DL, Capodice JL, Anastasiadis AG, et al. Zyflamend, a unique herbal preparation with nonselective COX inhibitory activity, induces apoptosis of prostate cancer cells that lack COX-2 expression. *Nutr Cancer* 2005;52[2]:202–212.

104. Chendil D, Ranga RS, Meigooni D, et al. Curcumin confers radiosensitizing effect in prostate cancer cell line PC-3. *Oncogene* 2004 Feb 26;23[8]:1599–1607.

105. Dorai T, Cao YC, Dorai B, Buttyan R, Katz AE. Therapeutic potential of curcumin in human prostate cancer. III. Curcumin inhibits proliferation, induces apoptosis, and inhibits angiogenesis of LNCaP prostate cancer cells in vivo. *Prostate* 2001 Jun;47[4]:293–303.

106. Shukla Y, Singh M. Cancer preventive properties of ginger: a brief review. *Food Chem Toxicol* 2006 Nov 12; epub ahead of print: http://dx.doi.org/10.1016/j.fct.2006.11.002, accessed 12/24/06.

107. Bemis DL, Capodice JL, Gorrochurn P, et al. Anti-prostate cancer activity of a beta-carboline alkaloid enriched extract from Rauwolfia vomitoria. *Int J Oncol* 2006;29[5]:1065–1073.

108. Wasserman TH, Brizel DM. The role of amifostine as a radioprotector. *Oncology* 2001;15[10]: 1349–1354.

109. Hellmann K. Anthracycline cardiotoxicity prevention by dexrazoxane: breakthrough of a barrier-sharpens antitumor profile and therapeutic index. *J Clin Oncol* 1996;14[2]:332–333.

110. Klein P, Muggia FM. Cytoprotection: shelter from the storm. *Oncologist* 1999;4[2]:112–121.

111. Dorr RT. Cytoprotective agents tor anthracyclines. *Semin Omul* 1996;23[4 Suppl 8]:23–34.

112. Ciaccio M, Tesoriere L, Pintaudi AM, et al. Vitamin A preserves the cytotoxic activity of adriamycin while counteracting its peroxidative effects in human leukemic cells in vitro. *Biochem Mol Int* 1994;34[2]:329–335.
113. Ripoll EA, Rama BN, Webber MM. Vitamin E enhances the chemotherapeutic effects of adriamycin on human prostatic carcinoma cells in vitro. *J Urol* 1986;136[2]:529–531.
114. Shimpo K, Nagatsu T, Vamada K, et al. Ascorbic acid and adriamycin toxicity. *Am J Clin Nutr* 1991: 54[6 suppl]:1298S–1301S.
115. Geetha A, Sankar R, Marar T, Devi CS. Alpha-tocopherol reduces doxorubicin-induced toxicity in rats-histological and biochemical evidences. *Indian J Physiol Pharmacol* 1990:34[2]:94–98.
116. Jotti A, Maiorino M, Paracchini L, Piccinini F, Ursini F. Protective effect of dietary selenium supplementation on delayed tardiotoxicity of adriamycin in rat: is PHGPX but not GPX involved? *Free Radic Biol Med* 1994:16[2]:284–288.
117. Myers CE, McGuire W, Young K. Adriamycin: amelioration of toxicity by alpha-tocopherol. *Cancer Treat Rep* 1976;60[7]:961–962.
118. Singal PK, Tong JG. Vitamin E deficiency accentuates adriamycin-induced cardiomyopathy and cell surface changes. *Mol Cell Biochem* 1988:84[2]:163–171.
119. Lenzhofer R, Ganzinger U, Rameis H, Moser K. Acute cardiac toxicity in patients after doxorubicin treatment and the effect of combined tocopherol and nifedipine pretreatmmt. *J Cancer Res Clin Oncol* 1983;106[2]:143–147.
120. Weilzman SA, Lorell E, Carey RW, Kaufman S, Stossel TP. Prospective study of tocopherol prophylaxis for anthracycline cardiac toxicity. *Curr Ther Res* 1980;28:682–686.
121. Wadsworth TL, Worstell TR, Greenberg NM, Roselli CE. Effects of dietary saw palmetto on the prostate of transgenic adenocarcinoma of the mouse prostate model (TRAMP). *Prostate* 2007 May 1;67[6]:661–673.
122. Yang Y, Ikezoe T, Zheng Z, Taguchi H, Koeffler HP, Zhu WG. Saw Palmetto induces growth arrest and apoptosis of androgen-dependent prostate cancer LNCaP cells via inactivation of STAT 3 and androgen receptor signaling. *Int J Oncol* 2007 Sep;31[3]:593–600.
123. Di Silverio F, Monti S, Sciarra A, et al. Effects of long-term treatment with Serenoa repens (Permixon®) on the concentrations and regional distribution of androgens and epidermal growth factor in benign prostatic hyperplasia. *Prostate* 1998;37:77–83.
124. Strauch G, Perles P, Vergult G, et al. Comparison of finasteride (Proscar®) and Serenoa repens (Permixon®) in the inhibition of 5-alpha reductase in healthy male volunteers. *Eur Urol* 1994;26:247–252.
125. Bonnar-Pizzorno RM, Littman AJ, Kestin M, White E. Saw palmetto supplement use and prostate cancer risk. *Nutr Cancer* 2006;55[1]:21–27.
126. In peer review as of October 2008.

41 Lung Cancer

Nutritional Support

Sheila George, M.D.

I. INTRODUCTION

This chapter informs primary care practitioners about what foods and nutrients are important for their patients with non-small cell lung cancer (NSCLC) in order to support the body's metabolic functions. It discusses nutritional approaches primarily based on seven strategies for cancer inhibition.[1]

II. EPIDEMIOLOGY

Lung cancer is the most common cause of cancer death in the United States with an average 5-year survival rate of approximately 16%.[2] Cigarette smoking is the number one risk factor with other risk factors being chemicals such as asbestos, radon gas, and chromium. Exposure to any of these toxicants can result in damage to various genes; and the inability to repair these genes can result in lung cancer.

Studies indicate that food and nutrients can affect gene alterations.[3] Consequently, we can use food and nutrients to assist in cancer inhibition, thus complementing existing therapy for patients with lung cancer.

III. PATHOLOGY

The two histologic types of lung cancer are small cell lung cancer (SCLC) and non-small cell lung cancer (NSCLC). The focus of this chapter is on tailoring a patient-specific nutritional plan for people with NSCLC, which is 75% to 80% of all lung cancer and includes adenocarcinoma (40%), squamous cell carcinoma (25%), and large cell carcinoma (10%).

IV. STRATEGIES FOR CANCER INHIBITION

Lung cancer is a result of an accumulation of genetic and epigenetic alterations caused primarily by exposure to toxins from smoking, asbestos, radon gas, and other toxic agents found in the workplace. Using food and nutrients to affect these pro-cancer events plays an important role in reversing or slowing down this process. The following are seven strategies to inhibit cancer progression as defined by John Boik in *Natural Compounds in Cancer Therapy* and how food and nutrients affect these strategies.[1]

1. Reduce genetic instability

    Production of reactive oxygen species (ROS) is a normal metabolic process, but excessive ROS production creates oxidative stress that can increase genetic instability. Fresh vegetables and fruits, which are rich in antioxidants, reduce the effects that oxidative stress has on cells and cellular DNA.

    Fresh vegetables and fruits also may help to restore normal DNA methylation.

    Epigenetic changes in DNA are primarily due to the attachment of methyl groups to specific locations on the cytosine base. Most genes in cancer cells tend to be hypomethylated, whereas tumor suppressor genes tend to be hypermethylated.[5]

    Antioxidants help protect DNA from oxidative damage. Therefore, they may help to reduce abnormal cytosine methylation. In addition, folate along with vitamin B12, and vitamin B6 assist in the production of S-adenosylmethionine (SAM), which helps to regulate DNA methylation.

2. Inhibit abnormal expression of genes

    Transcription factor proteins such as p53 protein, nuclear factor-κB (NFκB), and activator protein-1 regulate gene expression and thus control the expression and progression of cancer. P53 protein initiates repair of DNA and when it cannot, it will induce apoptosis. Certain food and nutrients increase normal p53 and decrease abnormal p53 proteins. NFκB, which promotes collagenases, inflammation, and angiogenesis, and activator protein-1 (AP-1), which promotes cell proliferation, are found in excess in cancer cells. Foods containing antioxidants and phytonutrients may help normalize transcription factor protein activity or down-regulate it by inhibition of signal transduction.

3. Inhibit abnormal signal transduction

    Signal transduction is a normal process that involves the movement of a signal from outside the cell toward the cell's nucleus, where it can stimulate proliferation. There is excess signal transduction found in cancer cells, which promotes unregulated proliferation and metastasis. Food and nutrients containing flavonoids such as apigenin, luteolin, and quercetin, curcumin, omega-3 fatty acids, selenium, and vitamin E can inhibit abnormal signal transduction.

4. Encourage normal cell-to-cell communication

    Normal cell-to-cell communication involves cell adhesion molecules (CAM), which are located on the outer cell membrane. It also involves intercellular communication via gap junctions. Cancer cells have altered CAM activity and a loss of gap junction communication, which promotes cancer proliferation. Foods with flavonoids such as apigenin and luteolin may inhibit NFκB and thus the up-regulation of CAM. In addition, food and nutrients consisting of various phytonutrients, omega-3 fatty acids, and selenium facilitate gap junction intercellular communication.

5. Inhibit tumor angiogenesis

    Although angiogenesis, the growth of new blood vessels, is a normal process in the body, cancer angiogenesis needs to be inhibited to prevent metastasis. Vascular endothelial growth factor (VEGF) stimulates angiogenesis and thus metastasis.[6] Nutrients such as omega-3 fatty acids and selenium may decrease VEGF and the resulting vascular permeability, thereby slowing down angiogenesis. COX-2 inhibitors also reduce angiogenesis. Alpha-lipoic acid and phytonutrients such as catechins, luteolin, proanthocyanins, and resveratrol may help chelate copper, which is needed for angiogenesis to take place.

6. Inhibit invasion and metastasis

Cancer cells must invade and digest the extracellular matrix (ECM) in order to spread. Food and nutrients that stabilize the extracellular matrix can be used to help decrease invasion and metastasis. Several phytonutrients have been found to inhibit enzymatic digestion of normal tissue around the tumor.

7. Increase the immune system

Cancer cells can evade immune attack by producing prostaglandin E2. Taking nutrients such as glutamine can enhance intracellular glutathione (GSH) and inhibit PGE2.[7] In addition, sufficient glutathione levels are required for activation of T-cells by interleukin-2.[8] Studies also show that nondenatured whey protein increases GSH levels in normal cells helping to detoxify carcinogens and other toxins, while it depletes GSH in cancer cells helping to inhibit their growth and proliferation.[9]

V. FOOD AND NUTRIENTS AS AN ADJUNCT TO THE TREATMENT OF NSCLC

Patients can use food and nutrients to powerfully affect multiple pro-cancer events on a daily basis while receiving cancer therapy.

VEGETABLES AND FRUITS

Vegetables and fruits are rich in vitamins, minerals, and phytochemicals that work synergistically to help inhibit the growth of cancer. They also contain soluble and insoluble fiber, which are important in controlling blood glucose levels and encouraging a healthful flora in the colon, respectively. This also helps inhibit the growth of cancer.

A clinical trial with vegetable supplements showed eating vegetables prolongs the life of people with advanced NSCLC.[10] Daily ingestion of selected vegetables prolonged survival and slowed normal progression of the disease.

Dark Green Leafy Vegetables

Dark green leafy vegetables (Table 41.1) are an excellent source of magnesium, potassium, folate, carotenoids, saponins, and flavonoids to support the functioning of a healthy metabolism.

Dark green leafy vegetables are a good source of beta-carotene, a carotenoid antioxidant that plays a role in blocking the development of cancer. Beta-carotene used as a concentrated supplement is harmful for smokers with lung cancer, as proven in the lung cancer chemoprevention trials.[11,12] But as part of a complex array of nutrients and phytochemicals in foods, it inhibits cancer growth.

The high amount of folate in dark green leafy vegetables is important for DNA replication and repair. Diets low in folate may increase the risk of lung cancer because without sufficient folate, there is a deficiency of methyl groups bound to cysteine in DNA, which promotes oncogenes.

TABLE 41.1
Dark Green Leafy Vegetables
- Spinach
- Dark green lettuce
- Swiss chard
- Chicory
- Collard greens
- Mustard greens
- Turnip greens
- Kale
- Bok choy

TABLE 41.2
Cruciferous Vegetables
- Arugula
- Bok choy
- Broccoli
- Brussels sprouts
- Cabbage
- Cauliflower
- Collard greens
- Horseradish
- Kale
- Kohlrabi
- Mustard greens
- Napa
- Radishes
- Rapini (broccoli rabe)
- Rutabagas
- Watercress

Cruciferous Vegetables (Table 41.2)

Cruciferous vegetables contain phytochemicals, isothiocyanates, and indole-3-carbinol, which have the ability to stop the growth of cancer. In particular, the isothiocyanates found only in cruciferous vegetables stimulate our bodies to break down potential carcinogens.

In a study of over 18,000 Chinese men in Shanghai, it was shown that subjects genetically deficient in the enzymes that quickly remove isothiocyanates from the body had a decreased risk of developing lung cancer.[13] They had more protection because the isothiocyanates remained in the body longer. Isothiocyanates induce phase II enzymes, thereby inactivating carcinogens and promoting their excretion.[14] They also induce apoptosis.

Berries

Berries have phytochemicals, including ellagic acid and flavonoids, that in lab studies work synergistically to stop the progression of cancer. The anthocyanins in berries are powerful antioxidant flavonoids that have anti-inflammatory properties and inhibit epidermal growth factor receptor on cancer cells. Berries also have the antioxidant vitamin C that helps to neutralize free radicals and ROS.

Grapes

Grapes have phytochemicals that work synergistically against DNA topoisomerase II, an enzyme necessary for the spread of cancer.[15] In addition, the skins of red and purple grapes have the polyphenol resveratrol. Resveratrol is a powerful antioxidant and anti-inflammatory, which helps inhibit angiogenesis.

WHOLE GRAINS

Whole grains such as millet, brown rice, oats, buckwheat, and quinoa are rich in fiber, vitamins, minerals (including selenium), and phytochemicals, all of which support the body's metabolism and prevent the promotion of cancer. Intact whole grains have a low glycemic index, which supports a noninflammatory state, while whole grain flour has nearly the same glycemic index as refined flour.

PROTEINS

Eating quality protein supports the body in building and repairing tissues and making essential components such as hemoglobin, enzymes, amino acids, and hormones. The minimum amount of daily protein an adult needs is 0.8 g/kg of body weight, but more is needed for patients with cancer based on their catabolic imbalance.

Eggs

Eggs are an excellent source of quality protein with very little fat. A large egg has a total of 5 g of fat with about 3.5 g being unsaturated. Unless a patient is "dietary cholesterol sensitive" or has allergies to eggs, they are an excellent source of protein. Almost all the absorbed nitrogen from egg protein can be retained and used by the body.

Fish

Fish is a good source of protein and easy to digest. In addition, fatty fish such as salmon, sardines, anchovies, trout, and herring are also rich in omega-3 fatty acids, which inhibit metastasis. However, avoid fish that is high in mercury. It can interfere with the proper functioning of the immune, nervous, and endocrine systems.

Whey Protein

If a patient is not allergic to whey protein, it is a good source for complete protein. In addition, low-temperature processed or nondenatured whey protein selectively depletes glutathione in cancer cells making them more susceptible to chemotherapy.

Legumes

Legumes, which include beans, lentils, and peas, are a good source of low-fat protein (though not a "complete" protein), fiber, vitamins, minerals, and antioxidants, which support the body and keep pro-cancer activity in check. They have phytochemicals such as saponins, protease inhibitors, and phytic acid, which inhibit cancer cells. In laboratory studies, saponins interfere with the replication of cancer cells and slow the growth of tumors, protease inhibitors inhibit tumors from releasing protease that destroys nearby cells, and phytic acid slows the progression of tumors.[1]

Beans have a low glycemic index, so there is a slow rise in blood glucose after eating them. This prevents hyperinsulinemia, insulin resistance, and inflammation that promote angiogenesis and the progression of cancer.

OMEGA-3 FATTY ACIDS

Foods such as sugar (cake, ice cream, soda, candy), junk food, fast foods, and high-fat meats are pro-inflammatory and stimulate the progression of cancer by stimulating angiogenesis, which is necessary for the survival and metastasis of lung cancer.

If omega-6 fatty acids are not excessive, omega-3 fatty acids inhibit inflammation by suppressing the synthesis of pro-inflammatory eicosanoids from arachidonic acid. Omega-3 fatty acids also promote normal activity of signal transduction molecules, which control cell growth, differentiation, and apoptosis.

It has been shown that omega-3 fatty acid supplementation improves the quality of life and survival of patients with end-stage cancer.[17]

The ideal ratio of omega-3 to omega-6 fatty acids is less than or equal to 1:4. The American diet typically consists of a ratio on average of greater than 1:15. Two and one-tenth (2.1) g of EPA and 1.9 g of DHA reduced production of PGE2 by intestinal cells in healthy subjects.[18]

In addition to omega-3 fatty acid supplements, coldwater fish is the best source for these fats. Flaxseed is the best plant source for alpha-linolenic acid (omega-3). Walnuts are also a good source of omega-3 fatty acids.

It is important to note as elaborated elsewhere in this text that high doses of flaxseed, flaxseed oil, and omega-3 fatty acids can interact with drugs that affect blood clotting.

Flaxseed

Flaxseed is a rich source of dietary lignans that has antiestrogenic properties and inhibits the aromatase enzyme. It is metabolized by the body into two major lignans, enterodiol and enterolactone. Enterolactone may produce an antiestrogenic effect by stimulating the production of sex hormone binding globulin in the liver and thus regulates the concentration of free sex hormones in the plasma.[19] And both enterolactone and enterodiol inhibit the aromatase enzyme, which is involved in estrogen synthesis.[20] Therefore, flaxseed may be beneficial to women over 65 with early NSCLC who have increased levels of estrogen receptor alpha on cancer cells and increased aromatase levels, which is associated with more aggressive disease.[21] In this scenario, flaxseed may help to slow the progression of the disease.

Selenium

Broccoli, brussels sprouts, and garlic grown in selenium-rich soil protect against lung cancer. These vegetables contain the most active form of selenium, selenium methylselenocysteine, which induces apoptosis independent of p-53 protein activity.[22] In addition to being an antioxidant that can neutralize free radicals, selenium inhibits prostaglandins and decreases the rate of tumor growth.

In NSCLC normal p-53 protein is suppressed while abnormal p-53 protein is expressed. Selenium activates normal p-53 protein, which induces DNA repair or apoptosis.

Daily doses of 100 to 200 μg of selenium inhibit genetic damage and cancer development in humans.[23]

Curcumin

Curcumin found in tumeric inhibits the cyclooxygenase-2 enzyme (COX-2 enzyme), which is up-regulated in lung cancer. COX-2 is typically undetectable or found in low amounts in normal tissue, but increases with the inflammatory process. And it is overexpressed and involved in the progression of NSCLC. Curcumin inhibits NFκB, which is activated by pro-inflammatory signals and up-regulates COX-2.[24]

Up-regulation of epidermal growth factor receptor (EGFR) is another factor implicated in the progression of NSCLC. Curcumin has also been found to inhibit EGFR intrinsic kinase activity and EGF-induced tyrosine phosphorylation of EGFRs.[25] In addition, curcumin increases the expression of normal p53 protein.[26]

Vitamin D

Vitamin D has anti-cancer properties. It can inhibit cell growth and angiogenesis and contributes to apoptosis and cell differentiation. It has been shown that a high vitamin D level is associated with prolonged survival in NSCLC.[27] Most people in the United States do not get enough sunlight, therefore, a 25-hydroxyvitamin D level is recommended to determine if supplementation is necessary.

VI.   EFFECT OF CHEMOTHERAPY AND RADIATION THERAPY ON NUTRITIONAL STATUS

Chemotherapy and radiotherapy affect the rapidly dividing cells of the gastrointestinal tract (GIT). This has an effect on digestion and absorption of nutrients. It also creates an environment for the development of food reactivities. Some patients have prior unrecognized food allergies that worsen with chemotherapy and radiation. Avoiding common allergens such as gluten and cow dairy and protecting and nourishing the cells of the GIT with glutamine can improve a patient's energy and well-being.

Chemotherapy can also upset the normal flora balance and create a dysbiosis, which can put an additional strain on the body. Small bowel overgrowth of microflora can interfere with the availability of nutrients. Probiotics and fiber-rich vegetables can help to maintain intestinal health and optimal absorption.

Because chemotherapy and radiotherapy kill tumor cells (and normal cells) this creates an increased toxic load for the body. Therefore, all the organs of elimination need to be functioning optimally. The liver must have all the necessary enzymes, vitamins, minerals, amino acids, antioxidants, and other nutrients required for phase I and II detoxification. The bowels must be open and moving regularly without dysbiosis. The patient must be well hydrated with pure water to facilitate the movement of intracellular and extracellular toxins out of the body and to optimize the functioning of the perspiration mechanism and urinary system. Daily dry skin brushing should be done to keep the toxic load in the lymphatic system moving toward the circulatory system, thus decreasing intercellular congestion and facilitating nutrients into the cells. Sinus cleansing should be done if the sinuses are not draining properly. In addition, moderate exercise helps with all the organs of elimination. Addressing the aforementioned will improve the overall health of the patient and the effectiveness of therapy.

The platinum and taxane chemotherapeutic drugs used for NSCLC can cause peripheral neuropathy. Acetyl-l-carnitine has been shown to improve damage done to the nervous system due to chemotherapy.[28] Also, B vitamins given IM are useful in decreasing the side effects of neuropathy. Moreover, starting both acetyl-l-carnitine and adequate B vitamins prior to chemotherapy may prevent the peripheral neuropathy commonly experienced. Cisplatinum can also cause electrolyte wasting. Foods such as celery juice and coconut water can help to maintain electrolyte balance.

Hyperglycemia and insulin resistance, which is a typical metabolic response in advanced cancer, can affect a patient's response to chemotherapy.[29] Proper diet, nutrients such as omega-3 fatty acids, alpha-lipoic acid, calcium, and magnesium, and stress reduction and exercise may help to improve insulin sensitivity and thus improve response to chemotherapy.

VII. FOOD AND NUTRIENTS AND COMORBID CONDITIONS

Cancer cachexia occurs in up to 80% of people with advanced cancer and is directly responsible for death in up to 20% of cases.[30] It is not fully understood, but the presence of the tumor leads to the persistent release of pro-inflammatory cytokines such as TNF alpha, interferon gamma, IL-1B, and IL-6 by the body. These cytokines coupled with the production of cytokines and the release of catabolic factors by the tumor such as lipid mobilizing factor (LMF) and proteolysis inducing factor (PIF) lead to tissue breakdown from both the fat and skeletal muscle compartments of the body.[31]

Melatonin decreases TNF production.[32] "In a randomized study of 70 patients with advanced NSCLC treated with cisplatin and etoposide, the addition of melatonin (at 20 mg/day, orally) increased the 1-year survival rate as compared to those receiving only chemotherapy (from 19% to 44%). In the group taking melatonin and chemotherapy, no cachexia was reported, but in the one taking chemotherapy only, 44% of patients experienced cachexia."[33]

Nutritional supplementation alone cannot reverse cachexia, but may be able to prevent or slow the process. EPA in large doses will down-regulate pro-inflammatory cytokines and PIF.[34] The intake of sufficient quality protein and glutamine will support protein synthesis. Melatonin will reduce TNF. So, the combination of EPA, highly absorbable and utilizable protein, glutamine, plus high-dose melatonin (20 mg at night) may help to slow down the progression of tissue wasting and the advancement of cachexia. Moreover, incorporating these nutrients early on may prevent cachexia altogether.

Fatigue is also a critical issue in patients with NSCLC. It can be due to multiple reasons such as the metabolic effects of the cancer itself, cancer therapy (chemotherapy or radiotherapy), endocrine dysfunctions, toxic overload in the body, poor assimilation of nutrients, depression, anemia, insomnia, shortness of breath, low-grade infection, and pain. Optimizing the diet, ensuring all the organs of elimination are functioning properly, addressing treatable causes of anemia and hormonal imbalances, incorporating relaxation techniques if insomnia is due to anxiety, treating any low-grade infections and pain, and incorporating mild to moderate exercise will help to mitigate fatigue.

VIII.   RECOMMENDATIONS

Assess Deficiencies

Laboratory tests to assess reversible nutrient and hormone deficiencies include:

- Essential amino acid profile
- Red blood cell mineral analysis
- Thyroid profile: TSH, free T3, and free T4
- Saliva for morning and evening cortisol levels
- 25-hydroxyvitamin D level
- Vitamin B12 level

Optimize the Function of Organ Systems

- Optimize digestive functioning with pancreatic enzyme support, if there is no history of gastritis.
- Supplement with iodine to achieve TSH levels in the optimal range.
- Utilize prebiotics and probiotics to maintain healthful microflora.
- Ensure phase I and phase II liver detoxification is balanced (Chapter 12, "Viral Hepatitis").
- Support adrenal glands as necessary based on stage of adrenal exhaustion (resistance or exhaustion stage).
- Keep all organs of elimination functioning properly.

Recommend Nutrients for Metabolic Support

- Cruciferous and dark green leafy vegetables, twice daily, plus a variety of other vegetables and fruits.
- Eggs, three to four times a week.
- Fish rich in omega-3 fatty acids, three to four times a week.
- Legumes and whole grains, which are free of gluten.
- Omega-3 fatty acid supplements with an EPA component of 2 g/day. Some patients may require supplemental GLA even though this is an omega-6 fat.
- Omega-3 fatty acids to omega-6 fatty acids should be maintained at a ratio of 1:4 or less.
- Selenium 200 µg/day.
- Calcium 1000 mg and magnesium 400 to 500 mg daily, with extra magnesium as needed.
- Multivitamins and minerals without iron and copper or beta-carotene.
- Vitamin D3, 1000 IU/day as a maintenance dose. Higher dosing may be necessary in some patients.
- Acetyl-l-carnitine, 500 mg twice a day between meals to protect the nervous system throughout the duration of chemotherapy.
- Glutamine swish and swallow between meals at a dose of 4 g twice a day.
- Melatonin, 20 mg a half hour before bed for advanced cancer. Caution should be taken with those patients on anticoagulants.
- Plenty of pure water.
- Nonallergic highly absorbable protein supplement, with amount based on deficiency of amino acids.
- Eating every 3 to 4 hours during the day.
- Avoiding processed sugar and junk food.
- Supplements should be taken with food unless otherwise specified.

Eating a variety of food and nutrients that support the body's metabolic functions while also inhibiting multiple aspects of pro-cancer activity in the body will improve the quality of life and survival of patients with NSCLC.

REFERENCES

1. Boik J. *Natural Compounds in Cancer Therapy*. Princeton, MN: Oregon Medical Press, 2001.
2. Jemal A, Siegal R, Ward E, Hao Y, Xu J, Murray T, Thun, MJ. Cancer statistics, 2008. *CA Cancer J Clin* 2008 Mar-Apr;58(2):71–96. Epub 2008 Feb 20.
3. Edited by Awad A, Bradford P. *Nutrition and Cancer Prevention*. Boca Raton, FL: CRC Press, Taylor & Francis, 2006.
4. Removed at proofs.
5. Ross SA. Diet and DNA methylation interactions in cancer prevention. *Ann NY Acad Sci* 2003;983:197–207.
6. Salven P, Manpaa H, Orpana A, et al. Serum vascular endothelial growth factor is often elevated in disseminated cancer. *Clin Cancer Res* 1997 May; 3(5):647–651.
7. Margalit A, Hauser SD, Zweifel BS, et al. Regulation of prostaglandin biosynthesis in vivo by glutathione. *Am J Physiol* 1998 Feb;274(2pt2):294–302.
8. Liang CM, Lee N, Cattell D, Liang SM. Glutathione regulates interleukin-2 activity on cytotoxic T-cells. *J Biol Chem* 1989;264(23):13519–13523.
9. Kennedy RS, Konok GP, Bounous G, Baruchel S, Lee TD. The use of a whey protein concentrate in the treatment of patients with metastatic carcinoma: a phase I-II clinical study. *Anticancer Res* 1995 Nov–Dec;15(6B):2643–2649.
10. Sun AS, Yeh HC, Wang LH, et al. Pilot study of a specific dietary supplement in tumor-bearing mice and in stage IIIB and IV non-small cell lung cancer patients. *Nutriton and Cancer* 2001;39:85–95.
11. Omenn GS, Goodman GE, Thornquist MD, Balmes J, Cullen MR, Glass A, Keogh JP, Meyskens FL, Valanis B, Williams JH, Barnhart S, Hammar S. Effects of a combination of beta carotene and vitamin A on lung cancer and cardiovascular disease. *N Engl J Med* 1996 May 2;334:1150–1155.
12. The effect of vitamin E and beta carotene on the incidence of lung cancer and other cancers in male smokers. The Alpha-Tocopherol, Beta Carotene Cancer Prevention Study Group. *N Engl J Med* 1994;330:1029–1035.
13. London SJ, Yuan JM, Chung FL, Gao YT, Coetzee GA, Ross RK, Yu MC. Isothiocyanates, glutathione S- transferase M1 and T1 polymorphisms, and lung-cancer risk: a prospective study of men in Shanghai, China. *Lancet* 2000;356:724–729.
14. Morris, ME, Telang U. Isothiocyanates and Cancer Prevention. In A Awad and P Bradford (Eds.), *Nutrition and Cancer Prevention*. Boca Raton, FL: CRC Press, Taylor & Francis, 2006, pp. 435–453.
15. Jo JY, Gonzalez de Mejia E, Lila MA. Effects of grape cell culture extracts on human topoisomerase II catalytic activity and characterization of active fractions. *J Agric Food Chem* 2005 Apr 6;53(7):2489–98.
16. Removed at proofs.
17. Gogos CA, et al. Dietary omega-3 polyunsaturated fatty acids plus vitamin E restore immunodeficiency and prolong survival for severely ill patients with generalized malignancy. *Cancer* 1998 Jan 15;82:395–402.
18. Bartram HP, Gostner A, Scheppach W, et al. Effects of fish oil on rectal cell proliferation, mucosal fatty acids, and prostaglandin E2 release in healthy subjects. *Gastroenterology* 1993 Nov;105(5): 1317–1322.
19. Adlercreutz H, Mousavi Y, Clark J, et al. Dietary phytoestrogens and cancer: In vitro and in vivo studies. *J Steroid Biochem Mol Biol* 1992;41(3–8):331–337.
20. Wang C, Makela T, Hase T, et al. Lignans and flavonoids inhibit aromatase enzyme in human preadipocytes. *J Steroid Biochem Mol Biol* 1994 Aug;50(3–4):205–212.
21. University of California—Los Angeles 2007, November 3. New Way To Predict Survival In Older Women With Lung Cancer. *Science Daily*.
22. Lu J, Jiang C, Kaeck M, et al. Dissociation of the genotoxic and growth inhibitory effects of selenium. *Biochem Pharmacol* 1995 Jul 17;50(2):213–219.
23. Whanger PD. Relationship of Selenium Intake to Cancer. In A Awad and P Bradford (Eds.), *Nutrition and Cancer Prevention*. Boca Raton, FL: CRC Press, Taylor & Francis, 2006, pp. 189–219.
24. Bremner P, Heinrich M. Natural products as targeted modulators of the nuclear-kB pathway. *J Pharm Pharmacol* 2002;54(4):453–472.

25. Korutla L, Cheung JY, Mendelsohn J, et al. Inhibition of ligand-induced activation of epidermal growth factor receptor tyrosine phosphorylation by curcumin. *Carcinogenesis* 1995 Aug;16(8):1741–1745.

26. Jee SH, Shen SC, Tseng CR, et al. Curcumin induces a p53-dependent apoptosis in human basal cell carcinoma cells. J *Invest Dermatol* 1998 Oct;111(4):656–661.

27. Zhou W, Suk R, Liu G, Park S, Neuberg DS, Wain JC, Lynch TJ, Giovannucci E, Christiani DC. Vitamin D is associated with improved survival in early-stage non-small cell lung cancer patients. *Cancer Epidomiol Biomarkers Prev* 2005 Oct;14(10):2303–9.

28. De Grandis, D. Acetyl-l-Carnitine for the treatment of chemotherapy-induced peripheral neuropathy: a short review. *CNS Drugs* 2007;21 Suppl 1:39–43; discussion 45–46.

29. Boyd, B. Insulin and cancer. *Integrative Cancer Therapies* 2003;2(4):315–329.

30. Tisdale MJ. Cachexia in cancer patients. *Nat Rev Cancer* 2002;2:862–871.

31. Gordon JN, Green SR, Goggin PM. Cancer cachexia. *Q J Med* 2005;98:779–788.

32. Lissoni P, Paolorossi F, Tancini G, et al. Is there a role for melatonin in the treatment of neoplastic cachexia? *Eur J Cancer* 1996;32A(8):1340–1343.

33. Lissoni P, Paolorossi F, Ardizzoia A, et al. A randomized study of chemotherapy with cisplatin plus etoposide versus chemoendocrine therapy with cisplatin, etopiside and the pineal hormone melatonin as a first-line treatment of advanced non-small cell lung cancer patients in a poor clinical state. *J Pineal Res* 1997 Aug;23(1):15–19.

34. Barber MD. Cancer cachexia and its treatment with fish-oil-enriched nutritional supplementation. *Nutrition* 2001;17:751–755.

Section IX

Reproductive Health

42 Pregnancy

Optimizing the *In Utero* Environment

Gary Chan, M.D.

I.   INTRODUCTION

Women with suboptimal nutrient levels may experience clinical symptoms consistent with deficiency syndromes during the high-nutrient demands of pregnancy. Delays in diagnosing nutrient deficiencies that arise during pregnancy can be costly to both maternal and fetal health. Recent technologic advances have allowed research into the consequences of a nutrient-compromised fetal environment. The fetal nutrient environment exerts measurable impact on the interpretation of genome. This chapter on the nutritional aspects of pregnancy presents research on the *in utero* environment, potential long-term implications, and strategies for mothers to improve their own nutrition during pregnancy. We will first review the effects of maternal nutrition, health status, and toxin exposure on the health of the fetus. We will then use the pathology of intrauterine growth restriction (IUGR) as a case example to illustrate how early nutritional deprivation in a fetus can exert long-term health consequences. Finally, we will conclude with a list of dietary recommendations for the pregnant woman aimed at maximizing the health of both mother and child.

II.   EPIDEMIOLOGY

Defined as the number of births per 1000 individuals, the birth rate has decreased from 16.7 in 1990 to 14 in 2005 [1]. There has been an increase in the percentage of infants born prematurely, less than 37 weeks gestation. Between 1990 and 2005, this percentage rose from 10.6% to 12.7%. Furthermore, this increase has been seen across multiple races since the year 2000. Some of this increase may be explained by an increased rate of multiple gestation pregnancies. Twin births rose from 22.6 in 1990 to 32.2 in 2005. However, it is important to note that an increase in premature births has also been noted in singleton pregnancies [1]. Another increasing trend is that of infertility. The underlying causes for these trends remain poorly understood, and maternal nutrition may be a contributing factor. A number of factors place women at an increased risk of infertility, including advancing age, polycystic ovarian syndrome (PCOS), and obesity. Of note, both PCOS and obesity have direct links to poor maternal nutrition.

III.   PATHOPHYSIOLOGY

Maternal Weight and Birth Outcomes

Appropriate weight gain during pregnancy has been associated with outcome. Weight gain comprises the changes in the mother's body and the products of conception: fetus, amniotic fluid, and placenta. More than 30 years ago, researchers [2] reported that the average weight gain during pregnancy for healthy primigravadas was 12.5 kg, a value still accepted as the norm. They estimated that the accepted 12.5 kg weight gain included: fetus (3400 g), amniotic fluid (800 g), placenta (659 g), blood volume expansion (1450 g), increased extracellular and extravascular water (1480 g), uterus (970 g), mammary tissue (405 g), and maternal fat (3345 g) [2].

Low gestational weight gain during pregnancy is associated with increased risk of intrauterine growth retardation (IUGR), low birthweight, and perinatal mortality. High gestational weight gain is associated with high birthweight but also with increased risk of complications during labor due to feto-pelvic disproportion. This complication is even higher in short-stature women [3]. The current Institute of Medicine recommendations for weight gain during pregnancy are shown in Table 42.1. The desirable weight gain in each pre-pregnancy weight-for-height category is that expected for delivery of a term infant weighing 3 to 4 kg. Higher weight gains are recommended for thin women. Lower weight gains are recommended for overweight and obese women to help minimize later maternal fat gain.

Pregnant obese women are at risk for perinatal complications. Women with a body mass index (BMI) greater than 30 kg/m^2 have a higher risk of gestational hypertension, diabetes, and fetal macrosomia compared with women with a BMI less than 30 kg/m^2. Also mothers with BMI 30 to 34.9 kg/m^2 have a 34% Cesarean section rate compared to 21% rate in mothers with a lower BMI. Obesity increases the operative complications such as excessive blood loss, anesthesia problems, increased operative time, wound infections, postpartum endometritis, and increased length of hospital stay [4].

Excessive weight gain during pregnancy increases the risk that the mothers will develop type II diabetes and obesity. The development of type II diabetes is affected by a multitude of factors, including ethnicity, age, obesity, and sedentary lifestyle, and whether the mother had pregnancy-induced diabetes. Obesity has been associated with the amount of weight gain during pregnancy and the time required to lose the pregnancy weight. Mothers who lost their pregnancy weight by 6 months only gained an average 2.4 kg later. However, those mothers who kept their pregnancy weight at 6 months postpartum weighed 8.3 kg heavier later in life [5]. Breastfeeding and exercise can help in weight loss but only if they are done for longer than 12 weeks.

TABLE 42.1
Recommended Total Weight Gain Ranges for Pregnant Women by Prepregnancy Body Mass Index (BMI)

Weight for Height	Recommended Total Weight Gain, Kg (lb)
Low (BMI < 19.8)	12.5 – 18 (28–40)
Normal (BMI 19.8 – 26)	11.5 – 16 (25–35)
High (BMI 26 – 29)	7 – 11.5 (15–25)
Obese (BMI > 29)	> 6 (15)

Adolescent and African American women should strive for gains at the upper end of the recommended range. Short women (< 157 cm or 62 in) should strive for gains at the lower end of the range. BMI is defined as weight in kilograms divided by height in meters^2.

Source: Institute of Medicine. Nutrition During Pregnancy (Washington, DC: The National Academies Press, 1990).

Maternal obesity also appears to impair the process of breastfeeding. While simple mechanical factors likely play a role in this, it appears that obesity reduces prolactin response. Rasmussen et al. studied the response to suckling in 40 women in the week following delivery [6]. Overweight and obese women exhibited a blunted prolactin response during lactation as compared to normal weight controls. The impaired milk production in overweight mothers may be the reason why they tend to breastfeed for shorter durations of time. As such, maternal obesity serves as a risk factor for inadequate lactation, often considered an extension of the *in utero* environment.

LACTATION, AN EXTENSION OF THE *IN UTERO* ENVIRONMENT

Further emphasizing the importance of breastfeeding on infant health, Von Kries [7] examined the association between breastfeeding and childhood obesity. This survey study evaluated 9357 5- and 6-year-old children. Results indicated that the prevalence of obesity (BMI > 97th percentile) was only 2.8% in children who were breastfed, versus 4.5% in nonbreastfed children. The prevalence of obesity steadily decreased with the longer duration of breastfeeding. This study indicates that post-partum women should be encouraged to breastfeed, as this may help decrease the number of obese children who become obese adults [8].

MATERNAL DIABETES

Diabetes during pregnancy presents higher mortality and morbidity for the mother and the fetus compared to nondiabetic mothers. The glucose control of the diabetic mother may become more difficult with increased risk of preterm labor and spontaneous abortions. The fetus has increased risk of developing malformations of the central nervous system, heart, gastrointestinal tract, renal system, and skeleton. Causes of these malformations have been related to the poor glucose control and impaired magnesium metabolism during the diabetic state [9]. Though stabilizing and controlling glucose levels during the diabetic pregnancy are critical, more research in this area is needed to improve the perinatal outcome in diabetic mothers.

MATERNAL IRON DEFICIENCY ANEMIA

Mothers with iron deficiency anemia are at risk for preterm delivery and low-birthweight infants. Anemia during the first trimester has been associated with preterm labor. This association may be due to the hypoxia from the anemia, stress, and/or maternal infection. More studies are needed to understand the basic pathophysiology between maternal anemia and the perinatal outcome [10].

MATERNAL PKU

Phenylketonuria (PKU) is an autosomal recessive genetic disorder characterized by a deficiency in an enzyme needed to metabolize the amino acid phenylalanine. Left untreated, the elevated phenylalanine can cause problems with brain development leading to mental retardation and seizures. Adults with PKU are generally not restricted in their phenylalanine intake. But, pregnant women who have PKU especially need to be on a low-phenylalanine diet so that their phenylalanine levels do not damage the developing fetal brain [11].

HYPERTENSION AND PREECLAMPSIA

High blood pressure may be a preexisting condition in the mother or develop during the pregnancy (preeclampsia). Hypertension has a major effect on the mother and fetus. For the mother, it may cause cardiovascular stress leading to cardiac failure and neurologic compromise leading to stroke and/or seizures. For the fetus, maternal hypertension will reduce uteroplacental blood flow, decrease placental growth and development, and compromise fetal oxygen and nutrient supply. Pharmacologic intervention remains the major treatment for maternal hypertension during pregnancy. The use of calcium supplementation for maternal hypertension is discussed later in this chapter.

MATERNAL EXPOSURE TO PHARMACOLOGIC AGENTS

Many commonly prescribed medications have the ability to impact the development of the fetus (Table 42.2). Drugs that affect the fetus do so by several mechanisms. First, the unique characteristics of the fetal circulation represent an important determination of drug distribution and disposition. A major part of umbilical venous blood flow enters via the ductus venosus, bypassing the liver, so the fetus is generally exposed to high levels of unmetabolized drug. Also, the fetal liver is immature and has relatively little drug-metabolizing capacity. The binding of the drug by fetal proteins is limited. Oxidative enzyme and conjugation systems appear to be deficient. Finally, the fetal excretory activity of drugs is limited. Renal excretion of drugs is limited in the fetus. The major clearance of drugs is by the fetal liver and placenta; this may be impaired from the drug itself or by placental impairment. Thus, the fetus may be exposed to high and prolonged drug levels [12, 13].

MATERNAL TOXIN EXPOSURE

Toxin exposure in the mother can have significant consequences for the fetus. One well-known example is that of maternal mercury exposure leading to a variety of neurological defects in the fetus. The tragic consequences of excessive mercury exposure were seen in Japan in the 1950s [14]. Thousands of people were exposed to high levels of mercury in their diets secondary to industrial dumping of chemicals, conversion of inorganic mercury into methylmercury by marine algae, and subsequent buildup of mercury stores within fish. Referred to as Minamata disease, the result of the exposure was a wide range of neurological illnesses and death in people of all ages. Fetal effects were likely compounded by the fact that the placenta may actually serve to concentrate mercury levels in the fetus by removing mercury from the maternal bloodstream.

Nishikido et al. studied the effects of selenium supplementation on pregnant mice who were exposed to varying levels of mercury [15]. He noted that relatively small amounts of selenium (one-tenth part per million) were able to prevent lethal fetal toxicity in mice whose mothers were fed mercury. Mercury levels did not vary between selenium supplemented and nonsupplemented

---

TABLE 42.2
Drugs Affecting Fetal Growth

Alcohol

Nicotine

Steroids

Illicit Drugs:

    Heroin

    Cocaine

    Marijuana

    Methadone

    Methamphetamine

    Opiates

    Phencyclidine

Immunosuppressive Drugs

Note: A variety of legal and illicit drugs have the potential to significantly alter fetal growth, thus making a thorough medication history essential when caring for the pregnant woman.

---

subjects, suggesting that selenium exerts its protective effect in a manner in addition to blocking mercury absorption.

INTRAUTERINE GROWTH RESTRICTION (IUGR)

Defining IUGR

Having reviewed the importance of maternal nutrition, health, and toxin exposure on the health of the fetus, let us turn to a specific cause of fetal nutritional deprivation to better understand how it affects the long-term health of the fetus. In generic terms, IUGR can be defined as the failure of a fetus to achieve its inherent growth potential. IUGR is the second leading cause of infant morbidity and mortality. Clinically, infants who are born at a weight less than the 10th percentile for their gestational age are often classified as IUGR [16], with those whose weight is less than the 3rd percentile being at increased risk for perinatal morbidity and death [17]. However, each of these definitions fails to distinguish between infants who are IUGR from those who are simply constitutionally small. The ability to make this distinction remains a difficult clinical and research problem. Despite this limitation, IUGR is a clinical risk factor for several medical conditions throughout life.

Multiple etiologies of IUGR exist, including problems inherent to the fetus itself such as genetic disorders, chromosomal abnormalities, and infectious diseases, as well as problems external to the fetus such as utero-placental insufficiency (UPI) and maternal malnutrition. The prevalence of different etiologies varies throughout the world, with UPI accounting for the majority of cases in the developed world [18].

The placenta is responsible for transporting all of the components of metabolism and nutrition to the developing fetus. Establishment of the placenta is a complex process beyond the scope of this review, but any disturbance to this process jeopardizes the ability of the placenta to effectively provide glucose, protein, fatty acids, oxygen, and other key elements to the fetus. It is important to note that, in up to one-third of twin pregnancies, the two fetuses share a common placenta. Therefore, twin studies that examine the effects of genetics on health outcomes face a significant confounding variable in that many of these subjects have also shared a similar intrauterine environment.

Since UPI and its associated deprivation of nutrient supply to the fetus is the leading cause of IUGR in the United States, examining the long-term health outcomes of IUGR infants provides an important insight into the role of intrauterine nutrition on health later in life. After briefly examining how IUGR impacts the nutritional status of the fetus, we will then discuss these long-term effects.

Glucose

Glucose serves as the primary energy source for the developing fetus. It is transported from the placenta to the fetus primarily through the actions of specific transporters in a concentration-gradient-dependent manner [19]. Along with amino acids, glucose stimulates the production of insulin, insulin-like growth factor (IGF)-1, and IGF-2, factors that play key roles in promoting fetal growth. As such, limitations in glucose supply have the ability to directly impair normal growth.

Once glucose delivery to the fetus drops below a critical level, fetal hypoglycemia ensues. This leads to a complex metabolic response in an attempt to compensate for inadequate fuel supplies for aerobic metabolism. Insulin secretion is inhibited and glucagon levels rise, which contributes to gluconeogenesis and release of limited hepatic glycogen stores [20]. Protein stores are broken down to provide substrates for gluconeogenesis [21]. In addition to adaptations directed toward normalizing plasma glucose levels, vital organs like the brain can utilize alternate sources of energy, such as lactate and ketones [22]. The net result of the compensatory measures is a relative normalization of glucose levels at the expense of glucose stores. As a result, IUGR infants are born with significantly depleted hepatic glycogen stores [23]. When the limited but continuous supply of glucose from the placenta is interrupted after birth, these infants are at increased risk for developing hypoglycemia and require frequent initial glucose monitoring. It is important to maintain a steady supply of glucose to the infant. It has been a standard of care to start parenteral nutrition of glucose and amino acids immediately after birth for preterm or IUGR infants.

Protein

In addition to leading to protein breakdown to generate the precursors of gluconeogenesis, IUGR adversely affects amino acid levels in the fetus in other ways. Per unit of body weight, IUGR infants exhibit decreased total body protein secondary to decreased muscle growth. Amino acids are transported across the placenta by transport systems that are specific for different types of amino acids [24]. In normal pregnancies, this active process leads to a greater fetal circulating pool of amino acids than that found in the maternal blood supply. Amino acids play key roles in helping to regulate insulin, IGF-1, and IGF-2 production, and are also necessary substrates for protein synthesis and muscle growth. For these reasons, early protein administration is considered the standard of therapy to prevent protein catabolism within the first 24 hours of life for preterm or IUGR infants.

Several studies have identified specific amino acid deficiencies in IUGR pregnancies [25]. While the underlying mechanism is not completely understood, decreases in amino acid transport from the placenta to the fetus may play a key role. The net decrease in amino acid transport and low fetal plasma levels contribute to growth deficiencies in the IUGR fetus.

Fatty Acids

Fatty acids are transmitted across the placenta by both simple diffusion and with specific binding proteins. These binding proteins enable higher levels of certain fatty acids within the fetal circulation relative to the maternal circulation. The vast majority of fat deposition occurs during the last 10 weeks of gestation [26]. This deposition serves as a significant source of postnatal energy stores. The combination of decreased fatty acid supply to the fetus as well as decreased insulin levels secondary to fetal hypoglycemia leads to impaired fat stores at birth in the IUGR infant.

In addition to being an important source of energy, fatty acids are key components to proper neurological and ocular development. In particular, two polyunsaturated fatty acids, arachidonic acid (AA) and docosahexaenoic acid (DHA), are thought to be integral to this function. Human studies demonstrate a decreased fetal-to-maternal serum ratio of AA and DHA in IUGR infants as compared to control infants [27]. While a causative link has not been established, this may play a role in the increased risk of neurological morbidity faced by IUGR infants.

Effects of IUGR on the Long-Term Health of the Fetus

What long-term consequences do these early nutritional insults have? Over the last 20 years, multiple large epidemiological studies have linked impaired intrauterine growth with several adult-onset metabolic morbidities. Barker et al. was the first to examine the association between birth weight and risk for ischemic heart disease [3]. In a retrospective study involving over 5600 men born in England between 1911 and 1930, subjects weighing less than 5.5 pounds were found to be at the highest risk for developing ischemic heart disease. In another large study involving a different population of more than 1500 men, Barker showed that IUGR, rather than simply low birth weight, was related to the increased risk of cardiovascular disease and mortality as an adult [28]. Additional studies have subsequently revealed that these increased risks are shared by small-for-gestational age (SGA) females as well [29].

In addition to the increased risks IUGR infants face for cardiovascular disease as adults, several studies have shown that these infants are more likely to suffer from impaired glucose tolerance and non-insulin-dependent diabetes mellitus as adults [30, 31]. For example, Ravelli compared glucose tolerance levels in adults who were prenatally exposed to the Dutch famine of the 1940s to adults who were conceived or born in the years prior to and following this period. As compared to subjects not exposed to famine conditions while *in utero,* exposed subjects had impaired glucose tolerance when challenged with an oral glucose load. Another study determined that ß-cell function in the pancreas becomes impaired secondary to nutritional deficiencies antepartum [32]. Further studies by Barker reported an increased risk of developing insulin resistance, observing that at age 50 years, subjects who had a birthweight of less than 2.5 kg had a 10-fold higher incidence of the insulin resistance syndrome than subjects with a birthweight greater than 4.5 kg.

Levy-Marchal et al. performed a case control study examining the association between insulin resistance and low birthweight. They compared 20-year-old subjects who were born with IUGR to age-matched controls of a normal birthweight. They measured peripheral glucose uptake under euglycemic hyperinsulinemic clamp and noted a significantly decreased peripheral glucose uptake in IUGR subjects [33].

The observation that IUGR leads to increased risks of both cardiovascular disease and impaired glucose metabolism led Barker and Hales to develop the "thrifty phenotype" hypothesis [34]. This hypothesis states that a fetus facing nutritional deprivation would divert nutrition to vital organs like the brain in preference to less vital organs like skeletal muscles and abdominal viscera. If this occurs during a critical stage of organ development, long-term alterations in organ function may result. This would allow a fetus to survive birth and prepare for a nutritionally restricted extrauterine environment. However, pathologies arise when the growth-restricted fetus enters a world not of nutritional deficit but rather nutritional excess. As these children grow into adults, adaptations in regulating metabolism meant for dealing with starvation may be maladaptive when calories are abundant. This then leads to increased risks for diabetes and cardiovascular disease. Indeed, studies have shown that, among SGA infants, those with the highest prevalence of diabetes are those that go on to develop obesity as adults [30]. For these reasons, parents of children with IUGR should be counseled regarding the increased adulthood risks for cardiovascular disease and diabetes and that a healthful diet and lifestyle is, therefore, of even more importance.

Pathophysiology of IUGR: Role of Epigenetics

What are the mechanisms by which IUGR, an insult that occurs prenatally, can give rise to adverse outcomes decades later? A growing body of literature suggests that IUGR leads to these changes via epigenetic modifications. Epigenetic modifications alter gene expression within cells without changing the underlying genome. Recall that all cells within a given person contain the identical DNA sequence, consisting of approximately 20,000 to 25,000 genes [35]. Despite possessing the information to express each of these genes, any given type of cell only expresses the genes needed for it to perform its specific functions. For example, the genes expressed by a cardiac cell vary greatly from those expressed by a neuron, despite the fact that each contains the same genetic information. Therefore, it is important for cells to "turn on" certain genes, while "turning off" others. This is accomplished by altering the chromatin structure of the DNA. This allows the transcriptional machinery responsible for generating mRNA and ultimately proteins to easily access some genes and bar others. In this way, within a given cell, certain genes will be more actively expressed.

Alterations in chromatin structure are achieved by chemical modifications of either the DNA itself or of the supporting proteins around which DNA is wrapped, known as histones. A variety of proteins have the ability to add methyl or acetyl groups to either DNA or histones. The addition of these groups alters the structure of the chromatin and either facilitates or inhibits a gene from being transcribed. Nutrients are known to affect the proteins responsible for making these modifications. For example, folate is needed for proper DNA methylation. It may be the case that folate deficiency during pregnancy leads to aberrant DNA methylation patterns and that this in turn plays a significant role in the increased risk for the development of neural tube defects in folate-deficient fetuses. Similarly, a growing body of literature has shown that IUGR alters the patterns of DNA and chromatin methylation and acetylation on specific genes. This may be the mechanism by which IUGR alters gene expression and ultimately leads to the pathologies seen in adult IUGR individuals.

Studies by Dolinoy et al. further support the argument that the nutritional status of the mother can alter gene expression in the fetus. Using a genetically altered mouse model, these researchers have shown that maternal exposure to bisphenol A (a toxic byproduct of plastic production) leads to hypomethylation of key genetic components in the offspring [36]. These alterations are visualized phenotypically by a change in fur color that results from the altered gene expression. Of striking importance, further supplementing the maternal diet with nutrients that serve as methyl donors (such as folic acid or genistein) negates the effects of bisphenol A by reducing the hypomethylation of these same genetic components. As such, this important work not only demonstrates that adverse nutritional exposures can alter gene expression, but that further nutritional interventions can counteract potential insults. This area of research offers exciting promise for future dietary recommendations to pregnant women.

IV.   MANAGEMENT RECOMMENDATIONS

EDUCATE

The primary care setting offers the opportunity to emphasize that the fetal environment, greatly influenced by nutrition, interprets the conferred genetic material.

ASSESS NUTRITIONAL STATUS

Assessment of a woman's nutritional status during pregnancy is more complicated than assessment of a nonpregnant woman. The physiological changes of pregnancy, including hormone-induced changes in metabolism, shifts in plasma volume, and changes in renal function and patterns of urinary excretion, result in alterations of nutrient levels in the tissues and fluids available for evaluation and interpretation [37]. Plasma concentrations of some nutrients show a steady decrease as pregnancy progresses, possibly a result of hemodilution. Concentrations of other nutrients, however, may be either unaffected or increased because of pregnancy-induced changes in the availability of carrier molecules.

The current recommended dietary reference intakes (DRIs) for pregnant, lactating, and nonpregnant adult women (ages 19–50 years) are shown in Table 42.3 [38]. Table 42.3 is based on the resources using the adequate intake (AI), which refers to the recommended daily average intake level, assumed to be adequate, that is based on either observed or experimentally determined estimates of nutrient intake by apparently healthy individuals; and the recommended dietary allowance (RDA), which refers to the average daily dietary nutrient intake level sufficient to meet the nutrient requirement of nearly all (97% to 98%) healthy individuals.

REVIEW NUTRIENT REQUIREMENTS

Energy

When compared with a nonpregnant woman, a pregnant woman requires an estimated average additional energy during the course of a term pregnancy of approximately 335 MJ (80,000 calories). This includes energy needed for the products of conception (0.2%), maternal fat stores (0.4%), and extra energy needed to maintain new tissues (0.5%) [2, 39]. Energy demands during pregnancy are affected by food intake, physical activity, diet-induced thermogenesis, and maternal fat storage. Thus the current recommended dietary reference intakes of an additional 340 kcal/day (1420 kJ/day) and 452 Kcal/day (1888 kJ/day) during the second and third trimesters, respectively, may not meet individual's energy needs. Interestingly, although the maternal basal metabolic rate rises throughout pregnancy in well-nourished women, it has been found to decrease in poorly nourished women until late in pregnancy, suggesting an energy-sparing metabolic flexibility that benefits the developing fetus [40].

TABLE 42.3
Recommended Daily Energy and Nutrients During Pregnancy and Lactation Compared to Nonpregnant Adults

| | Dietary Reference Intakes | | | % ≠ over Adult Women | |
Nutrient	Adult 19–50 y Women	Pregnant Women	Lactating Women	Pregnant Women	Lactating Women
Energy (Kcal)	No value	≠ 340 Kcal/d 2nd trimester ≠ 452 Kcal/d 3rd trimester	≠ 500 Kcal/d 0 – 6 m ≠ 400 Kcal/d 7 – 12 m	≠ —	≠ ≠
Protein, g	46	71	71	54.4	54.4
Vitamin C, mg	75	85	120	13.3	60
Thiamin, mg	1.1	1.4	1.4	27.3	27.3
Riboflavin, mg	1.1	1.4	1.6	27.3	45.5
Niacin, mg NE	14	18	17	28.6	21.4
Vitamin B6, mg	1.3	1.9	2	46.2	53.9
Folate, μg DFE	400	600	500	50	25
Vitamin B12, μg	2.4	2.6	2.8	8.3	16.7
Pantothenic Acid, mg	5	6	7	20	40
Biotin, μg	30	30	35	0	16.7
Choline, mg	425	450	550	5.9	29.4
Vitamin A, μg RE	700	770	1300	10	85.7
Vitamin D, μg	5	5	5	0	0
Vitamin E, mg TE	15	15	19	0	26.7
Vitamin K, μg	90	90	90	0	0
Calcium, mg	1000	1000	1000	0	0
Phosphorus, mg	700	700	700	0	0
Magnesium, mg	310	350	310	12.9	0
Iron, mg	18	27	9	50	50
Zinc, mg	8	11	12	37.5	50
Iodine, mg	150	220	290	46.7	93.3
Selenium, μg	55	60	70	9.1	27.3
Fluoride, mg	3	3	3	0	0

NE, niacin equivalents; DFE, dietary folate equivalents; RE, retinol equivalents; TE, tocopherol equivalents

Source: Institute of Medicine, *Nutrition During Pregnancy* (Washington, DC: The National Academies Press, 1990); Institute of Medicine, *Dietary Reference Intakes for Energy, Carbohydrate, Fiber, Fat, Fatty Acids, Cholesterol, Protein, and Amino Acids.* (Washington, DC: The National Academies Press, 2002); and MF Picciano, SS McDonald Nutrition requirements during pregnancy and lactation, in J Bhatia (Ed.), *Perinatal Nutrition Optimizing Infant Health and Development* (New York: Marcel Dekker, 2005, p. 22).

Protein

During pregnancy, the mother accumulates an estimated 925 g of protein, which is deposited in fetal, placental, and maternal tissues primarily during the second and third trimesters [37]. Protein requirements during the first trimester do not increase significantly. However, during the last two trimesters, the calculated protein RDA for a pregnant woman is 1.1 g/kg/day, equivalent to 25 g/day of additional protein for a pregnant 57 kg reference woman. This results in a recommended protein intake of 71 g/day for a pregnant woman compared with 46 g/day for a nonpregnant woman

[38]. However, studies show that women of reproductive age in the United States consume diets that provide mean protein intakes of about 70 g/day, well in line with the estimated pregnancy requirement [41]. It is recommended that pregnant women consume two or three servings of protein daily. A serving of protein is about 1 oz of cooked animal meat or fish, one-half cup of cooked dry beans, 1 egg, or 2 tablespoons of peanut butter.

Calcium

Calcium needs during pregnancy are increased because of the skeletal development of the fetus. There are no data showing that pregnancy causes a permanent negative effect on maternal calcium and bone metabolism. Dietary calcium requirements between pregnancy and nonpregnancy are not different since calcium intestinal absorption is increased during pregnancy. Requirements of calcium during pregnancy are 1200 mg/day for women aged 19 to 50 years and 1500 mg/day for women who are 18 years or younger. In a randomized controlled study, calcium supplementation of 1200 mg/d from dairy foods in adolescent mothers resulted in higher maternal vitamin D and folate levels and higher newborn weight and bone mineralization compared to controls [42]. Sources of calcium include dairy products, tofu, sesame seeds, and spinach. Most prenatal vitamins contain about 250 mg of calcium and therefore will fail to meet daily calcium requirements if used as the sole source.

Calcium metabolism is affected by eclampsia, preeclampsia, and pregnancy-induced hypertension. Mothers with preeclampsia have hypocalciuria, higher PTH concentrations, lower ionized calcium, and lower 1,25-dihydroxyvitamin D concentrations compared to mothers with normal pregnancies. Some investigators believe that low daily calcium intake may be the major cause of pregnancy-induced hypertension. Countries where the daily calcium intake is low have higher rates of eclampsia. Also, the risk of pregnancy-induced hypertension in American and Canadian women is higher among women with low milk intake (<1 glass/day) than among those with a moderate intake (1–2 glasses/day) [43, 44]. Results of calcium supplementation trials have been inconsistent, but they largely indicated a beneficial effect on pregnancy-induced hypertension and for pregnant mothers who have low daily calcium intake. It has been recommended to supply an extra 1000 to 2000 mg/day throughout the second half of pregnancy [45–50].

Calcium supplementation may also be beneficial in protecting both mothers and fetuses from toxic lead exposure. Lead can cause irreversible neurologic damage, negative renal effects, and reproductive toxicity. Lead is easily ingested through the GI tract and deposits largely in bones. As pregnancy results in increased bone turnover to mobilize calcium stores, lead can be released as well and potentially affect both the mother and the developing fetus's nervous system. Hernandez et al. conducted a randomized, double-blind placebo-controlled trial involving more than 600 lactating women [51]. They found that supplementation with 1200 mg of elemental calcium per day significantly decreased circulating lead levels, particularly in women who began the study with the highest lead level burdens. Calcium supplementation also lowers these levels in infants. Because similar increases in bone turnover can be seen during pregnancy, it seems likely that these results can be expanded to pregnancy as well.

To meet these needs, the pregnant woman needs to consume 1000 to 1500 mg calcium per day. Requirements can be met with various foods and/or supplemental calcium. Calcium supplements should be taken separately from prenatal vitamins or iron supplements, as iron absorption will be decreased. Additional information on calcium supplementation can be found in Chapter 32, "Metabolic Bone Disease." How the alkalinizing effect of fruits and vegetables reduces the metabolic demands for calcium is detailed in Chapter 31, "Osteoporosis."

Vitamin D

Vitamin D is necessary for increasing intestinal absorption of calcium, maintaining bone mineralization, and avoiding hyperparathyroidism (Chapter 17, "Hyperparathyroidisms"). Since vitamin D is generated from sunlight exposure, vitamin D synthesis is limited in the northern United States owing to the latitude and the decreased hours of daylight between October and March [52]. Recent studies indicate rates of vitamin D insufficiency to be as high as 40% [53, 54]. The best food sources of vitamin D are cod liver oil, fortified milk and other dairy products, and salmon. Mushrooms that have been exposed to UV light are under study as a potential nonanimal product food source of vitamin D. Requirement of vitamin D during pregnancy is 5 µg or 200 IU daily, though higher amounts may be needed for those mothers who have limited sunlight exposure.

It has been reported that despite taking prenatal vitamins that contain 200 to 400 IU vitamin D, 90% of pregnant women were still vitamin D deficient. Vitamin D deficiency during pregnancy has been associated with preeclampsia [55] and the development of newborn rickets. Whether vitamin D deficiency continues to be a clinical problem or public health issue and if the current vitamin D requirements need to be changed, warrant future research and studies.

Iron

Iron needs are increased during pregnancy because of the maternal increase in the mother's blood volume. A pregnant woman must take in an extra 700 to 800 mg of iron over the course of her pregnancy, most of which is needed during the last half of the pregnancy [56]. Since most women rarely start pregnancy with adequate iron stores, iron supplementation in the form of ferrous sulfate, gluconate, or fumerate may be necessary to prevent iron-deficiency anemia. Maternal iron-deficiency anemia has adversely affected both mother and infant outcomes, resulting in low gestational weight gain, premature delivery, low birthweight, and maternal hypothyroidism [57].

Iron requirements through diet alone during pregnancy are often not met, and therefore a supplement is required. The average prenatal vitamins contain 30 to 60 mg of iron, which is above the recommended daily requirement of 27 mg/day. Combining iron with vitamin C intake will improve iron absorption and may minimize GI intolerance. Excellent sources of iron include red meats, chicken, turkey, fish, and lentils. Additionally, cooking foods in an iron skillet may help to increase intake.

Folic Acid

Folic acid requirements increase during pregnancy in response to the demands of maternal erythropoiesis and fetal and placental growth [56]. Folate functions as a coenzyme in nucleic and amino acid metabolism. A deficiency in folic acid has resulted in neural tube defects in the fetus and poor pregnancy outcome. Therefore, it is recommended that all women of childbearing years and pregnant women should consume 400 µg of folic acid per day. Supplementation should begin 1 month before conception to ensure that vitamin levels are adequate at the time of neural tube closure [58]. Prenatal vitamins contain 1000 µg of folic acid, which is more than adequate to meet the daily requirements. Dietary sources of folate are fortified breakfast cereals, cowpeas (black-eye peas), spinach, liver, green vegetables, citrus fruits, juices, and whole wheat bread (see Chapter 38, "Cervical Cancer"). In addition to assuring that women consume adequate amounts of folate, it is important to note that several drugs interfere with folate metabolism. These include trimethoprim (commonly used to treat urinary tract infections), pyrimethamine (an antimalarial), methotrexate, and phenytoin. Other drugs may also disrupt folate utilization, and it is important to obtain a thorough medication history from any pregnant woman.

Essential Fatty Acids

Linoleic and alpha-linolenic acids are essential fatty acids, meaning that they come from diet. They are the nutrients that the body then further processes into gamma-linolenic acid, dihomo-gamma-linolenic acid, eicosapentaenoic acid, and docosahexaenoic acid to form the structural components of the central nervous system (Chapter 5, "Hypertension," Table 5.5). The requirements of these essential fatty acids are increased during pregnancy, especially in the last trimester. The daily requirements for linoleic acid and linolenic acid during pregnancy are 13 and 1.4 g/day, respectively.

Given the importance of essential fatty acids to fetal development, many studies have focused on a potential role for fatty acid supplementation in improving pregnancy outcomes. A recent Cochrane review pooled the results of several such studies in an attempt to better answer the question of whether such supplementation may lead to improved perinatal outcomes [59]. These studies focused on women whose pregnancies had not been complicated by preeclampsia or IUGR. The results of this review demonstrated that supplementation led to modest increases in length of gestation (2.6 days), decreased incidence of infants born prior to 34 weeks, and slight increases in birthweight. Functional nutritional assays and balanced essential fats supplementation approaches are discussed throughout this text.

Choline

Choline is a small molecule whose metabolites perform a wide array of functions in all cells throughout the body, including serving as structural components of cell membranes and trans-membrane signaling. Studies in rats have suggested that choline may be particularly important in neurological development [60–62]. These studies demonstrated that choline supplementation during critical periods of *in utero* neurological development improves memory function in rats as adults. While similar studies in humans have yet to be performed, this area of research may eventually support a role for choline supplementation in pregnant women, especially those who have undergone a cholecystectomy as they are at increased risk for developing choline deficiency.

Iodine

The demand for iodine increases during pregnancy commensurate with other minerals. Maternal goiter is a very late stage of iodine deficiency. Chapter 16, "Hypothyroidism," details methods of earlier detection and explains how certain foods and supplements can be goiterogenic.

AVOID TREND DIETS, SUPPLEMENT FADS, AND UNNECESSARILY RESTRICTING DIETS

Efforts to improve pregnancy outcomes by altering the nutritional intake of pregnant women through trend diets, supplement fads, and unnecessarily restrictive diets have met with limited success. Kramer performed a meta-analysis of 49 smaller trials looking at the effects of maternal energy and protein supplementation during pregnancy [63]. While augmenting energy and protein intake did lead to slightly larger fetal weight gain in general, the infants of undernourished women did not particularly benefit versus those of adequately nourished women. Furthermore, nutritional supplementation did not result in any long-term growth or neurodevelopment benefits. As such, this analysis concluded that simple energy or protein supplementation does not lead to improved maternal or fetal outcomes, and even more concerning, protein supplementation in particular may actually be associated with impaired fetal growth.

STRIKE A BALANCE ON CONTROVERSIAL FOODS

Tea

Tea is a good source of hydration that provides antioxidants and is low in calories and glycemic load. Furthermore, ginger teas help to reduce nausea associated with pregnancy. Despite these facts, the use of herbs and herbal supplements during pregnancy has not been recommended [64] out of concerns for imported teas, which are not regulated and for which the dosage and purity cannot be accurately determined. Some herbal products have been found to be contaminated with lead [65]. Many herbal supplements have been found to stimulate uterine contractions, which may increase the risk of miscarriage or preterm labor. The American Academy of Pediatrics recommends that pregnant women choose herbal teas in filter teabags and limit consumption to two 250 mL servings per day. Certain herbal teas such as citrus peel, ginger, lemon balm, linden flower, and rosehip are considered safe [58].

Fish

In many ways, fish represent an excellent food during pregnancy, being a good source of protein, fatty acids, vitamins, and minerals. However, ongoing concerns regarding mercury contamination limit the clinician's ability to recommend increasing fish intake by the pregnant woman. As a result of these concerns, the FDA has recommended that pregnant women avoid eating fish known to have high mercury levels (such as swordfish, shark, and king mackerel) and to limit consumption of other fish to no more than 12 ounces per week. Additionally, it is important to note that fish caught in local bodies of water may have highly variable mercury levels based upon the locale. It is important to counsel pregnant women to check local fish advisory services as to the levels of mercury in these fish. Dietary supplementation of selenium, a trace mineral found in most prenatal vitamins, may help to offset the damaging effects of mercury.

COUNSEL FAMILIES ON THE PROGNOSIS OF IUGR INFANTS AND OTHER INFANTS WITH A COMPROMISED *IN UTERO* ENVIRONMENT THAT THIS IS A RISK FACTOR FOR OBESITY AND INSULIN RESISTANCE

Unfortunately, while many children may have less than optimal fetal environments, this is seldom detectable at a preventable stage or later. IUGR is one postevent marker that the fetal environment was suboptimal and that a number of miscues may have occurred. When IUGR is detected, maximizing health in the postnatal environment, especially by focusing on the importance of healthful nutrition, becomes even more important.

ACKNOWLEDGEMENTS

Robert Langen, M.D., contributed to the development of the section on intrauterine growth restriction.

REFERENCES

1. Hamilton BE, Minino AM, Martin JA, Kochanek KD, Strobino DM, Guyer B. Annual summary of vital statistics: 2005. *Pediatrics* 119: 345–360, 2007.
2. Hytten FE. *The Physiology of Human Pregnancy.* Oxford: Blackwell Scientific Publications; 1971.
3. Barker DJ, Winter PD, Osmond C, Margetts B, Simmonds SJ. Weight in infancy and death from ischaemic heart disease. *Lancet* 2: 577–580, 1989.
4. American College of Obstetrics and Gynecology. ACOG encourages ob-gyns to address the health risks of obesity in women. September 30, 2005. Available from http://www.acog.org/from_home/publication/press_release.
5. Rooney BL, Schauberger CW. Excess pregnancy weight gain and long-term obesity: One decade later. *Obstet Gynecol* 100: 245–252, 2002.
6. Rasmussen KM, Kjolhede CL. Prepregnant overweight and obesity diminish the prolactin response to suckling in the first week postpartum. *Pediatrics* 113: e465–471, 2004.
7. Von Kries R, Koletzko B, Sauerwald T, von Mutuis E, Barnert D, Grunert V, von Voss H. Breast feeding and obesity: Cross sectional study. *Br Med J* 319: 147–150, 1999.
8. Koletzko B, von Kries R. Are there long term protective effects of breast feeding against later obesity? *Nutr Health* 15: 225–236, 2001.
9. Mimouni F, Tsang RC. Pregnancy outcome in insulin-dependent diabetes: Temporal relationships with metabolic control during specific pregnancy periods. *Am J Perinatol* 5: 334–338, 1988.
10. Allen LH. Biological mechanisms that might underlie iron's effects on fetal growth and preterm birth. *J Nutr* 131: 581S–9S, 2001.

11. Caulfield LE. Periconceptional nutrition and infant outcome. In Bhatia J (Ed.), *Perinatal Nutrition Optimizing Infant Health and Development.* New York: Marcel Dekker, 2005, p. 9.

12. Bell GL, Lau K. Perinatal and neonatal issues of substance abuse. *Pediatr Clin North Am* 42: 261–281, 1995.

13. Howell EM, Heiser N, Harrington M. A review of recent findings on substance abuse treatment for pregnant women. *J Subst Abuse Treat* 16: 195–219, 1999.

14. Harada M. Congenital Minamata disease: Intrauterine methylmercury poisoning. *Teratology* 18: 285–288, 1978.

15. Nishikido N, Furuyashiki K, Naganuma A, Suzuki T, Imura N. Maternal selenium deficiency enhances the fetolethal toxicity of methyl mercury. *Toxicol Appl Pharmacol* 88: 322–328, 1987.

16. Alexander GR, Himes JH, Kaufman RB, Mor J, Kogan M. A United States national reference for fetal growth. *Obstet Gynecol* 87: 163–168, 1996.

17. McIntire DD, Bloom SL, Casey BM, Leveno KJ. Birth weight in relation to morbidity and mortality among newborn infants. *N Engl J Med* 340: 1234–1238, 1999.

18. Brodsky D, Christou H. Current concepts in intrauterine growth restriction. *J Intensive Care Med* 19: 307–319, 2004.

19. Illsley NP. Glucose transporters in the human placenta. *Placenta* 21: 14–22, 2000.

20. Hubinont C, Nicolini U, Fisk NM, Tannirandorn Y, Rodeck CH. Endocrine pancreatic function in growth-retarded fetuses. *Obstet Gynecol* 77: 541–544, 1991.

21. Baschat AA. Fetal responses to placental insufficiency: An update. *BJOG* 111: 1031–1041, 2004.

22. Vannucci RC, Vannucci SJ. Glucose metabolism in the developing brain. *Semin Perinatol* 24: 107–115, 2000.

23. Shelley HJ, Neligan GA. Neonatal hypoglycaemia. *Br Med Bull* 22: 34–39, 1966.

24. Jansson T. Amino acid transporters in the human placenta. *Pediatr Res* 49: 141–147, 2001.

25. Cetin I, Marconi AM, Bozzetti P, Sereni LP, Corbetta C, Pardi G, Battaglia FC. Umbilical amino acid concentrations in appropriate and small for gestational age infants: A biochemical difference present in utero. *Am J Obstet Gynecol* 158: 120–126, 1988.

26. Haggarty P. Placental regulation of fatty acid delivery and its effect on fetal growth—AA review. *Placenta* 23 Suppl A: S28–38, 2002.

27. Cetin I, Giovannini N, Alvino G, Agostoni C, Riva E, Giovannini M, Pardi G. Intrauterine growth restriction is associated with changes in polyunsaturated fatty acid fetal-maternal relationships. *Pediatr Res* 52: 750–755, 2002.

28. Barker DJ, Osmond C, Simmonds SJ, Wield GA. The relation of small head circumference and thinness at birth to death from cardiovascular disease in adult life. *BMJ* 306: 422–426, 1993.

29. Osmond C, Barker DJ, Winter PD, Fall CH, Simmonds SJ. Early growth and death from cardiovascular disease in women. *BMJ* 307: 1519–1524, 1993.

30. Hales CN, Barker DJ, Clark PM, Cox LJ, Fall C, Osmond C, Winter PD. Fetal and infant growth and impaired glucose tolerance at age 64. *BMJ* 303: 1019–1022, 1991.

31. Ravelli AC, van der Meulen JH, Michels RP, Osmond C, Barker DJ, Hales CN, Bleker OP. Glucose tolerance in adults after prenatal exposure to famine. *Lancet* 351: 173–177, 1998.

32. Catalano PM, Kirwan JP, Haugel-de Mouzon S, King J. Gestational diabetes and insulin resistance: Role in short- and long-term implications for mother and fetus. *J Nutr* 133: 1674S–83S, 2003.

33. Levy-Marchal C, Jaquet D. Long-term metabolic consequences of being born small for gestational age. *Pediatr Diabetes* 5: 147–153, 2004.

34. Barker DJP. Fetal and infant origins of adult disease. *Monatsshr Kinderheilkd* 149:S2–S6, 2001.

35. International Human Genome Sequencing Consortium. Finishing the euchromatic sequence of the human genome. *Nature* 431: 931–945, 2004.

36. Dolinoy DC, Huang D, Jirtle RL. Maternal nutrient supplementation counteracts bisphenol A-induced DNA hypomethylation in early development. *Proc Natl Acad Sci USA* 104: 13056–13061, 2007.

37. Institute of Medicine. *Nutrition During Pregnancy.* Washington, DC: The National Academies Press, 1990.

38. Institute of Medicine. *Dietary Reference Intakes for Energy, Carbohydrate, Fiber, Fat, Fatty Acids, Cholesterol, Protein, and Amino Acids.* Washington, DC: The National Academies Press, 2002.

39. Kopp-Hoalihan LE, van Loan MD, Wong WW, King JC. Longitudinal assessment of energy balance in well-nourished, pregnant woman. *Am J Clin Nutr* 69: 697–704, 1999.

40. Prentice AM, Goldberg GR. Energy adaptations in human pregnancy: Limits and long-term consequences. *Am J Clin Nutr* 71: 1226S–32S, 2000.

41. McDowell MA, Briefel RR, Alaimo K, et al. Energy and macronutrient intakes of persons ages 2 months and over in the United States: Third National Health and Nutrition Examination Survey, Phase 1, 1988–91. *Adv Data* 1–24, 1994.
42. Chan GM, McElligott K, McNaught T, Gill G. Effects of dietary calcium intervention on adolescent mothers and newborns. *Obstet Gynecol* 108: 565–571, 2006.
43. Villar J, Repke J, Belizan JM, Pareja G. Calcium supplementation reduces blood pressure during pregnancy: Results of a randomized controlled clinical trial. *Obstet Gynecol* 70: 317–322, 1987.
44. Belizan JM, Villar J, Gonzalez L, Campodonico L, Bergel E. Calcium supplementation to prevent hypertensive disorders of pregnancy. *N Engl J Med* 325: 1399–1405, 1991.
45. Purwar M, Kulkarni H, Motghare V, Dhole S. Calcium supplementation and prevention of pregnancy induced hypertension. *J Obstet Gynaecol Res* 22: 425–430, 1996.
46. Lopez-Jaramillo P, Delgado F, Jacome P, Teran E, Ruano C, Rivera J. Calcium supplementation and the risk of preeclampsia in Ecuadorian pregnant teenagers. *Obstet Gynecol* 90: 162–167, 1997.
47. Lopez-Jaramillo P, Narvaez M, Weigel RM, Yepez R. Calcium supplementation reduces the risk of pregnancy-induced hypertension in an Andes population. *Br J Obstet Gynaecol* 96: 648–655, 1989.
48. Hofmeyr GJ, Roodt A, Atallah AN, Duley L. Calcium supplementation to prevent pre-eclampsia—a systematic review. *S Afr Med J* 93: 224–228, 2003.
49. Levine RJ, Hauth JC, Curet LB. Trial of calcium to prevent preeclampsia. *N Engl J Med* 337: 69–76, 1997.
50. Crowther CA, Hiller JE, Pridmore B, et al. Calcium supplementation in nulliparous women for the prevention of pregnancy-induced hypertension, preeclampsia and preterm birth: An Australian randomized trial. FRACOG and the ACT Study Group. *Aust N Z J Obstet Gynaecol* 39: 12–18, 1999.
51. Hernandez-Avila M, Gonzalez-Cossio T, Hernandez-Avila JE, Romieu I, Peterson KE, Aro A, Palazuelos E, Hu H. Dietary calcium supplements to lower blood lead levels in lactating women: A randomized placebo-controlled trial. *Epidemiology* 14: 206–212, 2003.
52. Webb AR, Holick MF. The role of sunlight in the cutaneous production of vitamin D3. *Annu Rev Nutr* 8: 375–399, 1988.
53. Holick MF. Sunlight and vitamin D: Both good for cardiovascular health. *J Gen Intern Med* 17: 733–735, 2002.
54. Hollis BW, Wagner CL. Vitamin D requirements during lactation: High-dose maternal supplementation as therapy to prevent hypovitaminosis D for both the mother and the nursing infant. *Am J Clin Nutr* 80: 1752S–8S, 2004.
55. Bodnar LM, Catov JM, Simhan HN, Holick MF, Powers RW, Roberts JM. Maternal vitamin D deficiency increases the risk of preeclampsia. *J Clin Endocrinol Metab* 92: 3517–3522, 2007.
56. Fagan C. Nutrition during pregnancy and lactation. In Mahan KL, and Escott-Stump S (Eds.), *Krause's Food, Nutrition, and Diet Therapy, 10th ed.* Philadelphia: The Curtis Center, 2000, pp. 167–195.
57. Zimmermann MB, Burgi H, Hurrell RF. Iron deficiency predicts poor maternal thyroid status during pregnancy. *J Clin Endocrinol Metab* 92: 3436–3440, 2007.
58. American Dietetic Association. Position of the American Dietetic Association: Nutrition and lifestyle for a healthy pregnancy outcome. *J Am Diet Assoc* 102: 1479–1489, 2002.
59. Makrides M, Duley L, Olsen SF. Marine oil, and other prostaglandin precursor, supplementation for pregnancy uncomplicated by pre-eclampsia or intrauterine growth restriction. *Cochrane Database Syst Rev* 3: CD003402, 2006.
60. Loy R, Heyer D, Williams CL, Meck WH. Choline-induced spatial memory facilitation correlates with altered distribution and morphology of septal neurons. *Adv Exp Med Biol* 295: 373–382, 1991.
61. Meck WH, Smith RA, Williams CL. Organizational changes in cholinergic activity and enhanced visuospatial memory as a function of choline administered prenatally or postnatally or both. *Behav Neurosci* 103: 1234–1241, 1989.
62. Meck WH, Smith RA, Williams CL. Pre- and postnatal choline supplementation produces long-term facilitation of spatial memory. *Dev Psychobiol* 21: 339–353, 1988.
63. Kramer MS. Effects of energy and protein intakes on pregnancy outcome: An overview of the research evidence from controlled clinical trials. *Am J Clin Nutr* 58: 627–635, 1993.
64. Gunderson EP. Nutrition during pregnancy for the physically active woman. *Clin Obstet Gynecol* 46: 390–402, 2003.
65. Mattison D. Herbal supplements: Their safety, a concern for health care providers, 2005. Available from http://search.Marchofdimes.com/cgibin/msmgo.exe. (September 6, 2007)

43 Male Infertility

Environmental Factors

Roger Billica, M.D.

I. INTRODUCTION

Numerous epidemiological studies in recent decades have documented a decline in male fertility. Many of these studies propose a link between the deterioration in fertility with growing exposure to environmental toxins such as anti-androgenic pesticides and fungicides (e.g., DDT and vinclozolin), plasticizers (e.g., bisphenol-A and dibutyl phthalate), water disinfection byproducts (e.g., dibromoacetic acid), heavy metals (e.g., lead, cadmium, and mercury), and common industrial contaminants in drinking water (e.g., benzene, phenol, and trichloroethylene). From a review of available literature, it is apparent that a variety of commonly used chemicals, now abundant in the environment, drinking water, and food chain, can have insidious and long-lasting effects on the male reproductive system.

The rising incidence of male infertility warrants a closer look at both preventable causes and potential solutions related to environmental and nutritional factors.

II. EPIDEMIOLOGY

Infertility is defined as the inability of a couple to achieve a pregnancy after 1 year of unprotected intercourse. Approximately 14% of couples are infertile, and in 40% to 50% of the cases, a male factor is a contributing cause of infertility [1, 2]. Therefore, an estimated 6% of men in their reproductive years are thought to be infertile.

In 1992 Carlsen and colleagues reported a significant global decline in sperm density between 1938 and 1990 [3]. A few years later Swan and colleagues revisited the same issue with an analysis of 101 studies published between 1934 to 1996 and concluded that there has been an overall decline in sperm density of approximately 1.5% per year in the United States and approximately 3% per year in Europe and Australia [4]. Their analysis controlled for variables such as abstinence time, age, percent of men with proven fertility, and specimen collection method. There was no decline trend in sperm density in non-Western countries, but the authors noted that data were very limited for these populations.

III. PATHOPHYSIOLOGY

There are many well-established known causes for male infertility which include [5]:

- Testicular disease (primary hypogonadism)
- Hypothalamic pituitary disease (secondary hypogonadism)
- Post-testicular defects (disorders of sperm transport)

- Alcohol and drug abuse (including anabolic steroid use)
- Smoking (known to decrease sperm count and sperm cell motility)
- Tight underwear (elevates scrotal temperature resulting in decreased sperm production)
- Malnutrition (inadequate vitamin C and zinc in the diet)
- Infection and disease (testicular atrophy caused by mumps, tuberculosis, gonorrhea, chlamydia, influenza, syphilis, brucellosis)
- Hypothyroidism
- Other endocrine imbalances (hyperprolactinemia, congenital adrenal hyperplasia, panhypopituitarism)
- Physical problems (erectile dysfunction, impaired sympathetic innervation of the genital tract, genital tract obstruction, ejaculatory dysfunction)

As epidemiological studies have recognized the declining trend in male fertility, the discussion of etiology has included possible involvement of environmental factors. Since both men and women require a proper balance of estrogens in order to be successful reproductively, some of the more obvious considered causes have included exposures to estrogens and xenoestrogens [6, 7]. These estrogen mimics are known to be endocrine disrupters and are found in everyday personal care products and as the breakdown products from plastics used in items such as water jugs and baby bottles. The estrogen-mimic bisphenol-A (BPA) is used in the manufacture of polycarbonate plastics and epoxy resins from which food and beverage containers and dental materials are made. Perinatal exposure to environmentally relevant doses of BPA has been shown to cause morphological and functional changes of the male genital tract and reduced fertility [8]. Dibutyl phthalate is used widely in production as a plasticizer, in cosmetics such as nail polish, and as an additive to adhesives and print inks. Dibutyl phthalate is considered to be an endocrine disrupter and has been shown to impair spermatogenesis and induce lesions in the reproductive system in animal models [9, 10].

Vinclozolin is a fungicide introduced in the 1970s and is used worldwide on fruits, vegetables, and vineyards, and thus is commonly ingested. Exposure to vinclozolin in rabbits during development stages induced presumably permanent changes in spermiogenesis and FSH secretion [11]. Exposure to the fungicides tebuconazole and epoxiconazole were investigated for reproductive effects in rats and found to have endocrine-disrupting effects including disturbances of key enzymes involved with the synthesis of steroid hormones [12].

Reproductive disorders including sperm abnormalities, hypospadias, and decreased fertility have been linked to pesticide exposure [13–16]. In addition to the direct endocrine disrupting effects of the various pesticides, there is also evidence that long-term exposure to pesticides can cause changes in antioxidant enzymes with harmful consequences not only on the immune and nervous system, but also with issues related to immunofertility [17, 18].

Another environmental concern with infertility is the negative impact of heavy metals on sperm quality and production. Occupational exposure to lead, mercury, and cadmium has been shown to cause significant decrease in male fertility [19–22]. Of course occupational contact with toxic metals is not the only risk of exposure due to the diffuse spread of these metals in the environment. Other studies have examined the impact of the presence of heavy metals [23]. For example, the mechanism of lead toxicity on the testis involves several areas including spermatogenesis, steroidogenesis, and the reduction-oxidation system. Chronic lead exposure can induce decreased testosterone synthesis, decreased germ cell population, and peritubular fibrosis [24].

Male infertility issues have also been linked with a variety of common industrial and household chemicals [25–27]. These include:

- Dibromoacetic acid (a water disinfection byproduct)
- Solvents such as trichlorethylene
- Phenol
- Chloroform

In the presence of such widespread exposure to potentially harmful toxins, there is some question as to why the impacts on male fertility are not even more widespread than noted. A reasonable explanation could be related to the concept of biochemical individuality, wherein the level of function of the detoxification and elimination pathways necessary for neutralization and removal of these chemicals and heavy metals varies from person to person. One study showed that individuals with impaired methylation due to genetic polymorphisms have frequent alterations in fertility [28]. Other studies have found that disruption of glutathione S-transferases (enzymes that detoxify electrophilic compounds) interferes with fertilizing ability of spermatozoa [29]. So whether an individual has genetic or acquired polymorphisms, changes in cellular detoxification functions appear to be an additional risk factor for environmental impacts on male fertility.

IV. PATIENT EVALUATION

In considering the possibility of environmental causes with a male patient diagnosed with infertility, a variety of testing is available. For example Accu-Chem Laboratories and US BioTek Laboratories offer various analyses for pesticides and common environmental and occupational chemicals including solvents and phthalates. Since blood testing for levels of heavy metals is only accurate for fairly recent exposure, most evaluations for heavy metals should more appropriately focus on testing that indicates tissue impact of past or chronic exposures. These tests would include urinary porphyrins 30 or a urine provocative challenge test using clinical dosing of the appropriate chelating agent (such as EDTA or DMSA). Many laboratories perform these tests and can provide the clinician with detailed guides for test administration and assistance with interpretation of the results. Testing for organophosphate pesticide exposure within a few months of exposure can be accomplished with red blood cell cholinesterase determination [31].

As with most diagnostic endeavors the clinician must take a careful history looking for potential exposures, family history of other potential manifestations of environmental toxicities (e.g., neurological and developmental disorders), and have a high index of suspicion. However, the chemicals and metals involved with increased risk of male infertility are so common and ubiquitous in today's world that it may not be necessary to find a specific or significant history of exposure. For example, one study demonstrated clinically significant human exposure to pesticides simply through the persistent presence of these chemicals on foods [32]. Another study demonstrated elevated pesticide urinary metabolites of children in farmworker households [33]. In many areas of the country households receive routine treatments with pesticides, and a number of communities have re-instituted pesticide spraying due to the recent concerns with the West Nile virus.

V. TREATMENT

While the various treatment approaches for the more typical causes of male infertility are detailed elsewhere, the successful clinical intervention for environmental causes requires that the clinician be familiar with three areas of priority: prevention, detoxification, and nutritional and biochemical support for male fertility.

PREVENTION

Prevention basically consists of avoidance of exposure to the offending agents. This is not only important for men of reproductive age, but also for women to prevent exposure to the fetus in utero and for children during growth and development. Due to the overwhelming presence of the identified chemicals and toxins in our environment, avoiding them may seem an impossible task.

However, there are simple, basic, and commonsense steps that any person or family can take to reduce their risk of exposure. For example:

- Knowing the source, quality, and content of household and workplace drinking water and if necessary, installing water filtration such as reverse osmosis sufficient to remove chemicals and heavy metals.
- Reducing exposure to pesticides and fungicides on fruits and vegetables (either through purchase of trustworthy organic produce or use of vegetable wash soaps prior to consumption).
- Being aware of and participating in efforts to reduce exposure to heavy metals that are still found in some vaccines, dental fillings, pharmacological agents, consumer products, certain fish and seafood, and other products.
- Finding nontoxic alternatives for the use of household pesticides and cleaning agents.
- Limiting exposure to plastics used in food preparation and storage. For example, use nonplastic containers and covers while heating food in microwave ovens. Discard scratched cookware with nonstick surfaces. Store food and beverages in glass instead of plastic containers.

DETOXIFICATION

Detoxification of offending chemicals and heavy metals may involve a variety of therapies. The basic principles of clinical detoxification remain important when dealing with either heavy metals, pesticides, plastics, or other chemical toxins. Especially important are the maintenance of tissue hydration and avoidance of constipation. Correction of underlying metabolic and nutritional deficiencies such as impaired methylation and hypothyroidism should precede any focused detoxification protocols.

Phospholipids and essential fatty acids: Because the area of toxic impact often involves disruption of the cell membrane bi-lipid integrity, steps to restore the balance of essential fatty acids in the cell membranes are a foundation for recovery. The health of the cell membrane is a key determinant of the function of the tissue, and therefore detoxification requires that the membrane of the cell be supported with balanced essential fatty acids and supportive phospholipids. Phosphatidylcholine (PC) is the most abundant phospholipid of the cell membrane and plays a key role in detoxification. In addition to phosphatidylcholine, a ratio of balanced essential fatty acids (4:1 omega-6 to omega-3 oil) provides the cellular nourishment for healthy membrane function [34–36]. Typical adult dosing for phosphatidylcholine in support of cell membrane repair and detoxification is in the range of 1200 to 2500 mg daily in two divided doses. Essential fatty acids can be found in a balanced ratio of 4:1 omega-6 (such as sunflower or safflower oil) and omega-3 (flax oil) and are recommended in a therapeutic dose range of 2 to 4 tablespoons daily. It is very important that these oils be organic, cold-pressed, and maintained in a refrigerated state to avoid rancidity. Foods that are high in phosphatidylcholine are those that provide lecithin, including eggs, soy, brewer's yeast, grains, legumes, fish, and wheat germ. A word of caution is prudent concerning the inclusion of soy products with men being treated for infertility due to the possible estrogenic effects of soy proteins. However soy-derived lecithin should not be an issue in this regard.

Glutathione (g-glutamylcysteinglycine [GSH]) performs a variety of vital physiological and metabolic functions within all cells affecting the preservation of tissue integrity. GSH plays a major role in detoxifying many reactive metabolites by either spontaneous conjugation or by a reaction catalyzed by the GSH S-transferases. As a result, its functions include a variety of areas such as:

- Maintenance of protein structure and function by reducing disulfide linkages of proteins, including metallothioneins (involved with heavy metal detoxification)
- Stabilization of immune function
- Protection against oxidative damage

- Detoxification of reactive chemicals
- Formation of bile
- Leukotriene and prostaglandin metabolism
- Reduction of ribonucleotides to deoxyribonucleotides

The elevation of cellular levels of glutathione provides a key defense against toxic products of oxygen, particularly in the mitochondria, and serves to up-regulate tissue detoxification [37, 38]. Various strategies exist for repleting cellular glutathione:

- Glutathione given orally has been demonstrated in vivo to raise plasma levels [39]. Recently available formulations of acetyl-glutathione appear to have good absorption and bioavailability with recommended dosing of 100 mg once or twice daily.
- Intravenous glutathione (push) in doses ranging from 1500 to 2000 mg has been combined in series with IV phosphotidylcholine as a therapy for various neurodegenerative disorders by various clinicians and is described in detail in the instructional manual *The Detoxx Book: Detoxification of Biotoxins in Chronic Neurotoxic Syndromes* by Foster, Kane, and Speight (2003).
- Glutathione precursors include n-acetyl-cysteine (NAC), l-methionine, l-glutamine, and l-taurine. Administration of precursors do not seem to raise glutathione levels if they are already in the normal range, but do appear to raise abnormally low GSH levels back to normal [40]. Following its intestinal absorption, NAC is converted to circulating cysteine and can effectively replenish GSH in depleted patients [41]. It is not recommended to use oral forms of plain l-cysteine because it is known to be highly unstable and potentially toxic. The activated counterpart of l-methionine, s-adenosylmethionine (SAMe), is well tolerated and has been shown to replenish erythrocyte GSH. Taurine is a sulfur amino acid that, given orally, can raise platelet GSH in healthy males [42].
- Alpha-lipoic acid (ALA) is a broad-spectrum, fat- and water-phase antioxidant with potent electron-donating capacity, and is another GSH repleter. Oral ALA raises GSH levels in HIV patients, and has been demonstrated to improve biliary excretion of heavy metals as transported by reduced glutathione [43, 44]. Typical therapeutic dosing is in the range of 100 to 300 mg twice a day.

Far infrared sauna is a broad-spectrum detoxification modality that is available for home and clinical use. Far infrared wavelength is a section of the natural band of light that is not visible to the human eye, but can be felt like heat. Rather than the traditional steam or dry saunas, far infrared saunas use that specific energy wavelength to penetrate the body tissues and stimulate cellular detoxification through the breakdown and release of fat-stored toxins and subsequent elimination through sweating. Although there are many claims regarding the ability of far infrared sauna to safely and effectively remove a variety of toxicants including heavy metals, there are few studies available to support these claims [45–47]. However, the data that are available suggest that this treatment warrants further attention and study given the scope of environmentally related illness.

Detoxification of heavy metals is performed using chelation agents such as EDTA (IV and oral) and DMSA (oral) according to clinically established protocols. Further training and certification in the treatment of heavy metals are available through the American College for Advancement in Medicine.

NUTRITIONAL AND BIOCHEMICAL SUPPORT

Nutritional and biochemical support for a healthy male reproductive system is an important adjunctive strategy in any attempts to help a patient recover fertility. The following nutritional therapies have shown promise in this area:

Arginine

The amino acid arginine is a precursor in the synthesis of putrescine, spermidine, and spermine, which are thought to be essential in sperm motility. A 1973 study by Schacter and colleagues demonstrated significant improvement in sperm count and motility in 74% of subjects after taking 4 g/day for 3 months [48]. Researchers in Italy evaluated the efficacy of arginine in 40 infertile men. After 6 months of therapy there was significantly improved sperm motility without any side effects [49].

Carnitine

In the epididymis, carnitine serves as an energy substrate for spermatozoa, enhancing transport of fatty acids into the mitochondria. In a study involving 124 infertile patients, a direct correlation between semen carnitine content and sperm motility was found [50]. Several other studies have demonstrated improvements in sperm health parameters following administration of carnitine in the ranges of 3 to 4 g/day [51, 52].

Zinc

The normal functioning of the male reproductive system requires this trace mineral. Zinc deficiency is associated with decreased testosterone levels and sperm count. An adequate amount of zinc ensures proper sperm motility and production, while deficient levels are often found in infertile men with diminished sperm count. Several studies have found supplemental zinc may be helpful in treating male infertility [53, 54].

Glutathione and Selenium

In addition to its role in detoxification as previously discussed, glutathione is vital to sperm antioxidant defenses and has demonstrated a positive effect on sperm motility [55]. Selenium and glutathione are essential to the formation of an enzyme present in spermatids that is necessary for spermatozoa maturation. Deficiencies in either substance can lead to defective sperm motility [56]. A variety of studies have shown improvement in male fertility parameters following administration of glutathione (600 mg daily IM) or selenium (200 µg/day) [57, 58].

Vitamin C

Studies have shown the concentration of ascorbic acid in seminal fluid directly reflects dietary intake, and that lower levels of vitamin C may lead to infertility and increased damage to the sperm's genetic material [59]. One study demonstrated significant improvements in sperm count in previously infertile but otherwise healthy men following administration of 1000 mg of vitamin C daily [60].

Vitamin B12

The synthesis of RNA and DNA as part of cellular replication requires vitamin B12, and deficiency states have been associated with decreased sperm count and motility. Studies have administered doses in the range of 1000 to 6000 µg/day (the average dose being 1500 µg daily) and have consistently shown improvements in sperm production [61, 62].

Antioxidants

Key components of the sperm cell include polyunsaturated fatty acids and phospholipids, which are susceptible to oxidative damage. As with all cells, sperm metabolism results in production of reactive oxygen species, which can result in free-radical-induced damage. Various reports indicate that supplementation with additional antioxidants such as vitamin E and CoQ10 may provide improvement to sperm cell function.

VI. SUMMARY

The decline in male fertility has been attributed in part to an increasing incidence of exposure to environmental factors such as pesticides and fungicides, heavy metals, plastics, and industrial and household chemicals. As part of a workup with patients who suffer from infertility, these environmental factors should be taken into consideration by the clinician. Testing for exposure could include:

- Urine panels for environmental pollutants and chemical exposures
- Heavy metals testing using urine porphyrins and provocation with chelation agents
- Red blood cell cholinesterase determination for pesticide exposure

Treatment for these environmental factors in male infertility focuses first on prevention, with avoidance of exposures. Remediation of the toxicity can involve:

- Proper hydration and bowel elimination
- Correction of underlying nutritional and metabolic deficiencies
- Providing a therapeutic balance of phospholipids and essential fatty acids
- Administration of glutathione and glutathione precursors
- Removal of heavy metals via chelation
- Far infrared sauna

Nutritional support for a healthy male reproductive system includes:

- Arginine
- Carnitine
- Zinc
- Glutathione and selenium
- Vitamin C
- Vitamin B12
- Antioxidants

Male infertility involves a variety of factors and contributing causes. Since a large percentage of male infertility cases are due to unknown causes of deficient sperm production, environmental factors and nutritional considerations should be a standard part of the evaluation and therapeutic considerations. Occupational exposures, diet and lifestyle choices, pesticide residues, and xenoestrogens adversely affect spermatogenesis. Therefore exposure avoidance and clinical management of these issues are indicated, including proper detoxification and nutritional support strategies.

REFERENCES

1. MacLeod J. Human male infertility. *Obstet Gynecol Surv* 26:335 (1979).
2. Purvis K, Christiansen E. Male infertility: current concepts. *Ann Med* 24:258–272 (1992).
3. Carlsen E, Giwercman A, Keiding N, Skakkebaek N. Evidence for decreasing quality of semen during past 50 years. *Br Med J* 305:609–613 (1992).
4. Swan S, Elkin E, Fenster L. The question of declining sperm density revisited: an analysis of 101 studies published 1934–1996. *Env Health Pers* 108:961–966 (2000).
5. Matsumoto A. The Testis. In: Felig P and Frohman L, eds. Endocrinology and Metabolism. 4th ed. New York, McGraw Hill; 2001: 635–705.
6. Sharpe R, Skakkebaek N. Are oestrogens involved in falling sperm counts and disorders of the male reproductive tract? *Lancet* 341:1392–1995 (1993).
7. Toppari J et al. Male reproductive health and environmental xenoestrogens. *Environ Health Perspect* 104:741–803 (1996).

8. Maffini M, Rubin B, Sonnenschein C, Soto A. Endocrine disruptors and reproductive health: the case of bisphenol-A. *Mol Cell Endocrinol* 25:254–255:179–86 (2006).

9. Higuchi T, Palmer J, Gray L, Veeramachaneni D. Effects of dibutyl phthalate in male rabbits following in utero, adolescent, or postpubertal exposure. *Toxicol Sci* 72:301–313 (2003).

10. Lee S, Veeramachaneni D. Subchronic exposure to low concentrations of Di-n-butyl phthalate disrupts spermatogenesis in Xenopus laevis frogs. *Toxicol Sci* 84:394–407 (2005).

11. Veeramachaneni D, Palmer J, Amann R, Kane C, Higuchi T, Pau K. Disruption of sexual function, FSH secretion, and spermiogenesis in rabbits following development exposure to vinclozolin, a fungicide. Society for Reproduction and Fertility (paper) 2006.

12. Taxvig C, Hass U, Axelstad M, Dalgaarad M, Boberg J, Andeasen H, Vinggaard A. Endocrine-disrupting activities in vivo of the fungicides tebuconazole and epoxiconazole. *Toxicol Sci* 100(2):464–473 (2007).

13. Frazier L. Reproductive disorders associated with pesticide exposure. *J Agromedicine* 12(1):227–237 (2007).

14. Peiris-John R, Wickremasinghe R. Impact of low-level exposure to organophosphates on human reproduction and survival. *Trans R Soc Trop Med Hyg* 102(3):239–245 (2008).

15. Fernandez M, Olmos B, Granada A, Lopez-Espinosa M, Molina-Molina J, Fernandez J, Cruz M, Olea-Serrano F, Olea N. Human exposure to endocrine-disrupting chemicals and prenatal risk factors for cryptorchodism and hypospadias: a nested case-control study. *Environ Health Perspect* 115:8–14 (2007).

16. Veeramachaneni D, Palmer J, Amann R, Pau K. Sequelae in male rabbits following developmental exposure to DDT or a mixture of DDT and vinclozolin: cryptorchidism, germ cell atypia, and sexual dysfunction. *Reproductive Toxicology* 23:353–365 (2007).

17. Lopez O, Hernandez A, Rodrigo L, Gil F, Pena G, Serrano J, Parron T, Villanueva E, Pla A. Changes in antioxidant enzymes in humans with long-term exposure to pesticides. *Toxicol Lett* 171(3):146–153 (2007).

18. Palan P, Naz R. Changes in various antioxidant levels in human seminal plasma related to immunofertility. *Arch Androl* 36:139–143 (1996).

19. Shiau C, Wang J, Chen P. Decreased fecundity among male lead workers. *Occup Environ Med* 61(11): 915–923 (2004).

20. Gennart J, Buchet J, Roels H, et al. Fertility of male workers exposed to cadmium, lead, or manganese. *Am J Epidemiol* 135:1208–1219 (1992).

21. Weber R, de Baat C. Male fertility: possibly affected by occupational exposure to mercury. *Ned Tijdschr Tandheelkd* 102(12):495–498 (2000).

22. Dickman M, Leung C, Leung M. Hong Kong male subfertility links to mercury in human hair and fish. *Sci Total Environ* 214:165–174 (1998).

23. Sinawat S. The environmental impact on male fertility. *J Med Assoc Thai* 83(8):880–885 (2000).

24. Martynowicz H, Andrzejak R, Medras M. The influence of lead on testis function. *Med Pr* 56(6):495–500 (2005).

25. Veeramachaneni D, Palmer J, Amann R. Long-term effects on male reproduction of early exposure to common chemical contaminants in drinking water. *Hum Reprod* 16(5):979–987 (2001).

26. Feichtinger W. Environmental factors and fertility. *Hum Reprod* 6(8):1170–1175 (1991).

27. Veeramachaneni D. Impact of environmental pollutants on the male: effects on germ cell differentiation. *Anim Reprod Sci* (2007), doi:10.1016/j.anireprosci.2007.11.020.

28. Dhillon V, Shahid M, Husain S. Associations of MTHFR DNMT3b 4977 bp deletion in mtDNA and GSTM1 deletion, and aberrant CpG island hypermethylation of GSTM1 in non-obstructive infertility in Indian men. *Mol Hum Reprod* 13(4):213–222 (2007).

29. Hermachand T, Gopalakrishnan B, Slaunke D, Totey S, Shaha C. Sperm plasma-membrane-associated glutathione S-transferases as gamete recognition molecules. *J Cell Sci* 115:2053–2065 (2002).

30. Geier D, Geier M. A prospective assessment of porphyrins in autistic disorders: a potential marker for heavy metal exposure. *Neurotox Res* 10(1):57–64 (2006).

31. Nigg H, Knaak J. Blood cholinesterases as human biomarkers of organophosphate pesticide exposure. *Rev Environ Contam Toxicol* 163:29–111 (2000).

32. Rivas A, Cerrillo I, Granada A, Mariscal-Arcas M, Olea-Serrano F. Pesticide exposure of two age groups of women and its relationship with their diet. *Sci Total Environ* 382(1):14–21 (2007).

33. Arcury T, Grzywacz J, Barr D, Tapia J, Chen H, Quandt S. Pesticide urinary metabolite levels of children in eastern North Carolina farmworker households. *Environ Health Perspect* 115(8):1254–1260 (2007).

34. Kalab M, Cervinka J. Essential phospholipids in the treatment of cirrhosis of the liver. *Cas Lek Ces* 122:266–269 (1983).

35. Kuntz E. The "essential" phospholipids in hepatology—50 years of experimental and clinical experiences. *Gastroenterol* 29(2):7–19 (1991).
36. Rottini E, Brazzanella F. Marri D, et al. Therapy of different types of liver insufficiency using "essential" phospholipids. *Med Monatsschrift* 17:28–30 (1963).
37. Martensson J, Meister A. Mitochondrial damage in muscle occurs after marked depletion of glutathione and is prevented by giving glutathione monoester. *Proc Natl Acad Sci USA* 86(2):471–475 (1989).
38. Ketterer B, Coles B, Meyer D. The role of glutathione in detoxification. *Environ Health Perspect* 49:59–60 (1983).
39. Lomaestro B, Malone M. Glutathione in health and disease: pharmacotherapeutic issues. *Annals Pharmacother* 29:1263–1273 (1976).
40. Tateishi N, Higashi T, Naruse A, et al. Relative contributions of sulfur atoms of dietary cysteine and methionine to rat liver glutathione and proteins. *J Biochem* 90:1603–1610 (1981).
41. Traber J, Suter M, Walter P, et al. In vivo modulation of total and mitochondrial glutathione in rat liver. *Biochem Pharmocol* 43:961–964 (1992).
42. Kidd P. Glutathione: systemic protectant against oxidative and free radical damage. *Altern Med Rev* 1:155–176 (1997).
43. Fuchs J, Schofer H, Milbradt R, et al. Studies on lipoate effects on blood redox state in human immunodeficiency virus infected patients. *Arzneimittelforschung* 43:1359–1362 (1993).
44. Gregus Z, Stein A, Varga F, Klassen C. Effect of lipoic acid on bililary exretion of glutathione and metals. *Tox and Applied Pharmacol* 114:88–96 (1992).
45. Cecchini M, Root D, Rachunow J, Gelb P. Use of the Hubbard sauna detoxification regimen to improve the health status of New York City rescue workers exposed to toxicants. *Townsend Ltr* 273:58–65 (2006).
46. Henderson G, Wilson B. Excretion of methadone and metabolites in human sweat. *Res Comm Chem Path Pharmacol* 5(1):1–8 (1972).
47. Masuda A, Munemoto T, Tei C. A new treatment: thermal therapy for chronic fatigue syndrome. *Nippon Rinsho* 65(6):1093–1098 (2007).
48. Schachter A, Goldman J, Zukerman Z. Treatment of oligospermia with the amino acid arginine. *J Urol* 110:311–313 (1973).
49. Scibona M, Meschini P, Capparelli S, et al. L-arginine and male infertility. *Minerva Urol Nefrol* 46:251–253 (1994).
50. Menchini-Fabris G, Canale D, Izzo P, et al. Free L-carnitine in human semen: its variability in different andrologic pathologies. *Fertil Steril* 42:263–267 (1984).
51. Vitali G, Parente R, Melotti C. Carnitine supplementation in human idiopathic asthenospermia: clinical results. *Drugs Exp Clin Res* 21:157–159 (1995).
52. Costa M, Canale D, Filicori M, et al. L-carnitine in idiopathic astheno-zoospermia: a multi-center study. Italian Study Group on Carnitine and Male Infertility. *Andrologia* 26:155–159 (1994).
53. Madding C, Jacob M, Ramsay V, Sokol R. Serum and semen zinc levels in normozoospermic and oligospermic men. *Ann Nutr Metab* 30:213–218 (1986).
54. Tikkiwal M, Ajmera R, Mathur N. Effect of zinc administration on seminal zinc and fertility of oligospermic males. *Indian J Physiol Pharmacol* 31:30–34 (1987).
55. Lenzi A, Lombardo F, Gandini L, et al. Glutathione therapy for male infertility. *Arch Androl* 29:65–68 (1992).
56. Hansen J, Deguchi Y. Selenium and fertility in animals and man—a review. *Acta Vet Scand* 37:19–30 (1996).
57. Lenzi A, Culasso F, Gandini L, et al. Placebo-controlled, double blind, cross-over trial of glutathione therapy in male infertility. *Hum Reprod* 8:1657–1662 (1993).
58. Scott R, MacPherson A, Yates R, et al. The effect of oral selenium supplementation on human sperm motility. *Br J Urol* 82:76–80 (1998).
59. Dabrowski K, Ciereszko A. Ascorbic acid protects against male infertility in teleost fish. *Experientia* 52:97–100 (1996).
60. Dawson E, Harris W, Rankin W, et al. Effect of ascorbic acid on male fertility. *Ann N Y Acad Sci* 498:312–323 (1987).
61. Kumamoto Y, Maruta H. Ishigami J, et al. Clinical efficacy of mecobalamin in the treatment of oligospermia—results of double-blind comparative clinical study. *Hinyokika Kiyo* 34:1109–1132 (1988).
62. Sandler B, Faragher B. Treatment of oligospermia with vitamin B-12. *Infertility* 7:133–138 (1984).

Index

Page numbers followed by f indicate figure; those followed by t indicate table.